医療英会話
キーワード
辞典

そのまま使える
16000例文

森島祐子
仁木久恵
Flaminia Miyamasu

Medical
English for
Hospital Staff

医学書院

著者略歴

森島　祐子（もりしま　ゆうこ）
　米国生まれ．筑波大学在学中，カナダのマギル大学，マックマスター大学にて Clinical Clerkship を行う．医学博士．米国内科学会フェロー（FACP）．現在，筑波大学医学医療系准教授．専門分野は呼吸器内科学．

仁木　久恵（にき　ひさえ）
　米国テキサス大学大学院にて M.A. 取得後，津田塾大学大学院博士課程修了．元 NHK ラジオ基礎英語講師．聖路加国際大学・明海大学教授を経て，聖路加国際大学名誉教授．

Flaminia Miyamasu（フラミニア　みやます）
　英国出身．リバプール大学卒業後，米国ジョージア大学大学院にて M.A. 取得（ロマンス諸語）．現在，筑波大学医学医療系准教授．専門分野は医学英語教育法．

医療英会話キーワード辞典—そのまま使える 16000 例文

発　行　2019 年 4 月 1 日　第 1 版第 1 刷©
著　者　森島祐子・仁木久恵・Flaminia Miyamasu
発行者　株式会社　医学書院
　　　　代表取締役　金原　俊
　　　　〒113-8719　東京都文京区本郷 1-28-23
　　　　電話　03-3817-5600（社内案内）
印刷・製本　三美印刷

本書の複製権・翻訳権・上映権・譲渡権・貸与権・公衆送信権（送信可能化権を含む）は株式会社医学書院が保有します．

ISBN978-4-260-02813-4

本書を無断で複製する行為（複写，スキャン，デジタルデータ化など）は，「私的使用のための複製」など著作権法上の限られた例外を除き禁じられています．大学，病院，診療所，企業などにおいて，業務上使用する目的（診療，研究活動を含む）で上記の行為を行うことは，その使用範囲が内部的であっても，私的使用には該当せず，違法です．また私的使用に該当する場合であっても，代行業者等の第三者に依頼して上記の行為を行うことは違法となります．

JCOPY〈出版者著作権管理機構　委託出版物〉
本書の無断複製は著作権法上での例外を除き禁じられています．複製される場合は，そのつど事前に，出版者著作権管理機構（電話 03-5244-5088，FAX 03-5244-5089，info@jcopy.or.jp）の許諾を得てください．

序

　社会のグローバル化が進むなかで，外国人が医療機関を受診するケースが増えている．医療の現場では，情報の収集，検査・治療方針の説明，ケアなど，多方面にわたる患者支援のために，言語コミュニケーションは欠かすことのできないツールである．もしコミュニケーションが適切に行われなければ，疾病の診断や治療が円滑に進まず，患者に身体的・心理的不利益が生じてしまう．

　先に医学書院より発刊した『そのまま使える　病院英語表現5000』は，幸いにも多くの読者からご支持をいただいた．しかし，同書では用例を診療の時系列や領域別に沿って配置しているために，系統的な検索には有用である一方で，一つの語彙から派生する英語表現の検索には向いていない．そこで，同書の初版を出版した2006年に，「現場で使いやすい医療英会話用例辞典を作ろう」というコンセプトのもとに本書の執筆を開始した．手探りで始めた辞書作りではあったが，医学英語教育に携わるFlaminia Miyamasu，多くの一般英和・和英辞典や看護英和辞典の執筆を手掛けてきた仁木久恵，臨床医学に身をおく森島祐子の3人がタッグを組むことで，これまでにない実用性の高い医療英会話辞典が完成した．本書は日本で外国人の診療を行う際に役立つことはもちろんのこと，海外での診療，さらには英語で症例報告をするような場面でも活用することができる．

　必要な語彙や例文がすぐに探せる本書が，医師や看護師をはじめとする医療スタッフ，将来医療に従事する医学生や看護学生たちの必携の一冊としてお役に立てれば幸いである．

　10年余の歳月を要してようやく上梓の日を迎えるにあたり，その間，お世話くださった医学書院の方々に心からお礼を申し上げる．

2019年3月

著者を代表して　**森島祐子**

凡例

■ 編集方針

- 日常の臨床現場において使用頻度が高いと考えられる一般用語，医療用語などを収集した．
- 見出し語の主体は名詞，形容詞であるが，動詞や副詞も加え，そのまま使えるよう，語義や用例を記載した．
- 見出し語は検索しやすいように，かな見出しを採用し，五十音順で掲載した．
- 米国と英国で表記が異なる場合は米国式を優先し，必要に応じて《英》として英国式も併記した．
- 医療用語の表記法や読みなどは主要関連学会の用語集などを参考にした．

■ 構成

　本書は，見出し語の読み，和文表記，語義の分類，英文表記，発音記号，参照見出し語，用例（和文，英文），注釈，複合語（和文，英文）で構成されている．

【見出し語】

配列順序

- 清音→濁音→半濁音の順に配列した
　　例：ヘッド→ベッド→ペット

- 直音→促音（っ）・拗音（ゃ）の順に配列した
　　例：しつけ→しっけ（湿気）　　しよう（使用）→しょう（小）

- ひらがな→カタカナの順に配列した

- 長音記号（ー）は，それぞれの母音に置き換え配列した
　　例：マーカー→マアカア　　ポリープ→ポリイプ
　　　　アメーバ→アメエバ　　コード→コオド

- 「ヴァ，ヴィ，ヴェ，ヴォ」は「バ，ビ，ベ，ボ」に置き換えた
　　例：バルサルバ洞 Valsalva sinus　　レビー小体 Lewy body

- 同音異義語は，別の見出し語として右肩に番号をつけて配列した

> **は¹　刃** （刀身）blade（刃先）edge　◆鋭利な刃で指を切る cut *one's* finger with a sharp blade
> **は²　波** wave
> **は³　歯** tooth（複teeth 形dental 腰歯 が生える teethe /tíːð/）

- 英語表記の見出し語は，カタカナに置き換えて示した

> **アールアイ** RI, radioisotope ☞放射性同位元素
> **アールエイチ** Rh （アールエイチ因子）Rh factor, Rhesus factor /ríːsəs-/ ◆あなた

発音記号

- 発音記号は，使用頻度が高く発音が難しいと思われるものについてのみ記載した．原則として，国際音声字母を用いた

語義・注釈

- ニュアンスが異なる英文表記については，（　）内にその状況を示した
- 通例複数形で用いるもの，狭義・広義の意味など，使う際に注意が必要な英文表記については★に続けて注釈（注意事項）を記載した

> **たて** 縦(の) （垂直の）vertical （縦方向の）longitudinal （幅・距離が長い）long ★英語では長いほうを縦，短いほうを横とする． ◆縦方向 a vertical[longitudinal] direction

- 語義によって使い方が変わる場合は，《　》内にその語義を示し，用例もそれぞれ分けて掲載した

> **あたたかい** 暖かい・温かい
> 《温度などが》warm /wɔ́ːm/ （気候が温和な）mild ◆きょうはとても暖かですね It's nice and warm today, isn't it? ◆今年の冬は暖かです We're having a mild[warm] winter this year. ◆温かいお茶はいかがですか(熱い)How about a cup of hot tea? ◆暖かいひざ掛け a warm lap throw [robe]
> 《人柄が》warm ◆彼女は気さくで心の温かな人です She is a friendly and warm-hearted person.

解説文

- 一部の見出し語では，その内容を表す英文表現をイタリック体で記載した

> **アカラシア** achalasia : *a condition that affects the muscles of the esophagus and causes difficulties in swallowing* ◆食道アカラシア esophageal achalasia

その他

- 人名の末尾に付くアポストロフィ・エス（'s）は，原則として省略した
- 略語は，日本国内および国際的に広く常用されているものを原則として採用した

【用例】

- ◆に続けて和文とともに対応する英語表現を記載した
- 用例は，臨床の場でそのまま使える平易な表現を心掛けた
- 注意が必要な表現には★に続けて注釈を記載した
- 表現が似ている用例（別表現）は，スラッシュ / で区切り，ニュアンスが異なる場合には小括弧（ ）内にその状況を示した

> **おつかれさま** **お疲れ様** ★このねぎらいの表現は状況に応じて使い分ける．◆さあ，終わりました．お疲れ様〈よくやりましたね〉That's it. All finished. Well done! ◆今日はここまでにしましょう．お疲れ様〈見事にやり遂げましたね〉That's all for today. You did a good job![Good job! / You did well.] ◆お疲れ様〈疲れすぎてないといいのですが〉I hope you're not too tired. / I hope we didn't make you too tired. /〈お疲れになったでしょう〉You must be tired. ◆お疲れ様〈ありがとう〉Thank you! / Thank you for your patience. ◆お疲れ様〈さようなら〉See you! / See you tomorrow morning! / See you next time!

- （ ）で囲んだ英文表記は，省略可能である

> **スポーツ** sport（略運動競技の athletic）☞運動 ◆何かスポーツをしていますか Do you play any sports? ◆どんなスポーツをしますか What (kind of) sports do you play[do]?

- ［ ］は，同じ意味の表現で言い換え可能な語句を示した
- 〈 〉は，異なる意味の表現で言い換え可能な語句を示した
  なお，［ ］や〈 〉内を複数の語で言い換える場合，該当フレーズの先頭箇所に＊を付記した．ただし，文頭からのフレーズとの言い換えはその限りではない
- 略語のピリオドは原則として付けていない（例：Dr Mr am pm）

> **しんり** **心理** （心の状態）state of mind, mental state （精神的傾向）mentality（略mental）（心理学的課程・心の働き）psychology /saɪkálədʒɪ/（略psychológical）☞精神 ◆このような心理状態はどのくらい続いていますか How long have you been in this state of mind? ◆職場でいつもより多く心理的な圧力〈ストレス〉を受けていますか Have you been under more psychological[mental] pressure〈stress〉than usual at work? ◆音楽を聴くと心理的な効果があってリラックスできます Listening to music can *have a psychological effect [affect you psychologically] and will help you relax.

【複合語】

- 見出し語を含む複合語は ◀ または ▶ に続けて記載した
- ◀は別の語＋見出し語で構成される複合語を示す
- ▶は見出し語＋別の語で構成される複合語を示す
- ただし頻度が高く，用例などを含む重要語については，☞に続けて記載し，別見出し語とした．

> **さん** **酸** acid（略acid）◀胃酸 stomach [gastric] acid 脂肪酸 fatty acid 制酸薬 antacid 胆汁酸 bile acid 乳酸 lactic acid 尿酸 uric acid；UA ▶酸塩基平衡 acid-base balance 酸塩基平衡異常 acid-base imbalance 酸逆流 acid reflux 酸損傷 acid injury 酸熱傷 acid burn ☞酸化，酸性，酸味

【囲み記事】

- 見出し語に関連して役立つ表現，参照すべき用語，日本と欧米でニュアンスが異なる表現，注意点などを囲み記事として掲載した
  - 例：「体位」の箇所（438頁）で，囲み記事「体位・動作の指示」

【巻末付録】（759頁）

- 「悪い診断結果を伝える時」「訊きにくい質問のコツ」「単位の換算」「あいさつ」「電話応対の表現」「病院関係者」の項目を設けた

【記号】

( )　①（ ）で囲んだ英文表記は，省略可能であることを示す

　　　②（ ）で囲んだ和文表記は，語義・用例のニュアンスや状況を示す

　　　③その他，参照すべき項目（異なる読み，複数形，対義語，商品名，掲示，囲みなど）で使用する

　　　例：りょうはし 両端 ☞両端（りょうたん），foot（複 feet），start（↔ stop），（商標名）Band-Aid,（掲示）Lost and Found (Office)，流動食《☞食事（囲み）》

[ ]　同じ意味の表現で言い換え可能な語句であることを示す

〈 〉　異なる意味の表現で言い換え可能な語句であることを示す

《 》　①語義が異なる場合には改行し，《 》ごとに用例を分けた

　　　②米国と英国で表記が異なる場合は米国式を優先し，《英》として英国式を併記した

↔　　対義語

☞　　参照

◆　　用例の開始

/　　表現が似ている用例（別表現）や，言い換え可能な語句の区切り

*　　[ ]や〈 〉内を複数の語で言い換える場合，該当フレーズの先頭箇所に付けた

◀ ▶　複合語の開始

★　　注意が必要な英文表記や英語表現

略号　图 名詞　　圏 形容詞　　動 動詞　　副 副詞　　接頭 接頭辞　　接尾 接尾辞
　　　単 単数形　　複 複数形

■参考文献

1) Baile, W.F., et al.: SPIKES—A six-step protocol for delivering bad news ; application to the patient with cancer. Oncologist 5 : 302-311, 2000.

2) Goldmann, D.R. and Horowitz, D.A.（eds）: American College of Physicians ; Home Medical Adviser. DK Publishing Inc., 2002.

3) Longman's English-Japanese Dictionary『ロングマン英和辞典』. Pearson Education, 2007.

4) Stedman's Medical Dictionary 28th ed. Lippincott Williams & Wilkins, 2005.

5) The U. S. National Library of Medicine : Medline Plus.（http://medlineplus.org）

6) Venes, D., et al.（eds）: Taber's Cyclopedic Medical Dictionary 23rd ed. F.A. Davis Co., 2017.

7) Iverson, C., et al.: AMA Manual of Style-a Guide for Authors and Editors 10th ed. Oxford University Press, 2007.

8) 石田名香雄 編：医学英和辞典 第2版. 研究社, 2008.

9) 伊藤正男・井上裕夫・高久史麿 編：医学書院 医学大辞典 第2版. 医学書院, 2009.

10) 井上永幸・赤野一郎 編：ウィズダム英和辞典 第3版. 三省堂, 2013.

11) 金澤一郎・永井良三 編：今日の診断指針 第7版. 医学書院, 2015.

12) カルペニート, リンダ J.・浅倉稔生：医師とナースのための問診とフィジカルアセスメントの英語—Bedside English for doctors and nurses. 医学書院, 1998.

13) 高久史麿 監：ステッドマン医学大辞典—英和・和英 改訂第6版. メジカルビュー社, 2008.

14) 竹林滋・小島義郎・東信行・赤須薫 編：ルミナス英和辞典 第2版. 研究社, 2005.

15) 仁木久恵・森島祐子・F. Miyamasu：そのまま使える医療英会話. 医学書院, 2010.

16) 仁木久恵・Nancy Sharts-Hopko・助川尚子：臨床看護英語 Let's Listen, Speak and Learn 第5版. 医学書院, 2012.

17) 日本医学会：医学用語辞典 WEB 版.（http://jams.med.or.jp/dic/mdic.html）

18) 日本呼吸ケア・リハビリテーション学会, 他 編：呼吸リハビリテーションマニュアル—運動療法 第2版. 照林社, 2012.

19) 日野原重明 監訳：診察術マニュアル—問診-診察-記録. 医学書院, 1982.

20) 森島祐子・仁木久恵・Nancy Sharts-Hopko：そのまま使える病院英語表現 5000 第2版. 医学書院, 2013.

21) 山岸勝栄 監：スーパー・アンカー和英辞典 第3版新装版. 学習研究社, 2015.

22) 福井次矢・高木誠・小室一成 編：今日の治療指針—私はこう治療している 2018 年版. 医学書院, 2018.

ご注意

　用語やその使い方は, 医療のニーズや社会情勢に応じて常に変化しています. 著者, 出版社として, 本書に収録されている情報が正確であるように最善の努力を払っております. ただし, 収録情報の誤りにより発生するいかなる事故, 損害に対してもその責を負いかねますのでご了承ください.

株式会社　医学書院

あ

あ— 亜— sub- ▶亜区域 subsegment 亜脱臼 subluxation ☞亜急性

アー ah ◆口を大きく開けて，「アー」と言って下さい Please open your mouth wide. Say "ah."

ああ oh ◆ああ，そうですか Oh, is that so? / Oh, really? ◆ああ，よかった，血圧が正常値以下まで下がりましたね Oh, good [great], your blood pressure has dropped to below normal.

アーノルド・キアリきけい —奇形 Arnold–Chiari malformation

アールアイ RI, radioisotope ☞放射性同位元素

アールエイチ Rh （アールエイチ因子）Rh factor, Rhesus factor /ríːsəs–/ ◆あなたはB型で，アールエイチは陰性です You have type B Rh[Rhesus] –negative blood. ◆アールエイチ陰性の女性 an Rh-negative woman ▶Rh血液型 Rh[Rhesus] blood type　Rh不適合 Rh incompatibility　Rh陽性 Rh positive

アールエスウイルス RSV, RS virus, respiratory syncytial virus

あい 愛 love （動love） （穏やかな親愛の情）affection ◆親の愛に飢えている be hungry for parental love ◆母親の愛 a mother's love for her child / motherly [maternal] love ◆愛する人の死を悲しむ grieve the death of a loved one ◀異性愛 heterosexuality / heterosexual love　性愛 sexual love　同性愛 homosexuality / homosexual love

アイウエオじゅん —順 ◆アイウエオ順に in a-i-u-e-o order / in the order of the Japanese （kana） syllabary

あいかわらず 相変わらず （今もなお）still （いつものように）as usual, as always ◆お仕事は相変わらずお忙しいですか Are you still busy at work? ◆今日も相変わらず暑いですね Today is hot as usual, isn't it?

◆彼は担当医の忠告を無視して相変わらずタバコを吸っています He keeps on smoking against the advice of his physician. ◆彼女は危機的な状況にあっても相変わらず落ち着いていました She remained calm in times of crisis.

あいき 噯気 burp, belch ☞げっぷ

アイキュー IQ, intelligence quotient ☞知能

アイコンタクト eye contact ☞視線

あいさつ 挨拶する greet （図greeting） ☞巻末付録：あいさつ ◆患者に笑顔で挨拶する greet patients with a smile ◆…と挨拶を交わす exchange greetings with …

アイシーユー ICU, intensive care unit ☞集中治療室 ▶ICU症候群 ICU syndrome

あいしょう 相性 ◆彼女は同室の患者との相性がいいです She gets along[on] well with her roommate.

あいじょう 愛情 love, affection ☞愛

アイシング icing ◆怪我をした部位にアイシングする apply ice or a cold pack to the injured area / ice the injured area

あいず 合図 （光・ブザー音などによる合図）signal （身振りによる合図）sign ◆合図しますので，それまで動かないで下さい Please don't move till *I say "OK"[I give you the signal].

アイスキューブ ice cube

アイスクリームずつう —頭痛 ice cream headache

アイスパック ice pack

アイゼンメンゲルしょうこうぐん —症候群 Eisenmenger syndrome

あいそ(う) 愛想 ◆愛想のいい人 *a sociable[a friendly / an amiable] person ◆彼は自分の愚かな行動に愛想をつかしています（うんざりしている）He is simply disgusted by his own foolish behavior.

アイソザイム isozyme, isoenzyme

アイソトープ isotope ◀ラジオアイソトープ radioisotope

アイソメトリックうんどう —運動 isometric exercise

あいだ 間

あいだ　《時間》between, for, during, while　（以内に）in, within　（…まで）till, until　◆この薬は食事と食事の間に服用して下さい Please take this medication between meals.　◆数日の間，自宅療養をして下さい Please stay at home for several days to recuperate. / Please recuperate at home for several days.　◆夏休みの間にどこか外国へ行きましたか Did you go anywhere abroad[overseas] during the summer vacation?　◆夜寝ている間に汗を大量にかきますか Do you sweat *a lot[profusely] while sleeping?　◆平日の面会時間は午後3時から8時までの間です Visiting hours are *between 3 pm and 8 pm[from 3 pm till 8 pm] on weekdays.　◆私が戻ってくるまでの間，ここでお待ち下さい Please wait here till[until] I get back.　◆この検査は15分も経たない間に済みます This test won't last more than fifteen minutes. / This test will be over in less than fifteen minutes.　《空間・場所》between, among　★通例，2つの場合は between，3つ以上の場合は among.　◆歯の間に歯垢がたまっています You have plaque between your teeth.　◆正面玄関とエレベーターホールの間に車椅子が用意してありますので，ご自由にお使い下さい Wheelchairs are available in the space between the main entrance and the elevator hall. Please feel free to use them.　《関係・間柄》between, among　★通例，2人の場合は between，3人以上の場合は among.　◆医師と患者の間の良好なコミュニケーションは治療を成功させるための鍵になります Good communication between doctors and patients is the key to successful treatment of a disease.　◆その感染症は高齢者の間に急速に広まっています That infectious disease is spreading rapidly among elderly[older] people.　◆臨床道化師は子供達の間に人気があります Clini-Clowns[Hospital clowns] are popular with[among] children.

あいちゃく　愛着　attachment, bond
◆母子間の愛着 the attachment[bond] between (a) mother and (her) child / the mother-child bond[attachment]　◆今の職場や仕事に愛着を感じていますか Do you feel a sense of attachment to your workplace or job?

あいづち　相づち　◆相づちを打つ（軽くうなずく）nod slightly /　（受け答えする）use short utterances during conversation (to show that *one* is listening carefully)

相づちは会話をスムーズに進めるための潤滑剤になるが，日本人はとかく「話を聞いていますよ」という意味で半ば無意識に Yes, Yes などと頻繁に相づちを打つ．外国人の患者さんは医師や看護師が自分の話に同意しているものと誤解しかねないので注意したい．英語では，相手が話している間黙って聞いていて，ある程度の区切りのところで軽く Uh-huh /əhʌ́/, Really?, I see. などと言葉をはさむ．その場合，ワンパターンにならないように気をつける．

あいて　相手　◆相談相手がいますか Do you have anyone you can go[turn] to for advice? / Do you have someone you can talk to?　★Yes という答えを期待する時には someone を用いる．　◆話し相手が欲しいですか Would you like to have someone to talk to[with]?　◆大切なのは相手に伝わるように話すことです It's important to speak[communicate] in a way that will make sure you are understood.　◆相手の表情を読み取る read the facial expressions of the person *one* is talking with　◆性行為の相手 *one's* sexual partner

アイデア　idea　☞考え　◆それはいいアイデアですね That's a good idea!

アイディーカード　ID (card), identification card, identity card

アイディーばんごう　―番号　ID number, identification number, identity number

アイディーバンド　ID band, identification [identity] band　（手首の）ID wristband　（足首の）ID ankle band　（腕輪の）ID bracelet　（札）ID tag　◆ID バンドを手首につけましょう Let me attach your ID band to your wrist.　◆入院中はこの ID バンドをはずさないで下さい Please don't remove this ID band during your hospital stay.

あいている 空いている ☞空く(あく)

アイデンティティ **identity** ◆彼はアイデンティティの危機に瀕しています He is having[going through / experiencing] an identity crisis. ◆アイデンティティを確立する establish a sense of identity

あいとう 哀悼 **condolences** ☞お悔やみ

アイドナー **eye donor**

あいにく ◆あいにく火曜日は休診です Unfortunately, the office is closed on Tuesdays. ◆あいにく今度の土曜日は予定が入っています I'm sorry, but *I've got another appointment[I'm not free] this coming Saturday.

アイバンク **eye bank**

アイピーエスさいぼう iPS 細胞 **iPS cell** (人工多能性幹細胞)**induced pluripotent stem cell**

あいべや 相部屋 **shared room** ◆ほかの患者さんと相部屋でかまいませんか Do you mind sharing a room with another patient? ▶2 人部屋 semiprivate[two-bed] room / room for two　4 人部屋 four-bed room / room for four　大部屋 shared[multiple occupancy] room / room shared by several patients

あいまい 曖昧(な) (不確かな)**unclear**, **obscure** (漠然とした)**vague** (多義的な)**ambiguous** ◆曖昧な点があれば何でも訊いて下さい If there's anything you don't understand, don't hesitate to ask me. ◆起こった出来事について曖昧な記憶しかない have only *a vague[an ambiguous] memory of what happened

あいよう 愛用(の) **favorite** ◆入院の際には，CD プレイヤーやクロスワードパズルなど愛用している物をいくつかお持ちになるとよいでしょう You could bring a few of your favorite things, such as a CD player or crossword puzzles, with you when you are admitted to the hospital. ◆愛用の杖 *one's* own cane

アイルランド **Ireland** (アイルランドの・アイルランド人の)**Irish**) ☞国籍 ▶アイルランド人(男性)Irishman / (女性)Irishwoman

あう¹ 会う (会って話をする)**see** (日時を約束して会う)**meet** ◆では，また後で〈明日の朝〉お会いしましょう See you later〈tomorrow morning〉. ◆午後 3 時に私のオフィスでお会いしましょう I'll meet you in my office at three in the afternoon. ◆(再診の時などに)またお会いしてうれしく思います Nice to see you again. ★すでに面識のある人には meet ではなく，see を用いる。

あう² 遭う (困難な事態を経験する)**have**, **meet** (with) (巻き込まれる)**get[be, become] involved** (in) ◆その事故にあったのはいつですか When did you have[meet with] the accident? / When were you involved in the accident? ◆あまり無理をしすぎるとひどい目にあいますよ You'll have a hard time of it if you overdo things.

あう³ 合う (サイズなどが合う)**fit** (意見・食べ物が合う)**agree** (with) (目的などに合う)**suit** ◆眼鏡〈入れ歯〉が合わないと感じますか Do your glasses〈dentures〉feel like they don't fit? / Do you feel that your glasses〈dentures〉don't fit? ◆レンズの度が合っていませんね The lenses are not the right strength for your eyes. ◆ご自分に合わない食べ物がありますか Are there any foods that don't agree with you? ◆あなたの症状にこの薬が合うか試してみましょう Let's try this medication to see if it suits your symptoms. ◆病院食はお口に合いますか (How) do you like the hospital food?

あえぐ 喘ぐ (息遣いが荒い)**breathe hard [heavily]** /brí:ð-/ (はあはあと息を切らす)**pant** (for air), **gasp** (for breath) ◆階段を上る時喘ぐことがありますか Do you ever breathe hard[heavily] going up stairs? ◀喘ぎ呼吸 gasping[panting] breathing [respiration]

あえて 敢えて ◆あえて来院する必要はありません．お電話で結構です You don't need to bother to come to the hospital. A phone call will do. ◆あえて申し上げますが，焦らないほうがいいですよ Excuse me for saying so, but you shouldn't be so impatient. ◆あえて外泊をご希望でした

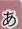

ら，月曜日の朝10時までに必ず戻ってきて下さい If you insist on going home for the night, just remember that you have to be back by ten o'clock Monday morning.

あえん 亜鉛 zinc ▶亜鉛欠乏(症) zinc deficiency

あおあざ 青あざ （打撲による内出血斑）bruise /brúːz/, black-and-blue mark （蒙古斑）blue spot, bluish spot ☞あざ ◆足になかなか消えない青あざがある have a bruise on *one's* leg that won't go away

あおい 青い blue （青白い）pale （青みがかっている）bluish ☞青黒い，青白い，青味 ◆お子さんは泣くと顔が青くなりますか Does your child turn blue when he⟨she⟩ cries? ◆唇が青くなる *one's* lips turn blue[bluish] / *one's* lips become blue [bluish]

あおぐろい 青黒い （怪我・打撲などによる皮下出血の色調）black-and-blue （あざなどの色調）livid, dark blue-and-gray ◆皮膚の表面に青黒い痕がある There is a black-and-blue mark on the surface of the skin. ◆足に青黒いあざがある have livid[dark blue-and-gray] bruises on *one's* leg

あおじろい 青白い pale ◆顔色はいつもより青白いですか Has your face color become paler than usual? ◆胸が痛む時，顔が青白くなると人から言われたことがありますか Have you ever been told that you turn pale or bluish when you have chest pain? ◆青白く見える look pale ◆青白い肌 pale skin ◆青白い顔色 a pale complexion

あおみ 青味(を帯びた) bluish （緑色を帯びた）greenish

あおむけ 仰向け(に) on *one's* back (↔on *one's* stomach) ☞背臥位 ◆診察台の上に仰向けに寝て下さい Please lie (down) on your back on the exam table. ◆息切れは仰向けに寝るとひどくなりますか Do you find breathing more difficult when you're lying flat on your back? ◆仰向けに倒れる fall on *one's* back ◆ごろりと仰向けになる turn[roll] onto *one's* back

あおやさい 青野菜 （dark) green vegetables ★複数形で．☞野菜

あか 垢 （汚れ）dirt （耳垢）earwax ◆お風呂で垢を落とす take a bath and *wash oneself* clean[wash off the dirt] ◆爪の垢 dirt under the fingernails

あかあざ 赤あざ red birthmark, strawberry mark

あかい 赤い red （赤味を帯びている）reddish （赤く擦りむけている）raw /rɔ́ː/ ☞赤味 ◆全身に赤い発疹が出る get[have] red spots all over the body ◆皮膚が赤く擦りむけている the skin is raw ◆目が赤い the eyes are red / （充血している）the eyes are bloodshot, have bloodshot eyes ◆手の赤紫色の斑点 reddish purple spots on *one's* hand ◆赤くなった皮膚 reddened skin

あかぎれ cracks （略cracked), chaps （略chapped) ★いずれも通例，複数形で．

あかぐろい 赤黒い dark red-and-gray

あかさびいろ 赤さび色(の) reddish brown ◆赤さび色の痰 reddish brown phlegm

アカシジア akathisia, acathisia ; *inability to sit still*

あかちゃん 赤ちゃん baby ◆赤ちゃんをしっかり抱っこして下さい Please hold your baby firmly. ◆男〈女〉の赤ちゃん a baby boy⟨girl⟩

あかはな 赤鼻 （酒皶性痤瘡）acne rosacea

あかぶどうしゅようけっかんしゅ 赤ぶどう酒様血管腫 port-wine stain[hemangioma]

あかみ[1] 赤身(の) red-fleshed ◆赤身のマグロには蛋白質が豊富に含まれています Red-fleshed tuna is rich in protein.

あかみ[2] 赤味(を帯びた) reddish ◆赤味を帯びた便〈尿〉reddish stools⟨urine⟩

あからがお 赤ら顔 ruddy face （顔色）ruddy complexion

アカラシア achalasia ; *a condition that affects the muscles of the esophagus and causes difficulties in swallowing* ◀食道アカラシア esophageal achalasia

あかり 明かり light ☞光 ◆明かりを消

しましょうか Shall I turn off the light? ◆明かりをつける turn on the light ◆明かりを落とす turn down the light ★turn up は照明をもっと明るくするの意.

あがりおり　上がり下りする　go up and down, walk up and down ◆階段の上がり下りはつらいですか Do you have difficulty going up and down stairs?

あがる　上がる

《上へゆく》**go up**（↔go down）（登る）**climb** （物などの上に乗る）**get onto** ◆息切れしないで階段が上がれますか Can you *go up [climb] stairs without getting short of breath? ◆診察台に上がって下さい Please get onto the exam table.

《向上する》**improve** ◆最近この病気の治療効果はかなり上がっています Treatment for this disease has significantly improved recently.

《数値が増す》**go up, rise, increase** ◆今朝, 彼女の体温は 39℃に上がりました Her temperature *went up[rose] to thirty-nine degrees Celsius this morning. ◆塩辛いものばかり食べると血圧が上がります Your blood pressure will *go up[rise] if you eat salty foods all the time. ◆血糖値が上がる *one's* blood sugar level *goes up [rises / increases]

《速くなる》**quicken, become fast** ◆パニックが起こると息が上がる breathing quickens[becomes faster] during a panic attack ◆脈拍が上がる the pulse quickens[becomes faster]

《どきどきして落ち着きを失う》 ◆人前であがる *one's* heart pounds when *one* is with people

《終わる》 ◆月経があがる stop menstruating / *one's*（menstrual）periods end / menstruation ends

あかるい　明るい

《十分な光量がある》**bright**（よく日の差す）**light** ◆部屋が明るすぎて眠れません Is it because the room is too bright that you can't sleep? ◆明るい病室 a bright[well-lit / well-lighted] room

《精通している》 ◆彼は日本の医療事情に明

るい He knows a lot[He is well informed] about the medical situation in Japan.

◆あなたは日本の音楽に明るいですね You're familiar with Japanese music, aren't you?

《見通しが楽観できる》 ◆物事〈人生〉の明るい面に目を向ける look on[at] the bright side of things〈life〉

アカントアメーバ　acanthamoeba ▶アカントアメーバ角膜炎 acanthamoeba keratitis

あかんぼう　赤ん坊 ☞赤ちゃん

あき　空き（の）　vacant /véɪkənt/, **unoccupied, empty** ◆空きベッド *a vacant [an unoccupied / an empty] bed ◆忙しくて空き時間（割ける時間）がありません I'm so busy that I don't have time to spare.

あきゅうせい　亜急性（の）　subacute ▶亜急性硬化性全脳炎 subacute sclerosing panencephalitis；SSPE　亜急性甲状腺炎 subacute thyroiditis

あきらか　明らか（な） （明白な）**clear, obvious, apparent** （違いがはっきりした）**distinct** （確実な）**definite** （根拠が確かな）**evident** ☞はっきり, 明確 ◆この陰影は明らかに異常です（I'm afraid）This shadow is clearly[obviously / definitely] abnormal. ◆この 2 つの方法の間には明らかな違いがあります There is a distinct difference between these two techniques. ◆この検査によって診断が明らかになるでしょう This test will confirm the diagnosis. ★confirm は「立証する」の意. / The diagnosis will become definite[clear] from the results of this test. ◆喫煙が肺に悪影響を及ぼしていることは明らかです It is obvious[clear] that smoking *is bad for[badly affects] your lungs.

あきらめる　諦める （断念する）**give up** （放棄する）**abandon** ◆諦めないで下さい Please don't give up. ★最後までという意味で until the very end を付けると, 最後は諦めてもよいというニュアンスになるので注意. ◆リハビリを諦めてはだめですよ Don't give up on your rehabilitation! ◆その治療法は

諦めざるをえません I'm afraid that we have to give up with the treatment. ◆彼女は有効な治療を模索するのを諦めかけました She almost abandoned any hope of finding an effective treatment. ◆眠るのを諦める give up *getting any sleep[trying to get some sleep]

あきる 飽きる get[be, become] tired (of) ◆病院食に飽きましたか Are you tired of (eating) the hospital food? ◆お子さんはゲームで遊んでもすぐに飽きてほかの新しいことをやりたがりますか Does your child quickly get tired of playing games and want to move on to something new?

アキレスけん ―腱 Achilles tendon / əkíli:z-/ ◆アキレス腱が切れています You've ruptured your Achilles tendon. / Your Achilles tendon *has ruptured[is cut / is torn]. ▶アキレス腱断裂 Achilles tendon rupture アキレス腱反射 Achilles tendon reflex；ATR / ankle jerk[reflex] アキレス腱縫合術 Achilles tendon repair

あきれる 呆れる （驚いている）be amazed at[by] （ショックを受けている）be shocked at[by] ◆彼の軽率な行動に呆れています We're amazed[shocked] at his thoughtless behavior.

あく¹ 開く open （図open） ☞開く（ひらく） ◆初診の受付は午前8時に開きます The registration counter[desk] for new patients opens at eight in the morning.

あく² 空く 《空いている》empty, vacant, unoccupied ◆申し訳ありませんが，空いているベッドはありません I'm sorry, but there are no empty[vacant] beds available. / I'm sorry, but all the beds are occupied. ◆空いている椅子にお座り下さい Please find an empty seat and sit down. 《暇である》free ◆今週の土曜日の午後は空いています I'm free this Saturday afternoon.

あくい 悪意 （悪感情）ill will （敵意）hostility ◆…に対して悪意を抱く bear ill will toward[against] … ◆私の言葉を悪意に

とらないで下さい，よかれと思って言ったのですから Please don't take *my words wrong[what I said the wrong way]. I meant well.

あくえいきょう 悪影響 bad influence （図悪い影響を与える badly affect） （直接的な悪影響）harmful effect ☞影響 ◆妊娠中の喫煙はあなたと赤ちゃんに悪影響があります Smoking during pregnancy *is bad for [badly affects] you and your baby. ◆睡眠不足は体全体に悪影響を及ぼします Lack of sleep *is harmful to[has a harmful effect on] the whole body. ◆過度の飲酒に伴う悪影響 the harmful effects of excessive drinking

あくえきしつ 悪液質 cachexia ◀がん性悪液質 cancerous cachexia

アクシデント accident ☞事故

あくしゅう 悪臭 （嫌なにおい）bad smell, offensive odor （むかつくようなにおい）foul smell /fául-/ （図foul-smelling） ◆分泌物は悪臭がしますか Does the discharge have a bad smell? ◆痰は悪臭がしますか Is the phlegm foul-smelling?

あくじゅんかん 悪循環 vicious circle [cycle] ◆悪循環に陥る *lead to[result in / end up in] a vicious circle ◆ストレスの悪循環を断ち切る break the vicious circle of stress ◆悪循環から抜け出す break *out of[away from] a vicious circle

あくじょうけん 悪条件 （悪い条件）bad condition （不利な条件）unfavorable condition ◆悪条件が重なる a series of bad conditions happen[occur] / unfavorable conditions happen[occur] one after another

あくせい 悪性（の） malignant /məlígnənt/ （図malignancy） （伝染力が非常に強い）virulent （悪い型の）a bad type (of) （悪質な・有害な）pernicious ◆生検の結果，悪性細胞が認められました Your biopsy showed signs of malignant cells. ◆残念ながら腫瘍は悪性です Unfortunately, your tumor is malignant. ▶悪性関節リウマチ malignant rheumatoid arthritis；MRA 悪性（胸膜）中皮腫 malignant (pleural) mesothelioma　悪性黒色腫 malignant melanoma　悪性腫瘍 malignant tumor　悪性リンパ腫 malignant lymphoma

アクセス　(利用の便)**access** (**to**)　(利用しやすさ)**accessibility**　◆医療情報へのアクセス access to medical information　◆介護サービスへのアクセス accessibility to care services　◆最寄りの保健所はアクセスがよい〈悪い〉ですか Is your local public health center conveniently〈inconveniently〉located?

あくせんくとう　悪戦苦闘する **struggle**　◆あなたは体重のコントロールに悪戦苦闘しているのですね You are struggling to keep your weight under control, aren't you?　◆彼はリハビリに悪戦苦闘しています He is struggling hard with his rehabilitation training.

あくだまコレステロール　悪玉コレステロール **bad cholesterol,** ***low-density lipoprotein**[**LDL**] **cholesterol**

あくび　欠伸　**yawn** /jɔ́ːn/　◆あくびを抑える stifle[suppress] a yawn　◆大きなあくびをする give a big yawn　◀生あくび small[half / slight] yawn

あくへき　悪癖　**bad habit**　◆早食いの悪癖は直したほうがいいですよ You should break your bad habit of *eating too fast [eating on the run].

あくむ　悪夢　**bad dream**　(恐ろしい夢)**nightmare**　◆悪夢にうなされる have a *bad dream[nightmare]

あぐら　◆床にあぐらをかいて坐る sit cross-legged on the floor　▶あぐら座位 sitting crossed-legged / crossed-leg position

あくりょく　握力　(手の強さ)**hand strength**　(握る強さ)**grip strength**　◆握力が強い have a strong grip　◆握力がない(しっかりつかめない)be unable to grasp things　▶握力計 hand grip strength meter / hand dynamometer

あけがた　明け方　**dawn, daybreak** (圖**very early in the morning**)　◆明け方にひどく咳き込みますか Do you cough a lot very early in the morning?　◆明け方近く冷え込みますので, 風邪を引かないように気をつけて下さい It gets cold toward dawn[daybreak], so be careful not to catch (a) cold.

あげく　挙げ句　◆何日も迷ったあげく彼女は手術を受けないことに決めた After hesitating for several days, she finally decided not to have the surgery.

あげさげ　上げ下げ　**raising and lowering**　◆腕の上げ下げに問題はありますか Do you have any difficulty raising and lowering your arms?

あげもの　揚げ物　**deep-fried foods**　★複数形で.　◆揚げ物の摂取はなるべく控えて下さい Please try to avoid eating deep-fried foods as best you can. / Please do your best not to eat deep-fried foods.

あける¹　開ける　**open** (圏**open**)　☞開く(ひらく)　◆目〈口〉を開けて下さい Please open your eyes〈mouth〉.　◆目が開けにくいですか Do you have difficulty opening your eyes?　◆目を開けて真っ直ぐ前を見て下さい Keep your eyes open and look straight ahead.　◆口を大きく開けて「アー」と言って下さい Open your mouth wide and say "ah."　◆このガウンは前を開けて着て下さい Please put this gown on with the front left open.　◆ドアは開けたままにしておきましょうか Should I leave the door open?　◆カーテンを開ける open the curtains

あける²　空ける　**empty**　(場所を)**make room for**　(経路を)**make way for**　◆屑かごの中身をこのビニール袋の中にあけて下さい Please empty the contents of the wastebasket into this plastic bag.　◆車椅子を置くための場所をあけて下さい Please make room for wheelchairs.　◆担架を通すための道をあける make way for the gurney

あける³　明ける　◆もうすぐ夜が明けます It will be morning soon / The sun will be rising soon.　◆明けましておめでとう Happy New Year!

あげる　上げる・挙げる　《高くする》**raise**　(持ち上げる)**put up, lift up**

（引っ張り上げる）pull up ◆右腕を上げて下さい Please raise[lift] your right arm. ◆手を上げて頭の上に載せて下さい Please lift up your hands and put them on your head. ◆両手を上に高く上げて下さい Please raise both hands high above your head. ◆下着のシャツの裾をたくし上げる pull up *one's* undershirt ◆ベッドの頭を上げる際にはこのボタンを押して下さい To raise the head of the bed, push[press] this button. ◆ブラインドを上げる pull up the (window) shade

《与える》give ◆熱を下げるためのお薬を出してあげましょう I'm going to give you a medication to bring down the fever. ◆この血圧手帳をあなたにあげましょう This blood pressure diary is for you.

《人のために何かをする》 ◆私が彼を心電図室へ連れて行ってあげます I'll take him to the EKG room. ◆この車椅子を貸してあげますよ You can use this wheelchair.

《数値を上げる》raise ◆室温を摂氏23℃に上げる raise the room temperature to twenty-three degrees Celsius ◆ストレスは血圧を上げます Stress will raise your blood pressure.

《例を示す》give ◆典型的な例を挙げましょう Let me give you some typical examples. / Here are some typical examples.

あご　顎　jaw /ʤɔː/　（下あごの先端）chin ◆あごをこの台の上に載せて，額をヘッドサポートに付けて下さい Please place your chin on this rest and your forehead against the head support. ◆あごがはずれる dislocate *one's* jaw / have a dislocated jaw ◆あごが痛む have (a) pain in *one's* jaw ◆あごを動かすとカクカクという音が聞こえますか Do you hear clicking sounds when you move your jaw? ◀上〈下〉あご upper〈lower〉jaw ▶あご当て chin rest　あご骨 jawbone

あさ　朝　morning ◆朝は何時に起きますか What time do you get up in the morning? ◆診察時間は朝9時から正午まで，午後は2時から4時までです The office hours are nine to twelve in the

morning, and two to four in the afternoon. ◆では，月曜日の朝にお会いしましょう I'll see you on Monday morning. ◆朝のこわばりがありますか Do you have morning stiffness? ◆明日の朝 tomorrow morning ◆毎朝 every[each] morning ◆朝6時頃 about[around] six o'clock in the morning ☞朝寝坊

あざ　痣　（打撲による内出血斑）bruise /brúːz/　（飀bruise）　（目のまわりの内出血斑）black eye　（先天性の色素沈着）birthmark　（皮膚の変色）skin discoloration ◆あざがありますか Do you have any bruises? ◆あざができやすいですか Do you bruise[get bruises] easily? ◆気づかないうちに黒や青いあざができることがありますか Do you ever get *black or blue spots [bruises / skin discoloration] for no obvious reason? ◆手足に紫色のあざが出る get purple bruises[（大きな斑点）patches] on *one's* hands and legs ◀青あざ（打撲による内出血斑）bruise, black-and-blue mark /（蒙古斑）blue[bluish] spot　赤あざ red birthmark / strawberry mark　黒あざ mole / pigmented nevus

あさい　浅い

《眠りが》shallow, light (↔deep, sound) ◆眠りが浅いですか Are you a light sleeper? / Do you sleep poorly? ◆眠りが浅いと翌朝体が休まった感じがしないでしょう You probably don't feel rested the morning after (you've had) a shallow sleep, do you?

《傷などが》superficial, shallow, slight ◆潰瘍は浅い The ulcers are superficial[shallow]. ◆浅い傷 a slight[superficial] injury[wound]

《呼吸が》shallow ◆呼吸が浅い The breaths are shallow. / The breathing is shallow. ◆浅く息を吸ったり吐いたりして下さい Take shallow breaths in and out.

《月日が》short ◆彼女は日本に来てからまだ日が浅い It's only been a short time since she came to Japan. / She hasn't been in Japan long.

《経験・知識が》shallow, superficial, limited

◆彼女はその問題について浅い知識しかもっていない She has only a shallow [superficial] knowledge of the subject. ◆彼はまだ経験が浅い He has limited experience. / He still lacks experience.

あさごはん 朝ご飯 breakfast ☞朝食
あさって 明後日 the day after tomorrow
あさねぼう 朝寝坊する〈寝過ごす〉oversleep〈遅くまで寝ている〉get up late ◆よく朝寝坊して朝食を抜きますか Do you often oversleep and skip breakfast?
あざやか 鮮やか(な)
《はっきりした》bright, vivid ◆血痰〈血便〉の色は鮮やかな赤ですか Is the blood in your phlegm〈stools〉bright red? ◆鮮やかな画像 a vivid image
《見事な》skillful, excellent ◆鮮やかな腕前の外科医 a skillful surgeon
あさんかちっそ 亜酸化窒素 nitrous oxide 〈笑気〉laughing gas
あし 足・脚〈下肢〉leg〈足首から下の部分〉foot〈複feet〉〈太もも〉thigh /θáɪ/〈膝〉knee /níː/〈向こうずね〉shin〈ふくらはぎ〉calf〈足首・くるぶし〉ankle〈かかと〉heel
《部位の表現》◆足の裏 the sole (of the foot) ◆足の甲 the instep ◆足の指 a toe ◆足の指先 the tip of one's toe / one's toe tip ◆足の付け根[股関節]a hip joint
《診察の基本表現》◆足に何か問題がありますか Do you have any problems with your legs〈feet〉? ◆足を見せて下さい Now, let me see[examine] your leg〈foot〉. ◆足に怪我をしたことがありますか Have you ever had a leg〈foot〉injury? ◆足がむくんだことがありますか Have you noticed any swelling in your feet or legs? ◆右足はどういう時に痛みますか In what situations do you get the pain in your right leg〈foot〉? / When does your right leg〈foot〉usually hurt? ◆いつから足がしびれていますか How long has it been since you lost the feeling in your legs〈feet〉? ◆足を少し開いて立ってみて下さい Please stand with your feet slightly apart. ◆ここに横になって左足を上げて下さい Please lie down here and raise your left leg.
《症状の表現》◆足が痛む one's legs〈feet〉*feel painful[hurt / ache] ◆足が痒い one's legs〈feet〉feel[are] itchy / one's legs〈feet〉itch ◆足がむず痒い one's legs feel[are] itchy and creepy-crawly / have itchy, crawly legs ◆足がだるい one's legs feel tired[sluggish / weak / heavy] ◆足がつる have[get] leg cramps / have[get] cramps in one's leg ◆足がぴくぴく動く have twitchy legs ◆足がむくむ have swollen legs / one's legs are swollen / have swelling in one's legs ◆足が弱い be weak in the legs / have weak legs ◆足を引きずる shuffle /〈片足を引きずる〉limp ◆足を小刻みに引きずって歩く walk with short, quick, and shuffling steps
《受傷の表現》◆スケートをしていて足を骨折しましたか Did you break your leg (while) skating? ◆階段を降りる時に足を踏み外す miss one's step going down the stairs ◆足が折れている have a broken leg ◆足をくじく[足をひねる]twist one's ankle ◆足を捻挫する sprain one's ankle
《動作の表現》◆足を伸ばす stretch one's legs〈knees〉◆足を曲げる bend one's legs〈knees〉

◀摺り足 shuffle 垂れ足 footdrop / drop foot ☞足置き, 足音, 足型, 足首, 足腰, 足白癬, 足踏み, 足元, 足湯

あじ 味 taste〈動taste〉◆甘い味がする It has a sweet taste. / It tastes sweet. ◆苦い味 a bitter taste ◆酸っぱい味 a sour taste ◆酸味 an acidic taste ◆辛い味 a hot taste ◆塩辛い味 a salty taste ◆味が薄い It tastes weak[thin]. ◆どんな味でしたか What did it taste like? ◆お味はいかがですか How does it taste? / How do you like it? ◆味がわからなくなっていますか Do you think you are losing your sense of taste? ◆薄味の物を食べるように心がけて下さい〈塩分の少ない食べ物を食べる〉You must try to eat *lightly salted[low-salt] foods. /〈塩を入れ過ぎないようにする〉You should try not to put too much salt in your foods. ◆あっさりした味の食べ物 plain[simple] food ◆薄い味付けの食べ物 lightly-seasoned food ◆濃い味付けの食べ物 well-seasoned[highly seasoned] food ◆口の中が酸っぱい味がする have a sour taste in *one's* mouth ◆味の感覚が鋭い have *a keen[an acute] sense of taste

あしおき　足置き　footrest, footstool
◆この足置きに左足を乗せて下さい Please put your left foot on this footrest.

あしおと　足音　footstep　◆夜になると廊下の足音が神経にさわりますか Do the footsteps in the hall grate[get] on your nerves at night?

あしがた　足型・足形　footprint（▥footprint）　◆看護師が赤ちゃんの足型をとります The nurse will get your baby's footprint. / The nurse will footprint your baby.

あしからず　悪しからず　◆当院は完全予約制になっておりますので，悪しからずご了承下さい I'm sorry, but[I'm sorry to say that] we see patients by appointment only in this hospital.

あしくび　足首　ankle　◆足首をひねる twist *one's* ankle　◆足首を捻挫する sprain *one's* ankle　◆足首がむくむ have swollen ankles / have swelling in *one's* ankles / *one's* ankles swell　▶足首サポーター ankle support

あじけない　味気ない　boring, dull　◆生活が味気ないと感じていますか Do you feel that your life is boring[dull]?

あしこし　足腰　lower body　◆スクワットで足腰を鍛える strengthen *one's* lower body by doing squats

アシスタント　assistant

アジソンびょう　―病　Addison disease；*an endocrine disorder caused by insufficient production of steroid hormones by the adrenal cortex*

あした　明日　tomorrow　◆では，また明日 See you tomorrow.　◆明日の午後1時にお電話を下さい Please call me at one tomorrow afternoon.

あじつけ　味付けする　season　☞味
◆濃い味付けの食べ物がお好みですか Do you like well-seasoned[highly seasoned / strongly seasoned] foods?

アシドーシス　acidosis；*a disorder of the acid-base balance of the body with a condition of increased acidity of the blood*　◀腎尿細管性アシドーシス renal tubular acidosis；RTA　代謝性アシドーシス metabolic acidosis　代償性アシドーシス compensatory acidosis　乳酸アシドーシス lactic acidosis

あしはくせん　足白癬　athlete's foot（▤feet）, ringworm of the foot, tinea pedis

あしぶみ　足踏みする　march on the spot, step　◆目を閉じて50歩その場で足踏みをして下さい Please close your eyes and march on the spot for fifty steps.　▶足踏み検査 stepping[step] test

あしもと　足元　◆足元にお気をつけ下さい Please watch your step.　◆足元がふらつきますか Do you feel unsteady[shaky] on your feet?

あしゆ　足湯　foot bath

あじわう　味わう
《味を楽しむ》**taste**　◆お食事はゆっくり時間をかけて味わいながら召し上がって下さい Please take time to eat slowly and taste your food.
《体験する》**go through, experience**　◆夫を亡くして彼女は経済的苦難を味わっています Since her husband's death, she has been *going through[experiencing] some financial difficulties.

あす　明日　tomorrow　☞明日(あした)

あずける　預ける　leave　◆貴重品はご家族の方にお預け下さい Please leave your valuables with a family member.

アスピリン　aspirin /ǽspərɪn/　◆低用量のアスピリンは血管の詰まりを予防してくれます Low-dose aspirin helps prevent blood from clotting.　▶アスピリン喘息 aspirin-induced asthma；AIA / aspirin-sensitive asthma

アスベスト　asbestos　◆これまでにアスベストに曝されたことがありますか Have

you ever been exposed to asbestos? ◆これまでにアスベストを吸い込んだことがありますか Have you ever inhaled asbestos（fibers）? ▶アスベスト肺 asbestos lung / pulmonary asbestosis　アスベスト曝露 asbestos exposure

アスペルガーしょうこうぐん ―症候群
Asperger syndrome；AS　☞自閉

アスペルギルス *Aspergillus* ◀侵襲性肺アスペルギルス症 invasive pulmonary aspergillosis　肺アスペルギルス症 pulmonary aspergillosis　慢性進行性肺アスペルギルス症 chronic progressive pulmonary aspergillosis；CPPA

アスペルギローマ　aspergilloma ◀肺アスペルギローマ pulmonary aspergilloma

あ せ　汗 sweat /swét/　（圏sweat 厖sweaty）, perspiration（圏perspire） ◆いつもより汗をたくさんかきますか Do you sweat more than usual[（以 前 より）you used to]?　◆汗が出にくいですか Do you sweat very little?　◆汗 を か き 始め る break into[out in] a sweat　◆汗ばんでじっとりする become[get] slightly sweaty and clammy　◆汗をかいている be in a sweat　◆大量に汗をかく sweat heavily[a lot]　◆汗臭い smell sweaty ◀脂汗greasy[oily] sweat　冷や汗 cold sweat ☞寝汗

アセスメント　assessment（圏assess） ◆退院後自立生活の可能性についてアセスメントを行う assess[make an assessment of] *a patient's* ability to live independently after discharge from the hospital ◀リスクアセスメント risk assessment フィジカルアセスメント physical assessment

アセチルサリチルさん ―酸 acetylsalicylic acid　☞アスピリン

アセトアミノフェン acetaminophen

アセトン acetone ▶アセトン血症 acetonemia　アセトン血性嘔吐（症）acetonemic vomiting　アセトン尿症 acetonuria

あせも 汗疹 prickly heat, heat rash ◆背中にあせもができる have *prickly heat[a heat rash] on *one's* back

あせる 焦る get[grow, become] impatient ◆なかなか回復しないので彼は焦り始めています He is getting[growing] impatient with the slow pace of his recovery.　◆焦らないで下さい．手術後は体を十分に休ませる必要があります Take it easy[Don't be in a rush]. To recover from the surgery, your body needs a good rest.

あそび 遊び （動作）play （活動）playing activity （ゲーム）game （気晴らし）pastime （楽しみ）pleasure ◆お子さんはどんな遊びが一番好きですか What activities does your child like to play at the most?　◆遊びを通して学ぶ learn through play　◆たまには遊びも必要ですよ You need to relax and have fun sometimes too. ★have fun は「楽しむ」を意味する． / You should enjoy a pastime once in a while too.　◆日本へいらっしゃったのは仕事ですか，それとも遊びですか Did you come to Japan for business or pleasure? ▶遊び時間 playtime 遊び道具（玩具）toy　遊び友達 playmate 遊び場 play area

---

子供の遊び　プレイルームで

- ●ごっこ遊びをする play make-believe, play pretend
- ●ゲームをする play a game
- ●トランプする play cards
- ●おままごとをする play house
- ●鬼ごっこする play tag
- ●かくれんぼする play hide-and-seek
- ●物を作る make things
- ●絵を描く draw（a picture）
- ●塗り絵をする do some coloring
- ●おままごとをしよう Let's play house!
- ●トランプで遊ぼう Let's play cards!
- ●ブロックで高いタワーを作ろう Let's make a tower with blocks!
- ●クマさんと遊びたい? Do you want to play with（your）teddy?
- ●塗り絵（お絵かき）をしたい? Do you want to do some coloring〈drawing〉?
- ●ジグソーパズルをやりたい? Do you want to do a jigsaw puzzle?

■遊び道具

●人形 doll, dolly ●ぬいぐるみのクマ teddy bear, teddy ●ぬいぐるみのおもちゃ stuffed toy, soft[cuddly] toy ●レゴ (商標名)Lego ●積み木 blocks ●ジグソーパズル jigsaw puzzle ●お話の本 storybook ●絵本 picture book ●塗り絵 coloring ●お絵かき drawing ●ボードゲーム board game ●列車セット train set ●茶器セット tea set

あそぶ　遊ぶ

《楽しむ》play, enjoy *oneself*, have a good time ◆息子さんは他の子供達と遊びますか，それともひとりで遊ぶほうが好きですか Does your son play with others or by himself? ◆友達と遊ぶ play with friends ◆積み木で遊ぶ play with blocks ◆ビデオゲームで遊ぶ play a video game ◆遊ぶ暇がない have no time to enjoy *oneself*

《無為に過ごす》idle *one's* time away, loaf around ◆彼は定職につかず遊んで暮らしています He doesn't have a steady job, but is *idling his time away[loafing around] with nothing to do.

あたい　値する　be worth ◆糖尿病に関するこの記事は，一読に値します This article on diabetes is worth reading.

あたえる　与える　give (引き起こす)cause (影響を及ぼす)do ☞あげる, 供給

◆外泊の許可を与える give *a patient* permission to go home for the night ◆乳製品がアレルギーの原因と考えられるので，お子さんに与えないように注意して下さい Milk[Dairy] products are probably causing your child's allergic reaction, so please don't give them to him〈her〉anymore. ◆妊娠中の喫煙は胎児に悪影響を与えます Smoking during pregnancy is *bad for[harmful to] the unborn baby. ◆患者に無用な不安を与える give [cause] unnecessary anxiety to patients / make patients unnecessarily anxious

◆苦痛を与える cause distress ◆損害を与える damage / harm / cause[do] dam-

age ◆損傷を与える injure / harm / cause injury

あたたかい　暖かい・温かい

《温度などが》warm /wɔ́ɚm/ (気候が温和な)mild ◆きょうはとても暖かですね It's nice and warm today, isn't it? ◆今年の冬は暖かです We're having a mild[warm] winter this year. ◆温かいお茶はいかがですか(熱い)How about a cup of hot tea?

◆暖かいひざ掛け a warm lap throw [robe]

《人柄が》warm ◆彼女は気さくで心の温かな人です She is a friendly and warm-hearted person.

あたためる　温める　warm /wɔ́ɚm/, apply heat ◆このスープを電子レンジで温めなおしましょうか Shall I warm up this soup in the microwave? ◆傷が腫れている時は温めないで下さい Please don't apply heat to an injury when it is swollen.

◆血流を良くするために温める apply heat to increase blood flow

あだっきゅう　亞脱臼　subluxation, incomplete dislocation, partial dislocation

あたま　頭　head　★英語では首から上の部分すべてを含む. ☞頭部

《診察の基本表現》☞痛み，頭痛 ◆頭に何か問題がありますか Do you have any problems with your head? ◆頭が痛いのですか Do you have a headache? ◆頭はどのように痛みますか What's the headache[pain in the head] like? / Can you describe the headache[pain in the head] for me? ◆頭の痛みはどのくらいの間続いていますか How long have you had the headache[pain in the head]? ◆頭全体が痛みますか Does it hurt all over your head? ◆頭に怪我をしたことがありますか Have you ever had a head injury?

《症状の表現》◆頭が重い *one's* head feels heavy / have a heavy feeling in the head ◆頭がくらくらする(めまいがする) feel dizzy ◆頭がふらっとする(気が遠くなる) feel faint / (めまいがする) feel light-headed ◆頭がぐるぐる回る feel like *one's* head is spinning ◆頭がずきずき痛

あたま　　　　　　　　　　　　　　13　　　　　　　　　　　　　　あたる

む one's head is throbbing / have a throbbing headache[pain in one's head]　◆頭が割れるように痛む have a splitting headache

《受傷の表現》　◆頭から落ちる fall headlong (into)　◆頭をぶつける hit one's head on　◆転んで頭を床にぶつける fall down and hit one's head on the floor　◆頭にこぶができる get[have] a bump on the head　◆頭を怪我する injure[hurt] one's head

《動作の表現》　◆頭を洗う wash one's hair　◆頭を下げる bend[lower] one's head　◆頭を反対方向に向ける turn one's head in the opposite direction　◆頭を反対の肩のほうに傾ける tilt one's head to[toward] the opposite shoulder

《その他の慣用表現》　(悩み・苦労がある)　◆病院の支払いのことで頭が痛いのですか Does it give you a headache just thinking about how to pay the hospital fees? / Are you worried[concerned] about paying the hospital fees?　◆彼女は退院後の生活設計のことで頭がいっぱいになっています She's full of her plans for what she's going to do after getting out of the hospital.　◆彼女は子供の暴力のことで頭を抱えています She has no idea what to do about her child's violent behavior.　(感心する)　◆あなたの粘り強さには頭が下がります I really admire you for your patience.　(頭脳)　◆お子さんは頭がいいですね Your child is really smart[clever].　◆パズルやクイズで頭の体操をするとよいでしょう You should *give your brain a workout [exercise your brain] with puzzles and quizzes.　(性格・考え方)　◆彼は頭が固くて自分のやり方に固執します He's stubborn[He's inflexible] and sticks to his way of doing things.　◆頭の柔らかい人 a flexible person / a person who deals with situations flexibly　(意識)　◆いい考えが頭に浮かびました I (suddenly) had [thought of] a good idea.　(冷静になる)　◆頭を冷やしてから話し合いましょう Let's talk after we've calmed[cooled] down a bit. / Let's calm[cool] down a bit before carrying on with our talk.　(その他)　◆息子さんを頭ごなしに叱らないで下さい You shouldn't scold your son without first listening to what he has to say.

アタマジラミ　head lice (圏louse)　★通例，複数形で．　▶アタマジラミ症 pediculosis capitis

アダムス・ストークスほっさ　―発作 Adams-Stokes attack

あたらしい　新しい　(新たな・新しくできた) new　(新鮮な)fresh　(清潔な)clean　(最新の) the latest　◆新しい生活を始める start a new life　◆新しいシーツをベッドに敷く put clean[fresh] sheets on the bed　◆新しい情報 the latest information

あたり　辺り
《近辺》　◆この辺りにはコンビニがありません There are no convenience stores *around here[in this area / near this hospital].
《おおよその位置・時刻など》　◆来週辺りご都合はいかがですか Is sometime next week convenient for you?

あたりまえ　当たり前(の)　(妥当な)reasonable　(自然な)natural　(最も適切な) right　(普通の・通常の)normal　◆あなたの要求は当たり前です I think your request [demand] is quite reasonable.　◆こうした困難な状況の下では強いストレスを感じるのは当たり前のことです It's natural that you feel extremely stressed under such difficult circumstances.　◆私は当たり前のことをしたまでです I only did *what anyone would have done[what was right].　◆看護師に助けを求めるのは当たり前のことです It's normal to ask the nurses for help.　◆このような出来事は病院ではごく当たり前に起こります Such an event happens every day in hospitals. / Such an event is a normal part of everyday hospital life.

あたる　当たる
《ぶつかる》hit　◆テニスのボールが目に当たったのですか Did a tennis ball hit you in the eye? / Did you get hit in the eye by a

tennis ball?

《該当する》 ◆あなたの国の言葉で"Good morning"に当たる言葉は何ですか How do you say "Good morning" in your language?

《中毒になる》 ◆昨夜食べた物の何かに当たったと思いますか(体に合わない物を食べた) Do you think you ate something that didn't agree with you last night?

《天気に曝される》expose ◆日光に当たり過ぎないように気をつけて下さい Be careful not to *expose your skin to too much sunlight[spend too much time in the sun]. ◆薬は直射日光が当たらない場所に保管して下さい Please keep medications *out of[away from] direct sunlight. / Don't store medications in direct sunlight. ◆この病室は南向きなので日がよく当たります This room faces south, so it gets plenty of sunshine.

《打診する》sound out ◆この件については他の医師に当たってみます I'm going to *sound out another doctor[seek out another doctor's opinion] on this matter.

あちら (あそこ)**over there** (その方向)**that way** ◆トイレはあちらにあります The restroom[The toilet] is over there. ◆あちらでお待ちします I'll be waiting for you over there. ◆あちらへどうぞ Go that way, please.

あつい¹ 熱い・暑い (温度が高い)**hot**, **very warm** (熱した)**heated** ◆熱い風呂に入る take a hot bath ◆熱いものを飲むと胸焼けがしますか When you drink something hot, do you get heartburn?

あつい² 厚い (厚みがある)**thick** (函**thicken**) (重い)**heavy** ◆プラークがたまって血管の壁が厚くなっています The walls of the blood vessels have become thick due to a buildup of plaque. ◆動脈は加齢で厚くなる傾向があります Arteries tend to thicken with age.

あっか 悪化する **get worse** (重くなる)**become more serious** ☞増悪 ◆痛みは悪化していますか Is the pain getting worse? ◆痛みを悪化させるものがありま

すか Is there anything that makes the pain worse? ◆頭痛を悪化させるものは何ですか What makes the headache worse? ◆頭痛は軽快傾向ですか, 悪化傾向ですか, 変化なしですか Is your headache getting better, getting worse, or is there no change? ◆彼は今朝容体が急激に悪化しました He took a sudden turn for the worse this morning. ◆彼女の病状が悪化しています Her condition has become more serious.

あつかう 扱う
《使用する》**use** (手で扱う)**handle** ◆吸入器を扱ったことはありますか Have you ever used an inhaler before? ◆この器具の扱いは十分に気をつけて下さい Please handle this device with great care. ◆酸素濃縮装置の扱い方を説明する explain how to handle the oxygen concentrator

《対処する》**deal** (**with**), **treat** ◆扱いにくい人 a person who is hard to deal with / (満足させるのが難しい人)a person who is hard to please

《受け付ける》**accept** ◆残念ですが, 当院ではあなたの旅行保険は扱えません I'm afraid that we can't accept your travel insurance at this hospital.

《物品などを扱う》**carry** ◆当院ではその薬は扱っていませんので, 代替薬を処方いたします We don't carry that medication in this hospital, so I'm going to prescribe an alternative medication for you.

あつかく 圧覚 **pressure sense[sensation]**

あつがり 暑がり ◆暑がりですか Are you sensitive to (the) heat?

あつぎ 厚着 ◆赤ちゃんには厚着をさせないほうがいいでしょう You should not clothe your baby too heavily. ◆厚着しすぎる wear too much clothing / be too heavily clothed

あっこんふしゅ 圧痕浮腫 **pitting edema**

あつさ 暑さ **heat** ◆暑さは頭痛を悪化させますか Does heat[hot weather] make your headache worse?

あつざそんしょう 圧挫損傷 **crush injury**

あっさり

《くどくない》(味が淡白な)plain (薄い味付けの)lightly-seasoned ◆あっさりした食べ物のほうがお好きですか Do you prefer plain[lightly-seasoned] food?

《即座に》readily ◆彼は飲酒をあっさり認めました He readily admitted that he had been drinking alcohol.

アッシャーマンしょうこうぐん ―症候群
Asherman syndrome

あっしゅく 圧縮する compress (圧圧縮された compressed) ☞圧迫

あっせん 斡旋 ◆申し訳ありませんが,当院ではご家族の宿泊施設の斡旋はいたしておりません I'm sorry, but we can't assist with finding accommodation for family members.

あっつう 圧痛 tenderness ◀反跳圧痛 rebound tenderness ▶圧痛点 tender point

あっぱく 圧迫 (圧力)pressure (圧press) (圧縮)compression ◆胸に圧迫感を覚えることがありますか Do you feel any chest pressure? / Do you feel any pressure in [on] your chest? ◆少し圧迫感を覚えるかもしれません You may feel some pressure. ◆これから腹部を圧迫しますので痛みがあれば教えて下さい I'm going to press on your abdomen. If it hurts, let me know. ◆圧迫されるような痛み a pressure-like pain ◀胸骨圧迫心マッサージ chest compression cardiac massage 神経根圧迫 nerve root compression 脊髄圧迫(spinal) cord compression 壁外性圧迫 extrinsic compression ▶圧迫骨折 compression fracture 圧迫固定 pressure dressing 圧迫帯 tourniquet 圧迫包帯 pressure[compression] bandage

あつはんしゃ 圧反射 baroreflex

あつふか 圧負荷 pressure overload

アップルコアちょうこう ―徴候 apple core sign

あつまる 集まる

《集合する》gather (会合する)meet ◆家族全員が彼のベッドの周りに集まりました The family all gathered around his bed.

◆アルコール依存症患者の自助グループは毎週金曜日に集まりますので,どうぞご出席下さい The self-help group for alcoholics meets every Friday, so you're welcome to attend it. ◆皆さんがお集まりになったら,すぐに始めます(着いたら)We'll begin as soon as everyone *gets here[(現れたら)shows up].

《集中する》focus (on) ◆最近,分子標的治療に注目が集まっています Much attention has recently been focused on molecularly targeted therapy.

あつめる 集める

《収集する》(集める)collect, gather (手に入れる)get, pick up ◆データを集める collect[gather] data ◆清掃係が毎朝ごみを集めます The cleaners collect the trash every morning. ◆院内の図書室でその病気についての情報を集めることができます You can get[pick up] some information about the disease in the hospital library.

《人の目を引く》attract, draw ◆この新しい治療法は国際的にも注目を集めました This new treatment has attracted[drawn] international attention.

あつらえる 誂える ◆装具はあなたに合わせて誂えます You can have a prosthesis made specially for you. / You can have a custom-made prosthesis.

あつりょく 圧力 pressure ◆精神的圧力 psychological[mental] pressure

あて¹ 宛 ☞宛てる ◆あなた宛のお手紙ですよ Here's a letter *for you[addressed to you]. ◆紹介状はどなた宛にお送りしましょうか Who shall I send the referral letter to? / To whom should I address the referral letter?

あて² 当て ◆当てになる親戚や友人はいますか(頼りにできる)Do you have any relatives or friends you can *count on[rely on / depend on]? ◆インターネットの情報は当てにならないものもありますので,注意して下さい(信頼できないかもしれないので)Information on the Internet may not be reliable[dependable], so be careful about using it.

アテトーシス athetosis ▶アテトーシス様運動 athetoid movement

アデノイド adenoids /ǽdənɔ̀ɪdz/ ★通例，複数形で． ◆アデノイドが腫れています Your adenoids are swollen． ◆アデノイドを切除する remove *a person's* adenoids / take *a person's* adenoids out ◆アデノイドを切除する必要があります（切除してもらう）You need to have your adenoids out[taken out / removed]． ▶アデノイド切除術 adenoidectomy

アデノウイルス adenovirus ▶アデノウイルス感染症 adenovirus infection

アデノシンデアミナーゼ adenosine de-aminase；ADA ▶アデノシンデアミナーゼ欠損症 adenosine deaminase deficiency

あてはまる 当てはまる apply ◆当てはまる項目の番号を○で囲んで下さい For each item, please circle the number that applies to you.

あてる¹ 宛てる address /ədrés/ ◆家庭医に宛てた紹介状を書く write a referral letter（addressed）to a family doctor

あてる² 当てる
《あてがう》（置く）put, place（くっつける）attach ◆切り傷にガーゼを当てる put a piece of gauze over the cut / cover the cut with gauze ◆胸，腕，足に電極を当てる *place the electrodes on[attach the electrodes to] a person's* chest, arms, and legs ◆額に手を当てる put *one's* hand on the forehead
《曝す》expose ◆この薬を直射日光に当てないで下さい Please don't expose this medication to direct sunlight. / This medication should not be exposed to direct sunlight.
《ぶつける》hit, bump ◆ここの天井は低くなっています．頭を当てないよう注意して下さい The ceiling ahead is low, so take care you don't hit[bump] your head. / Watch out for the ceiling. It's low, so mind your head. / （掲示）Low ceiling. Mind your head.
《的中させる》（言う）tell（推測する）

guess ◆これから5つの品物を見せて隠しますので，それから何があったかを当てて下さい I'm going to show you five items and then hide them, and after that I want you to tell me what they were.

アテローム atheroma ★日本ではアテロームを粉瘤の意味で使用するが，欧米では一般に動脈硬化性の弱腫を意味するので注意する． ☞プラーク ◆アテロームが動脈の壁にたまると，血管の内腔が狭くなって血液の流れを悪くします When atheroma builds up on the arterial walls, it causes narrowing of the insides of the arteries and, therefore, reduces blood flow. ▶アテローム血栓 atherothrombosis アテローム血栓性梗塞 atherothrombotic infarction アテローム血栓性塞栓 atherothrombotic embolism アテローム性動脈硬化 atherosclerosis

アテンダント attendant

あと¹ 後
《より遅く・以降》later（圏圏after） ◆後でそちらに参ります I'll be there later. ◆手術後は集中治療室へ移ります You'll be taken to the *intensive care unit[ICU] after the surgery. ◆食事の後はゆっくり休んで下さい Take a good rest after meals[eating]. ◆それは後回しでよいでしょう That can wait. / You can do that later.
《後ろ》 ◆私の後についてきて下さい Please follow me. ◆お子さんはあなたの後を追いますか Does your child follow after you? ◆私の後に繰り返して言って下さい Please repeat after me.
《他のこと・残り》the rest ◆後のことは私達に任せて下さい Just leave the rest to us.
《さらに》 ◆あと2，3分お待ち下さい Please wait a few more minutes. ◆あと10分で終わります We'll finish[It'll be over] in ten minutes. / Ten more minutes to go.
《過去》 ◆もう後戻りできませんから，現時点でできる最善の方法を考えましょう We can't turn back now[It's too late to turn back], so let me think what's the best option we've got now for treating your condition.

あと² 痕・跡 （傷跡）scar （しみ・印）mark （斑点）spot （存在した形跡）trace （証拠・印）sign ◆この傷はかなり深いので痕が残るかもしれません This cut is very deep, so it may leave a scar. ◆右足にやけどの痕がある have a scar from a burn on *one's* right leg ◆引っ掻いた痕がある have scratch marks ◆胃に潰瘍の（治った）痕があります You have traces[signs] of a stomach ulcer that has healed. ◆蚊に刺された痕 a mosquito bite ◀爪痕 nail mark[引っ掻き傷]scratch] にきび痕 acne spot[(へこみ)pit]

あとざん 後産 afterbirth ☞後産（こうさん）

アトニー atony ◀胃アトニー gastric atony 子宮アトニー uterine atony 膀胱アトニー vesical atony

アドバイス advice ☞助言，勧める，忠告

アトピー atopy /ǽtəpi/ （圏atópic）(↔nonatopic) ◆アトピー性皮膚炎になる get atopic dermatitis[eczema] ◀非アトピー性喘息 nonatopic asthma ▶アトピー遺伝子 atopic gene アトピー性結膜炎 atopic conjunctivitis アトピー性疾患 atopic disease アトピー性喘息 atopic asthma アトピー素因 atopic predisposition / atopic diathesis

アドレナリン adrenaline （圏adrenergic） ▶アドレナリン拮抗薬 adrenergic antagonist アドレナリン作動薬 adrenergic drug[agent / agonist] アドレナリン遮断薬 adrenergic *blocking agent[blocker]

あな 穴・孔 hole （穿孔）perforation ☞穿孔 ◆あなたの右肺に穴が開いて気胸になっています Pneumothorax has occurred because of a hole that developed in your right lung. / You've got[suffered] a collapsed lung because of a hole in your right lung. ◀毛穴 pore

アナフィラキシー anaphylaxis （圏anaphylactic） ◀運動誘発性アナフィラキシー exercise-induced anaphylaxis ▶アナフィラキシー反応 anaphylactic reaction ☞アナフィラキシーショック

アナフィラキシーショック anaphylactic shock ◆アナフィラキシーショックは，深刻なアレルギー反応が全身に及ぶ緊急を要する状態です Anaphylactic shock is an emergency condition in which a severe allergic reaction involves the entire body. ◆(人が)アナフィラキシーショックを起こす develop[go into] anaphylactic shock ◆(アレルゲンとなる食べ物や薬などが)アナフィラキシーショックを引き起こす induce[trigger] anaphylactic shock

アナフィラクトイドしはんびょう ―紫斑病 anaphylactoid purpura

アナライザー analyzer

あに 兄 （older, big, elder）brother ★英語では通例 brother のみでよい．

アニサキス *Anisakis* ▶アニサキス症 anisakiasis

アニリン aniline ▶アニリン中毒 aniline poisoning / anilinism

あね 姉 （older, big, elder）sister ★英語では通例 sister のみでよい．

アパート （一世帯）apartment,《英》flat （建物全体）apartment building[house],《英》block of flats ◆住んでいる家はアパートですか，一戸建てですか Do you live in an apartment or a house? ◆あなたのアパートは何階ですか What floor is your apartment on? ◆アパートにはエレベーターがありますか Is there an elevator in your apartment building?

アパシー apathy, lack of interest ◀学生アパシー student apathy

あばた pockmark （圏pockmarked）

あばれる 暴れる （もがく）struggle （暴力をふるう）become violent, behave violently ◆息子さんは思い通りにならないと暴れますか Does your son become violent when he can't get his own way?

アビウムイントラセルラーレコンプレックスがたこうさんきん ―型抗酸菌 *Mycobacterium avium-intracellulare* complex；MAC

あびる 浴びる （風呂・シャワーを浴びる）take, have （曝される）be exposed （to） （覆われる）be covered （with） ◆今日のと

ころはシャワーを浴びるのを控えて下さい You should not take[have] a shower today. / Please refrain from taking[having] a shower today. ◆通常 X 線検査で浴びる放射線は身体に影響が出るほどの量ではありません The amount of radiation in an X-ray is usually so small that it isn't considered dangerous to the body.

アブ　horsefly　▶アブ刺咬症 horsefly bite

アプガースコア　Apgar score　◆アプガースコアは出生時の赤ちゃんの身体の状態を評価するテストです The Apgar score is a test for evaluating an infant's physical condition at birth.

アフガニスタン　Afghanistan　（形Afghan）　☞国籍　▶アフガニスタン人（の）Afghan

アフタ　aphtha　（形aphthous）　▶アフタ性口内炎 aphthous stomatitis / aphthous ulcer / canker sore / mouth sore　アフタ様潰瘍 aphthoid ulcer

アフターケア　aftercare

あぶない　危ない　（危険な）dangerous, risky　（危篤状態の）critical　（不安定な）unsteady　◆手術後すぐにひとり歩きするのは危ないですよ It's dangerous for you to walk *by yourself[without any support] soon after the surgery.　◆彼はまだ危ない状態にあります He is still in (a) critical condition.　◆彼女は足元が危ない She is unsteady on her feet.

あぶみ　（産婦人科用の）stirrups　★複数形で.　◆足をこのあぶみに入れて下さい Please put your feet into these stirrups.

アブミこつ　―骨　stapes, stapedes　★複数形で.

あぶら　脂・油　（油脂）grease　（液体の油）oil　☞脂汗, 脂性, 脂っこい, 脂肪

あぶらあせ　脂汗　greasy sweat, oily sweat　☞汗　◆脂汗が出る break out in *a greasy[an oily] sweat　◆脂汗をかいている be in *a greasy[an oily] sweat

あぶらしょう　脂性（の）　greasy, oily　◆脂性の肌をしている have greasy[oily] skin　◆肌は脂性ですか Is your skin greasy[oily]?

あぶらっこい　脂っこい　（脂身の多い）fatty　（脂っぽい）greasy, oily　◆脂っこい物をたくさん食べましたか Have you eaten large amounts of fatty[greasy] food?　◆脂っこい食べ物は痛みを悪化させるでしょう Fatty[Greasy] foods will make the pain worse.

アフリカけいアメリカじん　―系アメリカ人　African American

アブレーション　ablation　◀高周波（カテーテル）アブレーション radiofrequency (catheter) ablation；RFA

あふれる　溢れる　《流れ出る》overflow, run over　◆理由もなく涙があふれますか Do your eyes overflow with tears for no apparent reason?　◆洗面台があふれないように忘れずに蛇口をひねって水を止めて下さい Please remember to turn off the tap so the sink doesn't overflow[run over].　《いっぱいになる》be filled with, be full of　◆この病棟は笑い声と笑顔にあふれています This ward is *filled with[full of] laughter and smiling faces.　◆彼女は息子にあふれんばかりの愛情を注いでいます She showers her son with love.

アプローチ　approach　◆新しいアプローチをする take[adopt] a new approach

アヘン　阿片　opium　（アヘン剤）opiate

アポイント　appointment　☞予約　◆受付に行って次回のアポイントを取って下さい Please go to the reception desk and make an appointment for your next visit.

アポクリンせん　―（汗）腺　apocrine sweat gland

アポトーシス　apoptosis；*programmed cell death*

あまい　甘い　《味・匂い》sweet　◆甘い物をよく食べますか Do you often eat sweet things?　◆甘い香りの花 sweet-smelling flowers　《考え方・姿勢》（楽天的な）optimistic　（自由放任の）permissive　（寛大な）indulgent, lenient　◆この病気を甘くみてはいけません（軽々しく考えてはいけない）Don't take this illness too lightly. / Don't be too optimistic about this illness.　◆甘すぎる親

overly permissive[indulgent] parents / parents who pamper their children too much

あまえ 甘え （関心を引こうとする行為）attention-seeking （behavior） （依存心）emotional dependence ◆甘えっ子 an attention-seeking child / a child who wants to be the center of everybody's attention

あまやかす 甘やかす pamper, spoil, overindulge ◆子供を甘やかす pamper [spoil / overindulge] one's child ◆甘やかされた子供 a spoiled child

あまり 余り
《残り》the remainder, the rest （食べ物の残り）leftovers ★複数形で。 ◆100から7を引くと余りはいくつになりますか What's seven from one hundred? / If you take [subtract] seven from one hundred, what's the remainder? ◆坐薬を使用したら，余りは冷蔵庫にしまって下さい After using a suppository, store the rest in the refrigerator. ◆食事の余りはこの容器に入れて下さい Please put （any） leftovers in this container.
《…と少し》over …, more than … ◆彼女は寝たきりになってから2年あまりになります She has been bedridden[confined to bed] for *over two years[more than two years].
《過度に》too, excessively ◆あまり無理をしないで下さい Please don't work too hard. / Please don't overdo things. ◆甘い物をあまり食べないように気をつけて下さい Be careful not to eat too many sweets [sweet things]. ◆サプリメントはあまり摂り過ぎるとかえって害になります Taking too many supplements can do you more harm than good.
《あまり…ない》not … very, not … much ◆彼女の容体はあまりよくありません Her condition isn't very good. ◆日本食はあまりお好きではないのでしょう You don't seem to like Japanese food very much. / You don't like Japanese food very much, do you? ◆手術日まであまり時間がありません There isn't much time before the day of your surgery. ◆あまり長くお話しする時間がないのですが I'm afraid I can't talk with you for long. / I'm afraid I can't spare much time to talk with you. ◆寝てばかりいてあまり体を動かさないでいると足の筋力が落ちてしまいます If you stay in bed all the time not moving much, the muscles in your legs will become weak.

あみだす 編み出す （作り出す）develop, create （考え出す）work out, think out ◆肺がんに関する新しい検査技術〈治療法〉を編み出す develop[create] a new *diagnostic technique〈treatment option〉for lung cancer

アミノさん ―酸 amino acid ▶必須アミノ酸 essential amino acid ▶アミノ酸代謝異常 disorder of amino-acid metabolism

アミラーゼ amylase

アミロイド amyloid ▶アミロイド腎臓 amyloid kidney　アミロイドニューロパチー amyloid neuropathy　アミロイド斑 amyloid plaque　アミロイド変性 amyloid degeneration

アミロイドーシス amyloidosis ◀心アミロイドーシス cardiac amyloidosis　腎アミロイドーシス renal amyloidosis　全身性アミロイドーシス systemic amyloidosis　透析アミロイドーシス dialysis-related amyloidosis；DRA　肺アミロイドーシス pulmonary amyloidosis

アメーバ ameba, amoeba （形 amebic） ◀肝アメーバ症 hepatic amebiasis　赤痢アメーバ *Entamoeba histolytica* ▶アメーバ症 amebiasis　アメーバ性肝膿瘍 amebic liver abscess　アメーバ性大腸炎 amebic colitis　アメーバ赤痢 amebic dysentery

アメニティ amenity

アメリカ America （形 American） （アメリカ合衆国）the United States of America, the United States；the USA, the US ★ピリオドを付けて the U.S.A., the U.S. とも書く。 ◀北アメリカ North America　中央アメリカ Central America　南アメリカ South

America ▶アメリカ英語 American English ☞アメリカ人

アメリカじん 一人 American (圏American) ☞国籍 ◆彼女はアメリカ人です She is (an) American. ◀アフリカ系アメリカ人 African American アラブ系アメリカ人 Arab American 韓国系アメリカ人 Korean American 先住アメリカ人 Native American 中国系アメリカ人 Chinese American 日系アメリカ人 Japanese American

あやうく 危うく （ほとんど）almost, nearly ◆彼はアレルギー反応で危うく命を落とすところでした He almost[nearly] died from the allergic reaction. ★ほぼ同じ意味に用いられるが，nearly のほうが「かろうじて助かってよかった」という意味合いが強い．

あやぶむ 危ぶむ doubt ◆彼女が薬を指示どおりに飲むかどうか危ぶんでいます I doubt that she'll take the medication exactly as directed. ◆彼の病状から考えると，来月の旅行は危ぶまれます Considering his condition, *I doubt whether[it's doubtful if] he can *go on[take] a trip next month.

あやまち 過ち mistake, error （過失・落ち度）fault ☞誤り

あやまった 誤った （事実と異なった）false （間違った）wrong, mistaken （圏意図せず accidentally 間違って by mistake） ☞誤り，間違う ◆誤った思い込みをする make a false[wrong / mistaken] assumption ◆誤って硬貨を飲み込む accidentally swallow a coin

あやまり 誤り （間違い・失敗）mistake, error （過失・落ち度）fault ☞誤った，間違い，ミス ◆誤りを犯す make a mistake / make[commit] an error ◆誤りを認める admit one's mistake[error] ◆誤りを正す correct *a mistake[an error] ◆判断の誤り *a mistake[an error] of judgment ◆明らかな誤り an obvious mistake[error] ◆重大な誤り a serious mistake[error] ◆不注意による誤り a careless mistake[error] ◆よくある誤り a common mistake[error]

あやまる 謝る （すまなく思う）be[feel] sorry （すまないと言う）say sorry （謝罪する）apologize ☞すみません，申し訳，詫びる ◆お待たせしたことを謝ります．ごめんなさい I'm sorry to have kept you waiting. / I apologize for keeping you waiting. ◆謝れば彼女は許してくれますよ I'm sure that if you say sorry, she'll forgive you. ◆（患者が失敗した時などに）謝らなくていいんですよ．慣れていますから You don't have to apologize. I'm used to it.

あゆみよる 歩み寄る （妥協する）compromise, make a compromise ◆問題解決のために歩み寄る try to compromise[make a compromise] to solve the problem

アラーム alarm ▶アラームシステム alarm system

あらい¹ 荒い violent, rough ◆彼女は気が荒い She has a violent temper. ◆彼はいつも荒い口調で話します He always speaks in a rough tone. ◆彼女は呼吸が荒くなっています（苦しそうに息をしている）She is breathing hard[heavily]. / （喘いでいる）She is panting for breath.

あらい² 粗い 《ざらざら・ごつごつしている》rough, coarse ◆このタオルは手触りが粗い This towel feels rough[coarse]. 《細かくない》◆粗く刻んだ食事を提供する give roughly chopped[minced] foods ★mince は特に「みじん切りにする」ことを意味する．

あらう 洗う wash （洗浄・消毒する）cleanse /klénz/ （髪を洗う）shampoo /ʃæmpúː/ ◆傷口を石鹸とぬるま湯でそっと洗って下さい Please wash the incision gently with soap and warm water. ◆手をきちんと〈丁寧に〉洗う wash one's hands properly〈thoroughly〉 ◆髪を洗う shampoo one's hair ◆洗い流す wash away

あらかじめ 予め in advance, beforehand, ahead of time ◆来院なさる時はあらかじめお電話下さい Please call us *in advance[beforehand / ahead of time] before coming to the hospital. ◆薬や食べ物にアレルギーがある時はあらかじめお

あらかじめ　　　　　21　　　　　ある

知らせ下さい If you have any medication or food allergies, let us know in advance.

あらそい　争い　（論争）dispute, conflict
（口げんか）**quarrel**　（不和・いざこざ）**trouble**
◆医療事故をめぐる患者と医療従事者の争いを解決する settle a dispute[conflict] between a patient and medical professionals concerning a medical accident　◆患者とその妻の間では争いが絶えない The patient and his wife are always quarreling [fighting].

あらためて　改めて　（もう一度）again　（別の機会に再び）**another time, some other time**　◆検査結果が出てから改めてお話しいたします I'll talk with you again when the test results come in.　◆では改めて参ります I'll come again later.　◆今週はスケジュールが詰まっています．日を改めておいで下さい My schedule is pretty tight this week. Please come and see me *another time[some other time].

あらためる　改める　（変える）change, make a change　（部分的に変える）**alter**
（改善する）**improve**　（修正する）**modify**
◆生活習慣を改めて下さい You need to make some changes to your lifestyle.
◆職場環境を改める improve the work environment　◆考えを改める change one's ideas　◆衣服を改める change one's clothes

アラブじん　―人　Arab　（㉑Arab）　◆アラブ系アメリカ人 Arab American

あらゆる　（可能な限りの・ある限りの）every
（すべての）**all**　◆彼女を助けるためにあらゆる手を尽くします We'll do everything we possibly can to save her. / We'll try every possible means to save her.　◆その病気について入手可能なあらゆる情報を集める collect all the information available on the disease

あらわす　表す　（示す）show　（表現する）**express**　（文字・図などを意味する）**represent, stand (for)**　◆検査結果は鉄分の不足を表しています The test result shows that *you have an iron deficiency[you're low in iron].　◆感情を表す show one's

emotions[feelings]　◆考えを言葉で表す express one's ideas in words　◆彼女の死に遺憾の意を表す express one's regret(s) over her death　◆感謝の気持ちを表す show one's gratitude　◆あなたが描いた図は何を表しているのですか What does your drawing represent[stand for]?

あらわれる　現れる　appear, make one's appearance　（効果が出る）**work, have an effect**　☞出現　◆この薬の効果はゆっくりと現れます The effects of this medication will appear slowly. / This medication will work slowly.　◆この薬はすぐに効果が現れます This medication will *have an immediate effect[start working right away].　◆治療の効果が現れるにはしばらく時間がかかります It will take some time before *you feel the effects of the treatment[the effects of the treatment become apparent].

ありがとう　Thank you., Thanks.　☞感謝
◆どうもありがとう Thank you so[very] much.　◆長い間お待ちくださってありがとう Thank you for waiting so long.　◆ご協力ありがとうございます Thank you very much for your cooperation. / I appreciate your cooperation.

ありのまま　（率直に）frankly, plainly　（正確に）**exactly**　（実際に・現に）**actually**　◆経験したことをありのままにお話し下さい Please tell me *frankly about your experience[exactly what you experienced].
◆それがありのままの事実です That's the plain fact.　◆ありのままの自分を見て自信をもって下さい Please try to see yourself as you actually are and feel confident about yourself.

ありゅうさん　亜硫酸　sulfurous acid
▶亜硫酸ガス中毒 sulfur dioxide poisoning

ある　a, an, some, certain　◆ある意味で彼女の言うことは正しいかもしれません I think she may be right *in a sense[in a way].　◆この治療はある程度の効果をあげるはずです This treatment should *have some effect[be effective to a certain degree]. ◆ある種の薬は副作用として便秘を起こすかもしれません Constipation may be a side effect of certain medications. / Certain medications may have constipation as a side effect.

あるがまま ◆あるがままを受け入れる accept reality[one's life] as it is

アルカリ alkali (圏alkaline) ▶アルカリ中毒 alkaline intoxication　アルカリ尿 alkaluria / alkaline urine　アルカリホスファターゼ alkaline phosphatase

アルカロイド alkaloid

アルカローシス alkalosis ◀代謝性アルカローシス metabolic alkalosis　代償性アルカローシス compensatory alkalosis

アルギニノコハクさんにょう 一酸尿（症）argininosuccinic aciduria

あるきまわる 歩き回る　walk around [about]（通路や室内を行ったり来たりする）**walk up and down**（徘徊する）**wander about** ◆疲れなければ院内を自由に歩き回っていいですよ As long as you don't get tired, you may walk around the hospital freely.

あるく 歩く　walk ☞歩行 ◆歩きにくいですか Do you have difficulty walking? ◆休まないで何メートル歩けますか How many meters can you walk without taking any rest? ◆歩くのがつらい時にはこの車椅子を使って下さい Please use this wheelchair when you have difficulty walking. ◆このトレッドミルの上を歩いて下さい Please walk on this treadmill. ◆手術後看護師が歩くのをお手伝いします Your nurse will assist you with walking after the surgery. ◆歩く訓練をする practice walking ◆早足で歩く walk quickly ◆真っ直ぐ歩く walk straight ◆大またで歩く stride ◆よたよた歩く waddle / walk with faltering steps ◆よちよち歩く toddle ◆足を引きずって歩く shuffle / walk with short, quick, and shuffling steps ◆片足を引きずって歩く limp ◆手すりにつかまって伝い歩きする walk holding on to the handrail / walk with the support of the handrail ◆ひとり歩きする

walk without support[help] / walk unaided ◆介助なしで歩く walk without help[assistance] ◆職場に歩いて通う walk to work

アルコール alcohol /ǽlkəhɔ̀ːl/（圏alcoholic）（酒）alcohol（蒸留酒）liquor, spirits ★通例，複数形で．☞飲酒，酒 ◆アルコールにアレルギーはありますか Are you allergic to alcohol? ◆（採血の前などで）アルコール綿での消毒は大丈夫ですか Is it *all right[safe] to use alcohol wipes (on your skin)? ◆アルコールで傷口を消毒する swab the wound with alcohol ◆アルコール消費量は徐々に増えましたか Has your alcohol consumption gradually [steadily] increased? ◆ご自分はアルコールに依存していると思いますか Do you feel you are dependent on alcohol? / Do you have a drinking problem? ◆これはアルコールによって引き起こされる症状です This is an alcohol-induced symptom. ◆この薬を飲んでいる間はアルコールを控えて下さい You should not drink alcohol while you are taking this medication. / Please refrain from drinking（alcohol）while you are taking this medication. ◆アルコールを大量に摂取する drink alcohol heavily / have a heavy intake of alcohol ◀エチルアルコール ethyl alcohol　血中アルコール濃度 blood-alcohol level[concentration]　消毒用アルコール rubbing alcohol　ノンアルコール飲料 nonalcoholic drinks　非アルコール性脂肪性肝炎 nonalcoholic steatohepatitis；NASH　非アルコール性脂肪性肝疾患 nonalcoholic fatty liver disease；NAFLD　非アルコール性慢性膵炎 nonalcoholic chronic pancreatitis　メチルアルコール methyl alcohol

▶アルコール依存 alcohol dependence [addiction] / alcoholism / alcohol abuse /（アルコール使用障害）alcohol use disorder　アルコール依存者 alcoholic　アルコール臭 alcohol（breath）odor　アルコール消毒 alcohol-based antiseptics　アルコール性

肝炎 alcoholic hepatitis　アルコール性膵炎 alcoholic pancreatitis　アルコール度数 alcohol strength[content]　アルコール離脱症候群 alcohol withdrawal syndrome
☞アルコール中毒

アルコールちゅうどく　—中毒 （アルコール依存）alcoholism　（酩酊による中毒）alcohol intoxication[poisoning]　◆ごく短時間に大量の飲酒をすると急性アルコール中毒を起こします Acute alcohol intoxication [poisoning] can occur after drinking too much alcohol too quickly.　▶アルコール依存症患者 alcoholic　アルコール依存症者更生会 Alcoholics Anonymous；AA

アルゴン　argon　▶アルゴンレーザー argon laser

アルゼンチン　Argentina （⨂**Argentinian**）☞国籍　▶アルゼンチン人（の）Argentinian

アルツハイマーびょう　—病　Alzheimer disease；**AD**　◀若年性アルツハイマー病 early-onset Alzheimer disease　▶アルツハイマー型認知症 dementia of the Alzheimer type；DAT

アルデヒド　aldehyde　▶アルデヒド脱水素酵素 aldehyde dehydrogenase

アルドステロン　aldosterone　◀レニン-アンギオテンシン-アルドステロン系 the renin-angiotensin-aldosterone system　▶アルドステロン産生腺腫 aldosterone-producing[aldosterone-secreting] adenoma / aldosteronoma　アルドステロン症 aldosteronism

アルドラーゼ　aldolase

アルバイト （仕事）**part-time job** （パートの労働者）**part-time worker, part-timer** （パートの学生）**part-time student**　◆彼女はレストランでアルバイトをしています She works part-time in a restaurant. / She has a part-time job in a restaurant.

アルファ　alpha　▶αグロブリン alpha globulin　α遮断薬 alpha-blocking agent / alpha blocker　α胎児性蛋白質 alpha fetoprotein；AFP　α波 alpha wave　α₁アンチトリプシン欠損（症）alpha-one antitrypsin deficiency

アルファベット　the alphabet /ǽlfəbèt/ （⨂**alphabétical**）　◆名前をアルファベット順に並べる list[arrange] names alphabetically[in alphabetical order]

アルブミン　albumin　◀血清アルブミン serum albumin　低アルブミン血症 hypoalbuminemia　ラクトアルブミン lactalbumin　卵白アルブミン ovalbumin　▶アルブミン / グロブリン比 albumin / globulin [A / G] ratio

アルブミンにょう　—尿　albuminuria　◀偶発性アルブミン尿 accidental albuminuria　微量アルブミン尿 microalbuminuria

アルポートしょうこうぐん　—症候群　Alport syndrome

アルミニウム　aluminum /əlúːmənəm/, 《英》**aluminium** /ǽljəmíniəm/　◀水酸化アルミニウムゲル aluminum hydroxide gel　▶アルミニウム骨症 aluminum-related bone disease　アルミニウム脳症 aluminum encephalopathy　アルミニウム肺 aluminum lung

あれしょう　荒れ性（の） （乾燥した）**dry** （⨂**dry**）（ひび割れた）**chapped** （⨂**chap**）（ざらざらな）**rough**　◆彼女は肌が荒れ性だ Her skin dries[chaps] easily. / Her skin is dry and tends to get rough.

あれた　荒れた 《荒廃している》（ざらざらな）**rough** （ひび割れた）**chapped**　◆口〈舌〉は荒れていますか Does your mouth〈tongue〉feel rough?　◆唇が荒れている *one's* lips are rough [chapped]　◆荒れてかさかさになった手 a rough and chapped hand　◆胃が荒れています（胃壁が炎症を起こしている）Your stomach (lining) has become inflamed [irritated].
《すさんでいる》**wild**　◆彼はかなり荒れた生活をしています He lives[leads] a pretty wild life.
《穏やかでない》　◆きょうは天気が荒れそうですね Today's weather seems stormy [rough], doesn't it?

アレルギー　allergy /ǽlədʒi/ （⨂**allergic** /əláːdʒɪk/）　◆アレルギーは何かありますか

Do you have any allergies? / Are you allergic to anything? ◆食べ物〈薬〉にアレルギーはありますか Are you allergic to any foods〈medications〉? ◆どの薬に対するアレルギーですか Which medications are you allergic to? ◆これまでに造影剤〈化粧品〉でアレルギー反応を起こしたことがありますか Have you ever had an allergic reaction to *a contrast material〈cosmetics〉? ◆どんなアレルギー反応を起こしましたか What happened to you when you had the allergic reaction? ◆アレルギー反応を起こす化粧品は避けて下さい You should avoid cosmetics that can cause allergic reactions. ◆カビ〈牛乳〉にアレルギーがある have an allergy to mold〈milk〉/ be allergic to mold〈milk〉 ◆卵を食べた直後にアレルギー症状が出る symptoms of the allergy start[appear / come on / develop] soon after *one* has eaten eggs ◆アレルギー性の発疹が出る break out in an allergic rash ◆アレルギー体質がある be prone to allergies / have a tendency toward allergies / have an allergic predisposition[constitution] ◆アレルギーで苦しむ suffer from allergies ◆アレルギー反応を抑える suppress an allergic reaction

◀Ⅰ型アレルギー反応 type 1 allergic reaction 海産食品アレルギー seafood allergy かびアレルギー mold allergy 眼アレルギー eye[ocular] allergy 寒冷アレルギー cold allergy 季節性アレルギー seasonal allergy 牛乳アレルギー milk allergy 金属アレルギー metal allergy 抗アレルギー薬 antiallergic (medication / drug / agent) 口腔アレルギー症候群 oral allergy syndrome；OAS 小麦アレルギー wheat allergy 職業性アレルギー occupational allergy 食物アレルギー food allergy スギ花粉アレルギー *sugi*[Japanese cedar] pollen allergy 接触アレルギー contact allergy 遅延型アレルギー delayed-type allergy 通年性アレルギー year-round[perennial] allergy 動物の毛アレルギー allergy to animal fur ハウス

ダストアレルギー house dust allergy 鼻アレルギー nasal allergy 光アレルギー性接触皮膚炎 photoallergic contact dermatitis 皮膚アレルギー skin[cutaneous] allergy 物理的アレルギー physical allergy ペニシリンアレルギー penicillin allergy 薬物アレルギー drug allergy ▶アレルギー検査 allergy test アレルギー疾患 allergic disease アレルギー症状 allergic symptom[reaction / condition] アレルギー性気管支肺アスペルギルス症 allergic bronchopulmonary aspergillosis；ABPA アレルギー性結膜炎 allergic conjunctivitis アレルギー性紫斑病 allergic purpura アレルギー性肉芽腫性血管炎 allergic granulomatous angiitis；AGA アレルギー性鼻炎 allergic rhinitis アレルギー性皮膚炎 allergic dermatitis アレルギー専門医 allergist アレルギー体質 allergic predisposition[constitution] アレルギー反応 allergic reaction

アレルゲン allergen /ǽlədʒən/ ◆皮膚パッチテストを行ってアレルギー反応を引き起こすアレルゲンを調べましょう I'm going to[Let me] do a (skin) patch test to find out which allergens are causing the allergic reaction. ◀花粉アレルゲン pollen allergen 食物アレルゲン food allergen 放射性アレルゲン吸着試験 radioallergosorbent test；RAST ▶アレルゲン除去食品 allergen-free food アレルゲンテスト allergen test

アロエ aloe

アロマテラピー aromatherapy

あわ 泡 《液体表面の気泡》foam (形foamy), froth (形frothy) 《1つ1つの気泡》bubble ◆泡状の痰 foamy[frothy] phlegm ◆泡状の分泌物 foamy[frothy] discharge ☞泡風呂

あわい 淡い 《明るめの》light 《暗めにほのかな》pale ◆淡い黄色の尿 light yellow urine

あわせる 合わせる 《1つにまとめる》《くっつける》put … together 《合計する》sum up 《足す》add up 《協力する》work together, cooperate (with) ◆両

手を合わせるのが難しいですか Do you have difficulty putting your hands together? ◆合わせて3種類の薬を処方いたします I'm going to prescribe three kinds of medications altogether[in all]. ◆問題解決のために力を合わせる work together to solve the problem
《焦点を合わせる》focus, adjust the focus ◆遠くにある小さな物にピントを合わせる focus[adjust the focus] on a distant small object
《調合する》mix (図mixture) ◆この錠剤は2種類の降圧薬を合わせたものです This tablet contains a mixture of two kinds of antihypertensives. / This tablet contains two kinds of antihypertensives mixed together.
《適合させる》 ◆薬の量を患者の年齢や体重に合わせて調節する adjust the dosage according to the age and weight of the patient

あわてる （急ぐ）hurry （狼狽する）panic, get upset ◆あわてないで下さい There's no need to hurry. / （ゆっくり時間をとって）Take your time. / （パニックに陥らないで）Please don't panic. / （のんびりして）Take it easy.

あわぶろ 泡風呂 （気泡浴）bubble bath

あんい 安易（に） （軽々しく）lightly, all too easily （衝動的に）on impulse ◆この症状を安易に考えてはいけません Don't take this symptom lightly. / （深刻に考えるべきだ）You should take this symptom seriously. ◆安易に決めると後で後悔するかもしれません If you make a decision *without giving it much thought[on impulse], you may regret it later.

あんがい 案外 （予想外に）unexpectedly （驚くほど）surprisingly （かなり）fairly ◆膝の手術からの回復は案外早かったですね You've made a quicker recovery from the knee surgery than we expected. / Your recovery from the knee surgery was unexpectedly[surprisingly] early. ◆彼女の日本語は案外上手です She speaks Japanese fairly well.

あんかっしょく 暗褐色（の） dark brown ◆彼の尿は暗褐色を呈しています His urine is dark brown.

あんかんせつ 鞍関節 saddle joint

あんき 暗記する memorize ☞記憶 ◆暗記は得意ですか Are you good at memorizing things? ◆暗記は苦手である be weak[poor] at memorizing things / be not good at memorizing things

アンギオテンシノゲン angiotensinogen

アンギオテンシン angiotensin ◀レニン-アンギオテンシン-アルドステロン系 the renin-angiotensin-aldosterone system ▶アンギオテンシン変換酵素阻害薬 *angiotensin-converting enzyme[ACE] inhibitor

アンケート questionnaire /kwèstʃənéɚ/ ◆このアンケートに答えて下さい Please answer this questionnaire. ◆アンケート用紙に記入する fill out a questionnaire ◆患者満足度調査に関するアンケートを行う conduct a questionnaire-based survey of patient satisfaction

あんざん¹ 安産 easy delivery, easy birth

あんざん² 暗算 mental arithmetic, mental calculation ◆暗算して下さい Do the sums in your head. / Calculate the numbers in your head. ◆暗算が得意である be good at mental arithmetic[calculation] ◆暗算が苦手である be weak[poor] at mental arithmetic[calculation] / be not good at mental arithmetic[calculation]

あんじ 暗示 suggestion （動suggest 形影響を受けやすい suggestible）, hint, clue ◆彼は暗示にかかりやすい He is easily influenced by other people. / He is highly suggestible. ◆暗示を与える give[drop] a hint / provide a clue ◀自己暗示 autosuggestion ▶暗示療法 suggestion therapy

あんじゅんのう 暗順応 dark adaptation （↔light adaptation）

あんしん 安心する ◆ご安心下さい（心配しないで）Please don't worry. / （心配なこと

はない）There's nothing to worry about. /（気分を楽にして）You can relax now. ◆手術はうまくいきましたのでご安心下さい I'm glad to tell you that *the surgery went well[everything went well with the surgery], so don't worry. ◆彼女はもう安心です（危機を脱している）She is now out of danger. ▶安心感（安全が保証される感じ）sense of security /（ほっとする感じ・気楽さ）sense of ease

あんずる 案ずる worry（about）, be anxious（about）, be concerned（about）☞心配 ◆簡単な検査ですから案ずることは何もありません It's a simple test, so there's nothing to worry about.

あんせい 安静 rest（動rest）, bed rest（動stay[rest] in bed）◆安静時にも痛みますか Do you have pain even when you are resting[at rest]? ◆約1週間の安静が必要です You need about a week's rest. / You need to stay in bed for about a week. ◆トイレに行く時以外は安静にしていて下さい Don't get out of bed except to use the toilet. ◆お父様は現在絶対安静の状態です Right now your father is on complete bed rest. ◀床上安静 bed rest 絶対安静 complete bed rest；CBR / absolute bed rest；ABR ▶安静時エネルギー消費量 resting energy expenditure；REE 安静時狭心症 angina（pectoris）at rest / rest angina（pectoris）安静時胸痛 chest pain during[at] rest 安静時呼吸困難 dyspnea during[at] rest 安静時振戦 tremor[shaking] during[at] rest / resting[rest] tremor 安静度 level[degree] of bed rest（needed by a patient）

あんせきしょく 暗赤色（の） dark red ◆暗赤色の血液 dark red blood

あんぜん 安全 safety（形safe）（警備上の）security（形secure）◆この薬は安全です This medication is safe to take. ◆安全のために貴重品は病院に持ってこないで下さい For your own safety and security, please don't bring any valuables to the hospital. ◆安全用の手すりにつかまる hold on to the safety rail ▶安全基準

safety standards 安全装置 safety device 安全対策 safety[security] measure(s)

アンダーシャツ undershirt （下着）underwear

アンダーソン・ファブリびょう ─病 Anderson-Fabry disease, Fabry disease, alpha-galactosidase deficiency

あんち 安置 ◀遺体安置所（hospital）morgue

あんてい 安定（した）stable（图stability 動stabilize）（↔unstable）, steady（↔unsteady）, secure（↔insecure）◆彼女の病状は安定しています She is now in a stable condition. ◆彼の呼吸は安定しています His breathing remains steady. ◆この薬は血圧を安定させます This medication will *stabilize your blood pressure[make your blood pressure stable]. ◆安定した仕事〈収入〉a secure job〈income〉◆情緒の安定 one's emotional stability ◀精神安定薬 tranquilizer ▶安定期 stable period 安定狭心症 stable angina（pectoris）

あんてん 暗点 scotoma, blind spot ◀閃輝暗点 scintillating scotoma 中心暗点 central scotoma 中心暗点計 scotometer 輪状暗点 annular[ring] scotoma

アンドロゲン androgen

あんない 案内する（示す）show （連れて行く）take（图情報 information 手引き guide 指示 instruction）◆病室をご案内しましょう I'll show you to your room. ◆病棟をご案内しましょう I'll show you around the floor[ward / unit]. ◆スタッフが検査室までご案内します One of our staff will take you to the laboratory. ◀総合案内 general information counter[desk] 入院案内 guide for inpatients / admission instructions ▶案内所 information counter[desk]

案内の表現

● レントゲン室への行き方をご説明いたしましょう Let me explain how to get to the X-ray room.

● エレベーターに乗って3階に行って下さい Please take the elevator to the third

floor.
- エスカレーターをご利用下さい Please use the escalator.
- CT検査室は2階〈地下〉にあります The CT scan room is *on the second floor 〈in the basement〉.
- エレベーターを降りたら青い線に沿って歩いて下さい When you *get off[get out of] the elevator, *walk along[follow] the blue line.
- 2つめの角を右〈左〉に曲がって下さい Turn right〈left〉at the second corner.
- 20メートル直進して下さい．右〈左〉側にあります Go straight for twenty meters, and you'll find it on your right〈left〉.
- 超音波室の隣です It's next to the ultrasound room.
- 廊下の突き当たり〈角を曲がった所〉にあります It's *at the end of the hallway 〈around the corner〉.
- ここ〈そこ／あそこ〉にあります It's here 〈there／over there〉.
- ご案内しましょう．ご一緒にどうぞ I'll show you where it is. Please come (along) with me.

あんび 鞍鼻 saddle nose
アンビューバッグ Ambu bag
アンフェタミン amphetamine ▶アンフェタミン中毒 amphetamine intoxication[poisoning]
アンプル ampule, 《英》ampoule
あんぽう 罨法 compress, pack ☞湿布
あんまマッサージしあつし ─指圧師 shiatsu practitioner, massage and finger pressure practitioner 〈男性の〉masseur 〈女性の〉masseuse
あんみん 安眠 sound sleep, good sleep (動sleep well[soundly]) ☞睡眠
アンモニア ammonia ◆アンモニアのにおい ammonia smell
あんらくし 安楽死 euthanasia /jùːθənéɪʒə/, mercy killing 〈医師の手を借りた安楽死〉physician-assisted suicide ☞尊厳死 ◆積極的な〈消極的な〉安楽死 active〈passive〉euthanasia ◆(患者の意思によ

る)自発的な安楽死 voluntary euthanasia
あんりょくしょく 暗緑色(の) dark green

い

い 胃 **stomach** /stʌ́mək/ (🏥**gastric**)
★stomach は狭義では「胃」をさすが，広義では「腹」を意味する．そこで stomachache は広義では腹痛，狭義では胃痛となるが，胃と腸を区別しないで腹部全体の痛みとみなすことが多い．横隔膜から骨盤までを含む腹部をさす医学用語は abdomen．幼児は胃や腹部を区別せず tummy を使う．

《症状の表現》 ◆胃が重苦しい have a heavy feeling in *one's* stomach / *one's* stomach feels heavy / feel heavy in *one's* stomach ◆胃が締め付けられる have knots in *one's* stomach / *one's* stomach is in knots ◆胃がむかむかする have an upset[unsettled] stomach / *one's* stomach is churning ◆胃がむかつく(吐き気がする) have a nauseous feeling in *one's* stomach / feel sick to the stomach ★feel sick … は「ショックを受けている」「怒っている」という比喩的な意味でも用いられる．◆胃がもたれる have a heavy[sinking] feeling in *one's* stomach ◆胃の具合が悪い have stomach trouble / have problems with *one's* stomach ◆胃をこわしている have something wrong with *one's* stomach / have a stomach disorder[upset] ◆胃の不快な症状 symptoms of stomach discomfort ◆胃の不調 a stomach upset / an upset stomach ★stomach upset は「胃が不調である」「胃がむかむかする」など，広い意味で用いられる．

《診察の基本表現》 ◆胃の調子はどうですか How is your stomach? ◆胃に何か問題がありますか Do you have any problems with your stomach? ◆胃が痛みますか Do you have any pain in your stomach? / Do you have a stomachache? ☞痛み ◆空腹〈満腹〉の時に胃の痛みは悪化しますか Does *the stomachache[the pain in your stomach] get worse when your stomach is empty〈full〉? ◆食べ物で胃が

もたれますか Does your food sit[feel] heavy on your stomach? ◆胃がもたれるような食事をする eat a heavy meal ◆何か胃薬は飲んでいますか Are you taking any stomach medication? ◆今までに胃の病気にかかったことがありますか Have you ever had any stomach disease before? ◆胃の異常を指摘されたことがありますか Have you ever been told that you have a problem with your stomach? ◆胃を診察しましょう I'm going to examine your stomach.

《所見・治療の表現》 ◆胃が荒れています(炎症を起こしています)Your stomach (lining) has become inflamed[irritated]. ◆胃に小さいびらんの徴候が認められます There are signs of a small erosion in your stomach. ◆胃潰瘍のようですね I think you probably have a stomach ulcer. / I think it's probably a stomach ulcer. ◆胃を刺激するような食べ物は避けたほうがよいでしょう You should avoid foods that irritate your stomach. ◆胃酸を抑えて痛みをコントロールする薬を処方しますので，しばらくそれで様子をみましょう I'm going to prescribe a medication that will lower the amount of acid in your stomach and control the pain, so let's wait a while and see *what happens[if it helps]. ◆胃を部分的に切除する remove part of the stomach ◆胃を全摘出する remove *all of the stomach[the entire stomach]

☞胃亜全摘術，胃アトニー，胃アニサキス症，胃液，胃炎，胃潰瘍，胃拡張，胃管，胃がん，胃吸引，胃空腸吻合術，胃薬，胃憩室，胃痙攣，胃検診，胃酸，胃重感，胃・十二指腸潰瘍，胃出血，胃静脈瘤，胃食道逆流症，胃切除術，胃腺，胃穿孔，胃腺腫，胃洗浄，胃疝痛，胃全摘術，胃大腸反射，胃腸，胃痛，胃底腺，胃内視鏡，胃内容物，胃粘膜，胃バリウム検査，胃壁，胃泡，胃膨満，胃ポリープ，胃抑制性ペプチド，胃瘻

いあぜんてきじゅつ 胃亜全摘術 **subtotal gastrectomy**

いあつ 威圧(的な) **domineering**, **controlling** ◆威圧的な親 a domineering[controlling] parent ◆子供に対して威圧的な

態度をとる be domineering[controlling] toward[with] *one's* child

いアトニー　胃アトニー　gastric atony

いアニサキスしょう　胃アニサキス症 gastric anisakiasis

イー　◆「イー」と言ってみて下さい Please say "e."

いい

《よい》(望ましい・有益な)**good, nice**　(適切な)**right**　(容易な)**easy**　☞良い

◆ウォーキングは健康にいい Walking is good for your health.　◆いいですよ，その調子で! Good. That's the way!　◆いい判断をなさいましたね You've made the right decision.　◆消化にいい食べ物 food that is easy to digest

《許可・確認》**all right, okay[OK], may**　(かまわないか)**mind**　◆話をボイスレコーダーにとってもいいですか Is it all right to use this voice recorder? / Do you mind if I use this voice recorder?　◆窓を開けてもいいですか May I open the window?　◆来週の月曜日にお会いしましょう．いいですか I'll see you next Monday, *all right[okay / OK]?

《承諾・礼への返答》**Sure., Certainly., That's [It's] all right., You're welcome.**　◆「お願いがあるのですが」「いいですよ，何ですか」"Would you do me a favor?" "Sure[Certainly]. What is it?"　◆「なんとお礼を申しあげてよいか」「いいんですよ」"I cannot thank you enough." "Oh, that's all right. / You're welcome."　★Don't mention it. / It's a pleasure. などともいう.

《忠告》**should, had better**　◆十分に休息をとったほうがいいですよ You should get plenty of rest.　◆タバコはやめたほうがいいですよ You should[You'd better] stop smoking.　★You should は軽い忠告だが，You had better[You'd better] は命令的な口調になることに注意.

《好み》◆朝食は何がいいですか What would you like to eat for breakfast?

いいあやまり　言い誤りをする　make a slip of the tongue, slip *one's* tongue　☞言い間違い

いいえ　no　★英語の受け答えの Yes と No は日本語の「はい」と「いいえ」と微妙に異なるので注意．英語では返事の内容が肯定文のときは Yes，否定文のときは No で答える．◆「予約は火曜日ですか」「いいえ，木曜日です」"Is my appointment (on) Tuesday?" "No, it's (on) Thursday."　◆いいえ，結構です(婉曲的な拒絶)No, thank you.　◆「チョコレートはお好きではないのですか」「いいえ，好きです」"Don't you like chocolate?" "Yes, I do."　★No で答えると「好きではない」という意味になる．◆「病室でお酒を飲んでもいいですか」「いいえ，申し訳ありませんがそれは困ります」"Do you mind if I drink alcohol in my room?" "Yes, I do mind. Sorry."　★No で答えると「飲んでもよい」という意味になる．

イーエスさいぼう　ES 細胞　ES cell　(胚性幹細胞)**embryonic stem cell**

いいかえる　言い換える　say … (in) *a different[another] way, put … (in) *a different[another] way, rephrase　◆それを別なことばに言い換えていただけませんか Could you say that (in) a different way? / Could you rephrase that[what you just said]?　◆Rubella「風疹」は言い換えると German measles のことです 'Rubella' is just another way of saying 'German measles.'　◆言い換えると，うつ病は色々な要素が引き金になります To put it differently[In other words], depression can be triggered by many factors.

いいかた　言い方　way of speaking[saying]　◆物の言い方に気をつけないと，意図せずに人を傷つけてしまいます If you aren't careful about *the way[how] you say things, you might hurt *someone without meaning to[someone's feelings unintentionally].　◆彼は言い方はきついけれど，根は優しいですよ He is rough-spoken, but he is really kind at heart.　◆ていねいな言い方をする speak in a polite way / speak politely　◆厳しい言い方をする speak in a harsh and critical way / have a sharp tongue　◆アスリートフットは足白癬の別の言い方です Athlete's foot is also called tinea pedis. / Another name for athlete's foot is tinea pedis. ◆言い方を変えると In other words, … ☞言い換える

いいかねる　言いかねる (確かには言えない) can't say for sure, can't tell exactly ◆お腹の赤ちゃんの性別は，今の時点でははっきりとは言いかねます I can't say for sure now what the sex of your baby is. / At this moment I'm afraid I can't tell exactly what the baby's sex is.

いいきかせる　言い聞かせる (話す) tell (納得させる) convince ◆息子さんに廊下を走り回らないよう言い聞かせて下さい Please tell your son not to run around in the corridor. ◆私は同じ間違いをしないように自分に言い聞かせています I'm trying to tell[convince] myself not to make the same mistake again.

いいすぎる　言い過ぎる　say too much (度を越す) go too far ◆言い過ぎました．ごめんなさい I said too much[I went too far when I said that]. I'm sorry.

いいつける　言い付ける (頼む) ask (命じる) tell (告げ口をする) tell on ◆看護助手に私用を言い付けるのはご遠慮下さい Please don't ask the nursing assistants to run personal errands. ◆彼女はしょっちゅう同室の患者のことを看護師に言い付けます She often tells on her roommates to the nurses. ◆(小児患者に)お母さんに言い付けたりしないから，自分自身のことについて何でも話してごらん I won't tell your mom, so you can tell me whatever you want about yourself.

イートン・ランバートしょうこうぐん　―症候群　Eaton-Lambert syndrome, Lambert-Eaton myasthenic syndrome

いいにくい　言いにくい (気の毒に思う) be sorry to tell[say] (言うのがためらわれる) hesitate to tell[say] (言い難い) find (it) hard to tell[say] ◆大変言いにくいのですが，お嬢さんの白血病が再発しました I'm so sorry to tell you this, but your daughter's leukemia has come back. ◆医師に言いにくいことは，医療ソーシャルワーカーに相談に乗ってもらうとよいでしょう If you have anything you hesitate[find

(it) hard] to say to your doctor, *you should talk about it with a medical social worker[a medical social worker is a good person to go to for advice]. ◆言いにくそうに話す(ためらいながら) speak hesitantly / (自信なさそうに) speak falteringly ◆言いにくい問題(微妙な) a delicate problem[matter]

いいのこす　言い残す (伝言を残す) leave a message ☞言い忘れる ◆他に何か言い残すことはありませんか Do you have anything else (you want) to say? ★肯定文で訊く． ◆ご家族に何か言い残すことがありますか(私がかわりに伝えること) Is there anything you'd like me to tell your family (from you)? / Is there any message you'd like to leave for your family?

イービーウイルス　EBV, EB virus (エプスタイン・バーウイルス) Epstein-Barr virus

いいぶん　言い分　what one has to say ◆あなたの言い分を聞かせて下さい Let me hear[I'd like to hear] what you have to say.

いいまちがい　言い間違いをする (誤った語を使う) use the wrong words (うっかり口を滑らせる) make a slip of the tongue ◆彼女はよく言い間違いをしますか Does she often use the wrong words? ◆言い間違いをして不正確なことを言ってしまいました．ごめんなさい Sorry, that was a slip of the tongue. What I said was incorrect. I do apologize.

イーメール　Eメール　email, e-mail, E-mail ☞メール ◆Eメールアドレスは何ですか What's your email address?

いいわけ　言い訳　excuse (詫び) apology ◆それは喫煙の言い訳にはなりません That's no excuse for smoking. ◆遅れてすみません．ちょっと言い訳させて下さい I'm sorry I'm late, but let me say a few words by way of apology.

いいわすれる　言い忘れる　forget to tell[mention] ◆きょう，岡本先生がお休みであることを言い忘れました．すみませんでした I forgot to tell you that Dr Okamoto is off today. I'm sorry. ◆もう少しで一番大

いいわすれる　31　**いがい**

切なことを言い忘れるところでした I almost forgot to mention the most important thing I have to tell you.

いいん¹ 医院　(診療所)clinic, doctor's office

いいん² 医員　member of the medical staff, staff physician　(レジデント)resident

いいんかい 委員会　committee　(委員会の会議)committee meeting　◆委員会を設置する form[organize] a committee　◆委員会を開く hold a committee meeting　◆委員会に出席する attend a committee meeting　◀苦情処理委員会 complaints[grievance] committee　調査委員会 fact-finding committee　倫理委員会 ethics committee　倫理審査委員会 ethical[ethics] review board；ERB

いう 言う　(口をきく)say, speak, talk　(伝える・知らせる)tell　◆自分の考えを遠慮せずに言って下さい Please don't hesitate to say what you think.　◆もっとゆっくり言って下さい Could you speak more slowly? / Please speak more slowly.　◆もっと大きい声で言って下さい Could you speak louder? / Speak up, please.　◆もう一度言って下さい(聞き返す時)I beg your pardon? / Pardon? / Could you say that again? ★上昇調で言う。　◆私の言うことが聞こえますか Can you hear me?　◆彼女は頭が痛いと言っています She says she has a headache. / (訴える)She complains of a headache.　◆私の言うことをよく聞いて下さい Please listen to me carefully.　◆この薬は言われた通りに飲んで下さい Please take this medication as directed. / Please take this medication as the doctor told you. ☞言い誤り，言い換える，言い方，言いかねる，言い聞かせる，言い過ぎる，言い付ける，言いにくい，言い残す，言い分，言い間違い，言い訳，言い忘れる，言うまでもなく

いうまでもなく 言うまでもなく　(まして…でない)let alone　(もちろん)of course　(言う必要もなく)needless to say　◆睡眠不足は言うまでもなく，過度の睡眠も体によくありません Too much sleep is not good for your health, let alone not enough sleep.

◆言うまでもなくあなたの要求に応じます Of course, we'll do as you request.　◆言うまでもありませんが，この薬は指示通りに飲んで下さい Needless to say, you should take this medication exactly as directed.

いえき 胃液　gastric juice, digestive juice　☞胃腸　◆食道裂孔ヘルニアがあるために胃液が食道に逆流しやすいのです Because you have a hiatal hernia, it's easy for gastric juice to come up into the esophagus.　▶胃液分泌 stomach[gastric] secretion

イエローカード　(黄熱病の予防注射接種証明書)yellow card

いえん 胃炎　gastritis /gæstráitis/；*inflammation of the stomach lining*　◀萎縮性胃炎 atrophic gastritis　急性胃炎 acute gastritis　出血性胃炎 bleeding[hemorrhagic] gastritis　表層性胃炎 superficial gastritis　びらん性胃炎 erosive gastritis　慢性胃炎 chronic gastritis

いおう 硫黄　sulfur, (英)sulphur　◀二酸化硫黄 sulfur dioxide

イオンこうかんじゅし ―交換樹脂　ion-exchange resin

いか 異化　catabolism　(形catabolic)　▶異化作用 catabolism

―いか ―以下　◆10 以下 ten or less / (10 未満)less than ten　◆熱は 38℃以下に下がっています The temperature has dropped to below[less than] thirty-eight degrees Celsius. ★厳密に 38℃を含める場合には The temperature has dropped to 38℃ or below[less]. という。　◆平均以下である(平均未満)be below average

いがい 意外(な)　(予想外な)unexpected　(驚くような)surprising　◆それは意外な結果でした It was *a surprising[an unexpected] result.　◆今日は意外に暖かいですね It's unexpectedly warm today, isn't it?　◆彼女の行動はまったく意外でした Her behavior was quite unexpected. / We were very surprised by her behavior.　◆この運動は意外に簡単です This exercise is easier than you might think. / This exercise is surprisingly easy.

―いがい　―以外

《…を除いて》except …, except for … ★通例, 入れ替えて用いることができる. (…のほかに) other than …, besides … ◆日曜日以外はほとんど毎日病院にいます I'm in the hospital almost every day except (on) Sundays. ◆私は月曜日と水曜日の朝以外であればいつでも結構です Any time is fine with me except Monday and Wednesday mornings. / Any time other than Monday and Wednesday mornings is fine with me. ◆毛布以外に欲しい物はありませんか Isn't there anything else you want *other than[besides] a blanket? ◆医療関係者以外立ち入り禁止 (掲示)Staff Only / Authorized Medical Personnel Only / Restricted Area―Do Not Enter

《…の外で》outside … ◆指定の喫煙所以外では禁煙になっております Smoking is not permitted outside the designated smoking area. / Smoking is permitted only in the designated smoking area.

いがいがする　irritated, scratchy ☞いがらっぽい

いかいよう　胃潰瘍　stomach ulcer, gastric ulcer ◆胃潰瘍ですね It's[You have] a stomach ulcer.

いかが

《具合》how ◆今日はご機嫌いかがですか How are you today? ◆ご気分はいかがですか How are you feeling now? / How do you feel now? ◆この前診察してから具合はいかがでしたか How have you been since I last saw you? ◆お食事はいかがでしたか How did you like the food?

《提案・勧誘》would you like (to), how about, what about ◆お風呂はいかがですか Would you like to take a bath now? ◆院内を散歩なさってはいかがですか How about[What about] taking a walk in the hospital? ◆日本茶はいかがですか How about[What about] some Japanese green tea?

いかがく¹　医科学　medical science
いかがく²　医化学　medical chemistry
いがく　医学　medicine (略medical), med-

ical science ◀核医学 nuclear medicine 家庭医学 family medicine 基礎医学 basic medical sciences 産業医学 occupational[industrial] medicine 周産期医学 perinatal medicine 精神医学 psychiatry 西洋医学 Western medicine 中国医学 Chinese medicine 東洋医学 Oriental [Asian / Eastern] medicine 熱帯医学 tropical medicine 法医学 forensic[legal] medicine 予防医学 preventive medicine 臨床医学 clinical medicine ▶医学会 medical society / (会議)medical conference[meeting] 医学生 medical student 医学図書 medical book 医学博士 PhD in medical sciences 医学用語 medical term[terminology / language / vocabulary] 医学倫理 medical ethics ☞医学部

いかくちょう　胃拡張　stomach dilatation, gastric dilatation

いがくぶ　医学部　school of medicine, medical school ◆私は T 大学医学部を卒業しました I graduated from the T University School of Medicine. ◆医学部5年生の井上と一緒に診察させていただいてもよろしいですか Is it all right if Mr Inoue, a fifth-year medical student, sees[examines] you with me?

いかす　生かす・活かす　(活用する)make good use of, put … to good use ◆今回の経験を次に生かす make good use of this experience for the next time ◆これまでの経験を生かして最善を尽くします I'm going to put my previous experience to good use and do all I can do.

いかだいがく　医科大学　medical university[school / college] ☞医学部

いかなる ◆いかなる時でも決してあきらめないで下さい(たとえ何が起ころうとも)No matter what happens, never give up. ◆暴力はいかなる場合も許されません(どんな事情でも)Violence will not be tolerated under any circumstances.

いかに　how　(たとえどんなに…とも)no matter how ◆いかに強い痛みでも薬で制御することは可能ですので, 我慢しなくて結

構ですよ No matter how severe the pain, we can control it with medication, so you don't have to put up with it.

いかにして　how　◆喘息の治療はいかにして発作を予防するかが重要です How we prevent asthma attacks is crucial to the treatment of asthma.

いカメラ　胃カメラ　gastroscope, gastro-camera　☞胃内視鏡

いがらっぽい　（ひりひりして痛む）**irritated**（ちくちくする）**scratchy**　◆喉がいがらっぽいですか Do you have an irritated throat? / Does your throat feel irritated?　◆2, 3日喉がいがらっぽいかもしれません Your throat may feel[be] scratchy for a few days.

いかり　怒り　anger（団get angry, feel angry）（激しい怒り）**rage, fury**（団get furious, feel furious）　◆怒りを表す express[show] one's anger　◆怒りを抑える control one's anger　◆怒りを鎮める calm one's anger　◆患者の怒りに対処する cope with a patient's anger

いかん¹　如何　◆人種・宗教・国籍・経済状況のいかんを問わず，患者さんには平等に接します We treat all patients equally regardless of race, religion, nationality, or financial means.　★treat は「扱う・対応する」，「治療する」という両方の意味で使用できる。

いかん²　胃管　stomach tube, gastric tube　◆胃管が喉の奥まできたら飲みこんで下さい Please swallow the (stomach) tube when it reaches the back of your throat.　◀経鼻胃管 nasogastric tube　経鼻胃管栄養 nasogastric feeding ; *providing nutrition through a tube that passes through the nose and into the stomach*

いかん³　遺憾　regret（団regret）　◆このような結果になって本当に遺憾に思います I really regret this outcome.　◆遺憾なことにがんが再発しています（残念ながら）Unfortunately,[I'm sorry to say that] your cancer has returned.　◆その事故に遺憾の意を表す express one's regret(s) about[over] the accident

いがん　胃がん　stomach cancer, gastric cancer　◀スキルス胃癌 scirrhous gastric carcinoma　▶胃がん検診 stomach cancer screening[checkup]

いかんせんせい　易感染性(の)　**compromised**　▶易感染性宿主［免疫不全宿主］compromised[immunocompromised] host

いき　息　breath /bréθ/（動breathe /bríːð/）　☞呼吸　◆息を吸う breathe in / take a breath / inhale　◆息を吐く breathe out / let out a breath / exhale　◆鼻〈口〉で息をする breathe through the nose〈mouth〉

《口臭の表現》　◆息がにおいますか Do you have bad breath? / Does your breath smell?　◆息が酒臭い smell alcohol on the breath　◆息はアンモニア臭がする have ammonia-smelling breath　◆息は便のにおいがする have breath with fecal odor / have fecal breath

《息苦しさの表現》　◆息をするのが苦しいですか Do you have difficulty breathing?　◆彼女は鼻が詰まっていて息ができない Her nose is stuffed up, so she can hardly breathe.　◆彼女は息が荒い She is breathing hard[heavily]. / She has difficulty breathing. / She is panting for breath.　◆息が詰まる（物が気道をふさいで）choke / （酸素不足で）suffocate　◆息がぜいぜいする wheeze / gasp for breath　◆息が切れる・息を切らす get[become] *short of breath[out of breath]* / get[become] breathless　◆肩で息をする gasp[pant] for breath / breathe hard

《診察の基本表現》　◆口を開けて普通に息を吸ったり吐いたりして下さい With your mouth open, please breathe normally.　◆深く［大きく］息を吸って，止めて下さい Take a deep[big] breath in, and hold.　◆ゆっくり息を吸う〈吐く〉breathe in〈out〉slowly　◆軽く息をする breathe lightly / take shallow breaths　◆できるだけ勢いよく息を吐く（強く速く）breathe out as hard and fast as one can

《その他の慣用表現》　◆息を引き取る pass away / breathe one's last　☞死ぬ, 亡くな

い

る ◆息を吹き返す come back to life / be revived ☞息切れ，息苦しい，息む

いぎ　**意義**　**significance**（形**significant**）☞意味 ◆食事療法の意義を認める realize the significance of diet[dietary] therapy ◆意義のある結果 a significant result

いきいき　**生き生き(した)**　（活気に満ちた）**full of life**[**spark**]（元気のよい・陽気な）**lively** ◆生き生きしていますね．最近何かよいことがあったのですか You look *full of life[full of spark / lively]. Did something good happen (to you) lately?

いきおい　**勢い**
《動作などの強さ》**force** ◆尿線に勢いがなくなっていますか Have you noticed any decrease in the force of your stream? / Has your stream gotten smaller? ◆できるだけ勢いよく息を吐いて下さい(強く速く) Please breathe out as hard and fast as you can.
《事の成り行き上》◆彼は酔った勢いで電柱に車をぶつけて大怪我を負いました He was under the influence of alcohol when he crashed his car into a telephone pole and was seriously injured.

いきがい　**生き甲斐** ◆生き甲斐がある〈ない〉have something〈nothing〉to live for

いきかた　**生き方**　（生活様式）**lifestyle**（暮らし方）**way of life**[**living**] ◆健康的な生き方をする have a healthy lifestyle

いきぎれ　**息切れする**　**get**[**become**] ***short of breath**[**out of breath**]（名**shortness of breath, breathlessness**）☞息苦しい ◆息切れしますか Do you get short of breath? ◆息切れしないで階段を上がることができますか Can you climb stairs without getting out of breath? ◆息切れを感じたことがありますか Have you ever had [experienced] shortness of breath? ◆息切れと同時に咳が出ますか Do you also cough when you're short of breath? / Is the shortness of breath accompanied by coughing? ◆仰向けに寝ると息切れしますか Do you become short of breath when you lie down[flat]?

いきぐるしい　**息苦しい**　**have difficulty breathing**（息切れする）**get**[**become**] **short of breath**（形物が気道を塞いで **choking** 酸素不足で **suffocating** 鼻・胸などが詰まって **stuffy**）☞息切れ ◆夜間に〈早朝に〉息苦しくて目が覚めることがありますか Do you wake up *at night〈early in the morning〉*because of[with] difficulty breathing? / Does breathing difficulty ever cause you to wake up *at night〈early in the morning〉? ◆息苦しいと感じるのはたいていいつの時間帯ですか What time of day do you usually get short of breath? ◆どんな時に息苦しいと感じますか In what situations do you get short of breath? ◆何かが喉に詰まったような息苦しさがある have a choking feeling[sensation] as if something is stuck in *one's* throat ◆暑くて息苦しい feel suffocated by the heat / find the heat suffocating ◆鼻が詰まって息苦しい have difficulty breathing due to a stuffy nose

いきごみ　**意気込み**　（熱烈な気持ち）**enthusiasm**（形**enthusiastic**）（熱心さ）**eagerness**（形**eager**） ◆あなたの意気込みはわかりますが，結論を急がないで下さい I understand your enthusiasm[eagerness], but you shouldn't jump to conclusions. ◆体重を減らそうと意気込んでいますが，運動をやり過ぎると結局は挫折しますよ Although you're eager to lose weight, too much exercise will only cause you frustration in the long run.

いきさつ　**経緯**　（詳細）**details** ★通例，複数形で．（副どんな事情で **how**）◆その出来事のいきさつを話して下さい Could you tell me *the details of what actually happened[how you got to be that way]? ◆どういういきさつで今日本にいるのですか How did you *come to be in Japan[get to be here in Japan]?

いきしょうちん　**意気消沈する**　**feel**[**be**] **depressed** ☞がっかりする，気落ち ◆意気消沈していると感じることはありますか Do you ever feel depressed? ◆彼女は妊娠できないと知って意気消沈しています

She's feeling depressed because she realizes that she can't get pregnant.

いきすぎ　行き過ぎ　too much, too far（略 **too much**　過剰の **excessive**）　◆あなたの食事制限は少し行き過ぎですよ You're restricting your diet a bit too much. / Your dietary restrictions are going a little too far.　◆行き過ぎた運動はよくありません Too much[Excessive] exercise is not good for you.

いきち　閾値（境界・基準）**threshold**（値）**threshold value**　◆痛みに耐えられる閾値を超えている be above[over] one's pain threshold　◀感覚閾値 sensory threshold　反応閾値 reaction threshold　無酸素閾値 anaerobic threshold；AT

いきちがい　行き違い（誤解）**misunderstanding**　☞誤解　◆私たちの間には何か行き違いがあったようです There seems to have been a misunderstanding between us. / We seem to have had a misunderstanding.

いきづかい　息遣い　breathing　☞息

いきとどく　行き届く　◆入院中何か行き届かない点がございましたでしょうか(不都合な事・問題を経験したか)Did you experience any inconvenience during your hospital stay? / (ニーズを満たさなかったか)Did we in any way fail to meet your needs during your hospital stay?

いきなり　suddenly　◆退院したからといって，いきなりきつい運動をしてはいけません Just because you *were discharged from the hospital[are out of the hospital now] doesn't mean you can suddenly take up strenuous exercise.

いきむ　息む（トイレで）**strain**（**on the toilet**）（分娩時）**push, bear down**　☞力む　◆排尿する時息みますか Do you strain when you urinate?　◆指示があったら息んで下さい Please push when I tell you.

いきゅういん　胃吸引　gastric aspiration

いきょく　医局（場所）**medical office**（組織）**department**　◆医局で術前カンファレンスを行う have a preoperative conference in the medical office　◆原先生と私

は同じ医局です Dr Hara and I work together in the same department.　▶医局員 member of the medical staff

イギリス（略称）**(Great) Britain**（略 **British**）★Northern Ireland は含まない．（連合王国）**the United Kingdom (of Great Britain and Northern Ireland)；the UK**　★England, Wales, Scotland, Northern Ireland から構成される。かつては England（イングランド）でイギリスを代表させていたが、最近は使われなくなってきている。　◆イギリス英語 British English　◆彼女はイギリス人です She is British. / She is from Britain.　☞国籍　★an Englishman, an Englishwoman はイングランド[英国の南部地区]の人を指し、スコットランド人，ウェールズ人，北アイルランド人は含まない．

いきる　生きる
《生存・生活する》**live**（命がある）**be alive**☞生存　◆90 歳まで生きる live to be ninety　◆生きている限り as long as one lives　◆生き続ける stay alive　◆人工呼吸で患者を生き続けさせる keep the patient alive *by means of artificial respiration[on a ventilator]
《有効な》**valid**　◆あなたのビザは今でも生きていますか(有効な)Is your visa still valid? / Do you have a valid visa?

いく　行く
《移動する》（自分を中心にして離れていく）**go**（相手のほうへ行く）**come**　◆もう行かなくてはなりません Well, I must be going now.　◆散歩に行く go for a walk　◆歯医者に行く go to see a dentist　◆（患者に呼ばれて）すぐ行きます I'm coming.　★この場合 I'm going. は使えない。 / I'm on my way.　◆すぐそちらに行きますから，ちょっとお待ち下さい I'll be right there, so could you wait just a few moments?
《物事が進行する》**go**　◆手術はすべてうまくいきました Everything went well with the surgery.

いくうちょうふんごうじゅつ　胃空腸吻合術　gastrojejunostomy

いくじ　育児　child care, childcare（動 **take care of** one's **child**）（特に乳幼児の）**infant care**　◆ご主人はあまり育児に協力的では

ないのですか Doesn't your husband *help you take care of your child[help you with your child]? ◆1年の育児休暇をとる take one year's child-care leave ◆育児休暇中である be on child-care leave ▶育児室 nursery 育児ストレス child-care stress 育児手当 child benefits / family allowance 育児ノイローゼ postpartum [postnatal] depression 育児放棄 child neglect

いぐすり 胃薬 stomach medication[medicine] ◆胃薬を飲む take a stomach medication / take medicine for *one's* stomach

いくど 幾度 how often, how many times ☞何回 ◆幾度吐きましたか How many times did you vomit? ◆幾度かけても彼に電話がつながりません No matter how many times I try, I can't get through to him on the phone. ◆幾度となく関節炎の再燃を繰り返す have repeated arthritis flare-ups

いくにち 幾日 how many days, how often ☞何日 ◆今の段階ではアレルギー症状が消えるまで幾日かかるかわかりません Right now[At this stage], I can't tell you for sure how many days it will take for your allergy symptoms to *go away [clear up]. ◆幾日も経たないうちに退院できます You'll be able to leave the hospital in a matter of days.

いくぶん (ちょっと) a little (いくらか) somewhat ☞少し ◆今日は熱も下がっていますし，顔色もいくぶんいいですね Your fever has come down, and you look *a little[somewhat] better today.

いくもう 育毛 hair restoration ▶育毛剤 hair restorer

いくら
《金額》how much ◆会計係が退院前日までに入院費がいくらかかったか概算してくれます The cashier will *estimate roughly how much your hospital expenses will be [give you a rough estimate of your hospital expenses] by the day before your discharge.

《どんなに》no matter how, however ◆いくら説得しても彼女は聞き入れてくれません No matter how[However] hard I try to persuade her, she won't listen to me. ◆食べ物にはいくら注意しても注意し過ぎることはありません You can't be too careful about what you eat.

いけい 異型 (非定型) atypia (形atypical 他の・反対の) heterotypical, heterotypic) (変種) variation (形variant) ◀細胞異型 cellular atypia ◆異型狭心症 variant angina (pectoris) 異型細胞 atypical cell 異型上皮 atypical epithelium 異型肺炎 atypical pneumonia 異型リンパ球 atypical lymphocyte

いけいしつ 胃憩室 gastric diverticulum, stomach diverticulum

いけいせい 異形成 dysplasia (形dysplastic) ◀高度異形成上皮 severe dysplasia 骨髄異形成症候群 myelodysplastic syndrome；MDS

いけいれん 胃痙攣 stomach cramp, stomach spasm, gastrospasm ★cramp は激しい腹痛．月経痛，胆石や尿路結石などの痛みにも用いる． ◆胃痙攣を起こす have stomach cramps[spasms] / have cramps [spasms] in *one's* stomach

いけない
《よくない・困る》(悪い) bad (間違った) wrong ◆微熱があるのですか．それはいけませんね You've had a slight fever? That's too bad. ◆私たちの何がいけないのかを教えて下さい Could you please tell us *what we're doing wrong[what it is that we're not getting right]?
《行為の抑制・禁止》don't (do not) (すべきではない) shouldn't (should not) (禁止する) mustn't (must not) ◆検査後すぐに車を運転してはいけません Don't drive immediately after the test. / You mustn't drive immediately after the test. ◆そんなにお酒を飲んではいけません You shouldn't drink so much alcohol.

いけん 意見 (考え) opinion (見解) view (助言) advice ☞見解，説 ◆治療のことであなたのご意見をお聞きしたいのですが I'd like to hear your opinion[view] about the treatment. / Please let me know what you think about the treatment. ◆特に意見はありません I don't have any particular opinion. ◆その点ではあなたの意見に賛成です I'm[I agree] with you on that point. ◆残念ながらあなたとは意見が違います I'm afraid that you and I don't see things the same way. / I'm afraid that we have different opinions. ◆私の(個人的な)意見では In my (personal) opinion ◆客観的〈主観的〉な意見 *an objective〈a subjective〉opinion ◆血液内科医の意見を聞いてみましょう Let's get some professional advice from a hematologist.

いけんしん　胃検診　stomach[gastric] screening, stomach[gastric] checkup

いげんせい　医原性(の)　iatrogenic；*relating to any abnormal condition caused by a medical procedure* ▶医原性感染 iatrogenic infection[transmission]　医原性気胸 iatrogenic pneumothorax　医原性甲状腺機能低下症 iatrogenic hypothyroidism

いご　以後　after ◆夜の12時以後は何も口にしないで下さい Don't eat, drink, or chew anything after midnight. ◆この手術以後, 普通の生活ができます You'll be able to live[lead] a normal life after this surgery. ◆以後, 転ばないように気をつけて下さい(これからは)From now on you need to be careful not to fall down. ◆この前の診察以後, 具合はいかがでしたか How have you been since I last saw you?

いこう¹　意向　(考え)thought　(希望)wish ☞要望 ◆この件についてご意向をお聞かせ下さい I'd like to know your wishes[thoughts] on this matter. / Could you tell me what you want *to do[to be done] about this matter? ◆申し訳ありませんが, ご意向に添うことができません I'm sorry, but we're not able to do that for you.

いこう²　移行する　(変わる)turn　(into)　(進展する)develop (into), progress (to)　(図transition　図transitional) ◆この種のポ

リープはがんに移行することがあります This type of polyp has the potential to turn[develop] into cancer. ▶移行期 transition / transitional stage　移行上皮癌 transitional cell carcinoma　移行乳 transitional milk

いさい　委細　details ★通例, 複数形で. ☞詳細 ◆委細は金曜日の面談でお話しいたします I'm going to discuss[I'll go over] the details (with you) in our interview on Friday.

いさん　胃酸　stomach acid, gastric acid ☞胃液 ◆胃酸を抑える薬を出しましょう I'm going to give you something to reduce the stomach acid. ▶胃酸過多 gastric hyperacidity / excessive acid in the stomach

いざん　遺残　remnant　(図remnant) ▶胆嚢管遺残症候群 cystic duct remnant syndrome　尿膜管遺残 urachal remnant ▶遺残組織 remnant tissue

いし¹　石　stone　(砂利)gravel　(結石)stone, calculus　(腰calculi) ☞結石 ◆胆嚢内に石があります You have gallstones. / There are stones stuck in your gallbladder. ◆石のサイズは1cm以下です The stone is smaller than one centimeter. ◆尿に石が出る have stones[gravel] in *one's* urine ◆尿管の石を取り除く remove[get rid of] stones in the ureter ◆腎臓の石を細かく砕く crush a kidney stone ◆小さい石を溶かす dissolve small stones

いし²　医師　doctor, Dr, Dr.　(学位)medical doctor, MD, M.D. ★日本ではMD, M.D.は6年制の医学課程を修了し, 国家試験に合格した医師をさす. ☞巻末付録：病院関係者 ◆医師に診てもらう see[visit] a doctor ◆乳腺外科専門の医師に相談する consult a breast surgeon ◆かかりつけの医師を呼ぶ call *one's* regular[family] doctor ◀一般開業医 general practitioner；GP　オンコール医師 on-call doctor / doctor on call　かかりつけ医 regular[family] doctor　眼科医 eye doctor / ophthalmologist　外科医 surgeon　歯科医 dentist　専門医 specialist　内科医 physician　病院勤務医

hospital doctor[physician] ▶医師会 medical association　医師-患者-家族関係 physician[doctor]-patient-family relationship　医師-患者関係 physician[doctor]-patient relationship　医師国家試験 The National Examination for Medical Practitioners　医師免許証 medical license / physician's license

いし³　意思・意志　(決意)decision(動decide), will　(意向)intention, intent(動intend)　(希望)wish(動wish)　◆ご自分の意思で決めるのは難しいですか Do you have difficulty[trouble] making your own decisions? / Is it hard for you to decide things by yourself?　◆彼女は意志が強い She has a strong will. / She is strong-willed[strong-minded].　◆自分の意思に反して against one's will　◆患者の意思を尊重する respect the wishes[intentions] of the patient　◆患者の意思を確認する confirm the wishes[intentions] of the patient　◆臓器提供の意思を表明する state[express] one's intent to be an organ donor / state[express] one's wish to donate one's organs　◆仕事に復帰する意志はありますか Do you intend to *go back[return] to work? / Are you planning on *going back[returning] to work?　◆日本語で意思を伝えるのは難しいですか Is it hard for you to make yourself understood in Japanese?　◆患者と意思の疎通を図る communicate with patients　◆生前の意思表示 living will / advance (health care) directive[decision]　◀臓器提供意思表示カード organ donor card；a card that indicates one's wish to donate one's organs　▶意思決定 decision-making　意思決定過程 decision-making process　意思決定者 decision maker

いし⁴　遺志　final wishes, last wishes, dying wishes, wishes of a deceased person　★通例，複数形で. deceased person は故人を意味する.　◆彼の遺志を尊重する respect his final wishes

いし⁵　縊死　death by hanging(動hang

oneself)

いじ¹　医事　medical affairs, medical matters　★いずれも複数形で.　▶医事課 section[department] of medical affairs

いじ²　意地　(意思)will　◆意地がある have a will of one's own　◆意地を張る(頑固である)be stubborn / be obstinate　◆意地が悪い be nasty

いじ³　維持　maintenance(動keep, maintain)　(支持)support　◆健康を維持する keep healthy / stay in good health / maintain good health　健康維持 health maintenance　生命維持 life support　▶維持透析 maintenance dialysis　維持量 maintenance dose[dosage]　維持療法 maintenance therapy[treatment] / support therapy[treatment]

いじ⁴　遺児　orphan

いしき　意識　consciousness(形conscious↔unconscious)　◆救急車で搬送されてきた時彼はまだ意識がありました He was still conscious when the ambulance brought him to the hospital.　◆彼の意識は2, 3分のうちに戻りました His consciousness returned within a couple of minutes.　◆彼女はまだ意識がはっきりしていません She's not conscious yet.　◆彼女は意識が混乱してはっきりしていません She's still confused.
《意識状態の基本表現》　◆意識状態 a state of consciousness　◆意識が回復する one regains consciousness / one's consciousness returns / one becomes conscious again　◆意識が混濁する be delirious / one's consciousness is cloudy　◆意識が遠のく feel faint　◆意識がない be unconscious / (昏睡状態の)be in a coma　◆意識がもうろうとする(意識が完全に戻っていない)be not fully conscious / (半ばぼうっとしている)be only half conscious / (意識が混乱している)be confused / (見当識がない)be disoriented　◆意識を失う lose consciousness / be[fall] unconscious / (昏睡状態に陥る)fall into a coma / (めまいなどで一時的に意識を失う)faint[black out / pass out]
《診察の基本表現》　◆意識の有無を調べる

check to see if *the patient* is conscious or not ◆意識がなくなったのですか Did you lose consciousness? /（一時的に）Did you faint[black out / pass out]? ◆どのくらい長く意識を失っていましたか How long were you unconscious? ◆怪我や事故で意識を失ったことがありますか Have you ever lost consciousness because of an injury or an accident?

《認識》awareness（圏aware）, consciousness（圏conscious） ◆彼は自分の病状を意識しているようには見えません He doesn't seem to be aware[conscious] of his own condition. ◆糖尿病コントロールに対する彼女の意識は高い She is fully aware of the importance of diabetes control.

《意図》◆私は意識的にそのような行動をとったわけではありません，誤解しないで下さい（そのつもりではなかった）I didn't mean to act that way. Please *don't misunderstand[don't take it the wrong way]. /（故意ではなかった）I didn't do that *on purpose[deliberately]. Please don't get me wrong.

◀一時的意識消失 temporary loss of consciousness / fainting[blackout] 危機意識 sense of crisis 自意識 self-consciousness 潜在意識 subconscious awareness[mind] 被害者意識 feeling of being victimized[treated unfairly] ▶意識消失 loss of consciousness / unconsciousness 意識低下（傾眠）drowsiness /（低下した意識）impaired consciousness 意識レベル level of consciousness ☞意識混濁，意識障害，意識不明

いしきこんだく　意識混濁　（せん妄）delirium（圏delirious）　（鈍った意識）clouded consciousness, consciousness clouding （意識の混乱状態）confusion（圏confused） ◆入院した時彼には意識混濁がありました He was delirious[confused] when he was admitted to the hospital.

いしきしょうがい　意識障害　consciousness disorder[disturbance], confusion ☞意識混濁，意識不明

いしきふめい　意識不明（の）　unconscious（圏unconsciousness）　◆彼女はまだ意識不明です She is still unconscious. ◆意識不明に陥る fall into a coma / fall unconscious ◆意識不明の状態 a state of unconsciousness

いしつぶつ　遺失物　lost article[property] ▶遺失物取扱所（掲示）Lost and Found (Office) /《英》Lost Property Office

いじめる　bully /bóli/（圏bullying）（からかう）pick on ◆彼女はクラスの友達からいじめを受けています She is being bullied by her classmates. ◆彼は職場でいじめに遭っていました He was bullied *at work[in the workplace]. / He was picked on at work. ◆いじめ問題にもっと注意を払う必要があります We need to pay more attention to the problem of bullying. ◆いじめっ子 a bully ◆いじめられっ子 a bullied child ◆いじめの事例 a bullying case

いしゃ　医者　doctor　☞医師

いしゃりょう　慰謝料　compensation（money）（圏慰謝料を払う compensate） ◆外科手術のミスで患者に慰謝料を支払う pay compensation（money）to a patient for suffering resulting from a surgical error / compensate a patient for an injury sustained due to a surgical error

いしゅいしょく　異種移植　heteroplasty, heterologous transplant[transplantation]

いしゅう　異臭　（変なにおい）strange smell[odor]　（嫌なにおい）bad[offensive] smell　☞悪臭

いじゅうかん　胃重感　sinking feeling in the stomach, heavy feeling in the stomach

いじゅうにしちょうかいよう　胃・十二指腸潰瘍　gastroduodenal ulcer

いしゅく　萎縮　atrophy /ǽtrəfi/（圏atrophic）　◆CTで脳の萎縮がみられます The CT scan showed *brain atrophy[shrinking of the brain]. ◆萎縮した皮膚 atrophic skin ◆人前に出ると萎縮してしまい思ったことが言えないのですか（恥ずかしくて緊張してしまう）Do you become so shy and nervous in front of people that you can't say what you're thinking? ◀筋萎縮

muscular atrophy　廃用性萎縮 disuse atrophy　▶萎縮腎 atrophic[contracted] kidney　萎縮性胃炎 atrophic gastritis　萎縮性腟炎 atrophic vaginitis

いじゅつ　医術　the art of medicine　☞医学

いしゅっけつ　胃出血　gastric bleeding [hemorrhage], bleeding[hemorrhage] of the stomach

いしょ[1]　遺書　（遺言書）will　（お別れの書き置き）farewell note　（自殺の書き置き）suicide note

いしょ[2]　医書　medical book

いじょう[1]　移乗　transfer　▶移乗介助 transfer assistance　移乗動作 transfer activity[movement]

いじょう[2]　異常・異状　（解決すべき問題）problem　（故障・困難）trouble　（不調・障害）disorder　（正常からの逸脱）abnormality, aberration　（異形）anomaly　（㊐正常ではない abnormal　具合が悪い wrong　普通ではない unusual　異形の anomalous　㊥㊦dys-）
◆胃に異常を感じているのですか Have you noticed any stomach problems[trouble]?　◆便通に何か異常がありましたか Have you ever had any problems[trouble] with your bowel movements?　◆健診で何か異常な所見はありましたか Did they find anything wrong with you at your health checkup? / Did they tell you at your health checkup that you have a problem?　◆検査結果に少し異常がありますので，もう1つ別の検査を受けて下さい You have a slightly abnormal test result [Your test result is slightly abnormal], so you should have another test.　◆異常はありません There's nothing wrong with you. / Everything is all right with you.
◆異常な動悸を感じたらすぐ連絡して下さい Please call us if you have any abnormal palpitations.　◆異常に高い〈低い〉abnormally high〈low〉　◆異常に速い〈遅い〉abnormally fast〈slow〉　◆異常な動作をする move unusually / make unusual movements
◀健診異常 problem found at the checkup

脂質異常症 dyslipidemia　食行動異常 eating disorder　染色体異常 chromosome abnormality[aberration]　先天性異常 congenital abnormality[anomaly] / birth defect　▶異常陰影 abnormal shadow　異常感覚 dysesthesia　異常行動 abnormal behavior　異常呼吸音 abnormal breath sound　異常姿勢 abnormal posture　異常性格 abnormal character　異常増殖 abnormal multiplication　異常値 abnormal value /（統計の）outlier　異常妊娠 abnormal pregnancy　☞異状死

―いじょう　―以上
《…を含めてそれ以上》　◆5 以上 five or more　◆38℃以上になったらこの解熱剤を服用して下さい You can take this antipyretic when you have a temperature of thirty-eight degrees Celsius or more [higher].
《…を超えて》　◆5 以上（5 を含まない時）more than five　◆熱が37℃以上あります The temperature is over thirty-seven degrees Celsius.　◆お子さんの身長と体重は平均以上です Your child's height and weight are above average.　◆50 歳以上のすべての女性にマンモグラフィー検査をお勧めします I recommend *a mammogram to all women over the age of fifty [that all women over the age of fifty have a mammogram].　◆あなたは 10 年以上日本に暮らしているのですか Have you been living in Japan *for more than ten years[for over ten years]?
《…よりさらに》　◆予想以上によくなっています You are in better shape than we expected.　◆これ以上申し上げることはありません There's nothing else I can say. / That's all I can say.
《…であるからには》　◆入院している以上，規則に従って下さい As long as[While] you are in this hospital, please follow the regulations.

いじょうし　異状死　unnatural death, death from[by] an unnatural cause　☞変死

いじょうみゃくりゅう　胃静脈瘤　gastric varices　★通例，複数形で.

いしょく¹ 移植 transplant[transplantation]（㊖transplanted），graft[grafting]

★transplant と transplantation, graft と grafting の入れ替えが可能．transplant, graft は移植臓器・移植片としての意味でも用いられる．◆腎臓移植手術を行う perform a kidney transplant ◆右肺の移植を受ける have[undergo] a right lung transplant ◆移植された腎臓 transplanted kidney ◀異種移植 heteroplasty / heterologous transplant 角膜移植 corneal transplant / corneal graft 肝移植 liver transplant 骨移植 bone transplant 骨髄移植 bone marrow transplant；BMT 臍帯血移植 cord blood transplant 自家移植 autotransplant / autologous transplant 心臓移植 heart transplant 生体臓器移植 living-donor organ transplant 臓器移植 organ transplant 同種移植 homologous transplant / allotransplantation 脳死移植 organ transplant from a brain-dead donor [patient] 非血縁者間骨髄移植 unrelated bone marrow transplant；UR-BMT 皮膚移植 skin graft 末梢血幹細胞移植 peripheral blood stem cell transplant；PBSCT 遊離移植 free graft ▶移植患者 transplant patient 移植外科（the department of）transplant surgery 移植コーディネーター transplant coordinator 移植手術 transplant surgery[operation] 移植免疫 transplant immunity ☞移植片

いしょく² 異食〈症〉 pica

いしょくどうぎゃくりゅうしょう 胃食道逆流症 gastroesophageal reflux disease；GERD

いしょくへん 移植片 graft, transplant

◆移植片として足〈胸〉から血管を採取する take[remove] a section of a blood vessel from the leg〈chest〉as a graft ◀血管移植片 blood vessel graft 自家移植片 autograft 同種移植片 allograft 皮膚移植片 skin graft 伏在静脈移植片 saphenous vein graft；SVG ▶移植片対宿主病 graft-versus-host disease；GVHD

いしょせい 異所性（の）ectopic, heterotopic ▶異所性胃粘膜 ectopic gastric mucosa 異所性骨化 ectopic[heterotopic] ossification 異所性子宮内膜症 ectopic endometriosis 異所性心房頻拍 ectopic atrial tachycardia 異所性拍動 ectopic[heterotopic] beat 異所性ホルモン産生腫瘍 ectopic hormone-producing tumor

いしわた 石綿 asbestos ☞アスベスト

▶石綿肺 asbestos lung / asbestosis / pulmonary asbestosis

いす 椅子 chair （寝椅子）couch （丸椅子）stool ◆椅子に座る sit down on a chair ◆椅子から立ち上がる *get up [rise] from a chair ◆この椅子におかけ下さい Please sit on this chair. / Please take this chair. ◀補助椅子（予備の椅子）spare chair /（調節付きの椅子）adjustable chair リクライニング椅子 reclining chair / recliner ▶椅子便器 bedside commode

イスラエル Israel （㊖Israeli）☞国籍

▶イスラエル人（の）Israeli

イスラムきょう ─教 Islam （㊖Islamic）

▶イスラム教徒 Muslim

いずれ

《そのうち》《最終的に》eventually 《いつか》someday ◆いずれ彼女のリンパ腫は寛解期に入ると思います I believe her lymphoma will eventually go into remission. ◆いずれあなたの国に行ってみたいですね I hope I can visit your country someday. ◆いずれまた．どうぞお大事に See you later[Goodbye for now]. Please take care 《いずれにせよ》《とにかく》anyway, in any case ◆いずれにせよ，セカンドオピニオンをもらうほうがいいでしょう Anyway[In any case], you should get a second opinion.

いせい¹ 異性 the opposite sex, the other sex （㊖異性愛の heterosexual）◆彼は思春期に入って異性に関心を示しています He has reached puberty and is showing interest in the opposite sex. ▶異性愛 heterosexuality / heterosexual love

いせい² 遺精 emission, pollution ◀夜間遺精 nocturnal emission / wet dream

いせつじょじゅつ 胃切除術 **gastrecto-my** ▶胃切除(術)後症候群 postgastrec-tomy syndrome　胃切除(術)後貧血 post-gastrectomy anemia

いせん 胃腺 **gastric gland**

いぜん¹ 以前 **before** ☞前 ◆以前この病気にかかったことがありますか Have you ever had this illness before? ◆薬で治療する以前に，まず禁煙することをお勧めします Before you start taking any medica-tion, I recommend that you stop smok-ing. ◆以前ほどお腹がすきませんか Are you less hungry than you used to be? / Do you not get hungry like you used to?

いぜん² 依然 **still** ◆彼女は依然として危篤状態です She is still in critical condi-tion. / Her condition is still critical.

いせんこう 胃穿孔 **stomach perforation**, **gastric perforation**

いせんしゅ 胃腺腫 **gastric adenoma**

いせんじょう 胃洗浄 **gastric lavage**[irri-gation], **stomach pumping**

いせんせいはくしつジストロフィー 異染性白質ジストロフィー **metachromatic leukodystrophy**

いせんつう 胃疝痛 **colic, colicky pain**; *crampy abdominal pain*

いぜんてきじゅつ 胃全摘術 **total gas-trectomy**

いそう 移送 **transportation, transfer** ☞搬送

いそがしい 忙しい **busy** ◆仕事は忙しいですか Are you busy at work? ◆お忙しい中来て下さりありがとうございます Thank you for taking time out of your busy schedule to come and see me.

いそぐ 急ぐ **hurry** (up) 図**hurry** 圏急いで in a hurry 直ちに right away, immedi-ately すばやく quickly) ☞緊急 ◆急がなくていいんですよ，ゆっくりやって下さい There's no hurry[You don't need to hurry]. Take your time. ◆この手術は急ぐ必要はないでしょう You may not need this surgery *right away[immediately]. ◆この件はできるだけ急いで対処いたします I'll take care of this matter as quickly

as possible.

いぞく 遺族 **bereaved family** ▶遺族ケア grief[bereavement] care / care for the bereaved　遺族年金 Survivors Pension

イソフラボン **isoflavone**

いぞん 依存 **dependence** (圏**depend** (on [**upon**]) 圏**dependent**) (中毒)**addic-tion** 圏中毒 ◆ご自分はアルコールに依存していると思いますか Do you feel you are dependent on alcohol? / Do you feel you have a drinking problem? ◆睡眠薬への依存 one's dependence on sleeping pills ◆インスリン依存性の患者 an insu-lin-dependent patient ◀アルコール依存 alcohol dependence[addiction] / alco-holism　睡眠薬依存 dependence on sleeping pills / hypnotic dependence　ステロイド依存性喘息 steroid-dependent asthma　大麻依存 marijuana depend-ence　鎮静薬依存 sedative dependence　鎮痛薬依存 analgesic[painkiller] depend-ence　ニコチン依存 nicotine dependence　薬物依存 drug dependence[addiction] ▶依存性人格障害 dependent personality disorder

いたい¹ 遺体 (**dead**) **body, corpse** ◆彼の遺体は今朝浴室で見つかりました His body was found in his bathroom this morning. ◆遺体の引き取り手がいません No one has claimed the body. / There are no claimants for the body. ◆遺体を確認する identify a body ◆遺体を霊安室に搬送する transport[remove] the body to the morgue ◆霊安室で遺体と対面する view the body in the morgue ◆引き取り手のない遺体 an unclaimed body ▶遺体安置所(hospital) morgue

いたい² 痛い **have**[**feel**] (**a**)**pain** (圏**pain-ful**) (鈍い痛みがある)**ache** /éik/ (圏**ach-ing**) (傷・筋肉などが痛い)**become**[**be**] **sore** (触ると痛い)**become**[**be**] **tender** (体の一部が痛い)**hurt** 圏痛がる，痛み，痛む ◆背中が痛いのですか Do you have[feel] any pain in your back? / Does your back hurt[ache]? ◆足の筋肉が痛い the leg mus-cles are sore ◆触ると痛い be painful

いたい² 43 いたみ

to the touch / be tender

イタイイタイびょう ―病 **itai-itai disease** ◆イタイイタイ病はカドミウム中毒が原因の病気です Itai-itai disease is caused by cadmium poisoning.

いだいちょうはんしゃ 胃大腸反射 **gastrocolic reflex**

いたがる 痛がる ☞痛い, 痛み, 痛む ◆娘さんは足を痛がっているのですか Is your daughter complaining of leg pain? / Does your daughter say that her leg hurts? ◆彼は痛がって泣いています He is crying in[with] pain.

いたずら¹ ◆(子供に)この点滴をいたずらしてはいけませんよ Don't play with this IV drip.

いたずら² 徒(に) ◆いたずらにこの病気を恐れすぎてはいけません(理由なく)Don't be afraid of this illness for no real reason.

いただく
《受け取る》**have, accept** ◆できるだけ早くお返事をいただけますか Please let me have your answer as soon as possible. ◆患者様からご贈答品をいただくわけにはまいりません We really shouldn't accept gifts from our patients.
《…してもらう》 ◆電気を消していただけますか Could you turn off the light, please? ◆明日また来ていただきたいのですが I'd love to you to come again tomorrow. ◆来週のいつかこちらにお越しいただけますでしょうか Would you mind coming here sometime next week? / I wonder if you could come here sometime next week?

いたみ 痛み **pain** (鈍痛) **ache** /éik/ (傷・筋肉痛などによる痛み) **soreness** (圧迫・触った時の痛み) **tenderness** (動痛む **have** (a) **pain, ache** 体の一部が痛む **hurt**) ☞痛い, 痛がる, 痛む, 疼痛, 病歴(囲み:病歴聴取の基本表現)
《基本的な表現》 ◆痛みがある have[feel] (a) pain ◆胃の痛み(a) stomachache / (a) stomach pain ◆がんの痛み(a) pain caused by cancer ◆喉の痛み a sore throat ◆痛みを和らげる[軽くする]ease

[relieve] the pain ◆痛みを抑える control the pain ◆痛みに耐える[痛みをこらえる] endure[stand] the pain / put up with the pain ◆痛みのスケールを使って痛みの程度を説明する use a pain (rating) scale to describe the level[intensity] of pain / describe the degree of pain by using a pain (rating) scale ◆痛みを我慢しなくていいんですよ You don't have to put up with any pain. ◆痛かったら遠慮せずに言って下さい Don't hesitate to let me know if it hurts. ◆この検査は痛みがありません This test is painless. ◆手術中は痛みを感じませんよ You won't feel [have] any pain during the surgery. ◆痛みの数値評価尺度 *Numeric Rating Scale[NRS] for pain (measurement)
《症状について尋ねる》 ◆痛みがありますか Do you have any pain? ◆どこが痛みますか Where is the pain? / Where do you have[feel] the pain? / Where does it hurt? ◆痛みは胸のどこですか Where in your chest is the pain? / Where in your chest *do you have the pain[does it hurt]? ◆痛みのある場所を指で示して下さい Could you point to where you feel the pain? / Please point and show me where it hurts. ◆痛みは他の場所に移動しますか Does the pain move[spread] *to anywhere else (in your body) [to any other parts of your body]? ◆どんな痛みですか What is the pain like? / Can you describe the pain for me? ◆いつ痛みますか When does the pain come on? / When do you have the pain? ◆どの程度の痛みですか How severe is the pain? ◆痛みはひどいですか Is the pain very bad? / Does it hurt a lot? ◆(痛みのスケールを示しながら)0 から 10 の痛みスケールで, 最悪の痛みを 10 とすると, あなたの今の痛みの程度はどうですか On a scale of zero to ten, with ten being the worst pain you can imagine, how bad is the pain?
《経過について説明する》 ◆痛みがあってからどのくらい経っていますか How long *have you had[have you been having]

the pain? ◆痛みが出たのは最近ですか Did the pain *come on[start] recently? ◆痛みは悪化していますか Is the pain getting worse? ◆しばらくすれば痛みは和らぐでしょう The pain will ease after a while. ◆痛みはまもなく消えるでしょう The pain will go (away) soon. ◆2, 3日間は痛みが少しあるかもしれません You may have a slight pain for a few days. / There may be some soreness[tenderness] for a few days. ◆この薬が痛みを取ってくれるでしょう This medication will relieve the pain. ☞痛み外来, 痛み止め

痛みの表現

■痛みの部位
身体の部位＋pain[ache]で表す. ★「pain ＋in＋身体の部位」でも表すことができる.
(例)pain in one's chest
● chest pain (胸痛) ● backache, back pain (腰痛) ● stomachache, stomach pain (胃痛・腹痛) ● abdominal pain (腹痛) ● toothache, tooth pain (歯痛)

■痛みの程度
痛みなし no pain → 軽い[少しの]痛み mild pain → 我慢できる程度の痛み tolerable pain → 中程度の痛み moderate pain → 激しい[強い/ひどい]痛み severe [intense / strong / terrible / awful / horrible] pain → 耐えられない痛み unbearable[excruciating] pain
● スケールを使った痛みの程度の尋ね方 Please look at this scale of zero to ten. What's your pain level now?

0	1	2	3	4	5	6	7	8	9	10
no pain		mild		moderate			severe			unbearable

■痛みの起こり方
● 突然の痛み sudden pain ● 急性の痛み acute pain ● 慢性の痛み chronic pain ● 瞬時の痛み momentary[transient] pain ● 短い痛み brief pain ● 持続性の痛み constant[continuous / persistent] pain ● 間欠性の[発作的に繰り返す]痛み intermittent pain / pain that comes and goes ● 周期性の[繰り返す]痛み periodic pain

■痛みの領域
● 全身的な痛み pain all over one's body ● 表面的な痛み superficial[external] pain ● 深部の痛み deep[internal] pain ● 限局性の痛み localized pain ● 広範性の痛み generalized pain ● 放散性の痛み radiating[spreading] pain ● 移動性の痛み moving pain

■痛みの性状
★痛みの感じ方や表現には個人差があるので, 状況に応じて使い分ける.
● 鋭い痛み sharp pain ● 鈍い痛み dull pain ● 重苦しい痛み heavy pain ● 頑固な痛み stubborn[intractable] pain ● しくしくする[しつこい]痛み gnawing [nagging dull] pain ● ずきずきする痛み throbbing[pounding / pulsating] pain ● (傷などの)ひりひりする痛み smarting pain ● 焼けるようなひりひりする痛み burning pain ● 圧迫した時の痛み tender pain ● チクッとする痛み pricking pain ● ちくちくする痛み prickly[stinging / tingling] pain ● ピリピリッとくる痛み（電撃性の）electric shock-like pain ● ピーンと走るような鋭い痛み shooting pain ● 刺すような痛み stabbing pain ● ナイフで刺すような痛み knife-like, stabbing pain / sharp, knife-like pain ● (腹などが)きりきり差し込む痛み griping[colicky] pain ★激しい腹痛・月経痛は cramps という. ● (頭が)締め付けられるような痛み tightening band-like pain (around the head) ● 割れるような痛み splitting pain ● 締め付けられるような痛み tightening[squeezing / crushing] pain / tight [binding] pain ● 圧迫されるような痛み pressing[pressure-like] pain ● 引き裂かれるような痛み ripping[tearing] pain

いたみがいらい 痛み外来 pain clinic
いたみどめ 痛み止め pain medication [reliever], painkiller, analgesic ☞鎮痛薬

◆これは痛み止めの薬です This medication will help ease your pain. / This medication is for the pain. ◆痛み止めの注射をしましょう I'm going to give you a shot for the pain. ◆痛み止めがほしいですか Would you like to have some pain medication?

いたむ¹ 悼む （深く悲しむ）grieve （over） （嘆き悲しむ）mourn （for, over） ◆彼女は母親の死を悼んでいます She is *grieving over[mourning （for）] the death of her mother.

いたむ² 痛む have[get, feel] （a） pain （持続して痛む）ache （身体の一部が痛む）hurt （炎症などでひりひりする）get[become, be] sore （触ると痛む）get[become, be] tender （ずきずきする）throb （刺すように痛む） sting （ちくちく[ひりひり]する）tingle ☞痛い, 痛がる, 痛み ◆どこが痛みますか Where is the pain? / Where do you have [feel] the pain? / Where does it hurt? ◆痛む場所を指で示して下さい Please point with one finger to where it hurts. ◆ここを押すと痛みますか Does it hurt when I press here? ◆この辺りは押すと痛みますか Is this area tender? ◆初めて痛んだのはいつですか When did the pain first come on? / When did you first get the pain? ◆どのくらい長く痛んでいますか How long have you had the pain? ◆痛んだら教えて下さい Let me know *when it hurts[when you have the pain]. ◆切開したところがしばらく痛むかもしれません The incision may be sore for a while. ◆胃が少し〈ひどく〉痛む have （a） slight〈severe / bad〉pain in the stomach / have a slight〈severe / bad〉stomachache ◆歯が痛む have a toothache / one's tooth aches ◆頭が痛む have a headache / have （a） pain in one's head ◆喉〈舌〉が痛む have a sore throat 〈tongue〉/ have （a） pain in one's throat 〈tongue〉

いためる 痛める・傷める （障害を与える） hurt, injure （物理的に傷つける）damage ◆腰を痛めたのですか Did you hurt[in-

jure] your lower back? ◆乱暴に扱うとコンタクトレンズを傷める恐れがあります You may damage your contact lenses if you handle them roughly. ◆脊髄を傷める damage the spinal cord

いたらない 至らない ◆至らない点があれば遠慮なくおっしゃって下さい（不満な点があれば）Please don't hesitate to let us know if you have any complaints. / （快適に過ごせるようできることがあれば）Please don't hesitate to let us know if we can do anything to make your visit[stay] more comfortable.

イタリア Italy （㊙Italian） ☞国籍 ▶イタリア人（の） Italian

いち 位置 （姿勢・物の位置）position ◆体の位置[体位]を変えると楽になりますか Does changing your position help you? ◆まっすぐな位置に in an upright position ◆横の位置に in a horizontal position ▶位置感覚 position[body / posture] sense

いちあん 一案 good idea ◆セカンドオピニオンをお受けになるのも一案だと思います It might be a good idea to get a second opinion.

いちいち ◆答えたくない質問にはいちいち答えなくても構いません（すべての質問に答える必要はない）You don't have to answer every question if you don't want to. ◆細かいことがいちいち気になるほうですか Do you tend to worry about details[little things]?

いちいちきゅうばん 119番 ◆119番で救急車を呼ぶ dial[call] one-one-nine for an ambulance

いちいちぜろばん 110番 ◆110番で警察を呼ぶ dial[call] one-one-zero for the police ★0は /zíərou/ または /óu/ と読む.

いちがい 一概（に） （完全に）altogether （必ずしも）necessarily ◆飲酒は一概に悪いとは言えませんが，当面は控えたほうが無難です Drinking alcohol is not altogether [necessarily] bad, but it would be safer for you to stop drinking for the time being.

いちがた **1型・I型** **type 1, type I** （1度）**first degree** ▶I型アレルギー反応 type I allergic reaction　1型糖尿病 type 1 diabetes（mellitus）

いちがつ **1月** **January**；**Jan.** ◆インフルエンザの流行は冬季，特に1月や2月に多く見られます Flu outbreaks[Outbreaks of influenza] are more common in winter, especially in January and February. ◆当院は1月4日から診療を再開します We will reopen the hospital on January (the) fourth. ★「〇月に」は前置詞 in を用いる。「〇月×日に」は on を用いる． ◆外来に1月26日火曜日午前10時においで下さい Please come to the outpatient clinic[department] on Tuesday, January (the) twenty-sixth, at ten in the morning. ◆来年の1月に next January ◆昨年[この前]の1月に last January ★前置詞 in や on は付けない．

いちご **strawberry** ▶いちご舌 strawberry tongue　いちご状血管腫 strawberry mark[hemangioma]

いちじ¹ **一次（の）** （主な・初期の）**primary** （順番が最初の）**(the) first** （基本的な）**basic** ▶一次医療 primary medical[health] care　一次救急 primary emergency care　一次救命処置 basic life support；BLS　一次性徴 primary sex characteristic　一次予防 primary prevention

いちじ² **一時**
《しばらくの間》**for a while, for a time** ◆彼女は一時危険な状態でした She was in a critical condition for a while[time].
《臨時の》（短期の・仮の）**temporary** （暫定的な）**interim** （一過性の）**transient** ☞一過性 ◆一時的な処置を必要とする require temporary treatment ◆これで一時的に出血が止まるでしょう This will temporarily stop the bleeding. ◆治療を一時中断する discontinue the treatment temporarily ◆一時的な措置 *an interim[a temporary] measure
◀出産育児一時金 lump-sum birth allowance / childbirth and nursing allowance ▶一時帰国 temporary return to

one's home country　一時帰宅 temporary [brief] return to one's home　一時的意識消失 temporary loss of consciousness / fainting / blackout　一時的人工肛門 temporary stoma　一時的ペースメーカ temporary pacemaker

いちしきかく **1色覚** **achromatopsia, total color blindness** ☞色覚

いちじゅうもうまく **一絨毛膜（の）** **monochorionic** ▶一絨毛膜双胎 monochorionic twins　一絨毛膜二羊膜双胎 monochorionic diamniotic twins

いちじょ **一助** **help** （쿄help） ◆ソーシャルワーカーに相談していただければ，問題解決の一助となるかと思います I think if you *talk with[consult] our medical social worker, she〈he〉will help you solve this problem. / I'm sure our medical social worker is a good person to go to for advice on how to solve this problem.

いちじるしい **著しい** ☞顕著
《めざましい》**remarkable** ◆今日の血液検査の結果に著しい改善が見られます The blood test results we got today show a remarkable improvement.
《深刻である》**severe** ◆彼の内臓は著しく損傷しており，残念ながら回復は難しいと思われます His internal injuries are so severe that I'm afraid his recovery will be difficult.

いちたいいち **一対一** **one-on-one** （内密に）**in private** （2人だけで）**alone together** ◆折り入って一対一で話し合いたいのですが I'd like to talk with you *in private [alone together]. / I have something I'd like to talk with you about one-on-one.

いちど¹ **1度・I度** **(the) first degree** ▶I度熱傷 first-degree burn　1度房室ブロック first-degree atrioventricular[AV] block

いちど² **一度** （一回）**once** （一度に…ずつ）**a time, one time** （再び）**again** ☞1回 ◆週に一度 once a week ◆一度に2粒ずつ服用して下さい Please take this medication two tablets at a time. ◆もう一度やって下さい Do it once again[more]. /

Could you do that again? ◆もう一度言っていただけますか I beg your pardon? / Pardon ⟨me⟩? / Could you say that again?

いちどう　一同⟨の⟩　⟨全体の⟩ all, entire　◆職員一同を代表してお礼申し上げます On behalf of the entire staff I'd like to thank you.

いちにち　1 日　day, a⟨one, per⟩ day ⟨形 daily⟩　◆あなたの 1 日に必要なカロリーは 1,800 から 2,100 kcal です In your case, the amount of calories needed a[per] day is between one thousand eight hundred and two thousand one hundred kilocalories.　◆1 日中体がだるいのですか Do you feel tired all day long?　◆1 日 3 回薬を飲む take the medication three times a day　◆1 日おき every other day　◆1 日の終わり頃 later in the day　▶1 日人間ドック one-day comprehensive physical [health] checkup　1 日排泄量 daily output　1 日必要量 daily requirement　1 日量 daily dose

いちばん　一番⟨の⟩　⟨最初の⟩ the first ⟨副 first⟩　⟨最大の⟩ the most　⟨最もよい⟩ the best　☞最も　◆あなたにとって一番大切な事は何ですか What's the most important thing in life for you? / What's most important ⟨of all⟩ to you?　◆あなたの筋肉痛に一番必要なのは休息です Rest is the best thing for your sore muscles. / The best thing you can do for your sore muscles is rest.　◆あいにく夜間診療は行っておりませんので，明日の朝一番においで下さい I'm sorry, but our clinic is closed at night. Please come back first thing tomorrow morning.

いちびょうりつ　1 秒率　forced expiratory volume percentage in one[the first] second, the ratio of forced expiratory volume in one[the first] second to forced vital capacity；FEV$_{1.0}$／FVC

いちびょうりょう　1 秒量　forced expiratory volume in one[the first] second；FEV$_{1.0}$

いちぶ　一部　part ⟨形 partial⟩　◆だるいの

は体の一部ですか，それとも体全体ですか Do you feel tired in one part of your body or all over your body?　◀患者一部負担 partial copayment　▶一部介助 partial assistance

いちょう¹　医長　head doctor　◀外科医長 surgeon-in-chief　内科医長 physician-in-chief　★診療部長は medical director.

いちょう²　胃腸　stomach and⟨or⟩ bowels[intestines] ⟨形 gastrointestinal；GI　胃部の gastric⟩　☞胃，消化管，腸　◆胃腸の具合が悪いのですか Do you have any problems with your stomach or bowels?　◆胃腸が弱い⟨消化不良である⟩ have poor digestion　◀機能性胃腸症 functional dyspepsia　▶胃腸管[消化管] gastrointestinal tract　胃腸疾患 gastrointestinal disease／GI tract disorder　胃腸障害 stomach trouble／gastrointestinal disorder　胃腸症状 gastrointestinal symptom　胃腸病学 gastroenterology　胃腸薬 stomach medication[drug]／gastrointestinal medication[drug／agent]／⟨消化剤⟩ digestant　☞胃腸炎

いちょうえん　胃腸炎　gastroenteritis　⟨口語的に⟩ stomach flu[bug]　◀ウイルス性胃腸炎 viral gastroenteritis　急性胃腸炎 acute gastroenteritis

いちらんせいそうせいじ　一卵性双生児　identical twins, monozygotic twins, uniovular twins　⟨その 1 人⟩ identical twin　◆2 人は一卵性双生児です They're identical twins.

いちる　一縷⟨の⟩　faint　◆われわれとしてはこの新しい治療に一縷の望みを託しています This treatment gives us a faint ray of hope for a cure.

いつ　何時　when　⟨いつか⟩ sometime　⟨いまにも⟩ at any moment　◆痛み始めたのはいつですか When did the pain start?　◆次回の予約はいつがいいですか When is a good day for your next appointment?　◆いつ帰国されるのですか When are you going home?　◆いつから腫れているのですか Since when have you had the swelling? ◆いつから日本に住んでいますか（どれくらい長く）How long have you been in Japan? ◆彼の容態はいつ急変してもおかしくない状態です His condition is critical and could take a sudden turn for the worse at any moment. ◆来週のいつかお電話をいただけますか Could you give me a call sometime next week?

いつう 胃痛 stomachache, stomach pain, gastric pain, gastralgia ☞痛み, 腹痛 ◆胃痛がある have a stomachache / have (a) pain in the stomach ◆胃痛を起こす get a stomachache

いっかい 1回 once, one time ☞一度 ◆薬を1日1回飲む take the medication once a day ▶一回換気量 tidal volume；TV （薬の）一回分[量]（single) dose

いっかしょ 一箇所 （点）one spot （場所）one place ◆胸部X線写真で一箇所気になるところがあるので，CTで確認しましょう There's a spot on your chest X-ray that I'm concerned about, so let's get[have] it checked with a CT.

いっかせい 一過性（の） （臨時の）temporary （短期の）transient （一瞬の）momentary ☞一時 ◆脱毛は一過性のもので，髪の毛は2, 3か月で生えてくるでしょう The hair loss is temporary, so it will grow back within a few months. ◆痛みは一過性ですか，持続性ですか Does the pain come and go, or does it stay? ◆一過性の痛み (a) transient[momentary] pain ▶一過性健忘 temporary[transient] amnesia 一過性脳虚血発作 transient ischemic attack；TIA

いっかつばらい 一括払い lump sum payment ◆医療費は一括払いしていただけますか Could you please pay the medical expenses in one lump sum?

いっき¹ 一期・1期 （第1の段階）first stage （図1期的な one-stage） （1つの期間・時期）one period, one term ☞期 ▶一期的手術 one-stage surgery[operation]

いっき² 一気（に） （ひと呼吸に）in one breath （ひと飲みに）in one gulp （いっぺんに）in one go ◆大きく息を吸って，できる

だけ勢いよく一気に吐いて下さい Please take a deep breath, and blow out as hard and fast as you can in one breath. ◆コップの中身を一気に飲んで下さい Please empty the cup in one gulp. ◆一気飲みする down a drink (in one go) ★down は動詞.

いっきいちゆう 一喜一憂 ◆一喜一憂するのも無理ありませんが, 細かな数値の変動はさほど重要ではありません It is only natural for you *to be sometimes happy and sometimes disappointed[to swing back and forth between happiness and disappointment] with the results, but small changes in the test levels are not so important.

いっきゅう 一級（の） （評価）first rate [class] （レベル・程度）level[class] one ◆佐々木先生の手術の腕前は第一級ですので, どうぞご安心下さい Dr Sasaki is a first-rate surgeon, so please don't worry. ◆1級の身体障害者手帳を申請する apply for a level[class]-one physical disability handbook

いっけつはん 溢血斑 （網膜）blot bleeding[hemorrhage] （皮膚）ecchymosis

いっけん 一見 ◆関先生は一見不愛想に見えますが, 患者さん想いの優しい方ですので, 相談してみてはいかがですか Dr Seki looks[comes across as] unfriendly, but in fact he's〈she's〉really gentle and kind with patients. Why don't you ask him 〈her〉for advice?

いっこう¹ 一向（に） at all ★否定文で. ◆彼女の状態はいっこうに改善しません Her condition isn't improving at all. / Her condition isn't showing any (signs of) improvement.

いっこう² 一考 idea ☞考える ◆配置転換を願い出ることも一考に値します It may be a good idea to ask for a job transfer.

いっこく 一刻 ◆今は一刻を争います There is[We have] no time to lose. ◆お子さんは一刻も早く治療を始めなければなりません Your child should have the treatment as soon as possible. / （緊急に）Your child needs urgent medical attention [treatment].

いっさい 一切 （絶対に）absolutely ◆当院内での喫煙や飲酒は一切ご遠慮願います Please absolutely refrain from smoking or drinking alcohol inside the hospital.

いっさんかたんそ 一酸化炭素 carbon monoxide ▶一酸化炭素中毒 carbon monoxide poisoning

いっさんかちっそ 一酸化窒素 nitric oxide, nitrogen monoxide ◆呼気中の一酸化窒素を測定しましょう Let me check your level of exhaled nitric oxide.

いっしき 一式 complete set ◆これが当院の入院手続き書類一式になります This is the complete set of the hospital admission forms.

いっしょう 一生 one's life, one's lifetime ☞生涯

いっしょけんめい 一所懸命 ◆一所懸命にやる（精一杯努力する）try hard / （最善を尽くす）do one's best ◆一所懸命このリハビリに取り組めばずっとよくなります If you *try hard[do your best] with this rehab exercise, you'll be able to make a big difference. ◆お子さんを一所懸命お世話させていただきます We'll do our best to take care of your child.

いっしんいったい 一進一退 ◆これまでのところ彼女の病状は一進一退です（状態が不安定です）She's still in an unstable condition. / Her condition is still unstable[precarious].

いっそく 一側（の）unilateral ▶一側難聴 unilateral hearing loss 一側肺換気 one-lung ventilation

いったい on earth, whatever ◆これほどの怪我をするなんて，いったいどうなさったのですか How on earth *did you get such a serious injury[did you injure yourself so badly]?

いつだつ 逸脱 （規範からの逸脱）deviance （㊝deviant ㊌deviate） （型などからの脱出）extrusion （㊌extruded） （内臓器の脱出）prolapse ◀僧帽弁逸脱症 mitral valve prolapse；MVP ▶逸脱行動 deviant be-

havior 逸脱椎間板 extruded disk

いっち 一致する agree （with） （反映する）reflect ◆その点に関してはあなたと意見が一致しています I agree with you on that point. / You and I are of the same opinion on that point. ◆これらの検査データは病気の重症度とは必ずしも一致しません These test results do not necessarily reflect the severity of the disease.

いっちょういったん 一長一短 （利点・欠点）merit and demerit （有利な点・不利な点）advantage and disadvantage （よい所・悪い所）good point and bad point ◆お話しした治療法にはそれぞれ一長一短があります Each treatment option I told you about has *its merits and its demerits[its advantages and its disadvantages / its good points and its bad points].

いってい 一定（の）
《決まった》fixed, set （不変の）constant （規則正しい）regular ◆運動は規則的に，一定の時間を決めて行うと効果的です Exercise is effective if you always do it regularly at a fixed time. ◆一定の期間様子をみましょう Let's wait for a set period of time and see what happens. ◆血糖値は一定にする必要があります．高すぎても低すぎても体に悪影響を及ぼします You need a constant level of sugar in your blood because levels that are too high or too low can be harmful to the body. ◆陣痛は一定の間隔で来ていますか Are your contractions coming at regular intervals?
《ある程度》◆放射線治療は一定の効果はあったと考えています I believe the radiation therapy had the effect we were hoping for.

いつでも （どんな時でも）anytime （どんな日でも）any day （…する時はいつでも）whenever （常に）always （しょっちゅう）all the time ☞いつも ◆いつでもご都合のよい時においで下さい Please feel free to come and see me anytime[any day] that's convenient for you. ◆いつでもお手伝いしますよ We're here to help anytime. / We're always ready to help you. ◆ご用

のある時はいつでも遠慮しないでこのコールボタンを押して下さい Whenever you need any help, please don't hesitate to push [press] this call button. ◆彼はいつでもコンピュータゲームをしています He is always playing computer games. / He plays computer games all the time.

いつにゅう 溢乳 regurgitation of milk

いっぱい¹ 一杯 （コップ・グラス）a glass of （茶碗・カップ）a cup of ◆この薬はコップ一杯の水で飲んで下さい Please take this medication with a (full) glass of water. ◆お茶をもう一杯いかがですか Would you like another cup of tea?

いっぱい²
《幅》wide ◆目をいっぱいに見開いて下さい Please open your eyes wide.
《満杯》（溢れた）full （詰まった）stuffed ◆お腹がいっぱいになるほど食べてはいけません Please try to stop eating before you feel full[stuffed]. ◆心配ごとで頭がいっぱいになることはありますか（心配ごと以外考えられない）Do you ever feel as if you can't think about anything except your worries?

—いっぱい ◆外来の予約は今週いっぱいとれません（来週まで）I'm afraid there are no appointments available until next week.

いっぱく 一泊 overnight stay （動stay overnight[for a night]） ◆治療後に一泊の入院をお勧めします I recommend that you stay in the hospital overnight after the treatment. / I recommend overnight hospitalization[stay in our hospital] after the treatment.

いっぱん 一般（の）（総合的な）general （普通の）ordinary （日常の）everyday ►一般開業医 general practitioner；GP 一般概念 general idea 一般外来（general）outpatient clinic 一般外科 general surgery 一般語（単語）general[everyday] word 一般語（用語）general[everyday /（素人の）lay] term 一般事務職員（general office）clerk 一般食 ordinary meal 一般診療 general practice 一般診療所 general practice clinic 一般内科 general internal medicine 一般内科（診療科）the department of general internal medicine / the general internal medicine department 一般病院 general hospital 一般病床 general bed 一般名 generic name 一般用医薬品（市販薬）over-the-counter[OTC] drug

いっぽうか 一包化 ☞分包

いつまで ◆いつまで日本に滞在なさいますか（どれくらい長く）How long are you going to stay in Japan? / Until when are you going to be in Japan?

いつまでも ◆いつまでもこの治療を続けるわけにはいきません We can't continue this treatment indefinitely[forever]. ◆いつまでもお元気でね Stay well!

いつも
《常に・同じように》（しょっちゅう）all the time （必ず）always ☞いつでも ◆いつも痛みますか Does it hurt all the time? ◆喉がいつも渇いている感じがしますか Do you always feel thirsty?
《普段通り》as usual, usually, normally ☞通常，普段，普通 ◆食事はいつも通りですか Are you eating as usual? ◆楽な気持ちで，いつものように息をしていて下さい Just relax, and breathe normally.

いつりゅうせいにょうしっきん 溢流性尿失禁 overflow（urinary）incontinence

いつわり 偽り（嘘）lie （動lie）（事実についての虚偽）falsehood （形false） ◆偽りを言う tell a lie / do not tell the truth ◆偽りなく病状を伝える tell *the patient* the truth about his〈her〉condition / do not lie to *the patient* about his〈her〉condition ◆住所氏名を偽る give a false name and address

いていせん 胃底腺 fundic gland

いでん 遺伝（の）（遺伝性の）hereditary /hírédətèri/（图遺伝形質 heredity）（遺伝によって受け継がれた）inherited （動inherit 图遺伝形質 inheritance）（遺伝子の・遺伝学の）genetic /dʒənétɪk/ ◆あなたかご主人に何か遺伝性の病気がありますか Do you or your husband have any hereditary [genetic] diseases? ◆ご家族に遺伝性と思われる病気がありますか Is there any disease that seems to run in your family? ★run in *one's* family は家系に伝わる病気があるという意味．◆この病気はお子さんに遺伝しませんのでご安心下さい Your children will not inherit this disease from you[This disease is not hereditary], so don't worry. ◀X 連鎖優性〈劣性〉遺伝 X-linked dominant〈recessive〉inheritance　隔世遺伝 atavism　常染色体優性〈劣性〉遺伝 autosomal dominant〈recessive〉inheritance　発生遺伝学 developmental genetics　伴性遺伝 sex-linked inheritance　メンデル遺伝 mendelian inheritance[genetics] / mendelism　▶遺伝暗号 genetic code　遺伝因子 genetic factor　遺伝カウンセリング genetic counseling　遺伝学 genetics / genealogy　遺伝学者 geneticist　遺伝学的検査 genetic testing　遺伝疾患 genetic disease　遺伝性球状赤血球症 hereditary spherocytosis　遺伝性出血性末梢血管拡張症 hereditary hemorrhagic telangiectasia；HHT　遺伝性難聴 hereditary hearing loss　遺伝性ニューロパチー hereditary neuropathy　遺伝性非ポリポーシス大腸がん[リンチ症候群] hereditary nonpolyposis colorectal cancer；HNPCC　遺伝的特徴 genetic trait[characteristic] / hereditary trait[characteristic]　遺伝的変異 genetic variation　☞遺伝子，遺伝病

いでんし　遺伝子　gene /dʒíːn/（**genetic** /dʒənétɪk/）　◆乳がんの遺伝子 a breast cancer gene / a gene *for breast cancer[associated with breast cancer]　◆遺伝子を持っている carry a gene　◆遺伝子を受け継ぐ inherit a gene　◆遺伝子の異常 a genetic abnormality　◀がん遺伝子 cancer gene / oncogene　耐性遺伝子 resistance gene　抑制遺伝子 suppressor gene　▶遺伝子型 genotype　遺伝子組み換え食品 *genetically modified[GM] food　遺伝子検査 genetic[gene-based] testing / DNA-based testing　遺伝子工学 genetic engineering　遺伝子診断 genetic [gene] diagnosis　遺伝子操作 genetic

[gene] manipulation　遺伝子治療 gene therapy　遺伝子突然変異 gene mutation

いでんびょう　遺伝病　genetic disease, hereditary disease　◀X 連鎖遺伝病 X-linked genetic disease　常染色体性遺伝病 autosomal genetic disease　多因子遺伝病 multifactorial genetic disease

いと¹　糸　（ひと針の糸・縫い目）**stitch, suture**　（縫合糸）**surgical suture**　（縫い糸）**thread**　◆糸を抜く take out the stitches　◆糸を抜いてもらう have *one's* stitches（taken）out

いと²　意図　intention（動**intend**　形**intentional**　副故意に **on purpose, deliberately, intentionally**）　☞つもり　◆あなたを傷つける意図は全くありません I have no intention of hurting you at all.　◆彼女が何を意図しているのかわかりません I just don't understand what she intends to do.　◆意図的にやったわけではありません．まったくの不注意でした I didn't do it *on purpose [deliberately]. It was a careless mistake.

いどう¹　異動　change　☞転動　◆来週スタッフの異動があります There will be a change of staff next week.

いどう²　移動する　（動く）**move**（to）　（動き回る）**move**（around）　（歩き回る）**walk**（around）, **wander**　（広がる）**spread**　（搬送・護送する）**transfer, escort**（形移動式の **mobile** /móʊbaɪl/）　◆痛みは他の場所に移動しますか Does the pain move [spread] to another place?　◆病院内を自由に移動していいですよ Please feel free to move[walk] around the hospital.　◆明日の朝 8 時に手術室に移動していただきます You'll be transferred[escorted] to the operating room at eight o'clock tomorrow morning.　◆移動性の痛みがある have[get] a moving[wandering] pain　◀左方移動 shift to the left　▶移動診療所 mobile clinic　移動性盲腸 mobile cecum　移動図書室 bookmobile　移動用バー（つかまり棒）grab bar

いときりば　糸切り歯　（犬歯）**canine tooth**（形**teeth**）

いとこ　従兄弟・従姉妹　**（first**）**cousin**

―いない ―**以内** in, within (…より遅くなく) no later (than) (…より少なく) in less (than) (…より多くなく) in not more (than) ◆一時間以内に戻ってきます I'll be back in[within] an hour. ◆インフルエンザの治療は発熱してから48時間以内に始める必要があります Influenza treatment needs to be started *no later than [within] forty-eight hours after the first signs of fever.

いとようじ 糸ようじ dental floss

いないしきょう 胃内視鏡 gastroscope (検査) endoscopy of the stomach ◆正確な診断をするために胃内視鏡の検査をしましょう I'm going to[Let me] do[run] an endoscopy of your stomach for an accurate diagnosis. ◆胃内視鏡が喉まで来たら, ごくんと飲みこんで下さい Please swallow the gastroscope in one gulp when it reaches your throat. ▶胃内視鏡検査 gastroscopy / upper (GI) endoscopy

いないようぶつ 胃内容物 stomach contents, gastric contents ★通例, 複数形で.

いにょうしょう 遺尿症 enuresis ; *involuntary release of urine* ☞夜尿 ▶昼間遺尿症 diurnal enuresis 夜間遺尿症 nocturnal enuresis

イヌ 犬 dog ◆犬に手を噛まれたのですか Did a dog bite your hand? ◆犬が吠えるような咳 a barking cough ▶イヌ回虫症 toxocariasis イヌ糸状虫症 dirofilariasis 犬猫病院 pet clinic[hospital]

いねむり 居眠りする doze off, nod off ◆仕事中よく居眠りしますか Do you often doze[nod] off at work? ◆居眠り運転する fall asleep while driving

いねんまく 胃粘膜 gastric mucosa[mucous membrane], the mucosa of the stomach (形 gastric mucosal) ◀異所性胃粘膜 ectopic gastric mucosa 急性胃粘膜病変 acute gastric mucosal lesion ; AGML ▶胃粘膜下腫瘍 gastric submucosal tumor 胃粘膜保護薬 gastric mucosal protective medication[drug / agent]

いのち 命 life (形 命に関わる life-threatening 致命的な fatal) ☞寿命 ◆命を救う save *a person's* life ◆命を落とす lose *one's* life ◆命を絶つ(命を奪う) take *one's* own life / (自殺する) commit suicide ◆彼は朝まで命がもたないかもしれません I'm afraid he may not last[live] until the morning. ◆大怪我でしたが, 彼女の命に別状はありません She was severely injured, but her injury is not life-threatening. ◆このタイプのアレルギー反応は多くの場合命に関わります This type of allergic reaction is often life-threatening. ◆この病気は命に関わる心配はありません This disease is not fatal. ◆タバコの吸いすぎは命を縮めます Heavy smoking will shorten your life.

いのり 祈り prayer

いのる 祈る pray, offer a prayer ◆1日も早いご快復をお祈りしています I hope you *make a quick recovery[recover soon]. ◆彼が早くよくなるように祈る pray for his speedy[quick] recovery ◆彼女のご冥福をお祈りいたします I pray that *her soul[she] rests in peace. / May *her soul[she] rest in peace.

いバリウムけんさ 胃バリウム検査 barium swallow[meal], upper GI series

いはん 違反する (規則・法律などを破る) break, violate (規則などに従わない) disobey (前 規則などに反して against) ☞違法 ◆院内規則に違反する break[disobey] the hospital rules ◆その薬物の使用は法律に違反します It is against the law to use that drug. / The use of that drug is illegal.

いびき 鼾 snore (動 snore) ◆いびきをかくと人から言われたことがありますか Have you ever been told that you snore a lot? ◆大いびきをかく snore loudly while sleeping

いひろうせい 易疲労性 easy fatigability

いファイバースコープ 胃ファイバースコープ gastrofiberscope ☞胃内視鏡

いぶつ 異物 foreign object[body, matter, substance] ◆目の中に異物がある感じがしますか Do you feel as if *something is [you have something / there is some-

thing] in your eye(s)? ◆これから外耳道の異物を除去します I'm going to remove the foreign object from your ear canal.
◆異物を攻撃する attack a foreign body[substance] ◀眼内異物 foreign body in the eye(s) 気道内異物 foreign body in the airway / airway foreign body ▶異物反応 foreign body reaction ☞異物感

いぶつかん 異物感 **foreign body sensation** ◆喉に異物感がありますか Do you feel something strange and uncomfortable in your throat?

いふん 遺糞 **bowel incontinence, fecal incontinence, encopresis**

いへき 胃壁 **stomach wall, gastric wall**

いへん 異変 （異状）**something[anything] unusual, something[anything] wrong**
◆何か異変に気づいたら，すぐに連絡して下さい If you notice anything unusual[wrong], please *contact us[let us know] right away. ◆急に彼の病状に異変が起きました（病状が急に悪化した）His condition *has taken a sudden turn for the worse[has suddenly changed for the worse].

いぼ 疣 **wart, verruca** ☞疣贅 ◆首にいぼがある have a wart on the neck ☞疣痔

いほう¹ 胃泡 **gastric air bubble**

いほう² 違法（の）**illegal, unlawful** ◆日本では大麻を吸うことは違法です In Japan, *it is illegal[it is illegal] to smoke marijuana. ▶違法行為 illegal[unlawful] act 違法薬物 illegal drug[substance]

いぼうまん 胃膨満 **gastric fullness**

いぼじ 疣痔 （内痔核）**internal hemorrhoids, blind piles[hemorrhoids]** ★いずれも複数形で.

いポリープ 胃ポリープ **stomach polyp, gastric polyp**

いま 今
《現在》**now** （現時点で）**at the moment, at present** ☞これから，これまで ◆今のうちに手術をしたほうがよいでしょう You should have the surgery now[(手遅れになる前に)before it's too late]. ◆今のところ順調です Everything is going well at the

moment. ◆今までのところ何も問題はありません Up to now[So far], there has been no problem. ◆今からでも遅くはありません It's still not too late. / It's not too late yet. ◆今まで通りやっていただいて結構です It's *all right[okay] to carry on as usual[normal].
《直ちに》**right away, immediately, straightaway** ☞この場 ◆今すぐ行きます I'm coming! / I'll be there right away. ◆あなたは今すぐに入院する必要があります You need to be admitted to the hospital *right away[immediately].

いまひとつ 今一つ ◆治療効果は今一つのようです I'm afraid that the treatment is not quite working well enough. ◆彼女は手術に今一つ気が進まないようです（乗り気でない）She seems reluctant to undergo the surgery.

いみ 意味 **meaning** （圈**mean**） （特定の意味）**sense** （目的・意味）**point**
《言葉などの意味・意図》◆それはどういう意味ですか What do you mean by that? ◆この語の意味は何ですか What does this word mean? / Please tell me the meaning of this word. ◆ある意味であなたの言うとおりです In a sense, you're right.
《行為などの意義・価値》◆さらに治療を続けても意味がないでしょう There isn't much point[sense] in continuing the treatment. / It would be meaningless[pointless / useless] to continue the treatment. ◆新薬は患者さんの QOL を高めたという点で意味がありました The new drug was meaningful in that it improved the patient's quality of life.

イミグレーション （移住・入国管理）**immigration**

いみん 移民 （移住してきた人）**immigrant** /íməɡrənt/ （国外からの移住）**immigration** ◀不法移民 illegal immigrant

イメージ **image** ◀身体イメージ body image

イメージング **imaging** ◀三次元イメージング three-dimensional imaging

いもうと 妹 （**younger, little**）**sister** ★英

語では通例 sister のみでよい.

いもたれ 胃もたれ ☞胃重感

いもん 慰問する （慰める）comfort, console （元気づける）cheer up ◆患者を慰問する comfort[cheer up] a patient

いや 嫌(な) （におい・味などがむかつくような）foul /fául/ （不快な）bad, offensive, unpleasant ◆嫌なにおいの分泌物が出る have foul-[bad-] smelling discharge

いやがらせ 嫌がらせ harassment ◀性的嫌がらせ sexual harassment

いやがる 嫌がる （好かない）don't like （ひどく嫌う）hate （気が進まない）be reluctant (to) （拒否する）refuse ☞嫌う ◆彼女は学校を嫌がっています She *doesn't like[hates] school. / She doesn't want to go to school. ◆お子さんは水分をとるのを嫌がりますか Is your child reluctant to drink[take] fluids? / Does your child refuse fluids?

いやく 医薬 medicine （形medical) ▶医薬情報担当者 medical representative；MR 医薬分業 separation of physician and pharmacist functions / separation of the functions of the clinic and the pharmacy ☞医薬品

いやくひん 医薬品 medication, drug, medicine, pharmaceuticals ★複数形で. ☞薬, 薬剤, 薬品, 薬物 ◆医薬品でアレルギー反応を起こしたことがありますか Have you ever had any allergic reaction to medication? ◀一般用医薬品(市販薬) over-the-counter[OTC] drug 後発医薬品 generic drug[medication] / generics 指定医薬品 designated medication[drug] 同種医薬品 generic equivalent ▶医薬品等安全情報 drug safety information 医薬品副作用 adverse drug reaction；ADR

いやす 癒す （悲しみなどを）heal （渇きを）quench （病気を）cure ◆時間と家族の支えが悲しみを癒してくれるでしょう I hope that time and your family's support will help heal your sorrow. ◆心の傷を癒す heal *one's* *mental wound[emotional trauma] ◆喉の渇きを癒す quench *one's* thirst

イヤホン earphones ★通例, 複数形で. ◆イヤホンをする use[wear] earphones ◆イヤホンを付けて〈取って〉下さい Please *put on〈take off〉your earphones. ◆イヤホンを付けて音楽を聴く listen to music with earphones

いようこうがく 医用工学 medical engineering；ME

いよく 意欲 （意志）will （やる気）motivation ◆生きる意欲を失う lose the will to live ◆働く意欲を失う lose the motivation to work

いよくせいせいペプチド 胃抑制性(ポリ)ペプチド gastric inhibitory (poly)peptide；GIP

いらい 依頼 request （動request, ask) ◆そのようなご依頼に応じることはできません I'm sorry I can't meet[comply with] such a request. ◆依頼を断る *turn down [refuse] *a person's* request ◆往診を依頼する request[ask for] a house call

—いらい —以来 since ◆来日以来, 何年になりますか How long has it been since you came to Japan? / How long have you lived[been living] in Japan? ◆彼は昨年 4 月に心臓発作を起こしましたが, それ以来発作はありません He had a heart attack last April, but he hasn't had one since.

いらいら （苛立ち）irritation （形irritated) （はやる気持ち）impatience （形impatient) （欲求不満）frustration （形frustrated) ◆いらいら感がある feel irritated / have a feeling of irritation ◆よくいらいらしますか Do you often get[become] irritated? ◆隣室の音が気になっていらいらしているのですね You feel[You're] irritated by the noise from the next room, *don't you [aren't you]? / The noise from the next room is irritating for you, isn't it? ◆彼女は回復の遅さにいらいらし始めています She is getting[becoming] impatient[frustrated] with the slow pace of her recovery.

イラク Iraq （形Iraqi) ☞国籍 ▶イラク人(の) Iraqi

イラン Iran (㊟Iranian) ☞国籍 ▶イラン人(の) Iranian

いりぐち 入口 entrance ◀外来入口 outpatients entrance / entrance for outpatients 救急入口 emergency entrance 正面入り口 main entrance 夜間入口 night[nighttime] entrance

いりょう 医療 medicine (㊟medical) (ケア・治療)medical care[treatment] (医療業務)medical service (医療行為・臨床)medical practice ◆根拠に基づく医療 evidence-based medicine；EBM ◆生命倫理に基づく医療 ethics-based medicine ◀遠隔医療 telemedicine 緩和医療 palliative medicine 救急医療 emergency medical service；EMS / emergency medicine 公的医療保険 public health insurance 公費負担医療 publicly funded medical services 高齢者医療 medical care for elderly[older] people / medical elderly care 再生医療 regenerative[regeneration] medicine 在宅医療 home-based medical care / medical home care / medical services at *a person's* home 周産期医療 perinatal medical care 終末期医療 terminal (medical) care 先端医療 advanced medicine [medical care] / high-tech medicine 代替医療(代わりの) alternative medicine / (補足的な)complementary medicine 地域医療 community medicine[medical care] チーム医療 team *medical care [health care] テーラーメイド医療 tailor-made medicine 僻地医療 medical care in *remote areas[less populated areas] 包括医療 comprehensive medical care 保健医療サービス health care service 保健医療施設 health care facility ▶医療英語 medical English 医療過誤 medical malpractice[error / mistake] 医療過誤開示 medical malpractice[error / mistake] disclosure 医療活動 medical activity 医療観光 medical tourism 医療機器[器具] medical instrument [equipment] 医療技術 medical (care) technology 医療給付 medical (care)

benefits 医療記録 medical record 医療行為(業務)medical practice / (介入)medical intervention 医療サービス medical service 医療支援 medical support[assistance] 医療事故 medical accident 医療施設 medical facility[institution] 医療事務職員 medical clerk 医療スタッフ the medical staff / (個々のメンバー)member of the medical staff 医療センター medical [health] center 医療相談 medical counseling[consultation] 医療ソーシャルワーカー medical social worker；MSW 医療訴訟 medical (malpractice) lawsuit 医療チーム health-care[medical] team 医療通訳(通訳者)medical interpreter / (通訳・解釈)medical interpretation 医療廃棄物 medical waste / biomedical waste；BMW 医療ビザ medical visa / visa for medical treatment 医療品(機器)medical equipment / (製品)medical product / (必需品)medical supplies 医療福祉相談室 medical social work office[unit] / medical social services office[unit] 医療保険 health insurance 医療保障 medical security 医療補助者 paramedic / (総称的に)the paramedical staff 医療用ホッチキス medical[surgical] stapler 医療倫理 medical ethics ☞医療機関, 医療費

いりょうきかん 医療機関 medical institute[institution] (病院)hospital (診療所)clinic ◆この問題について他の医療機関で精密検査を受けたことがありますか Have you ever had a thorough examination for this problem at another clinic or hospital? ◀指定医療機関 designated medical institute[institution]

いりょうひ 医療費 (診療の)medical expenses[fees] (病院の)hospital fees ★いずれも通例, 複数形で. ◆医療費は3割負担となります You'll have to pay thirty percent of your medical expenses. ◆医療費は自己負担となります You'll have to pay *all your medical expenses[the full cost of your medical care]. / Your medical expenses are not covered by any health insurance. ◆医療費は総額5,000

円になります Your medical expenses *come to[will be] five thousand yen in total[all]. ◆医療費の控除を受ける receive a deduction for high medical expenses ◀高額医療費 high-cost medical-care expenses 難病医療費助成(制度) financial assistance for intractable diseases ▶医療費控除 tax deduction for high medical expenses

いれい 異例(の) **exceptional** ◆手術後異例の速さで回復する recover exceptionally fast from the surgery / make an exceptionally quick recovery from the surgery

イレウス ileus /íliəs/; *decreased motor activity of the digestive tract due to mechanical or nonmechanical causes* ◀絞扼性イレウス strangulation ileus 術後イレウス postoperative ileus 胆石イレウス gallstone ileus 麻痺性イレウス paralytic [adynamic] ileus 癒着性イレウス adhesive intestinal obstruction

いれずみ 入れ墨 **tattoo** ☞刺青

いれば 入れ歯 (一揃いの義歯)**dentures** ★複数形で. (個々の)**false tooth**, **artificial tooth** (圏**teeth**) ◆入れ歯をしていますか Do you wear dentures? ◆入れ歯の具合はいかがですか How are your dentures? ◆入れ歯が合わなくなったと感じますか Do you feel that your dentures don't fit you any more? ◆手術の前に入れ歯をはずしていただきます You need to remove[take out] your dentures before the surgery. ◆入れ歯をはめる put in *one's* dentures ◆入れ歯がぐらぐらする have loose dentures / *one's* dentures become loose ◀総入れ歯 complete dentures 部分入れ歯 partial dentures

いれる 入れる (中に設置する)**put … in [into]**, **place … in[into]** (挿入する)**insert** (入れておく)**keep … in** ◆これから腕に点滴を入れます Now, I'm going to put an IV in your arm. ◆栄養チューブを胃に入れる insert[put] a feeding tube into the stomach ◆ペースメーカを体内に入れる place[insert] a pacemaker inside *a per-*

son's body ◆坐薬をゆっくり直腸に入れて下さい Gently insert the suppository into your rectum[rectal opening]. ★anus (肛門)という語は患者に不快な思いを抱かせることがあるので避けたい. ◆この錠剤を溶けるまで舌の下に入れておいて下さい Keep this tablet under your tongue until it melts[dissolves] completely.

いろ 色 **color** ◆便はどんな色をしていますか What color are your stools? / What's the color of your stools? ◆色の区別がつきにくいですか Do you have difficulty distinguishing between colors? ◆分泌物の色は黄色味を帯びています The discharge is yellowish.

いろいろ (異なった)**different** (あらゆる種類の)**all kinds[sorts] of** (種々の)**various, a variety of** ☞様々, 種々 ◆毎日いろいろな果物と野菜を食べて下さい Please eat different[various] kinds of fruits and vegetables every day. ◆彼女に治療を受けてもらうためにいろいろと説得してみましたが駄目でした We tried all kinds of ways to persuade her to have the treatment, but she wouldn't listen to us. ◆奥さんが入院なさっていろいろと大変でしょう Now that your wife is in the hospital[With your wife in the hospital], things must be tough (for you).

いろう 胃瘻 **gastric fistula, gastrocutaneous fistula** ◆食べ物を通すために胃瘻チューブを挿入する insert a *gastrostomy tube[gastric feeding tube / G-tube] through which food can be supplied to the stomach ◀経皮経内視鏡的胃瘻造設術 percutaneous endoscopic gastrostomy ; PEG

いろん 異論 **different opinion** ◆この薬の効果については専門家の間でも異論のあるところです Different specialists have different opinions about the effects of this medication. / Specialists are divided in their opinions about the effects of this medication.

いわかん 違和感 ◆耳に違和感を覚える feel something strange in the ear(s) / feel like something is wrong with the ear(s) ◆胸が痛んだり違和感を覚えたら言って下さい Let me know if you have any chest pain or discomfort. ◆補聴器は少し違和感があるかもしれませんが，徐々に慣れるでしょう Your hearing aid may feel slightly strange and uncomfortable, but you'll gradually get used to it.

いんえい 陰影 shadow ☞影 ◀異常陰影 abnormal shadow 腫瘍陰影 tumor shadow 心陰影 heart[cardiac] shadow すりガラス陰影 ground-glass opacity 蝶形陰影 butterfly shadow 肺門陰影 hilar shadow

いんがい 院外（に・で） outside（the hospital）（圏外部の outside 病院外の out-of-hospital） ◆院外には何軒も薬局があり，どこでも調剤してもらうことができます There are several pharmacies outside the hospital, so you can have your prescription filled at any one of those. ◆院外心停止患者 a patient who has[had] an out-of-hospital cardiac arrest ▶院外処方箋 prescription to be filled at an outside pharmacy 院外薬局 outside pharmacy

いんがかんけい 因果関係 cause-and-effect relationship, causal relationship, relationship between cause and effect

いんかく 陰核 clitoris

いんかんさいぼう 印環細胞 signet ring cell ▶印環細胞癌 signet ring cell carcinoma

いんけい 陰茎 penis /pí:nɪs/（圏penile /pí:naɪl/） ☞ペニス ◆陰茎からの分泌物 drip from the penis ◀短小陰茎 small penis ▶陰茎海綿体 corpus cavernosum penis 陰茎部尿道上裂〈下裂〉 penile epispadias〈hypospadias〉 陰茎プロステーシス[人工陰茎] penile prosthesis

いんこう 咽喉 throat ☞喉 ◀耳鼻咽喉科学 otorhinolaryngology / otolaryngology 耳鼻咽喉科医 otorhinolaryngologist / ENT specialist ▶咽喉痛 sore throat 咽喉炎 pharyngolaryngitis

いんごのうよう 咽後膿瘍 retropharyngeal abscess

いんし 因子 factor ◀遺伝子因子 genetic factor インスリン様成長因子 insulin-like growth factor；IGF 顆粒球コロニー刺激因子 granulocyte colony-stimulating factor；G-CSF 顆粒球マクロファージコロニー刺激因子 granulocyte macrophage colony-stimulating factor；GM-CSF 冠疾患危険因子 coronary risk factor 緩和因子 palliating factor 危険因子 risk factor 凝固因子 coagulation[clotting] factor 共通因子 common factor 血管内皮成長因子 vascular endothelial growth factor；VEGF 決定因子 determinant 原因因子 causative factor 腫瘍壊死因子 tumor necrosis factor；TNF 上皮成長因子 epidermal growth factor；EGF 成長因子 growth factor 増悪因子 aggravating[provoking] factor 促進因子 promoting[precipitating] factor 耐性因子 resistance factor 内因子 intrinsic factor；IF 背景因子 background factor 発がん因子 carcinogenic[cancer-causing] factor 分化誘導因子 differentiation-inducing factor 放出因子 releasing factor 抑制因子 suppressor factor / repressor / inhibitor 予後因子 prognostic factor リウマチ因子 rheumatoid factor；RF

インシデントほうこく ―報告 incident report

いんしゅ 飲酒 drinking（alcohol）（動drink（alcohol）） ☞アルコール，酒 ◆飲酒量はどのくらいですか How much do you drink? ◆頭痛は飲酒で悪化しますか Does drinking alcohol make your headache worse? ◆病院内での飲酒は禁止されております You are not permitted to drink alcohol anywhere inside the hospital. ◆飲酒運転〈飲酒行為〉で逮捕される be arrested for drunk driving〈behavior〉 ▶飲酒運転 drinking and driving / driving under the influence（of alcohol）；DUI /（酔っ払い運転）drunk driving 飲酒問題 drinking problem

いんしょう 印象 impression ◆東京の第一印象はいかがでしたか What were your first impressions of Tokyo? ★通例，

複数形で. ◆日本の印象はいかがですか How do you like Japan? ◆よい〈悪い〉印象を与える make a good〈bad〉impression (on)

いんしょく　飲食 eating and[or] drinking ★語順が日本語と違うので注意. ◆検査後1時間は飲食しないで下さい After the test, please don't eat or drink anything for an hour. ◆飲食物 food and drink

いんしん　陰唇 labium (圏labia 圏labial) ◀小陰唇 labium minus　大陰唇 labium majus ▶陰唇癒合 labial fusion

インスリノーマ insulinoma

インスリン insulin /ínsələn/ ◆この病気はインスリン不足が原因です This disease is caused by insufficient insulin production. ◆このタイプのインスリンはおよそ8時間持続します This type of insulin will last about eight hours. ◆毎日インスリンの自己注射をする必要があります You need to *give yourself an insulin injection [self-inject insulin] every day. ◀強化インスリン療法 intensive insulin therapy　混合型インスリン mixed insulin　持効型インスリン long-acting insulin　速効型インスリン short-acting insulin　中間型インスリン intermediate-acting insulin　超速効型インスリン(ultra) rapid-acting insulin ▶インスリン過剰投与 insulin overdose　インスリン抗体 insulin antibody　インスリン自己注射 insulin self-injection　インスリンショック insulin shock　インスリン抵抗性 insulin resistance　インスリンポンプ insulin pump　インスリン様成長因子 insulin-like growth factor；IGF　インスリン療法 insulin therapy[treatment]

いんせい　陰性(の) negative (↔positive) ◆検査の結果は陰性でした The result of the test was negative. ◆あなたの血液型はA型で，Rhは陰性です You have type A Rh-negative[Rhesus-negative] blood. ◆Rh陰性の女性 an Rh-negative[Rhesus-negative] woman ◀偽陰性反応 false-negative reaction ▶陰性症状 negative symptom　陰性T波 negative T wave　陰性反応 negative re-

action

インターネット Internet, internet /íntə-nèt/ ☞ネット ◆パソコンでインターネットにアクセスする use a computer to access the internet ◆この病室にはインターネット接続の設備があります This room is equipped with internet access. / This room has internet access[facilities].

インターフェロン interferon
インターベンション intervention
インターロイキン interleukin；IL
インターン intern
いんたいしょうこうぐん　引退症候群 retirement syndrome
インチ inch；in ☞巻末付録：単位の換算
いんちょう　院長 president, director, hospital administrator ◀副院長 vice president
インデックス index ◀ボディマスインデックス body mass index；BMI
インド India (圏Indian) ☞国籍 ▶インド人(の) Indian
いんとう　咽頭 pharynx /fǽrɪŋks/ (圏pharyngéal) ☞喉(のど) ◀下咽頭 hypopharynx　耳管咽頭口 pharyngeal opening of the auditory tube　上咽頭 epipharynx　中咽頭 oropharynx　鼻咽頭エアウェイ nasopharyngeal airway　ワルダイエル咽頭輪 Waldeyer tonsillar ring / pharyngeal lymphoid ring ▶咽頭炎 pharyngitis　咽頭円蓋 pharyngeal fornix　咽頭がん pharyngeal cancer　咽頭結膜熱 pharyngoconjunctival fever　咽頭痛 sore throat / pharyngodynia　咽頭反射 pharyngeal reflex　咽頭扁桃炎 pharyngotonsillitis　咽頭扁桃切除術 adenoidectomy / adenotomy　咽頭扁桃肥大 enlarged adenoid
インドシアニングリーン indocyanine green；ICG ▶インドシアニングリーン蛍光造影 indocyanine green angiography
インドネシア Indonesia (圏Indonesian) ☞国籍 ▶インドネシア人(の) Indonesian
いんない　院内(に・で) in[inside, within] the hospital (圏(入院中にかかった)hospital-acquired, nosocomial) ◆院内では携

帯電話は指定の場所でご使用下さい Please use mobile phones in the designated area inside the hospital. ▶院内学級 hospital class　院内感染 hospital-acquired[nosocomial] infection　院内感染対策(管理・抑制) control of hospital-acquired[nosocomial] infection／(予防措置) preventive[precautionary] measures against hospital-acquired[nosocomial] infection　院内肺炎 hospital-acquired[nosocomial] pneumonia　院内薬局 hospital pharmacy

いんのう　陰嚢　scrotum (形scrotal)
◆陰嚢やペニスに何か変化がありますか Have you noticed any changes in your scrotum or penis?　◆陰嚢に痛みや腫れがありますか Do you have any pain or swelling in your scrotum?　◆陰嚢がかゆいのですか Is your scrotum itchy?　▶陰嚢腫脹 scrotal swelling／swelling of the scrotum　陰嚢水腫[陰嚢水瘤] scrotal hydrocele　陰嚢部尿道下裂 scrotal hypospadias　陰嚢ヘルニア scrotal hernia

インヒビター　inhibitor

いんぶ　陰部　genital region (陰部・大腿の) genitocrural region　(鼠径部) groin　(婉曲的に) private parts[areas]　★通例，複数形で．◆陰部はご自分で拭きますか Would you like to clean your private areas by yourself?　◀外陰(部)潰瘍 ulceration of the vulva　▶陰部湿疹 genital eczema　陰部剃毛 pubic hair shaving　陰部白癬 ringworm of the groin／tinea cruris／(インフォーマルに) jock itch　陰部[性器]ヘルペス genital herpes　陰部疣贅 genital[venereal] wart／(尖形コンジローマ) condyloma acuminatum

インフォームドコンセント　informed consent ☞同意，同意書　◆患者と家族からインフォームドコンセントを得る get[obtain] informed consent from the patient and his〈her〉family　◆HIV 検査のインフォームドコンセント informed consent for HIV testing

インフォメーション (情報) **information** (案内所) **information counter[desk]** ☞情報

インプラント　implant /ímplænt/ (動implánt) (歯の) **dental implant** ◆人工歯根をインプラントする implant an artificial tooth root

インフルエンザ　flu, influenza (軽いインフルエンザの口語表現) **flu bug** ◆今シーズン，インフルエンザの予防接種を受けましたか Have you had a flu shot this season?　◆職場でインフルエンザに罹る get[catch] (the) flu at *one's* workplace　◆インフルエンザ症状がある have flu symptoms　◆今インフルエンザが流行っています The flu is going around now.／There's a flu bug going around now.　◆インフルエンザの蔓延 a flu epidemic／(世界的流行) a flu pandemic　◀A 型〈B 型〉インフルエンザ human influenza type A〈B〉　季節性インフルエンザ seasonal influenza　新型インフルエンザ new strain[type] of influenza　鳥インフルエンザ bird flu／avian flu[influenza]　ブタインフルエンザ pig[hog] flu／swine flu[influenza]　▶インフルエンザ脳炎 influenza encephalitis　インフルエンザワクチン flu[influenza] vaccine

インフルエンザきん　―菌　*Haemophilus influenzae* ▶インフルエンザ菌 b 型[ヒブ]ワクチン *Haemophilus influenzae* type b vaccine／Hib vaccine

インポテンス　impotence (形impotent)

いんもう　陰毛　pubic hair ◆陰毛が薄くなりましたか Have you noticed any thinning of your pubic hair?

いんもん　陰門 (女性外陰) **vulva**

いんりょう　飲料　drink, beverage ◀スポーツ飲料 sports drink　清涼飲料水 soft drink　▶飲料水 drinking water

う

ういざん 初産 〈出産〉**first childbirth** 〈分娩〉**first delivery**

ウイスキー **whiskey**, 〈英〉**whisky**

ウィリスどうみゃくりん ―動脈輪 **Willis**〈**arterial**〉**circle, circle of Willis**

ウイルス **virus** /vάɪrəs/ 〈形 **viral**〉 ◆お子さんはインフルエンザウイルスに感染しています Your child has caught a *flu virus [viral flu infection]. / Your child has come down with a flu virus. ◆抗菌薬は感冒ウイルスには効果がありません Antibiotics have no effect against cold viruses. ◆B型肝炎ウイルスに免疫がある have immunity against hepatitis B virus / have hepatitis B virus immunity

◀RSウイルス respiratory syncytial virus；RSV EBウイルス Epstein-Barr virus；EBV エイズウイルス AIDS virus がんウイルス oncovirus / oncogenic virus 抗ウイルス薬 antiviral〈medication / drug / agent〉 弱毒化ウイルス attenuated virus 水痘帯状疱疹ウイルス chickenpox virus / herpes zoster virus / varicella zoster virus；VZV 脳炎ウイルス encephalitis virus ノロウイルス norovirus B〈C〉型肝炎ウイルス hepatitis B〈C〉virus B〈C〉型肝炎ウイルスキャリア hepatitis B〈C〉virus carrier ヒトTリンパ球向性ウイルス1型 human T-lymphotropic virus type 1；HTLV-1 ヒトパピローマウイルス human papillomavirus；HPV ヒトパルボウイルスB19感染症 human parvovirus B19 infection ヒトヘルペスウイルス human herpesvirus；HHV ヒト免疫不全ウイルス human immunodeficiency virus；HIV 病原性ウイルス pathogenic virus 風疹ウイルス rubella virus 変異ウイルス mutant virus ポリオウイルス poliovirus 麻疹ウイルス measles virus ムンプスウイルス mumps virus ▶ウイルス感染 viral[virus] infec-

tion ウイルス性胃腸炎 viral gastroenteritis ウイルス性疣贅 viral wart ウイルス性肝炎 viral hepatitis ウイルス性結膜炎 viral conjunctivitis ウイルス性出血熱 viral hemorrhagic fever ウイルス性心筋炎 viral myocarditis ウイルス性髄膜炎 viral meningitis ウイルス性脳炎 viral encephalitis ウイルス性肺炎 viral pneumonia

ウィルソンびょう ―病 **Wilson disease**

ウィルムスしゅよう ―腫瘍 **Wilms tumor**

ウール **wool** /wúl/ ◆ウールや化繊の肌着は避けたほうがよいでしょう You should avoid wearing underwear made from wool or synthetic fibers.

うえ 上：

《位置》〈表面に直接接触して〉**on** 〈直接接触しないで上に〉**above, over**〈↔below, under〉〈上方へ〉**up**〈↔down〉**, upward(s)**〈↔downward(s)〉 ◆あごをこの台の上に載せて下さい Please put your chin on this support. ◆診察台の上に仰向けに寝て下さい Please lie down on your back on the exam table. ◆手を頭の上にあげて下さい Please raise your hands above your head. ◆あなたの血圧は上が150で，下が95です Your blood pressure is one[a] hundred〈and〉fifty over ninety-five. ◆上を見て下さい Please look up[upward]. ◆ずうっと上まで見る look all the way up

《…した後で》**after** 〈いったん…してから〉**once** ◆心臓の専門医と相談の上で治療方針についてお話しします I'll talk with you about the course of treatment after I've consulted with a heart specialist. ◆それぞれの治療法のメリット・デメリットを十分に考慮した上でご判断下さい〈判断する前に考える〉Please carefully consider the advantages and disadvantages of each treatment option before you decide. ◆患者がリスクを納得した上で手術を行う perform surgery once the patient understands the risks involved

《…限りでは》**as far as … concerned** 〈…に関して〉**in terms of** ◆日常生活の上では特に

ご心配になることはありません As far as your everyday life is concerned, you don't have to worry about anything. / There's nothing to worry about in terms of your everyday life.

ウェゲナーにくげしゅしょう ―肉芽腫症 Wegener granulomatosis, （多発血管炎性肉芽腫症）granulomatous with polyangitis；GPA

うえこみがた 植え込み型（の） implantable ▶植え込み型除細動器 implantable (cardioverter) defibrillator；ICD 植え込み型ペースメーカ implantable pacemaker 植え込み型補聴器 implantable hearing aid

うえこむ 植え込む implant ☞埋め込む

うえじに 飢え死に ☞餓死

ウェステルマンはいきゅうちゅう ―肺吸虫 *Paragonimus westermani*

ウエスト waist /wéɪst/ ☞腹囲 ▶ウエストサイズ waist size ウエスト周囲径 waist circumference ウエスト測定 waist measurement

ウェストしょうこうぐん ―症候群 West syndrome

ウェットティッシュ wet wipe, （moist) towelette ☞ティッシュペーパー

うえむき 上向き（に） ☞仰向け

うえる 飢える （空腹に苦しむ・餓死する）be [go] hungry, starve （渇望する）be hungry for, crave ◆飢えた子ども a hungry [starving] child ◆その男の子は母親の愛情に飢えています That boy *is hungry for [craves] his mother's love.

ウェルシュきん ―菌 *Clostridium perfringens* ★旧称 *Clostridium welchii* ▶ウェルシュ菌食中毒 *Clostridium perfringens* food poisoning

ウェルドニッヒ・ホフマンびょう ―病 Werdnig-Hoffmann disease

ウェルニッケしつご ―失語 Wernicke aphasia

ウェルニッケちゅうすう ―中枢 Wernicke center, the sensory speech center

ウェルニッケのうしょう ―脳症 Wernicke encephalopathy

ウェルネス （健康）wellness ▶ウェルネス

センター wellness center

ウォーキング walking （for exercise) ☞散歩 ◆体重を減らすためにウォーキングをお勧めします I recommend walking as a good way to lose weight.

うおのめ 魚の目 （鶏眼）corn, clavus

ウォルフ・パーキンソン・ホワイトしょうこうぐん ―症候群 Wolff-Parkinson-White syndrome

うがい gargling （🔊gargle, rinse out *one's* mouth) ◆外出先から帰ったら必ずうがいをして下さい Please be sure to gargle after returning home. ◆ぬるま湯でうがいする gargle with lukewarm water ▶うがい薬 gargle / （口内洗浄の）mouthwash / （咽頭洗浄の）throat wash

うかがう

《質問する》ask ◆それでは，毎日の生活習慣についておうかがいします Now I'd like to ask you some questions about your daily routine. ◆うかがいたいことがあるのですが May I ask you some questions? 《行く》go[come] and see ◆用が済み次第おうかがいします I'll come and see you as soon as I finish my work. ◆今すぐうかがいます I'm coming right away.

うかぶ 浮かぶ

《空中・水面に》float ◆視野の中に黒い点がたくさん浮かんでいるのですか Do you see many black specks floating around in your field of vision?

《心に》 （心に浮かぶ）come to （*one's*) mind （頭をよぎる）occur ☞思い浮かぶ ◆この絵を見て心に浮かんだことを話して下さい Please tell me what comes to （your) mind when you look at this picture.

うきゃくブロック 右脚ブロック right bundle branch block；RBBB ◀完全右脚ブロック complete right bundle branch block；CRBBB 不完全右脚ブロック incomplete right bundle branch block；ICRBBB

うきょうしん 右胸心 dextrocardia

ウクライナ Ukraine （📐Ukrainian) ☞国籍 ▶ウクライナ人（の）Ukrainian

うけいれる 受け入れる accept （入院さ

せる)**admit** ◆重症患者を受け入れる ac-cept[admit] seriously ill patients ◆がんという事実を受け入れる accept the fact that *one* has cancer ◆死を受け入れる accept death

うけぐち　受け口 （反対咬合）**underbite**

うけこたえ　受け答えする　answer, reply, respond ◆彼女は受け答えに時間がかかります It takes time for her to answer [reply / respond]. ◆その子はしっかりした受け答えをします(返答が納得できる)That child answers convincingly. / (返答が信頼できる)That child gives a reliable answer.

うけつぐ　受け継ぐ （遺伝・相続する）**inher-it** （地位などを引き継ぐ）**take over, suc-ceed** ◆遺伝子を受け継ぐ inherit a gene ◆父の事業を引き継ぐ *take over [succeed to / inherit] *one's* father's busi-ness

うけつけ　受付 （受け付けること）**reception** （受付所）**reception counter[desk]** ◆お帰りになる前に受付で再診の予約をして下さい Please make a follow-up[revisit] ap-pointment at the reception counter [desk] before you go home. ◆当院では外来患者の受付は8時に始まります Out-patient reception at this hospital starts at eight in the morning. ◀外来受付 outpa-tient reception counter[desk]　再診受付 revisit counter[desk]　新患受付 new pa-tient registration counter[desk]　総合受付 general reception counter　入院受付 admissions counter[desk]　▶受付係 re-ceptionist　受付番号 check-in number　受付票 outpatient check-in slip / num-bered slip (given to patients in order of their arrival in the outpatient clinic)

うけつける　受け付ける （扱いを引き受ける）**receive, accept** （提供された物を受け取る）**take** （聞き入れる）**listen** (to) ◆外来患者は8時から受け付けます We start re-ceiving[accepting] outpatients at eight in the morning. ◆新患を受け付ける accept new patients ◆彼女は流動食も受け付けません She can't take even liquid food. / Her stomach rejects even liquid food.

◆彼は他の人達の言うことを受け付けません He won't listen to others.

うけとる　受け取る

《手に取る》**get, receive, accept** ◆先週あなたのかかりつけ医からの紹介状を受け取りました I received[got] your family doc-tor's referral letter last week. ◆患者さまやご家族の方からの贈り物は一切受け取ることができません(I'm sorry but) We are unable to accept gifts of any kind from a patient or patient's family.

《解釈する》**take** ◆彼女は私の言葉をどう受け取ったでしょうか How did she take what I said?

うけもち　受け持ち(の)　attending ☞受け持つ, 担当 ◆今日から受け持ちになった医師の佐藤です I'm Dr Sato and I'll be your doctor starting from today. ◆私の受け持ち患者 a patient assigned to me / a patient under my care ◆受け持ちのベッドを回る make the rounds of *one's* (as-signed) beds ▶受け持ち看護師 attend-ing nurse

うけもつ　受け持つ　take charge (of) （担当している）**be in charge** (of) ☞受け持ち, 担当 ◆今3人の患者を受け持っています I'm in charge of three patients now.

うける　受ける

《得る》**receive, get** ◆生活保護を受ける receive *public assistance[welfare]

《医療を施される》**have, undergo** ◆最近, 大きな手術を受けましたか Have you re-cently had any major surgery? ◆胆嚢の手術を受ける必要があります You need to have[undergo] surgery on your gallblad-der. ◆できるだけ早く胸の精密検査を受けて下さい Please have a thorough chest examination as soon as possible.

《苦痛や損害を被る》**suffer, have** ◆家庭内暴力による心の傷を受ける suffer the emo-tional trauma of domestic violence ◆ご家族の死別や離婚といった精神的ショックを受けたことがありますか Have you ever suffered an emotional shock such as a death in the family or divorce? ◆脳に損傷を受ける have some brain damage

◆彼女は母親が死んだと聞いてショックを受けています She is shocked at hearing *of her mother's death[that her mother passed away].

《経験する》experience ◆これまでに受けたことのない激しい痛みですか Is it an extreme pain such as you've never experienced before? ◆最近，いつもより多くストレスを受けていますか Have you been under more stress recently?

うこうとっき　烏口突起　coracoid process

うごかす　動かす　move ☞動く ◆頭を動かさないで Please don't move your head. / Please keep your head still. ◆体のどこかが動かしにくいですか Do you have difficulty moving any part of your body? ◆仕事中どのくらい体を動かしますか(肉体労働が必要か)How much physical labor does your work involve? ◆できるだけ体を動かすように心掛けて下さい Please try to move your body as much as possible. ◆もっと体を動かすとよいでしょう(運動する)You should try to get more exercise.

うごき　動き　movement ☞動作 ◆彼女は体の動きが遅い She moves slowly. / Her movement is slow. ◆身体の動き a body movement ◆筋肉の動き muscular movements ◆筋肉の細かい動き muscle twitching / fine muscle movements ◆目の動きを診る examine the eye movements ◆ぎこちない[ぎくしゃくした]動きをする(不器用な動きをする)move awkwardly[clumsily], have[make] awkward[clumsy] movements / (けいれん性の動きをする)move in a jerky manner, have[make] jerky movements / (協調がとれない動きをする)move in an uncoordinated fashion, have[make] uncoordinated movements

うごく　動く　move ☞動かす ◆楽にして動かないで下さい Please relax and don't move. ◆台がゆっくり動いていきます The table will move slowly. ◆息を止めて，動かないで(少しそのままで)Hold your breath and remain still for just a second. ◆痛みは他の場所に動きますか Does the pain move[(拡がる)spread] to another place? ◆手足が勝手に動きますか Do your hands, arms, or legs move involuntarily[by themselves / without your conscious control]? ◆急に動く move abruptly ◆動くと痛む be painful to move

うし　齲歯 ☞齲蝕，虫歯

ウシかいめんじょうのうしょう　─海綿状脳症　(狂牛病) bovine spongiform encephalopathy；BSE

うしつ　右室　right ventricle；RV (形right ventricular) ▶右室肥大 right ventricular hypertrophy

うしなう　失う　lose ◆買い物や家事など，ふだんやっていることに興味を失いましたか Have you lost interest in your usual activities, such as shopping or housework? ◆食欲を失う lose *one's* appetite ◆視力〈聴力〉を失う lose *one's* eyesight〈hearing〉 ◆記憶を失う lose *one's* memory ◆生きる意欲を失う lose the will to live ◆希望を失う lose hope ◆バランスを失う lose *one's* balance

うしょく　齲蝕　tooth decay, (dental) caries ☞虫歯 ◆歯根齲蝕 root caries　第1〈2〉度齲蝕 first-degree〈second-degree〉caries

うしろ　後ろ　the back (↔the front 形backward(s) (↔forward)) ◆痛むのは首の後ろですか Do you have the pain in the back of your neck? ◆この検査着は後ろを開けて着て下さい Please put on this gown with the opening in the back. ◆後ろを向いて下さい Please turn around. ◆体を後ろに曲げて下さい Bend backward, please. ◆後ろへさがって下さい Step back[backward], please. ◆首を後ろに傾ける lean *one's* head backward

うしん　右心　right heart, right-sided heart ▶右心バイパス right heart bypass　右心負荷 right heart overload　右心不全 right[right-sided] heart failure / right ventricular failure

うしんしつ 右心室 ☞右室

うしんぼう 右心房 right atrium；RA

うすい 薄い
《量・程度が少ない》light, little （↔heavy 圖 lightly, little） ◆塩分の薄いものを食べる eat lightly salted foods / eat foods with little salt ◆赤ちゃんを薄着にしてあげて下さい Please dress your baby lightly.
《濃さ・厚さが薄い》thin （↔thick）《飲み物が薄い》weak （↔strong）《色が淡い》light （↔dark）（希釈した）dilute （↔concentrated） ◆陰毛や腋毛が薄くなりましたか Have you noticed any thinning of your pubic or underarm hair? / Has your pubic hair or underarm hair become thin? ◆軟膏を薄く塗る apply a thin layer of the ointment ◆鼻水は薄くてさらさらしている The nasal discharge is thin. ◆薄いコーヒー weak coffee ◆薄茶色 light brown ◆薄い尿 dilute urine

うずく 疼く （傷口などがずきずき痛む）throb （継続的に鈍く痛む）ache ◆歯が疼きますか Is it a throbbing toothache?

ウズベキスタン Uzbekistan （圀Uzbek） ☞国籍 ▶ウズベキスタン人（の）Uzbek

うすめる 薄める （希釈する）dilute （液体などで薄める）thin （加える）add ... (to) ◆1目盛り分を約60mLの水で薄めて下さい Please dilute one unit of this solution in about sixty milliliters of water. ◆スープをお湯で薄める thin the soup with hot water / add hot water to the soup

うせつ 右折する turn right, make a right turn ◆バス停はコンビニの角を右折してすぐにあります Turn right[Make a right turn] at the corner where the convenience store is, and you'll find the bus stop right there.

うそ 嘘 lie ◆嘘をつく tell a lie / do not tell the truth ◆息子さんが嘘をつくのはあなたの注意を引きたいからかもしれません Your son is probably telling lies because he wants to get your attention. ☞偽り

うたがい 疑い （悪い可能性への疑惑）suspicion （圀suspect）（疑問）doubt （圀doubt） ◆胃潰瘍の疑いがあります I sus-pect you have a stomach ulcer. / You seem to have a stomach ulcer. ◆糖尿病の疑いがあります It may be diabetes. / You may have diabetes. / I suspect it's diabetes. ◆花粉症の疑いがあります I think you probably have hay fever. ◆妊娠の疑いがありますか Do you feel that you may be pregnant? ◆感染を疑う suspect an infection ◆疑いなく手術はうまくいきます I have no doubts about the success of the surgery. / No doubt[I'm sure] the surgery will succeed. ◆彼は疑い深い性格です He has a distrustful personality.

うたがわしい 疑わしい （不審な）suspicious （不確かな）questionable, doubtful ◆疑わしい組織を取って調べます We'll remove and examine some of the suspicious tissues. ◆このような場合ではステロイドの効果は疑わしい The effectiveness of steroids in a case like this is questionable[doubtful]. / It is questionable[doubtful] if steroids can be effective in a case like this.

うたがわれる 疑われる （示唆する）suggest ◆乳がん細胞診は悪性が疑われる所見です The breast cancer cytology findings suggest a malignancy. ◆MRI検査の結果、肝臓がんが疑われます Judging by (the results of) the MRI, *it could be[it's possibly] liver cancer.

うち 内
《一定の時間・期間・範囲内に》in, within （間に）while （…より前に）before ◆2, 3日のうちによくなるでしょう You'll get better in a few days. ◆リハビリは入院しているうちに始めます We'll start rehabilitation while you're still in the hospital. ◆症状がひどくならないうちに来院して下さい Please come and see me before your symptoms get worse.
《内側・内部》inside ☞内側（うちがわ，ないそく）

うちあける 打ち明ける （率直に言う）tell frankly （秘密などを話す）confide ◆胸の内を打ち明けて下さりありがとうございました Thank you for *telling me frankly [confiding to me] what was on your mind.

うちがわ　内側　the inside, the inner side ［part］　☞内側(ないそく)　◆右肘の内側が痛みますか Do you have any pain on the inside[inner side] of your right elbow?

うちき　内気(な)　(恥ずかしがりな)shy (内向的な)introverted (↔extroverted)　◆彼女はおとなしくて内気な患者です She is a quiet, shy[introverted] patient.

うちきず　打ち傷　bruise /brúːz/, contusion　☞あざ, 打撲傷

うちきん　内金　(支払額の一部)down payment, part payment (保証金)deposit　◆内金として1万円必要となりますが, よろしいですか You need to make a *down payment[deposit] of ten thousand yen. Is that all right with you?

うちとける　打ち解ける　(友好的に話す)talk in a friendly manner (心を開いて率直に話す)talk openly　◆職場の仲間とは打ち解けて話ができますか Can you talk to your colleagues in a friendly manner? / Can you talk openly with your colleagues?

うちみ　打ち身　bruise /brúːz/, contusion　☞あざ, 打撲傷　◆階段から転げ落ちて右腕に打ち身をつくる get a bruise on one's right arm from falling down the stairs

うちもも　内腿　inner thigh, the inside of the thigh

うちゅうせん　宇宙線　cosmic ray

うちわ　内鰐　pigeon toes　★複数形で.　▶うちわ歩行 toe-in[pigeon toe] gait

うつ¹　鬱　(うつ状態)depression (☞depressed)　☞うつ病, 憂鬱, 抑うつ　◆うつになる get[become] depressed　◆深刻なうつに陥る fall into a deep[serious] depression　◆うつ状態はどのくらい続いていますか How long have you been feeling [felt] depressed? / How long have you had this depressed mood[state of mind]?　◀抗うつ薬 antidepressant (medication / drug / agent)

うつ²　打つ　《叩く・ぶつける》hit, strike　◆転んで後頭部を打つ fall down and hit[strike] the back of one's head　《注射をする》give　◆注射を打ちましょう Let me give you an injection.　《感動させる》(感銘を受ける)be impressed (by) (称賛する)admire　◆リハビリに懸命に取り組まれているお姿に心を打たれました I was really impressed by how hard you worked on your rehabilitation.　《策を講じる》try means　◆現時点で打てる手はすべて打ちました We have tried every means possible at this point.　◆残念ですが手の打ちようがありませんでした I'm sorry, but there was nothing that could be done for him〈her〉.

うっけつ　うっ血　(体液の滞留)congestion (☞congested, congestive) (体液流の停止)stagnation, stasis　◆心臓のポンプ機能が低下して肺がうっ血しています Your lungs are congested because the pumping action of the heart has slowed down.　◀肺うっ血 pulmonary[lung] congestion　▶うっ血肝 congestive liver　うっ血性心不全 congestive heart failure ; CHF　うっ血乳頭 choked disk / papillary stasis

うつし　写し　copy　◆検査結果の写しは必要ですか Do you need a copy of the test results? / Would you like me to make a copy of the test results for you?　◆パスポートの写しを1部ご用意下さい Please have a copy of your passport ready.

うつす　移す　☞移動, 移る　《動かす》move, transfer　◆手術後患者をICU に移す move the patient into the *intensive care unit[ICU] after the surgery　◆患者を車椅子からベッドに移す transfer[move] the patient from a wheelchair into a bed　《感染させる》give, infect　◆インフルエンザを他の人に移さないように注意して下さい Please be careful not to give the flu to others.

うったい　うっ滞　(液体の停留・保持)retention (体液流の停止)stagnation, stasis　◆足の腫れはリンパ液のうっ滞によるものかもしれません The swelling in your legs may be caused by lymph fluid retention. ◆水分のうっ滞 water retention ◀胆汁うっ滞 cholestasis ▶うっ滞性乳腺炎 stagnation mastitis

うったえ　訴え　〈症状など苦痛の〉complaint 〈訴訟〉suit, lawsuit

うったえる　訴える
《苦痛・不満を述べる》〈症状などの苦痛を〉complain（of）〈苦情を言う〉complain（about）◆めまいを訴える complain of dizziness ◆機器の騒音のことで苦情を訴える complain about the noise of the machine
《告訴する》sue, bring a lawsuit（against）◆医療過誤〈過失〉で医師を訴える sue[file a suit against / bring a lawsuit against] the doctor for malpractice〈negligence〉

うつびょう　うつ病　depression（㊟depressed），depressive disorder ☞鬱，抑うつ ◆うつ病を患う suffer from depression ◆うつ病になる get[become] depressed ◆これまでにうつ病と診断されたことがありますか Have you ever been diagnosed with depression? ◆うつ病で今はつらい状態でも必ずよくなります You're suffering from depression, but no matter how hopeless you feel, I'm sure you can get better. ◀外因性うつ病 exogenous depression　仮面うつ病 masked depression　産後うつ病 postpartum depression　初老期うつ病 presenile depression　躁うつ病[双極性障害] manic-depressive illness[psychosis] / bipolar depression　大うつ病性障害 major depressive disorder；MDD / major depression / unipolar[monopolar] depression　退行期うつ病 involutional depression　反応性うつ病 reactive depression　引っ越しうつ病（house）moving blues / moving anxiety　不安うつ病 anxiety depression　老年期うつ病 senile depression / depression in elderly[older] people ▶うつ病患者 depressive

うつぶせ　うつ伏せ（に）　on one's stomach[face]（↔on one's back）☞腹臥位 ◆うつ伏せになって下さい Please lie on

your stomach. ◆うつ伏せに倒れる fall flat on one's face ◆乳幼児突然死の危険性を減らすには，赤ちゃんをうつ伏せではなく，仰向けに寝かせて下さい To reduce the risk of crib death, put your baby to sleep on his〈her〉back, not face down. ▶うつ伏せ寝 prone sleeping position / lying [sleeping] on one's stomach

うっぷん　鬱憤　〈欲求不満〉(pent-up) frustration 〈怒り〉(pent-up) anger ◆泣いて鬱憤を晴らす *let go of[release / vent (out)] one's frustrations[anger] by crying

うつる　移る　☞移動，移す
《移動する》move 〈搬送される〉be transferred ◆今日から外科病棟に移っていただきます You'll move[be transferred] to the surgical floor today. ◆別の病院に移る be transferred to another hospital
《感染する》〈人が〉catch 〈病気が人に〉be transmitted 〈感染力がある〉be infectious, be contagious ★contagious は通例，接触感染に用いる．〈広まる〉be spread ◆インフルエンザは職場で移ったのですか Did you catch the flu at your workplace? ◆この病気は抱き合ったりキスしたりでは移りません This disease can't be transmitted by hugging or kissing. ◆この病気は移りません This disease is not infectious[contagious]. ◆水痘は咳やくしゃみで移ります Chickenpox is spread by coughing and sneezing.

うつろ　虚ろ（な）　〈ぽかんとした〉blank 〈放心した〉vacant ◆彼は目が虚ろです He has a blank[vacant] look in his eyes. ◆虚ろな表情をしている have a blank[vacant] expression / have a blank[vacant] look on one's face

うで　腕　arm　〈肩と肘の間の部分〉upper arm
《動作の基本表現》◆腕を上げる raise one's arm ◆腕を下ろす lower one's arm ◆腕組みをする fold one's arms ◆腕を伸ばす stretch (out) one's arm ◆腕を曲げる bend one's arm ◆腕を回す rotate one's arm

《診察の基本表現》 ◆腕が痛みますか Do you have any pain in your arm? / Does your arm hurt? ◆腕に力が入らない感じがありますか Do your arms feel weak? ◆腕の力を抜いて下さい Please relax your arm. ◆右腕を肩の高さまで上げると肩が痛みますか Does your shoulder hurt when you raise your right arm to shoulder level? ◆腕を前に出して下さい Please hold your arms out straight. ◆腕をまくって下さい（袖を）Please roll up your sleeves.

《受傷の表現》 ◆腕にけがをする injure *one's* arm ◆腕を折る break *one's* arm ◆腕をひねる twist *one's* arm ◆骨折した腕 *one's* broken arm ◀利き腕 *one's* dominant hand[arm] ▶腕吊り(包帯)(arm) sling

うとい　疎い ◆すみません，その辺りの地理に疎いもので Sorry. I'm not familiar with that area. / Sorry. I don't know much about that area.

うながす　促す （強く勧める・迫る）**urge**, **press** （促進・誘発・刺激する）**promote, stimulate, induce** （強くする）**strengthen** （身振りで示す）**motion** ◆薬をすぐ飲むよう促す urge *a person* to take his⟨her⟩ medication promptly ◆便通を促すためには繊維を多く含む食品を摂る必要があります To promote[stimulate] regular bowel movements, you need to eat foods that are high in fiber. ◆生きる意欲を促す strengthen the will to live ◆身ぶりで椅子に座るよう促す motion *a person* to *take a seat[sit down]

うなされる ◆悪夢にうなされる have a *bad dream[nightmare]

うなじ　nape of the neck, the back of the neck ☞首筋

うのう　右脳　the right brain, the right hemisphere (of the brain)

うのみ　鵜呑み ☞無条件

うばぐるま　乳母車　stroller, baby buggy, 《英》**pushchair**

うぶぎ　産着　clothes for a newborn baby ★複数形で.

うぶげ　産毛　downy hair

うぶごえ　産声　the first cry (of a newborn baby)

うぶゆ　産湯　baby's first bath ◆赤ん坊に産湯を使わせる give a baby his⟨her⟩ first bath

うぼう　右房　right atrium：RA

うまい

《巧みな》good （圖**well**） ☞上手 ◆字がうまい⟨へただ⟩ *one's* handwriting is good⟨poor⟩ / *a person* has good⟨poor⟩ handwriting ◆文字がうまく書けないのですか Do you have any difficulty with handwriting? ◆人前に出ると緊張してうまく話せなくなりますか Do you become nervous in front of people so that you can't speak well?

《首尾よく》 （順調に行く）**go well** （成功する）**be successful** ◆すべてうまくいっていますよ Everything is going well. ◆禁煙しようとしたことがありますか．うまくいきましたか Have you tried to quit smoking? Did it go well? ◆手術はうまくいきました The surgery was successful. / Everything went well with the surgery.

うまれ　生まれ

《生年月日》 ◆何年生まれですか When[In what year] were you born?

《出生地》 ◆生まれはどちらですか Where were you born? / What's your place of birth? ◆生まれ故郷 *one's* hometown [home country]

うまれつき　生まれつき(の) （生得の）**natural, innate** （病気・障害が先天的な）**congenital** （圖**by nature**　出生時に **at birth**） ◆彼女は生まれつき陽気で社交的です She is naturally cheerful and sociable. / She is cheerful and sociable by nature. ◆生まれつきの体質 *a natural[an innate] predisposition ◆生まれつき心臓に異常がありましたか Were you born with a heart problem? / Do you have a congenital heart defect? ◆そのしこりは生まれつきのものですか Was the lump present *at birth[when you were born]?

うまれる　生まれる　be born ◆どこで生

まれましたか Where were you born? ◆生まれたばかりの子供 a newborn baby

うみ 膿 pus /pʌ́s/, purulence （國pus-like） （分泌物）discharge ☞膿む, 化膿 ◆傷口から膿が出ています The wound is oozing[producing] pus. / You have pus coming from the wound. ◆痰に膿が混じっていますか Is there any pus in your phlegm? / Have you noticed any pus in your phlegm? ◆傷が膿をもっています The wound has formed pus. ◆傷口に膿がたまっています The wound is filled with pus. / Pus has accumulated in the wound. ◆膿瘍を切開して膿を出す cut the abscess open and drain[let out] the pus ◆膿のような痰 pus-like phlegm

うむ¹ 産む have, give birth (to) ◆お子さんを何人産みましたか How many babies have you had? ◆彼女は未熟児を産みました She had a premature delivery. / She gave birth prematurely.

うむ² 膿む form pus, fester ☞膿（うみ）, 化膿 ◆傷は膿んでいます The wound has *formed pus[festered].

うむ³ 有無 （…かどうかを）whether （or not） ◆悪性腫瘍の有無を調べる check and see whether (or not) there is any malignant tumor / （存在を）check for the presence of a malignant tumor ◆この薬は症状の有無にかかわらず服用を続けて下さい（症状がなくなっても）Please continue taking this medication even if your symptoms go away. ◆配偶者の有無 marital status / whether *a person* is married or not

うめく 呻く groan, moan ◆患者は痛みで低く呻いています The patient is groaning[moaning] quietly in pain.

うめこむ 埋め込む （植え付ける・着床させる）implant （設置する）install ◆不整脈を治療するためにペースメーカを埋め込みます I'm going to implant[install] a pacemaker to treat your *irregular heart beat [arrhythmia]. ☞植え込み型

うらがえし 裏返し （逆・反対）reverse （別の形）another guise ☞裏腹 ◆息子さ

んの乱暴な振る舞いは寂しさの裏返しかもしれません Your son's violent behavior may be just his loneliness in reverse [another guise].

うらがえす 裏返す turn (over, up) （ひっくり返す）turn inside out ◆ID カードを裏返して機械に入れて下さい Please turn your ID card over and insert it into the machine. ◆上まぶたを裏返します I'm going to turn your upper eyelid inside out.

ウラけんさ ―検査 reverse typing （↔forward typing）

うらごしする 裏ごしする strain ◆裏ごしした野菜 strained vegetables

うらづけ 裏付け （支持・立証）support （國support, back 立証する prove） （事実に基づく根拠）evidence ◆この治療法は信頼できる研究成果で裏付けられています This treatment is supported[backed] by reliable research findings. ◆この病状に対してそのサプリメントの効果は医学的な裏付けがなされていません There is no medical evidence to suggest that the supplement is effective for this condition. / The effectiveness of the supplement for this condition has yet to be medically proven.

うらはら 裏腹（に） （正反対に）contrary (to) （…にかかわらず）in spite of ◆彼は陽気な人というイメージとは裏腹に不安な様子です Contrary to his cheerful exterior [In spite of the image he has of being cheerful], he seems worried[anxious]. ◆彼女は言っていることと裏腹な行動をします She says one thing and then does another[（逆のこと）the opposite].

うらむ 恨む feel bitter, hold a grudge (against) ◆彼女は父親を恨んでいました She *felt bitter toward[held a grudge against] her father.

ウラン uranium

うる 売る sell ◆院内の売店でパジャマを売っています They sell pajamas in the hospital shop.

うるおい 潤い （水分）moisture ◆クリームを塗って皮膚に潤いを与えて下さい You should apply cream to your skin to *give it moisture[moisturize it].

うるさい
《騒々しい》noisy　（気に障る）annoying（動annoy）☞騒々しい　◆廊下の足音がうるさくて眠れないのですか Can't you sleep well because the sound of the footsteps in the hall *is too noisy[annoys you]?
《しつこい》persistent　◆何度もうるさく言って恐縮ですが，禁煙をお勧めしますI hate to *keep saying it[be so persistent], but I recommend that you stop smoking.

うるし　（植物のウルシ属）*Rhus*　（ツタウルシ）poison ivy　（ウルシオール）urushiol　（漆塗料・漆器）lacquer　◆これまでにうるしにかぶれたことがありますか Have you ever had[gotten / developed] an allergic reaction to urushiol[lacquer / poison ivy]?
◆お子さんは恐らくうるしに触って湿疹ができたのです Your child has broken out into a rash because he〈she〉*probably touched[was probably exposed to] poison ivy.　◆うるしかぶれ a poison ivy rash / a rash from lacquer[poison ivy] / an allergic reaction to lacquer[poison ivy]　▶ウルシ過敏症 poison ivy hypersensitivity　ウルシ皮膚炎 *Rhus (toxicodendron)* dermatitis

ウレアーゼ　urease

うれしい　嬉しい　（好ましい）be nice　（喜ばしい）be glad　（満足である）be happy　◆（再診の時の挨拶）またお会いできてうれしく思います(It's) Nice to see you again. / (I'm) Glad to see you again.　◆お役に立てればうれしく思います I'm happy if I can be of any help to you.　◆今日は嬉しいお知らせがあります Today I have happy[good] news for you!

ウロビリノーゲン　urobilinogen

うわあご　上顎　upper jaw　☞顎(あご，がく)，上顎(じょうがく)

うわくちびる　上唇　upper lip　☞唇

うわごと　うわ言　delirious talk　◆うわごとを言う talk deliriously

うわば　上歯　upper tooth　（歯全体）the upper teeth　☞歯

うわまぶた　上まぶた　upper eyelid, top

eyelid　☞まぶた

うわまわる　上回る　（よりよい）be better　（より上である）be above　（超える）be beyond, exceed　（より以上の）be more than　◆今回の治療効果は予想を上回っています The effectiveness of this treatment *is better than we expected[has exceeded our expectations].　◆検査値が基準値を上回ったまま下がらないのが少し気になります I'm a little concerned that your test values are above the reference range and won't go down.　◆限界を上回るストレスがかかると身体や日常生活に支障が出てきます When you have more stress than you can endure[handle], it affects your body and your everyday life.

うわむき　上向き（に）　on *one's* back　☞仰向け

うわむく　上向く　take a turn for the better　◆体調がかなり上向いてきましたね It's good that your condition has taken a turn for the better, isn't it?

うんざりする　（退屈である）feel[be] bored with　（飽き飽きして嫌気がさす）get[be] fed up with　☞懲り懲り　◆リハビリは単調でうんざりなさるかもしれませんが，どうか根気よく続けて下さい You may *feel bored [get fed up] with the monotonous rehabilitation exercises, but please persevere and keep doing them.

うんち　poo-poo（動poop）, doodoo　☞便　◆うんちしたい？ Do you want to poop[do a poo-poo / go for a poo-poo]?　★大人には Do you want to go to the restroom? と声をかける.

うんてん　運転する　drive　◆今日は運転しないで下さい Please don't drive today.　◆運転しても結構です You can[may] drive.　◆この処置を受けた後少なくとも2時間は運転してはいけません You shouldn't drive for at least two hours following this procedure.　◆この薬を飲んでいる間は運転しないで下さい While taking this medication, please don't drive (your car).　◆居眠り運転する fall asleep while driving　◀居眠り運転 drowsy [dozing while] driving / driving (while) drowsy　飲酒運転 drinking and driving / driving under the influence (of alcohol)；DUI / (酔っ払い運転) drunk driving

うんどう　運動　〈健康のための訓練〉exercise（圏exercise, do［get］exercise）（スポーツ）sport（圏スポーツの）athletic（動き・動作）movement, motion（圏運動筋・運動神経の）motor）（動力学・動態）kinetics（圏kinetic）◆運動前に before you exercise　◆運動中に during exercise　◆運動後に after you exercise　◆ふだん運動していますか Do you usually do any exercise?　◆どんな運動をしていますか What (kind of) exercise［sports］do you do?　◆どのくらいの頻度で運動していますか How often do you exercise? / How frequently do you *(get) exercise［do sports］?　◆あなたは運動不足です You aren't getting enough exercise.　◆もっと運動して下さい Please try to get more exercise.　◆足の筋肉を鍛える運動をしたほうがよいでしょう You should do an exercise that will strengthen your leg muscles.　◆運動している時〈運動した後で〉痛みますか Do you get the pain *when you are exercising〈after you exercise〉?　◆今日は激しい運動は控えて下さい Please avoid hard［strenuous］exercise today. / You shouldn't exercise hard today.　◆あなたは運動を制限する必要があります You need to do less exercise.　◆定期的に運動する get regular exercise　◆軽い運動をする get some light exercise　◆適度の運動をする get some moderate exercise　◆彼女は運動神経がよい〈反射神経がよい〉She has good reflexes. / (運動能力がある) She has good athletic ability.

◀眼球運動 eye movement　協調運動 coordinated movement / coordination　筋肉運動 muscle exercise　準備運動 warm-up　上下運動 up-and-down movement［motion］　床上運動 bed exercise / exercise in bed　随意運動 voluntary movement　水中運動 underwater exercise　整理運動 cool-down　全身運動 whole body

exercise　線毛運動 ciliary movement　ピンクリボン運動 Pink Ribbon Campaign　不随意運動 involuntary movement　腹筋運動 sit-up (exercise)　有酸素運動 aerobic exercise / aerobics　リハビリテーション運動 rehabilitation exercise / exercise for rehabilitation　▶運動感覚 kinesthesia　運動器官 motor organ　運動機能 motor function　運動筋 motor muscle　運動亢進 hyperkinesis / hyperkinesia　運動失調性歩行 ataxic gait　運動障害 motor disorder［disturbance / impairment］　運動処方 exercise prescription　運動神経 motor nerve　運動神経伝導速度 motor nerve conduction velocity　運動制限 movement limitation　運動性失語 motor aphasia　運動性失調 motor ataxia / failure of muscle［muscular］coordination　運動性貧血 exercise anemia / exercise-induced anemia　運動生理学 exercise［sport(s)］physiology　運動中枢 the motor center　運動痛 pain on motion　運動低下 hypokinesis / hypokinesia　運動ニューロン疾患 motor neuron disease；MND　運動能力 motor ability / athletic ability　運動発達 motor development　運動範囲［可動範囲］range of motion；ROM　運動負荷試験 exercise stress［tolerance］test　運動不足 lack of exercise　運動麻痺 motor paralysis　運動野 motor area　運動誘発性アナフィラキシー exercise-induced anaphylaxis　運動誘発喘息 exercise-induced asthma；EIA　運動誘発電位 motor evoked potential　運動力学 kinetics　運動量 amount of exercise　運動療法 exercise therapy

え

え[1] 絵 （絵画）**picture** （絵具などを使った絵）**painting** （動**paint**） （鉛筆・ペンなどを使った線画）**drawing** （動**draw**） （挿絵）**illustration** （動**illustrate**）　◆絵がお上手ですね You can draw really well!　◆絵を描くのはお好きですか Do you like drawing [painting] pictures?

え[2] 柄 handle （形**handled**）　◆この長い柄のあるスプーンを使ってみて下さい Please try using this long-handled spoon.

エアウェイ airway ☞気道　◆経口エアウェイ oral[oropharyngeal] airway　経鼻エアウェイ nasal[nasopharyngeal] airway　食道胃管エアウェイ esophageal gastric tube airway；EGTA　食道閉鎖式エアウェイ esophageal obturator airway；EOA

エアコン air conditioner ☞冷房

エアバッグそんしょう ―損傷 airbag-associated injury, airbag-mediated injury

エアフィルター air filter

エアマット air mattress

エアロゾル aerosol ▶エアロゾル療法 aerosol therapy

エアロビクス aerobics （形**aerobic**）　◆エアロビクスをする do aerobics[aerobic exercise]

えいが 映画 movie,《英》**film**　◆映画を見るのはお好きですか Do you like watching movies?　◆最近何かいい映画を見ましたか Have you watched any good movies recently?

えいかいわ 英会話 （話し言葉の英語）**spoken English** （会話の英語）**conversational English** ★「英会話」の直訳は English conversation だが，英語圏では通例 spoken English または conversational English を用いる.　☞英語　◆私は英会話が苦手です I'm not good at spoken[conversational] English. / I can't speak English well.　◆英会話学校で教えているのですか Are you teaching at an English language school?

エイがた A型 （type）**A** （血液型）**blood type A, type A blood,**《英》**blood group A** ☞血液型　▶A型インフルエンザ influenza type A　A型肝炎 hepatitis A / type A hepatitis　A型性格 type A personality

えいきゅう 永久（の）**permanent** ☞永続　▶永久的人工肛門 permanent stoma　永久麻痺 permanent paralysis　永久免疫 permanent immunity ☞永久歯

えいきゅうし 永久歯 permanent tooth （複**teeth**） ☞歯　◆彼女は永久歯が生えかかっています She is cutting[getting] her permanent teeth. / Her permanent teeth are cutting in.

えいきょう 影響 influence （動**influence**） （直接的な影響）**effect** （動**affect**）　◆暴力的なテレビ番組は子供達に悪い影響を与えます Violent TV programs have a bad influence on children.　◆規則的に歩くことは体にとてもよい影響を与えます Walking, if done regularly, is very good for the body[health].　◆家庭や仕事上のストレスが呼吸に影響していますか Does stress at home or work affect your breathing?　◆妊娠中の喫煙は母子ともに悪い影響を与えます Smoking while pregnant can be harmful to both mother and baby.　◀悪影響 bad influence / harmful effect　好影響 good effect / （肯定的で好ましい影響）positive effect / （有益な影響）beneficial effect

えいぎょう 営業　◆院内のカフェテリアは平日のみの営業となっております The cafeteria in the hospital is open（on）weekdays only.

エイぐんようけつせいれんさきゅうきん A群溶血性連鎖球菌 group A hemolytic streptococcus, group A hemolytic strep；GAS ▶A群溶血性連鎖球菌感染症 group A hemolytic strep[streptococcus] infection

えいご 英語 English　◆私は英語がわかりません I don't understand English.　◆英語は得意ではないんです I'm not good at English.　◆英語が話せますか Do you speak English?　★Can を使うと相手の能力

を訊くことになり失礼になることがある. ◆英語の話せるスタッフを呼びますので，ここでしばらくお待ち下さい We'll *call for[(ポケベルで呼び出す)page] a member of staff who can speak English, so please wait here a while. ◆英語で書く write in English ◀アメリカ英語 American English イギリス英語 British English 医療英語 medical English

えいこく 英国 ☞イギリス

えいじゅう 永住 permanent residence
◆日本に永住する settle[live] permanently in Japan ▶永住外国人 permanent foreign resident 永住権 the right of permanent residence 永住ビザ permanent-resident[permanence-residence] visa

エイズ AIDS （後天性免疫不全症候群）acquired immunodeficiency syndrome ☞HIV ◆エイズに罹る get[have] AIDS ◆エイズを発症する develop AIDS ◆エイズによる症状がある have the symptoms of AIDS ◀薬害エイズ drug-induced AIDS /（汚染された血液製剤を介した）AIDS contracted from contaminated blood products, transfusion-transmitted AIDS /（非加熱血液製剤を介した）AIDS contracted from untreated blood products ▶エイズウイルス AIDS virus エイズ患者 AIDS patient エイズ関連症候群 AIDS-related complex；ARC エイズ関連日和見感染 AIDS-related opportunistic infection エイズ関連リンパ腫 AIDS-related lymphoma エイズ検査 HIV test エイズ治療薬 AIDS medication[drug / agent] エイズ認知症 AIDS dementia complex

えいせい 衛生 （環境・設備の）sanitation （㊑sanitary） （清潔さ・疾病予防の）hygiene / háidʒíːn/ （㊑hygienic） ◆台所用品の衛生にいつも気をつけていますか Are you always careful about keeping your *kitchen utensils[kitchenware] clean (and sanitary)? ◆調理済みの料理をそのまま放置するのは衛生上安全ではありません It's not hygienically safe to leave cooked food sitting out for too long. ◆ストレスを受け

過ぎるのは精神衛生上よくありません Too much stress is not good for your mental health. ◀環境衛生 environmental sanitation[health] 口腔衛生 oral[mouth] hygiene 公衆衛生 public health 産業衛生 industrial sanitation[hygiene] 歯科衛生士 dental hygienist 食品衛生 food hygiene[sanitation] ▶衛生状態 sanitary[hygienic] condition

えいぞく 永続(的な) permanent ☞永久 ▶永続性めまい permanent vertigo[dizziness]

エイチアイヴィー HIV （ヒト免疫不全ウイルス）human immunodeficiency virus ☞AIDS ◆HIV に感染している be infected with HIV ◆HIV 抗体が陽性である be HIV positive ◆HIV は握手, 抱擁, キスなどでは感染しません HIV is not transmitted through shaking hands, hugging, or kissing. ◀抗 HIV 薬 anti-HIV medication[drug / agent] ▶HIV 感染者 HIV-positive[HIV-infected] person HIV 感染症 HIV infection HIV キャリア HIV carrier HIV 抗原 HIV antigen HIV 抗体 HIV antibody ☞HIV 検査

エイチアイヴィーけんさ HIV 検査 HIV test （ヒト免疫不全ウイルス検査）human immunodeficiency virus test ◆HIV 検査を受ける get tested for HIV / get an HIV test ◆HIV 検査で陽性〈陰性〉と出ました You tested positive〈negative〉for HIV. / Your HIV test came back positive〈negative〉. ◆HIV 検査は感染の機会から少なくとも 3 か月以上経ってから行って下さい Please get tested for HIV at least three months after possible exposure to the virus.

エイティーエム ATM （現金自動預入引出機）automated teller machine, cash machine

えいてきがいしょう 鋭的外傷 penetrating trauma[injury, wound]

エイビーオーけつえきがた ABO 血液型 ABO blood type, ABO blood group, 《英》 blood group ABO ☞血液型

エイビーがた AB 型 (type) AB （血液

型）blood type AB, type AB blood,〈英〉blood group AB　☞血液型

えいみん　永眠する　(死ぬ) die　(婉曲的に) pass away　☞亡くなる　◆彼女は今朝5時に安らかに永眠されました She *passed away[died] peacefully at five (o'clock) this morning.

えいよう　栄養　(栄養摂取) nutrition　(形栄養のある nutritious, nourishing　栄養上の nutritional, nutritive　食生活上の dietary)　(滋養) nourishment　(栄養供給・授乳) feeding　◆あなたは栄養が不足しています You aren't getting[taking] enough nutrition.　◆栄養にもっと気をつけて下さい You should be more careful about your nutrition.　◆食事は栄養のバランスを考えて下さい Make sure that you take a balanced diet.　◆栄養のつく食べ物をとる eat nutritious food(s)　◆栄養をとる take nourishment　◆点滴で栄養を取る *be fed[receive nourishment] through an intravenous[IV] drip　◆栄養価の高い食物 (a) highly nutritious[nourishing] food　◆適切な〈不適切な〉栄養摂取 good 〈poor〉 nutrition

◀経管栄養 tube feeding　経口栄養 oral feeding　経腸栄養 enteral nutrition[feeding]　在宅経腸栄養法 home enteral nutrition；HEN　在宅静脈栄養法 home parenteral nutrition；HPN　静脈栄養 intravenous nutrition[feeding]　人工栄養 artificial feeding[nutrition]　成分栄養剤 elemental diet (mixture)　中心静脈栄養法 intravenous hyperalimentation；IVH /（完全静脈栄養）total parenteral nutrition；TPN　必須栄養素 essential nutrient　補充栄養 supplementary feeding　母乳栄養 breastfeeding[breast nutrition]　哺乳びん栄養 bottlefeeding /（調合乳による）formula (milk) feeding　▶栄養価 nutritive [nutritional] value　栄養学 nutritional science　栄養過多 excess nutrition / overnutrition　栄養管理部 the Department of Food and Nutrition Services / the Food and Nutrition Services Department　栄養血管 nutrient vessel　栄養指導 nutri-

tion education　栄養障害 nutritional[nutrition] disorder　栄養素 nutrient / nutritive element　栄養相談室 nutrition counseling room　栄養必要量 nutritional[dietary] requirement　栄養物[栄養分] nutrient　栄養不良 malnutrition　栄養補給剤 dietary[nutritional] supplement　☞栄養管，栄養士，栄養状態，低栄養

えいようかん　栄養管　feeding tube, nutritional tube　◆栄養管をお腹から直接胃に入れる insert[put] a feeding tube through the abdomen directly into the stomach　◀経鼻栄養管 nasal feeding tube

えいようし　栄養士　dietitian, nutritionist　◀学校栄養士 school dietitian[nutritionist]　管理栄養士 registered dietitian [nutritionist]

えいようじょうたい　栄養状態　nutritional state[status]　◆栄養状態が悪くなっています Your nutritional state is getting worse. / You aren't getting the right nutrition.　◆栄養状態を評価して改善する evaluate[assess] and improve *a person's nutritional status

えいん　会陰　perineum　(形perineal)　▶会陰部尿道下裂 perineal hypospadias　会陰裂傷 perineal tear[laceration]　☞会陰切開，会陰縫合

えいんせっかい　会陰切開(術)　episiotomy, perineotomy　◆会陰切開をする make an incision in the perineum / perform an episiotomy

えいんほうごう　会陰縫合(術)　episiorrhaphy, perineorrhaphy　◆会陰縫合する place stitches in the perineum

ええ　(肯定して) Yes　(確かに) Sure, Certainly　(相づちで) Uh-huh, Mm　◆ええ，もちろん Yes, of course.　◆「セカンドオピニオンをもらってもいいですか」「ええ，どうぞ」"May I have a second opinion?" "Sure [Certainly]."

エーテル　ether

ええと　(考えながら) Let me see, Let's see, Well　(間をとりながら) Er…

えがお　笑顔　smile　◆お母さんの笑顔が

お子さんには一番の薬です A mother's smile is the best medicine for her child. ◆笑顔で挨拶する *greet a person[say hello to a person] with a smile

えき　液　（液体）fluid, liquid　（分泌液）juice　（溶液）solution　☞液体　◆胃液 gastric juice　穿刺液 puncture fluid　ヨード液 iodine solution　▶液剤(水薬)liquid medication[drug / agent]

えきか　腋窩　armpit, underarm, axilla（㊓axillary）　☞腋の下　▶腋窩温 axillary temperature　腋窩腺 axillary gland　腋窩リンパ節 axillary lymph node

えきがく　疫学　epidemiology　▶疫学者 epidemiologist

エキシマレーザー　excimer laser　▶エキシマレーザー屈折矯正角膜切除(術) excimer laser photorefractive keratectomy

えきしゅう　腋臭　strong underarm odor, strong armpit odor　☞腋臭(わきが)

えきじょうべん　液状便　watery stool, liquid stool

えきせいめんえき　液性免疫　humoral immunity

えきたい　液体　liquid, fluid　☞液　◆吐いたものは透明な液体でしたか Did the vomit look like clear liquid?　◆合図するまでこの液体を口の中に含んでおいて下さい Please keep this liquid in your mouth till I say "OK."　▶液体酸素 liquid oxygen　液体窒素 liquid nitrogen　液体歯磨き mouthwash / dental rinse

エキノコックスしょう　―症　echinococcosis　◀肝エキノコックス症[肝包虫症] hepatic echinococcosis

えきもう　腋毛　underarm hair, axillary hair　☞腋毛(わきげ)

えくぼ　dimple　☞へこみ　▶えくぼ形成 the formation of dimples[dimpling]

エクリンせん　―(汗)腺　eccrine gland[apparatus], sweat gland[apparatus]

エコー　echo　☞超音波検査　◀肝腎エコーコントラスト hepatorenal echo contrast

エコノミークラスしょうこうぐん　―症候群　economy class syndrome

えし　壊死　necrosis（㊓壊死性の necrotiz-ing）　◀圧迫性壊死[床ずれ] pressure sore　乾酪壊死 caseous necrosis　腫瘍壊死因子 tumor necrosis factor；TNF　心筋壊死 myocardial necrosis　大腿骨頭壊死 femur head necrosis　▶壊死性筋膜炎 necrotizing fasciitis　壊死性血管炎 necrotizing angiitis　壊死性腸炎 necrotizing enterocolitis　壊死性リンパ節炎 necrotizing lymphadenitis

エジプト　Egypt（㊓Egyptian）　☞国籍　▶エジプト人(の) Egyptian

エスカレーター　escalator　◆神経内科はエスカレーターで2階に上がって右手になります Take the escalator to the second floor, and *you'll find the department of neurology on your right[the neurology department will be on the right].

エスじょうけっちょう　S状結腸　sigmoid colon

エストラジオール　estradiol

エストロゲン　estrogen　▶エストロゲン受容体 estrogen receptor　エストロゲン補充療法 estrogen replacement therapy；ERT

えそ　壊疽　gangrene（㊓gangrenous）　◆足の潰瘍は治療しないと壊疽を起こすことがあります Foot ulcers can turn gangrenous if they are not treated.　◀ガス壊疽 gas gangrene

エタノール　ethanol　（エチルアルコール）ethyl alcohol　◀経皮的エタノール注入療法 percutaneous ethanol injection therapy；PEIT

エックスきゃく　X脚　（外反膝）knock-knee

エックスせん　X線　X-ray, x-ray（㊓放射線の radiologic, radiological）　（撮影）radiography　☞放射線, レントゲン　◆X線検査が必要です You need to have an X-ray.　◆胸のX線を撮りましょう I'm going to[Let me] take an X-ray of your chest.
◀間接X線撮影 indirect radiography　単純X線撮影 plain radiography　デジタルX線撮影 digital radiography；DR　軟X線撮影 soft X-ray radiography　乳房X線検査 mammography　▶X線技師 X-ray

technician[technologist] / radiologic technician[technologist]　X線検査 X-ray examination[test]　X線照射 X-ray irradiation　X線所見 radiologic findings　X線診断 X-ray diagnosis　X線防御 X-ray protection　☞X線写真

エックスせんしゃしん　X線写真　**X-ray**, **x-ray**　☞レントゲン　◆一番最近胸のX線写真を撮ったのはいつですか When was your last chest X-ray? / When was the last time you had a chest X-ray?　◆胸部X線写真で右肺に結節影が見られます The chest X-ray shows a shadow of a nodule in the right lung.　◆胸のX線写真を撮る take an X-ray of *a person's* chest / X-ray *a person's* chest /（撮ってもらう）have *one's* chest X-rayed / have an X-ray taken of *one's* chest　◆乳房X線写真 mammogram

エックスせんしょくたい　X染色体　**X chromosome**

エックスれんさ　X連鎖（の）　**X-linked**　▶X連鎖遺伝 X-linked inheritance　X連鎖遺伝病 X-linked genetic disease

エナメルしつ　―質　**enamel**

エナメルじょうひしゅ　―上皮腫　**ameloblastoma, adamantinoma**

エネルギー　**energy** /énədʒi/　☞気力, 体力　◆エネルギーを供給する supply energy　◆エネルギーを消費する consume energy　▶運動エネルギー kinetic energy　▶エネルギー源 source of energy　エネルギー消費 energy consumption　エネルギー消費量 the amount of energy consumed　エネルギー代謝 energy metabolism　エネルギー必要量 energy requirement[allowance]

エピソードきおく　―記憶　**episodic memory**

エビデンス　**evidence**　☞根拠　▶エビデンスに基づく医療 evidence-based medicine；EBM

エピネフリン　☞アドレナリン　**epinephrine**

エフェクター　**effector**　▶エフェクター細胞 effector cell

エフェドリン　**ephedrine**

エブスタインきけい　―奇形　**Ebstein anomaly**

エプスタイン・バーウイルス　**Epstein-Barr virus**；**EBV**

エプロン　**apron**　◆エプロンを着ける put on an apron　◆エプロンを着けている wear an apron　◆鉛入りのエプロン a lead apron　◆防護エプロン protective apron　放射線防護エプロン X-ray[radiation] protective apron

エホバのしょうにん　―証人　（総称）**Jehovah's Witnesses**　（信者）**Jehovah's Witness**

エボラしゅっけつねつ　―出血熱　**Ebola hemorrhagic fever**

エムアールアイ　**MRI**　（磁気共鳴画像）**magnetic resonance imaging**　◆MRI検査が必要です You need to have an MRI.　◆頭部のMRI検査をしましょう I'm going to [Let me] get an MRI of your head taken.　◆MRI検査の結果, 肝臓がんが疑われます Judging by (the results of) the MRI, *it could be[it's possibly] liver cancer.　◆造影MRI検査 contrast-enhanced MRI

えらい　偉い　（勇気のある）**brave**　（強い）**strong**　（優れている）**good, great**　◆（子どもに）痛いのをがまんできて, えらかったね You put up with a lot of pain. You're very brave[Good for you]! / What a brave [strong] boy〈girl〉(you are) to put up with the pain!

エラスターゼ　**elastase**

エラスチン　**elastin**

えらぶ　選ぶ　**choose**　（より慎重に選択する）**select**　☞選択　◆前立腺がんの最適な治療を選ぶ choose[select] the most appropriate treatment for prostate cancer　◆乳房温存術と乳房切除術のどちらかを選ぶ choose between breast-conserving surgery and mastectomy

エリスロポエチン　**erythropoietin**

エリテマトーデス　**lupus erythematosus**；**LE**　◀全身性エリマトーデス systemic lupus erythematosus；SLE

える　得る　（手に入れる）**get, have**　（獲得す

る・許可を得る）**obtain** （稼ぐ）**earn, make**
◆よい検査結果を得ることができました We were able to get[obtain] a good test result. ◆外出は担当医の許可を得る必要があります You need to obtain[get] your doctor's permission before you *leave the hospital building[go out of the hospital]. ◆生活費を得る earn[make] a living

エルゴメーター **ergometer** ◀自転車エルゴメーター bicycle ergometer ▶エルゴメーター負荷試験（bicycle）ergometer stress test

エルディーエルコレステロール **LDL cholesterol, bad cholesterol**

エレベーター **elevator** /éləvèɪtə-/,《英》**lift**
◆エレベーターに乗って5階に行って下さい Take the elevator to the fifth floor.
◆アパートにはエレベーターがありますか Is there an elevator in your apartment building?

えん　円
《図形》**circle** ◆ここに円を描いて下さい Please draw a circle here. ◆親指と人指し指で円を作ることができますか Can you make a circle with your thumb and forefinger?
《通貨単位》**yen** ◆特別室の差額料金は1万円になります Special rooms cost ten thousand yen. / The charge for a special room is ten thousand yen.

えんい　遠位（の） **distal** ▶遠位型筋ジストロフィー distal muscular dystrophy；DMA　遠位型ミオパチー distal myopathy　遠位筋 distal muscle　遠位指〈趾〉節間関節 *distal interphalangeal[DIP] joint of the hand〈foot〉　遠位尿細管 distal（kidney）tubule；DT

えんいん　遠因 （間接的な原因）**indirect cause**

えんか　塩化 **chloride** ▶塩化アンモニウム ammonium chloride　塩化カリウム potassium chloride　塩化ベンザルコニウム benzalkonium chloride

えんがい　煙害 （汚染）**smoke pollution**
（被害）**damage caused by smoke**

えんかく　遠隔（の） **distant, remote** （接頭

tele-）▶遠隔医療 telemedicine　遠隔記憶 remote memory　遠隔治療 teletherapy / teletreatment　遠隔転移 distant metastasis

えんき　延期する **put off, postpone** ◆手術はしばらく延期することにしましょう We're going to *put off[postpone] the surgery for a while. ◆手術をあまり後に延期したくはありません We don't want to *put off[postpone] the surgery for too long. ◆予約を延期する *put off[postpone] one's appointment

えんぎせいじんかくしょうがい　演技性人格障害 **histrionic personality disorder**

えんきんかん　遠近感 **sense of distance**
◆遠近感に異常はありますか Do you have any problems with your sense of distance?

えんきんりょうようめがね　遠近両用眼鏡 **bifocals, bifocal glasses** ★複数形で.

えんげ　嚥下 **swallowing** （動**swallow**）, **deglutition** ☞飲み込む ◆嚥下に異常がありますか Do you have any problems （with） swallowing? ◀空気嚥下症 aerophagia / aerophagy ▶嚥下訓練 swallowing training　嚥下困難 difficulty[trouble]（with / in）swallowing / dysphagia　嚥下障害 impaired swallowing / swallowing[deglutition] disorder / dysphagia　嚥下食 dysphagia diet / diet for patients with a swallowing disorder　嚥下性肺炎 aspiration pneumonia　嚥下造影検査 barium swallow （test / examination）/ barium meal （test / examination）/ videofluoroscopic examination of swallowing　嚥下中枢 the swallowing[deglutition] center　嚥下痛 swallowing pain / painful swallowing / odynophagia　嚥下反射 swallowing[deglutition] reflex　嚥下不能 inability to swallow / aglutition

えんげい　園芸 **horticulture** （形**horticultural**）, **gardening** ▶園芸療法 horticultural therapy

えんけいだつもうしょう　円形脱毛症 **alopecia areata, spot baldness, patch baldness, patchy hair loss**

エンゲルけいすう ─係数 Engel's coefficient

えんさん 塩酸 hydrochloric acid （塩化水素）hydrogen chloride

えんし 遠視 farsightedness （↔nearsightedness）（📖farsighted），hyperopia （📖hyperopic） ◆遠視と言われたことがありますか Have you ever been told that you are farsighted? ◆遠視用の眼鏡をかけている wear glasses for farsightedness

えんじゃ 縁者 relative ☞親戚

えんじょ 援助 help （補助）assistance （励まし・支援）support （公的な援助）aid ☞支える，サポート，支援，助ける ◆援助をお望みですか Would you like some help[assistance]? ◆もし援助が必要でしたらこの番号におかけ下さい Please call this number if you need any help[assistance]. ◆退院後は日常生活に援助が必要になるでしょう You'll need help[assistance] with day-to-day life after leaving the hospital. ◆精神的な援助を必要とする need moral[mental / psychological] support ◆情動面の助けを必要とする need emotional support ◀医療援助[扶助] medical assistance[aid] 公的援助 public assistance 財政援助 financial help[assistance / aid] ▶援助計画 support plan 援助行動 helping behavior 援助ネットワーク support network

えんしょう 炎症 inflammation （📖炎症を起こした inflamed 炎症性の inflammatory）（ひりひりする痛み）irritation （📖irritated）
◆胸部 X 線写真を見ると肺に炎症があります Your chest X-ray shows there is an inflammation in your lungs. ◆傷は炎症を起こしています The wound is inflamed. ◆この炎症は 2, 3 日で治るでしょう This inflammation will *go away[clear up / subside] in a few days. ◆プールの水の過剰な塩素は眼や皮膚の炎症を起こします Excessive chlorine in pool water causes irritation of the eyes and skin. ◀抗炎症薬 antiinflammatory （medication / drug / agent） 癒着性炎症 adhesive inflammation ▶炎症性腸疾患 in-

flammatory bowel disease；IBD 炎症性ポリープ inflammatory polyp 炎症徴候 sign of inflammation 炎症反応 inflammatory reaction

えんしん 遠心（性の） centrifugal （神経などが）efferent ▶遠心性回路 efferent pathway 遠心性神経 efferent nerve 遠心分離機 centrifugal separator 遠心力 centrifugal force

えんすい 円錐 cone （📖conical, cone-shaped） ▶円錐角膜 keratoconus 円錐切除術 conization

えんずい 延髄 medulla oblongata （📖medullary），bulb （📖bulbar） ▶延髄呼吸中枢 the medullary respiratory center 延髄出血 bulbar bleeding[hemorrhage]

えんそ 塩素 chlorine ◆塩素系漂白剤はノロウイルスの消毒に使用できます Chlorine bleach can be used as a disinfecting agent against norovirus. ◀高塩素血症［高クロール血症］hyperchloremia 残留塩素 residual chlorine ▶塩素漂白 chlorine bleaching

えんたいきん 延滞金 late payment charge[fee] ◆お支払が遅れております．来月末までにお支払いいただけない場合には延滞金をいただくことになります I'm afraid that your payment is delayed. If you fail to pay your bill by the end of next month, we'll have to ask you to pay the late payment charge.

えんちゅう 円柱 （円柱型）cast （円筒）cylinder ◀顆粒円柱 granular cast 硝子円柱 hyaline cast 赤血球円柱 *red blood cell[erythrocyte] cast

えんちょう 延長
《長さ・期間を延ばすこと》extension （📖extend） 《更新》renewal （📖renew） ◆日本滞在を延長なさいますか Would you like to extend your stay in Japan? ◆治療を受けるにはビザの延長を申請する必要があります To have the treatment, you need to apply for a visa extension. ◆保険証は自動的に延長されませんので，毎月受付窓口で提示する必要があります Your insurance card is not renewed automatically, so you

must[have to] present it at the reception counter every month.

《一続きの物事》continuation (動continue)

◆今日の検査は昨日の検査の延長です Today's test is a continuation of yesterday's.

エンテロウイルス *Enterovirus*

エンテロコッカス *Enterococcus*

エンテロトキシン enterotoxin

エンテロバクター *Enterobacter*

えんてんか 炎天下 the (scorching) sun, the summer heat ◆炎天下で作業する work outside *in the sun[in the summer heat]

エンドトキシン endotoxin

えんぱい 円背 round back, rounding [bowing] of the back （脊柱後彎）kyphosis ★humpback や hunchback は侮辱的な響きがあるので使用を控えたい.

エンパシー （感情移入・共感）empathy

えんばんじょう 円板状(の) discoid
▶円板状エリテマトーデス discoid lupus erythematosus；DLE 円板状半月板 discoid meniscus

えんぴつじょう 鉛筆状(の) pencil-like ◆鉛筆状の便 pencil-like stools

エンプティネストしょうこうぐん 一症候群 （空の巣症候群）empty nest syndrome

えんぶん 塩分 salt (形salty), salt content ◆塩分を制限していますか Are you limiting your intake of salt? ◆塩分を摂りすぎていますよ You're getting too much salt. ◆塩分の摂取を控えて下さい Please be moderate in your intake of salt. ◆塩分を控えた食事の必要があります You need a low-salt diet. ◆塩分を減らす cut down on salt ◆減塩醤油にして塩分を減らす cut down on salt by using low-salt soy sauce ◆塩分の濃い食品を避ける avoid eating salty foods ◆塩分の薄い物を食べる eat lightly salted foods / eat foods with little salt ◆塩分の濃い食事 a salty meal ▶塩分制限 salt restriction 塩分摂取 salt intake

えんぽう 遠方 （遠い道のり）a long way （はるばる）all the way ◆遠方からのお越し

ありがとうございます Thank you for coming *a long way[all the way] to visit us.

◆遠方からの通院は大変ではないですか Don't you find it hard[difficult] coming such a long way to the hospital?

えんめい 延命 prolongation of life ◆もし不治かつ末期の症状になった場合に, 延命治療を希望なさいますか If you have an incurable, irreversible medical condition or if you have *a terminal[an end-stage] condition, would you like to *be put on life support[receive life support]? ◆延命治療についての要望はいつでも撤回や変更ができます You can cancel or change your (advance) directive about *life support[life-sustaining] treatment at any time. ★advance directive は事前指示書. / You can revoke[renounce] or change your wishes about *life support[life-sustaining] treatment at any time. ◆彼女は延命治療を望んでいません She doesn't want to be put on a life support (machine). / She refuses treatment to keep her alive. ▶延命医療 life-prolonging medical treatment 延命装置 life support system / (設備一式) life support equipment ☞生命維持装置 延命治療 life support treatment / (手段) life support measures

えんりょ 遠慮

《行為の抑制・ためらい》 ◆ご用のある時は, 遠慮しないでコールボタンを押して下さい(ためらわずに)If you need any help, don't hesitate to push[press] the call button.

◆何かご質問があったら遠慮せずに訊いて下さい(気軽に)If you have any questions, feel free to ask us.

《行為の中止・禁止》 （控える・がまんする）refrain from ☞控える ◆病室内での携帯電話のご使用はご遠慮下さい Please refrain from using mobile phones in your room. ◆すみませんが, 待合室でのタバコはご遠慮願います(やめてくれませんか)Excuse me, but would you mind not smoking in the waiting room? ◆ご家族の方以外の病棟内立ち入りはご遠慮いただ

いております Only family members may enter the unit[ward]. ◆入室はご遠慮下さい Please do not enter (the room)./Kindly refrain from entering (the room)./(掲示)Private[Do not enter].

お

おい 老い old age

おいかける 追いかける （動き・人を追う）
follow （走って後を追う）run after （追跡する）chase ◆目を大きく開けたままで，黒い点を追いかけて下さい Please keep your eyes open wide, and follow the black spot. ◆点滅する光を目で追いかける follow the flashing light with *one's* eye(s) ◆母親の後を追いかける *run after*[*follow*] *one's* mother ◆彼は逃げ出した犬を追いかけて車にはねられました He chased his runaway dog and got hit by a car.

おいしい good, tasty, delicious ◆食事はおいしく感じていますか Do you enjoy your food? / Do you find that the foods you eat taste good[delicious]? ◆おいしい食べ物と健康的な食べ物は同じではありません Tasty food and healthy food are not the same thing.

おいつめる 追い詰める corner ◆仕事の重圧で追い詰められた感じがしていますか Do you feel cornered by the pressure at work?

おいる 老いる get[become, grow] old ☞年(とし)

おう¹ 負う
《傷を被る》have, get injured[wounded] ◆額に切り傷を負う have a cut on the forehead ◆頭部に傷を負う have a head injury / get injured[wounded] in the head ◆自動車事故で重傷を負う get seriously injured in a car accident
《責任などを引き受ける》take, assume ◆事故の責任を負う take responsibility for the accident

おう² 追う run after, chase ☞追いかける

おうい 横位 transverse presentation

おうが 横臥 （横向きに寝る）lie on *one's* side （横になる）lie down

おうかくしんけい 横隔神経 phrenic nerve

おうかくまく 横隔膜 diaphragm /dáɪə-fræm/ （㊥diaphragmátic, phrenic） （上腹部分）midriff ◆腹式呼吸をするには横隔膜，すなわち胸とお腹の間にある筋肉を使います Abdominal breathing is breathing using your diaphragm, a muscle located between your chest and abdomen. ◀心横隔膜角 cardiophrenic angle ▶横隔膜下膿瘍 subdiaphragmatic[subphrenic] abscess 横隔膜痙攣 phrenospasm 横隔膜高位 elevation of the diaphragm 横隔膜呼吸[腹式呼吸] diaphragmatic breathing[respiration] / abdominal breathing [respiration] 横隔膜弛緩症 diaphragmatic relaxation / eventration of the diaphragm 横隔膜ヘルニア diaphragmatic hernia 横隔膜麻痺 diaphragmatic paralysis

おうき 嘔気 nausea ☞吐き気

おうきゅう 応急 （急場の処置）first aid （緊急）emergency ◆救急，緊急 ◆応急処置をする give a *person* *first aid*[emergency care / emergency treatment] ◆応急策を講じる take emergency measures

おうけい¹ 横径 transverse diameter

おうけい² 凹形 concave shape

おうこうけっちょう 横行結腸 transverse colon

おうこっせつ 横骨折 transverse fracture

おうじょう 凹状（の） concave (↔convex)

おうしょく 黄色（の） yellow （黄色っぽい）yellowish ▶黄色靱帯骨化症 ossification of the ligamentum flavum 黄色爪症候群 yellow-nail syndrome 黄色帯下 yellow[yellowish] discharge ☞黄色腫，黄色ブドウ球菌，黄色野菜

おうしょくしゅ 黄色腫 xanthoma ◀眼瞼黄色腫 xanthelasma 腱黄色腫 tendinous xanthoma ▶黄色腫症 xanthomatosis

おうしょくブドウきゅうきん 黄色ブドウ球菌 *Staphylococcus aureus* ◀メチシリン感受性黄色ブドウ球菌 methicillin-susceptible *Staphylococcus aureus*；MSSA メチシリン耐性黄色ブドウ球菌 methicillin-resistant *Staphylococcus aureus*；MRSA

おうしょくやさい 黄色野菜 **yellow vegetables** ★通例，複数形で．

おうじる 応じる
《相手の働きかけに応える》（質問に答える）**answer** （要求などを満たす）**meet, satisfy** （受諾する）**accept** ☞応対，対応 ◆ご質問があればいつでも応じます We're always ready to answer your questions. ◆残念ながら，ご要望に応じることはできません Unfortunately, we can't meet[satisfy] your request. ◆申し出に応じる accept an offer
《合わせる》◆治療はご希望に応じて変更いたします We can modify the treatment according to your request.

おうしん 往診 **house call, home visit**
◆往診する make a house call ◆往診を依頼する request[ask for] a house call ▶往診料 doctor's visiting fee

おうせい 旺盛（な） ◆彼は食欲が旺盛です He has a big[hearty] appetite. ◆息子さんは好奇心が旺盛なほうですか Is your son the type who's intensely curious about what's going on around him?

おうせっかい 横切開 **transverse incision**
おうせつしつ 応接室 **reception room**
おうせん 黄染 **yellowing, yellow coloring [discoloration]** （黄色っぽい変色）**yellowish coloring[discoloration]** ◆皮膚や眼球結膜の黄染を認めます I notice that your skin and the whites of your eyes have a yellow discoloration. / I notice that you have yellowing[a yellowish discoloration] of the skin and of the whites of the eyes.

おうたい¹ 黄体 **corpus luteum** （形容luteal 黄体化の **luteinizing**） ▶黄体期 luteal phase 黄体期維持療法 luteal phase support therapy 黄体機能不全 luteal insufficiency 黄体形成ホルモン luteinizing hormone；LH 黄体形成ホルモン放出ホルモン luteinizing hormone-releasing

hormone；LH-RH / gonadotropin-releasing hormone；GnRH 黄体ホルモン luteal hormone

おうたい² 応対する **attend** (to), **wait** (on)
☞応じる，対応 ◆英語の話せるスタッフがまもなく応対いたします One of our English-speaking staff[A member of our staff who can speak English] will *attend to [wait on] you soon. ◆当直医が応対します The doctor on (night) duty will see [attend to] you.

おうだん¹ 黄疸 **jaundice** /dʒɔ́ːndɪs/ （形容黄疸にかかった **jaundiced**） ◆黄疸が出現する[見られる] get[have] jaundice / be jaundiced ◆黄疸が強い have severe jaundice / have a severe form of jaundice ◆黄疸の徴候が見える show[have] signs of jaundice ◆黄疸で皮膚や白目が黄色くなっています The skin and the whites of the eyes have become yellow due to jaundice. ◆赤ちゃんに黄疸がみられます Your baby *is jaundiced[has jaundice]. ◆黄疸を治療するために赤ちゃんに光を当てますが，心配しないで下さい To treat the jaundice, we're going to place your baby under lights, but don't worry.
◀核黄疸 nuclear jaundice / kernicterus 肝性黄疸 hepatic jaundice 肝前性〈肝後性〉黄疸 prehepatic〈posthepatic〉jaundice 新生児黄疸 newborn[neonatal] jaundice / jaundice of the newborn 体質性黄疸 constitutional jaundice 閉塞性黄疸 obstructive jaundice 母乳性黄疸 breast milk jaundice 溶血性黄疸 hemolytic jaundice

おうだん² 横断（の） **transverse** （横断面の・横断的な）**cross-sectional** ◀体軸横断スキャン transverse axial scanning [scan] ▶横断性脊髄炎 transverse myelitis 横断的研究 cross-sectional study 横断面 cross section / transection

おうと 嘔吐 **vomiting** （動vomit, throw up）, **emesis** ☞吐き気，吐く ◀アセトン血性嘔吐症 acetonemic vomiting 悪心嘔吐 nausea and vomiting 習慣性嘔吐 habitual vomiting 周期性嘔吐 periodic vomiting　早朝嘔吐 morning vomiting　妊娠嘔吐 vomiting[emesis] of pregnancy　反復嘔吐 recurrent vomiting　噴出性嘔吐 projectile vomiting　▶嘔吐反射 vomiting reflex /（咽頭反射）gag reflex　☞嘔吐物

おうとう　応答　（反応）response（返答）reply, answer　◆アレルギー応答 allergic response　換気応答 ventilatory response　ストレス応答 stress response　生体応答 biological response　免疫応答 immune response

おうとつ　凹凸（の）　（反応表面が平らでない）uneven　◆表面にわずかな凹凸があります The surface is slightly uneven.

おうとぶつ　嘔吐物　vomit /vάmɪt/, vomi-tus　◆嘔吐物は何でしたか What did you vomit? / What did the vomit look like? / What was in the vomit?　◆嘔吐物はどんな色をしていましたか What color was the vomit?　◆嘔吐物は黄色〈緑色／黒色／コーヒーかすのような色／真っ赤〉でしたか Was the vomit yellow〈green / black / the color of coffee-grounds / bright red〉?　◆嘔吐物に血が混じっていましたか Did you notice any blood in the vomit?　◆嘔吐物は便のにおいがしましたか Did the vomit have a fecal odor? / Did the vomit smell like feces[stools]?　◀コーヒー残渣様嘔吐物 coffee-grounds vomit　黒色嘔吐物 black vomit　▶嘔吐物入れ emesis basin[bowl] / vomit bowl

おうねつ　黄熱（症）　yellow fever　▶黄熱ワクチン yellow fever vaccine

おうはん　黄斑　yellow spot（of the reti-na）, macula（of the retina）　（形macular）▶黄斑円孔 macular hole　黄斑症 macul-opathy　黄斑浮腫 macular edema　☞黄斑変性

おうはんへんせい　黄斑変性　macular degeneration　◀加齢黄斑変性症 age-re-lated macular degeneration；AMD

おうふく　往復する　walk back and forth, go and come back　◆この位置から廊下の端まで6分間歩いて往復し続けて下さい Please walk back and forth between this position and the end of the hallway for six

minutes. / Please go to the end of the hallway, turn around and come[walk] back to this starting position, and keep doing this for six minutes.

オウム　parrot　◆私の言葉をオウム返しに繰り返して下さい Please repeat after me. / Please repeat what I say.　▶オウム病 parrot fever / psittacosis　オウム病クラミジア Chlamydia psittaci

おうめん　凹面（の）　concave（↔convex）

おうもんきん　横紋筋　striated muscle, striped muscle　▶横紋筋腫 rhabdomyo-ma　横紋筋肉腫 rhabdomyosarcoma　横紋筋融解症 rhabdomyolysis

おうよう　応用　application（動apply）◆遺伝子治療の臨床への応用は，新しく発展性のある分野です Clinical application of gene therapy is a new and growing field.

おうりょくしょくやさい　黄緑色野菜　yellow and green vegetables　★通例，複数形で.　☞緑黄色野菜

おうレンズ　凹レンズ　concave lens（↔con-vex lens）

おえる　終える　finish, end, close　☞終わる　◆朝食は食べ終えましたか Have you finished your breakfast yet?　◆幸せな一生を終える end[finish] a happy life

おおい　多い　《分量が》（数が）*a lot[lots] of, many　（量が）*a lot[lots] of, much　（出血量などが）heavy　◆多く, 大量, 沢山, 多量　◆（月経の）出血量は普通ですか，多いですか Is your usual flow normal or heavy?　◆多い出血 heavy bleeding　◆おりものが多い have heavy vaginal discharge　《頻度が》（頻繁な）frequent（副frequently, often）（よくある）common　◆昼食を抜くことが多いですか Do you often[fre-quently] skip lunch?　◆月経の回数が多い have frequent periods　◆この病気は高齢者に多いです This disease is common in elderly[older] people.

おおう　覆う　cover, wrap　◆傷をガーゼで覆っておきますね Let me cover the wound with gauze.

オーガズム　☞オルガスム

オーがた　O型 (type) O　(血液型)blood type O, type O blood,《英》blood group O　☞血液型

オーガニックフード　organic food(s)

おおきい　大きい
《事態などが重大な》(病気などの程度が)**serious, major**　(負担が)**heavy**　☞大きく
◆これまでに何か大きな病気や怪我をしたことがありますか Have you ever had any serious[major] illnesses or injuries?
◆大きな手術 major surgery　◆仕事上の責任が大きな負担になりますか Does the responsibility of your job weigh heavily on you?
《物理的な量が》(形・数量・寸法が)**big, large, huge**　(音が)**loud**　◆このポリープのサイズはかなり大きいです This polyp is quite big[large].　◆この検査着はあなたには大きすぎます This (exam) gown is too big [large] for you.　◆もう少し大きな声で話して下さい Please speak a little louder.

おおきく　大きく　◆口を大きく開けて下さい(広く)Please open your mouth wide.
◆大きく息を吸って下さい(深く)Take a big [deep] breath in. / Breathe in deeply.
◆大きくなったら何になりたいの(成長したら) What do you want to be when you grow up?

おおきさ　大きさ　size　☞サイズ　◆レーズンくらいの大きさのポリープがあります You have a polyp about the size of a raisin.

オーきゃく　O脚　bowlegs, bow legs
★いずれも複数形で.　(内反膝)**genu varum**

おおく　多く(の)
《沢山の》(数が)***a lot[lots] of, many**　(量が)***a lot[lots] of, much**　☞多い, 大量, 沢山, 多量　◆必須ビタミンをとるために多くの野菜を食べる必要があります You need to eat a lot of vegetables to get essential vitamins.　◆彼には多くの友人がいます He has *a lot of[lots of / many] friends.
◆彼女は家族問題について多くを語りたがりません She doesn't like to talk much about her family problems.
《大部分の》**most**　◆多くの患者さんは手術を避けたいと思われるようです Most patients would prefer to avoid surgery.
◆批判の多くは誤解に基づいていると思います I think that many[most] of the criticisms are based on misunderstandings.

オーケー　OK, okay, all right　◆万事オーケーです Everything is *all right[OK].

おおけが　大怪我　serious injury, major injury　◆事故で大怪我を負う be seriously injured in an accident / sustain serious injuries in an accident

おおげさ　大げさ　exaggeration（動**exaggerate**）◆彼は大げさに症状を訴える傾向があります He tends to exaggerate his symptoms and complain about them.
◆大げさに考えなくても大丈夫ですよ(考え過ぎないで)Don't think too much about this. You'll be fine. / (くよくよしないで)Don't dwell on this too much. You're going to be all right.

オージオメーター　audiometer

おおすぎる　多すぎる　(量が)**too much**　(数が)**too many**　◆酒量が多すぎると思います I'm afraid that you drink too much.

オーストラリア　Australia（形**Australian**）☞国籍　▶オーストラリア人(の)Australian

オーストリア　Austria（形**Austrian**）☞国籍　▶オーストリア人(の)Austrian

おおたぼはん　太田母斑　nevus of Ota

オーティー　OT,　(作業療法士)**occupational therapist**

オートアナライザー　autoanalyzer

オートプシー　autopsy　(病理解剖)**clinical autopsy**　(司法解剖)**medicolegal[forensic] autopsy**　(剖検所見)**autopsy findings**

オーバー
《誇張する》**exaggerate**　☞大げさ　◆彼はいつもオーバーに表現します He always exaggerates.
《超過する》**exceed**　◆ベッド数はすでに定員をオーバーしています The hospital bed occupancy exceeds capacity.　◆標準体重を 12 kg オーバーしています You weigh twelve kilograms more than the standard body weight. / You're twelve kilograms

over[heavier than] the ideal body weight.

オーバーベッドテーブル overbed table

オーバーユースしょうこうぐん ―症候群
（使いすぎ症候群）overuse syndrome

オーバーラップしょうこうぐん ―症候群
overlap syndrome

オーバーワーク overwork ☞過労

おおはば 大幅（に） （かなり・相当に）**considerably, substantially** ◆検査データが前回から大幅に改善しています The test results have considerably[substantially] improved over the last ones.

おおべや 大部屋 multiple occupancy room, room shared by several patients
☞病室 ◆大部屋から個室へ移動すると1日1万円の差額が必要です We'll charge you an additional ten thousand yen a day if you move from a multiple occupancy room to a private room.

おおまか 大まか ☞おおよそ

おおめ¹ 大目 ◆お酒も多少であれば大目に見ましょう（反対しない）I won't object to your drinking if you put limits on how much you drink. / （見逃す）I'll overlook[（容認する）tolerate] your drinking alcohol if you only drink a little.

おおめ² 多め **a lot of, lots of, plenty of, much** ☞多い，十分，たっぷり ◆水分を多めに摂取するよう心掛けて下さい You should try to drink *lots of[plenty of] water.

おおよそ （だいたいの）**rough** （ほぼ正確な）**approximate** （圖圖約 **around, about**）
☞大体 ◆あなたへのおおよその治療計画はできました I've made[drawn up] *a rough[an approximate] treatment plan for you. ◆それについておおよその見当がついています I have a rough idea about it. ◆MRI検査をしたのはおおよそいつごろですか Around when did you have the MRI? ◆彼女は体重がおおよそ100 kgあります She weighs about one hundred kilos. ◆おおよそそんなところです That's just about right.

オーラル oral ☞経口，口腔 ▶オーラルケア oral care

オールマイティ almighty ◆どんながんにも効くオールマイティな薬は残念ながらありません I'm afraid to say *there's no miracle cure for cancer[there isn't an almighty medication that cures all types of cancer]. ★miracle cure は特効薬.

おかあさん お母さん mother ☞母

おかげ お蔭 ◆彼がここまで回復したのは彼の妻のお蔭です He owes much of his recovery to his wife.

おかしい
《普通でない》（具合が悪い）**wrong** （変な）**strange** （普通でない）**unusual** （とっぴな）**eccentric** （常軌を逸している）**abnormal**
◆胃の調子がおかしいのですか Is there something wrong with your stomach? ★疑問文では通例 anything を用いるが，この例の場合は相手の'Yes' という答えを予測しているので something を用いる. / Do you have stomach trouble? ◆彼女は言動が少しおかしい The way she talks and acts is somewhat strange[abnormal]. ◆彼は行動がおかしい He acts[behaves] strangely. ◆彼女が予約に遅れるのはおかしい It's unusual for her to be late for her appointment. ◆服装がおかしい wear eccentric clothing / wear unusual clothes
《面白い》**funny, amusing** ◆彼の話はいつもおかしい He's always so funny[amusing].

おかす 冒す・侵す （影響を及ぼす）**affect** （損傷する）**damage** （感染させる）**infect** （攻撃する）**attack** （侵略する）**invade** （行う）**take, run** ◆この病気は徐々に中枢神経を冒すかもしれません This disease may gradually affect[damage] the central nervous system. ◆両目が冒されています Both eyes are affected. ◆インフルエンザウイルスは鼻，喉，肺を冒します The influenza virus infects the nose, throat, and lungs. ◆体の免疫システムを冒す attack the body's immune system ◆近傍組織を侵す invade the neighboring tissues ◆危険を冒す take[run] a risk

おかね お金 money ☞金銭，現金

オカレンスレポート occurrence report

おかん　**悪寒**　**chills**　★通例，複数形で.
◆悪寒がする have[get / feel] the chills
▶悪寒戦慄 chills and shivering

—おき　◆2週間おきに来て下さい Please come every two weeks.　◆この薬は6時間おきに飲んで下さい Please take this medication every six hours.　◆便通は毎日ありますか，それとも1日おきですか Do you have bowel movements every day or every other day?　◆便通は何日おきにありますか How many days apart do you empty your bowels?

おきあがる　**起き上がる**　(上体を起こす)**sit up**　(立ち上がる)**get up, stand up, rise**
◆ベッドに起き上がってもいいですよ You can[may] sit up in bed.　◆(診察の後で)さあ，起き上がっていいですよ You can get up now.　◆2時間ごとに起き上がって歩いて下さい Please try to get up and walk every two hours.　◆自力で起き上がる sit up by *oneself*

おきかえる　**置き換える**　**replace**　☞換える，取り換える　◆移植で肝臓を置き換える以外に方法はありません The only option [form of treatment] is a transplant to replace the diseased liver with a healthy liver (from another person).　◆立場を置き換えて考えてみて下さい(異なる角度[観点]から)Please think about it from a different angle[point of view].

オキシダント　**oxidant**　◀抗オキシダント antioxidant　光化学オキシダント photochemical oxidant

オキシトシン　**oxytocin**；**OXT**

オキシメーター　**oximeter** /ɑksímətɚ/；*a device that measures the saturation of oxygen in the blood*　◆このオキシメーターで酸素レベルを測ります I'm going to measure[monitor] your oxygen level with this device, called an oximeter.
◀パルスオキシメータ pulse oximeter

おぎなう　**補う**　(補充する)**supplement**　(供給する)**provide**　(埋め合わせる)**make up (for), compensate (for)**　☞補給，補充
◆ビタミンDの不足を補う supplement a vitamin D deficiency / provide supplements for vitamin D deficiency　◆ビタミン剤で食事を補っているのですか Do you supplement your diet with vitamin pills?　◆閉経後の女性に女性ホルモンを補う provide women with female hormones after menopause /(ホルモン補充療法を処方する) prescribe hormone replacement therapy to postmenopausal women
◆睡眠不足を短い昼寝で補う make up for lack of sleep by taking a short afternoon nap

おきる　**起きる**
《目覚める》(目を覚ます)**wake up**　(眠らないでいる)**stay[be] awake**　◆夜，排尿のために何回起きますか How many times do you wake[get] up to urinate at night?
◆一晩中眠れないで起きている stay[be] wide awake all night
《起き上がる》(寝床から起き出る)**get up**　(上体を起こす)**sit up**　◆毎朝何時に起きますか What time do you usually get up in the morning?　◆スミスさん，起きる時間ですよ Mr Smith, it's time to get up.
◆ベッドの上で起きてもいいですよ You can sit up in bed.
《ある事態が生じる》**have, happen**　◆喘息発作はどのくらいの頻度で起きますか How often do you have asthma attacks?

おく¹　**奥**　(後ろ)**the back**　(突き当り)**the end**　(内部)**the inside**（國**inside**）　◆目の奥が痛む Does it hurt[Do you have (a) pain] at the back of your eye(s)?
◆喉の奥が痛む have (a) pain *down in[at the back of] one's throat　◆この廊下の奥にエレベーターがあります You'll find an elevator at the end of this corridor.　◆咳は胸の奥のほうから出始めますか Does the cough start deep inside the chest?

おく²　**置く**
《物を据える》**put, place, set**　◆花瓶はベッドサイドテーブルの上に置かないで下さい Please don't put a vase on the bedside table.　◆洗面器を下の棚に置く put the washbowl on the lower shelf　◆車椅子をベッドのわきに置く place[set] the wheelchair beside the bed

《残す・ある状態を保つ》leave, keep ◆彼は家族を国に置いて日本へ来ました He came to Japan, leaving his family (behind) in his country. ◆トレイはそのままにしておいて下さい Please leave the tray as it is. ◆ベッドランプをつけたままにしておく leave the bedside lamp on ◆酸素供給装置は火気から離しておく keep the oxygen supply equipment away from heat and flame sources

おくがい　屋外(で・の)　outside(副形**outside**), **outdoors**(形**outdoor**)　☞野外 ◆屋外で作業する際には熱中症予防のためこまめに水を飲んで下さい Whenever you work outside[outdoors], drink water as often as possible to prevent heat illness.　▶屋外駐車場 parking lot /《英》car park

おくさん　奥さん　(妻)wife　(夫人)Mrs ◆アダムズさん，奥さんにも同意書にサインをしていただきたいのですが Mr Adams, may I ask *your wife[Mrs Adams] to sign this consent form, too? / I'd like *your wife[Mrs Adams] to sign this consent form, too.

おくすりてちょう　―手帳　personal medication record[handbook] ◆おくすり手帳を持っていますか．お持ちでしたら見せて下さい Do you have your personal medication record? If you do, may I see it?

おくない　屋内(で・の)　inside(副形**inside**), **indoors**(形**indoor**)　◆病院の屋内は全面禁煙になっております Smoking is not allowed anywhere inside the hospital.　▶屋内駐車場 parking garage /《英》indoor car park　屋内プール indoor swimming pool

おくば　奥歯　back tooth　(大臼歯)molar (tooth)(複teeth)　☞歯

おくび　(曖気)belching, burping, eructation　☞げっぷ

おくやみ　お悔やみ　condolence /kəndóuləns/　◆お母さまのご逝去をお悔やみ申し上げます I'm very sorry about your mother's passing away. / Please accept my condolences on the death of your mother. ◆お悔やみを述べる express [offer] *one's* condolences

おくらせる　遅らせる　delay　(速度を落とす)slow (down)　(延期する)*put off, postpone ◆がんの進行を遅らせる delay [slow] the cancer's progression ◆予約を来週まで遅らせる *put off[postpone] the appointment until next week

おくりむかえ　送り迎え ◆ご家族またはお友達で病院への送り迎えのできる人はいますか Do you have someone in your family or a friend who can bring you to and from the hospital?

おくりもの　贈り物　gift, present ◆お志はありがたいのですが，贈り物はご遠慮申し上げます Thank you for the kind thought [I appreciate your kindness], but I *have to decline[can't accept] your gift.

おくる　送る

《発送する》　(手紙・メールなどを出す)send ◆ご要望のあった紹介状は今日中に送ります I'll send the referral letter you requested before the end of the day. ◆もし何か不明な点がありましたら，メールをお送り下さい If there's anything *you don't understand[you're unsure of], please *send me an email[email me].

《届ける》　(供給する)provide ◆胃瘻を通して栄養物を直接胃に送る provide nutrients directly into the stomach through a feeding tube

《暮らす》live, lead　(時を過ごす)spend ◆規則正しい生活を送る live[lead] a well-balanced[regulated] life / keep regular hours ◆安らかな余生を送る spend the rest of *one's* life peacefully / live the rest of *one's* days[life] in peace

おくれ　遅れる　(予定・進行が遅れる)be late (for), **be delayed　(図delay)**, **be behind** (進歩が遅い)**be slow　(月経・出産が予定日より遅くなる)be overdue** ◆遅れてすみません I'm sorry I'm late. ◆約束の時間に遅れる be late for *one's* appointment ◆彼女は月経が 10 日間遅れています Her (menstrual) period is ten days late[delayed]. ◆救急車を呼ぶのが遅れた There was a delay in calling the ambulance. ◆手術は1週間遅れる見込みです The surgery will be a week late[behind schedule]. ◆（掲示）混雑状況によっては遅れが生じることがあります Delays can be expected at busy times. ◆ピーター君は発達が少し遅れているようです Peter seems to be a little slow[behind] in his development. ◆分娩は予定日から2週間遅れています The delivery is two weeks overdue.

おこす　起こす ☞起こる
《目覚めさせる》**wake（up）** ◆（夜間見回りなどで）すみません，起こしてしまいましたか Sorry, did I wake you up?
《発症する》**have, get, become, develop** ◆心臓発作を起こす have a heart attack ◆てんかんの発作をよく起こしますか Do you often have epileptic seizures? ◆傷口が感染を起こしています The wound has got[become] infected. ◆食べ過ぎで消化不良を起こす get[have] indigestion from overeating ◆風邪から肺炎を起こしています Your cold has developed into pneumonia. ◆めまいを起こす feel[grow] dizzy ◆大量出血を起こす bleed massively[copiously] / lose a lot of blood
《原因となる》**cause** ◆問題を起こす cause a problem

おこたる　怠る　neglect ◆体調管理を怠らないで下さい You shouldn't neglect to take care of yourself. / （いくら注意しても注意しすぎることはない）You can't be too careful about your condition. ◆親の義務を怠る neglect one's duties as *a parent[parents]

おこなう　行う　do, perform, carry out, conduct ◆頭部外傷の緊急手術を行う do[perform / carry out] emergency surgery for a person's head injury ◆気管支鏡検査を行う do[perform / carry out] a bronchoscopic examination

おこりっぽい　怒りっぽい （いらいらしている）**irritable, irritated** ☞怒る ◆怒りっぽくなる get[feel] irritable ◆ご主人は最近怒りっぽいですか Is your husband easily irritated recently?

おこる¹　起こる ☞起こす，発症，発生
《発症する》**have, get, come on, develop** ◆痛みが起こるのはたいていいつですか When do you usually have[get] the pain? / When does the pain usually come on? ◆痛みの起こり方は突然でしたか，徐々でしたか Did the pain *come on[develop] suddenly or gradually? ◆痛みはどんな起こり方ですか How does the pain come on?
《ある事態が生じる》**occur, happen** ◆合併症が起こる可能性が少しあります There is a small chance[possibility] that complications will occur. ◆申し訳ありませんでした．今後このようなことが起こらないように注意いたします We're very sorry. We'll be very careful to make sure that this never happens again.
《あることが原因で生じる》**result（from）, be caused（by）, arise** ◆この症状は食べすぎ〈睡眠不足〉からよく起こります This symptom often results from overeating〈lack of sleep〉. ◆多くの子宮頸がんはヒトパピローマウイルスによって起こります Most cervical cancers are caused by the human papillomavirus. ◆その医療ミスは不注意から起こったものです That medical error arose from carelessness.

おこる²　怒る　get[be] angry （気分を害する）**get[be] upset** ◆何に怒っているのですか What are you at? ◆なぜそんなに怒っているのですか Why are you so upset[angry]? ◆誰があなたを怒らせるようなことを言いましたか Who said something to make you angry? ◆お願いですから，そんなに怒らないで下さい Please don't be so angry[upset].

おさえる¹　押さえる　hold（down） ◆（注射の後で）2, 3分ほどこのアルコール消毒綿を押さえておいて下さい Please hold this alcohol wipe down on your skin for a few minutes.

おさえる²　抑える （減らす）**reduce** （抑制する）**suppress** （コントロールする）**control, check, restrain** （止める）**stop** （最小限にする）**minimize** ◆胃酸の分泌を抑える

reduce[suppress] the secretion of stomach acid ◆アレルギー反応を抑える suppress the allergic reaction ◆感情〈怒り〉を抑える control[check / restrain] *one's* emotions〈anger〉 ◆吐き気を抑える薬 a medication to stop nausea / an antinausea medication ◆リスクを抑える minimize a risk

おさまる　治まる　（消える）go（away）, disappear, clear up　（症状が和らぐ）subside （止まる）stop　◆痛みは治まりましたか Has the pain gone（away）? ◆この薬で痛みが治まるでしょう The pain should disappear[go away] with this medication. / If you take this medication, the pain will disappear[clear up / stop]. ◆炎症は2, 3日で治まるでしょう The inflammation will subside in a few days. ◆彼女の咳の発作は治まりました Her coughing fit has stopped.

おさん　お産　（出産）childbirth　（分娩）delivery　（陣痛）labor　☞出産, 分娩　◆お産が軽い〈重い〉have *an easy*〈a difficult〉delivery　◆今回が初めてのお産ですか Is this your first childbirth[delivery]? / Is this the first time for you to give birth?

おしい　惜しい　◆惜しいですね，目標体重まであともう少しです What a pity [shame]! *You almost reached your target weight[You're so close to your weight-loss goal]. ◆惜しい人を亡くしました His〈Her〉death is a great loss to us all. He〈She〉was a wonderful[precious] person. ★「私たちにとって大きな痛手です．素晴らしい「大切な」人でしたから」という意味．

おじいさん　（祖父）grandfather　（高齢の男性）old man, elderly man　☞祖父

おしえる　教える

《指導する》teach　◆日本の学生に英語を教えているのですか Do you teach English to Japanese students?

《情報を伝える》tell, give, let *a person* know　☞知らせる　◆あなたの電話番号を教えて下さい Please tell[give] me your phone number. ◆便がどんな色をしているか教えて下さい What color are your

stools? / Please tell me what color your stools are. ◆痛かったら教えて下さい Let me know[Tell me] if it hurts.

おしたおす　押し倒す　push（over）◆彼は組みつかれて背後から押し倒された際に頭部を強打しました He got hit hard in the head when he was tackled and pushed over from behind.

おしっこ　pee, pee-pee, wee-wee　☞尿　◆おしっこしたい？ Do you want to *go pee[do a wee-wee]? ★大人には Do you want to go to the restroom? と声をかける

おしむ　惜しむ　◆友人との別れを惜しむ（悲しいと思う）feel sad when *one* has to part from *one's* friend(s) / （別れに気が進まない）be reluctant to part from *one's* friend(s)

おしめ　☞おむつ

おしゃぶり　（乳首の形をした）pacifier, dummy　（リング状の）teething ring

おしょうすい　お小水　urine　☞尿

おしるし　（お産の徴候）(bloody) show, sign of the onset of labor　◆おしるしがありましたか Have you noticed a bloody show? / Have you had your show yet?

おしん　悪心　nausea　☞吐き気

おす　押す　push　（圧を加える）press, apply pressure (to)　（ぎゅっと押し込む）squeeze　◆車椅子を押す push a wheelchair　◆ご用の時はこのコールボタンを押して下さい Please push[press] this call button when you want us. ◆ゆっくり息を吸い込むと同時に吸入器を押して下さい Breathe in slowly and push down on the inhaler at the same time. ◆この絆創膏を2, 3分押していて下さい Please hold this Band-Aid down and apply pressure for a few minutes. ◆むくみは押すとへこんだままですか Does a dent remain in the area if you press the swelling? ◆ここを押すと痛みますか Does it hurt here when I press it? / Is this area tender? ◆分泌物は押すと出ますか Does the discharge come out with pressure? ◆少し押される感じがするかもしれませんが，痛くはありません You may feel a little gentle pressure, but it's not painful. ◆乳頭を押すと分泌物が出る the discharge comes out *when *one* squeezes[when *one* applies pressure to] the nipple(s)

オスグッド・シュラッターびょう ―病
Osgood–Schlatter disease

オスラーけっせつ ―結節 Osler nodules
[nodes] ★通例，複数形で．

おすわり お座りする sit (up) ☞座る
◆お子さんはお座りができますか Is your baby[child] able to sit (up) without any support? ◆どうぞお座り下さい Please sit down. / Take a seat, please.

おせん 汚染 contamination (圏contaminated), pollution (圏polluted) ◆細菌による汚染 bacterial contamination ◆この病気は汚染された水が原因で起こります This disease is caused by contaminated water. ◆汚染された血液製剤 contaminated blood products ◀環境汚染 environmental pollution 光化学汚染 photochemical pollution 水質汚染 water pollution 大気汚染 air pollution 放射能汚染 radioactive contamination[pollution] ▶汚染物質 contaminant / pollutant / polluting substance

おそ 悪阻 vomiting, emesis ☞吐き気，嘔吐 ◀妊娠悪阻 excessive vomiting in pregnancy / hyperemesis gravidarum；HG

おそい 遅い
《時間が遅い》**late** (↔early) (圏late) ◆いつも遅くまで仕事をしますか Do you usually work late? ◆来るのが遅くなってすみません I'm sorry I'm late. ◆この治療を始めるのは今からでも遅くはありません It's still not too late to start this treatment.
《速度が遅い》**slow** (↔fast, quick) (圏slowly) ◆彼は動作が遅い He moves slowly. / He is slow in his movements.
◆反応が遅い be slow to respond ◆発達が遅い develop slowly ◆脈が遅い The pulse is slow.

おそかれはやかれ 遅かれ早かれ (いずれは)**sooner or later** ★日本語と語順が逆になる． (最後には)**eventually** (そのうちに)**in**

due course ◆彼女は遅かれ早かれ何が起こったかを知ることになるでしょう Sooner or later she's going to find out what happened. ◆遅かれ早かれ回復しますから，あせらないで下さい You will get better eventually[in due course], so don't be so impatient[restless].

おそらく 恐らく probably, likely (ややくだけた調子で)**maybe** ★可能性の一番高いのはprobably(十中八九)，一番低いのはmaybe．
◆この薬を飲めば恐らく気分がよくなるでしょう You'll probably feel better after taking this medication. ◆岸先生は恐らく明日の朝診察にお見えになります Dr Kishi *is probably coming to see you[will probably come and see you] tomorrow morning. ◆便秘は恐らく薬のせいでしょう Probably[Maybe] it's the medication *that has caused[that's causing] the constipation. ◆その痛みは恐らく2，3日で消えるでしょう The pain will probably go away in a couple of days. ◆現在満床なので，今日の入院は恐らく難しいと思います There are no empty beds available in the hospital at present, so I'm afraid it'll probably be difficult to accept new patients today. ★悪い結果を予想する時にI'm afraidを用いる．

おそれ 恐れ (可能性)**possibility** (心配)**fear** (危険性)**danger** (疑い)**suspicion** (圏suspect)** ☞疑い ◆転移の恐れがあるので，治療を続けましょう There's a possibility[danger] of the cancer spreading, so let's continue the treatment. / We can suspect metastasis, so let's continue the treatment. ◆肺炎を起こす恐れがあります There's some possibility of developing pneumonia. / Pneumonia may develop.
◆この病気が再発する恐れはほとんどありません There's little possibility of this disease recurring. ◆彼女には自殺の恐れがあります There's a danger that she might commit suicide. ◆失明する恐れはありません(心配する理由はない)There's no reason to worry about losing your sight.

おそれる 恐れる be afraid (of), fear

◆何を恐れているのですか What are you afraid of? ◆再発を恐れているのですか Are you afraid *that the disease may recur[of the disease recurring]? ◆お産を必要以上に恐れることはありません You don't have to be overly afraid of the delivery. ◆感染の拡大を恐れる fear the spread of infection

おそろしい 恐ろしい (ぞっとする)terrible (身の毛もよだつほど怖い)horrible ◆恐ろしい夢を見たのですか Did you have a terrible[bad / horrible] dream? / Did you have a nightmare? ◆この病気が恐ろしいのは，初期にはほとんどの人に自覚症状がないことです The terrible thing about this disease is that in its early stages most people *have no symptoms that they are aware of[have no subjective symptoms].

オゾン ozone

おだいじに お大事に ◆どうぞお大事に Please take (good) care of yourself. / Take care!

おだく 汚濁 (汚染)pollution (液体の混濁)turbidity ☞汚染

おたふくかぜ ☞ムンプス

おだやかな 穏やかな (温暖な)mild (静かな・くつろいだ)quiet, relaxing, relaxed (効き目がゆるやかな)mild (温厚な)gentle, mild (安らかな)peaceful ◆今日は晴れて穏やかなので，外でお散歩でもいかがですか It's sunny and mild today. How about taking a walk outside? ◆穏やかな気分でいる feel relaxed ◆ご家族と穏やかな一日を過ごされましたか Did you have a quiet[relaxing] day with your family? ◆この薬は穏やかに作用します This medication will have a mild effect on your body. ◆彼女は性格が穏やかです She has a gentle[mild] disposition. ◆穏やかな死を迎える die a peaceful death / die[pass away] peacefully

おちいる 陥る fall[get, go](into) (徐々に)lapse(into) (急に)be thrown(into) ◆昏睡状態に陥る fall[lapse] into a coma ◆パニックに陥る get[go] into a panic / be thrown into a panic ◆窮地に陥っている be in a very difficult situation

おちこむ 落ち込む feel[get, become] depressed, feel down ◆気分が落ち込むのはいつですか，朝ですか，それとも夕方ですか When do you feel depressed, in the morning or in the evening? ◆気分はいつから落ち込んでいますか How long have you felt depressed (like this)?

おちつかない 落ち着かない (そわそわした)restless (不安などでいらいらした)nervous (動揺した)unsettled ◆彼女は手術を前にして落ち着かない様子です She appears[looks] nervous[unsettled] ahead of the surgery. ◆落ち着かない(そわそわしている)be[feel] restless /(不安などでいらいらしている)be[feel] nervous /(じっとしていられない)be[feel] fidgety

おちつき 落ち着き calmness (㊌calm) (冷静さ)composure (㊌composed) ☞落ち着かない ◆その患者さんは落ち着きがあって，しかも思いやりもあります That patient appears[is] calm, and he〈she〉is considerate as well. ◆落ち着きを失う lose *one's* composure /(そわそわする)get [become] restless ◆落ち着きを保つ keep *one's* composure ◆落ち着きを取り戻す regain[recover] *one's* composure

おちつく 落ち着く 《心が穏やかになる》(平静になる)calm down (㊌calm, cool) (リラックスする)relax (㊌relaxed) ◆どうぞ落ち着いて下さい(興奮・動揺している相手に)Please calm down. /(相手が興奮・動揺しそうな話題を持ち出す時に)Please remain calm. /(不安そうな相手に)Please relax. / Please take it easy. ★take it easy はくだけた調子で言う。 ◆2，3回深呼吸をして下さい．落ち着きますよ Take a few deep breaths. It will calm you down. 《状態が安定した》stable ◆今のところ彼女の病状は落ち着いています Her condition is now stable. / She is in a stable condition for now.

おちる 落ちる 《落下する》fall ◆階段から落ちないように注意して下さい Please be careful not to fall down the stairs ◆ベッドから落ちる

fall out of (*one's*) bed　◆深い眠りに落ちる fall into a deep sleep

《機能などが衰える》**fail, decline**　☞衰える

◆視力〈腎機能／肝機能〉が落ちてきていますね Your eyesight〈kidney function / liver function〉is failing[declining].　◆納豆を食べるとワーファリンの効果が落ちますので，食べないようにして下さい（効果を低下させるので）Natto reduces the effect of warfarin, so please *don't eat it[refrain from eating it].

《比較して劣る》　◆この種類のがんは，ほかの種類と比べて抗がん剤による治療効果は落ちます Chemotherapy is usually not as effective in this type of cancer as it is in some other types.

おつうじ　お通じ　bowel movement
☞排便, 便, 便通

おつかれさま　お疲れ様　★このねぎらいの表現は状況に応じて使い分ける．　◆さあ，終わりました．お疲れ様（よくやりましたね）That's it. All finished. Well done!　◆今日はここまでにしましょう．お疲れ様（見事にやり遂げましたね）That's all for today. You did a good job![Good job! / You did well.]
◆お疲れ様（疲れすぎてないといいのですが）I hope you're not too tired. / I hope we didn't make you too tired. /（お疲れになったでしょう）You must be tired.　◆お疲れ様（ありがとう）Thank you! / Thank you for your patience.　◆お疲れ様（さようなら）See you! / See you tomorrow morning! / See you next time!

オッズひ　―比　odds ratio；OR

オッディかつやくきん　―括約筋　sphincter of Oddi

おっと　夫　husband　☞主人

おっぱい　(乳房)**breast**　(母乳)**breast milk, mother's milk**　☞乳房, 母乳

おつり　お釣り　change　◆300円のお釣りになります Here's your three hundred yen change. / That's three hundred yen in change.

おてあらい　お手洗い　(公共施設の)**restroom, lavatory,**《英》**toilet**　(個人の家の)**bathroom**　★浴室とトイレを兼ねる．☞トイレ

おでき　boil, furuncle　◆首におできができる get[have] a boil on *one's* neck　◆おできの膿を出す drain[let out] the pus from a boil

おでこ　forehead, brow /brάʊ/　☞額

おと　音　(一般的に物音)**sound**　(一定の高さの音・音色)**tone**　(雑音)**noise**　(心臓などの雑音)**murmur**　◆何か音が聞こえますか Do you hear anything?　◆どういう音が聞こえにくいですか What kind of sounds do you have difficulty hearing?　◆耳鳴りはどんな音ですか What kind of ringing sound do you hear in your ears?　◆テレビの音を小さく〈大きく〉する turn down〈up〉the sound on the TV　◆(検査で)機器がカチカチという音を出しますが，心配しないで下さい The machine makes a knocking noise, but don't worry.　◆それでは胸の音を聴かせて下さい Now, let me listen to your heart and lungs.　◆音を出す[立てる]make a sound[noise]　◆音の大きさ loudness　◆音の高さ pitch

音のいろいろ　☞耳鳴り
●高い音 high sound /（高音域の・かん高い）high-pitched sound /（音の調子が高い）high-pitched tone　●低い音 low sound /（低音域の）low-pitched sound /（音の調子が低い）low-pitched tone　●大きい音 loud sound　●小さい音 feeble sound　●鋭い音 piercing sound　●鈍い音 dull sound　●耳障りな音 unpleasant[harsh] sound　●がんがん響く音 banging[roaring] sound　●ゼイゼイする音 wheezing[wheezy] sound / wheeze　●ヒューヒューする音 whistling sound　●ブーンブーンする音 buzzing sound

おとうさん　お父さん　father　☞父

おとうと　弟　(younger, little) brother
★英語では通例，brother のみでよい．

おとがい　頤　lower jaw　(下あごの先)**chin**　☞顎

オトガイりゅうき　―隆起　mental protuberance

おどかす　脅かす　scare, frighten　◆脅か

すようですが，このまま放置すると失明する可能性があります I don't want to scare [frighten] you, but if we don't do anything, there's a possibility that you'll lose your sight.

おとこ　男　man（圏men）（男の子）**boy**（男の赤ちゃん）**baby boy**　☞男性　◆（分娩後に）おめでとうございます，男のお子さんですよ Congratulations! It's a boy.　▶男親 father / male parent　男きょうだい brother / male sibling

おとしもの　落とし物　**lost article, lost property**　☞遺失物

おとす　落とす
《物を落下させる》**drop**　◆よく物を落としますか Do you often drop things?
《減らす・失う》**lose, shed**　◆体重を10 kg落とす必要があります You need to lose [shed] ten kilos.　◆部屋の鍵を落とす lose *one's* room key　◆命を落とす lose *one's* life
《音・声を小さくする》**turn down, lower**　◆テレビのボリュームを落としていただけませんか Could you *turn down[lower] the volume on your TV?
《除去する》**take off, remove**　◆お化粧を落としていただいてもよろしいですか Could you please *take off[remove] your make-up?

おどす　脅す　scare, frighten　☞脅かす

おととい　一昨日　the day before yesterday

おとな　大人（成人）**adult**（子供からみた大人）**grown-up**　◆大人用の紙おむつは売店で売っています They sell disposable (absorbent) briefs[underwear / pads] at the hospital shop.　★おむつを adult diaper とも言うが，不快感を与えるので患者には用いないほうがよい．　◆大人になったら何になりたいの What do you want to be when you grow up?

おとなしい　大人しい（物静かな）**quiet**（温厚な）**gentle**（従順な）**obedient**　◆おとなしくしてね Be quiet! / (いい子にしてね) Be a good boy〈girl〉!　◆彼女はおとなしくて思いやりのある女性です She is a gentle,

caring woman.　◆彼はおとなしく担当医の指示に従いました He obediently followed his doctor's instructions.

おとる　劣る　be inferior（to）　◆ジェネリック薬はブランド薬に劣ると感じている人が多いようですが，決してそんなことはありません Many people feel that generic drugs are inferior to brand-name drugs, and this is simply not true.　◆この降圧薬の1日1回投与は1日2回投与に劣りません（同様に効果がある）This once-daily antihypertensive works just as well as the twice-daily one.

おとろえる　衰える（体力などが弱る）**become weak, weaken**（衰弱する）**decline**（記憶力・視力などが弱る）**fail**　☞落ちる，衰弱　◆筋力が衰えています The muscles have become weak.　◆免疫システムの衰え weakening of the immune system　◆彼は短期記憶が衰え始めています His short-term memory is beginning to fail[decline].

おどろく　驚く　be surprised（精神的な衝撃を受ける）**be shocked**（圏驚くべき・すごい **remarkable, astonishing**）　◆手術後の回復の速さにみんな本当に驚いています We're all really surprised at your quick [speedy] recovery from the surgery.　◆乳がんとわかってさぞ驚かれたことでしょう You must have been shocked to find out that you have breast cancer.　◆もう杖なしで歩けるとは驚くべき回復力ですね You no longer need a cane to walk. What a remarkable[astonishing] recovery you've made!

おなか　お腹（胃部・横隔膜から骨盤まで）**stomach**（腹部）**abdomen** /ǽbdəmən/（圏**abdóminal**）（腸）**bowels** /báʊəlz/（インフォーマルに）**belly**（幼児語）**tummy**　☞腹（はら），腹部　◆お腹がいっぱいだ be full / feel stuffed　◆お腹がすく get[be] hungry　◆いつもよりお腹が空かないのですか〈空いていますか〉Are you less〈more〉hungry than usual?　◆お腹が出ている have a pot[beer] belly
《症状の表現》　◆お腹が痛む have a

おなか　　　　　　　　　　　93　　　　　　　　　　おぼえる

stomachache / have (an) abdominal pain / have (a) pain in the stomach[abdomen]　◆お腹がキリキリ差し込むように痛む have (a) griping[spasmodic] pain in the abdomen　☞痛み　◆お腹がゴロゴロしている one's stomach is rumbling[growling / grumbling]　◆お腹に湿疹がある have a rash on one's abdomen　◆お腹をこわす upset one's stomach / get an upset stomach　◆お腹に痛みや不快感がある have (a) pain or discomfort in one's abdomen

《診察の基本表現》　◆お腹が張っていますか Do you feel heavy in the stomach? / Does your stomach feel bloated?　◆お腹を診察〈触診〉しましょう I'm going to examine 〈feel / palpate〉your abdomen.　◆ズボンを下げてお腹を見せて下さい Please lower your pants and show me your abdomen.　◆お腹の力を抜く relax one's abdominal muscles / release the tension in one's abdominal muscles　◆お腹をふくらませる *push out[inflate] one's abdomen　◆お腹をひっこめる suck[pull / draw] in one's abdomen

《所見・処置の表現》　◆お腹の風邪(ウイルス感染症) stomach flu / viral gastroenteritis　◆お腹の毛をそる shave a person's abdomen　◆お腹の手術をする(手術を受ける) have abdominal surgery / (手術を行う)do [perform / carry out] surgery on a person's abdomen

おなじ　同じ　(同一の)the same　(ほぼ同じの)similar　(まったく同一の)identical　☞同等，等しい　◆血圧はいつもと同じ条件で測って下さい Please take your blood pressure under the same conditions as usual.　◆以前にも同じ症状がありましたか Have you had similar symptoms before?　◆それでは同じことの繰り返しになりますよ That way[Then], you'll keep getting the same results.　◆一卵性双生児はほぼ同じ遺伝子をもっています Monozygotic twins have almost[nearly] identical genes.　◆その点に関して私の考えも同じです(賛成する)I agree with you on that.

オナニー　masturbation　☞自慰
おなら　gas　☞ガス　◆おならをする pass gas / break wind　◆(検査で)空気を入れますから，しばらくおならを我慢して下さい I'm going to insert air, so please don't pass gas for a while.

おねがい　お願い　hope　(実現の可能性が低い願い)wish　(強い願い)desire　(依頼)request　☞願い

おねしょ　bedwetting　(動wet the bed)，nocturnal[nighttime] enuresis　◆お子さんは現在もおねしょをしますか Does your child still wet the bed?

おばあさん　(祖母)grandmother　(高齢の女性)old woman, elderly woman　☞祖母

おはよう　◆ヒルさん，おはようございます Good morning, Mr Hill!　◆ナンシー，おはよう Morning, Nancy!　★"Morning"はインフォーマル.

おびえる　怯える　get[be] afraid (of)，get[be] scared (of)，get[be] frightened (of)　◆そのウイルスに怯える必要はありません．むしろ体調管理には十分に注意を払って下さい The virus is not something you need to be afraid[frightened] of. Instead[Rather], you should take good care of yourself.

オピオイド　opioid
おぶつ　汚物　(病院の廃棄物)medical wastes, hospital wastes　(人間・動物の排泄物)human wastes, excreta　★wastes, excreta は複数形で.　▶汚物入れ medical waste[sanitary] container　汚物処理室 dirty utility room / (尿・便などの)soiled (linen) utility room / (汚染物質の)utility room for contaminants

オブラート　wafer paper　◆この粉薬はオブラートに包んで飲んで下さい Please wrap this powder in wafer paper before swallowing[taking] it.

オペ　operation　☞手術　▶オペ室 operating room：OR
おぼえる　覚える
《学習する》learn　◆松葉杖の使い方を覚える必要があります You need to learn how to use crutches.

おぼえる　94　おもいあたる

《記憶する》remember　◆お父さんは昔のことを覚えていますか Does your father remember things that happened in the past?　◆これから３つの単語を言います．私が全部言い終わった後でその３つを復唱し，その後よく覚えておいて下さい I'm going to say three words. Please repeat the words after I've said all three, and then try to remember them.

《感じる》feel　◆背中に痛みを覚える feel (a) pain in *one's* back　◆ひどく疲れを覚える feel very tired

おぼれる　溺れる　（溺死する）**drown**/dráʊn/, **be drowned**　◆川で溺れて死ぬ drown[be drowned] in the river　◆溺れて死にかける be almost[nearly] drowned

おまたせ　お待たせ　◆お待たせして（本当に）申し訳ありません I'm (terribly / very) sorry to have kept you waiting. / I'm (terribly / very) sorry about the wait.　◆お待たせしました Thank you so much for waiting. / （患者さんから「お水をいただけませんか」などと頼まれて手渡しながら）Here you are.　★Here it is. とも言う．

おまる　bedpan

おむつ

《幼児用》diaper/dáɪəpɚ/, **《英》nappy**　（パンツ型の）**pull-up[pull-on] diaper**　◆お子さんはおむつを毎日何枚濡らしますか How many diapers does your child wet a day?　◆おむつを換える change a diaper　◆まだおむつをしている be still in diapers

《成人用》incontinence（absorbent）briefs[underwear], adult diaper　（パッド型の）**incontinence（absorbent）pad**　（パンツ型の）**adult pull-up[pull-on] briefs[underwear]**　★ほとんどの人が diaper という語に不快感をもつので，成人の患者には用いないほうがよい．話しかけるときには incontinence や absorbent を使わずに，briefs, underwear, pad などのみに言う．　◆おむつを換える change *a person's*（incontinence）briefs[underwear / pad]

◀紙おむつ（使い捨ての）disposable diaper /（成人用）disposable（incontinence）briefs

[underwear / pad] /（紙製の）paper diaper /（成人用）paper（incontinence）briefs[underwear / pad]　布おむつ cloth diaper　▶おむつカバー diaper cover　おむつかぶれ diaper rash　おむつ交換 diaper change /（成人）（incontinence）briefs[underwear / pad] change　おむつ皮膚炎 diaper dermatitis

おめでた　◆おめでたです．今妊娠５週目です You're expecting a baby. You're five weeks pregnant.

おめでとう　◆ご出産おめでとう Congratulations on the birth of your baby boy〈girl〉!　★Congratulations は常に複数形で．　◆お誕生日おめでとう Happy birthday (to you)!　◆ご退院おめでとうございます I'm glad you're leaving the hospital. Congratulations[Good for you]!

おもい　重い

《病状が重い》（深刻な）**serious**　（危篤状態の）**critical**　（痛みなどが激しい・ひどい）**severe**（↔mild）（程度が重大な・命に関わるような）**massive, major**（↔minor）　◆彼の病状はかなり重いです His condition is rather serious[critical].　◆重い症状がある have serious symptoms　◆重い心臓発作 massive[major / severe] heart attack

《心身が重苦しい》heavy　（気が滅入った）**depressed**　◆頭が重いのですか Do you have a heavy feeling in the head? / Does your head feel heavy?　◆気が重い feel depressed

《重量がある》heavy（↔light）　◆重い物を運んだり〈持ち上げたり〉しないで下さい Please don't carry〈lift〉heavy things.

《重要である》important　◆会社で責任の重い立場にあって，さぞストレスが溜まるのではありませんか Aren't you under a lot of stress, since you *hold an important position[have a lot of responsibility] in your company?

おもいあたる　思い当たる　（特定できる）**identify**　◆何か思い当たる誘因はありましたか Was there any cause that you could identify?　◆思い当たる原因がなく憂鬱になる（明白な理由がなく）feel depressed for no obvious reason

おもいうかぶ　思い浮かぶ　(思い出させる)
remind of　(考え付く)**think of**　(心に浮かぶ)**come to mind**　◆この図柄から何が思い浮かびますか What does this pattern *remind you of[make you think of]?
◆ぴったりした英語の表現が思い浮かびません I can't think of the right English expression. / The right English expression doesn't come to mind.

おもいきり　思い切り　◆このレバーを思い切り強く握って下さい(できるだけ力を込めて) Please grip this lever as firmly as possible.　◆合図と同時に息を思い切り吐いて下さい(できるだけ強く速く)Please breathe out as hard and fast as you can the moment *I say "Now"[I give you the signal].

おもいきる　思い切る　(決心する)**make up** *one's* **mind**　◆思い切って手術を受けてよかったですね You made up your mind and had the surgery. That's good!

おもいだす　思い出す　(覚えている)**remember**　(記憶をよみがえらせる)**recall, recollect**　◆彼女は最近のことが思い出せない She can't remember recent[short-term / new] things.　◆昔を思い出す remember[recall] the past

おもいつく　思いつく　think of　(心に浮かぶ)**come to mind**　☞思い浮かぶ

おもいつめる　思い詰める　(考え過ぎる)**think too much**　☞悩む　◆そう思い詰める必要はありません You're thinking too much. You shouldn't do that. / You don't have to think too much like that.

おもいで　思い出　(記憶)**memory, remembrance**　(思い出すこと)**recollection**　▶思い出話 reminiscences　★複数形で. / talking about the old days

おもいなやむ　思い悩む　have worries, be worried about　☞思い詰める，悩む

おもう　思う　(考える)**think**　(望む)**hope, want**　(期待する)**expect**　(不安に思う・恐れる)**be afraid**(of)**, fear**　(感じる)**feel**　(みなす)**consider, take, regard**　(推測する)**suppose**　(信じる)**believe**　☞思われる，考える

◆あなたはこのことについてどう思いますか What do you think about[of] this? / What's your opinion about[on] this?
◆おっしゃる通りだと思います I think you're right. / I think so, too. / That's what I think.　◆私はそうは思いません I don't think so. / I don't see it like that. / I disagree.　◆1，2週間で良くなると思います I hope you will get better in a week or so.　◆そんなに早く回復しないと思います I'm afraid[I fear] that you will not recover so soon.　◆私はそれが最善の方法だと思います I consider it to be the best option. / In my opinion, it's the best option.

おもくるしい　重苦しい　(胃にもたれる)**heavy**　(息が詰まるような)**stifling** /stáɪflɪŋ/　◆胃が重苦しい have a heavy feeling in *one's* stomach / *one's* stomach feels heavy　◆胸が重苦しい have a stifling sensation in *one's* chest　◆重苦しい雰囲気 a stifling atmosphere

おもさ　重さ　weight

おもしろい　面白い　(楽しむ・楽しく過ごす)**enjoy, have a good time**　(興味をそそる)**be interesting**　(とても愉快である)**have fun**
◆学校は面白いですか Do you enjoy school[college] (life)? / Do you have a good time at school?　◆お仕事に面白みを感じていますか Do you enjoy your work? / Do you find your work interesting?　◆そのテレビ番組は面白いですか Is that TV program interesting? / Do you enjoy watching that TV program? / (患者がテレビを観ている時に)Are you enjoying the program?　◆それは面白い見解ですね That's an interesting opinion[point of view / way of seeing things].　◆この雑誌はとても面白いですよ This magazine is really fun.　★fun は「楽しくさせてくれる物」という意味.

おもしろくない　面白くない　◆何か面白くないことでもあったのですか Did anything happen that you didn't like? / (不愉快な[嫌な]ことが起こったか)Did anything unpleasant[nasty] happen?

おもて　表

《戸外》the outside（쪮outside, outdoors）　◆お子さんはよく表で遊びますか Does your child often play outside?
《表面》the front（쮼外面的な outer）　◆紙の表と裏を区別する tell the difference between the front and the back of a sheet of paper　◆心の裏と表 inner and outer self　☞表玄関，オモテ検査

おもてげんかん　表玄関　（正面の入り口）the front door（主たる入口）the main entrance　◆表玄関から出入りして下さい Please use *the front door[the main entrance].

オモテけんさ ―検査　forward typing（↔reverse typing）

おもな　主な　main, chief（他と比較して大きな）major　☞主要　◆今日受診された主な理由を教えて下さい Please tell me your main[chief] reason *for coming to see me[you came to see me].　◆COPD の主な原因は喫煙です The main cause of COPD is smoking.　◆主な役割を果たす play a major role

おもに¹　主に　（主として）mainly, chiefly, predominantly　（ほとんど・大部分）mostly　◆咳が出るのは主に夜間ですか，それとも早朝ですか Do you cough[Do you have the cough] mainly at night or early in the morning?　◆この病気は主に子供に発症します This disease occurs mainly[predominantly] in children.　◆どんな音楽を主に聴いていますか What kind of music do you mostly listen to?

おもに²　重荷　burden, load　☞負担

おもゆ　重湯　rice gruel

おもらし　お漏らしする　wet　☞漏らす

おもわしくない　思わしくない　◆検査結果は思わしくありませんでした（期待はずれだった）The test results were not *what I'd hoped for[what I'd expected]. /（失望させるような）The test results were disappointing[not satisfactory].　◆ご主人の容体は思わしくありません（かなり深刻です）Your husband's condition is rather serious.

おもわれる　思われる　seem, appear　☞思う　◆この方法は役に立つと思われます This method seems to be useful.　◆この症状は遺伝子の異常からくるものと思われます This symptom appears to result from a genetic abnormality.

おや　親　parent（쮼parental）　（両親）parents　◆親が子供に干渉しすぎると親子関係がだめになるかもしれません Extreme interference from one or both parents may damage the parent-child relationship.　◆過保護な親 overprotective parent(s)　◆親の過干渉 overinterference[too much interference] from one's parent(s)　◀男親 father / male parent　女親 mother / female parent　里親 foster parent　一人親家庭 single-parent family　☞親兄弟・姉妹，親子

おやきょうだい　親兄弟・姉妹　parents and siblings, parents and brothers and sisters　（肉親）immediate family

おやこ　親子　parent(s) and child[children]　（肉親）immediate family　▶親子関係 parent-child relationship[relations]　親子鑑定 parentage test[diagnosis] /（父子関係の）paternity test[diagnosis]

おやしらず　親知らず　（智歯）wisdom tooth（쮼teeth）　☞智歯　◆親知らずが生える cut one's wisdom tooth　◆親知らずがある have *a wisdom tooth[wisdom teeth]　◆親知らずを抜く extract[pull out] a wisdom tooth /（抜いてもらう）have one's wisdom tooth（taken）out

おやすみ　◆お休みなさい Good night! / Sleep well! /（子供に）Night-night. Sleep tight!

おやつ　snack,《英》afternoon tea, tea　☞間食　◆軽いおやつくらいなら食べてもいいですよ It's all right if you eat light snacks. / As long as they're light snacks, you can have them.　◆おやつを食べすぎてはいけません You shouldn't eat too many snacks.

おやゆび　親指　（手の）thumb /θʌm/（足の）big toe, great toe　☞指　◆親指をしゃぶる suck one's thumb

およそ　☞おおよそ，大体

およぶ **及ぶ** (広がる)spread (続く)last
◆靱帯や骨にまで炎症が及んでいます The inflammation has spread to[into] the ligaments and bones. ◆がんの転移は複数の臓器に及んでいます The cancer has spread[(転移した)metastasized] to more than one organ. ◆彼女は10時間にも及ぶ手術に耐えました She endured[withstood] the surgery that lasted more than ten hours. ◆長期に及ぶ治療となりますが, ご一緒に頑張っていきましょう This treatment will be quite long, but let's *hang in there[stick with it] together.

およぼす **及ぼす** have an effect (on)
◆暴力的なビデオゲームは子供たちに悪影響を及ぼします Violent video games *have a negative effect on children[(害になる)are harmful to children].

オランダ the Netherlands, Holland (略オランダの・オランダ人の)Dutch) ★Holland は別称. ☞国籍 ▶オランダ人(男性)Dutchman / (女性)Dutchwoman

おり **折り** (時)time (場合)occasion (機会)opportunity, chance ☞機会

オリーブきょうしょうのういしゅくしょう ―橋小脳萎縮症 olivopontocerebellar atrophy；OPCA

オリーブゆ ―油 olive oil

オリエンテーション orientation ◀術前オリエンテーション preoperative orientation 入院時オリエンテーション admission (patient) orientation / (patient) orientation on admission

おりかえし **折り返し** ◆折り返しお電話いたします I'll call you back.

オリゴとう ―糖 oligosaccharide

おりたたむ **折り畳む** fold (up) ◆車椅子を折り畳む fold a wheelchair ◆紙を半分に折り畳んで三角形を作って下さい Fold the paper in half to make a triangle. ▶折り畳み式車椅子 folding wheelchair

おりもの (帯下)(vaginal) discharge /dístʃɑədʒ/ ◀帯下 ◆おりものが出ますか Do you have any vaginal discharge? ◆どんなおりものですか What does the (vaginal) discharge look like? ◆おりも

のはどんな色をしていますか What color is the (vaginal) discharge? ◆おりものの色は黄色味を帯びていますか, それとも透明ですか Is the (vaginal) discharge yellowish or clear? ◆おりものはにおいますか Does the (vaginal) discharge have any odor?
◆おりものが多い have heavy[frequent] (vaginal) discharge

おりものの性状

■色
●透明な clear, transparent ●白い white ●乳白色の milky white ●灰色の gray ●黄色の yellow ●黄色っぽい yellowish ●緑の green ●黄緑色の yellow-green

■性状
●さらっとした thin ●どろっとした thick ●濁った cloudy ●カッテージチーズ状の cottage cheese-like ●泡立った foamy, frothy ●膿のような pus-like ●水っぽい watery

■におい
●不快な unpleasant, bad-smelling ●魚臭い fishy ●かび臭い musty

おりる **下りる・降りる** (高い場所・乗り物から下りる)get *out of[off] (低い所に移動する)go down, come down, move down
◆ベッドから下りるのをお手伝いしましょう I'll help you (get) out of bed. ◆診察台から下りて立って下さい Please get off the exam table and stand up. ◆車椅子から下りる get out of a wheelchair ◆階段を下りる go down the stairs ◆赤ちゃんは下りてきています The baby is coming down.

おる **折る**
《骨折する》break ☞折れる ◆転ぶと骨を折る危険がありますから, 気をつけて下さい You could break[risk breaking] a bone if you fall, so be careful. ◆腕を折る break one's arm ◆足を折っている have a broken leg
《折り畳む・折り曲げる》fold (up) ◆この紙

を点線に沿って折って下さい Please fold this paper along the dotted line.

オルガスム orgasm ◆あなたはオルガスムに問題がありますか Do you have any difficulty reaching orgasm? ◆オルガスムに達する achieve[reach / have] an orgasm

おれい お礼 ☞感謝，礼

オレインさん 一酸 oleic acid

オレキシン orexin

おれみみ 折れ耳 folded ear

おれる 折れる
《骨折する》break ☞折る ◆この X 線写真を見ると，手首の骨が折れています This X-ray shows that your wrist is broken.
《譲歩する》give in ◆彼はついに折れて妻の要求を受け入れました He finally gave in to his wife's demands.

オレンジかわようひふ 一皮様皮膚 (橙皮状皮膚) orange peel skin

オレンジジュース orange juice

おろ 悪露 postpartum vaginal discharge, lochia

おろす 下ろす・降ろす (低い所に移動させる)lower, put down, bring down (引き下げる)pull down ◆では，腕を下ろして下さい Now, please lower your arms. / Now, please put your arms down. ◆車椅子に体をゆっくり下ろして下さい Please lower your body slowly into the wheelchair. ◆ブラインドを下ろす pull down the shades[blinds]

おろそか 疎かにする neglect ☞怠る ◆健康のためには歯のケアを疎かにしてはいけません To keep healthy, you shouldn't neglect to take proper care of your teeth.

おわび お詫び apology ☞謝る，詫びる

おわり 終わり end, close ◆それでは，今日はこれで終わりにしましょう All right! That's all for today. / OK! That'll be it for today. ◆初めから終わりまで from beginning to end ◆1 日の終わりに at the end of the day ◆1 日の終わり頃 later in the day

おわる 終わる be over, finish, be finished [done], end ☞済む ◆これで終わりまし

た It's over now. / Now, you're finished [done]. / That's all. ◆あと 2, 3 分で終わります It'll be over[finished] in a couple of minutes. / (Just) A couple more minutes and it'll be all over. ◆検査が終わったらこちらに戻って下さい When the tests are finished, please come back here. ◆手術は無事に終わりました The surgery went well[successfully].

おんあつ 音圧 sound pressure

おんいき 音域 sound[sound-frequency] range, audio[audio-frequency] range (声域)vocal range, voice range ◀会話音域 speech range

おんかく 温覚 warm sensation

おんがく 音楽 music ▶音楽療法 music therapy

おんきょう 音響 sound (胚acoustic) ▶音響学 acoustics 音響外傷 acoustic trauma

オンコール on call ◆彼女は今晩オンコールです She's on call tonight. ▶オンコール医師 doctor on call / on-call doctor

おんさ 音叉 tuning fork ◆この音叉を当てます I'm going to place this tuning fork on you.

おんしき 温式(の) warm ▶温式抗体 warm antibody 温式自己免疫性溶血性貧血 warm *autoimmune hemolytic anemia [AIHA]

おんしっぷ 温湿布 hot compress (温パック)hot pack, heat pack ☞湿布 ◆腰に〈痛むところに〉温湿布を貼る apply a hot compress *to the lower back〈where it hurts〉

おんしょう 温床 (繁殖地)breeding ground (楽園)haven ◆湿気があり暖かい台所は細菌の温床です。Damp and warm kitchens are *breeding grounds [havens] for germs.

おんすい 温水 warm water (ぬるま湯)lukewarm water ◆屋内温水プール heated indoor swimming pool

おんせい 音声 voice (発話)speech (胚phonetic) ◆CT 検査中は音声に従って息を吸ったり止めたりして下さい During the

CT scan, breathe in and hold when you're told to. ◀食道音声［食道発声］esophageal speech　代用音声 alternative voice　▶音声障害［発声障害］voice disorder / dysphonia　音声振戦 voice tremor　音声衰弱 phonasthenia　音声分析 phonetic analysis

おんせん　温泉　hot spring　（温泉地）spa　▶温泉病院 spa hospital　温泉療法 spa treatment / hot spring cure[treatment / therapy] / balneotherapy

おんぞん　温存　（保存）conservation（圓conserve　圀conservative）, preservation（圓preserve）　（修復・復旧）restoration（圓restore　圀restorative）　◀機能温存手術 function-preserving surgery　肛門温存大腸切除術 restorative proctocolectomy　乳房温存療法 breast-conserving treatment[therapy]；BCT

おんど　温度　temperature；T[temp]（圀熱性の thermal　熱量の caloric）　☞巻末付録：単位の換算　◆お部屋の温度は暑すぎますか, ちょうどいいですか Is the room temperature too hot or just right?　◆温度が上がる the temperature rises[goes up]　◆温度が下がる the temperature falls[goes down]　◆温度を測る take the temperature　◆温度を調節する adjust[control] the temperature　◀至適温度 optimum[optimal] temperature　摂氏温度計 Celsius thermometer　▶温度覚鈍麻 thermohypesthesia　温度感覚 temperature sensation[sense] / thermal sensation[sense]　温度眼振試験 caloric nystagmus test　温度計 thermometer　温度刺激 caloric stimulation

おんな　女　woman（圀women）　（女の子）girl　（女の赤ちゃん）baby girl　☞女性　◆（分娩後に）おめでとうございます, 女のお子さんですよ Congratulations! It's a girl.　▶女親 mother / female parent　女きょうだい sister / female sibling

おんねつ　温熱（の）　（温かい）warm　（熱の・熱性の）thermal　（有熱性の）febrile　▶温熱（感）覚 warm sensation　温熱蕁麻疹 febrile urticaria　温熱性損傷 thermal trau-

ma　温熱療法 heat[fever / hyperthermia] therapy

おんパック　温パック　hot pack, heat pack　☞湿布

おんよく　温浴　warm bath　◀高温浴 hot bath　微温浴 lukewarm[tepid] bath

おんりょう　音量　volume　◆テレビの音量を下げて〈上げて〉いただけませんか Could you please turn down〈up〉the volume on the television? / Could you please keep the television volume low〈up〉?

おんれいかく　温冷覚　sensitivity to heat and cold, hot and cold sensations　★通例, 複数形で.

か

か¹ 科 **department** ☞診療 ◆(受付で)何科の受診をご希望ですか What department would you like to visit? ▶科長 the head (of the … Department)

か² 蚊 **mosquito** /məskíːtou/ ◆蚊に刺される be bitten by a mosquito ◆蚊に刺されたのですか Have you been bitten by a mosquito? / Have you had a mosquito bite? ◆蚊によって媒介される be carried [transmitted / spread] by mosquitoes ◆蚊に刺された痕 a mosquito bite ◀防蚊剤 mosquito repellent ▶蚊アレルギー mosquito allergy 蚊媒介疾患 mosquito-borne disease

が 蛾 **moth** ◀チャドクガ tea tussock moth ドクガ poisonous[venomous] moth

ガーゼ **gauze** /gɔ́ːz/ ◆ガーゼを交換する change the gauze ◆ガーゼで傷口を覆う cover the wound with (a piece of) gauze ◆患部にガーゼを当てる place gauze over the affected area ◀滅菌ガーゼ sterile gauze ▶ガーゼ包帯 gauze bandage / (パッド)gauze pad / (ガーゼの巻き包帯)gauze roll

かあつたい 加圧帯 **cuff** ☞カフ

カーテン **curtain** ◆カーテンを閉めましょうか〈開けましょうか〉Shall I close〈open〉the curtains? ◆病室のベッドはすべてカーテンで仕切られています Beds in the hospital are all curtained off. ▶カーテン徴候 curtain sign

カート **cart** ◆正面玄関の近くに荷物運搬用のカートが配置してあります There is a load cart available for use near the main entrance. ▶救急カート emergency cart

カード **card** （クレジットカード）**credit card** （通行証）**pass** ◆お支払いはカードにしますか，現金にしますか Are you paying by credit card or in cash? ◆病院の費用をカードで支払う pay the hospital fees by credit card ◆申し訳ありませんが，当院ではカードをお使いになれません I'm sorry, but we don't accept credit cards. ◆ペースメーカを付けていることを示すカードを常に手元に所持して下さい Always carry your pacemaker ID card with you. ◀臓器提供意思表示カード(organ) donor card テレビカード prepaid TV card 糖尿病IDカード diabetic ID card / (腕輪) diabetic ID bracelet 訪問カード(面会許可証)visitor[visitors] pass / (面会用バッジ) visitor [visitors] badge 予約カード appointment card

ガードマン （security) **guard** ◆ガードマンを呼ぶ call a guard

ガーナ **Ghana** (㊥Ghanaian) ☞国籍 ▶ガーナ人(の) Ghanaian

かい¹ 回 （回数)**time(s)** （一連の治療に必要とされる回)**round** （周期)**cycle** ☞回数，クール ◆何回吐きましたか How many times did you vomit? ◆食事は1日3回食べていますか Do you eat three times a day? ◆1日1回 once a day ◆2回 twice[two times] ◆3回 three times ◆2, 3回 a few times ◆5, 6回 several times ◆何回も many times ◆4時間に1回 once every four hours ◆3日に1回 every three days ◆次回 (the) next time ◆前回(the) last time ◆毎回(すべての時に) every time / (1回1回に) each time ◆初回の化学療法 the first round [cycle] of chemotherapy

かい² 階 **floor** ◆(マンションの)何階に住んでいますか What floor do you live on? ◆1階にカフェテリアがあります There's a cafeteria on the first floor. ★1階は《英》では ground floor という.

かい³ 貝 **shellfish** ▶貝中毒 shellfish poisoning

がい 害 （人・物への危害)**harm** (㊥害のある harmful 害のない harmless) （物への物理的損害)**damage** ☞害する，有害 ◆害する (do[cause]) harm / (do[cause]) damage / (傷つける)injure / (特に感情を損なう) offend ◆高血圧は動脈に害を及ぼします High blood pressure can harm[damage]

がい 101 かいけい

your arteries. ◆お酒の飲み過ぎは健康を害します Too much drinking can be bad [harmful] for your health.

がいいん¹ 外因 external cause (形exter-nal 生体外の exogenous, exogenic 外部から生じた原因の extrinsic) ▶外因性感染 exogenous infection 外因性湿疹 exogenous eczema 外因性精神病 exogenous psychosis 外因性喘息 extrinsic asthma

がいいん² 外陰(部) vulva (形vulvar) ▶外陰異形成 vulvar dysplasia 外陰炎 vulvitis 外陰潰瘍 ulceration of the vulva 外陰がん vulvar cancer 外陰ジストロフィー vulvar dystrophy 外陰(部)疾患 vulvar disease 外陰搔痒症 vulvar itching [pruritus] 外陰腟カンジダ症 vulvovaginal candidiasis 外陰白斑症 vulvar leukoplakia 外陰パジェット病 Paget disease of the vulva

かいうんどうニューロン 下位運動ニューロン lower motor neuron；LMN ▶下位運動ニューロン疾患 lower motor neuron disease

かいが 絵画 picture (絵具などを使った絵)painting (鉛筆・ペンなどを使った線画) drawing (美術・芸術)art ▶絵画統覚検査 thematic apperception test 絵画療法[芸術療法] art therapy 絵画療法士 art therapist

かいがい¹ 回外 supination ▶回外筋 supinator muscle

かいがい² 海外(に) abroad, overseas (形overseas) ☞外国 ◆最近海外へ出かけましたか Have you been abroad[outside Japan] recently? ◆海外に旅行に出かける travel overseas[abroad] ◆海外からの訪問者 a visitor from overseas / an overseas visitor ▶海外傷害保険 overseas accident insurance 海外渡航歴 history of *one's* overseas[foreign] travel 海外旅行 overseas[foreign] travel 海外旅行保険 overseas travel insurance

がいかいてんじゅつ 外回転術 (胎児の) external version, abdominal version

かいかん (性の)快感 ☞オルガスム

がいかん 外観 appearance ☞外見

がいがんきん 外眼筋 extraocular muscle ▶外眼筋ミオパチー extraocular myopathy

かいき 回帰 (再発)relapse (動relapse), recurrence (動recur 形recurrent) (交換・往復運動)reciprocation (動reciprocate) (退行・逆戻り) regression (動regress) ◀房室回帰性頻拍 atrioventricular[AV] reciprocating tachycardia；AVRT ▶回帰性リウマチ palindromic rheumatism；PR 回帰熱 relapsing[recurrent] fever 回帰分析 regression analysis

かいぎ 会議 meeting (規模の大きい会議) conference ◆今日は3時から会議があります We have a meeting at three today. ◆斎藤先生は会議中です Dr Saito is in a meeting (right now). ◆会議に出席する attend a meeting[conference] ◆会議を開く hold a meeting[conference]

かいきょう 開胸(の) open-chest ◀非開胸式心マッサージ closed-chest heart [cardiac] massage ▶開胸式心マッサージ open-chest heart[cardiac] massage 開胸手術 thoracotomy / (心臓の)open heart surgery 開胸肺生検 open lung biopsy

かいぎょう 開業する practice ◆彼女は歯科を開業しています She practices dentistry. / She is a practicing dentist. ◆お近くの循環器科〈小児科 / 整形外科〉専門の開業医を紹介します I'm going to *refer you[give you a referral] to a nearby practitioner who specializes in cardiology 〈pediatrics / orthopedics〉. ▶開業医 practitioner / (一般開業医)general practitioner；GP

がいきよく 外気浴 sunbath, sunbathing (動sunbathe)

かいけい 会計 《支払い》payment (動pay) ◆会計は現金のみの取り扱いになります Hospital fees must be paid in cash. / We accept cash payments only. ◆会計はクレジットカードでも可能です You can pay by credit card. / We accept payments by credit card.

《会計係》cashier /kǽʃíə/ ◆1 階の会計窓口でお支払い下さい Please pay at the cashier counter[window] on the first floor.

◀外来会計 outpatient cashier　入院会計 inpatient cashier

がいけいじょうみゃく　外頸静脈　external jugular vein

がいけいどうみゃく　外頸動脈　external carotid artery；ECA

かいけつ　解決する　solve（図solution）（最終的に決着させる）settle（図settlement）

◆まず根底にある問題を解決しなければなりません We should solve the underlying problem first.　◆薬を変更すればめまいが解決するかもしれません Switching medications may solve your dizziness.
◆この問題は時が解決してくれるでしょう I hope time will solve[settle] this problem.

かいけつびょう　壊血病　scurvy, scorbutus　◆壊血病はビタミン C の欠乏によって起こります Scurvy is a disease caused by vitamin C deficiency.

がいけん　外見　（見かけ）appearance

☞姿　◆このポリープは外見では良性に見えますが，念のため組織を採って調べましょう This polyp appears[looks] benign, but I'm going to obtain a tissue sample to be sure.　◆外見で判断する judge by appearance(s)

かいご　介護　care（図care for, take care (of)）　☞介助，ケア，世話　◆自宅で介護する *care for[take care of] the patient* at home / give[provide] care at home
◆記憶障害のある人を介護する *care for [take care of]* a person with memory problems　◆彼女には 24 時間介護が必要です She needs twenty-four-hour care.
◆彼は要介護度 3 と査定されています He has been assessed as *requiring care (needs) level three[having level-three care needs].*　◆介護サービスを申請する apply[make an application] for long-term care services　◆訪問介護サービスを利用する have visiting home care / use the visiting home care services　◆要介護認定 4 を受ける be certified as requiring care (needs) level four / be certified as a person with level-four care needs　◆介護施設に入所する enter[be admitted to] a residential care home

◀患者中心介護 patient-centered care　公的介護制度 public care system　高齢者介護 elderly care / care of elderly[older] people　在宅介護 home-based care / care at one's home / in-home care　在宅介護サービス home care service　在宅介護（支援）センター home care (support) center[agency]　施設（居住）介護 institutional[residential] care / care in[at] a facility　終身介護 lifelong care　身体介護 physical care / care for physical needs　長期介護 long-term care；LTC　通所介護 day care　通所介護施設 day care facility　訪問介護 home-visit long-term care / （サービス）visiting home care service　夜間介護 night[nighttime] care　要介護（long-term）care needs / （long-term）care required[needed]　要介護者（介護保険利用者）long-term care insurance recipient / （長期介護を必要とする人）person requiring long-term care　要介護度 care (needs) level / the level of care needs　要介護認定 certification of (eligibility for) long-term care needs

▶介護休暇（family）care leave / dependent care leave　介護給付 long-term care benefits　介護犬 service[assistance] dog　介護査定 care needs assessment　介護支援サービス care (support) service　介護支援センター care (support) center　介護支援専門員 care manager / long-term care support specialist　介護施設 care facility　介護タクシー care taxi[cab]　介護認定審査会 certification committee of needed long-term care　介護福祉士 certified care worker　介護ベッド（nursing）care bed　介護保険 long-term care insurance　介護用品（nursing）care goods / （備品）care equipment　介護療養型施設 intermediate care facility / convalescent

かいご　103　かいしゃ

home　介護老人福祉施設 welfare facility for the elderly requiring long-term care　介護老人保健施設 health care facility for the elderly requiring long-term care　介護ロボット care[healthcare] robot ☞介護者

かいこう¹　開口　opening　▶開口期(分娩の) period of dilation / the first stage of labor　開口器 mouth opener[gag] / mouth[bite] prop　開口部 opening

かいこう²　開咬　open bite

かいごう　会合　meeting　☞会議

がいこう　外交(的な)　extroverted /ékstrəvɜːtɪd/ (↔introverted), extrovert (社交的な) outgoing　◆外交的な人 an extrovert / an outgoing person　◆外向的な性格 an outgoing[extroverted / extrovert] personality

がいこく　外国　foreign country (圖 abroad, overseas)　☞海外　◆夏休みには外国に行きますか Are you going abroad during the summer vacation? / Are you taking a trip overseas[outside Japan] during the summer vacation?　◆最近, 外国旅行をしましたか Have you recently traveled overseas[outside Japan]?　◆外国の保険 foreign insurance　▶外国語 foreign language　外国籍 foreign nationality　☞外国人

がいこくじん　外国人　foreigner (公式文書で) alien　★両語とも「よそ者」という否定的なニュアンスがあるので注意. 会話をする際には, アメリカ人, オーストラリア人など具体的な国名を言ったほうがよい. ☞国籍　◆定住外国人 permanent-resident foreigner　不法滞在外国人 illegal foreign resident　▶外国人観光客 foreign tourist　外国人患者 foreign[overseas] patient　外国人居住者 foreign resident　外国人登録 alien registration　外国人登録証明書(在留カード) residence card　外国人留学生 international [overseas / foreign] student　外国人労働者 foreign worker / (肉体労働者の) foreign laborer

かいごしゃ　介護者　(病院で) hospital attendant[care worker]　(男性の介護員)

(medical) orderly　(在宅で) home[in-home] care worker　(家族) family caregiver ☞介護

がいさん　概算　rough estimate　◆治療費は概算で5万円かかります Your medical expenses will be roughly[approximately] fifty thousand yen. / At a rough estimate, your medical fees will be fifty thousand yen.

かいさんしょくひんアレルギー　海産食品アレルギー　seafood allergy

かいし　開始する　(始める) start, begin (着手する) initiate　◆それでは麻酔を開始します Now, we're going to start giving you the anesthesia.　◆手術の開始時刻は朝9時です The surgery will start[begin] at nine in the morning.

かいじ　開示　(情報・身元の公表) disclosure (圖disclose), release (圖release)　◆透明性のある開示 transparent disclosure　◆患者さんの個人情報は本人の同意なく開示いたしません We will not disclose [release] patients' personal[private] health information without their consent.　◀医療過誤開示 medical error disclosure　カルテ開示 release of a patient's chart[medical records]

がいじ　外耳　external ear　▶外耳炎 external otitis / inflammation of the ear canal / (特に耳の中に水が残って起こる炎症) swimmer's ear　外耳道 external ear [auditory] canal

がいじかく　外痔核　external hemorrhoids[piles]　★通例, 複数形で.

がいじつりずむ　概日リズム　circadian rhythm(s)

かいしゃ　会社　company, firm　(仕事場) office, place of work, workplace　☞仕事　◆どちらの会社にお勤めですか What company do you work for?　◆朝8時に会社に行く *go to work[go to the office] at eight in the morning　◆会社を休む take some time off work　◆会社を辞める leave[resign from] *one's* job　◆会社を解雇される be dismissed[fired]　◀製薬会社 drug[pharmaceutical] company　▶会

社員 office worker / company employee

かいしゃく 解釈する **interpret** ◆彼の行動をどう解釈すべきでしょうか How should we interpret his behavior? / How should his behavior be interpreted? ◆その治療法の効果については解釈が分かれるところです The treatment effects can be interpreted in various ways.

がいしゃし 外斜視 **external strabismus[squint], divergent strabismus[squint], exotropia；XT**

がいしゃんと 外シャント **external shunt**

がいしゅつ 外出する **go out (of)** ◆外出する時には、必ず担当医の許可を得て下さい Before you go out of the hospital, be sure to check with your doctor and get his〈her〉permission. ◆無断で外出しないで下さい Please don't go out of the hospital without permission. ◆堀医師はただ今外出しております Dr Hori is out of the office right now. ◆平熱に戻ってからも2，3日は外出を控えて下さい Even after your temperature has returned to normal, please *stay home[don't leave your home] for *a couple of[two or three] days. ◆（病気・高齢で）外出できない人 a person confined to (the) home / a homebound[housebound] person ▶外出許可 permission to *go out[leave the hospital building]

がいしゅっけつ 外出血 **external bleeding[hemorrhage]**

かいじょ 介助する **help（図help）assist（図assistance 図assistive）** ☞介護，ケア ◆入浴はスタッフが介助しますのでご安心下さい Our staff will help you take a bath. So please don't worry. ◆彼女には食事の介助が必要です She needs help[assistance] with meals. ◆彼には排泄の介助が必要です He needs help[assistance] with using the toilet. ◆介助なしで歩けますか Can you walk without help[assistance]? ◀移乗介助 transfer assistance 一部介助 partial assistance 全介助 full assistance ▶介助運動 assistive exercise 介助犬 service[assistance] dog 介助者

caregiver / carer 介助用車椅子 attendant-controlled[attendant-propelled] wheelchair 介助ロボット care robot

がいしょう 解消する 《ストレスなどを》（取り除く）**get rid of …** （減らす）**reduce** （和らげる）**relieve** ◆どうやってストレスを解消しますか What do you do to *get rid of[reduce / relieve] stress? 《関係・契約などを》**cancel** ◆介護施設への入所契約を解消する cancel a contract to enter a care home

がいしょう 外傷 **(external) injury[wound], trauma（图traumatic）** ☞怪我 ◆頭に外傷を受けたことがありますか Have you ever had an injury to your head? ◆心の外傷となるような経験をする have a psychologically traumatic experience ◀鋭的外傷 penetrating trauma[injury] 音響外傷 acoustic trauma 眼外傷 ocular injury 交通外傷 traffic injury 心的外傷 psychological trauma スポーツ外傷 sport[athletic] injury 多発外傷 multiple injury[trauma] 頭部外傷 head injury [trauma] 頭部外傷後昏睡 coma after head injury 鈍的外傷 blunt trauma[injury] ハンドル外傷 handlebar injury ▶外傷外科 trauma surgery /（診療科）the department of trauma surgery / the trauma surgery department 外傷（専門）外科医 trauma surgeon 外傷後健忘 posttraumatic amnesia （心的）外傷後ストレス障害 posttraumatic stress disorder；PTSD 外傷性気胸 traumatic pneumothorax 外傷性くも膜下出血 traumatic subarachnoid bleeding[hemorrhage] 外傷性ショック traumatic shock 外傷性［外傷後］てんかん posttraumatic epilepsy 外傷性難聴 traumatic hearing loss 外傷性脳損傷 traumatic brain injury；TBI

がいしょうしゃ 外照射 **external irradiation**

がいしょく 外食する **eat out** ◆食事は外食が多いですか Do you often eat out?

かいしん 回診 **rounds** ★複数形で．◆まもなく医師の回診があります The

doctors will be making their rounds soon. ◆今佐藤先生は回診に出ています Dr Sato is out on his〈her〉rounds now. ◀教授回診 professor rounds　総回診 grand rounds　病棟回診 ward[floor] rounds　麻酔前回診 preanesthetic rounds

かいしんじゅつ 開心術　open heart surgery

かいすいよく 海水浴　swimming in the sea, sea bathing　▶海水浴皮膚炎 seabather's eruption

かいすう 回数　times　（頻度）frequency（形frequent）☞回　◆便通の回数はどのくらいですか How often[How many times] do you have a bowel movement? / How often[How many times] do you *move your bowels[（排便する）pass stools]?　◆便通の回数は増えていますか〈減っていますか〉Are your bowel movements more〈less〉frequent?　◆夜お手洗いに行く回数が多い（何回も起きてお手洗いに行く）get up to use the bathroom several times during the night / make frequent trips to the bathroom at night　◀換気回数 ventilation[ventilator] frequency　排尿回数 urinary frequency　排便回数 stool frequency

がいする 害する　（人を傷つける）injure, hurt　（物・機能を損傷する）damage　（人の感情を傷つける）offend　◆健康を害する injure[damage] *one's* health　◆気分[感情]を害する hurt *a person's* feelings / offend *a person*

がいせいしょくき 外生殖器　external genitals[genitalia, genital organs]　★いずれも複数形で.

かいせき 解析　analysis　（動analyze）◀画像解析 image analysis

かいせん¹ 回旋　rotation　▶回旋筋 rotator muscle　回旋枝 circumflex branch

かいせん² 疥癬　scabies /skéibiz/　◆疥癬に罹っているようです I think you have scabies.

かいぜん 改善する　（好転する・よりよくなる）improve, get better　（好転させる・よりよくする）improve, make … better　（和らげる）

relieve　◆症状が改善しない時は連絡して下さい Please call[contact] us if your symptoms do not improve.　◆肩の痛みは改善していますか Is the shoulder pain *getting better[improving]?　◆毎日の食事と生活習慣を改善する必要があります You need to improve[change] your everyday diet and lifestyle.　◆コミュニケーションは家族関係を改善する鍵になります Good communication is the key to improving family relationships. / Good communication can improve relationships *at home[within the family].　◆現在の症状を改善するには手術が必要です You need to have surgery to relieve these symptoms.　◀脳循環代謝改善薬 cerebral circulation and metabolism improver

がいせん¹ 外線　outside line　◆外線は9を回して下さい Please dial nine for an outside line.　◆外線にかける時は交換手を通して下さい Please make outside calls through the operator.

がいせん² 外旋　external rotation, lateral rotation, outward rotation

かいそう¹ 回想する　（思い出す）remember, recollect, recall　（振り返る）look back on　（遠い昔を回顧する）reminisce（図reminiscence）◆楽しかった昔の日々を回想する remember[recollect / recall] the good old days / look back on happy bygone days　▶回想法 reminiscence therapy；RT / life review

かいそう² 海藻　seaweed

かいそう³ 階層　class　◀社会階層 social class　社会的階層制 social hierarchy

がいそう 咳嗽　cough　☞咳　◀カプサイシン咳嗽試験 capsaicin cough test　痙攣性咳嗽 spasmodic cough　▶咳嗽失神 cough[tussive] syncope / cough fainting　咳嗽反射 cough reflex　咳嗽誘発試験 cough provocation test

かいそうき 開創器　retractor

かいそうじゅつ 開窓術　windowing, window operation, fenestration　◀気管開窓術 tracheal fenestration　心膜開窓術 pericardial fenestration　脳室開窓術

ventriculostomy

かいぞうりょく 解像力 resolving power, resolution

かいぞえ 介添え help, assistance ☞介助

がいそく 外側(の) lateral ☞外側(そとがわ) ◆外側面 the lateral surface ◆外側部 the lateral part[portion] ▶外側側副靭帯(膝関節の)lateral collateral ligament；LCL / lateral ligament of the knee

がいそけいヘルニア 外鼠径ヘルニア external inguinal hernia

かいぞん 開存(性の) patent ◀動脈管開存症 patent ductus arteriosus；PDA /(ボタロー管開存症)patent ductus Botalli 尿膜管開存症 patent urachus

かいたつ 介達(の) indirect ▶介達牽引法 indirect(skeletal)traction 介達骨折 indirect fracture

かいだん 階段 stairs (屋外の)steps ★いずれも複数形で. ◆階段を上る climb[go up](the)stairs ◆階段を下りる go down(the)stairs ◆階段や坂道を上る時，息切れしますか Do you get short of breath when you climb[go up]stairs or slopes? ◆アパートに入るのに階段を上る必要がありますか Do you need to climb steps to get to your apartment? ◆階段の上り下りに気をつけて下さい Please be careful when you go up and down stairs. ◆階段から落ちる fall down some stairs ◀非常階段 emergency stairs / fire escape マスター2階段テスト Master two-step(exercise)test ▶階段昇降 stair climbing 階段昇降機 stair lift 階段昇降用車椅子 stair-climbing wheelchair

かいちゅう 回虫 roundworm, *Ascaris lumbricoides* ▶回虫駆除薬 lumbricide 回虫症 roundworm disease / ascariasis

かいちゅうでんとう 懐中電灯 flashlight, 《英》torch

かいちょう 回腸 ileum /íliəm/ (形ileal) ◀終末回腸 terminal ileum ▶回腸疾患 ileal disease 回腸切除 ileectomy / ileal resection 回腸導管 ileal conduit；IC 回腸末端炎 terminal ileitis

回腸瘻造設術 ileostomy 回腸瘻バッグ ileostomy bag

かいてい 改訂する・改定する revise (形revision) ▶改訂版 revised edition[version]

かいてき 快適(な) (苦痛がなく安楽な)comfortable (心地よい)pleasant (満足のいく)satisfactory ◆快適なベッド a comfortable bed ◆お部屋の温度は快適ですか Is the room temperature *to your liking[comfortable]? ◆安全で快適な空の旅になりますように Have a safe and pleasant flight! ◆職場環境は快適ですか Do you have a comfortable working environment? / Is your work environment satisfactory?

がいてき 外的(な) (外部の・体外の)external (外側の)outer (外因の)extrinsic ◆外的環境 the external environment ◆外的要因 an external factor /(外因子)an extrinsic factor

かいてん 回転する turn(around) (速く回る)spin(around) (軸を中心に回る)rotate (形rotation 形rotary) ☞回る ◆めまいは回転する感じですか Do you have the sensation that you're turning or spinning[rotating]? ▶回転異常腎 malrotated kidney 回転性めまい rotary vertigo 胎児外回転術 external[abdominal]version

がいてん 外転 abduction, abducens (形abducent) ◀肩外転副子 airplane(shoulder)splint / shoulder abduction orthosis ▶外転位 abduction position 外転神経 abducent nerve

ガイド guide (形誘導された -guided) ◀超音波ガイド下生検 ultrasound-guided biopsy / ultrasonography[ultrasonically]-guided biopsy 超音波ガイド下穿刺術 ultrasound-guided puncture / ultrasonography[ultrasonically]-guided puncture

かいとう[1] 開頭 craniotomy, surgical incision into the skull ◆開頭手術を行う perform[do]a craniotomy[surgical incision into the skull] ◆開頭して血栓を除

去する make an opening in the skull and remove a blood clot / open up the skull to remove a blood clot ▶開頭減圧術 cerebral decompression

かいとう² 回答する （質問に答える・返答する）answer（図answer）, reply（図reply）（反応する・応答する）respond（図response）☞答える ◆アンケートに回答する answer a questionnaire /（用紙に記入する）fill out a questionnaire ◆文書で回答する reply [answer] in writing / reply[answer] in written form ◆よくある質問への回答 answers to *frequently asked questions [FAQs]

かいとう³ 解答する （試験問題などに答える）answer（図answer）（解決策を案出する）solve（図solution） ◆この引き算の問題に解答して下さい Please answer this subtraction question.

かいとう⁴ 解凍する thaw /θɔː/, defrost ◆冷凍した母乳はぬるま湯で解凍して下さい You should thaw[defrost] frozen breast milk in lukewarm water.

がいとうしん 外套針 trocar

かいどく 貝毒 shellfish poison[toxin], shellfish poisoning

がいどくそ 外毒素 exotoxin (↔endotoxin)

ガイドライン guidelines ★通例，複数形で． ◆ガイドラインに沿った治療をする follow medical treatment guidelines / treat according to the guidelines ◆安全に関するガイドライン guidelines on safety ◀診療ガイドライン clinical practice guidelines

かいない 回内 pronation (↔supination) ▶回内筋 pronator muscle

かいにゅう 介入する intervene（図intervention 図interventional） interfere（図interference） ◆彼女の個人的な問題には介入できません We can't intervene[interfere] in[with] her personal affairs. ◆家庭内暴力の徴候が見られる時には介入する必要があります We need to intervene when we see signs of domestic violence. ◀画像診断的介入治療 interven-

tional radiology；IVR 危機介入 crisis intervention ▶介入研究 intervention study

がいにょうどうこう 外尿道口 external urethral orifice[opening], external opening of the urethra

かいにん 懐妊 pregnancy ☞妊娠

がいねん 概念 （考え）idea, notion （論理的な見解）concept ◀一般概念 general idea 自己概念 self-concept 相対概念 relative concept ▶概念形成 concept formation

かいば 海馬 hippocampus

がいはく 外泊する go home for the night, stay home overnight ◆外泊の許可を与える give (the patient) permission to go home for the night / allow the patient to stay home overnight ◀無断外泊 staying home overnight without (one's doctor's) permission ▶外泊許可 (the doctor's) permission to *go home for the night[stay home overnight]

かいはくしつ 灰白質 gray matter ▶灰白質ジストロフィー poliodystrophy

かいはくしょく 灰白色（の） （白っぽい）whitish （粘土色の）clay-colored （薄い灰色の）light gray ▶灰白色便 whitish[clay-colored] stools

かいはくずいえん 灰白髄炎 poliomyelitis ◀急性灰白髄炎 acute poliomyelitis

かいはつ 開発する develop（図development） ◆パーキンソン病の新薬が目下開発されているところです They are now developing new medications to treat Parkinson disease. / New medications to treat Parkinson disease are now under [in] development. ◀研究開発 research and development

がいはん 外反 （四肢の）valgus (↔varus) （瞼・唇などの）ectropion ◀眼瞼外反症 ectropion of the eyelid ▶外反膝 genu valgum / knock-knees 外反足 talipes valgus 外反肘 cubitus valgus 外反扁平足 talipes planovalgus 外反母趾 hallux valgus

かいひ 回避する avoid（図avoidance），

evade（图evasion） ☞避ける ◀抗原回避 antigen avoidance ▶回避学習 avoidance learning 回避行動 avoidance behavior

がいび 外鼻 external nose ▶外鼻孔 nostril

かいびせい 開鼻声 rhinolalia aperta

かいふく¹ 回復する・快復する
《病気が治る》recover（from）（图recovery）, recuperate（from）（图recuperation）
（傷・怪我などが治る）heal （よくなる・好転する）get well[better], improve（图improvement） ☞治る, 持ち直す ◆彼の怪我は予想よりずっと早く回復しました He recovered from his injury *much earlier[more rapidly] than we expected. ◆彼女は回復の徴候を見せています She is showing signs of recovery. ◆彼女が回復する見込みは半々です I'm afraid she has a fifty-fifty[fifty percent] chance of recovery. ◆大丈夫，すぐに回復しますよ Don't worry. You'll soon get better. ◆彼は徐々に〈急速に〉回復しています He is *getting better[improving / recovering] gradually 〈rapidly〉. ◆回復には1か月ほど時間がかかるでしょう It'll take a month or so *to get better[till you feel well again]. ◆手術後彼女は順調に回復しています（順調に進んでいる）She's making good progress after her surgery. ◆残念ですが，これ以上回復は期待できません I'm sorry[Unfortunately], *there's nothing more we can do [we can't expect further improvement / （おそらく回復不能である）the condition is probably irreversible].
《失った体力・機能などを取り戻す》recover（图recovery）, regain, restore ◆毎朝，元気が回復していますか（休息した感じですか）Do you feel rested every morning? ◆体力を回復する recover one's strength ◆意識を回復する regain consciousness / become conscious again / come around ◆視力を回復する restore vision ◀機能回復 functional recovery / recovery of function 自然回復 spontaneous recovery 体力回復訓練 convalescent exercise ▶回復期 convalescence 回復期患者 convalescent 回復室 recovery room /（特に麻酔後の）postanesthesia [postanesthetic] care unit；PACU ☞回復不能

かいふく² 開腹 laparotomy, surgical incision into the abdomen ◆開腹手術を行う perform[do]（an）abdominal surgery ◆開腹手術を受ける have[undergo]（an）abdominal surgery ◀試験開腹 exploratory laparotomy

がいふくしゃきん 外腹斜筋 abdominal external oblique muscle, external oblique muscle of the abdomen

かいふくふのう 回復不能（な）irreversible ◆脳に回復不能な損傷が起こっています Irreversible damage has occurred to [in] the brain. / The brain has suffered irreversible damage. ◆彼女の脳への損傷はおそらく回復不能でしょう The damage to her brain is *likely to be[probably] irreversible. ◆彼は回復不能な昏睡状態にあります He's in an irreversible coma. / It's almost impossible that he'll come out of the coma.

がいぶしょうしゃ 外部照射 external irradiation

がいぶんぴつ 外分泌 external secretion, exocrine secretion ▶外分泌腺 exocrine gland

がいヘルニア 外ヘルニア external hernia

かいほう¹ 介抱 care ☞介護, 介助, ケア

かいほう² 快方 recovery, improvement ☞回復

かいほう³ 開放性（の）open（↔closed）▶開放隅角緑内障 open-angle glaucoma 開放骨折 open[（複雑な）compound] fracture 開放性結核 open tuberculosis 開放性損傷 open injury 開放性頭部外傷 open head injury[trauma] 開放性鼻声 rhinolalia aperta 開放創 open wound

かいぼう 解剖 （死因を究明するための）autopsy /ɔ́ːtɑpsi/, postmortem（examination）（解剖学上の）anatomy （生体構造を調べるための）dissection ◆解剖を行って

死因を特定する perform[do] *an autopsy [a postmortem] on the body to determine the cause of death　◆解剖の結果, 彼の死因は心筋梗塞でした The autopsy [postmortem] showed that *the cause of his death was myocardial infarction[he died of a myocardial infarction].　◀行政解剖 administrative autopsy　司法解剖 judicial[forensic] autopsy　人体解剖図 human anatomical chart　病理解剖 (pathologic) autopsy　法医解剖 medicolegal autopsy　▶解剖学 anatomy　解剖学者 anatomist

がいほう　**外包**　external capsule

かいみん　**快眠する**　have a good sleep, sleep well

かいめん¹　**海綿**　sponge （岡海綿状の spongy, spongiform　空洞の cavernous）　◀陰茎海綿体 corpus cavernosum penis　▶海綿骨 spongy bone　海綿状血管腫 cavernous hemangioma　海綿状組織 cavernous tissue　海綿状脳症 spongiform encephalopathy　海綿状ポリープ spongy polyp　海綿静脈洞 cavernous sinus　海綿腎 sponge kidney　海綿体 spongy[cavernous] body

かいめん²　**界面**　◀肺胞界面活性物質 alveolar surfactant　▶界面活性剤 surfactant / surface-active agent / detergent

がいめん　**外面**　the outer surface （↔the inner surface）, the outside （↔the inside）

かいもう　**回盲(の)**　ileocecal　◀回盲部 ileocecal region / ileocecum　回盲弁 ileocecal valve

かいよう　**潰瘍**　ulcer /ʌ́lsəⁱ/, ulceration （岡ulcerative）　◆口の中に潰瘍ができていますか Do you have any *ulcers in your mouth[mouth ulcers]?　◆胃に潰瘍がある have *a stomach ulcer[an ulcer in the stomach]　◆胃に潰瘍の治った跡がある have traces[signs] of an ulcer that has healed in one's stomach　◆潰瘍は深い〈浅い〉It's a deep〈shallow / superficial〉ulcer.　◀悪性の潰瘍 a malignant ulcer　◀アフタ性潰瘍 aphthous ulcer　アフタ様潰瘍 aphthoid ulcer　胃潰瘍 stomach[gastric] ulcer　外陰潰瘍 ulceration of the vulva　角膜潰瘍 corneal ulcer　抗潰瘍薬 antiulcer medication[drug / agent]　口腔潰瘍 oral ulcer　口唇潰瘍 canker sore　再発性潰瘍 recurrent ulcer　十二指腸潰瘍 duodenal ulcer　出血性潰瘍 hemorrhagic ulcer　消化性潰瘍 peptic ulcer　褥瘡性潰瘍 pressure[decubitus] ulcer　ステロイド潰瘍 steroid ulcer　舌潰瘍 tongue ulcer / ulcer of the tongue　穿孔性潰瘍 perforated[perforating] ulcer　難治性潰瘍 intractable ulcer　皮膚潰瘍 skin ulcer　吻合部潰瘍 stomal[anastomotic] ulcer　▶潰瘍性口内炎 ulcerative stomatitis　潰瘍性大腸炎 ulcerative colitis　潰瘍痛 ulcer pain

がいよう　**外用**　external use （岡局所用の topical）　◆この薬は外用薬としてのみ使います This medication is for external use only.　◀ステロイド外用薬 topical steroid　ステロイド含有外用薬 steroid-containing external medication

がいらい　**外来**　outpatient clinic[department]　（通院の）ambulatory clinic　◆外科の外来に4月15日月曜日, 午前9時においで下さい Please come to the outpatient surgery department[clinic] on Monday, April (the) fifteenth, at nine in the morning.　◆この手術は外来で行うことができます This surgery can be performed on an outpatient basis. / This surgery is an outpatient procedure.　◀痛み外来 pain clinic　一般外来 (general) outpatient department[clinic]　救急外来（救急部門）emergency (outpatient) unit[department] /（救急室）emergency room；ER　セカンドオピニオン外来 second opinion clinic　専門外来 special outpatient clinic　内科外来 outpatient internal medicine department　夜間外来入口 (hospital) night[nighttime] entrance /（救急の）emergency night[nighttime] entrance　▶外来入口 outpatient entrance / entrance for outpatients　外来受付 outpatient reception counter[desk]　外来会計 outpatient cashier　外来化学療法 outpatient chemotherapy　外来患者 outpatient / ambulatory patient　外来手術 outpatient[ambulatory] surgery　外来診療 outpatient treatment[care / service]　外来診療部門 outpatient department　外来リハビリテーション outpatient[ambulatory] rehabilitation

かいらく　**快楽**　(気晴らし)**recreation**　(形 **recreational**)　◆快楽用の薬物を使う use recreational drugs　◆日本では大麻など快楽用薬物の使用は違法です In Japan it's illegal to use recreational drugs such as marijuana. / The use of recreational drugs such as marijuana is prohibited by law in Japan.

かいり　**解離**　(遮断・隔絶)**dissociation**　(形 **dissociative**, **dissociated**)　(剝離・遊離)**dissection**　(形 **dissect**)　◀感覚解離 sensory dissociation　大動脈解離 aortic dissection　房室解離 atrioventricular[AV] dissociation　▶解離性感覚障害 dissociated sensory disturbance　解離性大動脈瘤 dissecting aortic aneurysm　解離性同一症[解離性同一性障害] dissociative identity disorder　解離反応 dissociative reaction

がいリンパ　**外リンパ**　**perilymph**　(形 **perilymphatic**)　▶外リンパ管 perilymphatic duct　外リンパ瘻 perilymphatic fistula

かいろ¹　**回路**　**circuit**　◀人工呼吸器回路 ventilator circuit

カイロ²　**懐炉**　**portable[pocket] body warmer**　◆携帯用カイロで指先を暖めると，レイノー症状は和らぐでしょう A portable body warmer over the tips of your fingers will relieve the symptoms of Raynaud's. / If you warm the tips of your fingers with a portable body warmer, the symptoms caused by Raynaud's will get better.　◀使い捨てカイロ disposable portable[pocket] body warmer

カイロプラクター　**chiropractor**

カイロプラクティック　**chiropractic**

カイロミクロン　**chylomicron**

かいわ　**会話**　**conversation**　(くだけた会話)**talk**　(話し言葉)**speech**　☞話　◆会話

をする have[carry on] a conversation　◆会話が聞き取りづらいですか Is it hard for you to hear what other people are saying?　▶会話音域 speech range　会話恐怖症 laliophobia

かいんとう　**下咽頭**　**hypopharynx**　(形 **hypopharyngeal**)　▶下咽頭がん hypopharyngeal cancer

かう¹　**買う**

《購入する》**buy, purchase**　◆入院に必要な品物は院内の売店で買うことができます You can buy[purchase] the things you need for your admission to the hospital at the hospital shop.

《価値・力などを認める》**recognize**　◆彼は手術の腕を買われています He is well recognized for his outstanding surgical skills.

《他の人から悪感情を抱かれる》　◆彼女の迷惑行為は他の患者のひんしゅくを買いました(顔をしかめられた)Her annoying behavior was frowned on[upon] by the other patients. / The other patients frowned at her annoying behavior.

かう²　**飼う**　(ペットを飼う)**have**　(家畜などを飼育する)**keep**　◆ペットを飼っていますか Do you have any pets?　◆ペットは室内・室外のどちらで飼っていますか Do you keep your pet indoors or outdoors?

カウザルギー　**causalgia**　(灼熱痛)**burning pain**

カウプしすう　**―指数**　**Kaup index**

ガウン　**gown**　◆服を脱いでこのガウンを着て下さい Please take your clothes off and put this gown on.　◀滅菌ガウン sterile[sterilized] gown

カウンセラー　**counselor**　◆悩み事をカウンセラーに相談する consult a counselor about *one's* troubles　◀学校カウンセラー school counselor　性専門カウンセラー sex counselor

カウンセリング　**counseling**　◆摂食障害のカウンセリングをする〈受ける〉give〈have / receive〉counseling for an eating disorder　◆カウンセリングは私のオフィスで3時から行います The counseling session will take place at three o'clock in my office. ◀遺伝カウンセリング genetic counseling　学校カウンセリング school counseling　グリーフカウンセリング grief counseling　心理カウンセリング psychological counseling　性カウンセリング sex counseling

かえいよう　過栄養　**overnutrition**

かえす　返す　**return, give back**　☞戻す
◆保険証〈診察券〉をお返しします I'm returning your *insurance card〈(hospital) ID card〉.　◆鍵は退院時に担当ナースにお返し下さい Please *return the key[give the key back] to your nurse at the time of your discharge.

かえって　（よりもっと）**more … (than)**　（すればするほどますます）**the＋比較級** …　◆励ましはかえって彼女を落ち込ませることになるので避けたほうがよいでしょう You should avoid *trying to cheer her up[saying words of encouragement to her] because it[they] might make her feel more depressed.　◆抗がん剤の治療によってかえって体力が低下してしまうことがあります Sometimes, chemotherapy does more harm than good because it drains *the patient's* energy levels.　◆掻くとかえって痒くなりますよ The more you scratch your skin, the itchier it will be.

かえる¹　替える・換える・代える　（一般的に）**change**　（交換する）**swap, switch, exchange**　（代用品と入れ替える）**replace**
☞代わる，交換　◆シーツ〈リネン〉を換えましょうか Shall I change your sheets〈bed linens〉?　◆包帯を換える change the bandage[dressing]　◆担当看護師を代えましょう We'll get you a different nurse. / We'll change your nurse.　◆病室を他の患者さんと換えていただけませんか Could you swap rooms with another patient?
◆濁った水晶体を取り除いて人工のレンズに替える remove the cloudy lens and replace it with an artificial one　◆ご飯をパンに替えることもできます You can have bread instead of rice.　◆ふつうの醤油を減塩タイプに替える use[have] low-salt soy sauce instead of regular soy sauce

かえる²　変える　（一般的に）**change**（図change）　（修正する）**revise, alter**　（移す）**shift**　◆変わる，変更　◆体の位置を変える change *one's* position /〈体重を〉shift *one's* weight　◆体の向きを変えて下さい Please change *your position[the position of your body].　◆Please try to move onto your other side.　◆薬を変えて様子を見ましょう Let's *change the medication[try a different medication] and see what happens.　◆散歩して気分を変えてはいかがですか How about taking a walk for a change of mind?　◆態度〈考え〉を変える change *one's* attitude〈mind〉　◆計画を変える revise[change / alter] a plan

かえる³　帰る　（自宅に帰る）**go home, return home**　（病院に戻る）**come back to the hospital, return to the hospital**　☞戻る
◆日曜日の午後までに病院に帰ってきて下さい Be sure to *come back[return] to the hospital by Sunday afternoon.

かえるがたしい　蛙型肢位　**frog-leg position**

かお　顔　**face**（図facial）　（目鼻立ち）**features**　★通例，複数形で.　（表情）**expression**　◆顔が少しむくんでいるようです Your face looks slightly bloated[swollen].　◆赤ら顔 a ruddy face[〈顔色〉complexion]　◆顔が青く〈紫色に〉なる *one's* face turns pale〈purple〉　◆顔がほてる have a flushed face / the face becomes flushed　◆顔中に発疹がある have a rash all over *one's* face　◆濡れたタオルで顔を拭く wipe *one's* face with a moist washcloth　◆顔の感覚 facial sensations　◆顔の部位 facial region　◆顔立ちの変化 change in *a person's* facial features　◆顔の特徴 facial features　◆顔の表情が乏しくなる have poor facial expression(s)
◆無表情な顔つき an expressionless appearance /（仮面のような）a masklike face /（ぼーっとした）a blank expression　◆嫌な顔をする frown / look displeased　◆怒った顔をする look angry[offended]　☞顔色

かおいろ　顔色
《皮膚の色》**complexion**　◆顔色がいい

かおいろ

have a good[healthy] complexion ◆青白い顔色 a pale complexion ◆人から顔色が悪いと言われたことがありますか Has anyone told you that *you look pale[your face looks pale]? ◆今朝は顔色がよくありませんね You don't look well this morning.
《機嫌》 ◆他人の顔色をうかがう(表情を注意深く見る)study a person's facial expression /(他人の気分を気にする)be sensitive to [about] other people's moods /(怒らせないように気をつける)take care not to offend [displease] others

かおり 香り smell ☞匂い

かおん 加温 heating ◀局所加温 local heat(treatment)

かがいしゃ 加害者 (暴行事件の)assailant, attacker (事故の)the person who caused the accident (犯罪の)perpetrator

かかえる 抱える have ◆彼は経済問題を抱えています He has financial problems [worries / burdens]. ◆仕事を抱えすぎていますか Do you have too much work (to do)? ◆右向きに寝て, 左膝を抱えて [曲げて]下さい Please lie on your right side with your left knee bent[flexed] (toward your chest).

かがく¹ 科学 science (形scientific)
◀医学 medical science 行動科学 behavioral science 自然科学 natural science 生命科学 life science /(生物上の)bioscience ▶科学技術 science and technology / scientific technique 科学的根拠 scientific evidence

かがく² 化学 chemistry (形chemical)
◀血液化学 blood chemistry 生化学 biochemistry 免疫化学 immunochemistry 有毒化学物質 poisonous[toxic] chemical ▶化学受容器 chemoreceptor 化学調味料 artificial seasoning 化学熱傷 chemical burn 化学反応 chemical reaction 化学物質 chemical(substance / agent) 化学物質過敏症 chemical hypersensitivity 化学名 chemical name 化学薬品 chemicals 化学薬品会社 chemical company ☞化学療法

かがく³ 下顎 lower jaw, mandible (形mandibular) ☞顎(あご, がく) ▶下顎挙上法 jaw-lift method 下顎呼吸 mandibular breathing[respiration] 下顎骨 *lower jaw[mandibular] bone 下顎前突症 mandibular protrusion 下顎反射 jaw [mandibular] reflex

かがくりょうほう 化学療法 chemotherapy (口語的に)chemo /kí:mou/ ◆化学療法は薬でがん細胞を破壊する治療法です Chemotherapy is a treatment using drugs that destroy cancer cells. ◆最初の化学療法は入院して行いましょう You'll need to be hospitalized[admitted to the hospital] for your first round of chemotherapy.
◆入院している間に化学療法の初回クールを受けていただきます You'll receive your first round of chemotherapy during your hospital stay. ◆化学療法の主な副作用は吐き気・嘔吐, 食欲不振, 血球減少, 脱毛です The most common[The main] side effects of chemotherapy include nausea and vomiting, loss[lack] of appetite, low blood cell counts, and hair loss. ◆化学療法を受ける have[receive / undergo] chemotherapy ◆化学療法を行う give[administer] chemotherapy (treatment) ◆2回目の化学療法を始める start *a person's* second round[cycle] of chemotherapy ◆化学療法の全コースを終える finish the full course of chemotherapy
◀外来化学療法 outpatient chemotherapy 術後化学療法 postoperative[adjuvant] chemotherapy 術前化学療法 preoperative[neoadjuvant] chemotherapy 大量化学療法 high-dose chemotherapy 多剤併用化学療法 combination chemotherapy 動注化学療法 intraarterial infusion chemotherapy ▶化学放射線療法 chemoradiotherapy / chemoradiation 化学療法薬 chemotherapeutic (medication / drug / agent) /(抗がん剤)anticancer medication[drug / agent] /(抗腫瘍薬)antineoplastic (medication / drug / agent)

かかせない 欠かせない ◆早期回復には

家族の励ましが欠かせません(絶対に必要です) Having family support is essential [crucial] to make a quick recovery.

かかつどう 過活動(の) **overactive**
▶過活動膀胱 overactive bladder；OAB

かかと 踵 heel ◆かかとにひび割れができる have *a cracked heel[cracked heels] ◆かかと膝試験 heel-knee test かかと歩行 heel gait

かがむ 屈む (上体を曲げる)bend (over, forward) (前かがみになる)stoop, bend down, lean forward (うずくまる)crouch ☞曲げる ◆腰をかがめると痛みを感じますか Do you feel the pain when you bend over[down]? ◆かがんだ姿勢で歩く walk with a stoop ◆かがみ姿勢(屈曲の) crouched posture

かかり 係 (担当者)clerk in charge, person in charge (受け持ち)charge ◆係の者にお尋ね下さい Please ask the clerk in charge. ◀受付係 receptionist 会計係 cashier

かかりつけ ◆かかりつけ医がいますか Do you have *a regular doctor[your own doctor]? ◆(紹介状を読みながら)かかりつけ医によると胸痛があるのですね. そのことについて話して下さい Your (family) doctor says you've been having trouble with chest pain. Please tell me about it. ▶かかりつけ医 regular doctor[physician] / (家庭医)family doctor[physician] かかりつけ薬局 regular pharmacy

かかる¹
《時間を要する》**take, require** ◆この点滴は約2時間かかります This (intravenous) drip will take about two hours. ◆この検査を済ますには30分かかります It'll take thirty minutes to complete this test. / This test will take thirty minutes. ◆完治には治療に数年かかります A complete recovery will require[take] several years of treatment.
《費用を要する》**cost** ◆この薬は1か月あたり5万円かかります This medication costs [will cost] fifty thousand yen a month. / The cost of this medication is[will be]

fifty thousand yen a month.
《医師の診察を受ける》**see, consult** ◆あなたは乳腺外科医にかかる必要があります You should see[consult] a breast surgeon. ◆ご自宅の近くではどこの病院にかかっていますか Which hospital[clinic] in your neighborhood are you being treated at?

かかる² 罹る (発症する)**have, get, develop** (感染する)**catch, contract** (病気で苦しむ)**suffer (from)** (病気が冒す)**affect** (感染しやすい)**be susceptible (to)** (疾病素因がある)**be predisposed (to, toward)** ◆現在, 何か病気に罹っていますか Do you currently have any medical conditions? ◆最近4週間以内に何か病気に罹りましたか Have you had any illness in the past four weeks? ◆これまでに肺の病気に罹ったことはありますか Have you ever had *any lung diseases? ◆喉の感染症によく罹りますか Do you often have[get] throat infections? ◆そのウイルスに罹ってからどのくらい経ちますか How long is it since you contracted the virus? ◆インフルエンザに罹る get[catch / have] (the) flu ◆肺炎に罹る have[get] pneumonia ◆保育園では多くの子供たちがその病気に罹ります The disease affects a lot of children at day care centers. ◆風邪に罹りやすい be susceptible to colds ◆彼女は乳がんに罹りやすい素因があります She may be predisposed to breast cancer.

かかわらず 拘らず
《…に関係なく》**regardless of** ◆この病気は年齢や性別にかかわらず誰でも罹ります Anyone can get this illness, regardless of age or gender.
《…であるのに》**despite, in spite of, though, although** ◆障害があるにもかかわらず彼女はとても活動的です Despite her disability, she is very active. / Even though she *has a disability[is disabled], she is very active.

かかわる 関わる
《関係・関与する》**concern** (関心をもつ)**be concerned, involve** (関わり合いをもつ)**be involved** ◆本来私たちが関わるべき問題

ではないかもしれませんが Under ordinary [normal] circumstances, this isn't a problem that concerns[involves] us, but … ◆その点について一切関わってはいません I'm not at all involved in that (matter). / (何の関係もない) I have nothing to do with that (matter). ◆あなたの治療は多くの医療スタッフが関わって決定されます Many members of the staff are working together closely in making decisions about your treatment. / Many members of the staff are involved in making decisions about your treatment. ◆当科は新薬の臨床試験に積極的に関わっています Our department is actively *involved in[(参加する) participating in] clinical trials of new drugs.
《影響する》 ◆この進行性の壊疽はできるだけ早く治療を開始しないと命に関わります If we don't start treating this progressive gangrene as quickly as possible, it could become life-threatening. ◆この決断は彼女の生死に関わる問題です This decision is a matter of life or death for her.

かかんき 過換気 hyperventilation, overventilation ☞過呼吸 ▶過換気症候群 hyperventilation syndrome

かがんけん 下眼瞼 lower eyelid

かかんしょう 過干渉 overinterference (動overinterfere) ☞過保護 ◆彼女は子供時代に母親の過干渉を受けていました As a child, she had an overinterfering mother. / Her mother was too interfering when she was a child.

かき¹ 火気 (火) fire (熱・火力) heat (炎) flame ◆酸素供給装置には火気を近づけないで下さい Please keep oxygen supply equipment away from heat and flame sources. ◆(掲示)火気厳禁 No Fire / (警告：可燃物) Caution Flammables / Danger Highly Flammable.

かき² 牡蠣 oyster ◆生牡蠣の食あたりが疑われます It's probably *raw oyster poisoning[raw oyster-borne infection].

かき³ 下記 the following ◆連絡先は下記を参照して下さい For contact numbers, please refer to the following. / Please see below for contact numbers. ◆詳細は下記の通りです Details are as follows：… ★通例，最後にコロン（：）を付ける。/ Please see below for details.

かぎ 鍵
《ドア・金庫の》key ◆これがロッカーの鍵です This is[Here's] the key to your locker. ◆貴重品は金庫に入れて鍵をかけて下さい Please lock your valuables in the safe. ◆ドアに鍵はかけないで下さい Please don't lock the door. ◆金庫の鍵を開ける unlock the safe ◆金庫の鍵を失くされたのですか Did you lose the key to your safe?
《秘訣・重要な点》key ◆訓練の継続がリハビリを成功させる鍵になります Continuing training is the key to successful rehabilitation. / The key to successful rehabilitation is to stick with it.

かきうつす 書き写す copy ◆その絵をこちらの紙に書き写して下さい Please copy the picture onto this paper.

かききず 掻き傷 scratch ☞傷

かききゅうか 夏季休暇 summer vacation[holidays] ☞休暇

かきことば 書き言葉 written language ◆日本語の書き言葉は理解できますか Do you understand written Japanese? / Do you read Japanese?

かきさん 過期産 (出産) postterm birth, postmature birth (分娩) postterm delivery, postmature delivery ▶過期産児 postterm[postmature] baby / postterm[postmature] infant

かきどう 下気道 lower airway, lower respiratory tract ▶下気道感染 lower airway [respiratory (tract)] infection

かきにんしん 過期妊娠 postterm pregnancy, prolonged pregnancy

かきねつ 夏季熱 summer fever

かきまぜる かき混ぜる (液体などをかき回す) stir (混ぜる) mix ◆この粉薬は水に溶かし，よくかき混ぜてからご使用下さい Please dissolve this powder in water and stir[mix] well before taking it.

かきむしる （爪などで引っ掻く）**scratch**（off） ◆かさぶたをかきむしる scratch the scab off

かぎゃく 可逆（性の） **reversible**（↔irreversible 图**reversibility**） ◀気道可逆性試験 airway reversibility test

かぎゅう 蝸牛 **cochlea**（图**cochlear**） ▶蝸牛管 cochlear duct　蝸牛神経 cochlear nerve

かきょうじんつう 過強陣痛 **uterine hypercontraction**

かぎる 限る
《制限する》（範囲を限定する）**limit**（規制する）**restrict** ☞制限 ◆アルコールを飲むのは1，2杯を週に数回に限ったほうがよいでしょう You should limit your alcohol consumption to one or two drinks a few times a week. ◆集中治療室にお入りになる人数を限らせていただいています We limit the number of people who are allowed to be in the intensive care unit. ◆ご面会はご家族に限らせていただきます Visiting is[Patient visitors are] restricted to family members. ◆電話受付は平日の9:00〜17:00に限ります We receive phone calls on weekdays from nine am to five pm only. ◆夜間の外出や週末の外泊は担当医が許可した場合に限ります(許可を必要とする)Patients need their doctor's permission if they wish to go outdoors or leave the hospital for an evening or weekend.
《最も良い・最も重要な》 ◆風邪を治すには十分睡眠をとるに限ります The most important thing you can do to cure a cold is to get a good sleep. /（十分な睡眠に勝る方法はない）There's no better way to cure a cold than to have a good sleep.

かく¹ 核 （cell）**nucleus**（图**nuclei** 图**nuclear, nucleic**） ◀視床核 thalamic nuclei ☞核医学，核酸，核磁気共鳴，核分裂

かく² 書く **write** ◆この紙にお名前とご住所を書いて下さい Please write your name and address on this paper. ◆黒のボールペンで書く write with a black ballpoint pen ◆名前を活字体で書く write one's name in block letters / print one's name

かく³ 描く （ペン・鉛筆などで）**draw** （絵具で）**paint** ◆ここに時計の絵を描いて下さい Please draw a clock here.

かく⁴ 掻く **scratch** ◆傷口を掻かないで下さい Please don't scratch the wound. ◆皮膚を掻かないで下さい Please avoid scratching your skin.

かぐ 嗅ぐ **smell**

がく 顎 **jaw** /dʒɔː/ （图上顎の **maxillary** 下顎の **mandibular**） ☞顎（あご），下顎，上顎 ▶顎顔面骨折 maxillofacial fracture　顎骨骨髄炎 osteomyelitis of the jaw　顎骨骨折 fracture of the jaw ☞顎下，顎関節

かくいがく 核医学 **nuclear medicine** ▶核医学検査 nuclear medicine test[testing] / radionuclide study

かくおうだん 核黄疸 **nuclear jaundice, kernicterus**

かくか 角化 **keratinization**（图**keratotic**） ◀脂漏性角化症 seborrheic keratosis ▶角化異常症 keratotic disorder　角化細胞 keratinocyte　角化症 keratosis

がくか 顎下（の） **submandibular** ▶顎下腺 submandibular gland　顎下リンパ節 submandibular lymph node

かくかぞく 核家族 **nuclear family**（↔extended family）

がくかんせつ 顎関節 **temporomandibular joint ; TMJ** ▶顎関節症 temporomandibular joint disorder　顎関節脱臼 jaw dislocation / dislocation of the jaw

がくぎょう 学業 **schoolwork** ◆その問題は学業に差し支えますか Does that problem interfere with your schoolwork? ◆学業を頑張る study[work] hard ▶学業成績 grades / school record　学業遅滞児 slow learner　学業不振 underachievement　学業不振児 underachiever

かくげつ 隔月 **every other month**

かくけつまくえん 角結膜炎 **keratoconjunctivitis** ◀乾性角結膜炎 dry eye / keratoconjunctivitis sicca；KCS　流行性角結膜炎 epidemic keratoconjunctivitis；EKC

かくさ 格差 （相違）difference （隔たり）gap

かくさん¹ 核酸 nucleic acid ◀デオキシリボ核酸 deoxyribonucleic acid；DNA リボ核酸 ribonucleic acid；RNA ▶核酸合成阻害薬 nucleic acid synthesis inhibitor 核酸増幅法 nucleic acid amplification technique 核酸代謝 nucleic acid metabolism

かくさん² 拡散する diffuse （図diffusion） ◀肺拡散能 pulmonary diffusing capacity ▶拡散障害 diffusion impairment

かくじききょうめい 核磁気共鳴 nuclear magnetic resonance；NMR ☞MRI ▶核磁気共鳴スキャン nuclear magnetic resonance scanning

かくじつ 隔日 every other day

かくしつそう 角質層 horny layer of epidermis, stratum corneum

かくしゅう 隔週 every other week

かくじゅう 拡充する expand （図expansion） ◆在宅診療部門の拡充を図る plan to expand the division of home-based care

がくしゅう 学習する （習得する・学ぶ）learn （図learning） （勉強する）study （図study） ◆あなたは日本語をどこで学習しましたか Where did you study Japanese? ◀回避学習 avoidance learning 問題基盤型学習 problem-based learning；PBL ▶学習困難 learning difficulty 学習症 learning disability[disorder]；LD 学習症児 child with a learning disability 学習能力 learning ability

かくしゅつじゅつ 核出術 enucleation

かくしん 確信する be sure[certain, confident]（of, about） ◆私はあなたが禁煙できると確信しています I'm sure[certain / confident] that you'll quit[give up] smoking. ◆残念ですが，その点に関しては確信が持てません I'm sorry, but I'm not sure about that.

かくす 隠す hide, conceal ◆隠さずに何でも話して下さい Please don't hide[keep] anything from me. / Please tell me anything without keeping[hiding / concealing] it from me.

かくせい¹ 覚醒する （麻酔などから離脱する）emerge （図emergence） （目覚める）wake up （目覚めている）be awake （図awakening, arousal） （意識清明である）be alert （図alertness） ◆麻酔から覚醒する emerge[wake up] from (the) anesthesia ◆検査〈処置 / 手術〉後は麻酔から十分覚醒するまで回復室で経過をみます After the examination〈procedure / surgery〉, you'll be monitored in the recovery room until you've fully *woken from[come out of] the anesthesia. ◀早朝覚醒 early morning awakening[arousal] 中途覚醒 awakening[arousal] from sleep ▶覚醒暗示 suggestion in the waking state 覚醒下手術 awake[wide-awake] surgery 覚醒時興奮 emergence excitement 覚醒状態 arousal state 覚醒遅延 prolonged awakening 覚醒反応 alerting[arousal] response / alerting[arousal] reaction

かくせい² 郭清 dissection ◀リンパ節郭清術 lymphadenectomy / lymph node dissection

がくせい 学生 student ◆彼女は東西大学の医学生です She is a medical student at the University of Tozai. ★前置詞は of ではなく at を用いる。 ◆彼は化学専攻の学生です He is a chemistry student[major]. ◆彼女は大学院の学生です She is a graduate student. ◀医学生 medical student 外国人留学生 international[overseas / foreign] student 看護学生 nursing student 歯科学生 dental student ▶学生アパシー student apathy 学生生活 student[college / university] life / campus life 学生ビザ student visa

かくせいいでん 隔世遺伝 atavism （図atavistic）

かくせいざい 覚醒剤 drugs, stimulants （違法薬物）(illegal) drugs （快楽を得るための薬物）recreational drugs ★通例，複数形で．（「ヤク」に相当する俗称）dope （メタンフェタミン）methamphetamine, （メタンフェタミンの俗称）meth ◆彼は覚醒剤中毒です

He is addicted to drugs. ◆覚醒剤を使用する take[use] drugs ◆覚醒剤を常用している be on drugs ▶覚醒剤中毒 stimulant addiction 覚醒剤中毒者 stimulant addict 覚醒剤取締法 Stimulants Control Act

かくだい　拡大する 《増大する》enlarge（図enlargement 形enlarged）《伸展・延長する》extend（図extension 形extended）《広がる》spread（図spread）《倍率などを拡大する》magnify（図magnification 形magnifying）☞拡張 ◆心臓が少し拡大しています Your heart is slightly enlarged. / You have a slightly enlarged heart. ◆湿疹の範囲が全身に拡大する the eczema extends[spreads] over *a person's* whole body ◆風疹が日本の成人の間に拡大しています Rubella is spreading among adults in Japan. ◆感染の拡大を防ぐ prevent the spread of infection / prevent an infection from spreading ◆X線の画像を拡大する magnify an X-ray image ◀感染拡大 spread of infection　強拡大（顕微鏡の）high-power field　弱拡大 low-power field　心（臓）拡大 heart enlargement / enlargement of the heart　脳室拡大 ventricular enlargement ▶拡大家族 extended family　拡大鏡 magnifying glass / loupe　拡大根治手術 extended radical surgery

かくたん　喀痰 sputum, phlegm ☞痰 ▶喀痰検査 sputum test[examination] 喀痰細胞診 sputum cytology　喀痰培養 sputum culture

かくちょう　拡張する 《血管・瞳孔などが広がる》dilate（図dilatation, dilation, ectasia, ectasis）《広がる》expand（図expansion）《膨らむ》distend（図distension）☞拡大 ◆血管が拡張しています The blood vessels have dilated. ◀胃拡張 stomach[gastric] dilatation　気管支拡張症 bronchiectasis 気管支拡張薬 bronchodilator　くも状血管拡張症 spider telangiectasia　血管拡張薬 vasodilator　膵管拡張 pancreatic duct dilatation　胆管拡張 bile duct dilatation バルーン拡張術 balloon dilatation　毛細血管拡張 telangiectasia ▶拡張型心筋症 dilated cardiomyopathy；DCM ☞拡張期

かくちょうき　拡張期 diastole（↔systole 形diastolic）, the diastolic period ▶拡張期血圧 diastolic blood pressure　拡張期高血圧 diastolic hypertension　拡張期雑音 diastolic murmur

かくっきょく　過屈曲 hyperflexion ▶過屈曲損傷 hyperflexion injury

かくてい　確定する decide (on)（図decision 形最終的な・決定的な definitive　明確な・確実な definite）◆手術日が確定しましたらお電話でご連絡いたします We'll call you once your surgery date is decided [scheduled]. ◆確定診断する make a definitive[definite] diagnosis ◆確定診断を行うために検査が必要です We need to run some tests to get a definitive[definite] diagnosis.

カクテル cocktail ▶カクテル療法 cocktail therapy

かくど　角度 《角の大きさ》angle ◆定位放射線治療では，さまざまな角度から腫瘍に照射します Stereotactic radiotherapy targets a tumor with beams delivered from multiple angles. ◆X線写真は何回か角度を変えて撮影を行います We'll take the X-ray from several angles. 《視点》point of view, viewpoint, angle ◆角度を変えてその問題を考えてみましょう Let's think about the problem from another[a different] *point of view[angle].

がくどう　学童 schoolchild（形若年性の juvenile）▶学童期側彎症 juvenile scoliosis　学童保育 after-school child care

かくとく　獲得する acquire ◆腫瘍がこの抗がん剤に対して耐性を獲得したと考えられます The tumor seems to have acquired resistance to this type of anti-cancer medication. ◆抗菌薬に対する耐性を獲得した細菌 bacteria that have acquired tolerance against an antibiotic ▶獲得免疫 acquired immunity

かくどけい 角度計 goniometer

かくにん 確認する （はっきり確かめる）
confirm （図confirmation 図confirmatory）
（照合・照会する）check （特定する）identify
◆要確認 confirmation required
[needed] ◆予約を確認する confirm the
appointment ◆（患者の）意思を確認する
confirm the wishes[intentions]（of the
patient） ◆（患者の）死亡を確認する confirm the death（of the patient） ◆まだ妊
娠をはっきり確認することはできません We
can't confirm your pregnancy yet. ◆お
名前を確認させて下さい Let me just confirm your name. ◆お名前と生年月日を確
認して下さい Please check your name and
birth date. ◆担当医に確認する check
with a person's doctor ◆原発腫瘍を確認
する identify the primary tumor ▶確認
強迫 compulsive rechecking[checking
and double-checking] 確認検査 confir-
matory test

かくひしょう 角皮症 keratoderma
◀掌蹠角皮症 palmoplantar keratoderma

がくぶ 学部 school, faculty, department
★およその規模は school＞faculty＞depart-
ment. ▶医学部 school of medicine /
medical school 看護学部 school[facul-
ty / department] of nursing / nursing
school[faculty / department]

かくぶんれつ 核分裂 （細胞核の分裂）nu-
clear fission （原子核の分裂）nuclear division, division of （the）nucleus

かくほ 確保する （固定・保持する）secure
◆気道を確保する secure the airway /（開
いた状態に保つ）hold the airway open
◀静脈確保 venous access / establishment of a venous route

かくまく¹ 角膜 cornea /kɔ́ɚ-niə/ （図cor-
neal 画kerat(o)-） ◆左目の角膜が炎
症を起こしています The cornea of your
left eye is inflamed. ◆角膜が傷ついたの
はコンタクトレンズの不適切な使用のため
です Corneal abrasion *is due to[is
caused by] inappropriate use of contact
lenses. ◆角膜の白濁 a nebula[faint
cloudy spot] in the cornea ◀全層角膜移

植 penetrating keratoplasty；PKP レー
ザー角膜切削形成術 laser-assisted in situ
keratomileusis；LASIK ▶角膜移植
corneal transplant[transplantation] /
corneal graft[grafting] 角膜異物 corneal
foreign body 角膜潰瘍 corneal ulcer 角
膜乾燥症 corneal xerosis 角膜矯正術 orthokeratology 角膜銀行 eye bank 角膜
計 ophthalmometer 角膜混濁 corneal
opacity[clouding] 角膜びらん corneal
erosion 角膜フリクテン corneal phlyctenule 角膜ヘルペス[疱疹] corneal herpes ☞角膜炎

かくまく² 隔膜 septum （図septa）

かくまくえん 角膜炎 keratitis, corneal
inflammation ◀強角膜炎 sclerokeratitis
単純ヘルペス性角膜炎 herpes simplex
keratitis 兎眼性角膜炎 lagophthalmic
[exposure] keratitis トラコーマ角膜炎
trachomatous keratitis フリクテン角膜炎
phlyctenular keratitis

かくやく 確約する promise for sure, definitely promise, make a definite promise
◆確約はできかねますが，ご希望に沿えるよ
う前向きに対処します I can't promise for
sure, but we'll try as hard as possible to
meet[follow] your request.

かくらん 撹乱 （中断・混乱）disruption （図
disruptive） （心身の動揺）disturbance
◀内分泌撹乱（化学）物質 endocrine dis-
ruptors / hormone-disruptive chemicals / endocrine-disruptive chemicals；
EDCs

かくり 隔離する （一般的に引き離す）iso-
late （図isolation） （感染拡大予防のために患
者を隔離する）quarantine /kwɔ́ːrənti:n/ （図
quarantine） ◆お子さんは麻疹ですので他
の患者さんから隔離する必要があります
Your child has measles, so he〈she〉needs
to be isolated from the other patients.
◆法定伝染病の疑いがある時には隔離させ
ていただきます You'll be quarantined[put
in quarantine] if you have a suspected
legally designated communicable[infec-
tious] disease. ▶隔離患者 isolated
[quarantined] patient 隔離期間 period

of isolation[quarantine] 隔離治療 isolation treatment 隔離病室 isolation[quarantine] room 隔離病棟 isolation[quarantine] unit[ward]

かくりつ¹ 確率 （見込み）**chance** （公算）**probability** （可能性）**likelihood** （胚**likely**） ◆手術が成功する確率は 95% です The surgery has a ninety-five percent chance of success. ◆あなたは他の人よりもこの病気に罹る確率が高いかもしれません You may have a higher chance of developing this disease than other people. ◆5 年以内に再発する確率 the chances of having a recurrence within five years ◆家族の他の人もインフルエンザに罹る確率は高いでしょう There's a high probability that other members of the family will get the flu. ◆この病気はウイルスが原因である確率が非常に高いです A virus is the most likely cause of this disease. ◀死亡確率 probability[likelihood] of death 生存確率 probability of survival

かくりつ² 確立する **establish** （図**establishment**） ◆この病気の有効な治療法はまだ確立されていません An effective treatment for this disease has not yet been established. ◆腹腔鏡下胆嚢摘出術は確立された手術法です Laparoscopic cholecystectomy is a well-established surgery.

がくれき 学歴 **educational background, academic background** ◆最終学歴を教えて下さい How far did you get in school? / （最後の教育機関）Please tell me the last educational institution you attended.

かくれる 隠れる **hide** ◆うつ病の隠れた徴候 hidden signs of depressive disorder ◆隠れてタバコを吸う（こっそり）*be a secret smoker[smoke secretly] / （気づかれずに）smoke a cigarette without being noticed[seen] by others

かげ 影 **shadow** ☞陰影 ◆（X 線写真を示しながら）ここに異常な影があります There's an abnormal shadow here.

かけい¹ 家系 （家柄）**family** （祖先からの血筋）**pedigree** ▶家系図 family tree / pedi-

gree chart

かけい² 家計 **family budget** ◆彼女は家計が大変苦しいのでパートに出ています She is working part-time because her family is on a very tight budget.

かけいせい 過形成 **hyperplasia** （胚**hyperplastic**） ◀下垂体過形成 pituitary hyperplasia 腺腫様過形成 adenomatous hyperplasia；AH 副腎過形成 adrenal hyperplasia ▶過形成性ポリープ hyperplastic polyp

かけなおす 掛け直す （電話を）**call back** ◆明日かけ直していただけませんか Could you please call (me) back tomorrow? ◆後でこちらからかけ直します I'll call you back later.

かけはなれる かけ離れる **be different (from), differ (from)** ◆その民間療法が謳う効果は現代医学の常識からかけ離れています The claims made about that folk remedy are quite different from what is generally understood in modern medicine.

かける¹ 欠ける （壊れる）**break** （物の一部が欠ける）**chip** （不足する）**lack** ◆歯が欠ける *one's* tooth breaks[chips] (off) / get a chipped tooth ◆歯が欠けている have a chipped tooth ◆彼は働く意欲に欠けている He lacks[doesn't have] the will to work. /（意欲を失った）He has lost the will to work.

かける² 掛ける

《椅子に座る》**sit, have a seat** ◆どうぞお掛け下さい Please sit down. / Please have a seat.

《かぶせる・装着する》**slip … over, put … over, put on** ◆この酸素マスクを口に掛けましょう Let me slip this oxygen mask over your mouth. ◆もう 1 枚毛布を掛けましょうか Shall I put another blanket over you? / Do you need another blanket? ◆眼鏡を掛ける put on glasses ◆眼鏡を掛けている wear glasses

《重みを加える》**put weight on** （増やす）**increase** ◆手足に体重を掛ける put *one's* body weight on *one's* hands and feet

◆荷重を掛ける increase the load
《戸締りする》 ◆鍵を掛ける lock
《注ぐ》 ◆お湯をかける pour hot water on [over]
《言葉をかける》 ◆声をかける say … (to) / speak (to) ◆ご用の時は声をかけて下さい If you need anything, *let me know [just give me a call].
《電話する》call ◆明日の午後電話をかけて下さい Please call me tomorrow afternoon.
《気遣う》 ◆気にかける care / be concerned (about)
《相手に負担を与える》 ◆心配をかける cause *a person* to worry ◆迷惑をかける trouble / cause a lot of trouble
《費やす》 ◆時間をかける spend time
―**かける** ◆先ほど何か言いかけていたようですが，よろしければ教えて下さい You *were going[were about] to say something a little while ago. If you don't mind, would you tell me what (it was) you were going to say? ◆忘れかけていた記憶 a memory *one* *was about to forget[was on the verge of forgetting]

かげん¹ **下限** **the lower limit** ◆赤血球数は正常下限値を下回っています Your red blood cell count is below the lower limit of normal.

かげん² **加減**
《体調》 ◆お加減はいかがですか How do you feel? / How are you doing[feeling]?
《程度》 ◆塩加減を控えめにして下さい Please reduce[cut down on] your salt intake. ◆お風呂の湯加減はいかがですか How is the bath? / Is the bath water hot enough?

かこ **過去** **the past** (📖past 圖以前に before) ☞昔 ◆過去にこのような発作を起こしたことがありますか Have you ever had these attacks before? ◆過去の診療記録 *one's* past medical record ◆過去の出来事を忘れる lose *one's* memory of past events ◆過去5年間にわたって over the past five years

かご¹ **過誤** ◆医療過誤 (medical) mal-

practice / medical error[mistake] 医療過誤開示 medical error disclosure 看護過誤 nursing malpractice[error / mistake]

かご² **籠** **basket** ◆所持品はこのかごに入れて下さい Please put your things in this basket.

かこう¹ **下降** **descent** (📖descend, go down), **depression** ◀ST下降 ST depression 児頭下降度 descent of the fetal head ▶下降感(妊娠後期の)lightening (sensation)

かこう² **下行(性の)** **descending** (↔ascending) ◀下行結腸 descending colon 下行大動脈 descending aorta

かこう³ **加工する** **process** (図processing) ◀防水加工 waterproofing ▶加工食品 processed food

かこうぎし **架工義歯** **(dental) bridge**, **bridgework**

がこうそう **鵞口瘡** **thrush**

かごうぶつ **化合物** **(chemical) compound** ◀有機化合物 organic compound 有機リン化合物 organophosphorus compound ヨウ素化合物 iodinated compound 類似化合物 analog / analogue

かこきゅう **過呼吸** **hyperventilation** (📖hyperventilate), **hyperpnea**, **abnormally deep breathing** ◆過呼吸で失神する faint from[due to] hyperventilation ◆ストレスで過呼吸になる hyperventilate because of stress ▶過呼吸症候群 hyperventilation syndrome

かごしゅ **過誤腫** **hamartoma**

かこむ **囲む** (丸で囲む)**circle** ◆(質問票の中で)当てはまる項目を丸で囲んで下さい Please circle the items (in the questionnaire) that apply to you.

かさ **傘** **umbrella** ◆傘をさす put up *one's* umbrella ◀日傘 sunshade

かさい **火災** **fire** ◀火災訓練 fire drill 火災警報 fire alert 火災報知器 fire alarm

かさかさ (ひび割れた)**chapped** (乾燥した)**dry** (ざらざらした)**rough** ◆唇がかさかさになっている the lips are chapped / have chapped lips ◆かさかさの肌 dry [rough] skin / (脱水状態の皮膚)dehydrated skin

かさねる　重ねる

《物を積み重ねる》**stack, pile（up）** ◆このブロックを1つずつ重ねていって下さい Please stack[place] these blocks one on top of the other.

《繰り返す》**repeat** ◆初めはうまくできなくても，練習の回数を重ねるにつれてできるようになりますよ Even though you can't do very well at the beginning, you'll improve by *repeating the same exercise[practicing the exercise over and over again].

◆重ねてご協力に感謝申し上げます Once again, I'd like to thank you for your cooperation.

カサバッハ・メリットしょうこうぐん　症候群　Kasabach-Merritt syndrome

かさぶた　scab（㊒scabby, scabbed）

◆2, 3日で傷口にかさぶたができるでしょう The wound will form a scab in a few days. / A scab will form over the wound in a few days. ◆かさぶたはまもなく取れます The scab will come[fall] off soon. ◆かさぶたを引っ掻かないで下さい Don't pick at the scab. ◆かさぶたをはがすと痕になります If you peel off the scab, it will *leave a scar[cause scarring]. ◆かさぶただらけの皮膚 scabby[scabbed] skin

かざる　飾る　decorate ◆病室にお花を飾っても構いません It's all right to[You can] decorate your hospital room with flowers. ◆着飾っている be dressed up

かさん　加算　addition（㊒割増しの additional, extra） ◆個室を利用される場合には料金が別途加算されます There *will be[is] an extra[additional] charge for a private room.

かさんか　過酸化　(過酸化物)peroxide ▶過酸化脂質 lipid peroxide　過酸化水素 hydrogen peroxide　過酸化窒素 nitrogen peroxide

かさんしょう　過酸症　hyperacidity, chlorhydria

かし¹　下肢　leg, lower limb[extremity] ▶下肢筋 lower limb muscle(s) / the muscle(s) of the lower limb(s)　下肢静脈瘤 varicose veins of the lower limbs [extremities] / lower limb varicose veins　下肢切断 lower limb amputation　下肢装具 lower limb orthosis

かし²　仮死　asphyxia ◆その子は仮死状態で生まれました The baby was apparently dead at birth. / The baby was born apparently dead. ◀新生児仮死 neonatal asphyxia　胎児仮死[機能不全] fetal distress

かし³　菓子　(総称的に甘いもの)sweets ★複数形で. 代表的な菓子類の表現：ケーキ類 cake, ケーキひと切れ a piece of cake, クッキー類 cookie, キャンディ類 candy. ◆菓子類を控える avoid[refrain from] eating sweets

かし⁴　華氏　Fahrenheit；F /fǽrənhàit/ ★華氏の換算式 °F = (℃×1.8) +32 ◆あなたの体温は華氏96度です Your temperature is[You have a temperature of] ninety-six degrees Fahrenheit. / On the Fahrenheit scale your temperature is ninety-six.

◆摂氏38度はおよそ華氏100.4度に相当します A temperature of thirty-eight degrees Celsius corresponds[is equal] to about one hundred point four degrees Fahrenheit. ▶華氏温度計 Fahrenheit thermometer

かじ　家事　housework ◆家事をすると疲れますか Do you feel tired when you do your housework? ◆軽い家事はしてもいいですよ You can do some light housework. ◆家事の負担を軽減する reduce [cut down on] one's housework load

がし　餓死　(飢え死に)death from starvation　(食事を与えないことによる死)death by starvation（㊒starve to death）

かしこうせん　可視光線　visible ray[light, radiation]

かしだす　貸し出す　lend（out）　(有料で)rent ◆当院の患者図書館では本を貸し出しております Our patients' library lends out books. / Patients are welcome to borrow books from the patients' library. ◆車椅子の貸し出しは行っておりません We don't rent（out）wheelchairs.

かしつ 過失 error, mistake ☞誤り，間違い，ミス

かじつ 果実 fruit

かしつき 加湿器 humidifier /hjuːmídəfàɪə/ ▶加湿器肺 humidifier lung

かじゅう¹ 果汁 fruit juice

かじゅう² 荷重 （重さ・重量）weight （重み・負荷）load ◆足首に少しずつ負荷をかけて荷重負荷運動をしていきましょう We'll gradually increase (the load of) your ankle weights for your weight-bearing exercise. ◆荷重をかける increase the load ◆荷重を減らす lighten the load ◀部分荷重 partial weight-bearing 荷重歩行 weight-bearing walking

かじゅくじ 過熟児 （過期産児）postterm baby[infant], postmature baby[infant]

かしょ 箇所 （場所）place （痛みなどの箇所）spot （全体の中の部分）part ◆ご覧下さい．ここが骨折している箇所です Look, this is (the place) *where the bone is broken[where you've broken the bone]. ◆頭を触ると特に痛む箇所がありますか If you touch your head, is there a spot where it's especially painful?

かしょう¹ 火傷 burn ☞火傷(やけど)，熱傷 ▶火傷死 death due to burns

かしょう² 過小 ☞過小評価

かしょう³ 過少（の） （数が）too few （量が）too little （腸瘍数・量が少ない olig(o)- より低い・少ない hypo-） ◆唾液過少 oligoptyalism 羊水過少症 oligohydramnios

かじょう 過剰（の） （数が）too many （量が）too much （余分な）supernumerary （過度の）excessive （腸瘍…を超えた over- より高い・より多くの hyper-） ☞過度，—し過ぎる，—過ぎる ◀水分過剰 overhydration ストレス過剰 overstress ビタミン過剰症 hypervitaminosis ▶過剰骨 supernumerary bone 過剰歯 supernumerary tooth 過剰適応 excessive adaptation / overadaptation 過剰投与 overmedication / overdose / overdosage 過剰反応 overreaction / overresponse / reacting too strongly 過剰防衛 excessive self-defense ☞過剰摂取

がしょう 臥床 （安静）resting in bed, bed rest （寝床に入っていること）lying in bed ◆家では臥床しがちですか Do you tend to rest[stay / lie] in bed a lot when you're at home?

かじょうせっしゅ 過剰摂取 overdose, excessive intake ◆サプリメントを過剰摂取する take an overdose of dietary supplements

かしょうひょうか 過小評価する underestimate （軽く受け止める）make light of ◆この病気を過小評価してはいけません You shouldn't underestimate[make light of] this illness.

かしょく 過食 overeating （動overeat），excessive eating （動eat too much），hyperphagia ◆強迫的な過食 compulsive overeating ◆過食症(神経性過食症)bulimia (nervosa)；BN / (むちゃ食い) binge eating / (むちゃ食いと嘔吐)binging and purging / (気晴らし食い症候群)binge-eating syndrome

かしん 過信する overestimate （自信を持ち過ぎる）have too much confidence (in) （依存し過ぎる）rely too much (on) ◆ご自分の体力を過信してはいけません Don't overestimate your own physical strength. / You shouldn't have too much confidence in your own physical strength. ◆サプリメントへの過信は禁物です Don't rely too much[Don't become too reliant] on supplements.

かしんてん 過伸展 hyperextension ▶過伸展損傷 hyperextension injury

かず 数 number ☞数える，数字 ◆りんごの数を数える count the (number of) apples ◆数が増える the number increases / increase in number ◆大きい〈小さい〉数 a large〈small〉number ◆3という数 the number three ◆数多くの細菌 *a large number[large numbers] of bacteria

ガス gas （動ガス［おなら］を出す pass gas） ☞おなら ◆ガスでお腹が張っていますか Do you feel as if your abdomen is bloated [distended] with gas? ◆お腹にガスが溜

まる have intestinal gas / have gas in *one's* bowels ◆ガスが出たら知らせて下さい Please let us know when you've passed gas. ◆血液ガス blood gas 呼気ガス expiratory gas 炭酸ガス carbonic acid gas 腸内ガス bowel gas 動脈血ガス分析 arterial blood gas analysis 排気ガス exhaust gas 腐敗ガス putrefactive gas フロンガス chlorofluorocarbon gas 麻酔ガス anesthetic gas 有毒ガス poison [toxic / poisonous] gas 遊離ガス（像）free air ▶ガス壊疽 gas gangrene ガス交換 gas exchange ガス自殺 gas suicide / suicide by inhaling gas ガス中毒 gas poisoning ガス麻酔薬 gas anesthetic ガス滅菌法 gas sterilization

かすい 下垂 （落下）drop （垂れ）drooping （脱出）prolapse （下降）descent （腰屈−ptosis） ◀眼瞼下垂 blepharoptosis / drooping eyelid 子宮下垂 uterine prolapse ▶下垂指 drop finger 下垂手 drop hand / （手首）drop wrist 下垂足 drop foot

かすいたい 下垂体 pituitary gland ◆下垂体は他の内分泌腺をコントロールする多くのホルモンを分泌します The pituitary gland is a gland that secretes many hormones that regulate other endocrine glands. ◀間脳下垂体系 the diencephalic-pituitary system ▶下垂体後葉ホルモン posterior pituitary hormone；PPH 下垂体腺腫 pituitary adenoma 下垂体前葉ホルモン anterior pituitary hormone 下垂体卒中 pituitary apoplexy ☞下垂体機能

かすいたいきのう 下垂体機能 pituitary function ◀汎下垂体機能低下症 panhypopituitarism ▶下垂体機能検査 pituitary function test 下垂体機能亢進症 hyperpituitarism 下垂体機能低下症 hypopituitarism

かすか 微か（な）（光・音などが弱い）faint, weak （うす暗くぼんやりした）dim （漠然とした）vague （わずかな）slight ◆かすかな光 a faint[dim] light ◆かすかな音 a faint sound[noise] ◆かすかな記憶 a dim[vague] memory ◆手術の成功にかすかな望みをつなぐ cling on to a faint

hope that the surgery will succeed[be successful]

ガストリノーマ gastrinoma
ガストリン gastrin

かすむ 霞む be blurred, be blurry ◆かすみ目 blurred[blurry] vision ◆物がかすんで見えますか Do things look blurry? ◆目がかすみますか Do you have blurred vision? / Is your vision blurred? ◆遠くの物がかすんで見える Distant things look blurry[blurred]. ◆左側の目がかすむ have blurred vision in *one's* left eye

ガスリーけんさ ─検査 Guthrie test；*a blood test for phenylketonuria*

かすりきず ─傷 （擦り傷）scrape, abrasion, abraded wound （軽い怪我）slight injury ☞傷

かすれる （しわがれる）get[become] hoarse （擦過音になる）get[become] scratchy ◆声がかすれますか Does your voice get hoarse[scratchy]?

かぜ 風邪 cold ◆普通の風邪 a common cold ◆お腹の風邪 stomach flu / viral gastroenteritis ◆風邪をひいていますか，最近ひきましたか Do you have or have you recently had a cold? ◆よく風邪をひきますか Do you often catch[get] colds? ◆風邪の症状はありますか〈ありましたか〉Do you have〈have you had〉any cold symptoms? ◆風邪をひいたようですね I think you've got a cold. ◆ひどい風邪をひいたのですか Did you have a bad cold? ◆風邪はもう治りましたか Have you recovered from your cold? ◆今，風邪が流行っています A cold has been going around. / There's a cold going around now. ◆風邪をひかないように気をつけて下さい Please take care not to catch a cold. ◆風邪をこじらせる *one's* cold gets worse ◀鼻風邪 head cold ▶風邪ウイルス cold virus 風邪薬 cold medication

かせい¹ 化生 metaplasia （化生metaplastic）◀腸上皮化生 intestinal metaplasia 扁平上皮化生 squamous cell metaplasia ▶化生性ポリープ metaplastic polyp

かせい² 仮性（の）（真性ではない）false

（接頭偽性の **pseud(o)-**） ▶仮性球麻痺 pseudobulbar palsy[paralysis]　仮性近視 false nearsightedness[myopia] / pseudomyopia　仮性クループ false croup / pseudocroup　仮性斜視 false strabismus / pseudostrabismus　仮性認知症 pseudodementia　仮性半陰陽 pseudohermaphroditism　仮性包茎 pseudophimosis

カセイソーダ　苛性ソーダ **caustic soda**

かせつ　仮説　**hypothesis** /haɪpάθəsɪs/（複 **hypotheses**）　◆仮説を立てる hypothesize / formulate a hypothesis　◆仮説を裏付ける confirm a hypothesis　◆仮説を検証する test a hypothesis

かそう¹　火葬　**cremation**　◆日本では亡くなった方は多くの場合火葬となります Cremation is performed in almost all cases in Japan. / Cremation is the most common form of funerary rite in Japan.　◆火葬許可証は市役所〈区役所〉で発行されます The cremation permit will be issued at the city〈ward〉office.　▶火葬場 crematorium / crematory

かそう²　仮想（の）　**virtual**　▶仮想記憶 virtual memory　仮想現実 virtual reality　仮想内視鏡 virtual endoscopy

がぞう　画像　（テレビ画面などの映像）**picture**　（カメラ・鏡などを通して見た像）**image**　（画像化）**imaging**　（フィルム）**film**　▶X線画像 X-ray image　磁気共鳴画像 magnetic resonance imaging；MRI　断層画像 scan[scanned] image　T1〈T2〉強調画像 T1〈T2〉-weighted image　デジタル画像 digital imaging　▶画像解析 image analysis　画像下治療 interventional radiology；IVR　画像処理 image processing　画像診断 diagnostic imaging

かぞえる　数える　**count**　☞数, 数字　◆ゆっくり1から10まで数えて下さい Please count slowly from one to ten.

かそく　加速する　**accelerate**（図**acceleration**）, **speed up**（↔slow down）　◆喫煙は肺機能の低下を加速します Smoking accelerates[speeds up] the decline in lung function.　◆がんの増殖を加速する accel-

erate the growth of a cancerous tumor / speed up the development[growth] of cancer　◀直線加速装置 linear accelerator；LINAC　▶加速歩行 festinating gait

かぞく　家族　**family**（複**family**　家族内・家族性の **familial**）　◆ご家族のことをうかがいます Let me ask you about your family. / Now, *tell me[I'd like to know a little] about your immediate family.　★immediate family は肉親の意味.　◆ご家族は全部で何人ですか How many people are there in your family?　◆ご家族は皆さんお元気ですか Are your family all in good health?　◆ご家族の中に高血圧や糖尿病など健康上の問題をもっておられる人はいますか Does anyone in your family have health problems, such as high blood pressure or diabetes?　◆ご家族の中にあなたと同じ症状の人はいますか Does anyone in your family have similar symptoms?　◆ご家族の中にこの病気の治療を受けた人はいますか Has anyone in your family been treated for this disease?　◆ご家族の中に原因不明で突然亡くなった人はいますか Has anyone in your family died suddenly of an unknown cause?　◆ご家族にアレルギーの人がいますか Does anyone in your (immediate) family have[suffer from] any allergies? / Do you have any family history of allergy?　◆そのことは私からご家族にお話ししましょうか Should I talk to your family about it?　◆治療についてはご家族で相談して下さい Please discuss the treatment with your family.　◆（家族の呼び出しで）ミラーさんのご家族の方はいらっしゃいますか Is there anyone here from Mr〈Mrs〉Miller's family?　◆その件について家族の了承をとる ask for *a person's* family members' consent[approval] on the matter　◆大家族を養う support[provide for] a large family

▶核家族 nuclear family　拡大家族 extended family　単親家族 single-parent family　扶養家族 dependent　▶家族会 family association[organization]　家族介護 family care　家族関係 family relationship[relations] 家族教育 family education 家族計画 family planning 家族指導 family guidance 家族集積性 familial [family] clustering 家族内感染 familial infection 家族療法 family therapy 家族歴 family history ☞家族性

かぞくせい　家族性(の)　familial ▶家族性高コレステロール血症 familial hypercholesterolemia　家族性大腸ポリポーシス familial polyposis coli；FPC

かそせい　可塑性　plasticity

かた¹　肩　shoulder ▶肩が痛みますか Does your shoulder hurt? / Do you have any pain in the shoulder(s)?　◆痛みは肩に放散しますか Does the pain spread[radiate] to your shoulders?　◆よく肩がこりますか Do you often have *stiff shoulders [a stiff neck]?　◆肩をすくめて下さい Please shrug your shoulders.　◆肩がはずれています Your shoulder has slipped out of joint. / You've dislocated your shoulder.　◆肩をもむ give a shoulder massage / massage *a person's* shoulders　◆肩の力を抜く relax *one's* shoulders　◆肩の上げ下げをする raise and lower *one's* shoulders　◆肩で息をする gasp[pant] for breath / breathe hard　◀五十肩 stiff and painful shoulder (due to old age) / fifty-year-old shoulder　水泳肩 swimmer's shoulder　凍結肩 frozen shoulder　動揺肩 loose shoulder　野球肩 baseball shoulder ▶肩押下げテスト shoulder depression test　肩外転副子 airplane (shoulder) splint / shoulder abduction orthosis　肩関節 shoulder joint　肩関節周囲炎 periarthritis of the shoulder / scapulohumeral periarthritis　肩関節脱臼 shoulder dislocation　肩骨折 shoulder fracture　肩吊り帯 shoulder suspension system ☞肩こり，肩幅

かた²　型　(種類)type　(パターン)pattern　(鋳型)mold　(歯などの印象)impression ☞パターン　◆血液型は何ですか What blood type are you? / What's your blood type?　◆あなたは A 型です You have type A blood.　◆行動の決まった型 a set

[fixed] behavioral pattern　◀足型 footprint　A⟨B⟩型インフルエンザ type A⟨B⟩ influenza　境界型 borderline type　緊張型 catatonic type　血液型 blood type / 《英》blood group　単純型 simple type　2 型糖尿病 type 2 diabetes (mellitus)　歯型 dental mold[impression]　分泌型 IgA secretory IgA　変異型 variant　偏執型 paranoid type

かた³　過多　excess　(医excessive)　(接頭… を超えた over‑　より多くの hyper‑, poly‑) ☞過剰(の)　◀胃酸過多 gastric hyperacidity / excessive acid in the stomach　栄養過多 excess nutrition / overnutrition　血中コレステロール過多 excessive blood cholesterol / hypercholesterolemia　脂肪過多 excess[excessive] fat / adiposis　分泌過多 hypersecretion　羊水過多症 polyhydramnios

かたあし　片足　one leg ◆目を閉じて片足で立って下さい Please stand on one leg with your eyes closed. / Please close your eyes and stand on one leg.

かたい¹　下腿(部)　lower leg ▶下腿義足 below-knee[BK] prosthesis　下腿骨 bone of the lower leg　下腿切断 below-knee[BK] amputation

かたい²　硬い・堅い・固い (物・体が)　(変形しにくい)hard　(医harden)　(固く引き締まった)firm, tight　(医tighten up)　(こわばった)stiff　(医get[become] stiff)　(厚くなった)thick　(医thicken)　◆便は硬めですか，軟らかめですか Have your stools been rather hard or soft?　◆血管が加齢で硬くなる the blood vessels harden[get hard] with age　◆乳房に硬いしこりがある have a firm[hard] lump in *one's* breast　◆体を硬くしないで下さい Please try not to tighten up. / Please let your muscles go quite relaxed.　◆目を固く閉じてください Please close your eyes tightly.　◆筋肉が硬い *one's* muscles are stiff[hard]　◆体が硬い *one's* body is stiff　◆硬くなった肩の筋肉のストレッチをする stretch *one's* stiff shoulders　◆以前より皮膚が硬くなった印象がありますか Do you feel your skin has become thicker than before? / Have you noticed any thickening of your skin?

《決意などが》（変わらない）firm （強い）**strong** ◆固い信念 a firm belief ◆彼は手術を受けないと固く決心しています He is determined not to have the surgery. / He has firmly decided against having the surgery.

かだい¹ 課題 （関心事）**concern** （解決すべき問題）**problem** （任務・仕事）**task** （研究などの課題）**assignment** ◆当面の課題は化学療法の間いかに体力を保つかです For the moment, our main concern is how to maintain your strength during the chemotherapy.

かだい² 過大 **too much** （圖あまりにも…すぎる too much 圀無理な unreasonable）◆治療にあまり過大な期待は禁物です Don't expect[You shouldn't expect] too much of the treatment. ◆過大な要求をする患者に対応する deal with a patient who makes unreasonable demands ☞過大評価

かだいじょうみゃく 下大静脈 **inferior vena cava ; IVC** ▶下大静脈フィルター IVC[inferior vena cava] filter

かだいひょうか 過大評価 **overestimate, make too much of** ◆この治療の効果を過大評価しないで下さい Please don't overestimate[make too much of] the effects of this treatment.

かたがき 肩書き （地位・身分）**position, status** （称号）**title** ◆よろしければお勤め先での肩書きを教えて下さい Would you mind telling me[If you don't mind, could you please tell me] your current position at work?

かたがわ 片側 **one side** （圀one-sided）☞片側（へんそく） ◆頭が痛むのは両側ですか，片側だけですか Do you have the pain on both sides or only on one side of your head? ▶片側検定 one-sided test

かたこり 肩凝り **stiff shoulder** （首の凝り）**stiff neck** （背中の張り）**stiff back** ◆肩凝りはありますか Do you have stiff shoul-

ders? / Do your shoulders feel stiff?

かたち 形 （物の外形）**shape** （形態）**form** ◆ポリープはサイズも形も様々です Polyps vary in size and shape. ◆丸い形〈卵の形〉をしている be round〈oval〉 in shape ◆サイズや形が変わる change in size and shape ◆研究がようやく形になってきました Our research is finally beginning to take shape. ◆薬をカプセルの形で処方します I'll prescribe the medication in capsule form.

かたづける 片付ける （整頓する）**tidy up, straighten up** （しまう・収納する）**put away** （テーブルの上などをきれいにする）**clear（away）** （捨てる）**get rid of** （持っていく）**take（away）** ◆お部屋の片づけをお手伝いしましょう Let me help you tidy [straighten] up your room. ◆おもちゃを片付ける put away the toys ◆床頭台の上を片付ける clear the bedside table ◆読み終わられた新聞を片付けましょうか Shall I get rid of the newspapers that you've finished reading? ◆（食事は）お済みになりましたか．トレーを片付けてもいいですか Are you finished? May I take away the tray?

かたて 片手 **one hand** （圀one-handed）◆片手用の道具 a one-handed tool

かたてしょうこうぐん 肩手症候群 **shoulder-hand syndrome**

カタトニー **catatonia** ☞緊張

かたはば 肩幅 **the width of *one's* shoulders, the breadth of *one's* shoulders** ◆彼は肩幅が広い〈狭い〉He has broad〈narrow〉shoulders. ◆足を肩幅に広げて立って下さい Please stand with your feet shoulder-width apart.

かたひざ 片膝 **one knee** ◆片膝を立てて座る sit with one knee up[raised]

かたほう 片方 **one** （一方の側面）**one side** ☞片側（かたがわ，へんそく）

かたまひ 片麻痺 **hemiplegia** ☞片麻痺（へんまひ）

かたまり 塊 （血などの塊）**clot** （集積した塊）**mass** （増大した塊）**build-up** （しこり・腫れ物）**lump** ◆便の中に血の塊がありまし

かたまり　127　―がち

たか Have you noticed any blood clots in your stools? ◆この症状は大脳動脈が血の塊で詰まって起こります This symptom results from *a blood clot blocking an artery in the brain[the blockage of an artery in the brain by a blood clot]. ◆プラークは脂肪性沈着物やコレステロールからなるネバネバした塊です Plaque is a sticky mass[build-up] of fatty deposits and cholesterol.

かたまる　固まる
《物が固まる》（形を成している）**be formed**（固くなる）**become hard, harden**　（血が凝固する）**clot, coagulate** ◆便は固まっていますか Are your stools well formed? ◆血が固まるのを防ぐ prevent *the clotting of blood[blood clotting] / stop blood from clotting
《決心が固まる》**make up** *one's* **mind** ◆手術を受ける意思が固まる make up *one's* mind to have the surgery /（最終決断をする）make a final decision to have the surgery

かたみ　肩身 ◆肩身が狭い（気が引ける・小さく感じる）feel small（恥ずかしく思う）be [feel] ashamed ◆肩身が広い be[feel] proud ◆外国人ということで肩身の狭い思いをすることはありますか Do you ever *feel you're not good enough[feel small] because you're a foreigner? ◆彼は生活保護を受けているので肩身の狭い思いをしています He is ashamed of[to be] receiving public assistance payments.

かたみみ　片耳　one ear ◆音が聞こえにくいのは片耳ですか，両耳ですか Do you have difficulty hearing in one or both ears?

かたむける　傾ける（曲げる）**lean**（物・首などを片方に傾ける）**tilt** ◆頭を後ろに傾けて下さい Please lean your head backward. ◆首を左〈右〉に傾ける tilt[put] *one's* head to the left〈right〉 ◆彼女は物を見る時首を傾けますか Does she tilt her head to see things? / Does she put her head to one side to see things? ◆これから検査台を傾けます Now, I'm going to tilt the exam table.

かため　片目　one eye ◆片眼をつぶってこれを見て下さい Please look at this with one eye closed. / Please close one eye and look at this.

かたよる　偏る
《アンバランスである》**be unbalanced** ◆まず栄養の偏った食事を考え直す必要があります The first thing you have to do is to think again about your unbalanced diet.
《偏見をもっている》**be prejudiced (against)** ◆同性愛者たちに偏った考えをもつ *be prejudiced[have a prejudice] against *homosexual men and women [LGBT]

カタラーゼ　catalase

カタル　catarrh（[形]**catarrhal**）◀胃カタル gastric catarrh　春季カタル spring catarrh / vernal keratoconjunctivitis ▶カタル期 the catarrhal stage　カタル性結膜炎 catarrhal conjunctivitis　カタル性扁桃炎 catarrhal tonsillitis

カタルシス　catharsis /kəθάːsɪs/（[形]**cathartic**）

カタレプシー　catalepsy（[形]**cataleptic**）

かたん　加担する　take sides (with, in) ◆私どもはあくまでも中立で，どちら側にも加担しない立場です We remain neutral no matter what, and won't take sides with any party.

かち　価値　worth（[動]**be worth**）, **value**（[動]**value, be valuable**）◆その治療はやってみる価値があると思います I think that the treatment is worth trying[a try]. ◆人生において最も価値を置いている事柄は何ですか What *do you value[are the things you value] (the) most in your life? ▶価値観 sense of values

―がち（病気などになりやすい）**be prone to**（傾向がある）**tend to**　☞傾向 ◆便秘がちですか Are you prone to constipation? / Do you often[Do you tend to] get constipated? ◆若い頃から病気がちですか Have you been prone to illness since childhood[a young age]?

カチカチ

カチカチ 《音》tick (圖tick) ◆カチカチという耳鳴りがする hear a ticking sound[noise] in *one's* ear(s) ◆機械がカチカチ音をたてる The machine makes a ticking sound[noise].
《固さ》◆便がカチカチになっている The stools are hard and dry.

カチッ click (圖click) ◆カチッカチッという耳鳴りがする hear a clicking sound[noise] in *one's* ear(s) ◆(吸入指導などで)このつまみをカチッと鳴るところまで右に回して下さい Turn this knob to the right until it clicks.

かちょう 科長 the head ◆神経内科科長 the head of the Neurology Department

かちょうかんまくどうみゃく 下腸間膜動脈 inferior mesenteric artery

ガチョウのくびへんけい ―首変形 goose-neck deformity

かつえき 滑液 synovial fluid ▶滑液包 synovial bursa 滑液包炎 bursitis

がっかい 学会 (学術団体)society (学術会議・大規模な集会)conference (会合・集まり)meeting ◆医学会 medical society ◆看護学会 nursing society ◆関先生の学会出席のため明日は休診です Due to attendance at a conference, Dr Seki will not accept patients tomorrow. ◆学会発表する present[give] a paper at a medical conference[meeting] ◀日本医学会 the Japanese Association of Medical Sciences

かっかする get[be] excited (激怒する) get[be] furious ☞興奮

がっかりする (落胆する)be[get, become] discouraged (失望する) be disappointed ☞意気消沈, 気落ち, 失望 ◆血糖の数値が正常値を超えていても, そうがっかりなさる必要はありません There's no need to be[You shouldn't be] so discouraged [disappointed] just because your blood sugar count is above normal. / You don't have to let (having) high blood sugar *get you down[discourage you].

がっきゅう 学級 class ◀院内学級 hos-pital class 特別支援学級 special needs [education] class / class for children with special needs / special class for children with disabilities 母親学級 childbirth class for expectant mothers 両親学級 childbirth and parenting class ▶学級崩壊 classroom chaos[collapse] ☞学級閉鎖

がっきゅうへいさ 学級閉鎖 class closure ◆インフルエンザのため学級閉鎖になっています Classes are temporarily closed due to the flu.

かっけ 脚気 beriberi /bèribéri/ ◆脚気になる get[develop] beriberi ▶脚気心 beriberi heart 脚気ニューロパチー beriberi neuropathy

かっけつ 喀血 hemoptysis (血を吐く) spitting up blood (咳き込んで)coughing up blood ◆喀血する spit up blood / cough up blood

がっこう 学校 school ◆どこの学校に行っているのですか Where do you go to school? / (学校名を知りたい場合)Which school do you go to? ◆何日学校を休みましたか How many days *were you absent [did you stay home] from school? ◆学校教育はどのくらい受けましたか How much schooling did you have? / How far did you go in school? ◆学校で最近感染症にかかった人がいますか Has anyone at school recently had any infections? ◀看護学校 nursing school / school of nursing 専門学校 vocational school[college] 特別支援学校 special needs[education] school / school for children with special needs / special school for children with disabilities 盲学校 school for the blind and visually impaired ▶学校医 school doctor[physician] 学校栄養士 school dietitian[nutritionist] 学校カウンセラー school counselor 学校感染症 school infectious disease / infectious disease in school 学校給食 school lunch [meal] / (プログラム)school lunch program 学校恐怖症 school phobia 学校健康診断 school health checkup / health checkup at school　学校歯科医 school dentist　学校保健師 school nurse　☞学校閉鎖

がっこうちゅうしょう　顎口虫症　gnathostomiasis

がっこうへいさ　学校閉鎖　school closure　◆その小学校はインフルエンザの感染拡大で学校閉鎖になっています The elementary school is temporarily closed due to the spread of influenza.

かつじたい　活字体　（ブロック体）block letters　★複数形で．◆お名前を活字体で書いて下さい Please write your name in block letters. / Please print your name.

かっしゃしんけい　滑車神経　trochlear nerve

かっしょく　褐色（の）　brown　◀赤褐色 reddish brown　◆褐色細胞腫 pheochromocytoma

かっせい　活性　activity（📖active）　◆この薬には広範囲の抗菌活性があります This medication has a broad-spectrum antibacterial activity.　◀界面活性剤 surfactant / surface-active agent / detergent　酵素活性 enzyme activity　生物活性 biological activity / bioactivity　レニン活性 renin activity　▶活性酸素 active oxygen / oxygen（free）radical / reactive oxygen species / ROS　活性炭 activated charcoal　☞活性化, 活性型

かっせいか　活性化する　activate（📖activation　📖活発な・活性のある active　活性化した activated）　☞賦活　▶活性化酵素 activating enzyme　活性化物質 activator　活性化部分トロンボプラスチン時間 activated partial thromboplastin time；APTT　活性化プロテインC　activated protein C；APC

かっせいがた　活性型（の）　active　▶活性型ビタミンD active vitamin D

かつだつ　滑脱（した）　sliding, slipped　▶滑脱型（食道）裂孔ヘルニア sliding（esophageal）hiatal hernia　滑脱ヘルニア sliding[slipped] hernia

かって　勝手　勝手なことをする do as one pleases[likes]　◆院内では自分勝手な行動を慎んで下さい Please don't do just

as you please in the hospital, but be respectful of others. / (他の人たちに気を配って下さい)Please be mindful of others *in the way[in how] you behave in the hospital.

かっとう　葛藤　conflict（📖conflicted）, dilemma　◆心の葛藤 one's emotional conflict　◆内面の葛藤 one's inner[internal / mental] conflict　◆対人関係について葛藤がある be[feel] conflicted about one's relationships with others

かつどう　活動　activity（📖active）　◆どんな活動をすると疲れますか What kind of activity causes you to feel tired?　◆活動を少し制限して下さい You should restrict your activities slightly.　◆体に負担のかかるような活動を避ける avoid doing strenuous activities　◆活動的な生活 an active life　◆非活動的な生活スタイル(体を動かさない)physically inactive lifestyle / (座りがちな)sedentary lifestyle　◀グループ活動 group activity　身体活動 physical activity　生活活動指数 index of living activity　精神活動 mental activity　ボランティア活動 voluntary work / volunteer activities　野外活動 outdoor activities　余暇活動 leisure activities　▶活動亢進 hyperactivity / hyperactive behavior　活動制限 activity restriction　活動低下 hypoactivity　活動範囲 scope[field] of activities

カットオフち　―値　cutoff value

かっぱつ　活発（な）　（元気のよい）lively（積極的な）active（📖促進する promote　刺激する stimulate）　◆活発なお子さんですね Your child is really lively[active], isn't he〈she〉?　◆乳がんのサポートグループは活発に活動しています The breast cancer support group is now very active.　◆食物繊維は腸の働きを活発にします Dietary fiber helps promote regular bowel function. / Dietary fiber helps to stimulate bowel activity.

カップ　cup　◀採尿カップ urine collection cup

カップル　couple　◀不妊カップル infertile couple

がっぺいしょう　合併症　complications
★通例，複数形で．☞併発　◆前回の手術後に合併症を起こしましたか Did you experience any complications after your previous surgery? / Did any complications develop after your previous surgery?　◆この処置に伴う合併症としては薬剤によるアレルギーや感染があります There are possible complications involved with this procedure, such as allergic reactions to the medications and infection.　◆血糖値を正常に維持して糖尿病をコントロールしないと様々な合併症を起こす可能性があります If you don't control your diabetes by maintaining normal sugar levels, you may develop a variety of complications.　◆この治療による合併症はめったに起こりません Complications from this treatment *are rare[rarely occur].　◆糖尿病の合併症を防ぐ prevent[avoid] diabetic complications　◆非常に重い合併症 very serious complications　◀術後合併症 complications after surgery / postoperative complications　糖尿病合併症 diabetes[diabetic] complications / complications of diabetes　妊娠合併症 pregnancy complications / complications of pregnancy　麻酔合併症 complications of anesthesia

がっぺいせつじょ　合併切除　combined resection

かつまく　滑膜　synovial membrane
▶滑膜炎 synovitis　滑膜切除術 synovectomy　滑膜肉腫 synovial sarcoma

かつやくきん　括約筋　sphincter　◀オッディ括約筋 sphincter of Oddi　下部食道括約筋 lower esophageal sphincter；LES / gastroesophageal sphincter　肛門括約筋 anal sphincter　尿道括約筋 urethral sphincter　膀胱括約筋 vesical sphincter　▶括約筋再建術 sphincter reconstruction　括約筋修復術 sphincter repair　括約筋障害 sphincter disorder[disturbance]

かつら　(頭全体のかつら)**wig**　(ヘアピース)**hairpiece**　◆かつらを使っていますか Do you use a wig?　◆かつらをつける put on

a wig　◆かつらをつけている wear a wig　◀部分かつら partial wig

かつりょく　活力　(生命力)**vitality**　(スタミナ)**stamina**　(エネルギー)**energy**　◆活力がある be full of vitality[energy] / have stamina　◆活力がない lack vitality[stamina]　◆活力をつける develop[build up] *one's* stamina　▶活力不足 lack of vitality [energy]

かつれい　割礼　circumcision　(動circumcise)　◆割礼していますか Are you[Have you been] circumcised?

かてい¹　家庭　home　(形home, domestic)　(家族)**family**　(形family)　☞家族　◆ご家庭に同じ症状の人はいますか Does anyone around you have similar symptoms at home?　◆ご家庭に何か問題がありますか Do you have any problems at home?　◆家庭の事情で家族と別れて暮らす live apart from *one's* family for family reasons　◀共働き家庭 dual-income family　ひとり親家庭 single-parent family　父子家庭 motherless[father-child / father-children] family　母子家庭 fatherless [mother-child / mother-children] family　▶家庭医 family doctor[physician]　家庭介護 home[family] care　家庭環境 family background[environment]　家庭血圧 home blood pressure　家庭生活 family[home] life　家庭内暴力 domestic violence；DV　家庭分娩 home birth[delivery]　家庭崩壊 family breakdown　家庭問題 domestic[family] problem

かてい²　過程　(物事の進行・道程)**process**　(経過)**course**　◆老化の過程で in the process of aging　◆死に至る過程 the dying process　◆化学療法の過程で in the course of the chemotherapy　◀意思決定過程 decision-making process　心的過程[意識過程] mental process　心理過程 psychological process　成長過程 growth process　老化過程 aging process

かてい³　課程　program　(特定科目の課程)**course**　(全教育課程)**curriculum**　◆両親学級の全課程の受講をお勧めします I recommend that you take the entire program [course] in childbirth and parenting. ◀修士課程 master's program　博士課程 doctoral program

かてい⁴　仮定する (推測する)suppose (図supposition)　(見なす)assume (図assumption)　(仮説を立てる)hypothesize (図hypothesis　図hypothetical) ◆このまま喫煙し続けると仮定すると，確実に肺機能が低下します Supposing that you keep smoking, your lung function will definitely decline[get worse].　◆仮定の話をしても仕方がありませんので，検査結果が出てから治療方針のご相談をしましょう It's no use talking about what could happen hypothetically, so let's discuss the treatment plan after getting the test results.

カテーテル　catheter /kǽθətɚ/ (術・法)catheterization ◆尿を出すためのカテーテルを膀胱に入れる insert[put / place] a catheter into the bladder to drain the urine ◀吸引用カテーテル suction catheter　経鼻カテーテル transnasal catheter　静脈カテーテル法 venous catheterization　心臓カテーテル cardiac catheter　スワン・ガンツカテーテル法 Swan-Ganz catheterization　中心静脈[CV]カテーテル central venous[CV] catheter　尿管カテーテル ureteral catheter　尿道カテーテル urethral catheter　ネラトンカテーテル Nélaton catheter　肺動脈カテーテル pulmonary artery catheter　バルーンカテーテル balloon catheter　フォガーティカテーテル Fogarty catheter　フォリイカテーテル Foley catheter　膀胱カテーテル bladder catheter　留置カテーテル indwelling catheter ▶カテーテル合併症 catheter complications　カテーテル感染 catheter-associated infection　カテーテル焼灼術 catheter ablation　カテーテル尿 catheterized urine

カテコールアミン　catecholamine
カテランしん　―針　Cathelin needle
かでんずけんさ　蝸電図検査　electrocochleography
かど¹　角 (曲がり角・物の隅)corner　(端)edge ◆待合室は角にあります The waiting room is on[at] the corner. ◆作業療法室は角を曲がった所にあります The occupational therapy room is just around the corner. ◆角を曲がる turn the corner ◆2つめの角を左に曲がる turn left at the second corner ◆口の角がただれている have sores in[at] the corners of *one's* mouth / have sores at the edge of *one's* mouth

かど²　過度(の) ☞―し過ぎる，―過ぎる　(多すぎる)too much　(度を越した)excessive ◆この症状は過度の飲酒が原因で起こります This is a symptom caused by *too much[excessive] drinking. ◆過度のダイエットは危険です Excessive dieting is dangerous. / It's dangerous to diet to excess.

かとう　果糖　fruit sugar, fructose ▶果糖不耐症 fructose intolerance
かどう　可動(性) (動き・動作)motion　(移動性)mobility (図移動式の mobile, movable) ▶関節可動域
カドミウム　cadmium ▶カドミウム腎症 cadmium nephropathy　カドミウム中毒 cadmium poisoning
カトリックきょうと　―教徒　Catholic
ガドリニウム　gadolinium
かなう　適う・叶う
《適する・合う》suit (図suitable, appropriate　筋の通った reasonable) ◆あなたの症状にかなった治療計画を立てましょう Let's make a treatment plan that's suitable [appropriate] to your symptoms. ◆彼女の行為は実に道理にかなっています Her behavior is quite reasonable.
《実現する》come true, realize ◆いつか彼の夢がかないますように！ Let's hope[I hope] his dream comes true some day!

かなしい　悲しい　sad (図sadness　強い悲しみ sorrow　死別などによる深い悲しみ grief) ◆残念ですが，悲しいお知らせです I'm sorry, but I've got sad news for you. ◆特に理由もないのに悲しい気分になることはありますか Do you ever feel sad for no apparent[obvious] reason?

かなしむ　悲しむ　be[feel] sad (悲嘆に暮

れる）grieve

カナダ Canada （㊤Canadian） ☞国籍
▶カナダ人（の）Canadian

カナマイシン kanamycin ▶カナマイシン耐性 kanamycin resistance　カナマイシン難聴 kanamycin hearing loss

かならず 必ず （確実に）**definitely, certainly, surely** （㊤必ず…する be sure to …）（いつも）**always** ☞きっと　◆会議の後必ず戻ってきます I'll definitely[I promise to] come back after the meeting.　◆必ずよくなりますよ（私は確信している）I'm sure that you'll get better. / You'll certainly get better.　◆新たな薬を服用する時には，必ず主治医に確認して下さい Always check with your doctor before starting any new medication.　◆運動を始める前には必ず医師にご相談下さい Please be sure to consult your doctor before you begin any exercise program.

かなり **pretty, fairly, rather** ★会話の中では pretty が最も一般的に用いられ，rather は fairly よりもやや意味が強い．（相当な程度に）**considerably** （著しく）**significantly** ☞相当
◆血圧がかなり高いです Your blood pressure is pretty[rather / quite] high. / Your blood pressure has *gone up[risen] considerably.　◆白血球数がかなり下がっています Your white blood cell count is pretty[rather] low. / Your white blood cell count has fallen considerably.　◆傷口からかなりの量の血が出ている lose a considerable amount of blood from *one's* wounds　◆今年のスギ花粉の飛散はかなり多いという予測です The *sugi*[Japanese cedar] pollen levels in the air this year are predicted to be fairly[considerably] high.　◆今日はかなり気分がよさそうですね You're looking much better today, aren't you? / You look much better today, don't you?

かにゅう 加入する （メンバーになる）**become a member** (of) （入る）**join**　◆乳がん患者会に加入しませんか Won't you join the patients' association of breast cancer? / How about becoming a member of

the patients' association of breast cancer?　◆国民健康保険に加入していますか Do you have National Health Insurance?

カニューラ cannula ◀気管カニューラ tracheal cannula　酸素カニューラ oxygen cannula　鼻カニューラ nasal cannula

かねつ 加熱する **heat** (up) （熱処理する）**heat-treat**　◆ビタミン C は加熱処理で容易に壊れます Vitamin C is easily destroyed during[by] heat treatment.　◀非加熱血液製剤 untreated[non-heat-treated] blood product　▶加熱血液製剤 heat-treated blood product　加熱滅菌 heat sterilization

かねんちゅうどしょうこうぐん 過粘稠度症候群 **hyperviscosity syndrome**

かのう¹ 化膿する （膿を持つ）**form pus, fester, suppurate** （㊤suppuration, ㊤suppurative） （細菌により炎症を起こす）**get [become, be] infected** （㊤pyogenic, purulent, septic） ☞膿（うみ），膿む　◆傷口が化膿しています The wound has *formed pus[become infected / become purulent].　◆化膿を防止する薬 medication to prevent suppuration　◀肺化膿症 pulmonary suppuration　▶化膿菌 pyogenic bacteria　化膿性関節炎 pyogenic[septic] arthritis　化膿性感染症 pyogenic infection ☞化膿止め

かのう² 可能（な）**possible** （㊤possibility 腰尾-able） ☞可能性　◆点滴をするために毎日通院することは可能ですか Is it possible for you to[Can you] come to the hospital every day to have a drip?　◆早期のがんであればこの手術で根治可能でしょう If the cancer is in its early stages, with this surgery *you'll have a good chance of being[there's a good possibility that you'll be] completely cured.　◆可能な限りの手を尽くします We'll do[try] everything possible.　◆もし可能ならば入院を来週の月曜日まで延長しましょう If (at all) possible, we'll extend your hospital stay until next Monday.　◀睡眠時無呼吸症候群は治療可能な病気です Sleep apnea syndrome is a treatable disorder.　◆除去

可能な皮下のしこり a removable lump under the skin / a lump under the skin that can be removed　◆外科手術で切除可能な腫瘍 a surgically resectable tumor

かのうせい　可能性　possibility（圏**possible**）（見込み）**chance**　☞可能，一かもしれない　◆妊娠なさっている可能性はありますか Is there any possibility that you're pregnant? / Could you be pregnant?　◆他の可能性を除外するために検査をしましょう I'd like to rule out other possibilities. So let's do[run] some tests.　◆合併症が起こる可能性が少しあります There's a small chance[possibility] that complications will occur.　◆彼女が回復する可能性は十分あります There's a good chance[possibility] she will recover.　◆発作がまた起こる可能性があります Further attacks are possible. / You could have further attacks.　◆ポリープががん化する可能性があります There's some possibility that your polyp will turn[change] into cancer. / Your polyp may turn[change] into cancer.　◆残念ですが，回復する可能性は低いです I'm sorry, but the possibility of his〈her〉recovering is slim.　◆高い可能性 a strong[definite] possibility　◆低い可能性 a slight[slim / remote] possibility　◆根治する可能性 curability

かのうどめ　化膿止め（抗生物質）**antibiotics**　★通例，複数形で．（圏**antibiotic**）**antisuppurative, medication to prevent suppuration, medication for suppuration**　◆化膿止めを処方しましょう I'll prescribe[give you] some antibiotics.　◆化膿止めの軟膏を塗る apply an antibiotic ointment

カバー　cover　◆おむつカバー diaper cover　ベッドカバー bedspread　便座カバー(toilet) seat cover　枕カバー pillowcase

かはんしん　下半身　the lower half[part] of the body, lower body　◆下半身の服を脱いで下さい Please take your clothes off from the waist down.　◆彼女は自動車事故で下半身が麻痺しています The lower

part of her body is paralyzed[She is paralyzed from the waist down] as a result of an automobile accident.　◆下半身を鍛える strengthen *one's* lower body

かひ　痂皮　scab　☞かさぶた

かび　mold（圏**moldy**　かび臭の **musty**）　◆かびアレルギーがある be allergic to mold　◆かびの生えた食べ物 moldy food　◆かび臭いおりもの musty vaginal discharge

かびん　過敏（化学薬品・食品などに対する敏感さ）**sensitivity**（圏**sensitive**），**hypersensitivity**（圏**hypersensitive**）（炎症性の鋭敏さ）**irritability**（圏**irritable**）（活動亢進状態）**hyperactivity**（圏**hyperactive**）（精神的な不安・緊張）**nervousness**（圏**nervous**）　☞敏感　◆肌は過敏なほうですか Do you have very sensitive skin?　◆ペニシリンに過敏に反応する have *a sensitivity[an allergy] to penicillin / be hypersensitive[allergic] to penicillin　◆彼女は神経が過敏になっています She has become very nervous.

◀気道過敏性(試験) airway hyperreactivity（test）　夏型過敏性肺炎 summer-type hypersensitivity pneumonitis / Japanese summer-type allergic alveolitis　光過敏性てんかん photosensitive epilepsy；PSE　▶過敏性血管炎 hypersensitivity vasculitis　過敏性腸症候群 irritable bowel syndrome；IBS　☞過敏症

かびんしょう　過敏症　hypersensitivity

◀化学物質過敏症 chemical hypersensitivity　光線過敏症 photosensitivity / hypersensitivity to light　知覚過敏症 hyperesthesia　聴覚過敏症 hyperacusis / hyperacusia　ヨード過敏症 iodine hypersensitivity　ラテックス過敏症 latex hypersensitivity

かふ¹　寡婦　widow

かふ²　寡夫　widower

カフ　cuff　◆腕にこのカフを巻きましょう Let me put this cuff on your arm.

かぶ　下部　the lower part　◆背中の下部の痛み(a) pain in the lower back /（a）lower back pain　▶下部消化管 lower gastrointestinal[GI] tract　下部消化管造

影検査 barium enema / lower gastrointestinal［GI］series　下部食道 lower third of the esophagus　下部食道括約筋 lower esophageal sphincter；LES / gastroesophageal sphincter　下部尿路 lower urinary tract

カフェイン　**caffeine**　◆カフェインを含む飲み物は控えたほうがよいでしょう You should avoid *drinks containing caffeine［caffeinated beverages］.　◆カフェイン抜きのコーヒー decaffeinated coffee　◆カフェイン抜きのソフトドリンク caffeine-free［decaffeinated］soft drinks　▶カフェイン中毒 caffeine poisoning［intoxication］

カフェオレはん　―斑　**café-au-lait spots**　★通例，複数形で．

カフェテリア　**cafeteria**

かふか　過負荷　**overload**　☞負荷

ガフキーごうすう　―号数　**Gaffky scale（number）**

かふくつう　下腹痛　**lower abdominal pain, pain in the lower abdomen**　(痙攣痛)**lower abdominal cramps**　★複数形で．

かふくぶ　下腹部　**the lower abdomen**　(骨盤の部位)**the pelvic region**　◆痛みは下腹部に移動しますか Does the pain move to your lower abdomen?

カプサイシン　**capsaicin**　▶カプサイシン咳嗽試験 capsaicin cough test

かぶせる　被せる　**cover, wrap**　☞覆う，掛ける

カプセル　**capsule** /kǽpsl/　◆1回にカプセル2個，1日に3回飲んで下さい Please take two capsules three times a day.　▶カプセル剤 capsule　カプセル内視鏡 capsule endoscope

カプラン・マイヤーほう　―法　**Kaplan-Meier method［analysis, estimate］**

かぶる
《覆う》(身に着ける)**put on**　(身に着けている)**wear**　◆この帽子をかぶって下さい Put this hat［cap］on.　◆外出にはかつらを着けるにしても，家では帽子をかぶると簡単で楽ですよ Even if you wear a wig when you go out, you'll find it easier and more comfortable to wear a hat around the house.
《浴びる》　◆熱湯をかぶって火傷を負う get burned from boiling water

かぶれる　(発疹が出る)**get［have, break out in］a rash**　(アレルギー反応を起こす)**get［have］an allergic reaction（to）**　☞発疹　◆アルコール綿で皮膚がかぶれたことがありますか Have you ever had a (skin) rash from using alcohol wipes?　◆薬でかぶれる get a (skin) rash from a medication　◆おむつかぶれ(a) diaper rash　◆うるしかぶれ(a) poison ivy rash / *a rash from［an allergic reaction to］poison ivy / (塗料によるもので)a rash from lacquer poisoning　◆化粧品かぶれ a cosmetics［make-up］allergy / a rash caused by cosmetics

かふん　花粉　**pollen**　◆スギ花粉にアレルギーがある〈アレルギーを起こす〉have〈develop〉an allergy to *sugi*［Japanese cedar］pollen　◆今年は花粉の飛散が多い〈少ない〉The pollen levels in the air this year are high〈low〉. / The pollen count is high〈low〉this year.　▶花粉アレルゲン pollen allergen　花粉情報 pollen forecast［information］　☞花粉症

かぶんかつしょうしゃほう　過分割照射法　**hyperfractionation**

かぶんきょく　過分極　**hyperpolarization**

かふんしょう　花粉症　**hay fever, pollen allergy, pollinosis**　☞花粉　◆花粉症の季節です It's hay fever season.　◀スギ花粉症 Japanese cedar pollen allergy / *sugi* pollen allergy

かべ　壁　**wall**　(障害物)**barrier**　◆言葉の壁 a language barrier　◆文化の壁 a cultural barrier

かへいじょうしっしん　貨幣状湿疹　**coin-shaped eczema, nummular eczema**

かへきこうそく　下壁梗塞　**inferior wall infarction**

がほう　芽胞　**spore**

かぼうちょう　過膨張　(肺の)**overinflation**

かほご　過保護　**overprotection**　(動**overprotect**　形**overprotective**)　☞過干渉　◆過保護な母親 an overprotective mother

かほご ◆過保護に育てられた子供 an overprotected child ◆彼女は両親に過保護に育てられました She was brought up by overprotective parents. / She grew up (being) overprotected by her parents.

カポジすいとうようほっしんしょう　―水痘様発疹症 Kaposi varicelliform eruption

カポジにくしゅ　―肉腫 Kaposi sarcoma；KS

かまう　構う（気にする）**mind** ◆個人的なことをお聞きしても構いませんか Do you mind if I ask you a personal question? ◆この薬はいつ飲んでいただいても構いません This medication can be taken at any time. / (いつ飲むかは重要ではない)It doesn't matter when you take this medication. ◆窓を開けても構いませんか May I open the window? / Would you mind if I open the window?

ガマしゅ　―腫 ranine tumor, ranula

かまじょうせっけっきゅう　鎌状赤血球 sickle cell ▶鎌状赤血球症 sickle cell disease；SCD　鎌状赤血球貧血 sickle cell anemia

がまん　我慢する☞辛抱
《耐える》(辛抱する)**be patient, have patience**（不平を言わずに耐える）**put up with, stand, bear**（園我慢できる）**bearable, tolerable**（長期にわたって耐える）**endure**（園**endurance**）◆少し痛むかもしれませんが，ちょっと我慢して下さい This might hurt a little bit, but please be patient just a moment. ◆痛かったら我慢しなくていいんですよ You don't have to put up with any pain. ◆我慢ができなくなったら教えて下さい Please let me know when you can't stand[take] it any longer. / If the pain gets too much for you, let me know right away. ◆我慢できない痛み an unbearable pain ◆我慢できる痛み a tolerable pain ◆3年以上もこのつらい痛みを我慢していたのですか Have you endured [put up with] this severe pain for more than three years?
《持ちこたえる》(保つ)**hold**（踏みとどまる）**hold on** ◆尿意を我慢することができます

か Can you hold your urine? ◆ゲップを我慢して下さい Hold on without belching. / Please don't belch. / Don't let any air out.

かみ[1]　紙　paper ◆1枚の紙 a sheet [piece] of paper ◆紙切れ a slip of paper ◀ボール紙 cardboard ▶紙コップ paper cup　紙ナプキン paper napkin ☞紙おむつ

かみ[2]　髪　hair ☞毛, ヘア ◆薬の副作用で髪の毛が抜けるかもしれません As a side effect of the medication *you may lose some of your hair[some of your hair may fall out]. ◆治療が終わればほとんどの場合髪の毛はまた生えてきます Usually, your hair will start growing back after the treatment. ◆髪を洗う wash one's hair ◆髪を乾かす dry one's hair ◆髪を染める dye one's hair ◆髪をとかす comb [brush] one's hair ◆髪を整える do one's hair ◆髪を傷める damage one's hair ◆髪を抜く癖がある have a habit of pulling one's hair

かみあわせ　噛み合わせ（咬合）(**dental**) **bite, occlusion of the teeth**（歯列の整合性）**teeth alignment, alignment of the teeth** ◆彼の歯は噛み合わせが悪い He has a bad bite. / His teeth don't meet properly when he bites. ◆噛み合わせを見ましょう I'm going to look at the alignment of your teeth. ◆噛み合わせの異常 an abnormal alignment of one's teeth / (不正咬合)malocclusion

かみおむつ　紙おむつ（使い捨ての）**disposable diaper**（成人用）**disposable (incontinence) briefs[underwear, pad]**（紙製の）**paper diaper**（成人用）**paper (incontinence) briefs[underwear, pad]** ☞おむつ

かみそりまけ　かみそり負け　razor rash [burn] ◆よくかみそり負けを起こしますか Do you often get *a razor rash[a rash after shaving]?

かみん　仮眠する　take a nap, take short sleep breaks

かみんしょう　過眠症　hypersomnia

◀周期性過眠症 periodic hypersomnia

かむ¹ 噛む （咀嚼する）**chew** （かじる）
bite ☞咀嚼 ◆物が噛みにくいですか Do
you have any difficulty[trouble] chewing? ◆物を噛む時に痛みますか Does it
hurt when you chew （something）? /
Does chewing hurt? ◆この錠剤は噛んだ
り飲み込んだりしないで下さい Don't chew
or swallow this tablet. ◆食事はよく噛ん
で食べるようにすると満腹感が得られます
If you chew your food well, your stomach
will feel full and satisfied. ◆お子さんは
爪を噛みますか Does your child bite his
〈her〉 nails? ◆唇を噛む bite *one's* lip
◆犬に噛まれる be bitten by a dog

かむ² （鼻を）かむ **blow *one's* nose**

ガム （**chewing**）**gum** ◆ガムを噛む chew
gum ◆ニコチンガム nicotine gum

カメラ **camera** ◀胃カメラ gastroscope / gastrocamera 眼底カメラ fundus camera ガンマカメラ gamma camera

かめん 仮面 **mask** （㊇**masked**） ◆仮面
をかぶったような顔 a masklike face ▶仮
面うつ病 masked depression 仮面高血圧
masked hypertension 仮面様顔貌 masklike face

―かもしれない （可能性がある）**may**,
might ★might のほうが控えめな言い方.
（悪い事態が予測される）**I'm afraid** （疑いがあ
る）**I suspect** ☞可能性 ◆急性胃炎かもし
れません. It may[might] be acute gastritis. ◆膀胱炎かもしれません You may
[might] have cystitis. ◆治療は長引くか
もしれません I'm afraid the treatment is
going to take a long time. ◆肺炎を起こし
ているかもしれません I suspect you've developed[got] pneumonia.

かゆ 粥 （食）**rice porridge** （diet）, **semisolid diet** ◆普通に炊いたご飯とお粥とど
ちらがいいですか Which would you like,
regular rice or rice porridge?

かゆい 痒い **itchy** /ítʃi/ （㊇図**itch**） ☞痒
み ◆かゆいところはありますか Do you
feel itchy anywhere? ◆目〈耳〉がかゆい
ですか Do your eyes〈ears〉feel itchy? /

Are your eyes〈ears〉itchy? ◆かゆい所を
掻かないで下さい. 掻けば掻くほどもっとか
ゆくなりますよ Don't scratch the itchy
area. The more you scratch, the itchier it
will become. ◆背中がかゆい have an
itchy back / *one's* back *is itchy[itches]
◆かゆくて赤い発疹が出る have itchy, red
spots ◆少しかゆい be slightly[mildly]
itchy ◆発疹がかゆいと訴える complain
of an itchy rash ◆痛かゆい painful and
itchy

かゆみ 痒み **itch** （㊇**itchy**）, **itching**, **itchiness**, **pruritus** （㊇**pruritic**） ☞痒い ◆かゆ
みがありますか Do you feel itchy? ◆かゆ
みの程度はどのくらいですか How bad is
the itching? ◆かゆみはとれたり，また痒
ゆくなったりしますか Does the itching
clear up and then come back? ◆目にか
ゆみがある have itchy eyes ◆広範囲のか
ゆみが出た時には，直ちにこの薬の服用を
中止して下さい If you get itchy over a
wide area, please stop this medication at
once. ◆かゆみが強い The itchiness is
intense. ◆かゆみを和らげる relieve itching[itchiness] ◆かゆみを止める stop
[prevent] itching[itchiness] ◆膣のかゆ
み vaginal itching

かゆみどめ 痒み止め **medication for
itching**, **antiitch medication**, **antipruritic**
（**medication**, **drug**, **agent**） （軟膏）**antiitch
ointment[cream]** ◆かゆみ止めを飲む
take medication to relieve[stop / prevent] the itching ◆かゆみ止めを塗る
apply an antiitch ointment ◆かゆみ止め
の塗り薬 topical antipruritic （medication / drug / agent）

かよう¹ 過用 **overuse** ▶過用症候群
overuse syndrome

かよう² 通う （訪れる）**go**, **visit** （場所に着
く）**get to** （通学・通勤する）**commute** ◆歯
科医へ定期的に通っていますか Do you *go
to[visit] the dentist regularly? ◆会社へ
はどうやって通っていますか How do you
get[commute] to work? ◆近くの病院に
通う go to a nearby hospital ◆リハビリに
通う go for rehabilitation

かようせい　可溶性(の)　**soluble**　▶可溶性抗原 soluble antigen

かようび　火曜日　Tuesday；**Tue.**, **Tues.**
◆火曜日に on Tuesday　◆火曜日ごとに on Tuesdays

から　空にする　《中身を空ける》**empty**（⇔ **empty**）　《きれいにする》**clear**　◆胃の中を長く空にしてはいけません．少しずつ頻繁に食べて下さい You shouldn't have an empty stomach for too long. Try to eat a little and often.　◆腸の中を空にする empty[clear] one's intestines

カラー　collar　◆カラーを着ける put on a collar　◆カラーを着けている wear a collar　◀頸椎カラー neck[cervical] collar

カラードプラちょうおんぱけんさ　―超音波検査　color Doppler ultrasound[ultrasonography]

からい　辛い
《辛味がある》《香辛料の利いた》**spicy**　《口内がひりひりする》**hot**　◆最近，辛い食べ物をたくさん食べましたか Have you eaten large amounts of spicy food recently?　◆辛い食べ物を制限する limit spicy foods　◆辛い味 hot taste
《塩辛い》**salty**　◆塩辛い食べ物を避ける avoid salty foods

ガラガラごえ　―声　hoarse voice, raspy voice　☞声　◆ガラガラ声で話す speak in a hoarse[raspy] voice

ガラクトースけつしょう　―血症　galactosemia

ガラス　glass　◀耐熱ガラス heat-resistant glass　▶ガラス板法 slide precipitation test

からせき　空咳　dry cough　《痰がからまない咳》**nonproductive cough**　☞咳　◆空咳が出る have a dry cough

からだ　体
《身体》**body**　☞身体　◆体全体に all over one's body　◆体の一部に in a[one] part of the body　◆発疹は体中ですか，一部のみですか Do you have the rash all over your body or just in one part?　◆体の力を抜いて下さい Please relax (your muscles). / Please let your body go

limp.　◆体の向きを変える change one's position / turn around　◆体を動かす move one's body / (運動する) get some exercise(s), exercise one's body　◆(寝ている状態から)体を起こす sit up / rise from a lying position　◆体を横たえる lie down　◆体をまっすぐにして立つ stand (up) straight　◆体を使う仕事 physical work[labor]
《健康》**health**　☞具合, 体調, 調子　◆お体に気をつけて下さい Please take care of yourself. / Take care!　◆喫煙はあなたの体によくありません Smoking is not good for your health.　◆お体はいかがですか How do you feel? / How are you feeling [doing]? / How is your health?　◆休みなく働きすぎると体を壊します You'll damage your health if you overwork[work too hard] without taking a break. / Overworking without taking a break will damage your health.

からのすしょうこうぐん　空の巣症候群　empty nest syndrome

かり　仮(の)　《臨時の》**temporary**（↔permanent）　《試験的な》**tentative**（↔definite）　《暫定的な》**provisional**　◆仮の処置をしておきましょう I'm going to give you a temporary treatment.　◆この措置は仮のものです This is only a temporary measure.　◆仮の計画 a tentative plan　◀仮診断 provisional[tentative] diagnosis　仮包帯 temporary bandage　☞仮歯

カリウム　potassium　◀塩化カリウム potassium chloride　高カリウム血症 hyperkalemia / hyperpotassemia　シアン化カリウム potassium cyanide　低カリウム血症 hypokalemia / hypopotassemia　ヨウ化カリウム potassium iodide　▶カリウム制限食 potassium-restricted[low-potassium] diet　カリウム保持性利尿薬 potassium-sparing diuretic

ガリウム　gallium　▶ガリウムシンチグラフィ gallium scintigraphy

カリエス　caries　◀脊椎カリエス spinal caries

カリニはいえん　―肺炎　《ニューモシスチス

肺炎）Pneumocystis pneumonia；PCP

かりば　仮歯　temporary crown（暫間義歯）temporary dentures　▲通例，複数形で．　◆仮歯がとれる a temporary crown falls off

カリフラワー　cauliflower　▶カリフラワー耳 cauliflower ear　カリフラワー状腫瘤 cauliflower-like tumor

かりゅう　顆粒　granule（形granular）　◀分泌顆粒 secretory granule　▶顆粒円柱 granular cast　顆粒剤 medication in granular form／granules

かりゅうきゅう　顆粒球　granulocyte　▶顆粒球減少症 granulocytopenia　顆粒球コロニー刺激因子 granulocyte colony-stimulating factor；G-CSF　顆粒球マクロファージコロニー刺激因子 granulocyte-macrophage colony-stimulating factor；GM-CSF

かりゅうよく　渦流浴　whirlpool bath

かりょう¹　加療　medical treatment［care］　☞治療　◆あなたの病気は1週間の入院加療が必要です Your disease requires a week's hospitalization（and treatment）. ／You need to receive［undergo］a week's treatment in the hospital.　◆現在加療中である be currently receiving［undergoing］medical treatment

かりょう²　過量（多すぎる）too much（薬など）overdose　☞過剰

かるい　軽い（重さ・負担が）light（↔heavy）（病気・症状がひどくない）mild（↔severe）（程度が重大ではない）minor（↔major）（程度がわずかな）slight（楽な）easy　☞軽く，軽度　◆軽い運動をする必要があります You need to do some light exercises.　◆軽い食事をとる have a light meal　◆軽い痛みがある have a mild［slight］pain　◆軽い脳卒中を起こす have a minor［mild］stroke　◆事故で軽い傷を負う be slightly injured in an accident　◆この薬の副作用は軽いでしょう The side effects of this medication are rather mild.　◆軽いお産 an easy delivery

かるく　軽く　☞緩和，和らぐ，和らげる　◆この四脚杖は怪我をした足への負担を軽くしてくれます（減らす）This quad cane will decrease the load on the injured leg.　◆頭痛を軽くするものがありますか（和らげる）Is there anything that relieves［eases］the headache？／Is there anything that makes the headache better？　◆その痛みは軽くなっていますか Is the pain getting better？　◆この軟膏は軽くすり込んで下さい（優しく）Please rub this ointment in gently.

カルシウム　calcium /kǽlsiəm/　◆カルシウムを多く含む食べ物を摂って下さい Please eat foods that are rich［high］in calcium.　◆カルシウムサプリメントを飲む take calcium supplements　◀高カルシウム血症 hypercalcemia　高カルシウム尿症 hypercalciuria　シュウ酸カルシウム結石 calcium oxalate stone　炭酸カルシウム結石 calcium carbonate stone　低カルシウム血症 hypocalcemia　乳酸カルシウム calcium lactate　補正カルシウム値 corrected［adjusted］calcium level　▶カルシウム拮抗薬 calcium antagonist　カルシウム結石 calcium stone　カルシウム摂取量 calcium intake　カルシウム代謝障害 calcium metabolism disorder

カルジオリピンしけん　—試験　cardiolipin test

カルシトニン　calcitonin

カルタゲナーしょうこうぐん　—症候群　Kartagener syndrome

カルチノイド　carcinoid　▶カルチノイド症候群 carcinoid syndrome

カルチノーマ　☞がん

カルチャーショック　culture shock　◆カルチャーショックを受ける experience culture shock

カルテ（medical）chart（診療記録）medical record　◆当院では日本の法律に則ってカルテを開示しております We will release patients' medical records in accordance with Japanese law.　◆書面による本人の許可がなければ，ご本人以外にはカルテを開示いたしません We will not release information from your chart to anyone other than yourself without your

カルテ 139 **かわり**

written permission. ◀電子カルテ electronic medical record；EMR／computer-based patient record／electronic health record；EHR

カルンクル (小丘)**caruncle**

かれい 加齢 **aging**，《英》**ageing**（圏加齢性の **age-related, age-associated**） ☞老化 ◆白内障は加齢に密接に関係しています Cataracts are closely *related to[associated with] aging. ◆血管は加齢で硬くなります The blood vessels harden[get hard] *with age[as we age]. ◆加齢による目の問題 age-related[age-associated] eye problems ◆加齢の徴候 signs of aging ▶加齢黄斑変性症 age-related macular degeneration；AMD 加齢白内障 age-related cataract

かれる 嗄れる **get[become, be] hoarse** ◆声がかれますか Does your voice get hoarse? ◆声がかれていますか Is your voice hoarse?／Do you feel hoarse? ◆風邪で声がかれる get[become] hoarse from a cold ◆声の使い過ぎで声がかれる get[become] hoarse from excessive use of *one's* voice

カレンダー **calendar** /kǽləndə-/ ◆カレンダーに月経の印を付けていますか Do you mark your periods on a calendar? ◀妊娠カレンダー pregnancy calendar

かろう 過労 **overwork**（圖**overwork**） ◆過労は避けて下さい Please try not to overwork yourself.／Please try to avoid overworking. ◆過労が原因で病気になる get sick from overwork ◆過労死を予防する prevent death from overwork ◆過労死と認定される be recognized as a victim of death from overwork

かろくぶ 下肋部 **hypochondriac region**

カロテン **carotene**

カロリー **calorie** /kǽləri/；**cal**（圏**calóric**） ◆この食べ物はカロリーが高い This food is high in calories.／This food contains a lot of calories. ◆野菜はカロリーが低い Vegetables are low in calories. ◆カロリー計算をする count calories ◆カロリーに気をつける watch *one's* calories ◆カロリーを

減らす cut back on calories ◆カロリーを消費する burn off calories ◆カロリー摂取量を1,800 kcal に制限する restrict *one's* *caloric intake[calories] to one thousand eight hundred kilocalories ◆1日 2,000 kcal の食事をする eat[consume] two thousand kilocalories a day ◆1日に必要なカロリー量 the amount of calories needed a[per] day ◆極端なカロリー制限は子供の成長や発達にとって危険です Cutting caloric intake by too much[Extreme calorie restriction] can be dangerous for the growth and development of children. ◀キロカロリー kilocalorie；kcal, Cal 高カロリー食 high-calorie diet；HCD／high-calorie food 高カロリー輸液 hyperalimentation／(経静脈高カロリー輸液) intravenous hyperalimentation；IVH／(完全静脈栄養) total parenteral nutrition；TPN 低カロリー low calorie／(脂肪分の少ない)light calorie 低カロリー食 low-calorie diet；LCD／calorie-restriction[calorie-reduction] diet／low-calorie food

かわ 皮 **skin** ☞皮膚

がわ 側 **side** ◆頭の右側が痛む have (a) pain in the right side of *one's* head ◀片側 one side 左側 left side 右側 right side 両側 both sides

かわかす 乾かす **dry** ◆髪を乾かす dry *one's* hair ◆体を乾かす dry *oneself* (off)

かわく¹ 乾く (乾いた)**dry** ☞乾燥 ◆口が乾く have a dry mouth／*one's* mouth is [gets／becomes] dry ◆乾いた咳 a dry cough

かわく² 渇く **get thirsty, feel thirsty**（圏 **thirst**） ◆喉はよく渇きますか Do you often get[feel] thirsty? ◆喉の渇きを癒すために角氷をあげましょう I'm going to give you some ice cubes to quench your thirst.

かわさきびょう 川崎病 **Kawasaki disease**

かわり 代わり (別の選択肢)**alternative**（圏 **alternative**） (代用・代理の)**substitute**（圖

substitute (📖**instead of**) ☞代わる ◆代わりの治療を提案いたします I'd like to propose an alternative treatment. ◆砂糖の代わりに人工甘味料を使うとよいでしょう You can substitute (an) artificial sweetener for sugar. / You can use (an) artificial sweetener instead of sugar. ◆極端な食事制限をする代わりにウォーキングや軽い運動をなさったほうが効果的に減量できます You can lose weight more effectively by walking or doing light exercise than by *going on an extreme diet[strictly limiting your diet]. ◆この薬はよく効く代わりに高価です This medication works very well, but it's expensive. ◆私が代わりに車椅子を押してあげましょう Let me push the wheelchair for you.

かわる¹ 代わる・替わる・換わる (他のものに取って代わる)**replace** (交換する・交替する)**exchange, swap** (代理を務める)**substitute, take the place** (of) ☞代わり ◆治療法が新しいものに代わっています We've replaced the old treatment with a new one. / A new treatment has replaced the old one. ◆すみませんが彼女とベッドを換わっていただけませんか I'm sorry, but would you mind exchanging[swapping] beds with her? ◆私の代わりに診察するのはベテラン医師ですからご安心下さい An experienced[expert] doctor will substitute for me, so please don't worry. ◆今日は佐藤先生がお休みなので，私が代わって診察します Dr Sato *is off[took the day off] today, so I'll examine you *in his ⟨her⟩ place[instead of him⟨her⟩]. ◆日本語のできる方と代わっていただけますか (日本語を話せる人と話をさせて下さい)Could you please let me speak to someone who can speak Japanese?

かわる² 変わる (変化する)**change** ☞変える，変化，変更 ◆今日からお薬が変わります Starting today your medication will change[be changed]. / Starting today you'll have a different kind of medication. ◆今月から担当医が変わります You'll have a new doctor from this

month. ◆この前の診察からお変わりありませんか How have you been since I last saw you? ◆(入院患者などへの声かけ)お変わりありませんか How are you feeling today? ◆痛みは軽くなっていますか，お変わりませんか Is the pain getting better or is it just the same? ◆気が変わる change *one's* mind ◆気分が変わる(気分変動がある)have mood swings

かん¹ 管 (導管)**duct, canal, conduit** (チューブ・筒状の管)**tube** (物が通過する管)**tract** (脈管)**vessel** (トンネル状の管)**tunnel** ☞チューブ，管(くだ) ◆栄養管(食べ物を与えるための管)feeding[nutritional] tube 血管 blood vessel 手根管 carpal tunnel 消化管 digestive tract 足根管 tarsal tunnel 胆管 bile duct 排液管 drainage tube リンパ管 lymph[lymphatic] vessel 涙管 tear duct[canal] / lacrimal duct

かん² 冠 **crown** ◆金属冠 metal crown 歯冠(dental / tooth) crown

かん³ 肝 (肝臓)**liver** (📖**hepatic**) ☞肝臓 ◀うっ血肝 congestive liver 脂肪肝 fatty liver ☞肝アメーバ症, 肝萎縮, 肝移植, 肝エキノコックス症, 肝炎, 肝芽腫, 肝管, 肝がん, 肝機能, 肝吸虫症, 肝区域切除, 肝血管腫, 肝血流量, 肝硬変, 肝後性黄疸, 肝再生, 肝細胞, 肝疾患, 肝周囲炎, 肝周囲膿瘍, 肝腫大, 肝腫瘍, 肝障害, 肝静脈, 肝小葉, 肝腎エコーコントラスト, 肝腎症候群, 肝性, 肝生検, 肝切除, 肝前性黄疸, 肝損傷, 肝動脈, 肝内, 肝嚢胞, 肝膿瘍, 肝庇護療法, 肝不全

がん **cancer** (📖**cancerous**) (上皮性の悪性腫瘍)**carcinoma** /kὰ:sənóumə/ (📖**carcinómatous**) (肉腫)**sarcoma** ☞腫瘍 ◆がんに罹る have[get / develop] cancer ★cancerには通例，冠詞 a を付けない。 ◆がんと診断する diagnose cancer ◆がんの早期発見 early detection of cancer ◆がんと闘う fight against cancer / struggle with cancer / battle cancer ◆がんを克服する beat[conquer] cancer

《告知に関する表現》☞巻末付録：悪い診断結果を伝える時 ◆がんを告知する inform the patient that he⟨she⟩ has cancer / inform the patient about[of] his⟨her⟩ cancer

◆がんの診断結果が出たら告知を望みますか Do you want to be told if it's[the diagnosis is] cancer? ◆がんの疑いがあります I suspect[think] you may have cancer. ◆胃にがんがあります You have *stomach cancer[(悪性腫瘍)a malignant tumor in the stomach]. ◆甲状腺にがんが見つかりました We found cancer in your thyroid gland. ◆残念ですが，彼女はがんが再発しました I'm sorry to tell you that her cancer has come back. / Unfortunately, her cancer has relapsed. ◆がんが脳に転移しています The cancer has spread[metastasized] to the brain. ◆がんがすでにリンパ節に転移しています The cancer has already entered[spread to] the lymph nodes. ◆がんの骨転移が見つかりました We found (a) metastasis to the bone. / We found that the cancer has metastasized[spread] to the bone.

《治療・予後に関する表現》 ◆がんを取り除く remove the cancer ◆この種のがんの90％以上は，早期に治療すれば治ります If treated early, this type of cancer has a cure rate of more than ninety percent. / This type of cancer is curable in more than ninety percent of patients if treated early. ◆がん性疼痛治療ラダーを用いて鎮痛薬を調整していきましょう Let's adjust the pain medication *in line with[following] the cancer pain (relief) ladder. ◆がんが小さくなっています The cancer is shrinking. ◆このポリープはがん化する恐れはほとんどないでしょう This polyp is not likely to *turn into cancer[become cancerous]. / There's little possibility of this polyp *turning into cancer[becoming cancerous]. ◆彼のがんは予後が大変悪いのです His cancer has a very poor prognosis. / He has a cancer with a very poor prognosis.

《進展度》 ◆前がん precancer ◆前がん期 precancerous stage ◆早期がん early [early-stage] cancer / cancer in its early stages ◆進行がん(進行性の) progressive cancer / (症状が進行した) advanced cancer ◆末期がん terminal[terminal-stage / end-stage] cancer

《病理学的分類》 ◆印環細胞癌 signet ring cell carcinoma ◆基底細胞癌 basal cell carcinoma ◆巨細胞癌 giant cell carcinoma ◆高分化癌 well-differentiated carcinoma ◆小細胞〈非小細胞〉癌 small cell〈non-small cell〉carcinoma ◆上皮内癌 carcinoma in situ；CIS ◆髄様癌 medullary carcinoma ◆スキルス[硬性]癌 scirrhous carcinoma ◆腺癌 adenocarcinoma ◆大細胞癌 large cell carcinoma ◆低分化癌 poorly differentiated carcinoma ◆粘液癌 mucinous carcinoma ◆扁平上皮癌 squamous cell carcinoma ◆未分化癌 undifferentiated[anaplastic] carcinoma ◆類上皮癌 epidermoid carcinoma ◆濾胞癌 follicular carcinoma

《臓器別》 ★部位＋cancer もしくは cancer＋of＋部位で表す． ◆胃がん stomach cancer / cancer of the stomach ◆肝がん liver cancer ◆甲状腺がん thyroid cancer ◆喉頭がん laryngeal cancer ◆子宮がん uterine cancer ◆子宮頸がん cervical cancer ◆食道がん esophageal cancer ◆膵臓がん pancreatic cancer ◆前立腺がん prostate cancer ◆大腸がん(結腸の) colon cancer / (結腸・直腸の) colorectal cancer ◆重複がん double cancer ◆乳がん breast cancer ◆肺がん lung cancer ◆皮膚がん skin cancer ◆卵巣がん ovarian cancer

《併発症》 ◆がん性悪液質 cancerous cachexia ◆癌性胸膜炎 carcinomatous pleurisy[pleuritis] ◆癌性心膜炎 carcinomatous pericarditis ◆がん性疼痛 cancer pain ◆がん性腹水 cancerous ascites[ascitic fluid] ◆癌性腹膜炎 carcinomatous peritonitis ◆癌性リンパ管症 carcinomatous lymphangitis

◀原発がん primary cancer 転移がん metastatic cancer ▶がん遺伝子 cancer gene / oncogene がんウイルス oncovirus / oncogenic virus がん化学療法 cancer chemotherapy がん患者 cancer patient /

patient with cancer　がん恐怖症 cancerophobia　がん検診 cancer screening [checkup]　がん5年生存率 the five-year survival rate for cancer　がん細胞 cancer cell　がんセンター cancer center　がん専門医 cancer specialist /〈腫瘍専門医〉oncologist　癌胎児性抗原 carcinoembryonic antigen；CEA　がん疼痛管理 cancer pain management　がん登録 cancer registration　がんマーカー cancer marker　がん抑制遺伝子 tumor suppressor gene / antioncogene　☞がん化

がんあつ　眼圧 intraocular pressure；IOP, eye pressure, ocular tension　◆眼圧が高い the pressure within *one's* eye is high / *one's* intraocular pressure is high [elevated]　◆眼圧を測りましょう Let me measure[check] the pressure within your eyes.　◆眼圧が正常より高いので下げる薬を処方しましょう Your eye pressure is higher than normal, so I'll prescribe a medication to lower it.　◀正常眼圧緑内障 normal-tension glaucoma；NTG　▶眼圧計 tonometer　眼圧測定 tonometry

がんアメーバしょう　肝アメーバ症 hepatic amebiasis

がんアレルギー　眼アレルギー ocular allergy

がんい　眼位 eye position　▶眼位計 phorometer　眼位測定 phorometry

かんいしゅく　肝萎縮 atrophy of the liver

かんいしょく　肝移植 liver transplant [transplantation]　☞移植　◆肝移植を受ける have[undergo] a liver transplant / have[undergo] liver transplantation　◀生体肝移植 living (donor) liver transplant[transplantation]

がんいぶつ　眼異物 ocular foreign body

かんエキノコックスしょう　肝エキノコックス症 hepatic echinococcosis

かんえん　肝炎 hepatitis /hèpətáɪtɪs/　◆肝炎に罹っています I think you have hepatitis.　◆肝炎が進行して肝硬変を起こしかけているようです The hepatitis has progressed and it seems to be turning into

cirrhosis.　◀アルコール性肝炎 alcoholic hepatitis　ウイルス性肝炎 viral hepatitis　A〈B / C〉型肝炎 hepatitis A〈B / C〉/ type A〈B / C〉hepatitis　A〈B / C〉型肝炎ウイルス hepatitis A〈B / C〉virus / HAV〈HBV / HCV〉　A〈B〉型肝炎ワクチン hepatitis A〈B〉vaccine　急性肝炎 acute hepatitis　劇症肝炎 fulminant hepatitis　血清肝炎 serum hepatitis；SH　自己免疫性肝炎 autoimmune hepatitis　胆汁うっ滞性肝炎 cholestatic hepatitis　非アルコール性脂肪性肝炎 nonalcoholic steatohepatitis；NASH　慢性肝炎 chronic hepatitis　薬物性肝炎 drug-induced hepatitis　輸血後肝炎 posttransfusion hepatitis　▶肝炎ウイルスキャリア hepatitis virus carrier　肝炎患者 hepatitis patient / patient with hepatitis

がんえん　眼炎 ophthalmia, ophthalmitis　◀交感性眼炎 sympathetic ophthalmia　紫外線眼炎 photophthalmia

かんおう　陥凹 〈くぼみ〉depression 〈形depressed〉　〈引っ込み〉retraction 〈形retracted〉　〈埋伏〉impaction 〈形impacted〉　〈杯状のへこみ〉cupping 〈形cupped〉　☞陥没　◀乳頭陥凹〈視神経の〉optic disc cupping /〈乳房の〉nipple retraction　▶陥凹[陥没]骨折 depressed[impacted] fracture　陥凹性病変 depressed lesion　陥凹瘢痕 depressed scar

かんおんなんちょう　感音(性)難聴 sensorineural hearing loss[impairment]

がんか¹　眼科 the department of ophthalmology, the ophthalmology department　▶眼科医 eye doctor / ophthalmologist　眼科学 ophthalmology

がんか²　眼窩 eye socket, orbit 〈形orbital〉　▶眼窩筋炎 orbital myositis　眼窩腔 orbital cavity　眼窩骨折 orbital fracture　眼窩疾患 orbital disease

がんか³　がん化する become cancerous, turn into cancer　☞がん　◆がん化する恐れのあるポリープを切除する remove a polyp that is likely to *become cancerous [turn into cancer]

かんかい　寛解 remission；*a period when*

the symptoms of a serious illness lessen or are no longer evident ◆臨床的寛解に達する reach[achieve] (a) clinical remission ◆この病気に完治は望めませんが，部分寛解を得ることはできます There's no complete cure for this disease, but *partial remission is possible[you can achieve (a) partial remission]. ◆幸いにも，彼は1年以上寛解状態が続いています Happily, he has been in remission for over a year. ◆彼女の白血病は今寛解期にあります Her leukemia is now in remission. ◀完全寛解 complete remission　自然寛解 spontaneous remission　不完全寛解 incomplete remission　部分寛解 partial remission ▶寛解導入 remission induction

がんがいしょう　眼外傷　ocular injury

かんがえ　考え　（思い・思考）thought（題 think）（思いつき・アイデア）idea（意見）opinion（仮定・推測）assumption ☞考える ◆あなたの考えや気持ちを自由に話して下さい Please feel free to speak[talk] about *what you're thinking and feeling [your thoughts and feelings]. ◆それはいい考えですね That's a good idea. ◆素晴らしい考えが頭に浮かびました I've had a wonderful idea. / A wonderful idea *occurred to me[came to me]. ◆腫瘍専門医の考えを聞いてみましょう Let's listen to *what the oncologist thinks[the oncologist's opinions / the oncologist's ideas]. ◆私の考えをご説明しましょう Let me explain[tell you] what I think. ◆その考えは間違っているように思われます That assumption seems to be wrong [mistaken]. / That seems to be a wrong [mistaken] assumption. ◆この夏どこかに旅行される考えはありますか（旅行を計画しているか）Are you planning to go on a trip somewhere this summer? ◆その点に関して私の考えはあなたとは違っています（同意できない）I can't agree with you on that point.

かんがえる　考える　（思考する）think（of, about）（圏thought）（考慮に入れる・検討する）consider（圏consideration）（見なす）

regard（**A** as **B**）☞思う，考え ◆前向きな考え方をする think positively ◆あなたは放射線治療を受けることについてどう考えますか What do you think of[about] having radiotherapy? / What's your opinion on having radiotherapy? ◆私もそのように考えます I think so too. ◆私はそうは考えません I don't think so. ◆そのことは考えておきましょう I'll think about that. ◆いい解決法を考える think up[of] a good solution ◆私の提案を十分にお考え下さい I hope you'll think over my proposal carefully. / I hope you'll give my proposal full consideration. ◆よく考えてから決めて下さい Please *think carefully [give it lots of thought] before you decide. ◆その計画は慎重に考える必要があります The plan needs serious[careful] thought. ◆いくつか治療の選択肢を考えています I'm considering a number of treatment options for you. ◆喫煙は肺がんの主要な原因の1つと考えられています Smoking is *regarded as[considered to be] one of the primary[main] causes of lung cancer. ◆一般的に，子宮頸がんはヒトパピローマウイルスの性感染によると考えられています It is *generally believed [generally thought / commonly considered] that cervical cancer is caused by sexually transmitted human papillomavirus. ◆この薬であなたの症状は改善すると考えています（期待している）I expect that this medication will improve your symptoms. ◆あなたの頭痛は首の筋緊張によるものと考えられます（推測する）I suppose that your headache is caused by muscle tension in your neck.

かんかく¹　感覚　（五感から受ける印象）sensation, feeling（五感の1つ）sense（物の感じ方）sensibility（知覚・認識）perception, esthesia（圏感覚・知覚に関する sensory）☞感触 ◆感覚に異常はありましたか Have you noticed any abnormal sensation? ◆しびれやぴりぴりするような感覚はありましたか Have you noticed any numbness or tingling? ◆右手の感覚がな

い have no sensation in *one's* right hand / have lost all sensation in *one's* right hand ◆足指の感覚がなくなる lose (the) sensation[feeling] in *one's* toes /（感覚が麻痺する）*one's* toes go numb ◆味の感覚が鋭い have *a keen[an acute] sense of taste ◆触った感覚が過敏だ〈鈍い〉*one's* touch sensations are sharp〈dull〉 ◀異常感覚 dysesthesia　痛み感覚 pain sense[sensation]　温度感覚 temperature sense[sensation] / thermal sensation　時間感覚 time sense[perception]　触（感）覚 tactile sensation / sense of touch　振動（感）覚 vibration sense / pallesthesia　深部感覚 deep sense[sensation]　手袋靴下型感覚消失 glove and stocking anesthesia　表在感覚 superficial sense[sensation]　平衡感覚 sense of equilibrium[balance] / static sense　方向感覚 sense of direction　膀胱感覚 bladder sensation ▶感覚閾値 sensory threshold　感覚運動障害 sensorimotor disorder　感覚運動野 sensorimotor area　感覚解離 sensory dissociation　感覚過敏 hypersensibility　感覚器（官）sense[sensory] organ　感覚障害 sensory disorder[disturbance / impairment]　感覚消失 sensory loss / loss of sensation　感覚神経 sensory nerve　感覚性言語中枢 the sensory speech center　感覚性失語 sensory aphasia　感覚鈍麻 hypoesthesia / hypesthesia　感覚麻痺 sensory paralysis　感覚野 sensory area　感覚路 sensory tract

かんかく²　**間隔**　（時間の）**interval**　（空間の）**space** ◆陣痛の間隔 the intervals[time] between contractions ◆陣痛の間隔はどれくらいですか How close together are the contractions? ◆この薬は8時間の間隔で飲んで下さい Please take this medication every eight hours. ◆めまいの症状は3，4か月の間隔で再発しました The episodes of dizziness recurred at three-to-four month intervals. ◆一定の〈5分の〉間隔で at regular〈five-minute〉intervals ◆次の予防接種までは4週間以上間隔をあけて下さい You should wait at least four weeks before getting the next vaccination. ◆酸素濃縮装置と火気は少なくとも2ｍ間隔を空けて下さい Keep the oxygen concentrator at least two meters away from open flames or any source of heat. / Leave a space of at least two meters between the oxygen concentrator and open flames or other sources of heat. ◀授乳間隔 feeding interval

かんがしゅ　肝芽腫　hepatoblastoma

かんかん¹　汗管　sweat duct ▶汗管腫 syringoma

かんかん²　肝管　hepatic duct ◀総肝管 common hepatic duct

かんがん　肝がん　liver cancer, cancer of the liver　（肝細胞癌）hepatoma, hepatocellular carcinoma；HCC

がんがん　頭ががんがんする（割れるような頭痛）have a splitting headache /（ずきずきする頭痛）have a throbbing headache ◆がんがん響く音が聞こえる（ドンドン叩くような）hear a banging sound in *one's* ear(s) /（轟くような）hear a roaring sound in *one's* ear(s)

がんかんそう　眼乾燥（症）　dry eye

かんき　換気　ventilation （動ventilate 形ventilatory）◆換気のよい部屋 a well-ventilated room ◀一回換気量 tidal volume；TV[Vt]　一側肺換気 one-lung ventilation　過換気症候群 hyperventilation syndrome　間欠的強制換気 intermittent mandatory ventilation；IMV　経鼻間欠的陽圧換気 nasal intermittent positive pressure ventilation；nIPPV　拘束性換気障害 restrictive ventilatory impairment　呼気終末陽圧換気 positive end-expiratory pressure ventilation；PEEP　持続陽圧換気 continuous positive pressure ventilation；CPPV　人工換気 artificial[mechanical] ventilation　肺胞低換気症候群 alveolar hypoventilation syndrome　非侵襲的陽圧換気 noninvasive positive pressure ventilation；NPPV　分時換気量 minute ventilatory[ventilation] volume　閉塞性換気障害 obstructive ventilatory defect　補助換気 assisted

ventilation ▶換気応答 ventilatory response 換気回数 ventilation[ventilatory] frequency 換気血流比不均等 ventilation perfusion（ratio）inequality[mismatch] 換気装置 ventilator 換気調節 ventilatory regulation[control] 換気能 ventilatory capacity 換気不全 ventilatory insufficiency 換気モード mode of ventilation 換気量 ventilation volume

かんきけんいんし 冠危険因子 **coronary risk factor**

かんきつるい 柑橘類 **citrus fruits** ★複数形で．◆この薬はグレープフルーツなどの柑橘類と同時に服用しないで下さい Please don't take this medication with citrus fruits such as grapefruits.

かんきのう 肝機能 **liver function, hepatic function, function of the liver** ▶肝機能検査 liver[hepatic] function test 肝機能障害 liver[hepatic] dysfunction 肝機能不全 liver[hepatic] failure

がんきゅう 眼球 **eyeball, bulb of the eye**（形bulbar, ocular）▶眼球銀行 eye bank 眼球結膜 bulbar conjunctiva / conjunctival layer of the bulb 眼球振盪 nystagmus 眼球突出 exophthalmos / ocular proptosis / bulging[protrusion] of the eyes[eyeballs] 眼球内出血 intraocular bleeding[hemorrhage] 眼球偏位 eye[ocular] deviation ☞眼球運動

がんきゅううんどう 眼球運動 **eye movement** ◀急速眼球運動 rapid eye movement：REM 非共同眼球運動 disconjugate eye movement 輻輳眼球運動 convergence eye movement ▶眼球運動障害 eye movement disorder[disturbance]

かんきゅうちゅうしょう 肝吸虫症 **clonorchiasis**

かんきょう 環境 （生活・自然の環境）**environment**（形environmental）（人を取り巻く周囲の環境）**surroundings** ★複数形で．（暮らしなどの状況）**conditions** ★複数形で．（置かれた状況）**situation**（形situational）（背景にある事情）**background** ◆職場環境はストレスが多いですか Is your work envi-

ronment stressful? / Are your working conditions stressful? ◆環境に適応する adapt to the surroundings[environment] ◆環境に左右される be influenced by one's environment ◆新しい環境にすぐなじむ adapt[adjust] quickly to new surroundings ◆患者さんが心配なく治療を受けられるように環境を調整する adjust the environment so that patients can have[undergo] their treatment without any worries ◆環境を変える change one's environment ◆環境を改善する improve the environment ◆環境に優しい製品 environment-friendly[eco-friendly] products ◀家庭環境 family background[environment] 居住環境 residential[home] environment / housing conditions[situation] 社会環境 social environment 生活環境 home[living] environment / the environment one lives in /（暮らしの状況）living conditions 無重力環境 weightless environment 労働環境 working[work] environment[situation] ▶環境衛生 environmental sanitation[health] 環境汚染 environmental pollution 環境汚染物質 environmental pollutant 環境基準 environmental standards 環境制御 environmental control 環境整備 environmental improvement 環境破壊 environmental destruction 環境不適応 situational maladjustment 環境ホルモン environmental hormone

かんきん 桿菌 **bacillus, rod-shaped bacterium** ◀グラム陰性桿菌 gram-negative bacillus 肺炎桿菌 *Klebsiella pneumoniae*

がんきん 眼筋 **eye muscle, ocular muscle** ◀外眼筋 extraocular muscle ▶眼筋麻痺 ocular muscle palsy / ophthalmoplegia / paralysis of the ocular muscles 眼筋ミオパチー ocular myopathy

かんくいきせつじょじゅつ 肝区域切除術 **hepatic segmentectomy**

ガングリオン **ganglion**

かんけい 関係 (一般的な相互関係)relation (動relate) (より密な相互関係)relationship (一般的な事実関係) connection (動connect) ☞関連 ◆喫煙と喉頭がんの関係は明らかです The relationship[connection] between smoking and laryngeal cancer is obvious. / There is an obvious relationship[connection] between smoking and laryngeal cancer. ◆あなたの症状は食事と関係がありますか Is your symptom related to meals? / Is there any connection between your symptom and meals? ◆ストレスがあなたの今の症状に大いに関係しています Stress has a lot to do with your present symptoms. ◆皮膚の問題は食品に関係があると思いますか Do you think your skin problem has any relationship to food? ◆スミスさんとはどんなご関係ですか What relation is Mr〈Ms〉Smith to you? / How are you related to Mr〈Ms〉Smith? ◆親子の関係を改善する improve *the parent-child relationship[the relationship between parent(s) and child] ◆…と協力関係にある have a cooperative relationship with … ◆心と体の関係 relationship between mind and body ◆仕事上の関係 working relationship ◆信頼関係 relationship of trust / (ラポール)rapport ◆医師〈看護師〉患者関係 physician〈nurse〉-patient relationship / relationship between a physician〈nurse〉and a patient 因果関係 cause and effect relationship / relationship between cause and effect 家族関係 family relationship[relations] 血縁関係 blood relationship[relations] 宿主寄生体関係 host-parasite relationship 性的関係 sexual relationship[relations] 相互関係 reciprocal[mutual] relationship 対人関係 (個人的な相互関係)(human) relationship, interpersonal relationship / (一般的な相互関係)(human) relations, interpersonal relations 直接的関係 direct connection 夫婦関係 marital relationship[relations] 父子関係 father-child relationship[relations] 母子関係 mother-child relationship[relations] 用量反応関係 dose-response relationship[relations] ▶関係妄想 delusion of reference / reference delusion

かんげざい 緩下剤 ☞緩下薬，下剤

かんけつ¹ 簡潔(な) brief ◆これまでの経過を簡潔に話して下さい(どんな症状だったか，どんな問題を抱えていたか)Please tell me briefly *what kind of symptoms you've had[what problems you've been having].

かんけつ² 間欠(的な) intermittent /ìntəˈmítənt/ ◆痛みが間欠的でかなり強い The pain *is intermittent[comes and goes] and is very severe. ▶間欠性跛行 intermittent claudication 間欠痛 intermittent pain 間欠的強制換気 intermittent mandatory ventilation；IMV 間欠的腹膜透析 intermittent peritoneal dialysis；IPD 間欠的陽圧換気 intermittent positive pressure ventilation；IPPV 間欠熱 intermittent fever

かんけつ³ 観血(的な) (切開を伴う)open (手術の)surgical, operative (侵襲性の)invasive ▶観血的整復 open reduction 観血的治療 surgical treatment 観血的モニタリング invasive monitoring

かんけっかんかくちょうやく 冠血管拡張薬 coronary vasodilator

かんけっかんしゅ 肝血管腫 hepatic hemangioma[angiomatosis]

かんけっかんぞうえい 冠血管造影(法) coronary angiography[arteriography]；CAG；*X-ray recording of the coronary arteries after injection of a contrast medium*

かんけつりゅうりょう¹ 肝血流量 hepatic blood flow；HBF

かんけつりゅうりょう² 冠血流量 coronary blood flow；CBF

かんげやく 緩下薬 laxative /læksətɪv/；*medication that loosens the bowels* (便軟化剤)stool softener ☞下剤 ◆緩下薬を使う use[take] laxatives ◆市販の緩下薬を使う前には必ず私に相談して下さい Be sure to *consult (with) me[ask me] before using over-the-counter laxatives.

がんけん 眼瞼　eyelid, palpebra（咽頭）blephar(o)-）　☞瞼（まぶた）　◀下眼瞼 lower eyelid　上眼瞼 upper eyelid　▶眼瞼炎 blepharitis　眼瞼黄色腫 xanthelasma　眼瞼外反症 ectropion of the eyelid　眼瞼下垂 blepharoptosis / ptosis / drooping eyelid　眼瞼痙攣 eyelid twitching / blepharospasm　眼瞼結膜 blepharoconjunctiva

かんご 看護　nursing　（看護ケア）nursing care　◆彼女には 24 時間の看護が必要です She requires twenty-four-hour nursing care.　◆患者に手厚い看護を行う provide tender[（最大限の）the utmost] nursing care to patients　◀完全看護 comprehensive[twenty-four-hour] nursing care　在宅看護 home nursing[health] care　日本看護協会 Japanese Nursing Association　訪問看護 home-visit[visiting] nursing / home (care / health) nursing　▶看護学 nursing science　看護学生 nursing student　看護学部 school[faculty / department] of nursing / nursing school[faculty / department]　看護過誤 nursing malpractice[error / mistake]　看護学校 nursing school / school of nursing　看護教育 nursing education　看護業務 nursing service　看護記録 nursing (care) record　看護計画 nursing care plan　看護サマリー[看護要約] nursing summary　看護実習 nursing practicum　看護助手 nursing assistant / nurses' aide　看護診断 nursing diagnosis　看護スタッフ the nursing staff　看護大学 college of nursing / nursing university[college]　看護チーム nursing team　看護手順 nursing procedure　看護部 nursing department　看護目標 nursing goal[objective]　看護用品 nursing supplies[equipment]　☞看護師

がんこ 頑固（な）　（しつこい）stubborn, obstinate　（しつこく持続する）persistent　（扱いにくい）intractable　◆頑固な痛み *a stubborn[an intractable] pain　◆頑固な便秘に効く食事 a diet for stubborn[obstinate] constipation　◆頑固な咳に苦しむ suffer from persistent cough

かんこう¹ 汗孔　sweat pore

かんこう² 観光　sightseeing　◆日本へ来られた目的は観光ですか Have you come to Japan to do some sightseeing? / Is sightseeing the purpose of your visit to Japan?　◆今度のご旅行は観光ですか，それとも商用ですか Are you traveling for sightseeing or on business?　◀医療観光 medical tourism　外国人観光客 foreign tourist　▶観光ビザ tourist visa　観光旅行 sightseeing trip[tour]

かんこうへん 肝硬変　cirrhosis / sɪróʊsɪs /　◀アルコール性肝硬変 alcoholic cirrhosis　原発性胆汁性肝硬変 primary biliary cirrhosis；PBC　胆汁うっ滞性肝硬変 cholestatic cirrhosis

かんこく 韓国　(the Republic of) Korea, South Korea（㊡Korean）　☞国籍　▶韓国人(の) (South) Korean

かんごし 看護師　nurse　◆こんにちは，担当看護師の阿部です Hello, I'm your nurse, Ms〈Mr〉Abe. / Hello, I'm[my name is] Ms〈Mr〉Abe, and I'm your nurse.　◆ご用の時はいつでも看護師を呼んで下さい Please call the nurses anytime you need them.　◀夜勤看護師 night-duty nurse / nurse on night duty　▶看護師患者関係 nurse-patient relationship

---

看護師の名称

■免許・資格

●看護師 nurse　●専門看護師 certified nurse specialist；CNS　●認定看護師 certified nurse　●登録看護師《米》registered nurse；RN　●感染管理認定看護師 infection control nurse；ICN　●准看護師 associate[assistant] nurse　●看護助手 nursing assistant / nurse's aide

■管理職

●看護部長 director of nursing　●看護副部長 vice director of nursing　●看護師長 nursing[nurse] supervisor / nurse manager　●主任看護師 charge[head] nurse

■職分

●外来看護師 outpatient nurse　●手術室

看護師 surgical[scrub] nurse　●病棟看護師 ward[floor / unit / staff] nurse　●訪問看護師 visiting nurse

かんごせいおうだん　肝後性黄疸　post-hepatic jaundice

かんこつ　寛骨　hip bone, coxal bone　▶寛骨臼 the socket of the hip joint / acetabulum

かんさ　感作　sensitization （國感作された sensitized）　◀減感作療法 desensitization[hyposensitization] therapy　光感作物質 photosensitizer

かんさいせい　肝再生　liver regeneration

かんさいぼう¹　肝細胞　liver cell, hepatic cell, hepatocyte　▶肝細胞癌 hepatocellular carcinoma；HCC　肝細胞性黄疸 hepatocellular jaundice

かんさいぼう²　幹細胞　stem cell　◀人工多能性幹細胞 *induced pluripotent stem[iPS] cell　造血幹細胞 hematopoietic[blood-forming] stem cell　胚性幹細胞 *embryonic stem[ES] cell　▶幹細胞移植 stem cell transplant[transplantation]

かんさつ¹　間擦（の）　intertriginous　▶間擦疹 intertrigo　間擦性湿疹 intertriginous eczema

かんさつ²　観察する　observe （國observation 國observational）, watch, keep an eye（on）　◆お子さんは経過観察のために入院する必要があります Your child needs to be admitted to the hospital for observation.　◆私たちは彼女の病状を注意深く観察しています We're keeping a close eye on her condition.　◆彼は術後の経過観察中です He is now under observation after the surgery.　◆子供の行動を注意深く観察する observe[watch] the behavior of the child closely　◀顕微鏡的観察 microscopic observation　肉眼的観察 gross [macroscopic] observation / macroscopy　要観察 observation required / needs to be observed　▶観察研究 observational study　観察者 observer

かんさつい　監察医　medical examiner

がんサルコイドーシス　眼サルコイドーシス　ocular sarcoidosis

かんさんひょう　換算表　conversion table　☞巻末付録：単位の換算

かんし¹　鉗子　forceps　★複数形で.（留め金）clamp　▶血管鉗子 vascular forceps　生検鉗子 biopsy forceps　マギル鉗子 Magill forceps　▶鉗子分娩 forceps delivery　鉗子生検 forceps biopsy

かんし²　監視する　monitor （國monitor, monitoring）　watch … closely, keep watch（over）　◆この医療機器は心拍数，呼吸数などの状態を監視するものです This is a medical device that monitors your condition, such as your heart rate and respiration rate.　◀病床監視装置 floor monitor　分娩監視装置 tocomonitor　▶監視装置 monitor, monitoring device /（設備）monitoring equipment

かんじ　感じ　sensation, feeling　☞感覚, 感じる

がんし　眼脂　eye mucus[discharge], discharge from the eyes　☞目脂（めやに）

かんじくかんせつ　環軸関節　atlantoaxial joint

がんじくちょう　眼軸長　axial length of the eye

かんじくついだっきゅう　環軸椎脱臼　atlantoaxial dislocation

カンジダ　（学名）*Candida* （カンジダ症）candidiasis　◀外陰腟カンジダ症 vulvovaginal candidiasis　口腔カンジダ症（鵞口瘡）oral candidiasis / thrush　食道カンジダ症 esophageal candidiasis　爪カンジダ症 nail candidiasis　腟カンジダ症 vaginal candidiasis　皮膚カンジダ症 cutaneous candidiasis　▶カンジダ・アルビカンス *Candida albicans*　カンジダ血症 candidemia

かんしつ　間質　（間質）interstitium （國interstitial）　（支質）stroma （國stromal）　◀消化管間質腫瘍 gastrointestinal stromal tumor；GIST　▶間質細胞 interstitial cell　間質性腎炎 interstitial nephritis　間質性肺疾患 interstitial lung disease；ILD　間質性膀胱炎 interstitial cystitis

かんしっかん¹ 肝疾患 liver disease
◀アルコール性肝疾患 alcoholic liver disease 非アルコール性脂肪性肝疾患 nonalcoholic fatty liver disease；NAFLD

かんしっかん² 冠（動脈）疾患 coronary artery disease；CAD ▶冠疾患危険因子 coronary risk factor 冠疾患集中治療室 coronary care unit；CCU

かんしゃ 感謝する thank, be thankful （to）, be grateful（to）（図gratitude）, appreciate（図appreciation） ☞ありがとう ◆ご協力感謝します Thank you for your cooperation[help]. ◆お時間をいただき感謝します Thank you for your time. ◆感謝の気持ちを表す show one's gratitude

かんじゃ 患者 patient （医療などのサービスを受ける人）client ◆患者を診察する see [examine] a patient ◆手術に対する患者の理解を確認する confirm the patient's understanding of the surgery ◆患者の同意を得る obtain the patient's informed consent ◆気難しい患者 a difficult patient ◆歩行が可能な患者 an ambulatory patient ◆新型インフルエンザが疑われる患者 a patient with a suspected new strain of influenza ◀受け持ち患者 patient assigned to one / patient under one's care 外国人患者 overseas[foreign] patient 回復期患者 convalescent 外来患者 outpatient / ambulatory[day] patient 隔離患者 isolated[quarantined] patient がん患者 cancer patient / patient with cancer 救急患者 emergency patient 高齢患者 elderly[senior] patient 再診患者 follow-up patient 在宅患者 homebound patient / patient at home 重病患者 seriously ill patient 初診患者 new[first-visit] patient 待機患者 patient on the waiting list 透析患者 dialysis patient / patient on dialysis 入院患者 inpatient 寝たきり患者 bedridden patient 末期患者 terminal patient / patient with a terminal illness 模擬患者 simulated patient；SP 問題患者 problem patient ▶患者一部負担金 partial copayment 患者会 patients' association 患者教育 patient education

患者心理 patient psychology 患者中心医療 patient-centered medicine[health care] 患者中心介護 patient-centered care 患者調査 patient survey 患者登録 patient registration 患者ネットワーク patient（support / access）network 患者の権利 patient[patients'] rights 患者搬送 patient transport[transfer] 患者ファイル patient file 患者負担金 medical expenses borne[paid] by the patient 患者プロフィール patient profile 患者への説明 explanation to the patient 患者満足度 patient satisfaction

かんしゃく （temper）tantrum ◆お子さんはかんしゃくを起こしますか Does your child have tantrums?

かんしゅう 慣習 custom （しきたり）practice ☞習慣 ◆日本の慣習に従う follow Japanese customs ◆自分の国の慣習を守る keep[observe] the customs of one's own country

かんしゅういえん 肝周囲炎 perihepatitis

かんしゅういのうよう 肝周囲膿瘍 perihepatic abscess

かんじゅせい 感受性 （感度・過敏性）sensitivity（図sensitive） （影響の受けやすさ）susceptibility（図susceptible） ◀抗生物質感受性 antibiotic sensitivity[susceptibility] 放射線感受性 radiation sensitivity / radiosensitivity 薬剤感受性試験 drug susceptibility[sensitivity] test ▶感受性菌 sensitive bacteria 感受性訓練 sensitivity training

かんしゅだい 肝腫大 hepatomegaly, enlargement of the liver

かんしゅよう 肝腫瘍 liver tumor, hepatic tumor, tumor of the liver

かんしょう¹ 緩衝 buffer ▶緩衝液 buffer solution

かんしょう² 干渉する interfere（in, with）（図interference） ◆お子さんに対しては干渉しすぎないようにして下さい Please try not to be too interfering in your child's affairs. / Please try to put some space between yourself and your child. ◀過干

渉 overinterference

かんじょう¹ 感情 (気持ち・心持ち)**feelings** ★通例，複数形で．(情動・強い感情)**emotion** (麻**emotional** (専門用語として)**affective**) ☞情緒，情動 ◆感情面で最近何か問題がありましたか Have you had any emotional problems recently? ◆感情を表に出す show[express] *one's* feelings[emotions] ◆感情をコントロールする control[check / restrain] *one's* feelings[emotions] ◆感情の爆発(uncontrolled) emotional outbursts ◆季節的感情障害 seasonal affective disorder；SAD ▶感情移入 empathy 感情失禁 emotional incontinence 感情障害 affective disorder 感情鈍麻(無感情)apathy / lack of interest

かんじょう² 環状(の) **circular, annular** ◀包皮環状切除術 posthetomy / circumcision ▶環状紅斑 erythema annulare 環状切断術 circular amputation 環状肉芽腫 granuloma annulare

かんしょうがい 肝障害 **liver injury[damage], hepatic injury[damage]** ◀薬物性肝障害 drug-induced liver[hepatic] injury

かんじょうじょうみゃく 冠状静脈 **coronary vein**

かんじょうだん 冠状断 **coronal section** (前頭断)**frontal section**

かんじょうどうみゃく 冠状動脈 ☞冠動脈

かんじょうみゃく¹ 肝静脈 **hepatic vein**

かんじょうみゃく² 冠静脈 **coronary vein**

かんしょうよう 肝小葉 **hepatic lobule**

かんしょく¹ 感触 **feeling** (麻**feel**) (肌触り)**touch** ☞感覚 ◆感触に左右差がある feel a difference between *the left and right sides[the two sides] ◆彼女の容態は好転しているという確かな感触があります I feel sure[certain] that her condition is improving.

かんしょく² 間食する **eat between meals, have a snack between meals** ☞おやつ ◆日中または夜寝る前に間食しますか Do you eat between meals and before going to bed? ◆間食にはどんな物を食べますか What do you eat between meals? ◆間食は控えて下さい Please cut down on eating between meals.

かんじる 感じる **feel** ◆少し痛み〈圧迫〉を感じるかもしれません You may feel some pain〈pressure〉. ◆左右で同じように感じますか Does it feel the same on both sides? ◆疲労〈空腹〉を感じる feel tired〈hungry〉

かんしん¹ 汗疹 **prickly heat, heat rash** ☞あせも

かんしん² 関心 (興味)**interest** (麻**be interested** (in)) (気がかり)**concern** (麻**be concerned** (about)) ☞興味，心配 ◆新薬の臨床試験に関心がありますか Are you interested in (participating in) clinical trials of a new medication? ◆あなたの今の一番の関心事は何ですか What's your greatest concern at this moment? / (何が悩ませているか)What worries you most at this moment? ▶関心領域 area of interest

かんじん 肝心・肝腎(な) (重要な)**important** (不可欠な)**essential** ◆肝心なのは十分な睡眠をとることです The most important thing is to get enough sleep.

がんしん 眼振 **nystagmus**；*involuntary movement of the eyes* ◀温度眼振検査 caloric nystagmus test 眼性眼振 ocular nystagmus 耳性眼振 aural nystagmus 垂直眼振 vertical nystagmus 注視眼振 gaze nystagmus 頭位性眼振 positional [postural] nystagmus 頭位変換眼振 positioning nystagmus

かんじんエコーコントラスト 肝腎エコーコントラスト **hepatorenal echo contrast**

かんじんしょうこうぐん 肝腎症候群 **hepatorenal syndrome**

かんする (…に)関する (…について)**about** (特定の分野などについて)**on** (フォーマルに)**concerning, regarding, as regards** (関連して)**related to** ◆あなたの職場環境に関する情報がもっと必要です I need more information about[on] your

working environment. ◆その点に関して
はもう一度話し合いましょう Let's talk
about that again. ◆治療に関してはいく
つか選択肢があります We have several
options concerning[as regards] the treatment. ◆彼は薬物に関して問題があります
He has a problem related to drugs. / He
has a drug(-related) problem. ◆子育て
に関する問題をお持ちですか Do you have
any problems with taking care of your
child〈children〉? ◆新しい知見に関する
論文を学会誌に発表する publish a paper
on *one's* new findings in an academic
journal

かんせい¹ 肝性(の) **hepatic** ▶肝性黄
疸 hepatic jaundice 肝性昏睡 hepatic
coma 肝性脳症 hepatic encephalopathy

かんせい² 乾性(の) **dry** ▶乾性角結膜
炎 dry eye / keratoconjunctivitis sicca；
KCS 乾性湿疹 dry eczema 乾性咳 dry
[nonproductive] cough

かんせい³ 完成する・させる　(仕上げる)
complete　(図**completion**)　(終 え る) **finish** ◆以下の文を完成させて下さい
Please complete the following senten-
ces. ◆研究プロジェクトを完成するのにど
のくらい時間がかかりますか How long will
it take you to complete[finish] your
research project? ◆文章完成テスト sentence completion test；SCT

かんせいけん 肝生検 **liver biopsy**

がんせいしゃけい 眼性斜頚 **ocular torticollis**

がんせいひろう 眼精疲労 **asthenopia**
(目の疲れ・視覚疲労)**eye strain, eye fatigue**

かんせつ¹ 関節 **joint** (図**articular** 腰頭
arthr(o)-) ◆関節に痛みがありますか Do
you have *any joint pain[any pain in your
joints]? ◆どの関節ですか Which joints
are involved[affected]? ◆指の関節が腫
れて痛そうですね Your finger joints are
swollen and look painful. ◆肘の関節が
はずれています You've dislocated your
elbow joint. ◆関節の動きをよくする〈維
持する〉improve〈maintain〉*one's* joint
mobility ◀顎関節 temporomandibular

joint；TMJ 肩関節 shoulder joint 肩関
節周囲炎 stiff shoulder / periarthritis of
the shoulder / scapulohumeral periarthritis 肩関節脱臼 shoulder dislocation
環軸関節 atlantoaxial joint 胸鎖関節
sternoclavicular joint 股関節 hip joint
(手指の)指節間関節 finger joint / interphalangeal joint of the hand　(足指の)趾節間
関節 toe joint / interphalangeal joint of
the foot 膝関節 knee joint 手関節 wrist
joint 手根間関節 intercarpal joint 人工
関節 artificial joint 仙腸関節 sacroiliac
joint 足関節 ankle joint 多発関節痛
polyarthralgia 肘関節 elbow joint 動揺
関節 loose[flail] joint 変性関節疾患 degenerative joint disease；DJD 変形性関
節症 osteoarthritis；OA 変形性股関節症
hip osteoarthritis 変形性膝関節症 knee
osteoarthritis ▶関節位置覚 sense of
joint position 関節運動覚 sense of joint
movement 関節鏡 arthroscope 関節強
直 joint ankylosis / ankylosis of the joints
関節腔 joint[articular] cavity 関節拘縮
joint stiffness / articular contracture 関
節疾患 joint disease 関節周囲炎 periarthritis 関節穿刺 arthrocentesis 関節造
影 arthrography 関節脱臼 joint dislocation 関節置換術 joint replacement 関
節痛 joint pain[aches] / arthralgia 関節
内注射 intraarticular injection 関節包
joint capsule ☞関節炎, 関節可動域, 関節リ
ウマチ

かんせつ² 間接(の) **indirect** ◆間接的
な原因 an indirect cause ▶間接X線撮影
法 indirect radiography 間接感染 indirect (contact) infection 間接[受動]喫煙
indirect[passive] smoking / secondhand
smoking 間接クームス試験 indirect
Coombs test 間接蛍光抗体法 *indirect
fluorescent antibody[IFA] technique
間接照明 indirect illumination 間接対光
反射 indirect (papillary) light reflex 間
接ビリルビン indirect bilirubin

かんせつえん 関節炎 **arthritis** /ɑəθráɪ-
tɪs/ ◀化膿性関節炎 pyogenic[septic]
arthritis 多発性関節炎 polyarthritis 痛

風性関節炎 gouty arthritis

かんせつかどういき 　**関節可動域**　**range of motion**；**ROM** ◆関節可動域を広げる〈向上させる／維持する〉increase〈improve／maintain〉*one's* range of motion ▶関節可動域訓練 range-of-motion exercise　(関節)可動域制限 limited range of motion

かんせつじょ 　**肝切除(術)**　**hepatectomy**

かんせつリウマチ 　**関節リウマチ**　**rheumatoid arthritis**；**RA** ☞リウマチ ◆関節リウマチを発症したのはいつですか When did your rheumatoid arthritis start? ◆ご家族の中に関節リウマチの人はいますか Is there anyone in your immediate family that has rheumatoid arthritis?

かんせん¹ 　**感染**　**infection** (㊥感染性の **infectious**, **infective** 感染した **infected**) (接触による) **contagion** (㊥**contagious**) ☞伝染 ◆この病気は感染します This disease is infectious[contagious／(うつりやすい)catching]. ◆この病気は感染の危険性がかなり高いです The risk of infection with this disease is fairly high.／(強い感染力がある)This disease is highly infectious[contagious]. ◆感染してから2週間ほどで発症します You'll develop symptoms about two weeks after becoming infected. ◆感染の徴候が出たら直ちに知らせて下さい Please let us know at once if you have any signs of infection. ◆周囲への感染を防ぐために自宅でゆっくり休養して下さい Please stay at home and take a good rest to prevent the people around you from becoming infected. ◆血液を介して感染する get[become／be] infected through the blood ◆感染を疑う suspect an infection ◆感染の疑いのある患者 a patient with suspected infection ◀易感染 susceptibility to infection　易感染性宿主 compromised[immunocompromised] host　院内感染 hospital-acquired[nosocomial] infection　ウイルス感染 viral[virus] infection　家族内感染 familial infection　カテーテル感染 catheter-associated infection；気道感染 airway[respiratory tract] infection　細菌感染 bacterial infection　市中感染 community[community-acquired] infection　集団感染 mass infection　接触感染 contact infection　潜伏感染 latent infection　内因性感染 endogenous infection　二次感染 secondary infection　尿路感染 urinary tract infection；UTI　飛沫感染 droplet infection　日和見感染 opportunistic infection　不顕性感染 silent[asymptomatic／subclinical] infection　糞口感染 fecal-oral infection　母子感染 fetomaternal infection／mother-to-child transmission ▶感染経路 infection route　感染源 source of infection　感染者 infected person　感染性角結膜炎 infectious keratoconjunctivitis　感染性下痢 infectious diarrhea　感染性心内膜炎 infective endocarditis；IE　感染性腸炎 infectious enterocolitis　感染性廃棄物 infectious waste　感染巣 infection[infectious] focus　感染創 infected wound　感染対策 infection control measures　感染対策専門医 infection control doctor；ICD／infectious disease specialist　感染力 infectivity ☞感染症

かんせん² 　**汗腺**　**sweat gland** ◀アポクリン汗腺 apocrine sweat gland　エクリン汗腺 eccrine sweat gland ▶汗腺炎 hidradenitis

かんせん³ 　**乾癬**　**psoriasis** /səráɪəsɪs/ (㊥**psoriátic**) ◀尋常性乾癬 psoriasis vulgaris　膿疱性乾癬 pustular psoriasis ▶乾癬性関節炎 psoriatic arthritis　乾癬性紅皮症 psoriatic erythroderma　乾癬性脊椎炎 psoriatic spondylitis

かんぜん 　**完全(な)**　(すべて揃った・完了した)**complete** (↔incomplete)　(包括的・総合的な)**comprehensive**　(完璧な)**perfect**　(全面的な)**total**　(十分な)**full** ◆完璧, 全面的 ◆病気は完全には治っていません You haven't recovered completely.／Your disease has not been cured completely. ◆傷口は完全にふさがっています The wound has completely closed. ◆当院は完全看護です This hospital offers patients comprehensive[twenty-four-hour] nursing care. ◆それは完全な失敗でした It was a total failure. ◆彼女は澤先生のことを完全に頼りにしています She is putting herself totally in Dr Sawa's hands. ▶完全右脚〈左脚〉ブロック complete right 〈left〉 bundle branch block；CRBBB〈CLBBB〉 完全寛解 complete remission 完全主義 perfectionism 完全主義者 perfectionist 完全大血管転位 complete *transposition of the great arteries[TGA] 完全治癒 complete cure 完全房室ブロック complete atrioventricular[AV] block 完全麻痺 complete paralysis

がんせん 頑癬 ☞股部白癬

かんせんしょう 感染症 infectious disease, infection （接触による）contagious disease （伝染性の）communicable disease ☞感染 ◆耳の感染症によくかかりますか Do you often have ear infections? ◆あなたは最近感染症にかかった人のそばにいましたか Have you recently been around anyone with an infection? ◆お子さんのご家庭, 保育園, または幼稚園で最近感染症にかかった人がいますか Has anyone around your child had recent infections at home, or at the day care center or *nursery school[kindergarten]? ◀HIV 感染症 HIV infection 学校感染症 infectious disease in school settings / school infectious disease 検疫感染症 quarantine infectious disease 国立感染症研究所 the National Institute of Infectious Diseases 指定感染症 designated infectious[communicable] disease 上気道感染症 upper respiratory infection；URI / upper airway infection 新興感染症 emerging communicable[infectious] disease 人畜共通感染症 zoonosis 性（行為）感染症 sexually transmitted infection；STI / sexually transmitted disease；STD 尿路感染症 urinary tract infection；UTI 輸入感染症 imported infectious disease ▶感染症科 the department of infectious diseases 感染症患者 infectious[contagious] patient 感染症指定医療機関 designated medical institute

of infectious diseases 感染症専門医 infectious disease specialist 感染症対策 *infection control[infectious disease control] measures 感染症法 Infectious Disease Law 感染症予防 prevention of infectious diseases

かんぜんせいおうだん 肝前性黄疸 pre-hepatic jaundice

かんそう 乾燥（した）dry （動dry 名dryness）◆皮膚が乾燥していますか Is your skin dry? ◆口は乾燥した感じですか Does your mouth feel dry? ◆皮膚の乾燥を防ぐ prevent dry skin / prevent one's skin from drying ◆目の乾燥 dryness of the eyes ◀眼乾燥症 dry eye 口腔乾燥症 dry mouth / xerostomia 凍結乾燥 freeze-drying ▶乾燥感 feeling of dryness 乾燥症候群 sicca syndrome 乾燥肌 dry skin

かんぞう 肝臓 liver （形hepatic）☞肝 ◆今までに肝臓の病気に罹ったことがありますか Have you ever had any liver diseases before? ◆肝臓の異常を指摘されたことがありますか Have you ever been told that you have a problem with your liver? ◆肝臓の機能が低下しています Your liver is not functioning well. / Your liver function has declined. ◆少なくとも1週間に2, 3日は肝臓を休めて下さい Please give your liver a rest *a couple of days[two or three days] a week. ▶肝臓移植 liver transplant[transplantation] 肝臓がん liver cancer / cancer of the liver 肝臓病 liver disease

がんそうやく 含嗽薬 mouthwash, gargle ☞うがい

かんそく 患側 affected side （↔unaffected side）

かんそんしょう 肝損傷 liver injury

かんたい 間代 clonus （形clonic）▶間代性痙攣 clonic convulsion[seizure] 強直間代痙攣 tonic-clonic convulsion[seizure]

がんたい 眼帯 （目の遮蔽用）eye patch[pad, shield] （包帯）eye bandage ◆右目に眼帯をする put on *a patch[an eye patch] over *one's* right eye ◆眼帯をはずす take off an eye patch ◆眼帯をしている wear an eye patch ◆圧迫眼帯 pressure eye patch

かんたん 簡単(な) (単純な)simple (容易な)easy (短時間の・簡潔な)brief (即座の)ready ☞容易 ◆簡単な血液検査から始めましょう Let's start with a simple blood test. ◆この病気は検尿で簡単に診断できます A urine test can easily diagnose this disease. ◆治療はそんなに簡単ではありません The treatment is not that easy[simple]. / (考えるほどスムーズにはいかない)The treatment won't go as smoothly as you expect. ◆簡単な病気ではありません(治療が容易ではない)It's not an easy disease to treat. / (重篤な病気だ)It's rather a serious disease. ◆私の考えを簡単にご説明いたしましょう Let me explain briefly what I think. ◆その病気についての最新情報はインターネットで簡単に手に入れることができます Up-to-date information about the disease is readily accessible on the internet.

かんち 完治 complete cure (㊙cure completely), complete recovery (㊙recover completely) ◆病気が完治するには少なくとも半年はかかるでしょう It will take at least half a year for your disease to be completely cured. ◆この病気の完治は難しいでしょう Complete recovery from this disease *is probably difficult[probably can't be expected].

かんちょう 浣腸 enema /énəmə/ ◆便秘を解消するために浣腸が必要です To relieve the constipation, you need to have an enema. ◆浣腸薬は体温よりやや高めに温めて下さい Please warm the enema (solution) to slightly above body temperature. ◆それでは浣腸しましょう。できるだけ我慢して下さい Now, I'm going to give you an enema. Hold it in for as long as you can. ◆浣腸を使用する use enemas ◀グリセリン浣腸 glycerin enema

かんつい 環椎 atlas, first cervical vertebra

がんつう 眼痛 eye pain, aching eye, ophthalmalgia

かんてい 鑑定 (試験・検査)examination (㊙examine), test (㊙test) (分析)analysis (㊙analyze) (診断)diagnosis (㊙diagnose) ◆DNAの鑑定を専門家に依頼する ask a specialist to examine[analyze] *one's* DNA sample ◀親子鑑定 parentage test[diagnosis] / (父子関係の)paternity test[diagnosis] 精神鑑定 psychiatric examination[test] DNA鑑定 DNA test[testing / analysis] / DNA-based test

がんてい 眼底 eyegrounds, the fundus of the eye, the fundus oculi ◀蛍光眼底血管造影法 fluorescence fundus angiography 蛍光眼底撮影 fluorescence fundus photography ▶眼底カメラ fundus camera 眼底鏡 funduscope / ophthalmoscope 眼底検査 examination of the *eyegrounds[fundus of the eye] / ophthalmoscopy / funduscopy 眼底出血 fundus bleeding

かんてん¹ 観点 point of view, viewpoint ◆専門的な観点からは from a professional[scientific] *point of view[viewpoint]

かんてん² 寒天 agar ▶寒天培地 agar medium

かんでん 感電する be struck by an electric shock ▶感電死 death by (an) electric shock / electrical death

かんど 感度 sensitivity ◀測定感度 sensitivity of measurement

かんどうみゃく¹ 冠動脈 coronary artery ◀経皮経管的冠動脈形成術 percutaneous transluminal coronary angioplasty；PTCA 経皮的冠動脈インターベンション percutaneous coronary intervention；PCI 経皮経管的冠動脈再開通術 percutaneous transluminal coronary recanalization[revascularization]；PTCR ▶冠動脈狭窄 coronary artery stenosis 冠動脈形成術 coronary angioplasty 冠動脈血栓症 coronary artery thrombosis 冠動脈硬化症 coronary arteriosclerosis 冠動脈ステント術 coronary stenting 冠動脈造影法

coronary angiography[arteriography]；CAG 冠動脈バイパス手術 coronary artery bypass graft[grafting]；CABG 冠動脈閉塞 coronary occlusion 冠動脈攣縮 coronary artery spasm ☞冠疾患

かんどうみゃく2 **肝動脈** **hepatic artery** ▶経カテーテル肝動脈塞栓術(hepatic) transcatheter arterial embolization；TAE 経カテーテル肝動脈注入療法(hepatic) transcatheter arterial infusion；TAI

がんトキソプラズマしょう **眼トキソプラズマ症** **ocular toxoplasmosis**

かんとく **監督** (取り締まり)**supervision** (動**supervise**) (指揮・指導) **direction** (動**direct**) ◆研修医は指導医の監督の下で診療を行います Residents work[treat patients] under *the direction of medical supervisors[the supervision of senior medical doctors]. ▶監督者 supervisor / director

かんとん **嵌頓** **strangulation** (形**strangulated**), **incarceration** (形**incarcerated**) ▶嵌頓内痔核 strangulated[incarcerated] internal hemorrhoids 嵌頓ヘルニア strangulated[incarcerated] hernia 嵌頓包茎 paraphimosis / strangulation of the glans penis

かんない **肝内(の)** **intrahepatic** ▶肝内結石 intrahepatic gallstone[cholelithiasis] / hepatolithiasis 肝内胆管 intrahepatic bile duct 肝内胆管がん intrahepatic bile duct cancer 肝内胆汁うっ滞 intrahepatic cholestasis

がんない **眼内(の)** **intraocular** ▶眼内異物 foreign body in the eye(s) 眼内炎 endophthalmitis 眼内レンズ intraocular lens；IOL ☞眼(内)圧

がんないあつ **眼内圧** **intraocular pressure**；**IOP**, **eye pressure**, **ocular tension** ☞眼圧

がんなんこう **眼軟膏** **eye ointment**, **ophthalmic ointment**

かんにゅう **陥入・嵌入(の)** (埋伏した) **impacted** (くぼんだ)**depressed** (内向きに伸びた)**ingrown** ☞陥凹 ◀児頭嵌入 engagement (of the fetal head) ▶陥入骨折[陥没骨折] impacted[depressed] fracture 陥入爪 ingrown nail

かんねつめっきん **乾熱滅菌** **dry heat sterilization**

かんねん **観念** (考え)**idea**, **concept** (意識)**sense** ◀強迫観念 obsession / obsessional idea 固定観念 fixed idea / stereotype ▶観念運動失行 ideomotor apraxia 観念恐怖 ideophobia

かんのう **間脳** **diencephalon** (形**diencephalic**), **interbrain** ▶間脳下垂体系 the diencephalic-pituitary system

かんのうせいしんびょう **感応精神病** **induced psychosis**[**insanity**], **communicated psychosis**[**insanity**]

かんのうほう **肝嚢胞** **liver cyst**, **hepatic cyst**

かんのうよう **肝膿瘍** **liver abscess**, **hepatic abscess**

がんばる **頑張る** ◆仕事[学業]で頑張る work hard ◆つらかったでしょうが，よく頑張りましたね You had a hard time, but *you've made it[you got through it]. ◆さあ，終わりました．よく頑張りましたね It's all over. Well done! ◆私があなたをケアいたしますので，一緒に頑張りましょう I'll be in charge of your care throughout, so let's fight this together. / I'll be with you for your care, so let's work together. ◆頑張って！(踏ん張って)Hang in there! ◆リハビリ頑張ってね！(幸運・成功を祈る) Good luck with the rehabilitation[rehab]! ◆頑張り過ぎないで下さい Please don't push yourself too hard. ◆そんなに頑張らなくてもいいんですよ You don't have to work so hard. / You shouldn't *overdo things[push yourself] like that.

かんぱん **肝斑** **liver spot**, **age spot**, **senile lentigo**

かんひごりょうほう **肝庇護療法** **liver-supporting therapy**

かんぴしょう1 **柑皮症** **carotenosis**

かんぴしょう2 **乾皮症** **xeroderma**, **dry skin**

かんびょう **看病する** (看護する)**nurse** (面倒を見る)**look after**, **take care** (**of**)

か

☞介護，看護，世話

カンピロバクター *Campylobacter* ▶カンピロバクター食中毒 *Campylobacter* food poisoning　カンピロバクター腸炎 *Campylobacter* enterocolitis

かんぶ 患部 affected part[area] ◆患部を洗浄しましょう Let me clean[irrigate] the affected part. ◆患部に軟膏を塗る apply the ointment to the affected area

カンファレンス conference ☞会議 ◆術前カンファレンスを行う have a preoperative conference ◆カンファレンスに出席する attend a conference

かんふぜん¹ 冠不全 coronary failure[insufficiency]

かんふぜん² 肝不全 liver failure[insufficiency], hepatic failure[insufficiency]

かんぺき 完璧（な） perfect（図perfection）☞完全 ◆完璧を期する必要はありません You don't have to have everything perfect. / You don't have to be perfect at everything. ◆完璧な親はいません No parent is perfect. ▶完璧主義 perfectionism

かんべつ 鑑別する distinguish, differentiate（図differential） ◆腹部超音波検査では胆嚢ポリープと胆嚢がんとの鑑別は困難です It's difficult to distinguish[differentiate] between gallbladder polyps and gallbladder cancer（by）using abdominal ultrasound. ◀DNA鑑別法 DNA profiling ▶鑑別診断 differential diagnosis

かんぼう 感冒 cold ☞風邪 ◀総合感冒薬 common[general-purpose] cold medication　普通感冒 common cold

かんぼう¹ 汗疱 pompholyx, dyshidrosis（図dyshidrotic） ▶汗疱状湿疹 dyshidrotic eczema

かんぼう² 漢方 Kampo medicine；*the traditional herbal medicine of Japan, adapted from Chinese medicine* ◆漢方薬を使っていますか Are you using any Kampo medication? ▶漢方医 Kampo doctor　漢方薬 Kampo medication[medicine / drug]

がんぼう¹ 顔貌 （一般的に顔・表情）face

（ある特徴的な所見を示す顔貌）facies ◀アデノイド顔貌 adenoid face　仮面様顔貌 masklike face　パーキンソン顔貌 parkinsonian facies　満月顔貌 moon face

がんぼう² 願望 hope, wish ☞望み ◆落ち込んでいて，自殺願望がある feel depressed to the point of *being suicidal [wanting to kill *oneself*] ◀やせ願望 pursuit of thinness

カンボジア Cambodia（図Cambodian） ☞国籍 ▶カンボジア人（の）Cambodian

かんぼつ 陥没（した）（逆さになった）inverted（埋伏した）impacted　（くぼんだ）depressed　（引っ込んだ）retractive, retracted ☞陥凹 ◆乳首が陥没しています You have inverted[retracted] nipples. ▶陥没呼吸 retractive breathing[respiration] / inspiratory retraction　陥没[陥凹]骨折 impacted[depressed] fracture

ガンマ gamma ▶ガンマカメラ gamma camera　ガンマグロブリン gamma globulin　ガンマ線 gamma ray　ガンマナイフ gamma knife

がんマーカー cancer marker ☞腫瘍マーカー

かんまん 緩慢（な）（動作が遅い）slow（図slowness）（無気力な）lethargic（図lethargy）（ぐずぐずした）sluggish（図sluggishness）（鈍くのろい）dull（図dullness） ◆動作が緩慢で最初の一歩が踏み出せない be slow in *one's* movements and have difficulty taking the first step ◀運動緩慢[動作緩慢] slowness of（voluntary）movement / bradykinesia

かんみりょう 甘味料 sweetener ◀人工甘味料 artificial sweetener

かんむり 冠 （歯冠・頭頂）crown ☞冠（かん）

がんめん 顔面（の）facial ☞顔 ▶顔面位分娩 face presentation　顔面痙攣 facial spasm　顔面骨 facial bone　顔面骨骨折 facial fracture　顔面神経 facial nerve　顔面神経痛 facial neuralgia　顔面神経麻痺 facial nerve palsy[paralysis]　顔面損傷 facial injury　顔面チック facial tic　顔面痛 facial pain

かんもく 緘黙 （無言）silence, mutism

がんやく 丸薬 pill ▶丸薬丸め振戦 pill-rolling tremor

かんゆ 肝油 （タラ肝油）cod liver oil

がんゆう 含有する have （成分・栄養素などを含む）contain ☞含む ◆ホウレンソウは鉄分を豊富に含有しています Spinach has a high iron content. / Spinach is rich in iron. ◆ステロイド含有薬 steroid-containing medication ◀脂肪含有量 fat content ◀含有成分 component 含有量 content

かんよ 関与する involve （関わり合いをもつ）be involved ☞関わる，関係，関連

かんよう¹ 寛容 tolerance （形tolerant） ◀自己寛容 self-tolerance 免疫寛容 immunologic tolerance

かんよう² 間葉（の） mesenchymal ▶間葉系腫瘍 mesenchymal tumor 間葉系細胞 mesenchymal cell

かんらくえし 乾酪壊死 caseous necrosis

かんり 管理する （制御する）control （図control） （運営する）manage （図management） （データなどを監視する）monitor （図monitor, monitoring） （注意・世話する）take care（of）（図care），pay attention（to） （維持・保守する）maintain （図maintenance） （監督する）supervise （図supervision） ◆体重を管理する control[manage] one's weight ◆人工呼吸器を着けた患者の管理 management of a patient on an artificial respirator ◆糖尿病は血糖値の自己管理がとても重要です If you have diabetes, it's very important for you to self-monitor your blood sugar levels. ◆入院中，貴重品の管理には十分にご注意下さい Please *take good care of[pay close attention to] your valuables during your stay in the hospital. ◆危機管理 crisis[risk] management 健康管理 health care[management] 呼吸管理 respiratory care[management] 自己管理 self-monitoring / self-management 周術期管理 perioperative care[management] 術後管理 postoperative care[management] 術前管理 preoperative care[management] ストレス管理 stress management 全身管理 general care 疼痛管理 pain management[control] 病院管理業務 hospital administration 病棟管理 ward[floor / unit] supervision 病歴管理室 medical record management office 品質管理 quality control；QC 不安管理トレーニング anxiety management training 分娩管理 management of labor and delivery 米国疾病管理予防センター Centers for Disease Control and Prevention；CDC ▶管理栄養士 registered dietitian[nutritionist] 管理区域 controlled area 管理システム management system ☞管理職

かんりしょく 管理職 （職位）managerial position （管理者）manager, managing member （総称）management ◀中間管理職 middle management

かんりゅう 灌流 （特に血液の灌流）perfusion （胃などの洗浄）lavage ◀血液灌流 hemoperfusion 再灌流療法 reperfusion[recanalization] therapy

かんりょう 完了する complete （図completion），finish ☞終わる ◆リハビリテーションの完了 completion of rehabilitation

がんりょう 含量 content ☞含有

がんりんきん 眼輪筋 orbicular muscle of the eye

かんれい 寒冷（の） cold ▶寒冷アレルギー cold allergy 寒冷凝集素症 cold agglutinin disease；CAD 寒冷凝集素反応 cold agglutination reaction 寒冷刺激 low temperature stimulus 寒冷蕁麻疹 cold urticaria 寒冷赤血球凝集素 cold hemagglutinin

かんれん 関連する （具体的な相互関係がある）be related（to）（図relation, relationship） （結合・つながりがある）be associated（with）（図association） （一般的な事実関係をもつ）be connected（to, with）（図connection） （形（投射した）referred （提携している）affiliated ☞関係 ◆彼女の意識混濁は脱水に関連しているかもしれません Her delirium may be related to dehydration. ◆ストレスに関連した摂食障害 a stress-related eating disorder ◆加齢に関連した症状 an age-related symptom / a symptom associated with aging ◆眼精疲労とコンピュータ使用の関連 *an association[a relationship] between eyestrain and computer use ◀作業関連疾患 work-related disease　ストレス関連障害 stress-related disorder　日常生活関連動作(対応した動作)activities parallel to daily living；APDL　粘膜関連リンパ組織 mucosa-associated lymphoid tissue；MALT ▶関連痛 referred pain　関連病院 affiliated hospital

かんれんしゅく　冠攣縮　coronary vasospasm

かんわ　緩和する　(具合を良くする)make … **better**　(痛み・苦しみ・緊張をとる)**relieve** (図 **relief), ease, alleviate**　(根治ではなく症状を和らげる) palliate (形palliative /pǽlièɪtɪv/ 图palliation) ☞軽く，和らぐ，和らげる ◆症状を緩和するためのお薬をお出しします I'm going to give you a medication to make your symptoms better. / Let me give you a medication that will make you feel better. ◆胃の痛みを緩和する relieve *one's* stomachache ◆今後は彼女の痛みを緩和することを最優先していきます From now on, we'll make her pain relief our main[top] priority. / From now on, relieving her pain will be our main[top] priority. ◆緊張を緩和するには音楽を聴くといいですよ You can relieve[ease] tension by listening to music. / A good way to relieve[ease] tension is to listen to music. ◀終末期緩和ケア terminal palliative care　疼痛緩和 pain relief ▶緩和医療 palliative medicine　緩和因子 alleviating[palliating] factor　緩和ケア palliative care：*medical care that is meant to reduce the pain and relieve the symptoms rather than cure the disease*　緩和ケア病棟 palliative care unit；PCU　緩和処置のみ comfort measures only；CMO

き

き 期 (期間・時期)**period** (段階・病期)**stage** (局面)**phase** (年代)**age** ☞期間 ◆おたふく風邪の潜伏期 the incubation period for mumps ◆前立腺がんの初期です You have early-stage prostate cancer. ◆Ⅲ期の大腸がん *stage three [third stage] colon cancer ◆肺がんのⅣ期 the fourth stage of lung cancer ◆Ⅰ期の乳がん患者 a patient with stage one breast cancer

きあつ 気圧 (空気圧)**air pressure** (大気圧)**barometric pressure, atmospheric pressure** ◀内耳〈中耳〉気圧障害 inner〈middle〉ear barotrauma ▶気圧性副鼻腔炎 aerosinusitis / barosinusitis

キアリきけい ―奇形 Chiari malformation, Arnold-Chiari malformation

きい 奇異(な) paradoxical ◆奇異呼吸 paradoxical breathing[respiration] 奇異性塞栓症 paradoxical embolism

キーセルバッハぶい ―部位 Kiesselbach area

キーパーソン key person

きいろ 黄色(い) yellow (黄色味を帯びた)**yellowish** ◆皮膚の色がいつもより黄色いですか Has your skin become more yellowish than normal? ◆皮膚が黄色くなったことがありますか Has your skin ever turned yellow? ◆黄色味を帯びた痰 yellowish phlegm ◆淡い〈濃い〉黄色の尿 light〈dark〉 yellow urine

きいん 起因する (引き起こされる)**be caused (by)** ◆肺気腫はたいてい喫煙に起因しています Pulmonary emphysema is usually caused by smoking.

ぎいんせい 偽陰性(の) false-negative ◆偽陰性反応 a false-negative reaction

きえる 消える (なくなる)**go away, disappear** (薄れる)**fade** (症状・にきびなどが治る)**clear up** ◆この薬を飲むと痛みが消えます The pain will go away after you take this medication. ◆胸の写真の影は徐々に消えていくでしょう The shadows on your chest X-ray will disappear[fade] gradually. ◆手当をきちんとすればにきびは消えます Your pimples will clear up if treated properly.

きおう 既往 (past) **medical history** ◆痛風の既往はありますか Have you ever had gout? / Do you have a history of gout? ◆大きな病気の既往はありますか Have you ever had any major[serious] diseases[illnesses]? ▶既往症 past disease[illness] 既往歴 past (medical) history；PH / medical history

きおく 記憶 memory (動覚えている **remember** 暗記する **memorize**) ◆彼は過去の出来事をはっきり記憶していますか Does he have clear memories of past events? / Does he clearly remember past events? ◆彼女は記憶が衰え始めていますか Is her memory beginning to fail [decline]? ◆最近の出来事の記憶を失う lose *one's* memory of recent events ◆彼女は過去の記憶がすべて消えています Her memories of the past have all faded [disappeared]. ◆記憶を取り戻す recover *one's* memory ◆幼い頃に虐待された記憶がよみがえる memories of the abuse he〈she〉 suffered as a child come back ◆遠い過去の記憶を呼び戻す *bring back [recall] memories of the distant past ◆鮮明な記憶 a vivid memory ◆かすかな〈曖昧な〉記憶 a dim〈vague〉 memory ◆事故の前後についての記憶がありますか Do you remember what happened right before and after the accident? ◆これから3つの単語を言いますので記憶して下さい．(しばらくしてから)では，その単語をもう一度言って下さい I'm going to tell you three words, so please memorize them. Now, can you repeat the words? ◀短期記憶 short-term memory；STM　長期記憶 long-term memory；LTM　▶記憶障害 memory disorder[disturbance]　記憶喪失 memory loss / loss of memory / (記憶喪失症)amnesia　記憶範囲 memory span 記憶変調 memory change / change in memory ☞記憶力

きおくりょく 記憶力 memory, the faculty of memory[remembering] ◆彼女は年齢の割に記憶力がよい She has *a good [an excellent] memory *for her age[considering her age]. ◆記憶力が悪い have a poor[bad] memory ◆記憶力に変化が起こりましたか Have you noticed any changes in your ability to remember things? ◆最近記憶力が低下していますか(忘れやすくなったか)Have you recently become forgetful?

きおち 気落ちする be disheartened (by), feel down ☞意気消沈, がっかりする ◆お父上が亡くなられてさぞ気落ちなさっていることと思います You must *be really disheartened by[feel really down after] the death of your father.

きおん 気温 temperature ◆気温の変化 a change in temperature

きが 飢餓 starvation (空腹)hunger ◆飢餓で死亡する starve to death ▶飢餓死 death from starvation 飢餓療法 starvation[hunger] therapy

きかい¹ 器械 instrument (器具一式)apparatus ☞器具

きかい² 機械 machine /məʃíːn/ (㊟mechánical) ◆この機械はブーンという音を出しますが, 心配しないで下さい This machine makes a whirring noise, but don't worry. ◆これは機械の問題です This is a mechanical problem. ◆この機械には触らないで下さい Please don't touch this machine. ◆機械にスイッチを入れる start (up) a machine ◆機械のスイッチを切る turn off a machine ▶機械式人工呼吸 mechanical ventilation 機械的イレウス mechanical ileus 機械弁 mechanical (heart) valve

きかい³ 機会 (好機)opportunity, chance ★chance には偶然に与えられた機会という意味合いがある. (時)time (特定の時)occasion ◆この機会に精密検査をしましょう Let's take this opportunity[chance] to carry out a thorough examination. ◆この機会に食習慣を見直すことをお勧めします I recommend that you take advantage of this opportunity to reconsider your eating habits. ◆機会があり次第やってみます I'll try at the first opportunity. / I'll try it as soon as I get the chance. ◆手術をすることに決めたならば機会を逸しないことが大切です It's important not to miss the opportunity[chance] to have the surgery once you've decided on having it. ◆そのことは次の機会に話し合いましょう Let's discuss it next time. ◆お子さんに病気について話すには今が一番よい機会です This[Now] is the best time *to tell[for telling] your child about his〈her〉illness. ◆この機会にご協力に感謝させて下さい Let me take this occasion [opportunity] to thank you for your cooperation.

きがい 危害 (人・物への傷害) harm (動harm) (怪我)injury (動injure) (物への物理的損害)damage (動damage) ☞害 ◆ペットが危害を加えたのですか Did your pet harm[injure /(噛む)bite] you?

きがいしゅうしゅく 期外収縮 premature contraction[beat, complex, systole], extrasystole ◀上室期外収縮 supraventricular extrasystole 心室期外収縮 premature ventricular contraction;PVC / ventricular premature contraction;VPC 心房期外収縮 atrial premature contraction;APC / premature atrial contraction;PAC

きがえる 着替える change one's clothes (㊟change of clothes) ◆服を着替えて下さい Please change your clothes. ◆寝巻きに着替えて下さい Please change into your pajamas. ◆着替えとパジャマを2日分持ってきて下さい Please bring a change of clothes and pajamas for two days. ◆着替えを手伝いましょう(服を着るのを) Let me help you get dressed.

きがおもい 気が重い feel depressed ☞気が滅入る

きがかり 気がかり (不安材料)concern (動 be concerned about) (心配)worry (動

worry, be worried about）◆体調で気がか
りなことがありますか Do you have any
concerns about your health? ◆彼女は入
院費のことが気がかりなようです It seems
that she's worrying about the hospital
bill. / She seems to be worried about the
hospital expenses.

きがかわる　気が変わる　change *one's*
mind ◆（そのことで）気が変わったら教え
て下さい Please let me know if you
change your mind（about that）.

**きがすすまない　気が進まない　be reluc-
tant, be unwilling** ◆彼女は手術を受ける
ことに気が進まないようです She seems to
be reluctant[unwilling] to have the
surgery. / It seems she doesn't want to
have the surgery.

きがすむ　気が済む ◆手を洗うなど、ある
一定の動作を繰り返さないと気が済まない
ことがありますか Do you feel you need to
repeat certain behaviors[actions] such as
washing your hands? ◆気が済みました
か（気分がよくなったか）Do you feel better
now? / Does that make you feel better?

きがせく　気が急く（さっさとやる）**get on
with**（待ちきれない）**be impatient** ◆手術
をしたいと気が急くかもしれませんが，まず
放射線治療で手術前にできるだけ腫瘍を縮
小させましょう You may *want to get on
with having[be impatient to have] the
surgery, but first, let's shrink the tumor
as much as possible with radiation therapy.

きかせる　聞かせる　tell ◆子供の頃の話
を聞かせて下さい Tell me[I'd like to hear
all] about your childhood. ◆病院内では
静かにするようお子さんによく言って聞かせ
て下さい Please tell your child(ren) to be
quiet inside the hospital.

きちる　気が散る　feel distracted ◆気
が散って落ち着きませんか Do you feel distracted and restless?

きがつく　気がつく（意識する）**notice**（意
識を取り戻す）**regain consciousness, recover consciousness**（正気に戻る）**come to**
one's **senses** ☞気づく ◆そのしこりに初

めて気がついたのはいつですか When did
you first notice the lump? ◆他に気がつ
いたことがありますか What else did you
notice? ◆失神した後どのくらいしてから
気がつきましたか After you fainted
[blacked out], how long was it before you
*came to again[regained consciousness /
recovered consciousness]?

きがどうてんする　気が動転する（動揺す
る）**get[be] upset**（冷静さを失う）**lose**
one's **composure**

きがとおくなる　気が遠くなる（一時的に
ふらっとする）**feel faint, faint, feel giddy**（意
識を失う）**lose consciousness** ☞気を失
う ◆気が遠くなったのは，急に立ち上がっ
た時でしたか Did you feel faint when you
stood up too suddenly[quickly]? ◆震
え，発汗，動悸，気が遠くなるなどの症状が
現れたら，低血糖の可能性があります If
you have symptoms such as trembling,
sweating, pounding heart, or feeling faint,
*there's some possibility that your blood
sugar is too low[you may have low blood
sugar].

きがとがめる　気がとがめる ◆物事がう
まくいかないのは自分のせいだと気がとがめ
ることがありますか（自分を責めるか）Do you
blame yourself when things go wrong? /
（後ろめたく思うか）Do you ever feel guilty
about everything that goes wrong?

きかねつ　気化熱　the heat of vaporization

きがまぎれる　気がまぎれる ◆友達とお
国の言葉でおしゃべりしたら気がまぎれまし
たか（気分がよくなったか）Did you feel better
after you talked to a friend in your own
language? / （気持ちをそらしたか）Did talking to a friend in your own language take
your mind off things?

**きがみじかい　気が短い　short-tempered,
quick-tempered** ◆あなたは気が短いほう
ですか Do you tend to be short-tempered
[quick-tempered]? / Do you tend to
have a short[quick] temper?

きがむく　気が向く ◆気が向いたら散歩し
てみてはいかがですか How about going
out for a walk if you feel like it?

きがめいる　気が滅入る　feel[get, become] depressed, feel down　◆仕事のことを考えると気が滅入って出社できないことがありますか When you start thinking about your job, do you ever feel so depressed that you end up not going to work at all?

きがやすまる　気が休まる　(リラックスする) feel[become] relaxed, relax　(安心する) feel[be] at ease　◆最も気が休まるのはどんな時ですか When do you feel most relaxed?　◆忙しすぎて気が休まる時がないのですか Are you too busy to relax?　◆医療ソーシャルワーカーに話をしてみると気が休まるかもしれません It might put *your mind[you] at ease to talk to the medical social worker.

きがゆるむ　気が緩む　◆気が緩むと体重はすぐに増えます(十分注意しないと) If you're not careful enough[(ペースを落とすと) If you slacken off at all / (油断すると) If you let your guard down], you'll gain weight in no time.

きがらくになる　気が楽になる　feel easy　☞気を楽にする　◆その問題について今はだいぶ気が楽になりましたか Do you feel a lot easier about that now?

きがる　気軽(に)　◆何かご質問があれば気軽にお尋ね下さい(遠慮せず自由に) Please feel free to ask any questions.

きかん¹　気管　windpipe, trachea　(形 tracheal)　◆気管挿管する insert[place] a tube into the windpipe　◆気管から抜管する remove the tube from the windpipe　◆経口気管挿管 orotracheal intubation　経鼻気管挿管 nasotracheal intubation　▶気管(内)異物 tracheal foreign body　気管開窓術 tracheal fenestration　気管カニューラ tracheal cannula　気管気管支吸引 tracheobronchial suction　気管食道瘻 tracheoesophageal fistula　気管切開 tracheotomy / tracheostomy　気管挿管 tracheal[endotracheal / intratracheal] intubation　気管チューブ tracheal tube　気管分岐部 tracheal bifurcation

きかん²　器官　organ　◆運動器官 motor organ　感覚器官 sense[sensory] organ　実質器官[実質臓器] parenchymal organ　生殖器官 reproductive organ / genital[sex] organ / genitalia　聴覚器官 auditory organ　発音器官 speech[vocal] organ　▶器官形成期 organogenetic period

きかん³　期間　period　(継続期間・時間) duration　(時間的長さ) length　(形 副 long)　◆一定期間通院して下さい You must come to the outpatient clinic for a certain period of time.　◆この治療の期間中は激しい運動は避けて下さい Please avoid strenuous exercise for the duration of this treatment.　◆日本にはどのくらいの期間いらっしゃるご予定ですか How long are you going to stay in Japan?　◆貧血の治療はどのくらいの期間受けましたか How long were you treated for your anemia?　◆以前と比べると月経の期間は短い〈長い〉ですか Have your periods become shorter〈longer〉than before?　◆入院期間は1週間くらいでしょう You'll have to be in the hospital for about a week.　◀隔離期間 period of isolation[quarantine]　月経期間 menstrual duration　在胎期間 gestational age　在留期間 period of residence in Japan　試用期間 trial period　滞在期間 the length of *one's* stay　投与期間 dosing period　入院期間 the length of *one's* stay in the hospital　妊娠期間 length of pregnancy　不妊期間 infertility period

きかん⁴　機関　(施設) facility　(公共的な機関) institute, institution　(交通などの組織・手段) means　◀感染症指定医療機関 designated medical institute of infectious diseases　教育機関 educational institution　交通機関 means of transport[transportation]　公的医療機関 public medical facility[institution]

ぎがん　義眼　artificial eye, prosthetic eye

きかんし　気管支　bronchus, bronchial tube　◀アレルギー性気管支肺アスペルギルス症 allergic bronchopulmonary aspergillosis；ABPA　気管気管支吸引 tracheobronchial suction　区域気管支 segmental bronchus　経気管支肺生検 transbronchial lung biopsy；TBLB　細気管支炎 bronchiolitis　副鼻腔気管支症候群 sinobronchial syndrome；SBS　▶気管支(内)異物 bronchial foreign body　気管支炎 bronchitis　気管支拡張症 bronchiectasis　気管支拡張薬 bronchodilator　気管支鏡 bronchoscope　気管支収縮 bronchoconstriction　気管支洗浄 bronchial lavage　気管支喘息 (bronchial) asthma　気管支肺炎 bronchial pneumonia / bronchopneumonia　気管支肺胞洗浄 bronchoalveolar lavage；BAL　☞気管支鏡検査

きかんしきょうけんさ　気管支鏡検査 bronchoscopy, bronchoscopic examination　◆気管支鏡検査を行って，気管支を観察し，生検のために組織を採取します I'm going to perform a bronchoscopy to examine your bronchial tubes and take some tissue samples for a biopsy.

ぎかんせつ　偽関節 false joint, pseudarthrosis

きき¹　危機　(重大局面)crisis (圏crises 圏critical)　(危険)risk (圏risky)　☞危険，危篤　◆心不全を起こして危機的な状況にある be in a critical condition after suffering heart failure　◆危機は脱しました The crisis[critical stage] is over.　◆情緒的な危機を経験する go through an emotional crisis　◆アイデンティティの危機に直面している be faced with an identity crisis　◆中年の危機を乗り切る overcome [solve / handle] a midlife crisis　◀青春期危機 adolescent crisis　▶危機意識 sense of crisis　危機介入 crisis intervention　危機管理 crisis[risk] management

きき²　機器 equipment, device　☞器具　◀医療機器 medical equipment　福祉機器 assistive device[equipment]

ききて　利き手　dominant hand　(利き腕)dominant arm　◆利き手はどちらですか Which is your dominant hand? / Which hand do you use more often than the other?　◆利き手は右ですか，左ですか Are you right-handed or left-handed?

ききとる　聞き取る　(聞く)hear　(理解す

る)follow　(音を捉える)catch　◆特に高い音が聞き取りにくいのですか Do you have difficulty hearing, especially high[high-pitched] sounds?　◆すみません．おっしゃることが聞き取れないのですが Sorry, I can't follow[catch] what you're saying.

ききなれない　聞き慣れない　(なじみがない)not be familiar　◆寛解というのは聞き慣れない言葉でしょうが，これは病気の症状が一時的あるいは永続的に軽減することを意味します You may not be familiar with the word 'remission.' It means that the symptoms of a disease lessen temporarily or permanently.

ききめ　効き目　(効果)effect (圏effective 圏take effect, work)　(効能)efficacy, effectiveness　☞効く，効果　◆この注射の効き目はすぐ出ます This shot will *take effect [work] *right away[immediately].　◆この薬の効き目は速い〈遅い〉This medication works[acts] fast〈slowly〉.　◆この薬はめまいに効き目があります This medication is *effective against[good for] dizziness.　◆薬は彼には効き目がありませんでした The medication did not work for him. / The medication had no effect on him.

ききょう　気胸　pneumothorax /nùːmoʊˈθɔːræks/　(一般語)collapsed lung　◆気胸によって肺が縮んでいます Your lung has collapsed due to pneumothorax.　◆気胸のため，右胸腔内にある空気を抜きます You have pneumothorax, so I'm going to remove the air from your right pleural space.　◀医原性気胸 iatrogenic pneumothorax　外傷性気胸 traumatic pneumothorax　緊張性気胸 tension pneumothorax　血気胸 hemopneumothorax　自然気胸 spontaneous pneumothorax　人工気胸 artificial pneumothorax　両側気胸 bilateral pneumothorax

ぎきんし　偽近視　false nearsightedness [myopia], pseudomyopia

きく¹　聞く・聴く・訊く　《音・声が耳に入る》hear　(音を捕える)catch　◆私の声が聞こえますか Can[Do] you hear me (speaking)? ◆すみません．聞こえなかったのですが I'm sorry, I couldn't hear you. ◆耳が聞こえにくいですか Do you have difficulty hearing? ◆お名前が聞き取れなかったので，もう一度ゆっくり発音していただけませんか I didn't catch your name. Could you pronounce it more slowly? ◆お子さんは大きな音や聞き慣れない音に反応しますか Does your child respond to loud or unfamiliar noises?

《注意して聞く》listen (to) ◆心臓と肺の音を聴かせて下さい Let me listen to your heart and lungs. ◆私の言うことをよく聞いて下さい Please listen to me[what I'm saying] carefully. ◆イヤホンを付けてラジオを聴く listen to the radio with earphones

《訊く》ask ☞尋ねる ◆排便の習慣についてお訊きしたいのですが I'd like to ask you some questions about your bowel habits. ◆専門医の意見を訊いてみましょう Let's ask the specialists what they have to say. ◆わからないことがあったら遠慮せずに訊いて下さい If there is anything you don't understand, please feel free to ask me. ◆入院費については事務で訊いて下さい Please ask about your hospital bill at the business office. ◆ほかに何かお訊きになりたいことがありますか Is there anything else you'd like to ask?

きく² **効く** （作用する）**work** （**well**） （効果がある）**be effective** （**for, against**）, **have an effect** （**on**） （効果を表す）**take effect** （よい）**be good** （**for**） ☞効き目，効果 ◆その薬は効きましたか Did the medication *work well[help]? / Was the medication effective? ◆この薬はすぐに効きます This medication will take effect *right away[immediately]. ◆この湿布は肩こりに効きます This compress is good[effective] for stiff shoulders.

きぐ **器具** （装置・備品）**device, equipment** ★device は特定の機能をもった装置に用いられる． （道具）**instrument, appliance, tool** （器具一式）**apparatus** ◆器具の正しい使い方をご説明いたします I'm going to

[Let me] explain how to use the device properly. / I'm going to[Let me] explain the proper way to use the device. ◆この器具は血液中の酸素を測定します This device measures the levels of oxygen in your blood. ◆（検査で）この器具をつけますが痛くはありません I'm going to set up this equipment, but it won't hurt you. ◆器具をつける place[put] a *patient* on a device ◆器具を入れる *put in[insert] an instrument ◆明日器具を外します I'm going to remove[take off] the device [equipment] tomorrow. ◀医療器具 medical instrument[equipment] 計測器具 measuring instrument[device] 外科器具 surgical instrument 子宮内避妊器具 intrauterine (contraceptive) device；IUD / (リング状のもの) contraceptive ring 手術器具 surgical instrument[tool] 滅菌器具 sterilizer

きくう **気腔** **airspace**

ぎくう **偽腔** **false lumen**

きぐろう **気苦労** （心配事）**worry** （動**worry about**） ◆異国での生活は何かと気苦労が絶えないでしょう Since you *live away from your own country[live in a foreign country], you must always *have something or other to worry about[be worrying about one thing or another].

きけい **奇形** **abnormality, malformation, anomaly** ◀エブスタイン奇形 Ebstein anomaly キアリ奇形 Chiari[Arnold-Chiari] malformation 性器奇形 genital anomaly 精子奇形 abnormal spermatozoa 先天性奇形 congenital abnormality [anomaly] 多発奇形 multiple anomalies [malformations] 動静脈奇形 arteriovenous malformation 類奇形腫 teratoid tumor ▶奇形腫 teratoma

きけん **危険** （一般的な恐れ）**danger** （形**dangerous**） （行為に伴う危険）**risk** （形**risky**） （偶発的な危険要因）**hazard** （形**hazardous**） （危機的状況）**crisis** （複**crises** 形**critical**） ☞危機，リスク ◆転倒して骨折する危険がありますので注意して下さい There's a danger that you might fall and break a bone, so be careful. ◆今激しい運動をするのは危険です It's dangerous for you to do hard[strenuous] exercise now. ◆その手術には少し危険が伴います That surgery is slightly risky. / There is a slight[small] risk with that surgery. ◆現時点で手術をするのは危険すぎます It's too risky to operate now. ◆彼女は危険な状態です She is in critical condition. / She is critically ill. ◆彼女は危険な状態を脱しました She is no longer in critical condition. / She is out of danger now. ◆危険な状態に陥る lapse[fall] into (a) critical condition ◆心臓発作の危険性を減らす〈高める〉reduce〈increase〉the risk of a heart attack ◆危険を冒す take[run] a risk ◆高い〈低い〉危険性 a high〈low〉risk ◆職業上の危険に曝される be exposed to an occupational hazard ◆放射線障害の危険 a radiation hazard ◀手術危険度 surgical risk 相対危険度 relative risk；RR ▶危険物質 dangerous[hazardous] substance ☞危険因子

きげん¹ **期限** （制限時間）**time limit** （締め切り）**deadline** （契約などの期限）**term** ◆書類の提出に期限はありません There is no time limit for submitting the documents. ◆出生届書の提出期限は、（出生日を含めて）14日以内です The deadline for submitting a notice[notification] of birth is within fourteen days of the birth (including the date of the birth). ◆処方箋の有効期限は4日間です The prescription is valid for four days. ◆この塗り薬の使用期限は2019年11月です The expiration date of this ointment is November two thousand (and) nineteen. ◆ビザの期限が切れています Your visa has already expired. / Your visa is no longer valid. ◀使用期限 use-by date / expiration date

きげん² **機嫌** **mood** ☞気分 ◆今日はご機嫌いかがですか How are you feeling today? / How are you today? ◆お子さんの機嫌はどうでしたか How has your child's mood been? ◆機嫌がよい be in a good mood / be cheerful ◆機嫌が悪い be in a bad mood / be cross ◆機嫌が悪くふだんよりぐずる be in a bad mood and more fretful than usual ◆機嫌を損ねる（感情を害する）hurt *a person's* feelings / (怒らせる)offend *a person*

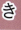

きけんいんし **危険因子** **risk factor** ◀冠疾患危険因子 coronary risk factor

きこう **気功** **qigong, Chinese breathing exercise** ◆気功を施す practice[do] qigong (breathing)

きごう **記号** **sign, symbol, mark** ★mark は○、×などの印をつける時に用いることが多い。

ぎこうし **技工士** **technician** ☞技師 ◀歯科技工士 dental technician

きこえる **聞こえる** **hear** ☞聞く

きこく **帰国する** **go back to** *one's* **country, return home** ◆帰国をご希望ですか Would you like[Do you want] to go back to your (home) country? ◆いつ帰国なさるご予定ですか When are you planning to *go back[return] to your (home) country? ◀一時帰国 temporary return to *one's* country

ぎこちない （不器用な）**awkward, clumsy** （硬くなった）**stiff** （ぎくしゃくした）**jerky** ◆ぎこちない動きをする move awkwardly[stiffly] / be stiff and awkward in *one's* movements

きこん **既婚(の)** **married** ☞結婚 ▶既婚者 married person

きさい **記載する** （必要事項を書き入れる・空欄を埋める）**fill out, fill in** （書類などに書き込む）**enter, write** ◆住所・氏名の記載は必須です Your name and address *must be filled out[（必要とされる）are required]. / You must[It is essential to] write[enter] your name and address. ◆記載漏れがないように必ずご確認下さい Please make sure that there are no omissions (or errors).

きざこきゅう **起坐呼吸** **orthopnea**；*difficulty breathing when lying down*

ぎし¹ **技師・技士** **technician, technologist** （特に機器などの技士）**engineer** ◀X線技師 X-ray technician[technologist] / radiologic technician[technologist] 診

療放射線技師 medical radiation[radiologic] technologist；MRT／radiographer
臨床検査技師 medical technologist；MT／medical laboratory scientist；MLS　臨床工学技士 clinical engineer；CE／medical engineer；ME

ぎし²　義肢 artificial limb, prosthetic limb ▶義肢学 prosthetics　義肢訓練 prosthetic training　義肢装具士 prosthetist and orthotist；PO

ぎし³　義歯 （一揃いの）dentures （各々の）false tooth, artificial tooth （閬teeth）☞入れ歯　架工義歯（dental）bridge／bridgework　不適合義歯 incompatible dentures

ぎじ　疑似（の） （疑いのある）suspected ◆コレラの疑似患者 a patient with suspected cholera ◆両親学級では，父親が妊婦の疑似体験をすることができます Fathers can experience what it's like to be pregnant by attending parenting classes. ▶疑似症例 suspected case

きしかん　既視感 ◆既視感がある have a sense[feeling] of déjà vu

ぎしき　儀式 ceremony ☞式

きしつ¹　気質 （気性）temperament, disposition （特徴・個性）personality ◆神経質な気質 a nervous temperament[disposition] ◆循環気質 cyclothymic personality／cyclothymia　分裂気質 schizothymic temperament

きしつ²　器質（の） organic （器質化の）organizing ▶器質性（心）雑音 organic (heart) murmur　器質性精神障害 organic mental disorder

きしむ　grate ◆関節を動かす時にきしむような音がしたり，きしむような感じがすることがありますか Do you sometimes hear a grating sound or feel a grating sensation when you move your joint(s)?

きしゃく　希釈 dilution （勖dilute） ◆このうがい薬は使用時に水で20倍くらいに希釈して下さい Please dilute this gargle with about twenty parts water when you use it.

ぎしゃし　偽斜視 false strabismus, pseudostrabismus

きしゅ　気腫 emphysema （圀emphysematous） ◀縦隔気腫 mediastinal emphysema　肺気腫 pulmonary emphysema　皮下気腫 subcutaneous emphysema

ぎしゅ　義手 （手）artificial hand, prosthetic hand （腕）artificial arm, prosthetic arm ◀上腕義手 above-elbow[AE] prosthesis　前腕義手 below-elbow[BE] prosthesis　肘義手 elbow disarticulation prosthesis　電動義手 electric arm

きじゅつ　記述する （書く）write （記録する）record, document （描写する）describe （圀description） ◆すべてはこの看護記録に記述してあります Everything has been *written down[recorded／documented] in this nursing (care) record.

ぎじゅつ　技術 （技法・手法）technique （特殊な技能）skill （科学技術）technology ◆新しい技術を用いる use a new technique ◆技術を習得する learn[acquire] a skill ◆心臓手術は技術面で以前よりずっと進歩しています Heart surgery is more technically advanced than before. ◀医療技術 medical (care) technology　科学技術 scientific technique[technology]　コミュニケーション技術 communication skills　診断技術 diagnostic technique　先進医療技術 advanced medical technology

きじゅん　基準 （標準）standard （判断の基準）criteria （圀criterion） ★通例，複数形で。（参照）reference ◆基準を設ける set *a standard[standards／criteria] ◆基準を満たす meet[satisfy／fulfill] the standards[criteria] ◀安全基準 safety standards　環境基準 environmental standards　看護基準 nursing standards　診断基準 diagnostic criteria／criteria of diagnosis　脳死判定基準 brain death criteria／criteria for the determination of brain death　労働基準監督署 Labor Standards Inspection Office ▶基準値 reference value

きしょう　起床する （一般的に起きる）get up （目を覚ます）wake up （ベッドから出る）get out of bed ◆朝は何時に起床しますか What time do you get up in the morning? ◆この薬は起床時に飲んで下さい

Please take this medication when you get up. ◆起床時にこわばりや痛みがありますか Do you wake up feeling stiff and sore?

キシリトール xylitol

キシレンちゅうどく ―中毒 xylene poisoning

キス kiss (圖kiss) ◆この病気は握手，軽いキス，抱擁などでは感染しません This disease is not transmitted through shaking hands, casual kissing, or hugging.

きず 傷
《身体の傷》 （一般的に）**wound** /wúːnd/ （怪我）**injury** /índʒəri/ （切り傷）**cut** /kʌ́t/ （打撲傷・打ち身）**bruise** /brúːz/ （手術などの切開傷）**incision** （重度の身体的外傷）**trauma** /trɔ́ːmə/ ☞傷つく，傷つける，怪我，損傷 ◆傷を見せて下さい Let me look at the wound. ◆これまで頭に傷を受けたことがありますか Have you ever had *an injury to your head[a head injury]? ◆傷は痛みますか Is the wound painful? / Does the wound hurt? ◆額の傷はどうなさったのですか(打撲傷)How did you get the bruise on your forehead? ◆傷が感染しています The wound has become infected. ◆傷が膿んでいます The wound has formed pus. ◆傷に膿がたまっています The wound is filled with pus. / Pus has accumulated in the wound. ◆この傷は治るのに時間がかかるかもしれません This wound may be slow to heal. / It may take some time for this wound to heal. ◆この傷はしばらく痛むかもしれません(切開傷) This incision may be sore for a while.
◆傷が治り次第退院できます Once the wound has healed satisfactorily, *you can leave the hospital[you can be discharged from the hospital]. ◆額に5cmの傷を負う(切り傷)have a five-centimeter cut on the forehead ◆傷がずきずき痛む the wound throbs with pain ◆傷がしみる the wound stings[smarts] ◆深い傷を負う be badly[deeply] injured[wounded]
◆浅い傷を負う be slightly injured [wounded] ◆傷の手当 treatment [dressing] for the wound ◆傷を消毒する(消毒液で)cleanse the wound with an antiseptic solution / (アルコールで) swab the wound with alcohol ◆傷を清潔に保つ keep the wound clean

《心の傷》**mental trauma, emotional trauma, psychological trauma**[**damage**] （心の傷跡）**mental scar** ◆家庭内暴力による彼女の心の傷が治るには時間がかかるでしょう It will take a long time for her to recover from the mental trauma of domestic violence. / It will take her a long time to heal from the mental scars of domestic violence.

◀掻き傷 scratch かすり傷 scrape / abrasion / abraded wound / (軽い怪我) slight injury 刺し傷(刺されて穴のあいた傷) puncture wound / (ナイフなどによる傷)stab wound / (ハチ・とげなどの刺し傷)sting / (虫によるかみ傷)bite 切開傷 incised wound / cut 生傷 fresh cut[(打ち身)bruise] ☞傷痕，傷口，切り傷

きずあと 傷痕・傷跡 **scar** (圖scar) ☞瘢痕 ◆切り傷が深いので傷痕が残るかもしれません The cut may leave a scar because it's very deep. ◆この手術では傷痕は残りません This surgery won't leave a scar. ◆顔に傷痕が残るかもしれません Your face may be left with a scar. ◆この傷痕は時間の経過とともに消えていくでしょう This scar will fade with time.

きずぐち 傷口 （open）**wound, wound's opening** （ぱっくり開いた傷口）**gaping wound** （切り傷の傷口）(open) **cut** （深い切り傷の傷口）**gash** （手術などによる切開傷）**incision** ◆傷口がじくじくしている(にじんでいる)The wound is oozing. / (湿ってねばねばしている) The wound is wet and sticky. ◆傷口からにおいのする分泌物が出ています You have a foul-smelling discharge from the wound. / The wound has produced a foul-smelling discharge.
◆縫った傷口が開く the stitches come open[undone] ◆傷口が感染したようです It seems that the wound has become infected. ◆傷口にかさぶたができる a

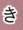

scab forms over the wound / the wound forms a scab ◆傷口がふさがる the wound *closes up[heals] ◆傷口がきれいになる(完全に治る) the wound heals completely ◆傷口から膿を出す drain [let out] the pus from the wound ◆傷口を3針縫う sew up the cut with three stitches[staples] / put three stitches[staples] in the cut ◆傷口をふさぐ close (up) the wound ◆傷口にガーゼを当てる cover the wound with (a piece of) gauze ◆傷口に絆創膏を貼る put *an adhesive tape[a Band-Aid] on[over] the wound ◆傷口に包帯をしましょう I'm going to bandage[dress] your wound. / Let me bind up the wound with a bandage.

きずつく 傷つく **get[be] hurt** ☞傷, 怪我 ◆彼女は見舞客の心ない言葉に傷ついて動揺しています She is upset because *she was[her feelings were] hurt by her visitor's thoughtless words. ◆お子さんはとても傷つきやすい年頃です Your child is at a very vulnerable age.

きずつける 傷つける (体の一部・心を痛める)**hurt** (危害を加える)**injure** (刃物などで傷つける)**wound** (ナイフなどでスーッと長く切る)**slash, slit** ☞傷, 怪我 ◆以前, 頭を傷つけたことがありますか(怪我を負ったことがあるか) Have you ever hurt[injured / wounded] your head before? ★hurt は injure や wound より軽い怪我に用いる. / Have you ever suffered a head injury [wound]? ◆手首を傷つける slash[slit] *one's* wrist(s) ◆自尊心を傷つける hurt *a person's* pride

きせい 規制する **regulate** (☞regulation) ◆この薬は30日を超える処方が規制されています According to drug regulations, doctors can prescribe only a thirty-day supply of this medication.

ぎせい 偽性(の) **false** (☞頭pseud-(o)-) ▶偽性貧血 pseudoanemia 偽性ヘルニア pseudohernia / false hernia

きせいちゅう 寄生虫 **parasite** (☞parasitic) ▶寄生虫(性)アレルギー parasitic

allergy 寄生虫感染症 parasitic infection 寄生虫検査 parasite examination 寄生虫卵 parasite egg

きせつ 季節 **season** (☞seasonal) ◆の症状はある決まった季節に起こりますか Does the symptom usually occur during a specific season? ◆インフルエンザ〈花粉症〉の季節です It's flu〈hay fever〉season. ◆季節の変わり目に with the change of (the) seasons ▶季節性アレルギー seasonal allergy 季節性アレルギー性鼻炎〈結膜炎〉seasonal allergic rhinitis 〈conjunctivitis〉季節性インフルエンザ seasonal influenza 季節性感情障害 seasonal affective disorder；SAD

きぜつ 気絶する (めまいなどで一時的に気を失う)**faint, pass out, black out** (意識を失う)**lose consciousness** ☞意識, 気を失う, 失神する

きせつこつ 基節骨 **proximal phalanx**

キセノン **xenon**

きそ 基礎 (土台)**base, basis, foundation** (基本)**(the) basics** ★複数形で. (☞basic, fundamental, basal 根底にある **underlying**) ☞基本 ◆基礎的な原理 the basic principle ◆疾病の基礎的な原因 the underlying cause of the disease ▶基礎医学 basic medical sciences 基礎研究 basic research 基礎疾患 underlying disease 基礎情報 basic[fundamental] information / (患者についてのデータベース) database 基礎代謝 basal metabolism；BM 基礎代謝率 basal metabolic rate；BMR ☞基礎体温

ぎそうかん 蟻走感 **formication, crawling sensation on the skin**

きそく 規則 《規則性》**regularity** (☞regular) ◆便通は規則的にありますか Are your bowel movements regular? / Do you have regular bowel movements? ◆月経は通常規則的ですか Are your periods usually regular? ◆規則正しい食生活をして下さい Please eat *at regular times[regularly]. ◆規則正しく運動する exercise regularly / do regular exercise

きそく　《決まり・秩序》（個人を規制する指針）rule（公的に強制力を持つ規則）regulation　◆病院の規則を守って下さい Please follow [abide by / observe] the hospital (rules and) regulations.　◆それは規則違反です That's a violation of the rules [regulations].　◆規則に違反する break [violate] the rules [regulations] / be against the rules [regulations]

ぎそく　義足　artificial leg, prosthetic leg（足首から下の部分）artificial foot, prosthetic foot　◆義足を着ける〈着けている〉*put on 〈wear〉 an artificial leg [foot]　◆義足を新調する have [get] *an artificial [a prosthetic] leg made　◀下腿義足 below-knee [BK] prosthesis　膝義足 knee disarticulation prosthesis　大腿義足 above-knee [AK] prosthesis

きそたいおん　基礎体温　basal body temperature ; BBT　◆毎朝，基礎体温をつけていますか Do you take your basal body temperature every morning?　▶基礎体温表 (basal body) temperature chart [record] / BBT chart [record]

きたい¹　奇胎　mole（🔲molar）　◀胞状奇胎 hydatidiform mole　▶奇胎妊娠 molar pregnancy

きたい²　期待する　（予想する）expect（🔲expectation）　（希望する）hope（🔲hope）☞希望，望み　◆ご期待に添うことが出来なくて残念です I'm sorry I couldn't meet [come up to] your expectation(s).　◆この治療は効果をあげるものと期待しています I hope [expect] that this treatment will work well.　◆腫瘍が縮小することを期待してまず化学療法を行います First, we'll start with chemotherapy in the hope of shrinking the tumor.　◆残念ながら薬の効果は期待外れでした I'm sorry, but the medication did not have the effect I was *hoping for [expecting]. / I'm sorry, but the effect of the medication was disappointing to me.　◆期待通りの検査結果が得られました We obtained the test result we had expected.　▶期待値 expected value / expectation

きたえる　鍛える　（強化する）strengthen（徐々に作り上げる）build up（訓練する）train（運動する）exercise　◆体を鍛える build up *one's body　◆トレーニングで足腰を鍛える strengthen *one's lower body through training　◆腹筋〈背筋〉を鍛える strengthen *one's abdominal 〈back〉 muscles

きたく　帰宅する　（家に帰る）go home, return home　（家に到着する）get home　◆帰宅はいつも遅いですか Do you always go home late (from work)?　◆（患者さんが）帰宅されたらすぐこちらに連絡をくださるようお伝え下さい When he〈she〉 gets home, please tell him〈her〉 to call us right away.　◀一時帰宅 temporary [brief] return to *one's home

きたす　来す　◆肺炎により呼吸不全を来しています The pneumonia has led to respiratory failure.

きたない　汚い　（汚れた）dirty　（非常に汚い）filthy　（尿・便などで汚れた）soiled　（乱雑な）messy　☞汚れた　◆汚くなったシーツを取り換えましょう I'm going to [Let me] change the dirty [soiled] sheets (for clean ones).

きちょう　貴重（な）　valuable, precious　◆貴重なご意見をいただきありがとうございます Thank you for your valuable comments.　◆貴重児 a precious [valuable] child　☞貴重品

きちょうひん　貴重品　valuables　★複数形で．　◆貴重品や多額のお金を病院に持ってこないで下さい Please do not bring valuables or large amounts of money to the hospital.　◆貴重品は病室に置かないで下さい Please don't keep your valuables in your room.　◆貴重品はロッカーに入れて下さい Please put your valuables in the locker.　◆貴重品は入院受付にお預け下さい Please leave your valuables in the admissions office.

きちょうめん　几帳面（な）　（細かいところまで正確な）precise　（細心の注意を払う）meticulous　◆あなたは几帳面な性格のほうですか Do you tend to be precise in everything you do? / Are you meticulous by

きちょうめん　　　　　　　　170　　　　　　　　きづく

nature?

きちんと

《正確に》　（正しく・正確に）**exactly**　（適切に）**properly**　（規則的に）**regularly**　（綿密に・丁寧に）**carefully**　☞必ず，几帳面，しっかり，ちゃんと　◆この薬は1日3回きちんと医師の指示どおりに服用して下さい Please be sure to take this medication three times a day exactly as directed by your doctor.
◆担当医の指示をきちんと守って下さい Please follow your doctor's instructions properly.　◆排便は毎朝きちんとありますか Do you have regular bowel movements every morning?　◆治療内容については入院時に改めてきちんとご説明します I'll explain the treatment (to you) again carefully at the time of your admission.
《整然と》　（小ぎれいに・見苦しくなく）**neatly**　（整理整頓して）**tidily, in order**　◆身辺はきちんと片付いていないと気が済まない性分ですか Do you feel that everything around you needs to be kept *neat and tidy[in order]?

きつい

《苦しい・激しい》**hard, strenuous**　☞苦しい，大変，辛い(つらい)　◆きつい運動はしないで下さい Please avoid hard[strenuous] exercise.　◆仕事はきついですか Is the work *too much[hard] for you?
《厳しい》**severe, harsh**　（批判的な）**critical**
◆きついことを言う say something severe[harsh / critical] / say severely[harshly / critically]
《窮屈な》**tight**　◆靴や指輪がきつい感じがしますか Do your shoes or rings feel tight?

ぎつうふう　偽痛風　pseudogout

きつえん　喫煙　smoking, smoke　(動smoke)　☞煙草　◆院内での喫煙はご遠慮下さい Please refrain from smoking in the hospital. / Smoking is not allowed in the hospital.　◆1日の喫煙量はどのくらいですか How much[How many cigarettes] do you smoke a day?　◆喫煙が肺に悪影響を及ぼすことは明らかです Smoking is definitely[clearly] bad for the lungs.　◆1

階に指定の喫煙所があります There is a designated smoking area[section] on the first floor.　◆間接喫煙 indirect smoking / secondhand smoke　受動喫煙 passive smoking　非喫煙者 nonsmoker
▶喫煙者 smoker

きつおん　吃音　stammer, stammering, stutter, stuttering　☞吃る　◆吃音を矯正する correct a stammer　▶吃音者 stammerer / stutterer

きづかう　気遣う　be concerned（about），be worried（about）　☞心配

きっかけ　（引き金）**trigger**（動trigger）（原因）**cause**（動cause）　◆症状を起こすきっかけがありましたか Was there any trigger for the symptom? / Did anything trigger the symptom?　◆発作のきっかけになったものがありますか Did anything bring on this attack?　◆下痢のきっかけに心当たりはありますか Do you have any idea what's caused the diarrhea?　◆過労をきっかけに症状がぶり返すことがありますので十分注意して下さい Overwork can sometimes cause[trigger] *a relapse of the symptoms[the symptoms to relapse], so you should be very careful.　◆あなたが日本に来ようとしたきっかけは何ですか What made you decide to come to Japan? / What brought you to Japan?

きつぎゃく　吃逆　hiccups　★通例，複数形で．**singultus**　☞しゃっくり

きづく　気づく　（意識する）**notice**　（認識する）**realize**　（知る）**be[become] aware（of）, know**　☞気がつく　◆その問題に初めて気づいたのはいつですか When did you first notice the problem?　◆そのほか何か気づいたことがあったら教えて下さい Please tell me if you noticed anything else.　◆リハビリを早く始めることの大切さに気づいてほしいですね I hope that you'll realize the importance of *early rehabilitation[starting rehabilitation early].　◆あなたはご家族や友人達から多くのサポートを受けていることに気づいていますか Do you notice[realize] that you're getting a lot of support from your family and friends?

きづく　　　　　　　　　　　　　　171　　　　　　　　　　　　　　きとく

◆おそらく喫煙のリスクに気づいていらっしゃることでしょう You're probably aware of the risk[dangers] of smoking.　◆気づかないうちに黒や青いあざができることがありますか(明白な理由なく)Do you ever get black or blue bruises for no apparent [obvious] reasons?

ぎっくりごし **―腰** **strained back**　(急性の腰痛) acute lower[low] back pain　◆ぎっくり腰になる have a strained back / strain one's back　◆ぎっくり腰を起こしている one's back is strained

きつご 吃語 **stammer, stutter**　☞吃音

きっこう 拮抗(する) **antagonistic**　(図 antagonism)　◆成長ホルモンにはインスリン拮抗作用があります Growth hormone has insulin-antagonistic effects.　▶拮抗筋 antagonistic muscle　拮抗(性)反射 antagonistic reflex　☞拮抗薬

きっこうやく 拮抗薬 **antagonist**　◀カルシウム拮抗薬 calcium antagonist　競合的拮抗薬 competitive antagonist　セロトニン(受容体)拮抗薬 serotonin (receptor) antagonist　ドパミン拮抗薬 dopamine antagonist　ニコチン拮抗薬 nicotinic antagonist　バソプレッシン受容体拮抗薬 vasopressin receptor antagonist　ヒスタミン(受容体)拮抗薬 histamine (receptor) antagonist　プリン代謝拮抗物質 purine antagonist　ムスカリン(受容体)拮抗薬 muscarinic (receptor) antagonist　モルヒネ拮抗薬 opioid antagonist　葉酸代謝拮抗薬 antifolate / folic acid antagonist　ロイコトリエン受容体拮抗薬 leukotriene receptor antagonist；LTRA

きっさしつ 喫茶室 **coffee shop**

キッチンドリンカー **alcoholic housewife, housewife with alcohol dependence**

きっと (確実に) **definitely, certainly, surely**　☞必ず　◆このリハビリ訓練を続けるうちにきっと歩けるようになります If you keep up this rehabilitation, you'll definitely[certainly] be able to walk again.　◆きっと治りますので, 諦めずに治療していきましょう(私は確信している)I know you're going to get better[I'm sure you'll get better], so

let's not give up with the treatment.

きてい¹ 規定　(個人を規制する指針) **rule**　(公的に強制力を持つ規則) **regulation**　(基準) **standard**　(調合) **formula**　◆規定に従う observe[follow / obey] the rules　◆規定を破る break[violate] the rules　▶規定食 formula[formulated / (処方された)prescribed] diet　規定料金 standard[regulation] charge

きてい² 既定(の)　(前もって打ち合わせた) **prearranged**　(すでに確立した) **established**　◆既定の計画に沿って治療する treat according to a prearranged plan

きていさいぼうがん 基底細胞癌 **basal cell carcinoma**

きと 企図　(意図) **intention**　(試み) **attempt**　(圏未遂の **attempted**)　◆自殺企図 attempted suicide　▶企図振戦 intention tremor

きとう 亀頭　(男性の) **head of the penis, glans penis**　(女性の) **head of the clitoris, glans clitoridis**　腰圏 balan(o)-　亀頭炎 balanitis　亀頭包皮炎 balanoposthitis / inflammation of the glans and foreskin of the penis

きどう 気道 **airway, respiratory tract**　◆気道を確保し呼吸を確認する open[secure] the airway and check for breathing / hold the airway open and assess for adequate breathing　◀下気道 lower airway[respiratory tract]　持続気道陽圧(呼吸) continuous positive airway pressure； CPAP　上気道 upper airway[respiratory tract]　▶気道可逆性(試験) airway reversibility (test)　気道確保 airway management[maintenance] / holding the airway open　気道過敏性(試験) airway hyperreactivity (test)　気道感染 airway[respiratory tract] infection　気道狭窄 airway narrowing[stenosis]　気道内異物 airway foreign body　気道熱傷 inhalation burn　気道閉塞 airway obstruction

きとく 危篤(の) **critical**　◎重症　◆彼女は危篤状態です She is[remains] in critical condition. / She is critically ill.　◆危篤に陥る fall into critical condition　◆危

篤状態を脱する come out of critical condition

きにいらない　気に入らない　(好まない) **not like**　(満足していない) **not be satisfied with**　☞気に障る　◆彼女は病院の食事が気に入らないようです It seems *she doesn't like[she's not satisfied with] the hospital food. / (不平・不満がある) She seems to have complaints about the hospital food.　◆何か気に入らないことがございましたでしょうか Is there anything you're not satisfied with? / Do you have any complaints?　◆彼は気に入らないことがあると怒鳴ることがよくありますか(思い通りにならないと) Does he often yell[shout] *when things aren't going the way he wants[(いらいらすると) when he's annoyed]?

きにいる　気に入る　(好む) **like**　(満足している) **be satisfied with**　(🏠大好きな **favorite**)　◆お仕事は気に入っていますか Do you like your work? / Are you satisfied with your work?　◆お気に入りの曲はなんですか What's your favorite (piece of) music?

きにかかる　気に掛かる　(不安に思う) **be concerned about**　(心配である) **be worried about**　☞気になる，心配　◆症状は治まりましたが，血液検査の結果が気に掛かっています Your symptoms have *gone away[cleared up], but I'm still concerned[worried] about the blood test results.

きにかける　気に掛ける　**care about**　☞気にする，心配　◆あなたのことを本当に気に掛けていますよ We really care about you.

きにさわる　気に障る　**hurt** *a person's* **feelings**　☞気に入らない　◆お気に障ったとしたら申し訳ありません I'm really sorry if I've hurt your feelings.

きにする　気にする　(悩む) **worry about**　(嫌だと思う) **mind**　◆他の人達の言うことは気にしないように Don't *worry about [mind] what others[people] say.

きになる　気になる　(心配である) **be worried about**　(不安に思う) **be concerned**

about　(困らせる・心配させる) **bother**　☞心配，不安　◆気になることがありますか Are you worried[concerned] about something? / Has something been bothering you?　◆気になる症状がある時は電話を下さい Please call us if you have any symptoms that you're worried[concerned] about.　◆何が気になっているのですか What's on your mind?　◆耳鳴りが気になりますか Is the ringing in your ear(s) bothering you?　◆血糖値が気になる be concerned about *one's* blood sugar level

きにやむ　気に病む　(心配する) **worry**　(悩ませる) **bother**　☞心配　◆将来のことを気に病む worry about the future　◆何をそんなに気に病んでいるのですか What's bothering you so much?

きにゅう　記入する　(必要事項を書き入れる・空欄を埋める) **fill out, fill in**　(書き留める) **write down**　◆この用紙に記入して下さい Please fill out[in] this form.

ぎにんしん　偽妊娠　false[imaginary, phantom] pregnancy, pseudopregnancy

キヌタこつ　―骨　incus, anvil-like bone, anvil-shaped bone

きのう¹　昨日　yesterday

きのう²　機能する　function　(🖼**function** 🏠**functional**)**, work**　◆彼女は腎臓がうまく機能していません Her kidneys are not functioning[working] well.　◆正常に機能する function normally　◆機能が衰える the function declines　◆機能を高める improve the function　◆肺機能の低下 decline in lung function　◀運動機能 motor function　肝機能 liver function　高次脳機能 higher brain function　甲状腺機能 thyroid (gland) function　残存機能 residual function　視機能 visual function　消化機能 digestive function　心機能 heart[cardiac] function　腎機能 kidney[renal] function　心肺機能 cardiopulmonary function　生殖機能 reproductive function　造血機能 hematopoietic[blood-forming] function / hematoopoietic capacity　造精機能 spermatogenic function 体温調節機能 thermoregulatory function 代償機能 compensatory function[mechanism] 肺機能 lung[pulmonary] function バリア機能 barrier function 膀胱機能 bladder function ▶機能温存手術 function-preserving surgery 機能回復 functional recovery / recovery of function 機能訓練 functional training[exercise] 機能亢進 hyperfunction 機能肢位 functional position 機能障害 dysfunction / functional disorder 機能性(心)雑音 functional (heart) murmur 機能装具 functional brace 機能代償 functional compensation 機能低下 hypofunction 機能的自立度評価表 functional independence measure；FIM 機能的電気刺激 functional electric stimulation 機能評価 functional assessment ☞機能検査, 機能不全

ぎのう　技能　skill（🔲skilled）◆田中先生は白内障の手術では熟練した技能を持っています Dr Tanaka is highly skilled in cataract surgery. / Dr Tanaka is a highly skilled cataract surgeon. ◀運動技能発達 motor skill development

きのうけんさ　機能検査　function test ◆めまいの原因を調べるために、平衡機能検査を行いましょう Let's do[run] a balance function test to find out what's causing your dizziness. ◀呼吸機能検査 respiratory function test 生理機能検査 physiologic function test 胎盤機能検査 placental function test 内分泌機能検査 endocrine function test 平衡機能検査 balance[equilibrium] function test

きのうしょう　気脳症　pneumocephalus
きのうふぜん　機能不全　(機能障害)dysfunction（🔲dysfunctional）, malfunction, insufficiency　(機能の遂行不能)incompetence（🔲incompetent）◆性機能不全である be sexually dysfunctional[incompetent] ◀黄体機能不全 luteal insufficiency 胎盤機能不全 placental dysfunction[insufficiency]

キノコ　mushroom　◀毒キノコ poisonous [toxic] mushroom ▶キノコ中毒 mushroom poisoning

きのせい　気のせい　(想像上の)imaginary（🔲imagine）◆耳鳴を気のせいとして片づけてしまうのは危険です It's dangerous to dismiss ringing in the ears as something *you're just imagining[that's just imaginary].

きのどく　気の毒　◆お気の毒に思います I'm (very / so) sorry. ◆お気の毒ですが、彼女は重症です I'm very sorry, but she is critically ill. ◆風邪ですって？ お気の毒に You've got a cold? That's too bad[I'm sorry to hear that].

キノホルム　chinoform, clioquinol　▶キノホルム中毒 chinoform poisoning

きはつげっけい　希発月経　oligomenorrhea, light or infrequent periods[menstruation]

きばらし　気晴らし　(息抜き)relaxation（🔲relax）(気分転換)change of pace　(娯楽)pastime, recreation ☞気分転換 ◆いいお天気ですから、気晴らしに散歩でもいかがですか It's a beautiful day. How about taking a walk *for relaxation[for a change (of pace)]?

きびしい　厳しい
《厳格である》(規則順守を旨とする厳しさ)strict　(柔軟性を欠いた厳しさ)rigid ☞厳重, 厳密 ◆厳しい規則 strict rules ◆厳しい塩分制限を受けている be under strict [rigid] salt restriction
《深刻である》serious　(重い)grave　(過酷な)severe ◆彼女の容体は依然として厳しい状況が続いています She remains in (a) serious[grave / severe] condition. ◆彼は経済的に厳しい問題を抱えています He has difficult[serious] financial problems. / He's in[He's having] financial difficulties[difficulty].
《実現が困難だ》difficult ◆1か月以内に仕事に復帰するのは厳しいでしょう It'll be difficult for you to go back to work in less than a month.

きふく　気腹　pneumoperitoneum
ギプス　ギプス(包帯)　(plaster) cast ◆腕にギプスをつける必要があります You

need to have your arm in a cast. / Your arm needs to be put in a cast. ◆今日ギプスをはずしましょう I'm going to take your cast off today. ◀長下肢ギプス包帯 long leg cast ; LLC　歩行ギプス包帯 walking cast

きぶん　気分 feeling （略feel）　（機嫌）mood
☞機嫌, 気持ち
《体調》 ◆気分がいい feel good[fine] /（前よりいい）feel better　◆気分がすぐれない not feel well　◆今日はご気分はいかがですか How are you feeling today? / How do you feel today?　◆気分が悪い〈悪くなる〉feel〈get〉 sick /（前より悪い）feel worse　◆診察中にご気分が悪くなったらおっしゃって下さい Please let me know if you start to feel sick[unwell] during the examination.
《心持ち, 精神状態》 ◆最近ご気分はどうですか How has your mood been recently?　◆気分が落ち込むのは朝ですか, それとも夕方ですか Do you usually feel [get / become] depressed in the morning or in the evening? / When do you feel depressed[down] —in the morning or in the evening?　◆どのくらい長くこんなふうに気分が落ち込んでいるのですか How long have you felt depressed like this?
◆気分が落ち着く feel relaxed　◆気分が楽になる feel relieved　◆気分が変動する have mood swings　◆気分を害する hurt *a person's* feelings / offend *a person*　◆気分を変える change the way *one* feels　◀不安気分 anxious mood　妄想気分 delusional mood　抑うつ気分 depressed [depressive] mood　▶気分安定薬 mood stabilizing medication[drug / agent]　気分障害 mood disorder　気分変調症 dysthymia / dysthymic disorder　☞気分転換, 気分変動

きぶんてんかん　気分転換　☞気晴らし
◆気分転換に音楽を聴く〈気分を楽にするために〉listen to music to relax /（たまには）listen to music for a change of pace

きぶんへんどう　気分変動　mood swings
★通例, 複数形で. ◆激しい気分変動がある have severe mood swings

きほう　気泡　air bubble　▶気泡浴 bubble bath

きほう　希望　（将来への期待）hope（略hope）　（願い・頼み）request（略request）
☞期待, 望み ◆手術がうまくいくという希望を持っています We hope the surgery will be successful.　◆希望を失う lose hope　◆できるだけご希望に添うようにいたします We'll try to meet[accommodate] your request to the best of our ability.　◆（予約などで）ご希望の日はありますか What days are good[best] for you? / What days do you prefer?　◆この病院での出産を希望されますか Would you like[Do you want] to have the birth[baby] at this hospital?

ぎほう　技法　technique　☞技術

きほん　基本　（基礎）basis（略basic）　（基礎的な事柄）fundamentals（略fundamental）
★通例, 複数形で. ☞基礎 ◆栄養は健康の基本です Good[Proper] nutrition is the basis of[to] good health. / Good [Proper] nutrition is fundamental[basic] to good health.　◆お子さんは基本的な生活技術を身につける必要があります I think your child needs to learn[acquire] basic life skills.　◆基本的にはそのような理解でよろしいかと思います Your understanding is basically right. / Basically, that's right.

ぎまく　偽膜　pseudomembrane（略pseudomembranous）, false membrane　▶偽膜性結膜炎 pseudomembranous conjunctivitis　偽膜性喉頭炎 pseudomembranous laryngitis　偽膜性腸炎 pseudomembranous enterocolitis

きまった　決まった　（特定の）specific, particular　◆咳はいつも決まった時間帯に出ますか Do you usually have the cough at a specific time of day?

きまる　決まる, 決定　（決定する）be decided　（日時・場所が定まる）be set, be fixed　（手配が整う）be arranged　◆決める, 決定
◆手術の日程が決まり次第お知らせします We'll let you know as soon as your surgery date has been set[fixed].　◆退院

は5月10日火曜日に決まりました The time for your discharge has been decided [fixed / arranged] for Tuesday, May (the) tenth. ◆消灯時間には特に決まりはありません There's no fixed[(特定の)particular] rule about *lights-out[when the lights are turned off].

―ぎみ 一気味 （軽めの）**a touch of, a little** (of) ◆風邪気味である have *a touch of cold[a slight cold] / (風邪をひきかけている)be getting a cold / feel a cold coming on ◆下痢気味である have a touch of diarrhea ◆少々お疲れ気味のようですね You look *a little[(ちょっとばかり)rather] tired.

きみどり 黄緑（の） **yellow-green, yellowish green**

きみゃく 奇脈 **paradoxical pulse**

きみょう 奇妙（な） （変な）**strange** （常軌を逸した）**odd** ◆奇妙な行動をする act [behave] strangely[oddly]

ぎむ 義務 **duty** （法律・道徳上の責任）**obligation** ◆結核は保健所に届け出る義務があります We have a legal obligation [We're under legal obligation] to report cases of tuberculosis to the health center. ◀守秘義務(医師・患者間の)doctor-patient confidentiality / (医療記録の) duty to keep patient records confidential 診療義務(legal) obligation to provide medical treatment 説明義務(legal) obligation to explain ▶義務感 sense of duty[obligation] 義務教育 compulsory education

きむずかしい 気難しい **difficult** ◆気難しい患者 a difficult patient

きめい 記銘 **memory, memorization** ☞記憶 ▶記銘力低下 memory disturbance / disturbance of memorization

きめつける 決めつける ◆もう治らないと決めつけてしまうのはよくありません It's no good deciding that you have no hope of recovering. / (即座に結論を出すべきではない)You shouldn't jump to the conclusion that you won't recover. ◆すべてあなたのせいだと決めつけているわけではありません I don't just assume that everything is your fault.

きめる 決める （決定する）**decide** (on) （図**decision**） （選択する）**choose** （図**choice**） （決心する）**make up** *one's* **mind** （結論を出す）**conclude** （図**conclusion**） （日時・場所を決める）**fix** ☞決定，定める ◆経過を見て今後の方針を決めましょう Let's see how things go[develop] before deciding *what to do next[the next step]. ◆あなたが決めて下さい It's up to you to decide. ◆その点はよく考えてから決めて下さい Please think about it carefully before you decide. ◆どうすることに決めましたか What have you decided? / What's your decision? ◆どちらに決めますか Which option will you choose? / Which have you decided on? ◆手術をするか否か，決めかねているのですね You just can't make up your mind about whether or not to have the surgery, can you? ◆次回はいつお会いするかを決めましょう Let's fix [decide on] a time for our next meeting.

きもち 気持ち
《気分》☞気分 ◆気持ちがよい(人が)feel good, feel refreshed[comfortable] / (場所・物などが)be comfortable, be pleasant ◆お風呂に入って気持ちがよくなりましたか Did you feel good[refreshed] after the bath? ◆気持ちのよい病室 a comfortable [pleasant] room ◆気持ちが悪い(人が)feel bad, feel uncomfortable / (場所・物などが)be uncomfortable, be unpleasant ◆汗を大量にかくとねばねばして気持ちの悪い感じがする have an uncomfortable, sticky feeling when *one* sweats a lot ◆気持ちを楽にして下さい Please relax. / (くだけた調子で)Please take it easy.

《具合》◆気持ちが悪い(吐き気がする)feel sick[bad] / (不快に感じる)feel uncomfortable ◆物を食べた後気持ちが悪くなりますか Do you feel sick[bad] after eating? ◆お腹が張って気持ちが悪いのですね You feel uncomfortable because your stomach is bloated, don't you?

《感情・思い》◆気持ちの変化 change in *one's* mood ◆お気持ちはわかりますが，

残念ながらご要望にお応えできません I know[understand] how you feel, but unfortunately, we cannot meet[satisfy] your request. ◆今のお気持ちを聞かせて下さい Please tell me what you're feeling and thinking. / Please tell me what's going through your mind (right) now. ◆お気持ちをお察しいたします I understand this must be a shock for you. 《厚意》 ◆感謝の気持ちを表す show *one's* gratitude ◆(謝礼に対して)お気持ちはありがたいのですが,いただくわけにはまいりません Thank you for your offer[gift], but I'm afraid we can't accept it.

ぎもん 疑問 (質問・問題)question (圏疑いの余地がある questionable) (疑念)doubt (圏doubt 圏doubtful) ◆疑問があれば何でも尋ねて下さい Feel free to ask (me) any questions. / Please ask me any questions you may have. ◆手術せずに治るかどうかはかなり疑問が残ります Whether you'll be able to recover without surgery is rather doubtful. / I doubt that you'll be able to recover without surgery. ◆それは有名な民間療法ですが,実際の効果についてはかなり疑問視されています That's a famous folk remedy, but its actual effectiveness is rather questionable[doubtful].

ぎゃく 偽薬 placebo ▶偽薬効果 placebo effect

ぎゃく 逆 (正反対)the opposite /ápəzɪt/ (反対)the contrary /kɑ́ntrəri/ (裏を表が反対)the reverse (位置が逆)inversion (圏opposite, contrary, reverse, inverse 副順序が反対に backward(s)) ▷反対 ◆検査結果は私が予期したものとはまったく逆でした The test result was quite the opposite [reverse] of what I had expected. / The test result was quite contrary to my expectation. ◆体を逆向きにして下さい Please turn your body to the opposite side. ◆100から数字を逆に数えて下さい Please count backward(s) from one hundred. ◆逆に言えば、入院は生活習慣を改善させるチャンスです(違う観点から考えれば) Thinking about it from a different angle, admission to the hospital is a good chance to improve your lifestyle habit. ☞逆位,逆効果,逆説,逆相関,逆転,逆方向,逆戻り,逆流

ぎゃくい 逆位 inversion : *abnormal arrangement[position] (of an internal organ)* ◀内臓逆位 visceral inversion / heterotaxia

ぎゃくこうか 逆効果 opposite effect (圏counterproductive) ◆運動しすぎは逆効果です Too much exercise has the opposite effect. / Too much exercise can be counterproductive. / (より悪化させる)Too much exercise will make the matter [symptom] worse.

ぎゃくせつ 逆説(的な) paradoxical ◆逆説的な結果を得る obtain a paradoxical result

ぎゃくそうかん 逆相関する (反対の)be inversely correlated (with) (圏inverse correlation) (負の)be negatively correlated (with) (圏negative correlation) ◆HDLコレステロール値と冠動脈疾患の罹患率は逆相関すると言われています HDL cholesterol and the incidence of coronary artery disease are said to be inversely correlated. / HDL cholesterol is said to be inversely correlated with the incidence of coronary artery disease.

ぎゃくたい 虐待 abuse /əbjúːs/ (圏abuse /əbjúːz/) ★名詞と動詞の発音の違いに注意. ◆身体の虐待を受けている be physically abused ◆虐待を疑わせる火傷〈青あざ〉を届け出る report suspected burns〈bruises〉 of abuse / report burns〈bruises〉suspicious for abuse ◀高齢者虐待 elder abuse / (放置)elder neglect 児童虐待 child abuse 身体的虐待 physical abuse 精神的虐待 emotional[psychological] abuse 性的虐待 sexual abuse 被虐待児 battered[abused] child 幼児虐待 infant abuse

ぎゃくてん 逆転する reverse ◆新生児は昼夜逆転することがよくあります Many newborn babies often have their days and nights reversed.

きゃくブロック 脚ブロック bundle branch block ◀完全右脚〈左脚〉ブロック complete right〈left〉bundle branch block；CRBBB〈CLBBB〉 不完全右脚〈左脚〉ブロック incomplete right〈left〉bundle branch block；ICRBBB〈ICLBBB〉

ぎゃくほうこう 逆方向 《反対方向》opposite direction[way] 《反対側》opposite side ◆心電図室は X 線室と逆方向にあります The EKG room is opposite[(向かい側に)across from] the X-ray room. ◆体を逆方向に向ける turn *one's* body to the opposite side

ぎゃくもどり 逆戻りする 《病気がぶり返す》relapse ◆ここで治療を中断したら元の状態に逆戻りしてしまいます If you stop the treatment now, *your condition will relapse（to how it was before）[you'll relapse to how you were before].

ぎゃくりゅう 逆流する flow back[backward(s)]（図backward flow）, regurgitate（図regurgitation）, reflux（図reflux）, reverse（図reversal） ◆胃酸が食道に逆流しているかもしれません Acid from the stomach may be *flowing backward[regurgitating] into the esophagus[gullet]. ◆血液の逆流 reversal[reflux] of blood flow / backward flow of blood ◆胃食道逆流症 gastroesophageal reflux disease；GERD 酸逆流 acid reflux 大動脈弁/僧帽弁/肺動脈弁/三尖弁)逆流症 aortic〈mitral / pulmonary / tricuspid〉(valve) regurgitation；AR〈MR / PR / TR〉 膀胱尿管逆流 vesicoureteral reflux；VUR ▶逆流性雑音 regurgitant murmur 逆流性食道炎 reflux esophagitis

きゃっかん 客観(的な) objective(↔subjective) ◆客観的な意見 an objective opinion ◆客観的な徴候や症状 objective signs and symptoms

ぎゃっこう 逆行・逆向(性の) retrograde ◀内視鏡的逆行性胆管膵管造影 endoscopic retrograde cholangiopancreatography；ERCP 内視鏡的逆行性胆管ドレナージ endoscopic retrograde biliary drainage；ERBD ▶逆向性健忘 retrograde amnesia 逆行性射精 retrograde ejaculation 逆行性腎盂造影 retrograde pyelography；RP 逆行性胆管造影 retrograde cholangiography 逆行性尿道造影 retrograde urethrography；RUG

ギャップ gap ◀カルチャーギャップ culture gap コミュニケーションギャップ communication gap 世代間ギャップ generation gap / gap[difference] between generations

キャリア carrier ☞保因者 ◀肝炎ウイルスキャリア hepatitis virus carrier ヒトTリンパ球向性ウイルス1型キャリア human T-lymphotropic virus type 1[HTLV-1] carrier 病原体キャリア disease carrier 無症候性キャリア silent[asymptomatic / healthy] carrier

キャンセル ─する cancel ◆歯医者の予約をキャンセルする cancel *one's* dental appointment

キャンピロバクター *Campylobacter* ☞カンピロバクター

きゅう¹ 灸 moxibustion ☞鍼灸(しんきゅう) ◆首筋に灸をすえる burn moxa on the nape of the neck / cauterize the nape of the neck with moxa ★moxa は灸に用いるもぐさを意味する. ▶灸師 moxibustion practitioner / moxa-cauterizer

きゅう² 急(な) 《突然》《突然の》sudden 《唐突な》abrupt ◆気を失ったのはおそらく急な血圧低下によるものでしょう A sudden drop in your blood pressure probably caused you to faint. ◆彼女の容態が急に悪化しました Her condition *took a sudden turn for the worse[suddenly took a turn for the worse / abruptly deteriorated]. ◆急に動く move abruptly

《急速・急性》《急速な》rapid, fast 《急性の》acute ◆彼女の血圧が急に下がっています Her blood pressure is falling rapidly. ◆胸が急に痛む(急性の)have (an) acute chest pain

《緊急》urgent ◆これは急を要する手術です This surgery is urgent. / This requires urgent surgery.

きゅういん 吸引 suction (▪suck), aspiration (▪aspirate) ▶吸い込む, 吸い出す ◆喉に吸引チューブを挿入する insert a suction tube down *a person's* throat ◀胃吸引 gastric aspiration　気管気管支吸引 tracheobronchial suction　持続吸引 continuous suction　痰吸引器 sputum aspirator ▶吸引器 (小型の) aspirator, suction pump / (大型の) suction machine [unit]　吸引性肺炎 aspiration pneumonia　吸引分娩 vacuum extraction delivery　吸引用カテーテル suction catheter

きゅうえん 救援 rescue, relief, aid ☞救護

きゅうか 休暇 vacation, holiday ★vacation は長期の休みに用いることが多い. (仕事を免除された休み) leave ▶休日, 休み ◆クリスマスの休暇には母国に帰りますか Are you going back to your country for your Christmas vacation?　◆病気休暇を取る take sick leave　◆有給休暇を一週間とる take a week's paid leave / take a week off with pay　◆育児休暇中である be on childcare leave　◆介護休暇 (family) care leave / (dependent) care leave　夏季休暇 summer vacation　忌引休暇 bereavement leave　出産休暇 maternity leave　病気休暇 sick leave　有給休暇 paid leave [vacation / holiday]

きゅうかく 嗅覚 sense of smell, smell sensation (▪olfactory) ◆嗅覚に変化がありましたか Have you noticed any changes in your *sense of smell [ability to smell]?　◆嗅覚を失う lose *one's* sense of smell　◆嗅覚が鈍る *one's* sense of smell becomes dull / *one's* smell sensations become dull ▶嗅覚過敏 hyperosmia　嗅覚幻覚 phantom smell / olfactory hallucination　嗅覚減退 hyposmia　嗅覚錯誤 parosmia　嗅覚障害 olfactory [smell] disorder [disturbance] / dysosmia　嗅覚測定検査 olfactometry

きゅうかん 急患 (患者) emergency patient　(症例) emergency case ◆時間外の急患については救急外来で対応いたします The staff members in the emergency room will help [assist] after-hours [off-hours] emergency patients. / After-hours [Off-hours] emergency services are available in the emergency room.

きゅうき 吸気 inspiration (↔expiration ▪inspiratory, inspired), inhalation (↔exhalation) ▶吸気圧 inspiratory pressure　吸気[吸入]酸素濃度 fractional concentration of inspiratory [inspired] oxygen；FiO₂　吸気性呼吸困難 inspiratory dyspnea

きゅうきゅう¹ 救急 emergency ☞救命, 緊急 ◀一次〈二次 / 三次〉救急 primary〈secondary / tertiary〉emergency care ▶救急医 emergency (room) doctor / ER doctor　救急入口 emergency entrance　救急医療 emergency medical services；EMS / emergency medicine [(health) care]　救急カート emergency cart　救急外来 (救急部門) emergency (outpatient) unit [department] / (救急室) emergency room；ER　救急患者 emergency patient　救急キット first aid kit　救急救命士 emergency medical technician；EMT / paramedic　救急蘇生バッグ Ambu bag　救急隊員 ambulance crew　救急当直医 doctor on duty in the emergency room　救急箱 first aid kit　救急搬送 emergency transport [(病院間の) transfer]　救急病院 emergency hospital　救急病棟 emergency unit [ward]　救急部 emergency and critical care unit [department / division] / emergency department；ED　救急呼び出し emergency call ☞救急車, 救急処置

きゅうきゅう² 嗅球 olfactory bulb

きゅうきゅうしゃ 救急車 ambulance ◆救急車を呼ぶ call an ambulance ◆119番で救急車を呼ぶ dial [call] one-one-nine for an ambulance　◆救急車で患者を近くの病院に運ぶ take [transport] the patient to a nearby hospital by ambulance　◆彼は救急車で運ばれてきました He was brought to the hospital by ambulance.　◆緊急の際には救急車を呼んで下さい In case of an emergency, please call an ambulance.

きゅうきゅうしょち 救急処置 emergency treatment[care] ◆救急処置を施す give emergency treatment[care]

きゅうぎょう 休業 leave ☞休暇

きゅうきん 球菌 coccus (圈cocci) ◀グラム陽性球菌 gram-positive cocci 腸球菌 *Enterococcus* 肺炎球菌 *Streptococcus pneumoniae* / pneumococcus B群連鎖球菌 group B streptococcus / GBS ブドウ球菌 *Staphylococcus* 連鎖球菌 *Streptococcus*

きゅうけい 休憩する ☞休む

きゅうげき 急激(な) sudden, abrupt, rapid, fast ☞急

きゅうご 救護 (救出・救助)rescue (救援)relief, aid ▶救護活動 rescue work / relief activities 救護所 first-aid station 救護班 rescue team[squad]

きゅうごししんけいえん 球後視神経炎 retrobulbar (optic) neuritis

きゅうさいぼう 嗅細胞 olfactory cell

きゅうし¹ 臼歯 molar ◀小臼歯 premolar (tooth) 大臼歯 molar (tooth)

きゅうし² 休止する stop (一時停止する) suspend ◆申し訳ありませんが，当院では分娩の取り扱いを休止しております We regret that[I'm sorry, but] maternity[obstetrics] services at this hospital have been suspended. ★掲示する場合には We regret to announce that … とする.

きゅうし³ 急死する die suddenly, pass away suddenly

きゅうじつ 休日 holiday (勤務のない日) day off ☞休暇, 休み ◆当院は週末, 休日および時間外の急患を受け付けております We offer emergency services[Emergency services are available] on weekends, public holidays, and *out of hours [after hours] in this hospital. ◆休日はどのように過ごしますか What do you usually do on your days off? / How do you spend your days off? ▶休日診療 out-of-hours [after-hours] outpatient services 休日診療所 out-of-hours[after-hours] clinic 休日当番医 out-of-hours[after-hours] (duty) doctor

きゅうしゅう 吸収する absorb (図absorption 図absorbent, absorbable) ☞吸う ◆この薬は皮膚から吸収されます This medication is absorbed through the skin. ◆栄養分を吸収する absorb nourishment ◆吸収性のパッド an absorbent pad ◀経皮吸収 percutaneous absorption 高吸収域[高濃度域] high-density area 骨吸収 bone resorption 再吸収 reabsorption 脂肪吸収試験 fat absorption study 消化吸収試験 digestion-absorption test 低吸収域[低濃度域] low-density area 糖質吸収 carbohydrate absorption 尿細管再吸収 tubular reabsorption 薬物吸収 drug absorption ▶吸収不良症候群 malabsorption syndrome 吸収性〈非吸収性〉縫合糸 absorbable〈nonabsorbable〉suture

きゅうじょ 救助 rescue ▶救助活動 rescue work[activities] 救助隊 rescue team 救助隊員 rescue worker

きゅうじょうせっけっきゅう 球状赤血球 spherocyte

きゅうしょく¹ 休職する take leave ☞休暇 ◆あなたは休職中ですか Are you on leave (from work)? ◀病気休職 sick leave

きゅうしょく² 給食 food service ◀学校給食 school lunch[meal] / (プログラム) school lunch program 病院給食 hospital food service

きゅうしん¹ 丘疹 papule ◀掻痒性丘疹 itching papule

きゅうしん² 休診 ◆当院は週末および祝祭日が休診です This hospital[clinic] *is closed[does not accept patients] on weekends and public holidays. ◆(掲示) 休診：日曜, 祝祭日, 土曜の午後 Closed: Sundays, National holidays, and Saturday afternoons

きゅうしんけい 嗅神経 olfactory nerve

きゅうしんせい 求心性(の) (同心・同軸の)concentric (特に神経が中枢へ向かう)afferent (↔efferent) ▶求心性収縮 concentric contraction 求心性神経 afferent nerve 求心性心肥大 concentric hypertrophy

きゅうすいなんこう 吸水軟膏 water-absorbing ointment

きゅうせい 急性(の) acute (↔chronic) ◆急性の病気 an acute disease[illness] ▶急性胃粘膜病変 acute gastric mucosal lesion；AGML 急性咽頭炎 acute pharyngitis 急性呼吸窮迫症候群 acute respiratory distress syndrome；ARDS 急性ストレス障害 acute stress disorder 急性転化(白血病の)blast crisis 急性肺損傷 acute lung injury；ALI 急性腹症 acute abdomen ☞急性期

きゅうせいき 急性期 acute stage [phase] ◆急性期の脳梗塞の処置 treatment of cerebral infarction during[in] the acute stage / treatment of acute-stage cerebral infarction ◆リハビリテーションは急性期に始めるとよいでしょう Rehabilitation should begin in the acute phase [stage]. ◆急性期の患者 a patient in the acute phase[stage] / an acute phase [stage] patient ▶急性期リハビリテーション acute phase[stage] rehabilitation

きゅうそく¹ 休息する take[have](a) rest, rest (*oneself*) ☞休む ◆体がだるいと感じたら十分な休息をとって下さい Please take *a good rest[plenty of rest] if you feel tired.

きゅうそく² 吸息 inspiration, inhalation ☞吸気

きゅうそく³ 急速(な) (速度がはやい)rapid, quick, fast (増減が急激な)sharp ☞急、速い ◆急速に快方に向かう recover rapidly[quickly] (from *one's* illness) ◆HIV 患者数の急速な増加 a sharp increase in the number of HIV-infected patients ▶急速導入 rapid induction

きゅうちゃく 吸着 adsorption (動adsorb 形adsorbent, adsorbable) ◆活性炭は様々な化学物質や毒物を吸着します Activated charcoal adsorbs various chemicals and toxins. ◀血液吸着 hemadsorption 血漿吸着 plasma adsorption 放射性アレルゲン吸着試験 radioal-

lergosorbent test；RAST 放射性免疫吸着試験 radioimmunosorbent test；RIST 免疫吸着法 immunosorbent technique

きゅうちゅう 吸虫 fluke ◀住血吸虫 schistosome / blood fluke 肺吸虫 lung fluke

ぎゅうとう 牛痘 cowpox

きゅうにゅう 吸入する inhale (↔exhale 反inhalation), breathe (in) ☞吸う ◆患者に酸素吸入を行う give the patient oxygen / have the patient inhale oxygen ◆気管支拡張薬を吸入する inhale a bronchodilator ◀酸素吸入療法 oxygen (inhalation) therapy 塵埃吸入 dust inhalation ▶吸入口 mouthpiece 吸入酸素濃度 fractional concentration of inspiratory [inspired] oxygen；FiO2 吸入ステロイド薬 inhaled corticosteroid[steroid]；ICS 吸入麻酔 inhalation anesthesia 吸入薬 inhalant 吸入療法 inhalation therapy ☞吸入器

ぎゅうにゅう 牛乳 (cow's) milk ☞ミルク ◀全(牛)乳 whole milk /《英》full-fat milk 脱脂(牛)乳 skim milk / one-percent milk /《英》skimmed milk 低脂肪(牛)乳 low-fat[light] milk / two-percent milk /《英》semi-skimmed milk ▶牛乳アレルギー milk allergy 牛乳不耐症 milk intolerance

きゅうにゅうき 吸入器 inhaler (インフォーマルに)puffer ◆吸入器を使ったことはありますか Have you ever used an inhaler before? ◆吸入器を使うお手伝いをしましょう I'll help you use an inhaler. ◆吸入器を軽く 3, 4 回振って下さい Please shake the inhaler gently three or four times. ◆ゆっくり息を吸い込みながら吸入器を押して下さい Please press the top of the inhaler down while breathing in slowly.

きゅうびょう 急病 sudden illness ▶急病患者 emergency patient

きゅうふ 給付 (保険の) benefits / bénəfits/ ★通例、複数形で. ◆医療給付を受ける receive medical (care) benefits ◆健康保険の給付 health insurance benefits ◀社会保障給付 social security benefits 出産給付金 maternity[childbirth] benefits 療養給付 medical treatment benefits

きゅうぶだいどうみゃく 弓部大動脈 aortic arch, arch of the aorta

きゅうへん 急変する take a sudden turn for the worse ◆今朝彼女の容体が急変しました Her condition took a sudden turn for the worse this morning.

きゅうまひ 球麻痺 bulbar palsy[paralysis] ◀仮性球麻痺 pseudobulbar palsy [paralysis] 進行性球麻痺 progressive bulbar palsy[paralysis]；PBP

きゅうめい¹ 救命 （延命措置）life support （人命救助）life-saving （🔁life-saving 🔁 save *a person's* life) ◀一次救命処置 basic life support；BLS 二次救命処置 advanced cardiac[cardiovascular] life support；ACLS ▶救命救急センター emergency and critical care center

きゅうめい² 究明する （調査する）investigate （追い求める）pursue ☞追究

きゅうよう¹ 休養 rest （🔁rest) ◆休み, 休む ◆しばらく仕事は休んで，休養して下さい You should take some time off work for a while and rest. / You should rest and not go to work for a while. ◆今のあなたに必要なのは十分な休養です What you need now is plenty of rest. / Good rest is the most important thing for you now. ◆数日十分な休養をとる take a good rest for several days

きゅうよう² 急用 emergency ◆急用ができたので失礼します An emergency has come up. Please excuse me.

ぎゅっと （固く・きつく）tight, tightly （しっかりと）firmly （力強く）hard ◆口をぎゅっと閉じて下さい Please shut your mouth tight[tightly]. / (すぼめて)Please squeeze your mouth shut. ◆私の手をぎゅっと握って下さい Please squeeze my hand firmly[hard]. ◆目をぎゅっとつぶる shut *one's* eyes tight[tightly]

きょう¹ 今日 today ◆(作業・リハビリ訓練の時など)今日はこれまでにしましょう That's all for today. / That'll be it for today. ◆今日は何曜日ですか What day (of the week) is it today? ◆今日は何日ですか What's today's date? / What day of the month is it today? ◆今日から1週間この薬を飲んで下さい Please take this medication for a week beginning from today. ◆今日の午後〈夕方〉this afternoon〈evening〉

きょう² 橋 pons （🔁pontine) ▶橋出血 pontine hemorrhage[bleeding] 橋中心髄鞘崩壊症 central pontine myelinolysis

きょうい¹ 胸位 （膝胸位）knee-chest position

きょうい² 胸囲 chest circumference （寸法）chest size[measurement]

きょういく 教育 education （🔁educational) （教えること）teaching （🔁teach, instruct) （訓練）training （🔁train) ◆医学教育〈看護教育〉を受ける receive[get] medical〈nursing〉education ◆新人スタッフを教育する teach[instruct / train] new members of staff ◆家族教育 family education 患者教育 patient education 現職教育 in-service[on-the-job] training 性教育 sex education 卒後教育 postgraduate education 訪問教育 visiting teaching (for sick[disabled] children) / visiting teacher service ▶教育入院 educational hospitalization 教育病院 teaching hospital

きょうか 強化する （強固にする）strengthen （🔁strength) （特徴・度を強める）intensify （🔁intensive, intense) （栄養価を増す）enrich ◆筋力を強化する strengthen *one's* muscles ◀ビタミン強化食品 vitamin-enriched food ▶強化インスリン療法 intensive insulin therapy

きょうかい 境界 border （境界線）borderline （🔁borderline) ◆あなたの血圧は正常と高血圧の境界にあります You have borderline high blood pressure. / Your blood pressure is borderline between normal and high. ▶境界型 borderline type 境界型糖尿病 borderline diabetes 境界(域)高血圧 borderline hypertension

境界病変 borderline lesion

ぎょうがい 仰臥位 supine position, face-up position ☞仰向け

きょうかく 胸郭 thorax（囲thoracic）, rib cage（胸部）chest ▶動揺胸郭 flail chest ▶胸郭出口症候群 thoracic outlet syndrome；TOS 胸郭バンド chest strap[binder] 胸郭変形 thoracic deformity

きょうがく 驚愕 startle ▶驚愕反射 startle reflex 驚愕反応 startle reaction

きょうかくだい 強拡大 （顕微鏡の）high-power field

きょうかくまくえん 強角膜炎 sclero-keratitis

きょうかん 共感する empathize（with）（囲empathy） ◆痛みのある患者に共感する empathize with a patient who is in pain

きょうかんかく 共感覚 synesthesia

きょうきゅう 供給する （補給する）supply（囲supply）（提供する）provide ◆安全な血液の供給 a safe and secure blood supply ◆患者に高度な医療サービスを供給する provide advanced medical care services to patients ◀酸素供給装置 oxygen supply equipment

きょうぎゅうびょう 狂牛病 mad cow disease （ウシ海綿状脳症）bovine spongiform encephalopathy；BSE

きょうきん 胸筋 pectoral muscle ◀大胸筋 pectoralis major / greater pectoral muscle 大胸筋皮弁 pectoralis major myocutaneous flap

きょうくう 胸腔 chest cavity, thoracic cavity ▶胸腔穿刺 thoracentesis / thoracic paracentesis 胸腔チューブ chest tube 胸腔ドレナージ chest[thoracic / intrathoracic] drainage ☞胸腔鏡

きょうぐう 境遇 surroundings, conditions, situation ☞環境

きょうくうきょう 胸腔鏡 thoracoscope（囲thoracoscopic）▶胸腔鏡下手術 thoracoscopic surgery 胸腔鏡検査 thoracoscopy

ぎょうけつ 凝血 （blood）coagulation, （blood）clotting （血の塊）（blood）clot

☞凝固

きょうけつしゃ 供血者 blood donor

きょうけんびょう 狂犬病 rabies ★複数形で. ▶狂犬病予防注射 rabies shot[vaccination]

ぎょうこ 凝固 coagulation（囲coagulate）, clotting（囲clot）◆血液の凝固を防ぐ prevent（blood）clotting[coagulation] / stop blood from clotting ◆血管内の血液凝固（the formation of）blood clots inside a blood vessel ◀血液凝固 blood clotting[coagulation] 抗凝固薬 anticoagulant （medication / drug / agent） 抗凝固療法 anticoagulant therapy 播種性血管内凝固 disseminated intravascular coagulation；DIC ビタミンK依存性凝固因子 vitamin K-dependent coagulation factor マイクロ波凝固療法 microwave coagulation therapy；MCT ▶凝固因子 coagulation factor 凝固時間 coagulation time 凝固線溶系 the coagulation and fibrinolytic system 凝固能亢進 hypercoagulability 凝固反応 coagulation reaction ☞凝固術

きょうこう 恐慌 panic ☞パニック

きょうごう 競合 competition（囲competitive）▶競合的拮抗 competitive antagonism 競合的遮断 competitive block 競合的阻害 competitive inhibition

ぎょうこじゅつ 凝固術 coagulation ◀高周波凝固術 radiofrequency coagulation レーザー光凝固術 laser photocoagulation

きょうこつ[1] 胸骨 breastbone, sternum（囲sternal）▶胸骨圧迫心（臓）マッサージ chest compression cardiac massage 胸骨正中切開 median sternotomy 胸骨穿刺 sternal puncture

きょうこつ[2] 頬骨 cheekbone, zygomatic bone, malar bone ▶頬骨骨折 zygomatic fracture

きょうこつばん 狭骨盤 contracted pelvis

きょうさいねんきん 共済年金 Mutual Aid Pension ☞年金

きょうさかんせつ 胸鎖関節 sternoclavicular joint

きょうさく 狭窄 （狭まること）narrowing （収縮）constriction （体内の管などの狭窄）stenosis, stricture （侵入による狭窄）encroachment ◀冠動脈狭窄 coronary artery stenosis 気道狭窄 airway narrowing[stenosis] 再狭窄 restenosis 視野狭窄 visual field constriction / narrowing of the visual field 椎間孔狭窄 foraminal encroachment

きょうさにゅうとつきん 胸鎖乳突筋 sternocleidomastoid[SCM] muscle

きょうさん 強酸 strong acid

きょうしきこきゅう 胸式呼吸 chest breathing[respiration], thoracic breathing[respiration], costal breathing[respiration]

きょうじゅ 教授 professor ◀准教授 associate professor

ぎょうしゅう 凝集 agglutination, aggregation ◀寒冷凝集反応 cold agglutination reaction ☞凝集素

ぎょうしゅうそ 凝集素 agglutinin ◀寒冷凝集素症 cold agglutinin disease：CAD 寒冷赤血球凝集素 cold hemagglutinin

きょうしんしょう 狭心症 angina (pectoris)／ændʒáɪnə péktərɪs／(⽫anginal) ◆狭心症は心臓への血液の供給が減ることによって起こります Angina is caused by a decrease in blood supply to the heart. ◀安静時狭心症 angina at rest / rest angina 安定狭心症 stable angina 異型狭心症 variant angina 血管攣縮性狭心症 vasospastic[coronary spastic] angina 抗狭心症薬 antianginal（medication / drug / agent） 梗塞後狭心症 postinfarction angina；PIA 不安定狭心症 unstable angina 労作性狭心症 effort[exertional] angina / angina of[on] effort ▶狭心症発作 anginal attack 狭心（症）痛 anginal pain

きょうしんやく 強心薬 heart stimulant, cardiotonic（medication, drug, agent）

きょうすい 胸水 fluid in the chest cavity, pleural fluid[effusion] ◆胸水がたまっています Excessive amounts of fluid have accumulated in your chest cavity. ◆胸水を抜く drain the fluid from the chest cavity / drain the pleural fluid ◀がん性胸水 cancerous pleural fluid[effusion] 血性胸水 bloody[hemorrhagic] pleural fluid[effusion] 滲出性胸水 exudative pleural effusion 漏出性胸水 transudative pleural effusion ▶胸水検査 pleural fluid examination[analysis]

きょうすいしょう 恐水症 aquaphobia, fear of water （恐水病）hydrophobia

きょうせい¹ 強制（の）（無理強いの・不自然な）forced （必須の）mandatory （強迫性の）obsessive ◆感染拡大予防のため患者を強制的に隔離する place *a patient[patients] in forced isolation to prevent the spread of infection ▶強制換気 mandatory ventilation 強制検査 mandatory test 強制呼吸 forced breathing[respiration] 強制泣き forced[obsessive] crying 強制利尿 forced diuresis 強制笑い forced[obsessive] laughing

きょうせい² 矯正する（調整する）correct （⽫correction ⽫corrective 調整した corrected）（まっすぐに直す）straighten ◆乱視を眼鏡で矯正する correct astigmatism with glasses ◆歯を矯正する straighten *a person's* teeth /（歯列矯正器をつけている）wear (dental) braces ◀角膜矯正術 orthokeratology 屈折矯正手術 refractive surgery 言語矯正 speech correction 歯科矯正学 orthodontics 歯科矯正装置 orthodontic appliance 視能矯正 orthoptics 歯列矯正 orthodontics / straightening of irregular teeth / teeth-straightening 胎位矯正 correction of malpresentation 徒手矯正 manual reposition[correction] 鼻中隔矯正術 septoplasty 美容矯正 cosmetic correction ▶矯正運動 corrective[correction] exercise 矯正具（歯の）arch wire 矯正歯科（診療所）orthodontics clinic /（病院の診療部門）the orthodontics department 矯正手術 corrective surgery 矯正視力 corrected vision[visual acuity] 矯正眼鏡 correcting glasses 矯正レンズ corrective lens

ぎょうせい 偽陽性（の） false-positive

◆偽陽性反応 a false-positive reaction
ぎょうせいかいぼう 行政解剖 administrative autopsy ★欧米では行政解剖と司法解剖を包括して medicolegal[forensic / judicial] autopsy ということも多い．
きょうせん 胸腺 thymus gland (🔁thymic) 胸腺腫 thymoma 胸腺退縮 thymic involution 胸腺摘出術 thymectomy
きょうだい 兄弟・姉妹 (男の)brother (女の)sister (男女を区別しないで)sibling ◆きょうだいはいますか Do you have brothers or sisters? ◆きょうだいは何人ですか How many brothers and sisters do you have? ◆お子さんのきょうだい関係は良好ですか Do your children get on well with each other? / Is your children's sibling relationship good?
ぎょうちゅうしょう 蟯虫症 enterobiasis, pinworm infection
きょうちょう¹ 協調 (共同作用・連携)coordination (🔁coordinate) (協力)cooperation (🔁cooperate 🔁cooperative) (調和)harmony ◆協調運動や平衡感覚に問題がありますか Do you have any problem with your coordination or balance? ◆彼女は周囲の人との協調性があります She works[cooperates] well with others. / She's a cooperative person. ◆彼は協調性に欠けています He's not cooperative enough. / He doesn't cooperate enough. ▶協調運動障害 coordination disorder[disturbance]
きょうちょう² 強調する emphasize (🔁emphasis) (重視する)stress (🔁stress) ◆糖尿病のコントロールには食事と運動が重要であることを強調します I would emphasize that diet and exercise are important for the management of diabetes. ◀T1〈T2〉強調画像 T1-weighted〈T2-weighted〉image
きょうちょく 強直 ankylosis (🔁強直性のtonic) ☞硬直 ◆関節強直 joint ankylosis / ankylosis of the joints 不全強直 partial ankylosis ▶強直間代痙攣 tonic-clonic convulsion[seizure] 強直性痙攣 tonic convulsion[seizure] 強直性脊椎炎 ankylosing spondylitis
きょうつい 胸椎 thoracic vertebra ▶胸椎椎間板ヘルニア thoracic disc hernia
きょうつう¹ 胸痛 chest pain ☞痛み(囲み：痛みの表現) ◆これまでに胸痛を起こしたことがありますか Have you ever had (any) chest pain? ◆今胸痛がありますか Do you have (a) chest pain now? / Do you have (a) pain in your chest now? ◆胸痛はどのような痛みですか〈でしたか〉What kind of chest pain do〈did〉you have? ◆胸痛は断続的な痛みですか Does the chest pain come and go? ◆胸痛の場所はどこですか Where is the chest pain (located)? ◆胸痛を起こすのは何か活動している時ですか Does any particular activity bring on the chest pain? / Does the chest pain come on with any particular activity? ◆胸痛が起こるのは普通に呼吸している時ですか，それとも深呼吸する時ですか Does the chest pain *come on [occur] when you're breathing normally or when you *take a deep breath[breathe deeply]? ◀安静時胸痛 chest pain at rest 心因性胸痛 psychogenic chest pain 労作性胸痛 exertional chest pain / chest pain *on exertion[during exercise]
きょうつう² 共通(の) common ◆共通因子 a common factor
きょうど 強度 (光・痛みなどの強さ)intensity (物理的な力)strength ◆胸痛の強度 the intensity of one's chest pain ◆光の強度 light intensity ◀運動強度 exercise intensity 労働強度 work[labor] strength ▶強度近視 high-level myopia / extreme nearsightedness
きょうどう¹ 共同(の) (協力・合同の)cooperative, collaborative, joint (相乗作用の)synergic (連合・結合の)conjugate ▶共同運動 synergic[conjugate] movement 共同研究 cooperative[joint] study 共同作業 group[collaborative] work
きょうどう² 協働(の) (専門職間の)interprofessional (協力・合同の)cooperative, collaborative ◀専門職間協働 interpro

fessional work；IPW　専門職間協働医療チーム interprofessional health care team

きょうどく　強毒(性の)　highly toxic[poisonous]　(危険度の強い)virulent　◆その化学物質は強毒性です That chemical is highly toxic[poisonous].　◆トリインフルエンザの強毒性の菌株 a virulent strain of avian flu

きょうはいぶ　胸背部　(the region of) the chest and back　☞胸部

きょうはく　強迫(的な)　(異常に執着する)obsessive, obsessional　(圏obsession 働obsess)　(行動などがやめられない)compulsive　(圏compulsion)　(不自然な・無理な)forced　◆彼女は手を洗うという強迫観念にとらわれています She is obsessed with the idea that she has to wash her hands.　◆強迫的な過食 compulsive overeating　◆強迫的な性格 a compulsive personality　◀確認強迫 compulsive rechecking [checking and double-checking]　▶強迫観念 obsession / obsessional idea　強迫行動 compulsive[obsessive] behavior / compulsion　強迫状態 obsessive-compulsive state　強迫神経症 obsessive-compulsive neurosis　強迫性障害 obsessive-compulsive disorder；OCD　強迫性人格障害 obsessive-compulsive personality disorder　強迫泣き forced[obsessive] crying　強迫笑い forced[obsessive] laughing

きょうひしょう　強皮症　scleroderma　◀全身性強皮症 systemic sclerosis；SSc

きょうふ　恐怖　(恐れ)fear　(強度の恐れ)terror, horror　(パニック)panic　(恐怖症)phobia　(接尾-phobia)　◆高い所に恐怖を覚える have a fear of heights　◆恐怖に襲われる be seized with fear / be panic-stricken　◀会話恐怖 laliophobia　学校恐怖 school phobia　がん恐怖 cancerophobia　観念恐怖 ideophobia　暗闇恐怖 nyctophobia　口臭恐怖 halitophobia　高所恐怖 acrophobia　視線恐怖 scopophobia / abnormal fear of being seen by others　疾病恐怖 nosophobia / pathophobia　社会恐怖 social phobia　醜形恐怖 dysmorphophobia　赤面恐怖 erythrophobia　先端恐怖 aichmophobia　対人恐怖 anthropophobia　他人恐怖 xenophobia　動物恐怖 zoophobia　広場恐怖 agoraphobia　不潔恐怖 mysophobia　閉所恐怖 claustrophobia

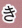

きょうぶ　胸部　chest, thorax　(圏thoracic)　☞胸　◆胸部に不快感がありますか Do you feel discomfort or have any unpleasant feeling in your chest?　◆胸部のX線を撮ります I'm going to take an X-ray of your chest.　▶胸部圧迫感 chest pressure (sensation) / feeling of tightness in the chest　胸部X線写真(検査) chest X-ray /(フィルム)chest film　胸部外科 thoracic surgery /(診療科)the department of thoracic surgery, the thoracic surgery department　胸部外科医 thoracic surgeon　胸部絞扼感 constriction in the chest　胸部損傷 chest injury [wound] / thoracic injury[wound]　胸部大動脈 thoracic aorta　胸部大動脈瘤 thoracic aortic aneurysm；TAA　胸部痛 chest pain　胸部誘導 chest lead

きょうへき　胸壁　chest wall, thoracic wall

きょうまく[1]　胸膜　pleura　(圏pleural)　▶胸膜腔 pleural cavity　胸膜中皮腫 pleural mesothelioma　胸膜播種 pleural dissemination　胸膜肥厚 pleural thickening　胸膜摩擦音 pleural friction rub　胸膜癒着術 pleurodesis　☞胸膜炎

きょうまく[2]　強膜　sclera；*the outer layer of the eyeball*　(圏scleral)　(一般語)the white of the eye　◀青色強膜 blue sclera　▶強膜炎 scleritis

きょうまくえん　胸膜炎　pleurisy, pleuritis　◀癌性胸膜炎 carcinomatous pleurisy [pleuritis]　結核性胸膜炎 tuberculous pleurisy[pleuritis]　細菌性胸膜炎 bacterial pleurisy[pleuritis]

きょうみ　興味　interest　(圏be interested in 圏interesting)　☞関心　◆どんなことに興味を持っていますか What are your interests? / What are you interested in?　◆普段やっていることに興味を失う lose interest in *one's* usual activities

ぎょうむ　業務　(仕事)**job, work, business**　(任務)**duty**　(専門的な業務)**service**　◆業務上の事故にあう have an on-the-job accident / have an accident while on duty　◀医療業務 medical service　看護業務 nursing service　▶業務上傷害 work-related[occupational / industrial] injury

きょうめんぞう　鏡面像　mirror image

きょうゆう　共有する　share　(形共同の**communal**)　◆患者と医療者間で臨床上の情報を共有する patients and physicians share clinical information (with each other)　◆この冷蔵庫は共有になります This is *a communal refrigerator for use by patients[a communal patient refrigerator].　▶共有スペース shared[communal] space

きょうようせい　強陽性(の)　**strongly positive**

きょうりょく¹　協力　cooperation　(動cooperate**(with)**　形cooperative)　◆私はほかの医療スタッフと密接に協力してやっています I'm working in close cooperation with the other medical staff.　◆ご主人は家事や子育てに協力的ですか Does your husband help you with the housework and taking care of your child? / Is your husband cooperative when it comes to doing the housework or taking care of your child?　◆ご協力感謝します Thank you for your cooperation[help]. / (お時間をとらせて)Thank you for your time.　◆院内での禁煙にご協力下さい Thank you for not smoking in the hospital.　▶協力関係 cooperative relationship[relations]

きょうりょく²　強力(な)　**powerful, strong**　(効果的な)**effective**　◆この薬の効き目は強力です This medication is quite powerful. / This medication is extremely effective.　◆強力な根拠 strong evidence

きょか　許可する　permit　(名permission)　(容認する)**allow**　◆外出許可(医師の)(the doctor's) permission *to go out[to leave the hospital building]　◆外泊許可(the doctor's) permission *to go home for the night[to stay home overnight]　◆外出する時には，必ず担当医の許可を得て下さい When you go out of the hospital, be sure to check with your doctor and get his〈her〉permission.　◆それには担当医の許可が必要です That will need your doctor's permission.　◆小さい〈12歳未満の〉お子さんの面会は許可されておりません Small children〈Children under the age of twelve〉are not allowed to visit patients.　◀火葬許可証 cremation permit　在留許可証 residence permit　▶許可外使用薬 unauthorized medication[drug / agent]　許可証 permit

ぎょかいるい　魚介類　(魚・甲殻類)**fish and shellfish**　(海産食品)**seafood**

きょぎせいしょうがい　虚偽性障害　factitious disorder

きょくざい　局在　localization　(形局在した**localized**　限局した**focal**)　◀機能局在 functional localization　▶局在関連性てんかん localization-related epilepsy　局在徴候 focal sign

きょくしょ　局所　area(of the body)**, part**(of the body)　(形局部的な**local, localized**　表面の**topical**)　◆まず局所を拭いてからこの軟膏を塗って下さい Please clean the area and then apply this ointment.　◆痛みは局所的ですか，それとも広範囲にわたりますか Is the pain localized or general? / Do you feel the pain in just one place or over a wider area of your body?　▶局所加温 local heat (treatment)　局所症状 local symptom　局所浸潤 local infiltration　局所性病変 local lesion　局所麻酔 local[topical] anesthesia　局所麻酔薬 local[topical] anesthetic　局所用ステロイド topical steroid　局所冷却 local cooling

きょくせん　曲線　curve, curved line　◀成長曲線 growth curve　体重曲線 weight curve

きょくど　極度(に)　**extremely**　◆極度の疲労を覚える feel extremely tired　◆極度に緊張する be extremely nervous

きょくぶ　局部　(陰部)**genital region**　(婉

きょくりょう 曲的に) private areas[parts] ★通例，複数形で． ▶局部サポーター(運動選手の)jockstrap / athletic supporter

きょくりょう 極量 maximum dose[dosage] ★dose は1回の摂取量，dosage は一定期間における摂取量をいう．

きょけつ 虚血 ischemia /ɪskíːmiə/；*deficiency of blood flow to a part of the body* (圏ischemic) ◀一過性脳虚血発作 transient ischemic attack；TIA 心筋虚血 myocardial ischemia 腸間膜虚血 mesenteric ischemia 脳虚血 brain[cerebral] ischemia ▶虚血時間 ischemic time 虚血性心疾患 ischemic heart disease；IHD 虚血性腸炎 ischemic enteritis 虚血性脳血管障害 ischemic cerebrovascular disorder 虚血性脳卒中 ischemic stroke 虚血性発作 ischemic attack

きょこつ 距骨 ankle bone, talus

きょさいぼう 巨細胞 giant cell ◀ランゲルハンス巨細胞 Langhans giant cell

きょじゃく 虚弱(な) (弱い) weak (もろくひ弱い) delicate ▶虚弱体質 weak[delicate] constitution

きょじゅう 居住 residence (圏residential) ◀外国人居住者 foreign resident 施設居住介護 residential care ▶居住型療養施設 residential treatment facility 居住環境 residential[home] environment 居住施設 residential facility 居住地 *one's* place of residence / the place where *one* lives

きょじょう 挙上 lift (圏lift), elevation (圏elevate) ◆足の浮腫は，下肢挙上で少し軽減するでしょう The swelling in your legs will *go down[decrease] if you keep your feet elevated. ◀下顎挙上法 jaw-lift method

きょしょく 拒食 food refusal, refusal to eat ▶拒食症 anorexia (nervosa)；AN ☞神経性やせ症

きょじんしょう 巨人症 gigantism, macrosomia ◀下垂体性巨人症 pituitary gigantism

きょせい 去勢 castration (圏castrate)

きょせきがきゅう 巨赤芽球 megaloblast (圏megaloblastic) ▶巨赤芽球性貧血 megaloblastic anemia

きょぜつ 拒絶する (申し出・要求などを強く断る) refuse (圏refusal) (却下・辞退する) turn down (きっぱりと拒む・拒絶反応を起こす) reject (圏rejection) ☞拒絶反応, 拒否, 断る

きょぜつはんのう 拒絶反応 rejection (動reject) ◆腎臓移植後は順調で拒絶反応は出ていません You are doing well after your kidney transplant and have not had any rejection problems. ◆彼女に拒絶反応の症状が出始めています She has begun to show some *symptoms of rejection [rejection symptoms]. ◆拒絶反応を引き起こす cause[trigger] a rejection ◆拒絶反応を防ぐ prevent a rejection

きょだい 巨大(な) huge (並外れて大きい) giant (腰頭mega-, macr(o)-) ◀先端巨大症 acromegaly ▶巨大結腸 giant colon / megacolon 巨大児 excessively large infant 巨大舌 macroglossia

きょだつ 虚脱 collapse ▶血管虚脱 vascular collapse 肺虚脱 pulmonary collapse

きょたんやく 去痰薬 expectorant；*a medication that helps bring up phlegm from the airway*

きょねん 去年 last year

きょひ 拒否する (申し出・要求などを強く断る) refuse (圏refusal) (却下・辞退する) turn down (きっぱりと拒む) reject (圏rejection) ☞断る ◆彼女は治療を拒否しています She refuses (medical) treatment. ◆医療ソーシャルワーカーの援助の申し出を拒否する *turn down[refuse / reject] a medical social worker's offer of help ◆生命維持装置を使うことを拒否する refuse life support / refuse use of a life support machine ◀出勤拒否 refusal to go to work 登校拒否 refusal to go to school / school[classroom] refusal 輸血拒否 refusal of (a) blood transfusion

きょよう 許容できる (容認できる) acceptable (差し支えない程度に認められる) permissible (我慢できる) tolerable (圏tolerance)

◆血糖値はやや高いものの許容範囲内です Your blood sugar levels are within the acceptable[permissible] range, though they're slightly high. ◆それは許容できる痛みですか Is it a tolerable pain? / Is the pain tolerable? ◆痛みの許容度が低い〈高い〉have (a) low〈high〉tolerance for pain ◀一日摂取許容量 acceptable daily intake；ADI （放射線の）最大許容線量 the maximum permissible dose；MPD 疼痛許容レベル pain tolerance level ▶許容限界 permissible[acceptable / tolerance] limit 許容量 permissible[tolerance] dose

きょり 距離 distance ◆2点間の距離 distance between two points ◆彼女は距離感がうまくつかめないようです She seems to have a poor[bad] sense of distance. / Her sense of distance seems to be poor[bad]. ◀焦点距離 focal distance[length] ▶距離感覚 sense of distance / distance perception

きょりゅう 居留 residence ☞在留

ぎょりんせん 魚鱗癬 ichthyosis, fish skin disease

きらう 嫌う not like, dislike （ひどく嫌う）hate ☞嫌がる ◆何か嫌いな食べ物がありますか Is there anything you don't like to eat? ◆体を動かすのが嫌いですか Don't you like[Do you hate] to exercise? ◀ミルク嫌い milk refusal

きらく 気楽にする （くつろぐ）relax, make *oneself* comfortable （のんびりする）feel at ease （遠慮しない）feel free ◆（検査などで緊張を解いてもらうために）どうぞ気楽にして下さい Please relax. / Please make yourself comfortable. ◆同郷の友人と一緒にいると気楽ですか Do you feel more at ease with friends *from the same country as yours[from your own country]? ◆ご用がある時には気楽にナースコールを押して下さい Feel free to push[press] the (nurse call) button whenever you need any help.

ギラン・バレーしょうこうぐん ―症候群 Guillain–Barré syndrome

きりきず 切り傷 cut （刃物による切り傷）slash （深い切り傷）gash ☞傷 ◆切り傷を受けたのですか Did you have any cuts? ◆切り傷を縫合する *sew up[suture] the cut(s)

きりきり （割れるような）splitting （締め付けられるような）squeezing （刺すような）stabbing （痙攣性の）griping, spasmodic ☞痛み（囲み：痛みの表現）

ギリシャ Greece （圀Greek） ☞国籍 ▶ギリシャ人（の）Greek

きりつ 起立（性の） （立位の）standing, stand-up, orthostatic （体位性の）postural ▶起立訓練 standing[stand-up] exercise 起立性失神 orthostatic syncope 起立性蛋白尿 orthostatic[postural] proteinuria 起立性調節障害 orthostatic dysregulation；OD 起立性低血圧 orthostatic[postural] hypotension / fall in blood pressure upon standing 起立台 standing table

きりゅうせいげん 気流制限 airflow limitation

きりょく 気力 （元気）energy （活力）vitality ◆気力の減退を感じますか Do you feel a decline in energy[vitality]? / Have you noticed any decrease in your energy levels?

きる[1] 切る
《刃物で切る》 （切断する）cut （細長い切り込みを入れる）slit （ざっくり切る）slash ◆ナイフで手首を切る cut[slit / slash] *one's* wrist(s) with a knife
《取り除く》take out, remove ◆いつ虫垂を切ったのですか When did you have your appendix (taken) out? ◆痰を切る remove[release / clear] phlegm
《断裂する》 （引き裂く）tear /té→/ （腱・血管などを断裂・破裂させる）rupture ◆アキレス腱を切る tear[cut / rupture] *one's* Achilles tendon
《回路や回線を止める》 （スイッチなどを）turn off （電話を）hang up ◆携帯電話の電源を切る turn[switch] off (the power on) *one's* mobile phone

きる[2] 着る （体に着ける）put on （着けてい

る〉wear （服を着る）get dressed　◆この検査着を着て下さい Please put on this exam gown.　◆では，服を着てもいいですよ You can get dressed now.

きれい
《美しい》beautiful　（目・耳に心地よい）pretty　◆お花がとてもきれいですね The flowers are[look] really beautiful. / What beautiful flowers (they are)!
《汚れがない》（清潔な）clean （圏clean）　（澄んだ）clear　◆手はきれいですか Are your hands clean?　◆フィルターを定期的にきれいにする clean[wash] the filter regularly　◆肺の音はきれいです Your chest sounds are clear.
《新鮮な》fresh　◆きれいな空気を吸う breathe fresh air
《完全に》completely, thoroughly, totally　◆傷がきれいに治るには2，3か月から1年かかるかもしれません It might take a few months to a year for the wound to heal completely.　◆胸のX線写真に見えた影はきれいになくなっています The shadow on your X-ray has completely[thoroughly / totally] disappeared.

きれじ　切れ痔　（裂肛）anal fissure　（出血性痔核）bleeding hemorrhoids[piles]　★複数形で．

きれつ　亀裂　（ひび）crack （圏cracked）　（割れ目）split （圏split）　（裂け目）tear /téə/ （圏tear）　（裂溝）fissure （圏fissured, furrowed）　◆爪に亀裂がよく入りますか Do your nails split easily?　◆骨に亀裂が入っている have a cracked bone　▶亀裂骨折 fissure fracture　亀裂舌[溝状舌] fissured[furrowed] tongue

―きれない　◆病院食は食べきれませんか Can't you eat[finish] all of your (hospital) food?　◆残念ですが，腫瘍を取りきれませんでした I'm sorry to say that we couldn't remove *the entire[the whole of the] tumor.

きれる　切れる
《刃物などの切れ味がよい》cut well　◆このハサミはよく切れます These scissors *cut well[are sharp].

《血管などが断裂する》burst, rupture　◆血管が切れています The blood vessel has burst [ruptured].
《息があがる》get[feel, be] short of breath, get[be] out of breath, get[be] breathless　◆階段を上る時息が切れますか Do you get[feel] *short of breath[out of breath / breathless] when you climb[go up] stairs?
《効力がなくなる》（有効期限を過ぎる）expire, run out　（効き目がなくなる）wear off　◆このビザの期限は切れています This visa has expired.　◆薬の効き目が切れ始めています The medication is starting to wear off.　◆麻酔が切れるのに1時間ほどかかります The anesthesia will take about an hour to wear off. / It will take about one hour for the anesthesia to wear off.　◆電池が切れています The battery is dead. / The battery has run down[out].
《電気回路が止まる》　◆この機器は10分後に自動的に切れます This instrument automatically turns itself off in ten minutes.

キロカロリー　kilocalorie；kcal, Cal　☞カロリー

きろく　記録　record /rékəd/ （圏record）　★名詞と動詞でアクセントが違うことに注意．（計器の数値）reading　◆この検査は運動中の心電図を記録します This test records your EKG during exercise.　◆毎日の体温を記録する record *one's* daily temperature　◆心臓の電気的活動を記録する record the electrical activity of the heart　◆血圧の記録を見せていただけませんか Could you show me your blood pressure reading?　▶看護記録 nursing (care) record　食事記録 diet record　診療記録 medical record　麻酔記録 anesthesia chart[record]

きろくぶ　季肋部　（下肋部）hypochondriac region

キログラム　kilo, kilogram；kg　◆あなたの体重は70 kgです You weigh seventy kilos[kilograms].　◆この1週間で何kg増えましたか〈減りましたか〉How many kilos did you gain〈lose〉in this week?

ぎろん　議論する　(話し合う)talk (about), discuss (図discussion)　(論争する)argue (図argument)　☞話し合う　◆私たちはその問題について真剣に議論しました We had a serious discussion about the matter. / We discussed the matter seriously.　◆この場合の治療方針については専門家の間でも議論のあるところです(異論がある)Different specialists have different opinions about the treatment plans in this case.

ぎわん　義腕　artificial arm, prosthetic arm

きをうしなう　気を失う　(めまいなどで一時的に失神する)faint, pass out, black out　(意識を失う)lose consciousness　☞意識, 失神　◆気を失いそうな感じがしますか Do you feel like you're going to faint[pass out]?　◆これまで気を失ったことはありますか Have you ever fainted[lost consciousness / blacked out]?　◆気を失っていたのはどれくらいの時間でしたか How long were you unconscious?

きをおとす　気を落とす　(動揺する)get upset　(失望する)get disappointed　(落胆する)get discouraged　◆大丈夫ですよ, 気を落とさないで It's all right. Don't get upset[disappointed]. / You're going to be just fine. (元気を出して)Cheer up!

きをつかう　気を遣う　◆どうぞ気を遣わないで下さい(ご心配なく)Please don't bother.

きをつける　気をつける　(注意して見る)watch　(用心・注意する)take care, be careful　◆足元に気をつけて下さい Please watch your step.　◆転ばないように気をつけて下さい Please take care (that) you don't fall.　◆では, お気をつけて！ Take care! / Take (good) care of yourself!　◆これからはもっと食事に気をつけて下さい Please be more careful about what you eat from now on.

きをらくにする　気を楽にする　(くつろぐ)relax　◆気を楽にしてもう一度やってみて下さい Please relax and try again.　◆お気を楽に Take it easy.

きをわるくする　気を悪くする　(批判的に考える)think badly[ill] of　(気分を害する)

get[be] offended　(動揺させる)upset　(傷つける)hurt　◆彼のことで気を悪くしないで下さい Please don't think badly[ill] of him. / Please don't get[be] offended by him.　◆私の言葉で気を悪くされたなら申し訳ありませんでした I'm sorry if I upset you by[with] what I said. / I'm sorry if *what I said[I] hurt your feelings.

きん¹　菌　(一般的に病原菌)germ　(細菌)bacteria (単bacterium)　(真菌)fungus (複fungi)　☞細菌　◆(細)菌の種類によって効く薬と効かない薬があります The effectiveness of medications[Whether (or not) a medication works] depends on the type of germs[bacteria] involved.　◆健康な人でも皮膚や体の中に多くの(細)菌が常在しています Even healthy people have a large number of different types of bacteria living on their skin and inside their body.　◆肺炎の原因菌を突き止めるために痰の培養検査を行いましょう Let's do a sputum culture to identify *the bacteria that are causing the pneumonia [which bacteria are causing the pneumonia].　◀化膿菌 pyogenic bacteria　感受性菌 sensitive bacteria　グラム陰性〈グラム陽性〉菌 gram-negative〈gram-positive〉bacteria　嫌気性〈好気性〉菌 anaerobic 〈aerobic〉 bacteria　弱毒菌 low-virulent bacilli　▶菌血症 bacteremia　菌交代現象 microbial substitution

きん²　筋　muscle (形muscular)　☞筋肉　◀運動筋 motor muscle　遠位筋 distal muscle　横紋筋 striated[striped] muscle　下肢筋 lower limb muscle / the muscle of the lower limb(s)　括約筋 sphincter　拮抗筋 antagonistic muscle / antagonist　共同筋 synergist / synergistic muscle　近位筋 proximal muscle　抗重力筋 antigravity muscle　呼吸筋 respiratory muscle　骨格筋 skeletal muscle　上肢筋 upper limb muscle / the muscle of the upper limb(s)　随意筋 voluntary muscle　背筋 back muscle　不随意筋 involuntary muscle　腹筋 abdominal muscle　平滑筋 smooth muscle　▶筋運

動 muscle exercise　筋痙縮 muscle spasticity　筋拘縮 muscle contracture　筋硬直 muscle stiffness[rigidity]　筋骨格系 the musculoskeletal system　筋細胞 muscle cell / myocyte　筋収縮 muscle contraction　筋生検 muscle biopsy　筋線維 muscle fiber　筋組織 muscle[muscular] tissue　筋損傷 muscle injury　筋断裂 muscle rupture　筋電計 electromyography；EMG　筋トレ muscle training　筋皮弁 myocutaneous[musculocutaneous] flap　筋疲労 muscle fatigue
☞筋萎縮，筋炎，筋緊張，筋痙攣，筋弛緩，筋ジストロフィー，筋腫，筋性，筋痛，筋電図，筋膜，筋無力症，筋力

きんい　**近位**（の）　**proximal**（↔distal）　▶近位筋 proximal muscle　近位指〈趾〉節間関節 proximal interphalangeal joint of the hand〈foot〉/ PIP joint of the hand〈foot〉　近位尿細管 proximal kidney tubule

きんいしゅく　**筋萎縮**（症）　**muscular atrophy, amyotrophy**（形amyotrophic）　◀頸椎症性筋萎縮症 cervical spondylotic amyotrophy　▶筋萎縮性側索硬化症 amyotrophic lateral sclerosis；ALS

きんえん[1]　**筋炎　myositis**　◆筋炎は様々な原因で筋肉に炎症をきたして筋肉の痛みや筋力の低下を起こします Myositis is inflammation of the muscles due to various causes, which results in muscle pain and weakness.　◀眼窩筋炎 orbital myositis　多発性筋炎 polymyositis；PM　皮膚筋炎 dermatomyositis；DM

きんえん[2]　**禁煙する　stop smoking, quit smoking, give up smoking**　◆禁煙したことがありますか Have you ever stopped smoking?　◆禁煙を試みたことがありますか Have you ever tried to stop[quit / give up] smoking?　◆いつ禁煙しましたか When did you stop smoking?　◆どんな方法で禁煙しましたか What method did you use to stop smoking?　◆薬を飲むより禁煙するほうが重要です It's more important to stop smoking than to take medications.　◆あなたの病状では禁煙が

必要です．決して遅すぎることはありませんから With your condition as it is, you should stop smoking. It's never too late.　◆院内は禁煙になっております Smoking is not allowed anywhere inside the hospital.　◆禁煙（掲示）No Smoking　▶禁煙指導 antismoking education　禁煙補助薬 antismoking[stop-smoking / quit-smoking] medication[drug / aid]

きんかん　**金冠　gold crown**（金歯）**gold-capped tooth**（形teeth）

きんがん　**近眼　nearsightedness, shortsightedness**　☞近視

きんき　**禁忌　contraindication**（形contraindicated）　◆この薬は妊娠している女性には禁忌です This medication is contraindicated for women who are pregnant.

きんきゅう　**緊急**　（切迫）**urgency**（形urgent）　（非常事態）**emergency**（形emergent）　☞救急　◆緊急に受診したい時にはお電話を下さい Please call us if you need to see me urgently.　◆緊急の際には救急車を呼んで下さい In case of an emergency[In an emergency], please call an ambulance.　◆緊急時用のカードを常に所持して下さい Please always carry your medical alert card with you.　◆緊急の対策を講じる take emergency measures　▶緊急検査 emergency test[examination]　緊急手術 emergency[emergent / urgent] surgery　緊急処置 emergency treatment[care]　緊急措置 emergency measures　緊急呼び出し emergency call　緊急呼び出しベル emergency *call bell[alarm]
☞緊急入院，緊急連絡先

きんきゅうにゅういん　**緊急入院　emergency admission[hospitalization], urgent admission[hospitalization]**　◆彼女は心臓発作で倒れて緊急入院しました She collapsed from a heart attack and was hospitalized for emergency treatment.

きんきゅうれんらくさき　**緊急連絡先　emergency contact number, phone number to contact in case of an emergency**　◆ここに緊急連絡先を書いて下さい Please write your emergency contact number here.

きんきゅうれんらくさき

◆緊急連絡先は何番ですか What's your emergency contact number? / Which phone number should we contact in case of an emergency? ◆緊急連絡先はどなたですか. その方のお名前, 電話番号, ご関係を教えて下さい Who should we contact in case of an emergency? Could you tell me the name and phone number, and your relationship to him or her?

きんきょりしりょくひょう 近距離視力表 near vision test chart

きんきんちょう 筋緊張 muscle tone[tension] (筋緊張症) myotonia (彫myotonic) ◆筋緊張を改善して柔軟性を高める improve the tone and increase the flexibility of a muscle ◆首の筋緊張 muscle tension in one's neck ▶筋緊張亢進 hypertonia / hypermyotonia 筋緊張性ジストロフィー myotonic dystrophy；MD 筋緊張性反応 myotonic reaction[response] 筋緊張低下 hypotonia / hypomyotonia 筋緊張低下児 floppy infant

きんけいれん 筋痙攣 muscle cramp [spasm]

きんけつしょう 菌血症 bacteremia

きんけんしりょく 近見視力 near visual acuity ▶近見視力障害 near visual disturbance

きんこ 金庫 safe ◆貴重品は病院備え付けの金庫に入れて下さい Please keep [put] your valuables in the hospital safe.

きんこう 均衡 (安定・調和)balance (↔imbalance 彫balanced) (釣り合い)proportion (↔disproportion), equilibrium (↔disequilibrium) ☞バランス, 平衡 ◆均衡を保つ keep one's balance ◆均衡を崩す lose one's balance ◆均衡状態で in balance [proportion / equilibrium](with) ▶均衡食 balanced diet

ぎんこう 銀行 bank ◆この銀行口座に10万円振り込んで下さい Please pay one hundred thousand yen into this bank account. ◀眼球[角膜]銀行 eye bank 血液銀行 blood bank 骨髄銀行 bone marrow bank 腎銀行 kidney bank 精子銀行 sperm[semen] bank 臓器銀行 or-

gan bank 組織銀行 tissue bank 皮膚銀行 skin bank 卵子銀行 egg[ovum] bank

きんし¹ 近視 nearsightedness (彫nearsighted), shortsightedness (↔farsightedness), myopia ◆あなたは近視ですか Are you nearsighted? ◆あなたは軽い近視です You have mild nearsightedness. ◆近視の度が進んでいます You're getting more nearsighted. / Your nearsightedness is getting worse. ◆強度の近視 extreme nearsightedness / high-level myopia ◆軽度の近視 mild nearsightedness / low-level myopia ◀仮性近視 false nearsightedness[myopia] / pseudomyopia

きんし² 禁止する (認めない)do not allow (公の権威によって禁じる)prohibit (規則で禁じる)forbid ★いずれも受身形で用いることが多い. ◆携帯電話は指定の場所以外では禁止されています The use of mobile phones is not allowed anywhere outside the designated area. ◆ここは駐車禁止ですので他に移動して下さい Parking is not allowed here[You cannot park your car here]. Please park somewhere else. ◆無断外泊は禁止です. Staying out all night without permission is forbidden. ◀駐車禁止(掲示)No Parking ▶禁止物質 prohibited substance 禁止薬物 prohibited [illegal / banned] drug[substance]

きんしかん 筋弛緩 muscle relaxation ▶筋弛緩薬 muscle relaxant

きんジストロフィー 筋ジストロフィー muscular dystrophy；MD ◀遠位型筋ジストロフィー distal muscular dystrophy；DMA 筋緊張性ジストロフィー myotonic dystrophy；MD 肢帯型筋ジストロフィー limb-girdle muscular dystrophy 進行性筋ジストロフィー progressive muscular dystrophy；PMD 先天性筋ジストロフィー congenital muscular dystrophy；CMD デュシェンヌ型筋ジストロフィー Duchenne muscular dystrophy；DMD ベッカー型筋ジストロフィー Becker muscular dystrophy；BMD

きんじち 近似値 approximate value

きんしつ 均質(の) homogeneous

(↔heterogeneous)

きんしゅ[1]　筋腫　myoma　◀子宮筋腫 uterine myoma　平滑筋腫 leiomyoma　リンパ脈管筋腫症 lymphangioleiomyomatosis；LAM　▶筋腫分娩 myoma delivery

きんしゅ[2]　禁酒する　stop drinking, quit drinking, give up drinking　▶妊娠中は禁酒して下さい Please *don't drink[stop drinking] alcohol while you're pregnant.

きんじる　禁じる　do not allow, prohibit, forbid　☞禁止

きんしん　近親(者)　close relative　(肉親) immediate family (member), blood relative　▶彼の近親者に至急連絡をとって下さい Please contact his close relatives immediately.　◆近親者の死 the death of a loved one　★loved one は配偶者やパートナーも含む.　▶近親(結)婚 consanguineous marriage / marriage between blood relatives　近親姦 incest

きんせい　筋性(の)　muscular　▶筋性眼精疲労 eyestrain / muscular asthenopia　筋性斜頸 muscular torticollis　筋性防御 muscular defense / muscle guarding

きんせいざい　金製剤　gold agent[compound]

きんせん　金銭　money　▶金銭問題 money problem /(経済的困窮)financial difficulties[worries]

きんぞく　金属　metal　(🔲metallic)　◆眼鏡や時計など金属の物はすべて外して下さい Please remove all metallic objects, such as glasses and watches.　◀重金属 heavy metal　重金属中毒 heavy metal poisoning　▶金属アレルギー metal allergy　金属音 metallic sound　金属冠 metal crown　金属製品 metal[metallic] product[object]

きんだんしょうじょう　禁断症状　(離脱症状)withdrawal symptom

きんちょう　緊張　tension (🔲tense, 🔲tense up)　(ストレス)stress (🔲stressful)　(不安)nervousness (🔲nervous)　▶頭痛は頭と背中にかけての筋肉が緊張して起こっているようです Your headache may be caused by *tension in[(こわばることで)tightening of] the muscles of the head and the shoulders.　◆彼は仕事上の緊張が高じて精神のほうが参ってしまったようです He seems to have built up so much stress at work that he had a nervous breakdown.　◆緊張しないで下さい Please don't *be so tense[tense up]. / Please relax.　◆緊張をほぐす release (nervous) tension　◆緊張を和らげる relax[relieve / ease / reduce] (nervous) tension　◆緊張がとれない have difficulty relaxing　◀心的緊張 psychological tension　▶緊張型統合失調症 catatonic schizophrenia　緊張性気胸 tension pneumothorax　緊張性頭痛 tension-type headache　☞筋緊張

きんつう　筋痛　muscle ache[pain], myalgia　◀線維筋痛症 fibromyalgia　リウマチ性多発筋痛症 polymyalgia rheumatica；PMR

きんでんず　筋電図　electromyogram；EMG　◀誘発筋電図 evoked electromyogram　▶筋電図検査 electromyography

きんとう　均等(な)　equal　(🔲equally)　◆左右の足に均等に体重を載せて立って下さい Please stand with your weight equally (distributed) on both feet[legs].

きんトーヌス　筋トーヌス　☞筋緊張

きんにく　筋肉　muscle /mΛsl/ (🔲muscular)　☞筋　◆筋肉の動き muscle[muscular] movement

《性状の表現》　◆筋肉質の体格をしている have a muscular[(がっしりした)sturdy] build　◆筋肉が落ちる muscles grow flabby /(筋力が低下する)muscles *become weak[weaken]　◆長らく寝たきりだったためすっかり筋肉が落ちてしまいましたね(衰える)Your muscles have become very weak because of your remaining[being] in bed too long.　◆筋肉の力が強い〈弱い〉ですね Your muscles are strong〈weak〉, aren't they?　◆筋肉をつける build up *one's muscles　◆筋肉が硬い〈やわらかい〉muscles are hard〈soft〉　◆筋肉が弛緩する muscles relax　◆筋肉が収縮する

muscles contract ◆筋肉が萎縮している muscles have shrunk[wasted away/atrophied]
《症状の表現》 ◆筋肉を痛める(無理に伸ばす) pull a muscle / (傷つける) injure a muscle ◆筋肉が痛む muscles ache / have *muscle pain[pain in *one's* muscles] ◆足の筋肉がどこか痛むのですか Are you having pain in any of your leg muscles? ◆筋肉は強直と弛緩を交互に繰り返しますか Do the muscles contract and relax by turns? ◆筋肉が硬直する have muscular stiffness[rigidity] ◆筋肉が突っ張る the muscles stiffen (up) ◆筋肉が勝手に動く muscles move without *one's* conscious control ◆筋肉がひきつる(激痛を伴って痙攣する) get a cramp / (ぴくぴく不随意に動く) have tics[spasms] / (急に突然ぴくっと収縮する) twitch ◆突然右足の筋肉がひきつったのですか Did the muscle in your right leg cramp up suddenly? / Did you have a sudden muscle cramp in your right leg?
《処置の表現》 ◆筋肉を刺激する stimulate *one's* muscles ◆お腹の筋肉を強化する strengthen *one's* abdominal muscles ◆筋肉をほぐす(緩める) loosen *one's* muscles / (リラックスさせる) relax *one's* muscles ◆筋肉をもみほぐす massage and loosen up *one's* muscles
▶筋肉増強剤 muscle-building drug / (アナボリックステロイド) anabolic steroid 筋肉(内)注射 intramuscular[IM] injection 筋肉トレーニング muscle training 筋肉疲労 muscle fatigue 筋肉労働 physical [manual] labor[work]

きんば 金歯 gold-capped tooth (圏 teeth), gold crown

ぎんば 銀歯 silver-capped tooth (圏 teeth), silver crown

きんぼうしりょく 近方視力 near visual acuity ☞近見視力

きんまく 筋膜 fascia (圏fascial) ▶筋膜炎 fasciitis 筋膜切開術 fasciotomy 筋膜皮弁 fasciocutaneous flap 筋膜弁 fascial flap

きんまんど (皮膚)緊満度 skin turgor

きんむ 勤務 (仕事)work (圏work) (交替制の勤務) shift (業務) service (任務) duty ◆勤務先はどちらですか Where do you work? / Who do you work for? ◆ここに勤務先の住所と電話番号を書いて下さい Please write your office[work] address and phone number here. ◆夜間の勤務につく work a night shift / work (on) the night shift ◆超過勤務する work overtime ◆超過勤務が多く疲れがたまりがちである fatigue tends to build up with overtime work ◆8時間の交代勤務 an eight-hour shift ◀交代勤務 shift work / (勤務時間) shift, rotation 交代勤務制 shift-work system 通常勤務 regular duty 日中勤務 day[daytime] work / day shift 夜間〈準夜/深夜〉勤務 night〈evening/late-night〉shift ▶勤務医 hospital doctor[physician] 勤務時間 working time[hours] 勤務体制(work) shift

きんむりょくしょう 筋無力症 myasthenia (圏myasthenic) ◀重症筋無力症 myasthenia gravis；MG 先天性筋無力症候群 congenital myasthenic syndrome ランバート・イートン筋無力症症候群 Lambert-Eaton myasthenic syndrome；LEMS ▶筋無力症クリーゼ myasthenic crisis

きんようび 金曜日 Friday；Fri. ◆金曜日に on Friday ◆金曜日ごとに on Fridays

きんりょく 筋力 muscle strength, muscular strength, muscle power[force] ◆筋力が衰える the muscles *become weak[weaken] ◆筋力を検査する check *a person's* muscle strength ◆筋力を測定する measure *a person's* muscle strength ◆筋力をつける build up *one's* muscle strength ▶筋力計 dynamometer 筋力増強訓練 muscle strengthening exercise 筋力低下 muscle weakness 筋力トレーニング muscle (strength) training

きんれんしゅく 筋攣縮 ☞筋痙攣

ぐあい 具合 ☞体調, 調子
《体調全般》 ◆今日の具合はいかがですか How do you feel today? / How are you feeling today? ◆この前診察してから具合はいかがでしたか How have you been since I last saw you? ◆具合はよくなりましたか Are you feeling better? ◆予防接種を受けて具合が悪くなったことがありますか Have you ever felt sick[unwell] after getting a vaccination? / Have you ever had any problems with previous vaccinations?
《病状》 ◆どこか具合が悪いのですか What's the matter? / Do you feel unwell[sick]? / Do you have any concerns about your health? ◆お腹の具合が悪いのですか Do you have any trouble[problems] with your abdomen? / Is there something wrong with your abdomen?
★疑問文では通例anythingを用いるが, この場合は相手から'Yes'という答えを予測しているのでsomethingを用いる. ◆どんな具合ですか What does it feel like? / What's the problem like? ◆痛みはどんな具合ですか What does the pain feel like? ◆具合が悪くなってからどのくらい経ちますか How long have you had the problem? ◆頭痛の具合がよくならない時には, もう一度来て下さい Please come back again if your headache hasn't improved.
《状態》 ◆入れ歯の具合はいかがですか How are your dentures?
《方法》 ◆こんな具合にやってみて下さい You should do it *(in) this way[like this]. ◆あなたの問題にはこういう具合に対応していきます This is how we approach your problem.

くいき 区域 （区分・ひと区切り・分節）segment （㊃segmental） （場所・空間・領域・範囲・地域）area （行政上の区画）district （建物内部の一画）section ◀亜区域 subsegment 管理区域 controlled area 喫煙区域 smoking section[area] 清潔区域 clean area ▶区域気管支 segmental bronchus 区域切除術 segmental resection / segmentectomy

くいちがい 食い違い （相違）difference （意見の不一致）disagreement （矛盾）inconsistency （㊃inconsistent） ◆前回伺ったお話と食い違っているようです What you're saying now seems to be inconsistent with what you said before. ◆退院後の介護についてご家族間の意見の食い違いを調整する必要があります As to your care after you're discharged, you should sort out any *differences of opinion[disagreements] that your family members may have.

くいとめる 食い止める ☞抑える, 止める
くいる 悔いる ☞悔やむ
クインケふしゅ ―浮腫 Quincke edema
くう 腔 cavity （空間）space ◀関節腔 joint[articular] cavity 胸腔 chest[thoracic] cavity くも膜下腔 subarachnoid space[cavity] 口腔 oral[mouth] cavity 骨盤腔 pelvic cavity 子宮腔 uterine cavity 腹腔 abdominal cavity
クウェート Kuwait （㊃Kuwaiti） ☞国籍 ▶クウェート人(の) Kuwaiti
ぐうかく 隅角 angle ◀前房隅角 anterior chamber angle ▶隅角鏡検査, 隅角緑内障
ぐうかくきょうけんさ 隅角鏡検査 gonioscopy ◆隅角鏡検査は緑内障を診断するための重要な目の検査です Gonioscopy is an important eye test used to *diagnose glaucoma[determine if you have glaucoma].
ぐうかくりょくないしょう 隅角緑内障 angle glaucoma ◀原発開放隅角緑内障 primary open-angle glaucoma；POAG 原発閉塞隅角緑内障 primary angle-closure glaucoma；PACG
くうかん 空間 space （㊃spatial） ◀視空間失認 visual-spatial agnosia 半側空間無視 hemispatial[unilateral spatial] neglect 閉鎖空間 confined space ▶空間

感覚 space sense[perception]

くうき 空気 air (喉頭aer(o)-) ◆胃の中に空気を入れますからゲップを我慢して下さい I'm going to pump air into your stomach (to expand your digestive tract), so hold on without belching. ◆窓を開けて空気を入れ替えましょうか Shall I open the windows and let in some fresh air? ▶空気圧 air pressure　空気嚥下症 aerophagia / aerophagy　空気感染 airborne infection　空気清浄器 air purifier　空気塞栓 air embolism

くうしょう 空床 empty (hospital) bed, vacant (hospital) bed, unoccupied (hospital) bed ◆現時点で空床はありません We don't have any empty beds right now. / There are no beds available right now. ◆空床がいくつかあります There are several empty beds available.

ぐうぜん 偶然(の) ☞偶然

くうちょう¹ 空腸 jejunum (形jejunal)

くうちょう² 空調 air conditioning ▶空調病 air conditioning disease

くうどう 空洞 cavity (形cavitary) ◆右肺に空洞がある have[show] a cavity in the right lung ◀脊髄空洞症 syringomyelia ▶空洞形成 cavity formation / cavitation　空洞性病変 cavitary lesion

くうないしょうしゃ 腔内照射 intracavitary irradiation

ぐうはつ 偶発(性・的の) (予期しない・過失による)accidental (図accident) (…に付随した)incidental (副たまたま by chance) ◆偶発的に見つかったがん cancer found by chance / incidental cancer ▶偶発事故 accident　偶発性アルブミン尿 accidental albuminuria　偶発性低体温 accidental hypothermia　偶発的発見 accidental[incidental] finding

くうふく 空腹 (飢え)hunger (形hungry) (空き腹)empty stomach ◆空腹時にお腹が痛みますか Do you get a stomachache *when your stomach is empty[when you're hungry]? ◆この薬は空腹時に飲んで下さい Please take this medication on an empty stomach. ◆空腹を感じる feel [be] hungry ◆空腹を満たす satisfy *one's hunger ▶空腹感 feeling of hunger　空腹時血糖値 *fasting blood sugar[FBS] level　空腹時痛 hunger pains　空腹時低血糖 fasting hypoglycemia

くうほう 空胞 vacuole (形vacuolar) ▶空胞形成 vacuolation / vacuolization　空胞変性 vacuolar degeneration

クームスしけん ─試験 Coombs test ◀直接〈間接〉クームス試験 direct〈indirect〉Coombs test

くうらん 空欄 blank ◆空欄にご記入下さい Please fill out[in] the blanks. ◆空欄にお名前と住所を書いて下さい Please write your name and address in the blanks.

クール (治療単位・経過)course (of treatment) ◆薬物療法の1クール a course of drug[medication] therapy ◆化学療法の1クール目 the first course of chemotherapy

クエンさん ─酸 citric acid

クオリティ quality ☞質

クオリティ・オブ・ライフ quality of life；QOL ☞生活の質

くがつ 9月 September；Sept. ☞1月

くけつたい 駆血帯 tourniquet /tɚ́ːnɪkət/, tight band ◆腕にこの駆血帯を巻きましょう Let me put this tourniquet [tight band] on your arm.

くさい 臭い smell (形bad smell) ☞悪臭, 臭い(におい) ◆息が臭い have (a) bad breath / *one's breath smells ◆息がアルコール臭い smell alcohol on *a person's breath

くさび 楔 wedge ▶楔状欠損 wedge-shaped defect

くさる 腐る (食べ物が傷む)go bad, spoil (形spoiled) (物が徐々に自然に腐ってゆく)rot (形rotten), decay (形decayed) ◆胸水は腐ったにおいがする The pleural fluid smells bad. ◆尿は腐った卵のようなにおいがする The urine smells like rotten eggs.

くし 櫛 comb /kóʊm/ (形comb)

くじく 挫く (捻挫する)sprain (ひねる)twist ◆転んで足首をくじく fall down

くじく | 197 | くすり

and sprain[twist] *one's* ankle

くしゃみ sneeze (図sneeze) ◆くしゃみがよく出ますか Do you sneeze a lot? ▶くしゃみ反射 sneeze[nasal] reflex

くしゅつ 駆出 ejection ▶駆出音 ejection sound 駆出期 ejection period 駆出雑音 ejection murmur 駆出時間 ejection time

くじょ 駆除する (除去する) get rid of, eliminate (図elimination) ◆回虫を駆除する *get rid of[eliminate] roundworms ◀回虫駆除薬 lumbricide

くじょう 苦情 complaint (國complain about[of]) (不当な扱いに対する不満) grievance ◆騒音についてのあなたの苦情には速やかに対処いたします We'll take some prompt measures to *deal with [handle] your complaints about the noise. ◆診察までの待ち時間の長さに苦情を言う complain about long wait times to see *one's* doctor ▶苦情処理委員会 complaints[grievance] committee 苦情処理手続き complaints[grievance] procedure

くしん 苦心 (努力)effort (面倒)trouble ☞苦労

くずかご 屑かご wastebasket

くすぐりかん ―感 tickling sensation, tickle sensation

クスマウルだいこきゅう ―大呼吸 Kussmaul respiration

くすり 薬 medication, medicine (國薬の・薬効のある medicinal) ★tablet (錠剤), pill (丸薬),powder(粉薬)など, いろいろな剤形の薬品の総称. 日常会話では medicine が一般的に使われる. (薬・薬物)drug ☞医薬品, 薬剤, 薬品, 薬物

《処方の説明》 (処方する) prescribe (a) medication (for) (投与する)give[administer] (a) medication (to *a patient*) (調合する) dispense[prepare] (a) medication ◆症状を和らげるための薬〈鎮痛剤〉をお出しします I'm going to[Let me] give you *some medicine〈a painkiller / an analgesic〉to relieve your symptoms.
◆いつもの薬を出しましょう I'll write you a prescription for your usual medication.
◆薬を変えて様子を見ましょう Let's *try a different medication[change the medication] and see what happens. ◆薬は水薬でお出しします I'm going to give you a liquid medication. ◆この薬は2週間分です This medication is for two weeks.
◆2種類の飲み薬が出ています You'll take two kinds of medicine. ◆これは薬の処方箋です This is a prescription for your medication. ◆薬を院外薬局でもらって下さい Please *pick up your medication [have your medication filled] at an outside pharmacy. ★院内薬局は the hospital pharmacy. ◆今日はお薬(の処方)がありません You don't need any medication today. ◆その薬は日本では手に入りません That medication is not available in Japan. ◆(入院中に)クロスさん, お薬ですよ Mrs Cross, here's your medicine.
《効能・効果の説明》 ◆関節炎の治療薬 a medication for (treating) arthritis ◆熱を下げる薬 (a) medication to *bring down [lower / reduce] fever ◆吐き気を和らげる〈軽減する / 止める〉薬 (a) medication to relieve〈reduce / stop〉nausea ◆細菌を殺す薬 (a) medication to kill bacteria
◆この薬は寝つきをよくしてくれます This medication will help you (to) fall asleep. / This is a medication to induce sleeping. ◆この薬はめまいに効きます This medicine is good[effective] for dizziness. ◆これは消化を助けるための薬です This medicine aids your digestion. / This medication is good[effective] for digestion. ◆この薬で痛みが治まるでしょう The pain should *go away[disappear] with this medication. / This medication should get rid of the pain. ◆この2つの薬は効き目という点で大きな違いはありません In terms of their effectiveness, there's not much difference between these two medications. ◆この薬は効果がすぐに現れるでしょう This medicine will take effect *right away[instantly].
◆この前の薬は効きましたか Did the last

medication work well?

《薬歴の聴取》 ◆現在何か薬を飲んでいますか Are you taking any medication(s)?/Are you on any medication(s)? ◆その薬は処方薬ですか，市販薬ですか Are they prescription medications or over-the-counter drugs? ◆お薬をお持ちでしたら見せていただけますか If you have the medications with you now, may I see them? ◆お薬手帳を持っていますか．持っていたら見せて下さい Do you have your personal medication record with you now? If you do, could I take a look at it, please? ◆(入院時に)現在飲んでいる薬をお持ち下さい Please bring any medications you are taking. ◆薬に対するアレルギーがありますか Are you allergic to any medications?/Do you have any drug allergies? ◆どの薬に対するアレルギーですか Which medications are you allergic to? ◆どんなアレルギー反応を起こしますか What happens to you when you have an allergic reaction?/What kind of allergic reaction do you have?

《用法・用量の説明》 (服用する) take (a) medication[medicine] (飲み込む) swallow (a) medication (使う) use (a) medication (軟膏を塗る) apply (an) ointment (吸入する) inhale (a) medication ◆お出しした薬の説明書です Here are the instructions for taking your medication. ◆この薬は指示通りに飲んで〈使って〉下さい Please take〈use〉this medicine exactly as directed[prescribed by your doctor]. ◆この薬は1日3回，2錠ずつ飲んで下さい Please take two of these tablets three times a day. ◆この薬は6時間おきに飲んで下さい Please take this medication every six hours. ◆この薬は1日2回朝晩食後に服用して下さい Please take this medication twice a day, in the morning and evening, after eating. ◆飲み忘れた時にはすぐに飲んで下さい If you forget to take your[this] medication[If you skip or miss a dose of this medication], take it as soon as you realize[remember]. ◆次の服用が近い時には，とばして次の服用まで待って下さい If it's almost time for your next dose, skip the last dose and wait until the time for the next dose. ◆飲み忘れても一度に2回分を飲まないで下さい If you skip[miss] a dose, please don't take *two doses[a double dose] at one time. ◆この薬は胸の痛みの症状が出始めたら飲んで下さい Please take this medication whenever you begin to feel chest pain. ◆この薬は必要に応じて飲んで下さい Please take this medication whenever you need it. ◆この薬は症状がなくなっても最後まで飲み続けて下さい Please continue taking this medication for the full course of treatment even if your symptoms disappear. ◆この薬は水かぬるめのお湯で飲んで下さい Please take this medication with water or lukewarm water. ◆薬を多めの水で飲む take the medication with *plenty of[a lot of] water ◆この薬は噛むか口の中で溶かしながら飲んで下さい This medicine should be chewed or allowed to dissolve in the mouth. ◆噛まずに薬を口の中で溶かして下さい Please let the medication dissolve in your mouth without chewing. ◆この薬は舌の下に入れて完全に溶かして下さい Please place this tablet[pill] under your tongue and let it dissolve completely. ◆この丸薬を飲み込めない時は砕いて食べ物や水，ジュースに混ぜて下さい If you can't swallow this pill, you can crush and mix it with[in] some food, water, or juice. ◆この粉薬を飲み込めない時はジュースやヨーグルトに混ぜて下さい If you can't swallow this powder, you can mix it with juice or yogurt. ◆この薬は25 mgです The dose of this medication is twenty-five milligrams. ◆薬の服用量を減らす decrease[lower] the dose[dosage] ◆薬の服用量を増やす increase the dose[dosage] ★doseは1回の摂取量，dosageは一定期間にわたり用いる摂取量をいう．

《副作用の注意》 ◆この薬はいくらか軽い副作用があります This medication has some

mild side effects. ◆まれですが，時に副作用が起こることがあります Side effects are rare, but they sometimes occur. ◆副作用には頭痛，むくみ，食欲不振などがあります Side effects include headaches, swelling, and loss of appetite. ◆この薬を飲むと，時には吐き気，嘔吐，脱毛などの症状が出るかもしれません With this medicine you may sometimes have symptoms such as nausea, vomiting, or hair loss.

◆この薬を飲むと眠くなるかもしれません This medication may make you sleepy.

◆この薬を飲んでいる間は運転しないで下さい Don't drive (your car) while taking this medication. ◆この薬は飲み続けると習慣性になります If you take this medication for a long time, it may[will] become habit-forming[addictive]. ◆この薬で何か予期しない副作用がみられる時は連絡して下さい Please call us and let us know if you notice any unexpected side effects.

◆副作用は体がこの薬に慣れるにつれて消えるでしょう The side effects will go away after your body gets used to this medication. ◆副作用はこの薬を飲み続ける間ずっと続くかもしれません The side effects may continue for as long as you take this medication. / (治療中ずっと) The side effects may continue throughout (your) therapy.

《相互作用の注意》 ◆薬物相互作用 medication[drug / drug-drug] interaction ◆薬物・食品相互作用 drug-food interaction

◆この薬は他の薬と相互作用を起こすかもしれません This medication may interact [cause (adverse) interactions] with other medications. ◆他の薬がこの薬の作用を弱めたり強めたりする〈遅らせたり速めたりする〉恐れがあります Other medications might *reduce or increase〈slow down or speed up〉the action of this medication.

◆この薬と一緒にグレープフルーツを食べたりグレープフルーツジュースを飲んだりしないで下さい Please don't eat grapefruit or drink grapefruit juice with this medication. ◆新しい薬を飲む前には必ず医師か

薬剤師にご相談下さい Please be sure to check with your doctor or pharmacist before taking a new medication. ◆処方された薬以外は医師に相談なく飲まないで下さい Please do not take any *nonprescribed medications[(市販薬) over-the-counter drugs] without consulting your doctor.

《保管上の注意》 ◆この薬は室温で保管して下さい Please keep this medication at room temperature. ◆この薬は冷蔵庫の中で保管して下さい Please keep this medication *in the refrigerator[refrigerated]. ◆直射日光を避け，涼しくて乾燥した場所に保管して下さい Please do not keep this medication in the sun, but keep it in a cool, dry place. / Please keep [store] this medication *away from[out of] direct sunlight, in a cool, dry place.

▶薬アレルギー medication[drug] allergy 薬代(一般的に) cost of medication / (処方箋の代金) prescription charge (お)薬手帳 personal medication record[history handbook] 薬箱 medicine cabinet / (救急のための) first aid kit 薬屋(薬局) pharmacy,《英》chemist / (化粧品・文房具など一般的な商品も売る店) drugstore

---

用法に用いられる表現

■回数・時間
●1日1回 once a day ●1日2回 twice[two times] a day ●1日3回 three times a day ●1時間ごとに every hour ●6時間ごとに every six hours ●週1回 once a week

■タイミング
●起床時に when you get up ●朝に in the morning ●昼に in the afternoon ●夜に in the evening / at night ●寝る前に before you go to bed ●就寝時に at bedtime ●運動の前に before (you) exercise ●空腹時に on an empty stomach ●必要に応じて as needed ●熱がある時 when you have a fever ●痛みがある時 when you have (a) pain ●吐き

気がある時 when you feel nauseous[like vomiting] ●便秘の時 when you are constipated ●下痢の時 when you have diarrhea ●医師の指示通りに as directed by *one's* doctor

■食事との関連
●食前に before meals ●食前30分に thirty minutes before eating ●食直前に right[immediately] before eating ●食事と一緒に with meals ●食後に after meals ●食直後に right[immediately] after eating ●食後30分に thirty minutes after eating ●食事の1時間前か2時間後に one hour before or two hours after eating ●朝食後に after breakfast ●昼食後に after lunch ●夕食後に after supper ●食間に between meals

剤形に関する表現

■内服薬 oral[internal] medication
●錠剤 tablet ●丸薬 pill ●カプセル剤 capsule ●粉薬 powder / powdered medication ●顆粒剤 medication in granular form / granules ●液剤[水薬] liquid medication ●シロップ syrup ●舌下錠 medication under *one's* tongue / sublingual tablet ●トローチ troche / (薬用ドロップ)(throat) lozenge

■外用薬
●湿布薬 compress / poultice ●温湿布 hot compress[pack / pad] / heat pack[pad] ●冷湿布 cold compress[pack / pad] / (氷の) ice pack[pad] ●貼付薬 patch ●スプレー薬 spray ●軟膏 ointment ●クリーム cream ●ローション lotion ●点眼薬 eye drops[lotion] ●点耳薬 ear drops ●点鼻薬 nose drops ●うがい薬 gargle / (口内洗浄の) mouthwash / (咽頭洗浄の) throat wash ●吸入薬 inhalant ●坐薬 (rectal) suppository ●浣腸 enema ●腟坐薬 vaginal suppository

■注射薬
●静脈注射 intravenous injection ●点滴 intravenous[IV] drip / drip infusion ●皮下注射 hypodermic injection / subcutaneous injection ●筋肉注射 intramuscular injection

薬効による分類

●降圧薬 antihypertensive (medication / drug / agent) / hypotensive (medication / drug / agent) ●抗菌薬 antibacterial (medication / drug / agent) / antibiotics ●風邪薬 cold medication ●鎮咳薬 cough suppressant / antitussive (medication / drug / agent) / (ドロップ) cough drop / (シロップ) cough syrup ●解熱薬 antipyretic (medication / drug / agent) ●鎮痛薬 painkiller / pain reliever / medication for pain / analgesic (medication / drug / agent) ●鎮痛解熱薬 analgesic-antipyretic (medication / drug / agent) / painkiller and medication for fever ●胃薬 stomach medication ●消化薬 digestive (medication / drug / agent) ●止瀉薬 diarrhea medication / antidiarrheal (medication / drug / agent) ●制吐薬 antiemetic (medication / drug / agent) / antinausea medication[drug / agent] ●下剤 laxative (medication / drug / agent) / purgative (medication / drug / agent) ●睡眠薬 sleeping pill ●止痒薬 (一般的に) medication for itching / medication to relieve[stop / prevent] itching / antipruritic (medication / drug / agent) / (軟膏) antiitch ointment[(クリーム) cream]

くすりゆび 薬指 ring finger, third finger ★親指を入れずに人差し指から数えて3番目の指になる. ☞指

ぐずる fret, get[become, be] fretful ◆子供がいつもよりぐずっています The child ⟨baby⟩ is more fretful than usual.

くせ 癖 habit ☞習慣 ◆爪を嚙む癖がある have a habit of *biting one's* nails[nail-biting] ◆髪の毛を抜く癖は直した方がよいでしょう You should break[get rid of] the habit of pulling out your hair. / You should try to overcome the[your] habit of pulling out your hair. ◆指しゃぶりは子供によくある癖ですから，あせらずに直してあげて下さい Thumb sucking is a common habit among children, so just take your time to cure[break] it. ◆この薬は長期間飲み続けると癖になるかもしれません If you take this medication for a long time, it may be habit-forming[addictive].

くだ　管　tube ☞チューブ ◆この管を膀胱に入れて尿を採ります Let me insert [put / place] this tube into your bladder to drain the urine. / I'm going to drain the urine from your bladder with this tube.
◆管をゴクンと飲んで下さい Please swallow this tube in one gulp. ◆この処置は管をお腹の壁を通して胃の中に入れるものです This is a procedure for inserting [putting / passing] a tube through the abdominal wall and into the stomach.
◆気管から管を抜く remove the tube from the windpipe

ぐたいてき　具体的（な） (明確な)**specific** (事実に基づいた)**concrete** ◆何が問題なのかをもう少し具体的にお話ししていただけますか（詳しく）Could you tell me about the problem in more detail? /（より明確に）Could you tell me more specifically about the problem? ◆具体的な証拠 concrete evidence

くだく　砕く　break (into pieces) (細かくつぶす)**crush** ◆胆石を砕く crush a gallstone

くだもの　果物　fruit ★fruit は通例，単数形で．◆新鮮な果物と野菜を食べる eat fresh fruit and vegetables

くち　口　mouth (圏oral) ◆口に何か問題がありますか Do you have any problems with your mouth?
《部位の表現》◆口の中に inside *one's* mouth. ◆口の周りに around *one's* mouth ◆口の角に at the corners[edges] of *one's* mouth
《動作の表現》◆口をもっと大きく開けて「アー」と言って下さい Please open your

mouth wider. Say "ah." ◆口を閉じて，いつも通りに鼻から呼吸して下さい Close your mouth and breathe through your nose normally. ◆息を鼻から吸って口から吐く breathe in through the nose and breathe out from the mouth ◆口で呼吸する breathe through *one's* mouth ◆口を閉じる shut[close] *one's* mouth ◆口をぎゅっと閉じる squeeze *one's* mouth shut / shut *one's* mouth tight[tightly] ◆口〈唇〉をすぼめる purse[pucker] *one's* mouth〈lips〉 ◆口を湿らせる moisten *one's* mouth ◆口を拭く wipe *one's* mouth ◆口をゆすぐ rinse out *one's* mouth
《所見・症状の表現》◆口が乾いていますか Do you have (a) dry mouth? / Is your mouth dry? / Does your mouth feel dry? ◆口がしびれていますか Is your mouth numb? / Does your mouth feel numb? /（周囲が）Do you feel numb around your mouth? ◆口を開けると痛みますか Does it hurt when you open your mouth? ◆口がにおう have bad breath / The breath smells bad. ◆口の中にただれ〈潰瘍〉がある have sores〈ulcers〉inside *one's* mouth.
☞口当たり, 口呼吸, 口すぼめ呼吸, 口に合う, 口にする, 口笛

くちあたり　口当たり ◆口当たりのよい食べ物（飲み込みやすいもの）food that is easy to swallow /（口になめらかな後味を残すもの）food that leaves a smooth taste in the mouth

くちこきゅう　口呼吸　mouth breathing, breathing through *one's* mouth

くちすぼめこきゅう　口すぼめ呼吸 pursed-lip breathing ☞呼吸(囲み：呼吸法)
◆口すぼめ呼吸をする breathe through pursed lips / breathe pursing *one's* lips
◆口すぼめ呼吸の練習をする do pursed-lip breathing exercises

くちにあう　口に合う ◆病院食がお口に合えばよいのですが I hope you'll like our hospital food.

くちにする　口にする ◆検査前 8 時間は

何も口にしないで下さい Please don't eat, drink, or chew anything for eight hours before the test.

くちびる 唇 lips ★通例，複数形で．
◆唇をすぼめてゆっくり息を吐いて下さい Purse[Pucker] your lips and breathe out slowly through your mouth．◆唇が荒れる have rough[chapped] lips ◆唇が腫れる have swelling of the lips / have swollen lips ◆唇が青く〈紫色に〉なる one's lips turn[become] blue〈purple〉 ◆唇を噛む bite one's lip ◆唇を湿らせる moisten one's lips ◆唇をなめる lick one's lips ◆乾いた唇 dry lips ◀上唇 upper lip 下唇 lower lip ▶唇形成術 cheiloplasty

くちぶえ 口笛 whistle (動whistle, give a whistle) ◆口笛を吹く時のように唇をすぼめて下さい Purse your lips as if to whistle.

くちゅうやく 駆虫薬 vermicide, anthelmintic

くつ 靴 shoes ★通例，複数形で．片方だけであれば a shoe．◆靴を脱ぐ take one's shoes off / take off one's shoes ◆靴を履く put one's shoes on / put on one's shoes ◆靴を脱いでこの体重計の上に乗って下さい Please take your shoes off and step[stand] on this scale．◆靴がきつくなりましたか Do your shoes feel tight? ◀整形靴 orthopedic shoes / (靴型装具)corrective shoes ☞靴下，靴擦れ

くつう 苦痛 (痛み)pain (肉体的・精神的な苦しみ)suffering ◆痛み，苦しむ ◆病気のために身体的に苦痛がある suffer physically from an illness ◆苦痛を訴える complain of (a) pain[suffering] ◆苦痛を和らげる relieve[ease] one's pain[suffering] ◆苦痛に耐える endure suffering ◀身体的苦痛 physical pain[suffering] 精神的苦痛 psychological pain[suffering]

くっきょく 屈曲 bending (動bend), flexion (動flex) ◀過屈曲損傷 hyperflexion injury ▶屈曲拘縮 flexion contracture 屈曲姿勢 flexed posture

くっきり (明瞭に)clearly (違いが明らかに)

distinctly ◆白内障の手術の後，物がくっきり見えるようになります After the cataract surgery you'll be able to see things clearly．◆足の血管がくっきり膨らんで見えるのに初めて気づいたのはいつですか When did you first notice the distinct swelling in the veins in your leg(s)?

くっきん 屈筋 flexor (muscle)

くつした 靴下 (短い靴下)socks (長い靴下)stockings ★いずれも複数形で．☞ストッキング，ソックス ◆靴下を脱いで下さい Please take your socks[stockings] off. ◀手袋靴下型感覚消失 glove and stocking anesthesia

クッション cushion

くっしん 屈伸 ◆膝の屈伸をする do knee bends / do knee-bending (and stretching)

クッシングしょうこうぐん —症候群 Cushing syndrome

クッシングびょう —病 Cushing disease

ぐっすり ◆昨夜はぐっすり眠りましたか Did you sleep well last night? ◆赤ちゃんはぐっすり眠っています Your baby is fast[sound] asleep.

くつずれ 靴擦れ (水疱)blister caused by one's shoe(s) ◆靴擦れができる get a shoe sore

くっせつ 屈折 refraction (形refractive) ▶屈折異常 refractive error / error of refraction / ametropia 屈折矯正手術 refractive surgery 屈折検査 refraction test / refractometry 屈折率 refractive index；RI

ぐったり ◆疲れてぐったりしているようですね You look tired out. / You look extremely[dead] tired．◆熱は下がっても彼はまだぐったりしています The fever has gone down, but he's still very weak and *without any energy[has no energy]．◆あまりの暑さにぐったりする feel weak and weary with the heat

くっつく stick (to) (粘りつく)adhere (to) ☞付着

ぐっと ◆このバリウムをぐっと飲み込んで

下さい Please swallow this barium mixture in one gulp. / Please swallow this barium mixture down as quickly as you can. ◆坐薬は抜け出てこないように直腸の中へぐっと押し込んで下さい Push[Insert] the suppository well[deeply] into the rectum（opening）so that it won't fall out. ★この場合，英語では肛門（anus）という語を避ける。◆上体をぐっと後ろに反らす lean[bend] back as far as *one* can

グッドパスチャーしょうこうぐん　―症候群　Goodpasture syndrome

くに　国　country　（母国）*one's*（own）country ◆お国はどちらですか Where are you from? / What country are you from? ◆夏休みはお国に帰るご予定ですか Are you planning to *go home[go back to your country] during the summer vacation? ◆お国での手術を希望しますか Would you like to have the surgery in your own country?

くび　首　neck　（頭部を含めて）head ◆首に何か問題がありますか Do you have any problems with your neck? ◆首を怪我したことがありますか Have you ever had a neck injury? ◆首を診察しましょう I'm going to feel[examine] your neck.
《部位の表現》痛むのは首の後ろ，横，あるいは前ですか Is the pain in the back, side, or front of your neck? ◆首の前〈後ろ〉the front〈back〉of *one's* neck ◆首の横 the side(s) of *one's* neck ◆首の周りに around *one's* neck
《動作の表現》◆首を右〈左〉に傾けて下さい Please tilt[lean / put] your head to the right〈left〉. ◆首を左右に傾ける tilt *one's* head from side to side ◆首を前後に曲げる bend *one's* neck[head] forward and backward ◆首を回す（水平に回旋する）turn *one's* head / （回転させる）rotate *one's* head
《所見・症状の表現》◆首を動かしにくいですか Do you have any difficulty moving your neck? / Is it difficult to move your neck? ◆首が痛みますか Do you have（any）*neck pain[pain in the neck]? / Is

your neck painful? ◆首が腫れたことがありますか Have you ever noticed any swelling in your neck? ◆首が以前より太くなっているように感じますか Does your neck seem larger than before? ◆首の両側にしこりがあります You have lumps on both sides of your neck. ◆首のリンパ節が腫れています The lymph nodes in your neck have swollen up. / You have swollen lymph nodes in your neck ◆（赤ちゃんの）首がすわる hold *one's* head up（steady）/ have good neck control ◆首が傾いている *one's* head tilts to one side ◆首が腫れる have a swelling in *one's* neck ◆首が凝る have a stiff neck / feel stiff in the neck / have stiffness and muscle tension in the neck ◆首を寝違える（首の筋肉が痙攣する）*get a crick[crick] in *one's* neck while sleeping / （首をひねる）twist *one's* neck while sleeping ◆首の骨を折る break *one's* neck

◀白鳥の首変形 swan-neck deformiy
▶首吊り（縊死）death by hanging ☞首筋，首周り

くびすじ　首筋　the back of the neck, the nape of the neck ◆首筋が痛い feel some pain *at the back[in the nape] of the neck ◆首筋を違える（首をひねる）twist *one's* neck / （首の筋肉が痙攣する）crick *one's* neck ◆首筋がこわばる have a stiff neck / feel stiff in the neck

くびまわり　首周り ◆首周りを測る measure *one's* neck size ◆首周りのサイズは前と比べて大きくなりましたか Has your collar size become larger?

くべつ　区別する　（一般的に見分ける）tell（違いを識別する）distinguish[make a distinction]（細かく比較して差異をつける）differentiate ◆色の区別がつきにくいですか Do you have difficulty *telling the difference[distinguishing] between colors? ◆良性のポリープと悪性のポリープを区別する distinguish[differentiate] a benign polyp from a malignant one

クボステックちょうこう　―徴候　Chvostek sign

くぼみ 凹み・窪み （乳房のくぼみ）dimple （⯂dimpled） （皮膚などのくぼみ）pit （⯂pitted） （穴）hole ☞凹み（へこみ） ◆いつ乳房のくぼみに気づきましたか When did you first notice the dimple in[on] your breast? ◆にきびの痕によるくぼみが気になりますか Are you worried[concerned] about pits[holes] being left on the skin by the pimples[acne]?

くま 隈 ◆目の下〈周り〉の隈 dark circles [rings] under〈around〉one's eyes ★複数形で.

くみあわせる 組み合わせる combine ◆治療効果を上げるため化学療法と放射線療法を組み合わせます We'll combine chemotherapy with radiation therapy to improve the effectiveness of the treatment. ◆この薬はこれまであなたが飲んでいる薬との組み合わせに問題がありません（相互に悪影響を及ぼさない）This medication does not have any adverse interactions with the medication that you've been taking.

くめん 工面 ◆もし治療費の工面が難しいようであれば当院のソーシャルワーカーに相談してみてはいかがですか If you're worried[concerned] about how you're going to pay the medical fees[bills], how about consulting with a social worker in the hospital?

くもじょうけっかんかくちょう 一状血管拡張 spider telangiectasia

くもじょうけっかんしゅ 一状血管腫 spider angioma, vascular spider

くもじょうゆび 一状指 spider finger, arachnodactyly

くもまく 一膜 arachnoid （membrane） ◀脊髄くも膜下麻酔 spinal anesthesia ▶くも膜下腔 subarachnoid space[cavity] くも膜下槽 subarachnoid cisterns くも膜嚢胞 arachnoid cyst ☞くも膜下出血

くもまくかしゅっけつ 一膜下出血 subarachnoid hemorrhage /sʌ̀bəræknɔɪd hémɔrɪʤ/；SAH, subarachnoid bleeding ◆脳動脈の破裂はくも膜下出血の主な原因になります Rupture of a cerebral aneurysm is a leading cause of subarachnoid hemorrhage. ◀外傷性くも膜下出血 traumatic subarachnoid bleeding[hemorrhage]

くもる 曇る （物がぼやける）get[become, be] blurred （レンズなどが濁る）get[become, be] cloudy[clouded] ◆視界が曇りますか Is your vision blurred? / Do you have blurred vision? ◆目のレンズが曇ってきています The lens in your eye(s) has become cloudy[clouded]. ◆白く曇る become milky （and cloudy） / become *cloudy white[a cloudy white color]

くもん 苦悶 agony ◆顔に苦悶の表情を浮かべる（the) agony shows in one's face / look as if one is in agony

くやくしょ 区役所 ward office

くやみ 悔やみ ☞お悔やみ

くやむ 悔やむ （後悔する）regret （⯂regrettable） （残念に思う）feel[be] sorry （for） ◆もっと早く腫瘍を発見できなかったことが悔やまれます We regret that the tumor was not detected earlier. ◆途中で治療を止めたことが悔やまれます It's regrettable [遺憾・不運な] unfortunate] that you stopped the treatment halfway. ◆40歳の若さでがんでお亡くなりになられたのが悔やまれます I feel sorry that he〈she〉died of cancer at the young age of forty.

クラーク clerk ◆この用紙を受付のクラークにお渡し下さい Please give this form to a clerk at the reception desk. ◀病棟クラーク ward[floor / unit] clerk / （取りまとめ役）unit coordinator

くらい 暗い dark （気分が落ち込んだ）depressed （気分が重苦しい）gloomy ◆暗い気持ちになる feel depressed[gloomy]

クライエント client ▶クライエント中心療法 client-centered therapy

クライオサージェリー （凍結手術）cryosurgery

クライシス crisis （⯂crises） ☞危機

クラインフェルターしょうこうぐん 一症候群 Klinefelter syndrome

クラウン¹ （冠・歯冠）crown

クラウン² （臨床道化師）hospital clown,

CliniClown

ぐらぐら loose ◆ぐらぐらしている歯がありますか Do you have any loose teeth?

くらくらする (めまいがする)feel dizzy (頭がふらふらする)*one's* head is swimming (ぐるぐる回る)*one's* head is spinning ☞めまい

くらす 暮らす (生活する)live (生計を立てる)make a living, earn a living ◆どなたと一緒に暮らしていますか Who lives with you? / Who do you live with? ◆退院後はどこで暮らしたいですか After you leave the hospital, where would you like to live [stay]? ◆英語を教えて暮らす make [earn] *one's* living by teaching English ◆年金で暮らす live on a pension ◆のんびり暮らす lead a quiet life / live leisurely / live a leisurely life

グラスゴーこんすいしゃくど 一昏睡尺度 Glasgow coma scale；GCS

クラッシュしょうこうぐん 一症候群 crush syndrome

クラッチ crutches ★複数形で．☞松葉杖

グラフト graft ☞移植片

くらべる 比べる compare (with) ☞比較

クラミジア chlamydia (㊟chlamydial) (学名)*Chlamydia* ◀性器クラミジア感染症 genital chlamydiosis ▶クラミジア感染症 chlamydial infection クラミジア頸管炎 chlamydial cervicitis クラミジア結膜炎 chlamydial conjunctivitis クラミジア・トラコマチス感染症 *Chlamydia trachomatis* infection クラミジア・ニューモニエ感染症 *Chlamydia pneumoniae* infection クラミジア尿道炎 chlamydial urethritis クラミジア肺炎 chlamydial pneumonia

グラム[1] gram；g ☞数字 ◆赤ちゃんの体重は 3,500 グラムです Your baby weighs three thousand five hundred grams. ◆1 錠の中には 50 ミリグラムの有効成分が含まれています Each tablet contains fifty milligrams of the active ingredient. ◀キログラム kilogram；kg ミリグラム milligram；mg マイクログラム

microgram；μg ナノグラム nanogram；ng ピコグラム picogram；pg

グラム[2] Gram, gram ▶グラム陰性桿菌 gram-negative bacillus グラム陰性菌 gram-negative bacterium グラム染色 Gram stain グラム陽性球菌 gram-positive coccus グラム陽性菌 gram-positive bacterium

くらやみきょうふ 暗闇恐怖(症) nyctophobia

グリアさいぼう 一細胞 glial cell, glia (cell), neuroglia (cell)

クリアランス clearance ◀腎クリアランス renal clearance 粘液線毛クリアランス mucociliary clearance

クリーゼ crisis ☞危機 ◀筋無力症クリーゼ myasthenic crisis 副腎クリーゼ adrenal crisis

グリーフ (悲嘆)grief ▶グリーフカウンセリング grief counseling グリーフケア grief care

クリーム cream ◆クリームをたっぷり患部に塗る liberally apply the cream to the affected area / lubricate the area with a generous amount of cream ◆日焼け止めのクリームを塗る *put on[apply] sun cream ◆市販のクリーム over-the-counter cream ◀スキンクリーム skin cream 洗顔クリーム facial cleansing cream 保護クリーム protective cream[ointment] 保湿クリーム moisturizing cream / moisturizer ▶クリーム剤 cream

クリーンルーム clean room, bioclean room

クリオグロブリンけつしょう 一血症 cryoglobulinemia

くりかえす 繰り返す repeat /rɪpíːt/ (㊟repetition /rèpətíʃən/ ㊟repétitive) (再発する)recur /rɪkə́ː/ (㊟recurrence ㊟recurrent) ◆周期的に繰り返す repeat periodically ◆断続的に繰り返す repeat intermittently ◆繰り返し説明する explain repeatedly[over and over / again and again] ◆私の言ったことを繰り返して下さい Please repeat what I've just said. ◆すみませんが，繰り返していただけますか

I beg your pardon? / Could you please repeat that? ★I beg your pardon? は聞き返す時の決まった言い方．上昇口調でいう．

◆リハビリには繰り返しが大切です Repetition is important in rehabilitation exercise. / Repetitive exercise is an important element of rehabilitation. ◆（禁煙・断酒など）ここで諦めてしまったら同じことの繰り返しになってしまいます If you give up at this stage, *you'll just find yourself repeating the process[you'll just have to repeat the same process] over again at a later stage. ◆繰り返し咳が出る have a recurrent cough ◆感染症を繰り返していますか Does the infection keep *coming back[recurring]? ◆下痢と便秘を交互に繰り返しますか Do you have alternating (bouts of) diarrhea and constipation? ◆周期的に繰り返す痛みがある have periodic pain

グリコーゲン glycogen ▶グリコーゲン病 glycogen storage disease

グリコヘモグロビン glycated hemoglobin

クリスチャン Christian

グリセリン glycerin ▶グリセリン浣腸 glycerin enema

グリセロールけんさ ―検査 glycerol test

クリック click (動click) ◆収縮期クリック systolic click ▶クリック音 clicking sound クリック徴候 click sign

クリッピング clipping ◀脳動脈瘤クリッピング cerebral aneurysm clipping ▶クリッピング術 surgical clipping

クリップ clip (動clip) ◆出血した血管をクリップで留める clip bleeding blood vessels / apply clips to stop the bleeding of blood vessels ◆鼻のクリップを付ける apply a nose clip ◆鼻のクリップを外す remove[take off] the nose clip ◆金属クリップ metal clip 手術用クリップ surgical clip 創縁クリップ wound clip

クリティカルパス critical pathway[path]

クリトリス clitoris

クリニカルパス clinical pathway[path]

クリニクラウン （臨床道化師）hospital clown, CliniClown

クリニック clinic ◀歯科クリニック dental clinic ペインクリニック pain clinic 訪問クリニック home-based health care clinic

クリプトコッカス cryptococcus (複cryptococcal) （学名）*Cryptococcus* ◀肺クリプトコッカス症 pulmonary cryptococcosis ▶クリプトコッカス髄膜炎 cryptococcal meningitis

クリミア・コンゴしゅっけつねつ ―出血熱 Crimean-Congo hemorrhagic fever

くる 来る

《到着する・訪れる・接近する》come ☞参る
◆担当の医師がもうすぐ来ます Your doctor will be[come] here soon. ◆いつ日本に来ましたか When did you come to Japan? ◆あとでまた来ます I'll come to see you later. ◆もう少し近くに来て下さい Please come a little closer. ◆来週もう一度診察に来て下さい Please come and see me again next week.

《由来する》（原因として起こる）be caused (by) （結果として起こる）result (from)
◆これらの症状は高血糖から来ています These symptoms are caused by high blood sugar (levels). / These symptoms result from high blood sugar (levels).

《…してくる》 ◆痛み止めが効いてきましたか Has the pain medication begun to work? / Has the painkiller begun to kick in? ◆痛みがひどくなってくるようなことがあったら知らせて下さい Let us know if the pain happens to get[become] worse.

クループ croup (複croupous) ◀仮性クループ false croup / pseudocroup 痙性クループ spasmodic croup 真性クループ true croup ▶クループ性喉頭炎 croupous laryngitis

グループ group ☞集団 ◆もっと情報を得るためにサポートグループに参加を希望しますか Would you like to join[attend] a support group to get more information? ◆友達と小さなグループで遊ぶ play with friends in a small group ◀支援グループ

support group 自助グループ self-help [peer support] group ▶グループ活動 group activity グループ訓練 group training[exercise] グループホーム group home グループ療法 group therapy

グルカゴン glucagon ▶グルカゴン・インスリン療法 glucagon-insulin[GI] therapy グルカゴン産生腫瘍 glucagonoma

ぐるぐる ◆頭がぐるぐる回る feel as if *one's* head is spinning ◆自分自身がぐるぐる回るような感じでしたか Did you feel as if you were spinning around? / Did you feel like you were spinning round and round? ◆部屋の中の物がぐるぐる回るようでしたか Did the objects in the room seem to be spinning?

グルコース glucose ☞ブドウ糖

くるしい 苦しい (痛い) painful (図pain) (不快な) uncomfortable (困難である) difficult, hard (呼吸が苦しそうな) difficult, labored (図difficulty) ◆胸が苦しい(痛む) have (a) pain in *one's* chest / (圧迫感がある)feel pressure in *one's* chest ◆息が苦しい have difficulty breathing ◆苦しいですか Are you uncomfortable? / (痛むか) Are you in pain? ◆苦しそうな息づかいをする have labored[difficult and uncomfortable] breathing ◆生活が苦しい find it difficult to make a living / be badly off (for money)

くるしむ 苦しむ suffer (from) (図苦痛) ◆激しい咳で苦しむ suffer from a violent cough ◆苦しまずに亡くなる die a painless death / pass away without feeling the slightest pain

グルタチオン glutathione

グルテン gluten ◀無グルテン食 gluten-free diet ▶グルテンアレルギー gluten allergy

くるびょう くる病 rickets ◀ビタミンD依存性くる病 vitamin D-dependent rickets ビタミンD欠乏性くる病 vitamin D-deficiency rickets ビタミンD抵抗性くる病 vitamin D-resistant[-refractory] rickets

くるぶし 踝 ankle ◆くるぶしをくじく sprain *one's* ankle ◆くるぶしをひねる twist *one's* ankle

くるま 車 car ☞自動車 ◆病院へは車で来ましたか Did you drive (your car) to the hospital? ◆今日は車の運転はしないで下さい Please don't drive today. ◆車を運転する drive a car ◆車に乗る get in the car ◆車を降りる get out of the car ◆車の事故にあう have a car accident ◆車にひかれる be run over by a car ◆車に酔う get carsick ☞車椅子, 車いす

くるまいす 車椅子 wheelchair ◆車椅子を押す push a wheelchair ◆車椅子の生活になる be a wheelchair user / use a wheelchair ◆ご気分が悪かったら車椅子を使って下さい Please use a wheelchair if you feel sick. ◆正面玄関の近くに車椅子が配置してありますので，ご利用下さい Please feel free to use one of the wheelchairs provided near the entrance. ◆車椅子に乗る〈車椅子から降りる〉お手伝いをしましょう Let me help you into〈out of〉the wheelchair. ◆この車椅子に乗って下さい Please get into this wheelchair. ◆この車椅子にゆっくりと体を移動させて下さい Please move yourself slowly into this wheelchair. ◆車椅子を自分で動かすことができますか Can you use a wheelchair by yourself? / Can you move[wheel] yourself around in a wheelchair? ◆当院には車椅子用のトイレが1階と3階にあります This hospital has restrooms with wheelchair access on the first and third floors. ◀折り畳み式車椅子 folding wheelchair 介助用車椅子 attendant-controlled[attendant-propelled] wheelchair 階段昇降用車椅子 stair-climbing wheelchair 手動車椅子 manual wheelchair / (自力推進式の) self-propelled wheelchair 電動車椅子 electric[electric-powered] wheelchair ▶車椅子利用者 wheelchair user 車椅子用入口 wheelchair access

くるまよい 車酔い carsickness

くるむ wrap ◆赤ちゃんをタオルや薄い毛布にくるんであげて下さい Wrap your

baby in a towel or thin blanket.

クレアチニン creatinine ▶クレアチニンクリアランス creatinine clearance；Ccr

クレアチン creatine ▶クレアチンキナーゼ creatine kinase；CK

グレーブスびょう ―病 Graves disease ◆グレーブス病は甲状腺ホルモンが過剰に分泌される自己免疫疾患です Graves disease is an autoimmune disorder in which the thyroid produces excessive amounts of hormone.

グレープフルーツ grapefruit ◆この薬と一緒にグレープフルーツを食べたりグレープフルーツジュースを飲んだりしないで下さい Please don't eat grapefruit or drink grapefruit juice *with this medication [while you're on this medication].

クレーム （苦情・文句）complaint （金銭などの請求）claim ☞苦情 ◆待ち時間についてクレームをつける complain[make complaints] about the *wait time[length of time spent waiting]

くれぐれも ◆くれぐれもお体を大切にして下さい Be sure to take good care of yourself.

クレジットカード credit card ☞カード ◆クレジットカードによる支払いに応じます We accept credit cards. / You can pay by credit card.

クレストしょうこうぐん ―症候群 CREST syndrome

クレゾール cresol ▶クレゾール石鹸液 saponated cresol solution

クレチンびょう ―病 congenital hypothyroidism, infantile hypothyroidism ★cretinism は不快な響きがあるため，一般的に使われなくなっている．

クレンザー cleanser

くろい 黒い black （黒ずんだ・黒っぽい）dark ◆便の色は黒い The stool color is black. ◆黒っぽい血を吐く vomit dark-colored blood ◆黒っぽい尿（黒褐色の尿）dark brown urine ◆目の前に黒い点が見えますか Do you see *a dark spot[dark spots] in front of your eyes? ◆皮膚の色が黒ずみましたか Has your skin become

darker? ☞黒ずむ，黒なます，黒目

クロイツフェルト・ヤコブびょう ―病 Creutzfeldt-Jakob disease；CJD

くろう 苦労 （困難）difficulty （㊀difficult） （苦難）hardship （㊀hard） （努力）effort （面倒）trouble ◆階段を上るのはひと苦労ですか Do you have a hard[difficult] time climbing stairs? / Do you find it hard [difficult] to climb stairs? ◆今タバコに手を出したらこれまでの苦労が水の泡になります If you start smoking again, all your efforts will *come to nothing[go down the drain]. ◆ご苦労の甲斐がありましたね Your efforts *were not wasted[were rewarded / paid off]. ◆ご苦労さまでした Thank you very much （for your trouble）.

クローニング cloning

クロール （塩素）chlorine ◀高クロール血症 hyperchloremia 低クロール血症 hypochloremia

クローンびょう ―病 Crohn disease ◆クローン病は消化管に炎症を起こす慢性疾患です Crohn disease is a chronic disorder that causes inflammation of the gastrointestinal[GI] tract.

クロストリジウム clostridium （㊀clostridial） （学名）*Clostridium* ▶クロストリジウム感染症 clostridium[clostridial] infection クロストリジウム・ディフィシル *Clostridium difficile* クロストリジウム・テタニ[破傷風菌] *Clostridium tetani* クロストリジウム・ボツリヌム[ボツリヌス菌] *Clostridium botulinum*

クロスマッチ （血液交差適合試験）（blood）crossmatching

くろずむ 黒ずむ turn[become] dark, turn [become] black ☞黒い

くろなまず 黒なまず （癜風）tinea versicolor

グロブリン globulin ◀ガンマグロブリン gamma globulin 免疫グロブリン immunoglobulin；Ig

クロム chromium ▶クロム親和性細胞腫 chromaffinoma / chromaffin tumor

グロムスしゅよう ―腫瘍 glomus tumor

くろめ 黒目 (虹彩)iris (and pupil) of the eye

くわえる 加える (付け足す)add (圏in addition (to) 圏additional) (含める)include ☞追加 ◆手術後，放射線治療にホルモン療法を加える予定です After the surgery, we're going to do hormone therapy in addition to radiation therapy. ◆血液検査に加えて，胸のX線検査が必要です In addition to blood tests, we need to take an X-ray of your chest. ◆検査結果によっては別の治療を加える必要があるかもしれません The test results may show that we need to do additional treatment. ◆もう少し詳しい説明を加えさせて下さい Let me explain in more detail.

くわしい 詳しい detailed (圏in detail) (それ以上の)further ☞詳細 ◆詳しい検査を行う carry out a detailed examination ◆詳しいことは看護師にお尋ね下さい If you need further information, please ask the nurse. ◆詳しいことはこの小冊子をお読み下さい For further details[information], please read this brochure. ◆詳しいことは後でお話ししましょう I'll give you the (full) details later. ◆治療方法について詳しくご説明いたしましょう Let me explain[tell you about] the treatment procedure in detail. ◆そのことについてもう少し詳しく話して下さい Please tell me more (about that). ◆どんな痛みでしたか，詳しく話して下さい What was the pain like? Could you describe it for me?

くわわる 加わる (参加する)join, take part (in), participate (in) (含む)include ◆私たちのグループに加わりませんか Would you like to join our group? ◆私たちの医療チームには緩和ケアの専門医が加わっています Our medical team includes palliative care specialists. / We have palliative care specialists in our medical team.

ぐんぱつ 群発 cluster ▶群発呼吸 cluster breathing 群発頭痛 cluster headache

くんれん 訓練 training (圏train) (練習)practice (圏practice) (運動)exercise (圏exercise, do exercise) ◆練習 ◆歩く訓練を廊下でしましょう Let's practice walking in the hallway. ◆日常生活に必要な作業が行えるよう患者を訓練する train the patient to perform important everyday tasks ◆訓練を行う give[provide] training ◆訓練を受ける get[receive] training ◀嚥下訓練 swallowing training (関節)可動域訓練 range of motion exercise 義肢訓練 prosthetic training 機能訓練 functional training[exercise] 起立訓練 standing[stand-up] exercise 強化訓練 strength training[exercise] / strengthening exercise 筋力増強訓練 muscle strengthening exercise グループ訓練 group training[exercise] 言語訓練 language[speech] training 呼吸訓練 breathing exercise 座位訓練 sitting exercise 社会生活技能訓練 social skills training；SST 職業訓練 vocational training 耐久力[持久力]訓練 endurance training[exercise] 他動運動訓練 passive exercise 聴能訓練 auditory training 動作訓練 movement exercise 日常生活動作訓練 activities of daily living training 排尿訓練(幼児の)toilet training /(排尿障害の)bladder training 排便訓練(幼児の)toilet training /(排便障害の)bowel training バランス訓練 balance training[exercise] 避難訓練(火災の)fire drill /(地震の)earthquake drill 歩行訓練 walking exercise[practice] / gait exercise[training] リハビリテーション訓練 rehabilitation training ▶訓練プログラム training program ☞訓練士

くんれんし 訓練士 (訓練指導者)trainer (療法士)therapist ◆療法士 ◀視能訓練士 orthoptist；ORT 聴能訓練士 auditory trainer[therapist]；AT

け

け 毛　(頭髪) hair (of the head)　(体毛)
(body) hair　(顔の毛) facial hair　(鼻毛)
nose[nostril] hair　(胸毛) chest hair　(腋
窩の毛) underarm hair　(陰部の毛) pubic
hair　(脚の毛) leg hair　★1 本の毛は a
hair.　☞髪, ヘア　◆毛が抜ける lose *one's*
hair / *one's* hair falls out　◆化学療法中は
おそらく毛が抜けるでしょう You'll prob-
ably lose your hair during chemotherapy.　◆化学療法が終われば通常 2, 3 か
月で毛が生えてきます Hair usually begins
to grow back two to three months after
the last chemotherapy treatment.　◆毛
は薄くなりましたか Has your hair been
getting thinner? / Have you noticed any
thinning of your hair?　◆毛は濃くなって
いますか Has your hair been getting
thicker? / Have you noticed any thickening of your hair?　◆毛を染める dye *one's*
hair　◆手術の準備のために胸の毛を剃り
ましょう To prepare for your surgery, let
me shave *your* chest hair[the hair off
your chest].　◀抜け毛(毛が抜けること)
hair loss / (抜けた毛) fallen hair　☞毛穴,
毛ジラミ

ケア　care (☞care for, take care of)　☞介
護　◆絶えずケアを必要とする need con-
stant care　◆毎日のケア daily care　◆長
期のケア long-term care　◀緊急ケア
emergency care　高齢者ケア elder care /
care of elderly[older] people　支持的ケ
ア supportive care　精神的ケア mental
[psychological] care　セルフケア self-
care　デイケア day care, daycare / (通所
施設) day care center　24 時間ケア
twenty-four-hour care　プライマリーケ
ア primary care　▶ケアチーム care team
ケアプラン care plan / plan of care　ケア
マネージメント care management　ケア
マネージャー care manager　ケアワーカー
care worker / professional caregiver

けあな　毛穴　pore

けい　系　system　◆呼吸器系 the respiratory system　◆消化器系 the digestive
system　◆免疫系 the immune system
◆日系アメリカ人 a Japanese American

ゲイ　gay man, (male) homosexual　☞同
性愛

けいい　経緯　(詳細) details　(一部始終)
complete account　◆事故の経緯について
聞かせて下さい Could you *tell me the
details[give me a complete account] of
the accident?

けいか　経過
《物事の》(進行) progress　(展開・推移)
development, course　(回復の速度) pace
of recovery　◆経過は順調です You're
doing well[fine].　◆彼の経過〈回復までの
経過〉はあまり思わしくありません His
progress〈The pace of his recovery〉 is not
*very good[what we'd like].　◆彼女の手
術後の経過は良好です She's making good
progress after her surgery.　◆もうしばら
く経過を見ることにしましょう Let's wait a
while and see how things go[develop]. /
We'll wait a while and see what happens. / (薬の効き目を見る) Let's see if[how]
the medication helps.　◆その後の経過は
どうですか How have you been? / How
have things been going? / How are you
recovering from your illness?　◆経過次
第で退院できるでしょう When you'll be
able to leave the hospital depends *on the
pace of your recovery[on how you're
doing].　◆術後の経過を評価する assess
the postoperative course
《月日・時間の》passage (☞pass)　◆術後 1
年が経過しています A year has passed
since the surgery.　◆時の経過とともに傷
の痛みは徐々に和らぐでしょう With the
passage of time the pain from the wound
will diminish gradually.　▶経過報告
progress report　☞経過観察

けいかい¹　軽快する　get better　◆めま
いは軽快傾向ですか, 悪化傾向ですか, 変
化なしですか Is your dizziness getting
better, getting worse, or is there no

change?

けいかい² 警戒する watch out (for), be alert, be on the alert ◆症状の急変を警戒する watch out for a sudden change in the symptom / be on the alert for a sudden change in the symptom

けいかかんさつ 経過観察 observation ◆経過観察のために入院する必要があります You need to *be hospitalized[be admitted to the hospital] for observation. ◆経過観察中である be under observation ◆腹部大動脈瘤の経過観察を行う monitor an abdominal aortic aneurysm with watchful waiting

けいかく 計画 plan (🔠計画された・予定の planned) (規模の大きい計画)project (設計・構図)design (治療・実験の計画)protocol ★protocol はフォーマルな語. (予定) schedule ◆ケア計画を作成する make[draw up] *a person's* care plan ◆喘息の長期治療計画を立てる make[develop / work out] a long-term treatment plan for asthma ◆ケア計画を実施する carry out a plan of care ◆計画を変える change[revise / alter] a plan ◆リハビリは計画通りにいっています Your rehabilitation is going according to plan. ◆援助計画 support plan 家族計画 family planning 仮計画 tentative plan 看護計画 nursing care plan 研究計画 research plan[project / design] 検査計画 test[examination] plan 退院計画 discharge plan 長期計画 long-term[long-range] plan 治療計画 treatment plan[program] / protocol 投与計画 dosage schedule リハビリテーション計画 rehabilitation plan ▶計画出産 planned childbirth[delivery]

けいカテーテルどうみゃくそくせん 経カテーテル動脈塞栓 transcatheter arterial embolization ；TAE

けいかん (子宮)頸管 cervical canal of the uterus, uterocervical canal ☞子宮頸管

けいがん 鶏眼 (魚の目)corn, clavus

けいかんえいよう 経管栄養 tube feeding

けいきかんしはいせいけん 経気管支肺生検 transbronchial lung biopsy；TBLB

けいけん 経験する experience (🔠experience), go through (…がある)have (🔠経験による・実証的な empirical) ☞体験 ◆このような痛みを経験したことがありますか Have you ever had[experienced] this kind of pain before? ◆これまでに経験したことのない激しい痛みですか Is this the first time for you to experience this kind of extreme pain? / Is it an extreme pain that you've never experienced before? ◆乳がん専門医の星先生に診てもらって下さい．彼女は経験が豊富ですから I'd like you to see Dr Hoshi, a breast cancer specialist. *She has a great deal of experience treating this disease[She's a doctor with years of experience]. ◆危機的な状況を経験する *go through[experience] a critical condition ◆不快な経験をする have an unpleasant experience ◆私の経験では in my experience ▶経験的投与 empirical administration

けいげん 軽減する (和らげる)relieve (減らす)reduce, cut down (on) ☞緩和 ◆ストレスを軽減する relieve[reduce] *one's* stress

けいこう¹ 蛍光 fluorescence (🔠fluorescent) ▶蛍光眼底血管造影法 fluorescence fundus angiography 蛍光眼底撮影法 fluorescence fundus photography 蛍光抗体法 fluorescent antibody technique[test] 蛍光透視検査 fluoroscopy 蛍光内視鏡検査 fluorescence endoscopy 蛍光免疫測定法 fluoroimmunoassay；FIA

けいこう² 傾向 tendency (🔠tend) (風潮)trend ◆食べ過ぎる傾向がありますか Do you tend[Do you have a tendency] to overeat? ◆痛みは食後悪化する傾向がありますか Does the pain tend to get worse after meals? ◆出血傾向がある bleed easily / have a tendency to bleed ◆転倒傾向がある fall easily / have a tendency to fall ◀自殺傾向 suicide[suicidal] tendency 嗜眠傾向 lethargic tendency 出血傾向 bleeding tendency / tendency to bleed 転倒傾向 tendency to fall 肥満傾向 tendency to obesity

けいこう³ 経口(の) oral 〔🔲by mouth, per os；PO 🔲or(o)-〕 ◀経口エアウェイ oral[oropharyngeal] airway 経口栄養 oral feeding 経口感染 oral infection 経口気管挿管 orotracheal intubation 経口血糖降下薬 oral hypoglycemic (medication/drug/agent) 経口ステロイド薬 oral steroid 経口避妊薬 the pill ★通例 the をつけて. / birth control pill / oral contraceptive 経口ブドウ糖負荷試験 oral glucose tolerance test；OGTT 経口補液 oral rehydration 経口補水剤 oral rehydration solution；ORS 経口薬 oral medication

けいこつ 脛骨 shinbone, tibia 〔🔲tibial〕 ▶脛骨骨折 tibial fracture 脛骨神経 tibial nerve

けいざい 経済 economy /ɪkánəmi/ 〔🔲経済の económic 財政上・金銭上の financial /faɪmǽnʃəl/〕☞財政 ◆経済的問題のことがご心配ですか Are you concerned about your financial problems? ◆経済上の理由で治療を中断する discontinue the treatment for financial[economic] reasons ◆患者の経済的な負担を軽減する lighten the patient's financial burden [load]

けいさつい 警察医 police physician[medical officer]

けいさん 計算する calculate 〔図calculation〕 (合計などを算出する)compute (数える)count (考慮に入れる)take … into account, take account of ☞考慮 ◆医療費を計算する calculate[compute] the medical expenses ◆計算力を失う lose the ability to calculate ◆出産予定日は10月1日の計算になります We've calculated your due date as October (the) first. / By our calculations, your due date is October (the) first. ◆輸血が必要な可能性も計算に入れなければなりません We have to take into account the possibility of a blood transfusion.

けいさんぷ 経産婦 (1人)primipara (2

人以上)multipara

けいしつ¹ 形質 (特徴・性質)character (遺伝的な特性)trait ◀劣性形質 recessive trait[character] ▶形質転換 transformation

けいしつ² 憩室 diverticulum 〔🔲diverticula〕 ◆大腸に憩室と呼ばれる小さな袋ができています You have small pouches, called diverticula, along your large intestine. ◀胃憩室 stomach[gastric] diverticulum 食道憩室 esophageal diverticulum 大腸憩室 diverticulum of the large intestine 膀胱憩室 bladder[vesical] diverticulum メッケル憩室 Meckel diverticulum ▶憩室炎 diverticulitis (多発性)憩室症 diverticulosis

けいしつさいぼう 形質細胞 plasma cell ▶形質細胞腫 plasmacytoma

けいしゃだい 傾斜台 tilt table, tilting table

けいしゅく 痙縮 spasticity

げいじゅつりょうほう 芸術療法 art therapy ◆芸術療法では，患者は芸術活動を通じて自らの感情を表現することにより生活の質の改善を図ります In art therapy, patients express their emotions through artistic means and thereby improve their quality of life.

けいしょう¹ 軽症 (病気)mild illness, slight illness (発作)mild attack (症例)mild case ◆あなたのうつ病は軽症ですから，必ずよくなります You have a mild form of depression, so you'll[it'll] definitely get better. / Your depression is still mild, so I'm sure you'll be able to get better.

けいしょう² 軽傷 slight injury[wound], mild injury[wound] ☞怪我 ◆軽傷を負う be slightly injured / have a slight injury

けいじょう 形状 form (外形)shape ▶形状記憶合金 shape-memory alloy

けいじょうとっき 茎状突起 styloid process

けいじょうほこう 鶏状歩行 ☞鶏歩

けいじょうみゃく¹ 頸静脈 jugular vein ◀外頸静脈 external jugular vein

けいじょうみゃく¹　内頸静脈 internal jugular vein　▶頸静脈圧迫試験 jugular compression test　頸静脈怒張 engorgement of the jugular vein

けいじょうみゃく²　経静脈（の）　intravenous；IV　▶経静脈栄養補給 intravenous feeding[alimentation]　経静脈高カロリー輸液 intravenous hyperalimentation；IVH

けいしょくどうしんエコーけんさ　経食道心エコー検査　transesophageal echocardiography

けいしんけい　頸神経　cervical nerve　▶頸神経叢ブロック cervical plexus block

けいずい　頸髄　cervical cord　▶頸髄症 cervical myelopathy　頸髄損傷 cervical cord injury

けいせい¹　形成　formation（動form）　◆この経験は彼の人格形成に役立つでしょう This experience will help form his character.　◆骨の形成を促す stimulate bone formation　◀えくぼ形成 dimple formation　概念形成 concept formation　過形成 hyperplasia　血栓形成 thrombus formation　空洞形成 cavity formation／cavitation　空胞形成 vacuolation／vacuolization　骨形成 ossification／bone formation　歯垢形成 plaque formation　歯石形成 tartar formation　肉芽形成 granulation　人間形成 character building[formation]　☞形成外科，形成術，形成不全

けいせい²　痙性　spasticity（形spastic, spasmodic）　▶痙性クループ spasmodic croup　痙性斜頸 spasmodic torticollis　痙性膀胱 spastic bladder　痙性歩行 spastic gait　痙性麻痺 spastic paralysis

けいせいげか　形成外科　plastic surgery（診療科）the department of plastic surgery, the plastic surgery department　▶形成外科医 plastic surgeon

けいせいじゅつ　形成術　plastic surgery（接尾–plasty）　◀血管形成術 angioplasty　口蓋形成術 palatoplasty　鼓室形成術 tympanoplasty　骨形成術 osteoplasty　乳房形成術 mammaplasty　噴門形成術 fundoplication／cardioplasty　弁形成術 valve repair（surgery）　弁輪形成術 valvuloplasty　幽門形成術 pyloroplasty

けいせいふぜん　形成不全　aplasia

けいそ　珪素　silicon

けいそうじょうたい　軽躁状態　hypomania

けいそく　計測　measurement（動measure）　☞測定，測る　◀密度計測 densitometry　▶計測器具 measuring device[instrument]

けいぞく　継続する　continue（名continuation）, go on（with）（形ongoing）（特定の期間続く）last　☞続く，続ける　◆化学療法を継続する continue[go on with] chemotherapy　◆慢性症状の継続治療 ongoing treatment for chronic symptoms　▶継続時間[期間] duration

けいたい¹　形態　（形状）form　（外形）shape　（物体）object　（接頭morph(o)–）　▶形態学 morphology　形態感覚 form sense[perception]　形態視覚 form[object] vision　形態失認 amorphagnosia

けいたい²　携帯（型の）　portable　▶携帯型心電図検査 portable[（歩行可能な）ambulatory] electrocardiography　携帯用酸素ボンベ portable oxygen cylinder　携帯用テレビ portable television[TV]　携帯用トイレ portable toilet／（便器）commode　☞携帯電話

けいたいでんわ　携帯電話　mobile phone /móʊbaɪl -/, cellphone　☞電話　◆ここでの携帯電話のご使用はご遠慮下さい Please refrain from using mobile phones here.　◆携帯電話は指定の場所でご使用下さい Please use mobile phones in the designated area.　◆携帯電話の電源を切る turn[switch] off *one's* mobile phone

けいちつ　経腟（の）　transvaginal, vaginal　▶経腟超音波検査 transvaginal ultrasound[ultrasonography／echography]　経腟分娩 vaginal delivery

けいちょう　傾聴する　listen attentively（to）　◆患者さんの訴えを傾聴する listen attentively to the patient's complaints

けいちょうえいよう　経腸栄養　enteral nutrition[feeding]　◀在宅経腸栄養法 home enteral nutrition；HEN　非経腸栄

養法 parenteral nutrition；PN

けいちょくちょうちょうおんぱけんさ
経直腸超音波検査 transrectal ultrasound [ultrasonography, echography]

けいつい 頸椎 cervical spine[verte bra(e)], backbone in the neck ▶頸椎カラー neck[cervical] collar, neck brace 頸椎牽引 neck[cervical] traction 頸椎症 cervical spondylosis 頸椎症性筋萎縮症 cervical spondylotic amyotrophy 頸椎症性脊髄症 cervical spondylotic myelopathy 頸椎損傷 cervical spine injury 頸椎脱臼 cervical dislocation 頸椎椎間板ヘルニア cervical disc hernia 頸椎捻挫 neck[cervical] sprain

けいど 軽度(の) (程度がわずかな)slight (病気・症状が軽い)mild, low-grade (程度が比較的大きくない)minor ☞軽い ◆軽度の熱がある have a slight[mild / low-grade] fever ◆軽度にかゆい be slightly[mildly] itchy ◆軽度のやけど a mild[minor] burn ◆胸部CTでは，腫瘍のサイズに軽度の変化が見られます The chest CT shows a slight change in the size of the tumor.

けいとう 系統 system (㊌systematic) ☞系 ◀神経系統 the nervous system ▶系統的脱感作 systematic desensitization

けいどうみゃく 頸動脈 carotid artery ◀外頸動脈 external carotid artery；ECA 総頸動脈 common carotid artery；CCA 内頸動脈 internal carotid artery；ICA ▶頸動脈小体 carotid body 頸動脈洞症候群 carotid sinus syndrome 頸動脈洞性失神 carotid sinus syncope 頸動脈洞マッサージ carotid sinus massage 頸動脈内膜切除術 carotid endarterectomy；CEA 頸動脈波記録 carotid pulse tracing；CPT

けいにょうどう 経尿道(的・の) transurethral ▶経尿道的前立腺切除術 transurethral resection of the prostate；TURP 経尿道的超音波検査 transurethral ultrasound[ultrasonography / echography] 経尿道的尿管砕石術 transurethral ureterolithotripsy 経尿道的膀

胱腫瘍切除術 transurethral resection of a bladder tumor；TURBT

けいねんてん 茎捻転 pedicle torsion, torsion of the pedicle

けいはい 珪肺 silicosis ▶珪肺結核 silicotuberculosis

けいひ 経皮(的・の) percutaneous, transcutaneous ▶経皮吸収 percutaneous absorption 経皮吸収薬 percutaneous medication[drug / agent] 経皮経肝胆汁ドレナージ percutaneous transhepatic biliary drainage；PTBD 経皮経肝胆道ドレナージ percutaneous transhepatic cholangio drainage；PTCD 経皮的冠(状)動脈インターベンション percutaneous coronary intervention；PCI 経皮経管的冠(状)動脈再開通術 percutaneous transluminal coronary recanalization[revascularization]；PTCR 経皮的心肺補助装置 percutaneous cardiopulmonary support；PCPS 経皮的穿刺 percutaneous puncture 経皮的電気神経刺激 transcutaneous electrical nerve stimulation；TENS 経皮的ペーシング transcutaneous pacing

けいび 経鼻(の) nasal, transnasal, pernasal ▶経鼻エアウェイ nasal airway 経鼻カニューラ nasal cannula 経鼻間欠的陽圧換気 nasal intermittent positive pressure ventilation；NIPPV 経鼻挿管 nasal intubation 経鼻内視鏡検査 transnasal[pernasal] endoscopy

けいびいん 警備員 security guard ◆警備員を呼ぶ call a security guard ▶警備員詰所 guardroom

けいぶ 頸部 neck, cervical region, cervix ◀臍帯頸部巻絡 umbilical cord around the neck 子宮頸(部) the cervix uteri / the uterine neck ▶項部硬直 cervical rigidity 頸部脊柱管狭窄症 cervical spinal canal stenosis 頸部脊椎症 cervical spondylosis 頸部痛 neck pain

けいふくへき 経腹壁(の) transabdominal (㊌across the abdomen, by the abdominal route) ▶経腹(壁)的腹膜前到達法 *transabdominal preperitoneal

[TAPP] approach

けいほ 鶏歩 steppage gait, drop foot gait

けいほう 警報 alert ◆警報を発する issue an alert ▶火災警報 fire alert 非常警報 emergency alert ▶警報器 alarm 警報装置 alarm system

けいみん 傾眠 drowsiness (㊟drowsy /dráuzi/), somnolence (㊟somnolent) ◆お子さんは異常なほど傾眠がちですか Is your baby abnormally drowsy? ◀日中傾眠 daytime drowsiness

けいらん 鶏卵 egg ☞卵

けいりゅう 稽留(の) (持続した)continued, sustained ▶稽留熱 continued[sustained] fever 稽留流産 (排出されない)missed abortion

けいれき 経歴 (略 歴)personal history (職業上の経歴)career

けいれん 痙攣 (体全体の)seizure, convulsive seizure, convulsion (㊟convulsive) ★一般的には seizure のほうが多く使われる. (筋肉の)spasm (㊟spastic, spasmodic) (筋肉の細かい動き)twitch (激痛を伴う痙攣)cramp ★複数形 cramps で激しい腹痛・月経痛をいう. ☞発作 ◆痙攣を起こしたことがありますか Have you ever had[suffered] seizures? / Have you ever suffered from convulsions[seizures]? ◆痙攣時に意識を失いますか Do you lose consciousness when you have a seizure? ◆痙攣の前〈間〉彼女はどんな様子でしたか What happened to her before〈during〉the seizure? ◆痙攣はどのくらい続きましたか How long did the seizure last? ◆彼女が痙攣を起こしたのは初めてですか Was this the first time she had a seizure? ◆足が痙攣する have[get] a cramp in the leg(s) ◆まぶたが痙攣する the eyelid twitches ◀胃痙攣 stomach cramps[spasm] 横隔膜痙攣 phrenospasm 眼瞼痙攣 eyelid twitching / blepharospasm 間代性痙攣 clonic convulsion[seizure] 顔面痙攣 facial spasm 強直間代性痙攣 tonic-clonic convulsion[seizure] 強直性痙攣 tonic convulsion[seizure] 筋痙攣 muscle cramp[spasm] 抗痙攣薬 anticonvulsant (medication / drug / agent) 喉頭痙攣 laryngeal spasm / laryngospasm ジャクソン痙攣 Jacksonian seizure[convulsion] 熱性痙攣 febrile seizure[convulsion] / fever seizure[convulsion] 憤怒痙攣(泣き入りひきつけ)breath-holding attack[spell] ▶痙攣性イレウス spastic ileus 痙攣性咳嗽 spasmodic cough 痙攣性チック convulsive tic 痙攣性腸閉塞 spastic ileus[bowel obstruction] 痙攣性発声障害 spasmodic dysphonia

けいろ 経路 (道筋)route (進路)course (目的達成のための道)pathway ◆その病気の感染経路はまだ判明していません The infection route of the disease *is not known yet[is still unknown]. ◀感染経路 infection route

けいろくしょうこうぐん 頸肋症候群 cervical rib syndrome

けが 怪我 (事故による怪我)injury /índʒəri/ (刃物などによる怪我)wound /wúːnd/ (重度の外傷)trauma /tróːmə/ ☞外傷, 傷, 損傷 ◆大きな怪我を負ったり, 事故を起こしたことがありますか Have you ever had any serious injuries or accidents? ◆頭に何らかの怪我を負ったことがありますか Have you ever had any type of *injury to your head[head injury]? ◆交通事故で大怪我〈軽い怪我〉をする be[become / get] seriously〈slightly〉injured in a traffic accident / suffer a serious〈slight〉injury in a traffic accident ◆全治3か月の怪我をする have an injury requiring three months *for complete recovery[to heal completely]

げか 外科 surgery (㊟surgical) (診療部門)the department of surgery, the surgery department ◆腎臓の結石を外科的に除去する remove the kidney stones surgically ◀移植外科 transplant surgery 一般外科 general surgery 外傷外科 trauma surgery 形成外科 plastic surgery 口腔外科 oral (and maxillofacial) surgery 呼吸器外科 thoracic surgery 消化器外科 gastroenterological surgery 小児外科

pediatric surgery　心臓血管外科 cardio-vascular surgery　整形外科 orthopedic surgery　乳腺・内分泌外科 breast and endocrine surgery　脳神経外科 neurosurgery　▶外科医 surgeon　外科外来 outpatient surgery department　外科学surgery / surgical medicine　外科器具 surgical instrument　外科手術 surgery / surgical procedure　外科助手 surgical assistant　外科的治療 surgical treatment　外科病棟 surgical ward[floor / unit]　外科部長 (the) head of the department of surgery

げかん　下疳　chancre /ʃǽnkɚ/　◀硬性下疳 hard sore[ulcer / chancre]　軟性下疳 soft sore[ulcer / chancre] / chancroid

げきしょうかんえん　劇症肝炎　fulminant hepatitis

げきつう　激痛　(激しい痛み)sharp pain, intense pain　(耐えがたい痛み)unbearable pain, excruciating pain　☞痛み

げきてき　劇的(な)　dramatic　◆劇的に回復する make a dramatic recovery　◆…に対して劇的な効果を上げる have a dramatic effect on …

げきどく　劇毒　deadly poison

げきぶつ　劇物　toxic substance[material]

げきむ　激務　hard work　◆激務からくるストレスで時に押しつぶされそうになることがありますか Do you sometimes feel overwhelmed by stress *from working hard [brought on by hard work]?

げきやく　劇薬　powerful medication[drug, agent]　(劇毒)deadly poison

げけつ　下血　bloody bowel discharge, melena　(黒色便)black stool　(タール便)tarry stool　◆下血がありますか Do you ever pass[notice] blood in your stools?

けさ　今朝　this morning

げざい　下剤　laxative /lǽksətɪv/, laxative medication[drug, agent], purgative, purgative medication[drug, agent]　◆検査前夜に下剤を服用して下さい Please take a laxative the night before the test.　◆腸の中を空にするための下剤を差し上げます

I'm going to give you a laxative to empty your bowels.　◆下剤を飲めばよくなるでしょう It may be helpful to take a laxative.

けしょう　化粧　makeup　◆化粧をする *put on[apply] makeup　◆化粧をしている wear makeup　◆化粧を落とす *take off[remove] one's makeup　◀死化粧 postmortem makeup　☞化粧品

けしょうひん　化粧品　cosmetic /kɑzmétɪk/ (㉿cosmetic)　◆最近ふだんと違う化粧品を使いましたか Have you recently used a different brand of cosmetics?　◆これまでに化粧品でアレルギー反応を起こしたことがありますか Have you ever had an allergic reaction to cosmetics?　◀薬用化粧品 medicated cosmetics　▶化粧品かぶれ allergy to cosmetics / rash caused by cosmetics　化粧品皮膚炎 cosmetic dermatitis

ケジラミ　毛ジラミ　(陰毛の)pubic lice (㉿louse), crab lice　▶毛ジラミ症 pediculosis pubis

けす　消す
《スイッチを切る》turn off, switch off　◆明かり〈テレビ〉を消す turn[switch] off the light〈TV〉
《除去する》get rid of, eliminate, remove　◆口臭を消す *get rid of[eliminate] bad breath

けずる　削る　(ドリルで穴を開ける)drill　(刃物で鋭くする)sharpen　(語句などを削除する)delete　◆歯を削る drill a tooth

けつあつ　血圧　blood pressure；BP　◆血圧を測りましょう I'm going to take [check] your blood pressure.　◆血圧は毎日同じ時間に同じ条件で測って下さい Please take your blood pressure at the same time and under the same conditions each day.　◆血圧はやや高めで，上が148，下が92です Your blood pressure is a little high. It's one[a] hundred (and) forty-eight over ninety-two.　◆血圧は正常です You have normal blood pressure. / Your blood pressure is normal.　◆血圧は正常値まで下がりました Your blood pressure has fallen[dropped / got down] to normal. ◆めまいは急な血圧低下によるものでしょう Your dizziness is probably caused by a sudden drop in blood pressure. ◆食事と生活習慣を変えることで血圧を下げることができます You can *bring down[lower] your blood pressure by making changes in your diet and daily habits. ◆血圧が上がる one's blood pressure *goes up[rises / gets high] ◆血圧を上げる raise[bring up] one's blood pressure ◆血圧が不安定である the blood pressure *is unstable[is not stable] ◆血圧を一定に保つ keep one's blood pressure steady ◆血圧を正常に維持する maintain normal blood pressure ◆上昇した血圧を正常にする normalize an elevated blood pressure ◀拡張期血圧 diastolic blood pressure 家庭血圧 home blood pressure 収縮期血圧 systolic blood pressure 随時血圧 casual blood pressure 正常血圧 normal blood pressure 早朝血圧 morning blood pressure 早朝血圧上昇 morning (blood pressure) surge[rise] 標準血圧 standard[normal] blood pressure 平均血圧 average[mean] blood pressure ▶血圧降下薬 antihypertensive (medication / drug / agent) 血圧測定 measurement of blood pressure / sphygmomanometry 血圧モニター blood pressure monitor ☞血圧計, 高血圧, 低血圧

けつあつけい 血圧計 **blood pressure measuring device[gauge] / sphygmomanometer** ◀自動血圧計 automatic blood pressure measuring device / automated sphygmomanometer

けつえき 血液 **blood** (語調**hem**(o)-) ☞血 ◆血液を採る collect[get] a blood sample from a person / do[get] a blood draw ◆痰に血液が混じっています The phlegm contains[is mixed with] blood. ◆血液の凝固を防ぐ prevent (blood) clotting[coagulation] / stop blood from clotting ◆血液の流れをよくする improve blood flow / facilitate the smooth flow of (the) blood ◆血液を送る pump blood ◆血液を提供する donate[give] blood ◆O 型の血液 blood type O / type O blood ◆微量の血液 a small amount of blood / (血痕)traces of blood ◀献血血液 donated blood 持続的血液濾過 continuous hemofiltration；CHF 循環血液量 circulating blood volume 循環血液量減少性ショック hypovolemic shock 代用血液 blood substitute 保存血液 stored [preserved / conserved] blood ▶血液化学 blood chemistry 血液学 hematology 血液ガス分析 blood gas analysis 血液灌流 hemoperfusion 血液吸着 hemadsorption 血液凝固 blood clotting [coagulation] 血液凝固因子 blood coagulation factor 血液交差適合試験 blood crossmatching (procedure) 血液疾患 blood[hematologic] disease 血液浄化 blood purification 血液成分 blood component 血液像 blood picture / hemogram 血液透析 hemodialysis；HD 血液内科 the department of hematology / the hematology department 血液脳関門 blood-brain barrier；BBB 血液培養検査 blood culture 血液バンク blood bank ☞血液型, 血液検査, 血液循環, 血液製剤

けつえきがた 血液型 **blood type**,《英》**blood group** ◆血液型は何ですか What blood type are you? / What's your blood type? ◆彼の血液型は A です He has type A blood. / He is blood type A. ◆血液型を調べる check[examine / determine] a person's blood type ◀ABO 式血液型不適合 ABO incompatibility 母児血液型不適合妊娠 incompatible pregnancy of maternal and fetal blood types / maternal and fetal blood type incompatible pregnancy ▶血液型検査 blood type test / blood typing 血液型不適合 blood type incompatibility 血液型不適合妊娠 blood-type incompatible pregnancy 血液型不適合輸血 incompatible blood transfusion

けつえきけんさ 血液検査 **blood test [examination]** ◆血液検査が必要です You need to have a blood test. ◆血液検

査をしましょう Let's do[run] a blood test. / I'm going to[Let me] take a blood sample. ◆(患者に)血液検査をする give *a patient* a blood test ◆血液検査を受ける have a blood test ▶血液検査項目 blood test item 血液生化学検査 biochemistry blood test 血液培養検査 blood culture

けつえきじゅんかん 血液循環 blood circulation ◆血液循環がよい〈悪い〉have good〈bad / poor〉blood circulation

けつえきせいざい 血液製剤 blood product ◆汚染された血液製剤を介して感染する contract the disease through contaminated blood products ▶加熱血液製剤 heat-treated blood product 非加熱血液製剤 untreated[non-heat-treated] blood product

けつえん 血縁 (close) blood relatives ★通例，複数形で．▶血縁関係 blood relationship[relations]

けっか 結果 (一般的に)result (成り行き・影響)consequence (効果・影響)effect (最終的な結果)outcome ☞効果 ◆今日の検査結果は次回の診察の時にお話しします I'll explain the results of today's test(s) at your next visit. ◆この症状は糖尿病の結果として起こります This symptom develops as a result of diabetes. ◆検査の結果はすべてが正常です Your tests show that everything is normal. ◆結果は思わしくありません I'm afraid things have not worked out well. / I'm afraid things have not turned out as we hoped. / The result is not quite satisfactory. ◆食事と運動で十分な結果が得られない時は薬を処方しましょう If diet and exercise alone don't produce sufficient results, I'll prescribe a medication. ◆肺気腫は長年にわたる喫煙の結果もたらされると考えられています Pulmonary emphysema is considered to be the result[consequence] of years of smoking. ◆この薬で少しはよい結果が得られるでしょう This medication should have some good[beneficial] effect. ◆タバコは手術の結果に悪影響を及ぼしますので禁煙して下さい Smoking *affects the

outcome of surgery negatively[has a negative effect on the outcome of surgery], so please stop smoking. ◆いい結果を得る get a good[successful] result ◆驚くような結果を出す achieve[produce] a surprising result ◆直接的な〈間接的な〉結果 *a direct〈an indirect〉result ◆最終的な結果 the final[end] result ◆原因と結果 cause and effect

けっかい 血塊 blood clot

けっかく 結核 tuberculosis /tʊbàːkjəlóʊsɪs/；TB (⟦形⟧tubérculous) ◆結核に罹る have[contract] tuberculosis ◆結核感染者に接触したことがありますか Have you ever been exposed to anyone with tuberculosis? ◆痰から結核菌が検出されたので，結核専門病院を紹介しましょう *Mycobacterium tuberculosis*[The bacterium that causes tuberculosis] was detected in your phlegm, so let me refer you to a hospital specializing in treating tuberculosis. ◆結核患者の医療費は免除あるいは減額されます．最寄りの保健所で公費負担申請をして下さい Medical fees for tuberculosis patients will be waived or reduced. Please go to the nearest public health center and apply for public assistance for your medical fees. ◆結核の症例を保健所に届け出る report cases of tuberculosis to the health center ▶開放性結核 open tuberculosis 活動性〈非活動性〉結核 active〈inactive〉tuberculosis 珪肺結核 silicotuberculosis 抗結核薬 antitubercular (medication / drug / agent) / tuberculosis medication 初感染結核 primary tuberculosis 潜在性結核 latent tuberculosis 粟粒結核 miliary tuberculosis 多剤耐性結核 multidrug-resistant tuberculosis；MDR-TB 腸結核 intestinal tuberculosis 肺外結核 extrapulmonary tuberculosis 肺結核 pulmonary tuberculosis / tuberculosis of the lung 非結核性抗酸菌 nontuberculous mycobacterium；NTM 非結核性抗酸菌症 nontuberculous mycobacterial disease 膀胱結核 bladder tuberculosis ▶結核患者 tuberculosis patient / patient with tuberculosis 結核腫 tuberculoma 結核性胸膜炎 tuberculous pleurisy[pleuritis] 結核性脊椎炎 tuberculous spondylitis 結核性膿胸 tuberculous empyema 結核性リンパ節炎 tuberculous lymphadenitis 結核予防法 the Tuberculosis Prevention Law

げつがく 　月額　◆CPAP は月額約 5,000 円の自己負担が必要となります You need to pay five thousand yen a month out of your own money for the CPAP machine.

けっかん 　血管　blood vessel 〔略vascular 頭angi(o)-, vas(o)-, vascul(o)-〕 ◆血管が切れて[破れて]出血しています The blood vessel has burst[ruptured] and is bleeding. /(出血は破れた血管による)The bleeding is due to a burst[ruptured] blood vessel. ◆脳の血管に瘤ができていて，それがいつ破れてもおかしくない状況です You have *an aneurysm in the brain[a bulge in a blood vessel in your brain], and it may burst[rupture] at any moment. ◆血管が硬くなっています Your blood vessels are hardening[getting hard]. ◆脳の血管が詰まっている The blood vessels in the brain are blocked[clogged]. ◆血管が詰まるのを予防する prevent the blood vessels from clotting ◆血栓が血管をふさぐ blood clots obstruct[block] a vessel ◆閉塞した血管 an obstructed[occluded] blood vessel ◆血管を拡げる dilate the blood vessels ◀栄養血管 nutrient vessel 血栓性血管炎 thromboangitis 心血管疾患 cardiovascular disease 人工血管 artificial blood vessel / prosthetic (vascular) graft / synthetic graft / vascular prosthesis[graft] 脳血管 *cerebral blood[cerebrovascular] vessel 毛細血管 capillary / capillary blood vessel ▶血管炎 vasculitis / angitis / angiitis 血管拡張薬 vasodilator 血管鉗子 vascular forceps 血管虚脱 vascular collapse 血管形成術 angioplasty 血管雑音 vascular murmur 血管収縮 vasoconstriction / constriction of the blood vessels 血管収縮薬 vasoconstrictor 血管神経性浮腫

angioneurotic edema / angioedema / Quincke edema 血管新生 angiogenesis 血管損傷 vascular injury 血管内凝固 intravascular coagulation 血管内溶血 intravascular hemolysis 血管壁 *blood vessel[vascular] wall 血管縫合 angiorrhaphy 血管迷走神経性失神 vasovagal syncope 血管迷走神経反射 vasovagal reflex 血管攣縮 vasospasm / angiospasm / vascular spasm 血管攣縮性狭心症 vasospastic[coronary spastic] angina ☞血管腫, 血管造影

けっかんしゅ 　血管腫　hemangioma ◀いちご状血管腫 strawberry mark[hemangioma] 海綿状血管腫 cavernous hemangioma 肝血管腫 hepatic hemangioma くも状血管腫 vascular spider ポートワイン状[赤ぶどう酒様]血管腫 port-wine stain[hemangioma]

けっかんぞうえい 　血管造影　angiography /ˌændʒiˈɑɡrəfi/ ◆冠動脈の血流を調べるために，冠血管の血管造影を行います I'm going to perform a coronary angiography to see how blood is flowing through the coronary arteries. ◀デジタル・サブトラクション血管造影 digital subtraction angiography；DSA ▶血管造影図 angiogram

けっききょう 　血気胸　hemopneumothorax ☞気胸, 血胸

けっきゅう 　血球　blood cell, (blood) corpuscle ☞赤血球, 白血球 ◀全血球計算 complete blood (cell) count ▶血球凝集反応 hemagglutination 血球数 blood cell count 血球成分 cellular component of blood 血球貪食症候群 hemophagocytic syndrome

けっきょう 　血胸　hemothorax ◆血胸は，胸腔内に血液が溜まっている状態のことです Hemothorax is a condition in which blood accumulates in the chest cavity.

けっきょく 　結局　after all, in the end, in the long run ◆結局どの治療を選択なさいましたか Which treatment option did you choose *after all[in the end]? ◆結局はそうしてよかったと思われるでしょう You'll think that you did the right thing in the long run. / In the end, you'll think that you did the right thing. ◆あらゆる手を尽くしましたが，結局意識は戻りませんでした We tried every possible means to revive her, but in the end, she did not regain consciousness.

けっきん 欠勤 **absence** (**from work**)
◆どのくらい長く欠勤していますか How long have you *been absent[stayed away] from work? ◀病気欠勤 absence from work *due to[because of] illness 無届け欠勤 absence without notice

げっけい 月経 (**menstrual**) **period, menstruation, menorrhea, menses** ★複数形で. ☞生理

《初経・閉経》 ◆今でも月経がありますか Are you still having (your) periods? ◆最初の月経があったのは何歳の時ですか How old were you when you had your first period? / How old were you when your periods started? ◆最後に月経があったのは何歳の時ですか How old were you when you stopped having periods? / How old were you when you had your last period?

《最終月経》 ◆最近の月経はいつでしたか When was your last period? ◆最終月経の初日はいつでしたか When was the first day of your last period? ◆その前の月経はいつでしたか When was your last period before that?

《月経周期・期間・規則性》 ◆月経周期は通常何日ですか How often do you get your periods? / How many days usually pass between your periods? ◆月経は通常何日続きますか How many days[How long] do your periods usually last? ◆月経は順調ですか Do you have regular periods? ◆月経は通常規則的ですか，不規則ですか Are your periods usually regular or irregular? ◆月経でない時に出血することがありますか Do you ever bleed between periods? ◆月経が3週間遅れている The period is three weeks late[delayed]. ◆月経周期がいつもより短い The menstrual cycle is shorter than usual. ◆月経がない do not have regular periods ◆月経がとぶ miss *one's* period ◆月経が止まる stop having periods

《出血量》 ◆月経の出血量は通常どうですか What's the flow of your period like usually? / What's your usual flow? ◆月経の出血量は毎月同じですか Is the amount of flow the same every month? ◆生理用ナプキンやタンポンを1日にどのくらい使いますか How many pads or tampons do you use a day? ◆月経の出血量が多い〈少ない / 普通〉have heavy〈light / normal〉periods ◆月経の出血量が増える〈減る〉the menstrual flow increases〈decreases〉

《月経痛》 ◆月経中にお腹が痛みますか Do you usually have cramps? ★cramps は月経痛. ◆月経中に痛みや不快感がありますか Do you have any pain[cramps] or discomfort during your periods?

◀過少月経 hypomenorrhea / excessively light[scanty] menstrual flow 過多月経 hypermenorrhea / menorrhagia / heavy periods / profuse menstruation 過短月経 too short menstruation / bleeding for too short a period 過長月経 prolonged menstruation / bleeding for too long a period 希発月経 oligomenorrhea / infrequent menstruation 早発月経 premature menstruation 遅発月経 delayed menstruation 頻発月経 polymenorrhea / abnormally frequent menstruation 無月経 amenorrhea / missed periods 無排卵性月経 anovulatory menstruation

▶月経異常 menstrual[menstruation] disorder 月経困難症 dysmenorrhea / painful menstruation[periods] 月経周期 menstrual cycle 月経前症候群 premenstrual syndrome；PMS 月経痛 painful menstruation[periods] / period cramps / the cramps 月経不順 irregular menstruation[periods] / menstrual irregularity 月経様出血 menstruation-like bleeding

けっこう¹ 血行 (循環) **blood circulation** (血流) **blood flow, bloodstream** ☞血流

けっこう¹

◆血行をよくする improve one's (blood) circulation / increase one's blood flow ◆血行が悪い have poor (blood) circulation ◆血行が悪くなっている the blood flow has *gotten worse[worsened] / the blood flow is *getting worse[worsening] ◀側副血行［循環］collateral circulation ▶血行再建 revascularization 血行障害 interruption of the blood flow / disturbed blood flow 血行性転移 hematogenous metastasis 血行動態 hemodynamics 血行不良 poor[bad](blood) circulation

けっこう²　結構

《十分である・よい》◆結構です．楽にして下さい Good[OK / Okay / Fine], please relax. ◆結構です．大変よくできました Great[Very good / Terrific]! *You did a good job[You're doing fine].

《許可》◆もう洋服を着て結構です You can get dressed now. / You can put your clothes back on now. ◆来週でしたらいつでも結構です You can come *any time [any day] next week. / I'm available *any time[any day] next week. ◆今回は結構ですが，次回の受診時に必ず保険証をお持ち下さい It's okay this time, but please be sure to bring your insurance card at your next visit.

《案外・かなり》◆1日10分軽く体を動かすだけでも結構違います It'll make quite a difference if you do some light exercise for ten minutes a day. ◆お仕事は結構きついですか Is your work quite hard?

けつごうそしき　結合組織　connective tissue ▶結合組織病 connective tissue disease

けっこん　結婚　marriage (圏get married (to), be married (to), marry 圏既婚の married　婚姻の marital) ◆結婚していますか Are you married? / (同棲相手がいますか)Do you have a partner? ◆これまでに結婚したことがありますか Have you ever been married before? ◆結婚してどのくらいになりますか How long have you been married? ◀近親［血族］結婚 consangui-neous marriage / marriage between blood relatives ▶結婚状況 marital status　結婚生活 married life　結婚歴 marital history

けっさつ　結紮する　ligate (圖ligature, ligation), **tie up, close off** ◀臍帯結紮 ligature of the umbilical cord　精管結紮 vasoligation　卵管結紮 tubal ligation ▶結紮糸 ligature

けっしきそ　血色素　hemoglobin ▶発作性夜間血色素尿症 paroxysmal nocturnal hemoglobinuria

けっして　決して ◆決してあきらめないで Never give up! ◆患部には決して触れないようにして下さい Be careful never to touch the affected part[area]. ◆社会復帰は決して不可能ではありません It's *not at all[by no means] impossible for you to go back to work.

けっしゅ　血腫　hematoma ◀硬膜外血腫 epidural[extradural] hematoma；EDH　硬膜下血腫 subdural hematoma　頭血腫 cephalohematoma

けつじょ　欠如 (不足)**lack** (圖lack) (存在しないこと)**absence** ◆お子さんは集中力が欠如しているのですか Does your child lack the ability to concentrate? / Does your child have a short attention span? ◆これまでの病歴に関する情報が欠如していると，的確に治療することは困難です I can't treat your illness properly if *information on your past medical history is lacking[you can't provide information on your past medical history]. ◆関心の欠如 lack of interest ▶欠如歯 missing tooth

けっしょう　血漿 (blood) **plasma** ◀循環血漿量 circulating plasma volume　新鮮凍結血漿 fresh frozen plasma；FFP　二重濾過血漿交換 double filtration plasmapheresis；DFPP ▶血漿吸着 plasma adsorption　血漿交換 plasma exchange / plasmapheresis　血漿浸透圧 plasma osmotic pressure　血漿蛋白分画 plasma protein fraction；PPF　血漿分画製剤 plasma derivatives[products]

けっしょうばん　血小板　(blood) platelet, thrombocyte　◀抗血小板薬 antiplatelet medication[drug / agent]　▶血小板凝集 platelet aggregation　血小板減少 thrombocytopenia　血小板数 platelet count　血小板増加 thrombocytosis　血小板無力症 thrombasthenia　血小板輸血 platelet transfusion

けっしょく　血色　(顔色)complexion　◆血色がよい〈悪い〉have a good〈poor〉complexion / look healthy〈pale〉

けっしん　決心する　(決定する)decide (on)　(⊠decision)　(心に決める)make up *one's* mind　▶決める，決断，決定　◆手術を受ける決心はつきましたか Have you decided to have the surgery?

けっしんてんかん　欠神てんかん　absence epilepsy

けっせい¹　血清　(blood) serum　(⊠serologic)　◀抗血清 antiserum　抗毒素血清 antitoxic serum　梅毒血清反応 serologic reaction (test) for syphilis；STS　ペア血清 paired serum　免疫血清検査 immunoassay　▶血清アルブミン serum albumin　血清学的検査 serologic test　血清学的診断 serologic diagnosis　血清肝炎 serum hepatitis；SH

けっせい²　血性(の)　bloody　(出血性の)hemorrhagic　▶血性下痢 bloody diarrhea　血性帯下 bloody discharge　血性腹水 bloody[hemorrhagic] ascites[ascitic fluid]

けつせいえきしょう　血精液症　hemospermia

けっせき¹　欠席する　be absent (from), stay away (from)　(出席し損なう)miss　◆昨日は欠席したのですか Were you absent from school yesterday? / Did you miss school yesterday?　◀病気欠席 absence *due to*[because of] illness　▶欠席届 notice of absence / absence note

けっせき²　結石　stone, calculus　(⊠calculi)　☞去　◆胆管結石の内視鏡的な〈外科的な〉除去 endoscopic〈surgical〉removal of a bile duct stone　◀カルシウム結石 calcium stone　肝内結石 intrahepatic

gallstone[cholelithiasis] / hepatolithiasis　コレステロール結石 cholesterol stone　サンゴ状結石 staghorn stone　シュウ酸カルシウム結石 calcium oxalate stone　腎盂結石 kidney[renal] pelvic stone　腎結石 kidney[renal] stone[calculus] / nephrolith　総胆管結石 common bile duct stone / choledocholithiasis　胆嚢結石 gallbladder stone / cholecystolithiasis　尿管結石 ureter stone　尿酸結石 uric acid stone　尿道結石 urethral stone　尿路結石 urinary stone　膀胱結石 bladder stone　無症候性結石 silent[asymptomatic] stone　▶結石摘出術 lithectomy / stone extraction / extraction[removal] of *a stone[stones]　結石溶解療法 stone dissolution (therapy)

けっせつ　結節　node, knot, tuber　(⊠tuberous)　(小結節)nodule　(⊠nodular)　▶結節影 nodular shadow　結節性黄色腫 tuberous xanthoma　結節性硬化症 tuberous sclerosis　結節性紅斑 erythema nodosum　結節性多発動脈炎 polyarteritis nodosa；PN　結節性痒疹 nodular prurigo

けっせん　血栓　blood clot, thrombus　(⊠thrombosed, thrombotic)　◆血栓が左足の静脈にできています Blood clots have formed in the veins of your left leg.　◆右足に血栓ができています You have developed blood clots in the veins of your right leg.　◆血栓が血流を移動して肺の血管を塞ぎます Blood clots move[travel] through the bloodstream and cause blockage in a vessel of the lungs.　◆血栓を溶かす dissolve blood clots　◆血栓を防ぐ prevent blood clot formation　◀心房血栓 atrial thrombus　肺血栓塞栓症 pulmonary thromboembolism；PTE　微小血栓 microthrombus　フィブリン血栓 fibrin thrombus　浮遊血栓 floating thrombus　壁在血栓 mural thrombus　▶血栓形成 thrombus formation　血栓除去術 thrombectomy　血栓性外痔核 external thrombosed hemorrhoids　血栓性血管炎 thromboangitis　血栓性血小板減少性紫斑

病 thrombotic thrombocytopenic purpura；TTP　血栓性静脈炎 thrombophlebitis　血栓溶解薬 thrombolytic (medication／drug／agent)　血栓溶解療法 thrombolytic therapy　☞血栓症

けっせんしょう　**血栓症**　**thrombosis**
◀冠動脈血栓症 coronary (artery) thrombosis　抗血栓症薬 antithrombotic (medication／drug／agent)　動脈〈静脈〉血栓症 arterial〈venous〉thrombosis　脳血栓症 cerebral thrombosis

けつぞく　**血族**　**blood relatives**　★通例，複数形で．（圏**consanguineous**）☞血縁　▶血族結婚 consanguineous marriage／marriage between blood relatives

けっそん　**欠損**　（欠陥）**defect**　（喪失）**loss**　（脱落）**deficit**　（圏抜けた **missing** 崩壊した **broken**）◀楔状欠損 wedge-shaped defect　歯牙欠損 tooth loss　視野欠損 visual field defect　脈拍欠損［結滞］missing heart beat／pulse deficit　▶欠損［崩壊］家庭 broken family　欠損歯 missing tooth　☞欠損症

けっそんしょう　**欠損症**　**deficiency, defect**　◀アデノシンデアミナーゼ欠損症 *adenosine deaminase[ADA] deficiency　心室中隔欠損症 ventricular septal defect；VSD　心房中隔欠損症 atrial septal defect；ASD

けったい　**結滞する**　（抜く・とぶ）**skip, miss**　（圏**skipped, dropped, missing**）◆脈が結滞することがありますか Do you ever feel your heart skipping beats?　◀脈拍結滞 missing heart beat／（脱落）pulse deficit　▶結滞脈 skipped heart beat／dropped beat［（断続的な）intermittent］pulse

けったん　**血痰**　**bloody phlegm［sputum］**　☞痰　◆血痰が出ますか Do you cough up bloody phlegm?　◆血痰を吐く cough [spit] up bloody phlegm

けつだん　**決断**　（firm）**decision**　（圏**decide, make a decision**）（実行への決意）**determination**　（圏**determine**）☞決める，決心，決定　◆あなたは決断するのが早いですね You're quick at making decisions, aren't you? ／You're a quick decision-

maker, aren't you?　◆その手術をするかどうかについてはご自分で決断すべきです You should decide for yourself[It's up to you to decide] whether you have the surgery.

けっちゅうにょうそちっそ　**血中尿素窒素**　blood urea nitrogen；BUN

けっちゅうのうど　**血中濃度**　**blood level ［concentration]**　◀薬物血中濃度 plasma drug level[concentration]　▶血中アルコール濃度 blood alcohol level[concentration]

けっちょう　**結腸**　**colon** /kóʊlən/　◀S状結腸 sigmoid colon　横行結腸 transverse colon　巨大結腸 giant colon／megacolon　上行〈下行〉結腸 ascending〈descending〉colon　▶結腸炎 colitis　結腸がん colon cancer　結腸憩室 colon diverticulum　結腸切除術 colectomy　結腸全摘術 total colectomy　結腸［大腸］内視鏡検査 colonoscopy　結腸瘻造設術 colostomy

けっちん　**血沈**　☞赤沈

けってい　**決定**　（複数の選択肢を考慮しての決定）**decision**　（圏**decide, make a decision**）（実行への決定）**determination**　（圏**determine**）（結論）**conclusion**　（圏**conclude**）（圏決定的な・明確な **definite, decisive**）☞決まる，決める，決心，決断　◆治療計画についてはまだ決定していません We haven't made a decision about the treatment plan yet.／We're still not definite about the treatment plan.　◆検査結果は治療方針を決定するのに重要な役割を果たします Test results play a crucial role in deciding [determining] treatment plans.　◆決定的な要因 a decisive factor　◀意志決定 decision-making　最終決定 final decision　▶決定因子 determinant

けってん　**欠点**　（悪い点）**bad point**　（弱点）**weak point**　（短所・不十分な点）**shortcoming**　（欠陥）**fault, defect**　（不都合）**drawback**　◆欠点を直す correct *one's* *bad points[weak points／shortcomings]　◆その治療の欠点 the drawback(s) of the treatment

けっとう 血糖 blood sugar[glucose]
◀空腹時血糖 fasting blood sugar；FBS 持続血糖測定 continuous glucose monitoring；CGM ▪血糖降下薬 hypoglycemic（medication / drug / agent） 血糖検査 blood sugar[glucose] test 血糖自己測定 self-monitoring of blood glucose；SMBG ☞血糖値, 高血糖, 低血糖

けっとうち 血糖値 blood sugar level, blood glucose level ◆血糖値を測りましょう I'm going to measure[check] your blood sugar level. ◆毎日定期的に血糖値を測り記録して下さい Please check and record your blood sugar regularly every day. ◆血糖値はやや高めで 130 mg/dL あります Your blood sugar level is slightly high. It's one[a] hundred（and）thirty milligrams per deciliter. ◆血糖値は正常です Your blood sugar level is normal. / You have a normal blood sugar level.
◆血糖値が正常値を超えています Your blood sugar level is above normal. ◆血糖値は正常値まで下がりました Your blood sugar level has fallen[dropped] to normal. ◆血糖値はできるだけ正常値に近づけるよう努力して下さい Please try to keep your blood sugar levels as close to normal as possible. ◆震えや冷や汗は血糖値が急に下がったからでしょう Your shakiness and cold sweats are probably caused by a sudden drop *in blood sugar[in your blood sugar level]. ◆血糖値が下がる *one's* blood sugar level *goes down[drops / falls / decreases] ◆血糖値が上がる *one's* blood sugar level *goes up[rises / increases] ◆血糖値を下げる *bring down[lower] *one's* blood sugar level ◆血糖値を上げる raise *one's* blood sugar level ◆血糖値をコントロールする control[maintain] *one's* blood sugar level / （一定に保つ）keep *one's* blood sugar level steady ◆血糖値をモニターする monitor *one's* blood sugar level ◀空腹時血糖値 *fasting blood sugar[FBS] level 随時血糖値 random[casual] blood sugar level ▶血糖値測定器 glucose meter /

glucometer

けつにょう 血尿 bloody urine, blood in the urine, hematuria ◆血尿が出ますか, 出たことがありますか Do you have or have you ever had *blood in your urine[bloody urine]? ◆血尿が出る have[pass] bloody urine ◀間欠的血尿 intermittent hematuria 顕微鏡的血尿 microscopic hematuria 腎後性血尿 postrenal hematuria 腎前性血尿 prerenal hematuria 肉眼的血尿 gross[macroscopic] hematuria / macrohematuria 無症候性血尿 asymptomatic hematuria

げっぷ burp（⑩burp）, belch（⑩belch）
◆げっぷはよく出ますか Do you often burp? ◆検査が済むまでげっぷを我慢して下さい Don't burp until the exam is over. / Hold on for a while without burping until the examination is completed. ◆赤ちゃんはげっぷをしなくても大丈夫ですよ It's OK even if your baby doesn't burp. ◆赤ちゃんにげっぷをさせる burp *one's* baby

けっぺい 血餅 blood clot

けっぺきしょう 潔癖症 rhypophobia
◆ご自分は潔癖症なほうだと思いますか Do you think[feel] that you're a little obsessive over cleanliness?

けつべん 血便 bloody stools, blood in *one's* stools ◆血便が出ますか, 出たことがありますか Do you have or have you ever had *blood in your stools[bloody stools]? ◆血便が出る have[pass] bloody stools ◆粘血便 bloody mucous[mucoid] stool

けつぼう 欠乏 （不足）lack （本質的な物の不足）deficiency ▶欠乏症状 deficiency symptom

けつまく 結膜 conjunctiva /kànʤʌŋktáɪvə/（⑪conjunctival） ◆結膜を見せて下さい Let me look at the conjunctiva of your eye(s). ◀眼球結膜 bulbar conjunctiva / conjunctival layer of the bulb 眼瞼結膜 palpebral conjunctiva ▶結膜疾患 conjunctival disease 結膜充血 conjunctival injection / congestion of the

けつまく　結膜出血 conjunctival hemorrhage　☞結膜炎

けつまくえん　結膜炎 conjunctivitis（流行性結膜炎の通称）pink eye　◆季節性のアレルギー性結膜炎 seasonal allergic conjunctivitis　◀ウイルス性結膜炎 viral conjunctivitis　カタル性結膜炎 catarrhal conjunctivitis　乾性角結膜炎 dry eye / keratoconjunctivitis sicca；KCS　偽膜結膜炎 pseudomembranous conjunctivitis　クラミジア結膜炎 chlamydial conjunctivitis　細菌性結膜炎 bacterial conjunctivitis　出血性結膜炎 hemorrhagic conjunctivitis　プール性結膜炎 swimming pool conjunctivitis　フリクテン結膜炎 phlyctenular conjunctivitis　流行性角結膜炎 infectious keratoconjunctivitis　濾胞性結膜炎 follicular conjunctivitis

けつまつ　月末 the end of the month　◆月末に at the end of the month　◆月末までに by the end of the month

けつゆうびょう　血友病 hemophilia（類 hemophiliac, hemophilic）　◆血友病は血液が固まりにくくなる遺伝性疾患です Hemophilia is a hereditary disorder in which the blood fails to clot properly.　◆血友病の患者 a hemophilia[hemophiliac] patient / a patient with hemophilia　▶血友病関節症 hemophilic joint

けつようび　月曜日 Monday；Mon.　◆月曜日に on Monday　◆月曜日ごとに on Mondays

けつりゅう　血流 blood flow, bloodstream　☞血行　◆血流をよくする薬を処方する prescribe a medication to improve *a person's* blood flow　◀肝血流 hepatic blood flow；HBF　冠血流 coronary blood flow；CBF　脳血流 cerebral blood flow；CBF　▶血流量 blood flow volume

けつろん　結論 conclusion（類conclude, make[draw] a conclusion）　◆結論を急がないで慎重に考えて下さい Please don't rush[jump] to conclusions, but think carefully.　◆ご家族と話し合ってどういう結論に達しましたか What conclusion did you come to after you talked with your family?　◆最終的な結論を出すのはまだ早すぎます It's too early for us to make a final conclusion.

ケトアシドーシス　ketoacidosis　◀糖尿病性ケトアシドーシス diabetic ketoacidosis；DKA

げどく　解毒 detoxification（類毒性を除く detoxify　毒を中和する counteract (a) poison）　◆解毒作用 detoxification / detoxifying effect　解毒薬 antidote

ケトン　ketone（類ケトンの・ケトンを含む ketonic　ケトン症の ketotic）　▶ケトン血症 ketonemia / ketosis　ケトン性低血糖症 ketotic hypoglycemia　ケトン体 ketone body　ケトン尿 ketonuria

げねつやく　解熱薬 fever reducer, antipyretic (medication, drug, agent), medication to bring a high fever down　☞熱　◀鎮痛解熱薬 analgesic-antipyretic (medication / drug / agent) / pain-fever medication

ゲノム　genome /dʒíːnoʊm/　▶ゲノムスクリーニング genome[genomic] screening　ゲノム創薬 genome drug development　ゲノム分析 genome analysis

けびょう　仮病 feigned illness[sickness], pretended illness[sickness]　◆仮病を使う pretend to be ill[sick] / play ill[sick]

ケブネルげんしょう　—現象 Köbner phenomenon

ケミカルピーリング　chemical peeling[peel]

ケラチノサイト　keratinocyte

ケラチン　keratin

ケラトアカントーマ　keratoacanthoma

げり　下痢 diarrhea /dáɪəríːə/, loose bowels　★複数形で。　◆下痢をしていますか Do you have diarrhea?　◆何回下痢しましたか How many times have you had diarrhea?　◆下痢は何日続いていますか How many days did you have the diarrhea?　◆食べ物が原因で下痢になったと思われますか Do you think you got the diarrhea from something you ate?　◆下痢と便秘を交互に繰り返しますか Do you have alternating (bouts of) diarrhea and constipation? ◆下痢気味である have a touch of diarrhea ◆下痢を止める stop the diarrhea ◀感染性下痢 infectious diarrhea 血性下痢 bloody diarrhea 抗生物質関連下痢 antibiotic-associated diarrhea 細菌性下痢 bacterial diarrhea 心因性下痢 psychogenic diarrhea 水様性下痢 watery diarrhea 難治性下痢 intractable diarrhea 乳児下痢症 infantile diarrhea 粘液性下痢 mucous diarrhea 旅行者下痢症 traveler's[travelers'] diarrhea ロタウイルス下痢症 rotavirus[rotaviral] diarrhea ▶下痢止め薬 antidiarrheal（medication / drug / agent）/ diarrhea medication 下痢便 watery[runny] stool

ゲル gel /dʒél/ ☞ゼリー

ケルススとくそう ―禿瘡 Celsus kerion

ケルニッヒちょうこう ―徴候 Kernig sign

ケロイド keloid /kíːlɔɪd/（❐keloid, keloidal）◆胸にケロイドの痕がある have keloid scars on *one's* chest ◀瘢痕ケロイド scar[cicatricial] keloid ▶ケロイド瘢痕 keloid scar

けん[1] 腱 tendon（❐tendinous）, sinew ◆アキレス腱を切る tear[cut / rupture] the[*one's*] Achilles tendon ◆あなたの右のアキレス腱は断裂しているようです Your right Achilles tendon seems to be ruptured. ▶腱炎 tendinitis / tendonitis 腱黄色腫 tendinous xanthoma 腱固定術 tenodesis 腱断裂 tendon rupture 腱縫合術 tendon suture / tenorrhaphy ☞腱反射

けん[2] 券 （カード）card （切符）ticket （紙片）slip ◀診察券 hospital[patient] ID card / consultation card 整理券（到着順を表した番号札）numbered ticket[slip] given to patients in order of their arrival 予約券 appointment card[slip]

げんあつ 減圧 decompression ◀開頭減圧術 cerebral decompression 内減圧術 internal decompression ▶減圧術 decompression surgery 減圧症 decompression sickness；DCS /（潜函病）divers'

disease, caisson disease

けんあん 検案 ☞検死 ◀死体検案書 death certificate

けんいやく 健胃薬 （消化薬）digestive （medication, drug, agent）（胃機能亢進薬）stomachic（medication, drug, agent）（炭酸水の一種）digestive tonic

けんいん 牽引 traction ◀頸椎牽引 neck[cervical] traction 骨盤牽引 pelvic traction 直達〈介達〉牽引 direct〈indirect〉(skeletal) traction 頭蓋牽引 skull traction ▶牽引反射 traction reflex 牽引療法 traction therapy

げんいん 原因 cause（🔲原因となる cause 🔲因果関係を示す causative）（誘発する）induce ☞要因 ◆下痢の原因に心当たりがありますか What do you think is the cause of your diarrhea? / What do you think is causing your diarrhea? ◆蕁麻疹の原因を調べるために皮膚のアレルギー検査を行いましょう Let's do[run] a skin allergy test to find out what's causing your hives. ◆検査で症状の原因がわかりました The test results show[tell us] what's causing your symptoms. ◆熱は喉の炎症が原因です The throat infection is causing your fever. ◆風邪が原因で気管支炎を起こしています The cold has developed into bronchitis. ◆この病気の原因はまだ十分にわかっていません The cause of this disease is not yet fully understood. ◆直接的な〈間接的な〉原因 *a direct〈an indirect〉 cause ◆根本的な原因 an underlying cause ◆ストレスが原因で起こる病気 an illness caused by stress / a stress-induced illness ▶原因因子 causative factor 原因菌 causative organism ☞原因不明

げんいんふめい 原因不明（の）（原因などが明らかでない）unknown （説明のつかない）unexplained （疑わしい）suspicious （特定されていない）undetermined ◆その症状はいまだに原因不明です The cause of the symptom remains unknown. ◆原因不明の熱 a fever of unknown origin；FUO ◆原因不明の死 *an unknown[an unexplained / an undetermined / a suspicious] (cause of) death

けんえき 検疫 quarantine (㋾quarantinable) ▶検疫感染症 quarantinable infectious disease 検疫所 quarantine office [station]

げんえん 減塩する cut down on salt, reduce *one's* salt intake ☞塩分 ▶減塩醤油 low-salt [low-sodium] soy sauce 減塩食 low-salt [low-sodium] diet / sodium-restricted diet

けんおん 検温する take *a person's* temperature ☞体温, 熱

けんかい 見解 opinion, point of view ☞意見 ◆それは面白い見解ですね That's an interesting opinion [point of view / way of seeing things]. ◆それは見解の相違です I guess we have different opinions [points of view] on that matter. / I guess we disagree with each other about that.

げんかい 限界 (限度)limit(s) (能力・活動などの限界)limitations ★通例, 複数形で. ◆その治療はよいのですが限界があります The treatment is good, but it has its limits [limitations]. ◆残念ですが, 現状ではこれが治療の限界です I'm sorry, but this is as far as we can go with treatment under the present conditions. / I'm sorry, but we've reached the limits of what we can do in terms of treatment. ◆彼女は我慢の限界に達しているようです She seems to have reached the limits of her patience. / It seems she's reached the point where she can't stand it anymore. ◆限界を設ける set limits (to) ◆限界を超える exceed [go over] a limit ◆体力の限界 physical limits ◀許容限界 permissible [acceptable / tolerance] limit 検出限界 limit of detection / detection limit

げんかく¹ 幻覚 hallucination (㋾hallucinate) ◆幻覚を見る hallucinate / have [suffer] hallucinations ◆幻覚に襲われる be *assailed by [overcome with] hallucinations ◀入眠時幻覚 hypnagogic hallucination ◀幻覚症 hallucinosis

げんかく² 厳格(な) strict, rigid ☞厳し

い, 厳重

けんがん¹ 検眼 eye examination (視力検査)eye[eyesight] test (検眼法)optometry ☞視力検査 ◆検眼しましょう Let's test[check] your eyes[eyesight]. ☞検眼鏡, 検眼士

けんがん² 献眼 eye donation ◆献眼する donate *one's* eyes

けんがんきょう 検眼鏡 ophthalmoscope ◀走査レーザー検眼鏡 scanning laser ophthalmoscope

げんかん 玄関 the entrance, the front door ☞表玄関

げんかんさ 減感作 desensitization, hyposensitization ◆減感作療法とは, アレルギーの原因物質を少量から徐々に投与することで体を慣れさせるための治療です Desensitization therapy is a treatment to help the body get used to an allergen by exposing it to gradually increasing amounts of the allergy-causing substance.

けんがんし 検眼士 optometrist

げんき 元気(な) well, fine (健康な)healthy (元気が回復した)rested (活力のある)energetic ◆お元気ですか How are you? ◆まもなく元気になりますよ I hope you *feel better[get well / recover] soon. ◆赤ちゃんは元気です The baby is healthy and well. ◆毎朝, 元気が回復していますか Do you feel rested every morning? ◆彼は元気そうに見える He looks well[healthy / energetic]. ◆ご家族は皆さんお元気ですか Are your family all in good health? ◆(退院する患者さんに)どうぞお元気で! Please take care of yourself! / Please look after yourself! ◆無理に彼女を元気づける必要はありません. ただそばにいてあげるだけでよいのです You don't have to cheer her up. All you need to do is to *stay by her side[be beside her]. ◆元気がない be in low spirits / be depressed / feel down ◆元気を回復する recover *one's* health ◆元気を出す take heart / cheer up ◆元気を失くす lose heart

けんきせいきん　嫌気性菌　anaerobic bacteria（圏**bacterium**）（↔aerobic bacteria）　▶嫌気性菌感染症 anaerobic bacterial infection

けんきゅう　研究　（一般的に）**study**（**of**）（学術的な研究）**research**（**into, on**）（圏**experimental, investigational**）　◆研究開発 research and development　◆乳がんの研究を行う *carry out[conduct / do] a study of breast cancer　◆アルツハイマー病の原因に関する研究 research into[on] the causes of Alzheimer disease　◆がん治療に関する最新の研究 *the most recent[the latest] research into[on] cancer treatment　◀横断的研究 cross-sectional study　応用研究 applied research　介入研究 intervention[interventional] study　観察研究 observational study　基礎研究 basic research　共同研究 cooperative[joint] study　症例対照研究 case-control study　事例研究 case study　予備研究 preliminary study　臨床研究 clinical study[research]　▶研究員 researcher / research fellow　研究計画 research plan[project / design]　研究集会 workshop　研究対象 research subject　研究対象者 research participant[patient]　★被験者が人間の場合には subject は避ける。　研究テーマ research theme　研究的治療 experimental[investigational] treatment[therapy]　研究分野 field of study

げんきゅう¹　幻嗅　olfactory hallucination

げんきゅう²　言及する　refer（**to**）**, mention**　☞言う，話す

けんきょう　検鏡　（顕微鏡検査）**microscopy, microscopic test[examination]**　☞顕微鏡

げんきょく　限局する　（範囲が限定している）**be confined**（**to**）　（身体の一部に局在化している）**be localized**（**to**）　◆痛みは1つの関節に限局していますか Is the pain confined[localized] to one joint?　◆がんは前立腺内に限局しているようです The cancer appears to be localized within the prostate.

げんきん　現金　cash　◆診療費の支払い

は現金でもクレジットカードでも可能です You can pay the hospital fees either by cash or by credit card.　▶現金自動預入引出機 ATM / automated-teller machine

けんけつ　献血　blood donation　◀成分献血 blood component donation　▶献血血液 donated blood　献血者 blood donor

げんご　言語　language　（発語）**speech**（単語）**word**（圏言葉の使用に関する **verbal**　言語に関する **linguistic**）　圏語，言葉，発話　◆彼女は今でも言語に障害があります She still has some difficulty speaking. / She still has speech problems.　◆言語の壁による誤解 a misunderstanding caused by a language barrier　◀身体言語 body language　発達性言語障害 developmental language disorder；DLD　非言語コミュニケーション nonverbal communication　▶言語矯正 speech correction　言語訓練 language[speech] training　言語検査 language test　言語行動 verbal behavior　言語症 language[speech] disorder / verbal[language / speech] impairment　言語中枢 the speech[language] center / the speech[language] area (of the brain)　言語聴覚士 speech-language-hearing therapist；ST　言語能力 language skills / linguistic competence /（言葉によるコミュニケーション技術力）verbal communication skills　言語発達 language[speech] development　言語明瞭性 word intelligibility　言語流暢性 speech fluency /（単語の）word fluency　☞言語療法

けんこう　健康　health（圏**healthy**）　◆健康上気がかりなことがありますか Do you have any concerns about your health?　◆健康を保つために何をしていますか What do you do to keep[stay] healthy?　◆その食べ物は健康によい〈悪い〉That food is good〈bad〉for your health.　◆過労で健康を損ねたのですね You ruined[damaged] your health through overwork[excessive work], didn't you? / Overwork damaged[ruined] your health, didn't it?　◆健康な赤ちゃんですよ He〈She〉is a healthy baby.　◆健康によいものを食べる

eat healthy food(s) ◆健康状態がよい〈悪い〉be in good〈poor〉health ◆健康を維持する keep[stay] healthy / maintain [stay in] good health ◆健康を取り戻す recover[regain] *one's* health ◆健康上の理由で for health reasons ◆健康的な生活 a healthy life[lifestyle] ◆健康的な皮膚 healthy[normal] skin ▶健康維持 health maintenance 健康管理 health care[management] 健康教育 health education 健康寿命 healthy life expectancy 健康食品 health food 健康増進センター fitness promotion center 健康相談 health consultation[counseling] 健康手帳 personal health record 健康法 way [how] to stay healthy 健康問題 health problem ☞健康状態, 健康保険, 健(康)診(断)

けんこうこつ 肩甲骨 scapula (形scapular), shoulder blade

けんこうじょうたい 健康状態 state of health, physical condition, health condition ◆これまでの健康状態はどうでしたか How has your health been up until now? ◆健康状態がよい be in good health / be healthy ◆健康状態が悪い be in poor[ill] health / be unhealthy

けんこうしんだん 健康診断 ☞健診

けんこうほけん 健康保険 health insurance ☞保険 ◆日本の健康保険がありますか Do you have Japanese health insurance? ◆国民健康保険に入っていますか Have you joined the National Health Insurance system? / Do you have National Health Insurance? ◆健康保険がないと全額自費診療になりますが，よろしいですか If you don't have health insurance, you'll have to pay *all your medical expenses[the full cost of your medical expenses yourself]. Is that all right? ◆この薬は日本の健康保険が適用されません This medication is not covered by Japanese health insurance. / Japanese health insurance does not cover this medication. ◀国民健康保険 National Health Insurance (system) ▶健康保険証 health insurance card[certificate] 健康保険組合 health insurance society

げんごりょうほう 言語療法 speech therapy ▶言語(療法)聴覚士 speech-language-hearing therapist；ST

けんさ 検査 (一般的に)test (動test), examination, exam (動examine) (特定の病気の検診)screening (動screen) (綿棒などによる粘膜の採取)swab (動swab) (分析)analysis (複analyses 動analyze) ◆血液検査をする do[run] a blood test ◆聴力の検査をする test[check] *a person's* hearing ◆前立腺がんの検査をする screen for prostate cancer ◆尿検査をする take a urine sample for a test / test *a person's* urine

《検査前》 ◆正確に診断するために検査をしましょう Let's do[run] some tests for an accurate diagnosis. / Let's do[run] some tests to help get an accurate diagnosis.

◆この検査は他の病気の可能性を除外するために行います This test is done[performed] to rule out the possibility of other disorders. ◆検査の前夜12時以後は，食べたり飲んだりしないで下さい Please don't eat or drink after midnight on the night before the day of the test.

◆この検査に特別な準備は必要ありません No special preparation is necessary for this test. ◆検査の15分前に検査室においで下さい Please come to the exam room fifteen minutes before the test. ◆この検査を行うためにはあなたの同意が必要です I need your consent to do this test. ◆この検査同意書をよく読んでサインして下さい Please read this consent form for the test carefully before signing it. ◆検査が終わったらここに戻ってきて下さい When the test is finished, please come back here.

◆この検査には一泊の入院が必要です. This test requires an overnight stay in the hospital. / For this test you need to stay overnight in the hospital.

《検査時》 ◆この検査は約10分かかります This test will take about ten minutes (to complete). / It'll take about ten minutes to complete this test. ◆この検査は 2, 3 分で終わります This test will be over in a few minutes. ◆検査は痛くありませんから心配しないで下さい The test is painless, so don't worry. ◆検査の間, 楽にしていて下さい Please try to relax during the test. ◆検査が済むまでじっとしていて下さい Please keep still until the test is finished.

《検査後》 ◆検査の結果はわかり次第お知らせいたします As soon as the results of the tests are available, we'll let you know. ◆検査の結果は 1 時間後に判明します You'll get the test results in one hour. ◆検査の結果は次回の外来の時にご説明します Let me[I'm going to] explain the test results next time you come to see me (in my office).

《検査の結果説明》 ◆検査の結果をご説明します Let me explain the test result(s). / Here's what we've found. ◆検査の結果貧血があります The test result shows[indicates / suggests] that you have anemia. ◆検査から判断すると, 胃炎のようです Judging from the tests, you seem to have gastritis. ◆検査結果に少し異常があります You have a slightly abnormal test result. / The test result is slightly abnormal. ◆検査の結果, 腎臓に異常は認められませんでした The tests confirm that nothing is wrong with[in] your kidney. ◆検査の結果は陰性〈陽性〉です The test results are negative〈positive〉.

◀X 線検査 X-ray examination[test] 緊急検査 emergency test[examination] 血液検査 blood test[examination] 再検査 reexamination CT 検査 CT scan 術前検査 preoperative test[examination] スクリーニング検査 screening test 精密検査 thorough[detailed] test[examination] 追加検査 further[additional] test[examination / testing] / another checkup 追跡検査 follow-up test[examination] 定期検査 regular[routine] test 内視鏡検査 endoscopy / endoscopic examination 尿検査 urine test[examination] / urinalysis；

UA 病理学検査 pathologic examination 便検査 stool test[examination] 臨床検査 clinical (laboratory) test[testing]

▶検査技師 medical technologist；MT / medical laboratory scientist；MLS 検査計画 test[examination] plan 検査項目 test item 検査食 special[prescribed] diet before the test[examination] 検査所見 examination[laboratory] findings 検査台 exam[examining] table 検査値 (lab) test value 検査データ test data 検査同意書 test consent form / consent form for the test 検査部位 the site[area] to be examined ☞検査着, 検査室

けんざい 健在(な) alive and well ◆ご両親はご健在ですか Are your parents still living[in good health]? / Are your parents alive and well?

けんさぎ 検査着 (exam) gown ☞ガウン ◆この検査着を着て下さい Please put this (exam) gown on. ◆検査着は後ろを開けて着て下さい Please put the gown on with the opening in the back.

けんさく¹ 検索 search (動search) ◆ウェブサイトで鳥インフルエンザの最新情報を検索する search the website for the latest information on avian influenza

けんさく² 腱索 tendinous cords ★複数形で. ▶腱索断裂 rupture of the tendinous cords

けんさしつ 検査室 laboratory /lǽbərətɔ̀ːri/, lab, examination[exam, screening] room ◀検体検査室 specimen laboratory 生理機能検査室 physiologic laboratory [examination room] 超音波検査室 ultrasound scanning room 内視鏡検査室 endoscopic examination room

けんし¹ 犬歯 canine tooth (複teeth)

けんし² 検死 (剖検) autopsy /ɔ́ːtɑpsi/ (死後解剖) postmortem examination (死因審問) inquest ◆死亡原因を突き止めるために検死をする perform an autopsy to determine the cause of *a person's* death ▶検死報告 autopsy report

けんし³ 絹糸 silk ▶絹糸縫合 silk suture

げんし¹ 幻肢 phantom limb ▶幻肢痛 phantom limb pain / pseudesthesia

げんし² 幻視 visual hallucination

げんじつ 現実 reality (圏really) (実際・実地) practicality (圏practically) (現状) actuality (圏actually) (事実) fact (圏factually) ☞現状, 実際 ◆ご自宅での介護は現実的には難しいですか Practically speaking, is it difficult to take care of him〈her〉at home? / Is it really[actually] difficult to take care of him〈her〉at home? ◆現実を受け入れる(現実と向き合う) face reality ◆現実を否定する deny reality ◆現実から逃避する escape from reality ◀仮想現実 virtual reality

げんしはんしゃ 原始反射 primitive reflex

けんしゅう 研修 (臨床の)(clinical) training ◆彼女は医学生で臨床研修をしています She's a medical student (who is) doing [undergoing] clinical training. ◀現場研修 on-site[on-the-job] training 卒後研修 postgraduate training ▶研修医 resident

げんじゅう 厳重(な) strict, rigid (極めて慎重な)very careful ☞厳しい, 厳密 ◆当分の間厳重な食事療法が必要です You have to follow a strict[rigid] diet for some time. ◆この薬の服用には厳重な注意が必要です. 指示通りに飲まないと予期しない副作用が現れることがあります You need to be very careful when you take this medication because you may have unexpected side effects if you don't take it exactly as directed.

げんじゅうしょ 現住所 present address, current address ☞住所

けんしゅしょうこうぐん 肩手症候群 shoulder-hand syndrome

けんしゅつ 検出する (一般的に見つける) find (検査で探り出す)detect ◆胃から毒物が検出されました A poisonous substance was detected in your stomach. / The results of the test showed a poisonous substance in your stomach. ▶検出限界 detection limit / limit of detection

けんしゅやく 嫌酒薬 alcohol deterrent

けんしょう 検証する (仮説などを調べる) test (点検する)inspect (確認する)verify ◆仮説を検証する test a hypothesis

げんしょう¹ 現症 present status

げんしょう² 現象 phenomenon (圏phenomena, phenomenons) ◀生理現象 physiologic phenomenon レイノー現象 Raynaud phenomenon 老化現象 signs and symptoms of aging / condition caused by aging

げんしょう³ 減少 (数量の低下)decrease (↔increase)(圏decrease) (失うこと)loss (↔gain)(圏lose) (枯渇) depletion 腰尾-penia ☞減る ◆白血球が少し減少しています Your white blood cells are down slightly. / There is a slight decrease in the number of white blood cells. ◆最近, 体重が減少しましたか Have you recently lost weight? ◀血小板減少 thrombocytopenia 好中球減少 neutropenia 体重減少 weight loss 尿量減少 oliguria / decreased[scanty] urinary output 表情減少 decreased expression リンパ球減少 lymphocytopenia / lymphopenia

げんじょう 現状 the present condition(s) [situation, circumstances], how things stand, the way things are ★circumstances, things は通例, 複数形で. ☞現実, 状況 ◆現状を維持する maintain the present condition(s)[situation] ◆現状を知る know *how things stand[the way things are] ◆現状を受け入れる take[accept] things as they are ◆現状をふまえる take the present conditions into consideration ◆現状では飛行機でのご旅行は難しいです Under the present conditions[circumstances], it's difficult for you to travel by plane. ◆あなたの症状の原因はまだわかっていないのが現状です For the moment[At this stage], I still don't know what's causing your symptoms.

けんしょうえん 腱鞘炎 tendovaginitis, tenosynovitis ◆コンピュータのキーボードやマウスの使い過ぎは腱鞘炎, すなわち腱とその周囲を覆う鞘の炎症を起こすことが

あります Overuse of a computer keyboard and mouse can lead to tendovaginitis, which means inflammation of a tendon and its surrounding sheath.

けんじょうしゃ 健常者 **person without disabilities, person without special health [care] needs**

けんじょうとっき 剣状突起 **xiphoid process**

げんしょく 幻触 **tactile hallucination**

けんしん[1] 検診 **screening (test), (medical) checkup** ◆大腸がんの検診を受けましたか Did you have a colon *screening test[checkup]? / Did you have a *screening test[checkup] for colon cancer? ◆乳がんの定期検診を受ける undergo *routine screening[a routine checkup] for breast cancer ◆検診で何か問題がありましたか Did they find anything wrong (with you) at the *screening test[checkup]? ◆次の検診日は3月10日月曜日です Your next checkup is Monday, March (the) 10th. ◀がん検診 cancer screening [checkup] 子宮頸がん検診 Pap smear test 集団検診 mass screening / *mass health[group medical] examination 婦人科検診 gynecologic screening[checkup]

けんしん[2] 健診 **(health) checkup, (physical) checkup, physical** ◆毎年健診を受けていますか Do you have[go for] an annual checkup[physical]? ◆健診はいつ，どこで受けましたか When did you have the checkup, and where? ◆健診で血糖値が高いと言われたのですか Were you told at the checkup that you have high blood sugar? ◆健診を行う perform a physical ◆生後4か月健診 the four-month health checkup after birth ◀学校健診 school health checkup / health checkup at school 就学児健診 school entry health checkup 住民健診 residents health checkup / health checkup for city〈town / village〉residents 定期健診 regular (health) checkup / periodic (health) checkup / routine (health) checkup 特殊健診 special physical[health] examination（of workers） 乳幼児健診 infant health checkup 妊婦健診 pregnancy [prenatal] health checkup 無料健診 free checkup ▶健診異常 problem found at the checkup 健診センター health screening center / comprehensive physical examination center

げんすうぶんれつ 減数分裂 **meiosis, successive cell division**

けんせい 顕性(の) (明白な)**apparent** (症状などが現れた)**manifest** (⇔silent, asymptomatic, subclinical, latent) ▶顕性感染 apparent infection 顕性斜視 manifest strabismus

げんそ 元素 **element** ◀必須元素 essential element 微量元素 trace element 微量元素欠乏症 trace element deficiency ▶元素記号 the symbol of an element

けんそく 健側 **unaffected side**

げんそく 原則 (一般的な規則)**general rule** (根本的な規則)**principle** ◆原則として外泊は許可しておりません As a general rule, staying out overnight is not allowed.

けんたい[1] 検体 **specimen, sample** ☞サンプル ◆血液〈組織〉の検体 a blood〈tissue〉specimen[sample] ▶検体検査室 specimen laboratory 検体採取 specimen collection / sampling[collecting] of the specimen

けんたい[2] 献体する (研究のために)**donate one's body to medical research**

げんたい 減退 (失うこと)**loss** (動lose) (減少・低下)**diminishment** (動diminish), **decline** (動decline) ◀嗅覚減退 hyposmia 食欲減退 loss of appetite 知覚減退 diminished sensation / hypesthesia / hypoesthesia

けんたいかん 倦怠感 **weariness, general tiredness, feeling of fatigue** (疲れなどからくる不快感)**malaise** ☞だるい ◀全身倦怠感 general malaise

げんちゅう 原虫 **protozoon** (複protozoan, protozoal) ◀マラリア原虫 malarial parasite ▶原虫感染症 protozoan

infection 原虫症 protozoal disease

けんちょ 顕著(な) (目立つ)marked (かなりの)significant (めざましい)remarkable ☞著しい ◆検査結果を見ると治療の効果が顕著に表れています The test results show a marked[significant] treatment effect. ◆白血球の増加が顕著です Your white blood cell counts have increased significantly.

げんちょう 幻聴 auditory hallucination ◆幻聴がありますか Do you hear imaginary voices or noises? / Do you hear voices or noises in your head?

けんてい 検定 ◆片側検定 one-sided test 両側検定 two-sided[two-tailed] test ログランク検定 log-rank test

げんど 限度 ☞限界

けんとう 検討する (考察する)examine (图examination) (調査・研究する)study (图study) (見直す)review (图review) (熟慮する)consider (图consideration) (原因を究明する)investigate (图investigation) ◆治療方針を検討する examine[review] the treatment plan ◆手術の適応についてさらに検討する必要があります I think we should give the matter further consideration before we decide whether or not to do the surgery ◆その問題に関してはまだ検討中です I'm still thinking about the problem. ◀再検討 review / reexamination 症例検討会 case conference

げんどう 言動 ◆最近彼女の言動がおかしい The way she's been talking and acting recently has been strange[abnormal]. / She's been talking and acting[behaving] strangely recently.

けんとうしき 見当識 orientation (图oriented) ◆意識は清明で見当識は保たれている be[remain] fully alert and oriented ◆見当識が障害される be disoriented ◆見当識障害 disorientation / orientation disturbance

けんにょう 検尿 urine test[examination], urinalysis (图urinalyses)；UA ☞尿, 尿検査 ▶検尿コップ urine[urinalysis] cup

けんばいようせき 犬吠様咳 barking cough

げんばくしょう 原爆症 atomic bomb disease, A-bomb disease

げんぱつ 原発(性・の) primary ▶原発がん primary cancer 原発腫瘍 primary tumor 原発性開放隅角緑内障 primary open-angle glaucoma；POAG 原発性硬化性胆管炎 primary sclerosing cholangitis；PSC 原発性胆汁性肝硬変 primary biliary cirrhosis；PBC 原発性肺高血圧症 primary pulmonary hypertension；PPH 原発巣 primary focus

けんはんしゃ 腱反射 tendon reflex ◆腱反射を調べましょう Let's check your tendon reflexes. ◆膝の腱反射を見ます Let me check your knee jerk[reflex]. ◆腱反射の減弱〈亢進〉decreased〈increased〉tendon reflexes / hyporeflexia 〈hyperreflexia〉of the tendon ◀アキレス腱反射 Achilles tendon reflex；ATR / ankle jerk 膝蓋腱反射 patellar tendon reflex；PTR / knee jerk[reflex] 深部腱反射 deep tendon reflex；DTR

けんびきょう 顕微鏡 microscope (图microscopic) ◆その組織を顕微鏡で調べる examine the tissue under[through] a microscope ◀光学顕微鏡 light microscope 細隙灯顕微鏡検査 slit lamp microscopy 電子顕微鏡 electron microscope ▶顕微鏡検査 microscopy / microscopic test[examination] 顕微鏡手術 microsurgery 顕微鏡的観察 microscopic observation 顕微鏡的血尿 microscopic hematuria 顕微鏡的多発血管炎 microscopic polyangiitis；MPA

けんびじゅせい 顕微授精 microinsemination, microfertilization

げんびょうれき 現病歴 present (medical) history, history of (the) present illness；HPI, history of (the) presenting complaint；HPC ☞病歴

けんべん 検便 stool test[examination] ☞便 ◆検便が必要です We need to do [run] a stool test. / We need *a sample of your stool[a stool sample]. / We need to examine your stool. ▶検便キット stool test kit

けんぼう 健忘(症) amnesia (形amnestic), memory loss, forgetfulness ◀一過性健忘 transient[temporary] amnesia　外傷後健忘 posttraumatic amnesia　逆向性健忘 retrograde amnesia　全健忘 total memory loss / total[global] amnesia　前向健忘 anterograde amnesia　部分健忘 partial *memory loss[amnesia] / (まだら) lacunar amnesia　▶健忘性失語 amnestic aphasia

げんみ 幻味　gustatory hallucination

げんみつ 厳密(な)　strict, rigid ☞厳しい, 厳重 ◆食事療法計画をあまり厳密に守ろうとすると挫折します If you follow your diet plan too strictly[rigidly], *it'll only end in frustration[it won't work out].

けんめい¹ 賢明(な)　wise ◆お酒を控えたのは賢明でしたね It was wise of you to refrain from drinking alcohol.

けんめい² 懸命(に)　☞一所懸命

けんり 権利　right ◆十分な説明と同意は重要な患者の権利です Informed consent is an important patient right. ◆患者は自分が受ける治療の選択肢を知る権利があります Patients have the right to know *what treatment options they have [their treatment options]. ◀患者の権利 patient[patients'] rights　患者の権利宣言 Patients' Bill of Rights

げんりょう 減量する　lose weight, reduce *one's* weight ◆減量が必要です You need to lose some weight. ◆5キロ減量する lose five kilograms ◆体重の減量 weight loss ▶減量食(体重の) weight-reduction[reducing] diet

こ

こ 子 child （圈children） （男の子）boy （女の子）girl ☞子供 ◆お子さんはいますか Do you have any children? ◆お子さんは全部で何人ですか How many children do you have? ◆（子供の患者に）いい子だね What a good boy〈girl〉!

ご 語 （単語）word （言語）language （用語）term ☞言語, 言葉 ◆家では何語を話していますか What language do you speak [use] at home? ◆（母語は何か）What's your *mother tongue[first language]? ◆この語の意味は何ですか What does this word mean? ◀一般語（用語）general[everyday / lay] term / （単語）general[everyday] word 専門語 technical term [word] 幼児語 baby talk / （小児語）child language

こい 濃い （色が）dark （↔light） （濃度・密度が）thick （↔thin） （味・匂いが）strong （↔weak） （濃縮した）concentrated （↔dilute, diluted） ◆濃い茶色の便 *dark brown[（コーヒーかす色）coffee-grounds, coffee-looking] stools / stools that look like coffee grounds ◆濃いサングラスをかけている wear dark sunglasses ◆濃いスープ thick soup ◆頭髪や体毛が前より濃くなっていますか Has your hair been getting thicker? ◆濃いコーヒー strong coffee ◆濃い味付けの食べ物を避ける avoid eating highly seasoned foods ◆塩分の濃い食品 salty food ◆濃い尿 concentrated urine

コイル coil ◆（カテーテルを通して）コイルを動脈瘤に留置し破裂を予防する fill in an aneurysm with a coil （inserted via a catheter） to prevent it from rupturing ◀脳動脈瘤コイル塞栓術 endovascular coil embolization of a cerebral aneurysm

ごいん 誤飲する swallow accidentally [by mistake] （気道内に吸い込む）aspirate （圖aspiration） ☞誤嚥 ◆お子さんは誤飲

したのですか Did your child accidentally *swallow something[put something in his 〈her〉 mouth]? ◆タバコの吸い殻を誤飲する swallow a cigarette butt accidentally [by mistake] ◆異物を誤飲する（気道内に）aspirate[breathe in] a foreign object accidentally

コインランドリー coin-operated laundry （商標名）《米》Laundromat

こう[1] 甲 （手の）the back of the hand （↔palm） （足の）instep, the upper side of the foot ◆手の甲を見せて下さい Let me look at the back of your hand(s). ◆爪の甲 the nail plate

こう[2] ☞このように

ごう 号 （番号）number ◆あなたの病室は 312 号室です Your room number is three hundred （and） twelve. / You'll be in room three hundred （and） twelve. ★312 は three-one-two ともいう. ☞数字

こうあくせいしゅようやく 抗悪性腫瘍薬 anticancer medication[drug, agent] ☞化学療法

こうあつ 高圧 high pressure （圈hyperbaric） ▶高圧酸素療法 hyperbaric oxygenation；HBO 高圧蒸気滅菌 high-pressure steam sterilization

こうあつやく 降圧薬 antihypertensive （medication, drug, agent）, hypotensive （medication, drug, agent）, medication for high blood pressure ◆血圧をコントロールするために降圧薬を飲む必要があります You need to take antihypertensives to control your blood pressure. ▶降圧利尿薬 antihypertensive diuretic （medication / drug / agent）

こうアレルギーやく 抗アレルギー薬 antiallergic （medication, drug, agent）

こうい[1] 行為 （一連の行動）action （1 回の行動）act （振る舞い・行い）behavior, conduct ☞行動 ◆彼の攻撃的な行為に皆が迷惑しています We're all annoyed by his aggressive behavior[actions]. / His aggressive behavior is annoying[bothering] us all. ◆職業倫理にかなった行為 professional conduct ◆倫理的行為 ethical conduct ◆反社会的な行為 antisocial behavior / an antisocial act ◆違法行為 illegal[unlawful] act 医療行為(業務)medical practice / (活動)medical activity / (介入)medical intervention 強迫行為 compulsive behavior / compulsion 自慰行為 masturbation 自殺行為 suicidal behavior[act] 自傷行為 self-destructive[self-injurious] behavior 性行為 sexual activity / (sexual) intercourse / sex act 暴力行為 violent behavior[act] / act of violence わいせつ行為 indecent behavior[act]

こうい² 校医 school doctor

こういしつ 更衣室 locker room, changing room

こういしょう 後遺症 aftereffect (長く続く影響)lasting effect ◆交通事故の後遺症はまだありますか Are you still suffering [Do you still have] the aftereffects of the traffic accident? ◆脳卒中の後遺症はありますか Do you have any lasting effects from the stroke? ◆この脳出血で後遺症が出るかもしれません This *bleeding in the brain[cerebral hemorrhage] may *have aftereffects[cause long-term damage later]. ◆事故の後遺症で腰から下が麻痺している as an aftereffect of an accident ◆心筋梗塞の後遺症に苦しむ suffer the aftereffects of myocardial infarction

こういせいそうてきじょじゅつ 高位精巣摘除術 high orchiectomy[orchidectomy]

こういそうはく 口囲蒼白 perioral pallor, circumoral pallor

こういまひ 後遺麻痺 residual paralysis

ごういん 強引 ◆子供を強引に登校させる force one's child to go to school against his⟨her⟩ will ◆強引な母親(高圧的な)a high-handed mother

こうウイルスやく 抗ウイルス薬 antiviral (medication, drug, agent)

こううつやく 抗うつ薬 antidepressant (medication, drug, agent)

こううん 幸運 good luck (㊤lucky), fortune (㊤fortunate) ☞幸せ ◆幸運に恵まれる have good luck ◆幸運をお祈りします(うまくいくように)Good luck (to you). / I wish you good luck. / (お幸せに)My thoughts and prayers are with you. / I pray for your happiness. ◆幸運にも彼女の手術はうまくいきました Luckily[Fortunately], her surgery was a success.

こうえんききゅう 好塩基球 basophil

こうえんしょうやく 抗炎症薬 antiinflammatory medication[drug, agent] ◀非ステロイド系抗炎症薬 nonsteroidal antiinflammatory drugs；NSAIDs

こうえんそけつしょう 高塩素血症 hyperchloremia

こうおん¹ 高音 high[high-pitched] sound (↔low[low-pitched] sound) (音色の) high[high-pitched] tone (声の) high[high-pitched] voice (高周波の)high frequency ☞音 ◆高音が聞こえにくい have difficulty hearing high[high-pitched] sounds ▶高音域障害型難聴 high-frequency[high-tone] hearing loss

こうおん² 高温 high temperature (↔low temperature) ◆直射日光や高温の所にいましたか(さらされたか)Have you been exposed to direct sunlight or high temperatures? ◆高温で殺菌する sterilize at a high temperature ◀超高温滅菌 ultra-high temperature sterilization ▶(基礎体温の)高温相 hyperthermic phase

こうおんしょうがい 構音障害 articulation disorder, dysarthria

こうか¹ 効果 effect (㊤effective ↔ineffective) (有効性)effectiveness (薬などの効能)efficacy, potency ☞効き目, 効く ◆薬は効果がありましたか Did the medication work[help]? ◆この薬は血圧を下げる効果があります This medication is effective[good] for lowering blood pressure. ◆この注射はすぐに効果が現れます This shot will *have an immediate effect [start working right away]. ◆この治療の効果はすぐには現れません You can't expect any immediate effects from this treatment. / The effects of this treatment won't be immediately apparent. ◆この薬の効果が出るまでにはしばらく時間がかかります It'll take some time before *the effects of this medication become apparent[you feel the effects of this medication]. ◆この薬の効果は患者によって異なります The effectiveness[efficacy] of this medication varies from patient to patient. ◆薬の効果を上げる〈下げる〉increase〈reduce〉the effect of the medication ◆望み通りの効果を挙げる get[obtain] the desired effect ◆効果的な治療 an effective treatment ◀偽薬効果 placebo effect　逆効果 opposite effect　心理的効果 psychological effect　造影効果 contrast enhancement　相加効果 additive effect　相乗効果 synergistic effect　蓄積効果 cumulative effect　遅発効果 delayed[late] effect　治療効果 therapeutic effect　鎮静効果 sedative effect　鎮痛効果 analgesic effect　ブースター効果 booster effect　併用効果 combined effect　抑制効果 inhibitory effect　冷却効果 cooling effect　▶効果器 effector

こうか²　硬化　hardening　（硬化症）sclerosis /sklɪróʊsɪs/　☞硬い ◀冠動脈硬化症 coronary arteriosclerosis　筋萎縮性側索硬化症 amyotrophic lateral sclerosis；ALS　結節性硬化症 tuberous sclerosis　骨硬化 osteosclerosis　耳硬化症 otosclerosis　粥状硬化症 atherosclerosis　腎硬化症 nephrosclerosis　巣状糸球体硬化症 focal glomerulosclerosis；FGS　多発性硬化症 multiple sclerosis；MS　動脈硬化症 arteriosclerosis / hardening[sclerosis] of the arteries　閉塞性動脈硬化症 arteriosclerosis obliterans；ASO　▶硬化性血管腫 sclerosing hemangioma　硬化像 consolidation　☞硬化療法

こうがい¹　口蓋　palate /pǽlət/　（圀palatine, palatal）◀硬口蓋 hard palate　軟口蓋 soft palate　軟口蓋裂 soft palate cleft　▶口蓋形成術 palatoplasty　口蓋垂 uvula / uvula of the soft palate　口蓋扁桃 palatine[faucial] tonsil　口蓋扁桃摘出術 tonsillectomy　☞口蓋裂

こうがい²　公害　（environmental）pollution　▶公害病 pollution(-caused) disease / illness caused by pollution / pollution-related disease　公害病認定患者 patient officially certified as having pollution-related disease / officially certified patient with pollution-related disease

こうかいようやく　抗潰瘍薬　antiulcer medication[drug, agent]

こうがいれつ　口蓋裂　cleft palate

こうかがく　光化学（の）　photochemical　▶光化学オキシダント photochemical oxidant　光化学汚染物質 photochemical pollutant　光化学スモッグ photochemical smog　光化学療法 photochemotherapy

こうかく　口角　the corners of the mouth, the angles of the mouth　◆口角に潰瘍がある have ulcers on[in] the corners of *one's* mouth　▶口角炎 angular cheilitis　口角びらん angular stomatitis

こうがく¹　工学　engineering　◀遺伝子工学 genetic engineering　生体工学 bioengineering　人間工学 human engineering / ergonomics　リハビリテーション工学 rehabilitation engineering　臨床工学 clinical engineering

こうがく²　高額　high cost（圀high-cost）, large sum of money　▶高額医療技術 high-cost medical technology　高額医療費 high medical expenses[costs]　☞高額療養費

こうがくけんびきょう　光学顕微鏡　light microscope　（検査）light microscopy

こうかくこうたい　抗核抗体　antinuclear antibody；ANA

ごうかくてん　合格点　（点数）passing score　（評価・成績）passing mark[grade]　◆これだけ達成できればリハビリで合格点をあげられます Once you can do this much, you'll have the passing score you need to finish rehabilitation. / Once you've achieved this much, I can give you the passing mark[grade] in rehabilitation.

こうがくりょうようひ　高額療養費　（給付

金）high-cost medical care benefits ★複数形で. ◆医療費が一定額を超えた場合, （申請により）超えた金額を高額療養費として受け取ることができます If your medical costs are above a certain level (and you submit the proper paperwork), you can receive[be reimbursed with] high-cost medical care benefits. ◆高額療養費の払い戻し金 reimbursement of high-cost medical care benefits

こうがしゅ 膠芽腫 glioblastoma

こうかしょう 硬化症 ☞強皮症

こうかっせいこうレトロウイルスりょうほう 高活性抗レトロウイルス療法 highly active antiretroviral therapy；HAART

こうかやく 降下薬 ◀血圧降下薬 antihypertensive（medication / drug / agent）血糖降下薬 hypoglycemic（medication / drug / agent）

こうカリウムけつしょう 高カリウム血症 hyperkalemia（形hyperkalemic），hyperpotassemia ▶偽性高カリウム血症 pseudohyperkalemia ▶高カリウム血性周期性四肢麻痺 hyperkalemic periodic paralysis

こうかりょうほう 硬化療法 sclerotherapy ◀内視鏡的硬化療法 endoscopic sclerotherapy

こうカルシウムけつしょう 高カルシウム血症 hypercalcemia

こうカルシウムにょうしょう 高カルシウム尿症 hypercalciuria

こうカロリー 高カロリー high calorie ▶高カロリー食 high-calorie diet；HCD / high-calorie food 高カロリー輸液（経静脈高カロリー輸液）intravenous hyperalimentation；IVH /（完全静脈栄養）total parenteral nutrition；TPN

こうかん 交換する （新しいものへの切り替え）change, switch （同種のものとの取り替え）exchange （交替・置換）replace （代用・補充）substitute （図change, switch, exchange, replacement, substitution） ☞換える，換わる ◆シーツを交換しましょう Let me change your sheets. ◆体位を交換する change one's body position ◆傷口の包帯を交換する change a wound dress-ing ◆傷口のガーゼを交換する change the gauze over a wound ◆薬を交換する change[switch] medications ◆電池を交換する replace[change] a battery ◆患者同士の情報交換 exchange of information among patients ◀イオン交換樹脂 ion-exchange resin おむつ交換 diaper change /（成人用）(incontinence) briefs[underwear / pad] change 血漿交換 plasma exchange

こうがん 睾丸 ☞精巣

ごうかん 強姦 rape （婉曲的に）assault ▶強姦被害者 rape victim

こうがんあつしょう 高眼圧症 ocular hypertension

こうがんざい 抗がん剤 anticancer medication[drug, agent] ☞化学療法

こうかんしんけい 交感神経 sympathetic nerve ◀副交感神経 parasympathetic nerve ▶交感神経作用薬 sympathomimetic（medication / drug / agent）交感神経遮断薬 sympatholytic（medication / drug / agent）交感神経切除術 sympathectomy 交感神経ブロック sympathetic nerve block ☞交感神経節

こうかんしんけいせつ 交感神経節 sympathetic ganglion ▶交感神経節切除術 sympathetic ganglionectomy 交感神経節ブロック sympathetic ganglion block

こうき¹ 好機 good chance[opportunity] ☞機会 ◆生活習慣を見直すまたとない好機です This is a good chance[opportunity] for you to change[improve] your daily habits. / Now is your best chance[opportunity] to change[improve] your daily habits.

こうき² 後期 the late stage[period] （後半）the second[latter] half ◀妊娠後期 the late stage of pregnancy /（妊娠第3期）the third trimester ▶後期高齢者（75歳以上）(elderly) person aged 75[seventy-five] years and older / senior senior /（総称的に）the old-old 後期流産 late abortion

こうきしん 好奇心 curiosity, inquisitiveness

こうきせいきん 好気性菌 aerobic bacteria（圏bacterium）（↔anaerobic bacteria）

こうきどかん 高輝度肝 bright liver

こうきのうじへいしょう 高機能自閉症 high-functioning autism ☞自閉

こうきゅう 恒久（的な） permanent, lasting ▶恒久的ペーシング permanent pacing

こうきょう 公共（の） public ▶公共サービス public services 公共施設 public facility[institution] 公共福祉 public welfare

こうぎょうこ 抗凝固（性の） anticoagulant ▶抗凝固薬 anticoagulant（medication / drug / agent） 抗凝固療法 anticoagulant therapy

こうきょうしんしょうやく 抗狭心症薬 antianginal（medication, drug, agent）

こうきん¹ 抗菌（性の）（抗細菌の）antibacterial（抗微生物の）antimicrobial ▶抗菌活性 antibacterial activity 抗菌作用 antibacterial[antimicrobial] action 抗菌スペクトラム antibacterial[antimicrobial] spectrum ☞抗菌薬

こうきん² 咬筋 masseter（muscle）▶咬筋間代 masseter clonus 咬筋反射 masseter[jaw / chin] reflex / jaw[chin] jerk

こうきん³ 拘禁 confinement（圏confined）☞拘束 ▶拘禁環境 confined environment 拘禁精神病 prison psychosis

こうきんやく 抗菌薬（抗生物質）antibiotics /æntibaiátiks/（圏antibiotic）, antibacterial（medication, drug, agent）☞薬 ◆最近，抗菌薬を服用しましたか Have you recently *been taking[been on] antibiotics? ◆抗菌薬を処方しましょう I'm going to *give you[prescribe] some antibiotics. ◆抗菌薬は症状がよくなり始めてもすべて飲みきって下さい You should finish a course of antibiotics, even if you start to feel better. ◆抗菌薬の効き目があるのは細菌であって，ウイルスには効果がありません Antibiotics are effective against bacteria, not against viruses. ◆抗菌薬の軟膏を塗る apply antibiotic ointment ◆抗菌

薬に対する耐性が生じる develop resistance to antibiotics ◆抗菌薬治療を受けている be on antibiotics ◀広域スペクトラム抗菌薬 broad-spectrum antibiotics ベータラクタム系抗菌薬 beta-lactam antibiotics ▶抗菌薬感受性試験 antibiotic sensitivity[susceptibility] test 抗菌薬関連下痢 antibiotic-associated diarrhea 抗菌薬抵抗性 antibiotic[antibacterial drug] resistance

こうくう¹ 口腔 oral cavity, mouth cavity, the inside of the mouth（圏oral）▶口腔アレルギー症候群 oral allergy syndrome；OAS 口腔衛生 oral[mouth] hygiene 口腔温 oral temperature 口腔潰瘍 oral ulcer 口腔がん oral cancer 口腔カンジダ症 oral candidiasis / thrush 口腔乾燥症 dry mouth / xerostomia 口腔ケア oral[mouth] care 口腔外科 oral（and maxillofacial）surgery /（診療科）the department of oral（and maxillofacial）surgery / the oral（and maxillofacial）surgery department 口腔外科医 oral surgeon 口腔習癖 oral habit 口腔錠 oral[mouth] tablet /（トローチ剤）troche /（薬用ドロップ）lozenge 口腔清浄 oral[mouth] cleaning 口腔底 oral floor 口腔内洗浄剤 mouthwash 口腔粘膜 oral[mouth] mucosa 口腔微生物叢 oral microbial flora

こうくう² 航空 aviation（圏頭 aer(o)-）▶航空中耳炎 aerotitis media 航空病 airsickness / aviation sickness 航空副鼻腔炎 aerosinusitis

こうくつ 後屈 retroflexion（圏retroflexed）◀子宮後屈症 uterine retroflexion / retroflexion of the uterus 頭部後屈法 head tilt method ▶後屈子宮 retroflexed uterus

こうクロールけつしょう 高クロール血症 hyperchloremia

ごうけい 合計 total（圏total）, sum ◆医療費は合計で 5,700 円になります Your medical expenses come to[The total cost of your medical expenses is] five thousand seven hundred yen. ◆処方された

お薬は合計 5 種類です There are five kinds of prescribed medications in all. / A total of five medications have been prescribed.

こうけいれんやく 抗痙攣薬 anticonvulsant（medication, drug, agent）

こうげき 攻撃（挑戦）aggression（國aggressive）（相手への攻撃）attack（國attack）◆周囲の人に対して攻撃的になる *behave aggressively[show aggression] toward the people around one ◆異物を攻撃する attack a foreign body[substance] ◆攻撃的な行動をとる take（an）aggressive action ◆攻撃的な性格である have an aggressive personality ◆言葉による攻撃 verbal aggression

こうけつ 硬結 induration ◀陰茎硬結 penile induration

こうけつあつ 高血圧（症）high blood pressure（↔low blood pressure），hypertension；HTN（↔hypotension 國hypertensive）☞血圧 ◆高血圧と言われたことがありますか Have you ever been told that you have high blood pressure? ◆高血圧の薬を飲んでいますか Are you taking any *medication for your high blood pressure[antihypertensive medication]? ◀境界（域）高血圧 borderline hypertension 抗高血圧薬 antihypertensive（medication / drug / agent）腎性高血圧 renal hypertension 妊娠高血圧症候群 pregnancy-induced hypertension；PIH 肺高血圧 pulmonary hypertension；PH 白衣高血圧 white-coat hypertension[high blood pressure] 本態性高血圧 essential hypertension ▶高血圧患者 hypertensive patient / patient with hypertension 高血圧性腎硬化症 hypertensive nephrosclerosis 高血圧性心疾患 hypertensive heart disease；HHD 高血圧性動脈硬化症 hypertensive arteriosclerosis 高血圧性脳症 hypertensive encephalopathy

こうけっかくやく 抗結核薬 antitubercular（medication, drug, agent）

こうけっしょうばん 抗血小板 antiplatelet ▶抗血小板薬 antiplatelet medication [drug / agent] 抗血小板療法 antiplate-let therapy

こうけっせい 抗血清 antiserum

こうけっせんしょうやく 抗血栓症薬 antithrombotic（medication, drug, agent）

こうけっとう 高血糖 high blood sugar, hyperglycemia（↔hypoglycemia）（國hyperglycemic）☞血糖 ◆高血糖を是正することが最優先です Your top priority should be to correct your high blood sugar levels. / You should make it your top priority to correct your high blood sugar levels. ◆高血糖を放置すると多くの重大な合併症が起こってきます Ignoring high blood sugar levels can lead to many serious complications. / If high blood sugar levels are left untreated, they can lead to many serious complications. ◀食後高血糖 after-meal hyperglycemia ▶高血糖性昏睡 hyperglycemic coma

こうけん 貢献する contribute（圖contribution）◆医学の進歩に大いに貢献する contribute greatly to the advancement of medicine

こうげん¹ 抗原 antigen /ǽntɪdʒən/ ◀癌胎児性抗原 carcinoembryonic antigen；CEA 前立腺特異抗原 prostate-specific antigen；PSA ヒト白血球抗原 human leukocyte antigen；HLA 表面抗原 surface antigen ▶抗原エキス antigen extract 抗原回避 antigen avoidance 抗原抗体反応 antigen-antibody reaction；AAR

こうげん² 膠原 collagen /kάlədʒən/（圖collágenous）▶膠原線維 collagen[collagenous] fiber ☞膠原病

こうげんびょう 膠原病 collagen disease

こうご 交互（に）（交替でかわるがわる）by turns（互い違いに）alternately（入れ替えて）interchangeably ☞交代 ◆筋肉が硬直と弛緩を交互に繰り返しますか Do the muscles contract and relax by turns? ◆下痢と便秘を交互に繰り返す have alternating（bouts of）diarrhea and constipation ▶交互脈 alternating pulse

こうごう 咬合 occlusion（of the teeth）

（🔲occlusal）　◀交差咬合 crossbite　反対咬合 reverse[opposite] occlusion　不正咬合 malocclusion / improper[abnormal] occlusion　▶咬合調整 occlusal adjustment

こうこうがい　硬口蓋　hard palate（↔soft palate）

こうこうしけつしょうやく　抗高脂血症薬　antilipemic（medication, drug, agent）

こうこうじょうせんやく　抗甲状腺薬　antithyroid（medication, drug, agent）

こうごしょうがい　構語障害　dysarthria

こうコリンやく　抗コリン薬　anticholinergic（medication, drug, agent）

こうコレステロールけつしょう　高コレステロール血症　hypercholesterolemia　◀家族性高コレステロール血症 familial hypercholesterolemia

こうさ　交差　cross（🔲cross　🔲crossed）（染色体の乗り換え）crossover, crossing-over　◆腕を胸のところで交差して下さい Please cross your arms over your chest.　▶交差感染 cross infection　交差咬合 crossbite　交差性片麻痺 crossed hemiplegia　（血液）交差適合試験 crossmatch / blood cross-matching（procedure）　交差反応 cross-reaction

こうさい　虹彩　iris /áɪrɪs/（🔲irid(o)-）▶虹彩炎 iritis　虹彩欠損 iridocoloboma　虹彩毛様体炎 iridocyclitis

こうサイトカインりょうほう　抗サイトカイン療法　anticytokine therapy

こうさつ　考察する（熟考する）consider（🔲consideration）（内容を検討する）examine（🔲examination）　◆この問題は様々な観点から考察する必要があります This problem needs to be considered[examined] from various angles.

こうさん　後産　afterbirth　▶後産期（分娩第3期）the third stage of labor　後（産期）陣痛 afterbirth pains / afterpains

こうさんか　抗酸化　antioxidation　▶抗酸化作用 antioxidation（effect）　抗酸化物質 antioxidant

こうさんきゅう　好酸球　eosinophil（🔲eosinophilic）　▶好酸球増加症 eosinophil-

ia　好酸球増加症候群 hypereosinophilic syndrome；HES

こうさんきん　抗酸菌　acid-fast bacteria, acid-resistant bacteria（🔲bacterium）, mycobacteria　◀非結核性抗酸菌 nontuberculous mycobacterium；NTM　▶抗酸菌症 mycobacteriosis

こうざんびょう　高山病　(acute) mountain sickness, altitude sickness

こうけつしょう　高脂血症　hyperlipemia, hyperlipidemia　▶抗高脂血症薬 antilipemic（medication / drug / agent）

こうじさぎょういん　工事作業員　construction worker

こうししょう¹　光視症　photopsia

こうししょう²　虹視症　iridopsia

こうしつコルチコイド　鉱質コルチコイド　mineralocorticoid

こうじのうきのう　高次脳機能　higher brain function　▶高次脳機能障害 higher brain dysfunction

こうしぼうしょく　高脂肪食　high-fat diet

こうしゅう　口臭　bad breath, halitosis　◆口臭が気になりますか Are you concerned about having bad breath?　◆自分で口臭を感じますか Do you smell the bad breath yourself? / Are you aware of having bad breath?　◆口臭がある have bad breath　◆口臭を消す *get rid of[eliminate] bad breath　▶口臭ケア oral[(bad) breath] care　口臭恐怖 halitophobia

こうしゅうえいせい　公衆衛生　public health

こうじゅうじじんたい　後十字靱帯　posterior cruciate ligament；PCL

こうじゅうじんたいこつかしょう　後縦靱帯骨化症　ossification of the posterior longitudinal ligament；OPLL

こうしゅうでんわ　公衆電話　public telephone, pay phone

こうしゅうは　高周波　radiofrequency；RF, high frequency　▶高周波（カテーテル）アブレーション radiofrequency（catheter）ablation；RFA / high frequency catheter ablation　高周波凝固術 radiofrequency coagulation

こうじゅうりょくきん 抗重力筋 anti-gravity muscle

こうしゅく 拘縮 contracture ◆可動域の運動は拘縮を予防します Range-of-motion exercises prevent contractures. ◀関節拘縮 joint stiffness / articular contracture　筋拘縮 muscle contracture　屈曲拘縮 flexion contracture　阻血性拘縮 ischemic contracture　瘢痕拘縮 scar[cicatricial] contracture　フォルクマン拘縮 Volkmann contracture　麻痺性拘縮 paralytic contracture

こうしゅようやく 抗腫瘍薬 antineoplastic（medication, drug, agent）☞化学療法

こうしょ 高所 height, high place （高度）high altitude ☞高地 ◆高所は苦手ですか Are you afraid[scared] of heights[high places]? ◆高所性赤血球増多症 high-altitude erythrocytosis　高所無酸素症 altitude anoxia　高所めまい height vertigo ☞高所恐怖

こうじょ 控除 deduction（㊣deduct　㊣控除できる deductible） ◆高額医療費の控除を受ける get high medical expenses deducted ◆高額医療費控除 tax deduction for high medical expenses

こうしょう¹ 咬傷 wound from a bite ◀舌咬傷 bite on the tongue　動物咬傷 animal bite　ヘビ咬傷 snake bite

こうしょう² 交渉する （話し合う）negotiate（㊣negotiation） ◆保険会社との交渉はご自身で行って下さい Please negotiate with the insurance company by yourself. ◆転院に関する交渉は当院のソーシャルワーカーが行います Our social worker will *negotiate your transfer to another hospital[help you with your transfer to another hospital].

こうじょう 工場 factory ◆工場で働く work in a factory ◆工場労働者 factory worker

こうじょうせん 甲状腺 thyroid（gland） ◆甲状腺の病気がありますか Do you have any thyroid disease? ◀抗甲状腺薬 an-tithyroid medication[drug / agent]　自己免疫性甲状腺疾患 autoimmune thyroid disease；AITD　腺腫様甲状腺腫 adenomatous goiter　無痛性甲状腺炎 painless[silent] thyroiditis ▶甲状腺炎 thyroiditis　甲状腺がん thyroid cancer　甲状腺刺激ホルモン thyroid-stimulating hormone；TSH　甲状腺刺激ホルモン放出ホルモン thyrotropin-releasing hormone；TRH　甲状腺腫 goiter　甲状腺シンチグラフィ thyroid scintigraphy　甲状腺切除術 thyroidectomy　甲状腺超音波 thyroid ultrasound　甲状腺ホルモン thyroid hormone；TH　甲状腺ホルモン補充療法 thyroid hormone replacement therapy　甲状腺マイクロソーム抗体 thyroid microsomal antibody ☞甲状腺機能

こうじょうせんきのう 甲状腺機能 thyroid（gland）function ◀下垂体性甲状腺機能低下症 pituitary hypothyroidism ▶甲状腺機能検査 thyroid（gland）function test　甲状腺機能亢進症〈低下症〉hyperthyroidism〈hypothyroidism〉

こうしょきょうふ 高所恐怖 acrophobia（㊣acrophobic）, fear of heights ◆高所恐怖症ですか Are you afraid[scared] of heights[high places]?

こうしん¹ 口唇 lip ☞唇, 口唇ヘルペス, 口唇裂

こうしん² 亢進する （上昇する・増す）increase（㊣increase）　（加速する）accelerate（㊣acceleration）（㊣機能亢進の overactive　㊣㊣hyper-）◆甲状腺の機能が亢進しています You have an overactive thyroid（gland）. / Your thyroid（gland）function is overactive. ◀運動亢進 hyperkinesis / hyperkinesia　活動亢進 hyperactivity / hyperactive behavior　機能亢進 hyperfunction　凝固能亢進 hypercoagulability　筋緊張亢進 hypertonia / hypermyotonia　腱反射亢進 increased tendon reflexes / tendon hyperreflexia　心悸亢進（速脈）rapid pulse, accelerated heart beat /（動悸）palpitations　蠕動亢進 hyperperistalsis　線溶亢進 excessive fibrinolysis

こうしん³　更新する　renew（図renewal）
◆ビザを更新する必要があります You need to renew your visa.

こうしんきん　抗真菌(性の)　antifungal, antimycotic　▶抗真菌薬 antifungal（medication / drug / agent）/ antimycotic（medication / drug / agent）

こうしんちょう　高身長　tall stature　☞身長，背

こうじんつう　後陣痛　afterbirth pain, afterpain　★通例，複数形で.

こうしんとうあつ　高浸透圧　hyperosmolarity（図hyperosmolar）　▶高浸透圧高血糖症候群 HHS　hyperosmolar hyperglycemic syndrome

こうしんヘルペス　口唇ヘルペス　cold sore, herpes labialis

こうしんりょう　香辛料　spice（図spicy）
◆最近，香辛料のきいた物をたくさん食べましたか Have you recently eaten large amounts of spicy food?　◆香辛料のきいた食べ物を制限する limit spicy foods

こうしんれつ　口唇裂　cleft lip

こうすい　香水　perfume　◆化粧品や香水をつけていますか Do you use cosmetics or perfumes?

こうせい¹　更生　rehabilitation, rehab
▶更生医療 medical rehabilitation service　更生施設 rehabilitation facility

こうせい²　構成　（構造）structure（図structural），construction（図constructional）（組成）composition　（組織）organization
◆あなたのご家族の構成を教えて下さい Tell me about *your family structure[the family members living at home].　◀家族構成 family structure / structure of the family　▶構成失行 constructional apraxia

こうせい³　硬性(の)　（硬い）hard　（硬くて曲がらない）rigid　（特に繊維成分の）indurated　（悪性腫瘍などの）scirrhous　▶硬性癌 scirrhous carcinoma　硬性下疳 indurated chancre / hard sore[ulcer / chancre]　硬性内視鏡 rigid endoscope

ごうせい　合成　synthesis（動synthesize 図synthetic）　▶核酸合成阻害薬 nucleic acid synthesis inhibitor　▶合成樹脂 synthetic resin / plastic　合成繊維 synthetic fiber　合成麻薬 synthetic narcotic

こうせいざい　抗生剤　☞抗菌薬

こうせいしんびょうやく　抗精神病薬 antipsychotic（medication, drug, agent）

こうせいしんやく　向精神薬　psychotropic（medication, drug, agent）

こうせいねんきん　厚生年金　Employees' Pension　☞年金

こうせいぶっしつ　抗生物質　☞抗菌薬

こうせいろうどうしょう　厚生労働省 the Ministry of Health, Labour and Welfare（of Japan）

こうせつれっとうじょうちゅう　広節裂頭条虫　broad tapeworm, fish tapeworm

こうせん　光線　（光・明かり）light　（光の筋）beam, ray　（放射線）radiation　☞光　◀可視光線 visible ray[light / radiation]　不可視光線 invisible ray[light / radiation]　レーザー光線 laser beam[light]　▶光線過敏症 photosensitivity / hypersensitivity to light　光線力学療法 photodynamic therapy；PDT　光線療法 phototherapy / light therapy

こうせんいしょく　高繊維食　high-fiber diet

こうぜんそくやく　抗喘息薬　asthma medication, antiasthmatic（medication, drug, agent）

こうせんようりょうほう　抗線溶療法　antifibrinolytic therapy

こうそ　酵素　enzyme /énzaɪm/　◀逸脱酵素 leaking enzyme　活性化酵素 activating enzyme　消化酵素 digestive enzyme　膵酵素 pancreatic enzyme　蛋白分解酵素 protease / proteolytic enzyme　変換酵素 converting enzyme　補酵素 coenzyme　薬物代謝酵素 drug metabolism enzyme　▶酵素活性 enzyme activity　酵素阻害薬 enzyme inhibitor　酵素免疫測定法 enzyme immunoassay；EIA / enzyme-linked immunosorbent assay；ELISA

こうそう　考想　☞考え，思考

こうぞう　構造　structure（図structural）

▶構造式 structural formula

こうそく¹ 拘束 （physical patient）restraint （🔲restrictive, constrictive） ◆点滴のチューブを抜かないよう彼の左手首にこのパッド入りの拘束をつけます．でも一時的なものですから心配しないで下さい I'm going to put this padded restraint on his left wrist so that he won't try to pull out his IV tube. But don't worry—it's just a temporary measure. ▶拘束衣 body holder / straitjacket / （チョッキ型）safety vest 拘束型心筋症 restrictive[constrictive] cardiomyopathy；RCM 拘束ストレス restraint stress 拘束性換気障害 restrictive ventilatory impairment 拘束性肺疾患 restrictive lung disease 拘束ベルト（腰の部分用）lap belt / （車椅子用）wheelchair belt

こうそく² 梗塞 infarction, infarct ◀（心臓の）下壁〈前壁 / 後壁 / 側壁〉梗塞 inferior〈anterior / posterior / lateral〉wall infarction 心筋梗塞 myocardial infarction；MI 脳梗塞 brain[cerebral] infarction 肺梗塞 pulmonary infarction ラクナ梗塞 lacunar infarction ▶梗塞後狭心症 postinfarction angina；PIA 梗塞後心室瘤 postinfarction heart aneurysm 梗塞後心臓破裂 postinfarction heart rupture

こうそく³ 高速 high speed （🔲highspeed, express, fast） ◆当病院は東京から高速バスで１時間の距離にあります It takes one hour from Tokyo to this hospital by express bus. / This hospital is one hour by express bus from Tokyo. ▶高速道路 highway / expressway / freeway /《英》motorway

こうそもうそう 好訴妄想 litigious paranoia, querulous paranoia

こうだ 叩打する tap, percuss ▶叩打法 percussion ☞叩打痛

こうたい¹ 交代・交替 （順番）turn （交代勤務）shift, rotation （交互）alternation （🔲alternating, alternative） （🔲交代する take turns 代わりをする take the place of 引き継ぐ take over） ☞交互 ◆私たちが交代で治療にあたります We're going to take turns treating you. ◆これから夜勤の看護師と交代します A night duty nurse will *take my place[take over from me] now. ◆交代（制）で in rotation ▶3交代制 three-shift system 世代交代 generational change / alternation of generations ▶交代視 alternative vision 交代斜視 alternating strabismus 交代性片麻痺 alternating hemiplegia 交代脈 alternating pulse ☞交代勤務

こうたい² 抗体 antibody /ǽntɪbɑ̀di/ ◆麻疹ウイルスに対する抗体を調べる check for antibodies against measles virus ◆HIV 検査は抗体が陽性化するまでに，感染後１〜３か月かかります The HIV antibody may take one to three months to become positive after infection. / It may take one to three months for the HIV antibody to develop. ◀蛍光抗体法 fluorescent antibody technique[test] 抗核抗体検査 *antinuclear antibody[ANA] test 抗原抗体反応 antigen-antibody reaction；AAR 自己抗体 autoantibody 沈降抗体 precipitating antibody 不規則同種抗体 irregular[unexpected] alloantibody 免疫抗体 immune antibody モノクローナル抗体 monoclonal antibody ▶抗体医薬 antibody medicine 抗体価 antibody titer

こうたい³ 後退する recede ◆歯肉が後退する the gums recede ◆後退した髪の生え際 a receding hairline

こうたいおん 高体温 hyperthermia, high temperature

こうたいきんむ 交代勤務 shift work （勤務時間）shift, rotation ◆8 時間の交代勤務で働く work an eight-hour shift ◆12 時間の交代勤務制を採っております We use[work on / adopt] a twelve-hour shift system at this hospital. ◆交代勤務を終える finish one's shift

こうだいのうどうみゃく 後大脳動脈 posterior cerebral artery；PCA

こうだつう 叩打痛 sensitivity to tapping ◆上背部に叩打痛がみられる the upper back is sensitive to tapping / have sensitivity to tapping on the upper back

こうたんさんガスけつしょう　高炭酸ガス血症　hypercapnia；*a condition in which one does not exhale[breathe out] enough carbon dioxide*

こうたんぱく　高蛋白　high (level of) protein (略high-protein)　◆高蛋白の食べ物 high-protein food(s) [diet]　▶高蛋白血症 hyperproteinemia

こうち　高地　high place　(高度)**high altitude** (略high-altitude)　☞高所　▶高地脳症 high-altitude encephalopathy　高地肺水腫 high-altitude pulmonary edema

こうちっそけつしょう　高窒素血症　azotemia, hyperazotemia

こうちゃ　紅茶　black tea　◆この薬と一緒に紅茶を飲まないで下さい Please don't drink black tea with this medication.

こうちゅう　鉤虫　hookworm　▶鉤虫症 hookworm infection / ancylostomiasis　鉤虫貧血 hookworm anemia

こうちゅうきゅう　好中球　neutrophil　▶好中球アルカリホスファターゼ neutrophil alkaline phosphatase；NAP　好中球減少症 neutropenia　好中球増多症 neutrophilia

こうちょう　高張(の)　hypertonic　▶高張食塩水 hypertonic saline solution　高張性脱水 hypertonic dehydration　高張尿 hypersthenuria

こうちょく　硬直　(筋肉などの凝り)**stiffness** (略stiff)　(体のこわばり)**rigidity** (略rigid)　(特に死後の)**rigor**　◆体が硬直しますか Does your body become stiff[rigid]?　◆硬直した筋肉 stiff[rigid] muscles　◀関節硬直 joint stiffness / ankylosis　筋硬直 muscle stiffness[rigidity]　項部硬直 nuchal[neck] stiffness　死後硬直 rigor mortis / stiffening of the body after death / postmortem[cadaveric] rigidity　除脳硬直 decerebrate rigidity　除皮質硬直 decorticate rigidity　腹部硬直 abdominal rigidity

こうつう　交通(の)　(自動車などの)**traffic**　(伝達・連絡の)**communicating**　▶交通外傷 traffic injury　交通機関 means of transport[transportation]　☞交通事故

こうつうじこ　交通事故　traffic accident　◆交通事故にあったのですか Did you have[Were you involved in] a traffic accident?　◆交通事故を起こす cause a traffic accident　◆交通事故で怪我をする get injured[hurt] in a traffic accident　◆交通事故の後遺症がある have the after-effects of a traffic accident　◆交通事故死 traffic accident death

こうてい　肯定する　(認める)**admit**　(はっきり断言する)**affirm** (略肯定的な **positive, affirmative**)　◆事実を肯定する admit[affirm] the fact　◆物事を肯定的に考える take a positive view of things　◆肯定的反応 positive feedback

こうていえき　口蹄疫　foot-and-mouth disease；FMD

こうてき　公的(な)　public　▶公的医療機関 public medical facility[institution]　公的医療保険 public health insurance　公的援助 public assistance　公的介護制度 public care system　公的介護保険 public long-term care insurance　公的年金 public pension

こうてん[1]　好転する　(よくなる)**get better**　(急によくなる)*take a turn[change] for the better**　(改善する)**improve**　◆彼女の病状は好転しています Her condition is *getting better[improving].

こうてん[2]　後天(性・的の)　acquired　◆後天的な病気(an) acquired disease　▶後天免疫 acquired immunity　☞後天性免疫不全症候群

こうてんかんやく　抗てんかん薬　epilepsy medication, antiepileptic (medication, drug, agent)

こうてんせいめんえきふぜんしょうこうぐん　後天性免疫不全症候群　acquired immunodeficiency syndrome；AIDS

こうど　高度(な)　(進歩・進行した)**advanced**　(高度に発達した)**high**　(症状などが重い)**severe, serious**　◆この手術は高度なテクニックが必要です This surgery requires *an advanced[a high-level] technique.　◆高度の意識障害 a severe consciousness disorder　▶高度障害 severe [serious] disorder　高度先進医療 highly advanced medical care / high-tech (medical) treatment

こうとう　喉頭　larynx（形laryngeal /ləríndʒiəl/）, the voice box　☞喉　◆喉頭部 the laryngeal region　▶喉頭炎 laryngitis　喉頭がん laryngeal cancer / cancer of the larynx　喉頭痙攣 laryngeal spasm / laryngospasm　喉頭ジフテリア laryngeal diphtheria　喉頭浮腫 laryngeal edema　喉頭ポリープ laryngeal polyp　喉頭麻痺 laryngeal paralysis　喉頭隆起 laryngeal prominence / （一般的に）Adam's apple　☞喉頭蓋，喉頭鏡

こうどう　行動　（一連の行為）action　（1回の行為）act　（振る舞い）behavior, conduct　（体の動き）movement（動act, behave　形behavioral）　☞行為　◆彼はいつもと違う行動をしますか Is he behaving[acting] differently from normal[usual]?　◆近頃彼女は行動がおかしい She's been acting odd recently. / She's behaving[acting] strangely these days.　◆問題行動を抑制する control[check / restrain] problem behavior　◆行動の自由を制限する restrict a person's freedom of movement [action]　◆暴力的な行動 a violent act / an act of violence / violent behavior　◀異常行動 abnormal behavior　逸脱行動 deviant behavior　援助行動 helping behavior　回避行動 avoidance behavior　強迫行動 compulsive[obsessive] behavior　攻撃的行動 aggressive behavior　食行動 eating[dietary] behavior / （授乳の）feeding behavior　食行動異常 eating disorder　ストレス対処行動 stress coping behavior　性行動 sexual behavior　逃避行動 escape behavior　認知行動療法 cognitive-behavioral therapy；CBT　排泄行動 eliminative behavior　病人役割行動 sick-role behavior　母性行動 maternal behavior　本能行動 instinctive behavior　レム睡眠行動障害 REM sleep behavior disorder　▶行動科学 behavioral science　行動障害 behavior disorder　行動パター

ン behavior pattern　行動評価 behavior assessment　行動変化 behavior change　行動療法 behavior therapy　行動力 energy / power of action

こうとうがい　喉頭蓋　epiglottis　▶喉頭蓋炎 epiglottitis

こうとうきょう　喉頭鏡　laryngoscope　◀マッキントッシュ型喉頭鏡 Macintosh laryngoscope　▶喉頭鏡検査 laryngoscopy

こうとうしんけいつう　後頭神経痛　occipital neuralgia

こうとうぶ　後頭部　the back of the head, the occipital region　◆後頭部が痛む have an ache in the back of one's head　◆後頭部にこぶができる have[get] a bump on the back of one's head

こうとうよう　後頭葉　occipital lobe

こうどくそ　抗毒素　antitoxin（形antitoxic）　◀ジフテリア抗毒素 diphtheria antitoxin　破傷風抗毒素 tetanus antitoxin　▶抗毒素血清 antitoxic serum

こうトリグリセリドけっしょう　高トリグリセリド血症　hypertriglyceridemia

こうないえん　口内炎　stomatitis, mouth ulcer, inflammation in the mouth　◆口内炎はよくできますか Do you often have mouth ulcers?　◀アフタ性口内炎 aphthous stomatitis　潰瘍性口内炎 ulcerative stomatitis　カタル性口内炎 catarrhal stomatitis　歯肉口内炎 gingivostomatitis　放射線口内炎 radiation stomatitis

こうないぼうりょく　校内暴力　school violence　（クラス内の）classroom violence　（大学内の）campus violence

こうナトリウムけっしょう　高ナトリウム血症　hypernatremia

こうにょうさんけっしょう　高尿酸血症　hyperuricemia

こうねつ　高熱　high fever　☞熱　◆数日前から高熱がある have had a high fever for the past few days　◆インフルエンザで高熱が出ている have a high fever *caused by[due to] influenza / have an influenza-related fever

こうねんき　更年期　the change of life, the

こうねんき climacteric （女性の） menopause / ménəpɔːz /, female climacteric （男性の） andropause, male climacteric （⑱menopausal, climacteric） ◆更年期の間にどんな問題がありましたか. 例えば, ほてり〈いらいら感 / 寝汗 / めまい / 気分の変動〉がありましたか Did you experience any problems during menopause, such as hot flashes〈irritability / night sweats / dizziness / mood swings〉? ◆それは更年期の症状の1つです It's one of the symptoms of menopause. ◆おそらく更年期が始まっているのでしょう Your menopause has probably started. ◆更年期が過ぎれば楽になるでしょう Things will *become easier[get better] when you're over [through] your menopause. ◆女性ホルモンであるエストロゲン減少のため更年期には骨からカルシウムが失われます Calcium is lost from the bones at menopause because of a decreased level of the female hormone, estrogen. ▶更年期愁訴 menopausal[climacteric] complaint 更年期障害 menopausal[climacteric] disturbance 更年期症状 menopausal[climacteric] symptom

こうねんしょさんぷ 高年初産婦 elderly woman giving birth to her first child, elderly primipara

こうのう 効能 efficacy, potency ☞効果 ▶効能書き leaflet with information on patient medication / prescribing information / statement of the effects of a medication

こうのうど 高濃度 high concentration ◆高濃度の大気汚染物質は喘息増悪の危険因子です High concentrations of air pollutants are a risk factor for *asthma exacerbation[exacerbation of asthma].

こうはいきん 広背筋 broadest muscle of the back, latissimus dorsi muscle

こうはつ¹ 好発する （頻繁に）occur most frequently （一般的に）occur most commonly ◆発疹はこのあたりの部位に好発します A rash most frequently occurs around here. / The most frequent site of a rash is around here. ◆この病気は40歳以上の人に好発します This disease most commonly occurs in people aged forty years and older. ☞好発年齢

こうはつ² 後発（の） delayed, late ▶後発[ジェネリック]医薬品 generic drug / generics 後発症状 delayed symptom

こうはつねんれい 好発年齢 （発症頻度が最も高い年齢）peak age ◆この病気の好発年齢は45歳から65歳です The incidence of this disease is highest in people aged forty-five to sixty-five years. / The peak age of this disease is from forty-five to sixty-five years.

こうはん¹ 紅斑 erythema （⑱erythematous） （斑点）red blotch[spot] ◆皮膚に紅斑が出ましたか Have you noticed red blotches[spots] on your skin? / Has your skin broken out in red blotches[spots]? ◀環状紅斑 erythema annulare 結節性紅斑 erythema nodosum 手掌紅斑 palmar erythema / red palm 多形滲出性紅斑 erythema multiforme exudativum 蝶形紅斑 butterfly erythema[rash] 伝染性紅斑 erythema infectiosum ▶紅斑性湿疹 erythematous eczema 紅斑性狼瘡[エリテマトーデス] lupus erythematosus；LE

こうはん² 広範（囲の）・広汎（性の） （全身の）generalized （↔localized） （幅が広い）wide, widespread （拡大した）extended （面積が大きい）large, big （広範囲をカバーする）comprehensive （大規模な）massive （根治的な）radical （びまん性の）diffuse （問題などが広範囲にわたる）pervasive ◆浮腫は局所的ですか, 広範囲ですか Do you have the edema[swelling] in just one place or over a wider area of your body? / Is the edema[swelling] localized or generalized[widespread]? ◆広範囲にかゆみがある have itchiness over a wide area of one's body / have extensive itchiness ◆広範囲の脳損傷 widespread damage throughout the brain ◆広汎性の痛み(a) generalized pain ▶広範囲照射 comprehensive field irradiation 広範囲熱傷 extensive burn 広汎性子宮全摘出

術 radical hysterectomy　広汎性脳損傷 diffuse brain injury　広汎性発達障害 pervasive developmental disorder；PDD　広範切除 wide resection

こうひ　公費　public expense　（助成金）public subsidy　◆結核治療は公費によって助成されます Tuberculosis treatment is subsidized by the government. / The cost of tuberculosis treatment is covered by public subsidies.　◆医療費の公費負担申請については市役所に問い合わせて下さい Please contact the municipal office about public financial assistance for medical expenses.　▶公費医療 publicly funded medical services / public medical financial assistance system

こうびくう　後鼻腔　postnasal space

こうびこう　後鼻孔　choana（㊫choanal），posterior nasal aperture　▶後鼻孔ポリープ choanal polyp

こうひじゅう　高比重　high density　▶高比重リポ蛋白 high density lipoprotein; HDL / good cholesterol

こうひしょう　紅皮症　erythroderma　◀乾癬性紅皮症 psoriatic erythroderma

こうヒスタミンやく　抗ヒスタミン薬　antihistamine, histamine antagonist

こうひょう¹　好評（な）（人気がある）popular　◆看護師の田中さんは親身に看護するので好評です Nurse Tanaka is very popular because of his tender[loving] care of patients.　◆そのリハビリプログラムは患者さん達に好評です That rehabilitation program is popular with patients. / That rehabilitation program is *thought of [judged] favorably by patients.

こうひょう²　公表する（公にする）make … public　（情報などを公開する）release　（印刷物などで発表する）publish　◆医療事故を公表する make medical errors public / release information about medical errors to the public　◆公表されているデータによると，女性の 11 人に 1 人が乳がんに罹患するとされています According to the published data, one in eleven women develops breast cancer.

こうびょうげんせいとりインフルエンザ　高病原性鳥インフルエンザ　highly pathogenic avian influenza

こうビリルビンけつしょう　高ビリルビン血症　hyperbilirubinemia

こうびろう　後鼻漏　postnasal drip；PND

こうぶ¹　口部　the oral region　▶口部ジスキネジア oral dyskinesia　口部失行 oral apraxia

こうぶ²　後部　the back（↔the front）

こうぶ³　項部　nape of the neck, nucha（㊫nuchal）　▶項部挙上 neck lift　項部硬直 nuchal stiffness　項部痛 nuchal pain

こうふあんやく　抗不安薬　antianxiety medication[drug, agent], minor tranquilizer

こうふか　後負荷　afterload

こうふく　幸福　happiness（㊫happy）　☞幸せ　◆幸福な結婚生活を送っている be happily married　◆幸福かどうかはご自分の心の持ちようです Happiness depends on your state of mind. / Happiness is all in the mind.

こうふくまく　後腹膜（の）　retroperitoneal（㊫behind the peritoneum）　▶後腹膜腫瘍 retroperitoneal tumor

こうふせいみゃくやく　抗不整脈薬　antiarrhythmic（medication, drug, agent）

こうプロラクチンけつしょう　高プロラクチン血症　hyperprolactinemia（㊫hyperprolactinemic）　▶高プロラクチン血症性無月経 hyperprolactinemic amenorrhea

こうふん　興奮　（わくわくすること）excitement（㊫get[be] excited）（動揺）agitation（㊫get[be] agitated）（刺激）stimulation　（易興奮性）excitability　（刺激による興奮）excitation　◆彼女は興奮しやすいですか Does she get easily excited[agitated]?　◆彼は興奮しています He's excited[agitated]. / He's in an excited[agitated] state.　◆そう興奮しないで下さい Please calm down. / Please don't get so worked up.　◀覚醒時興奮 emergence excitement　中枢神経興奮薬 central nervous system stimulant /（蘇生薬）analeptic（medication / drug / agent）　▶興

奮伝導系 the conduction system

こうぶんかいのうシーティー　高分解能 CT high-resolution CT［computed tomography］；HRCT

こうぶんかがん　高分化癌 well-differentiated carcinoma

こうへい　公平（な） fair　(平等な)equal
◆診察の順番は受け付け順に公平にお取り扱いしております Patients are treated equally and are seen in order of arrival. / We see patients fairly［equally］in order of their arrival.

こうぼ　酵母 yeast

こうほう　広報 (定期報告)bulletin　(広報活動)public relations；PR　◆市の広報で健診のスケジュールをチェックして下さい Please check the health checkup schedule in your city bulletin.

こうまく　硬膜 dura mater (慣dural)
◀代用硬膜 dural substitute　▶硬膜外血腫 epidural［extradural］hematoma　硬膜外出血 epidural［extradural］bleeding［hemorrhage］　硬膜外麻酔 epidural anesthesia　硬膜下血腫 subdural hematoma　硬膜下出血 subdural bleeding［hemorrhage］　硬膜穿刺 dural puncture

こうまひ　後麻痺 residual paralysis

こうもく　項目 item (動項目別に分ける itemize)　◆（問診票などで）あてはまる項目に印をつけて下さい Please check［mark］the items that apply（to you）.　◆項目別の一覧表を作る make an itemized list
◀血液検査項目 blood test item　▶検査項目 test item / item to be covered by the test

こうもん　肛門 anus /éɪnəs/ (慣anal 慣頭proct(o)-)　★anus（肛門）という語は患者に不快な思いを抱かせることがあるのでできれば避けたい. (口語で婉曲的に)bottom, back passage　◆この坐薬は肛門に挿入して下さい Please insert this suppository into your bottom［(直腸)rectum］.　◆（直腸診で）それでは肛門に指を入れます Now, I'm going to insert my finger into your *back passage［bottom］.　◀人工肛門 stoma / artificial anus　人工肛門造設術 colos-

tomy　▶肛門温存大腸切除術 restorative proctocolectomy　肛門科 the department of proctology / the proctology department　肛門科医 proctologist　肛門括約筋 anal sphincter　肛門鏡検査 anoscopy　肛門再建手術 reconstructive anal surgery　肛門指診 digital examination of the anus / digital anal examination　肛門周囲炎 periproctitis　肛門周囲膿瘍 perianal abscess　肛門出血 anal bleeding　肛門腺 anal gland　肛門掻痒症 anal pruritus［itching］/ (口語)itchy bottom　肛門ポリープ anal polyp

こうやく¹　絞扼 constriction, strangulation (慣strangulated)　◀胸部絞扼感 constriction in the chest　▶絞扼性イレウス strangulation ileus　絞扼性ヘルニア strangulated hernia

こうやく²　膏薬 (貼付剤)patch, plaster (軟膏)salve, ointment　◆肩に膏薬を貼る apply a patch［plaster］to the shoulder / put a patch［plaster］on the shoulder　◆傷口に膏薬を塗る apply an ointment to the wound

こうよう　効用 ☞効果, 効能

こうようかん　高揚感 heightened mood　◆このような高揚感は周期的に起こりますか Does this heightened mood occur［come on］periodically?

こうリウマチやく　抗リウマチ薬 anti-rheumatic (medication, drug, agent)

こうりつ¹　効率 efficiency (慣efficient)
◆背部痛に対する最も効果的で効率的な治療を見い出せるよう努めます We'll try to find the most effective and efficient treatment for your back pain.　◆効率的に検査を行い, できるだけ早く正確に診断する conduct examinations efficiently and make a correct diagnosis as quickly as possible　◀作業効率 work efficiency

こうりつ²　公立（の） public　▶公立病院 public hospital / (地方自治体の)municipal hospital

こうりにょうホルモン　抗利尿ホルモン antidiuretic hormone；ADH　▶抗利尿ホルモン不適切分泌症候群 syndrome of inappropriate ADH secretion；SIADH

こうりょ 考慮する consider, think over （考慮に入れる）take … into consideration [account] ◆手術を決める前に彼女の全身状態を考慮しなければなりません Before deciding[making a decision] about surgery, we'll have to *consider her general condition[take her general condition into consideration].

こうりょうほう 後療法 aftertreatment, aftercare

こうりょく 効力 ☞効果，効能

こうりんきん 口輪筋 orbicular muscle of the mouth

こうリンさんけつしょう 高リン酸血症 hyperphosphatemia

こうリンししつこうたいしょうこうぐん 抗リン脂質抗体症候群 antiphospholipid syndrome, antiphospholipid-antibody syndrome

こうれい 高齢 （advanced）age （圏aging, aged）, advanced years （圏elderly, senior）☞年（とし），年齢 ◆彼女は高齢のため手術のリスクが高い She is at high risk from surgery because of her age. ◆高齢で腰が曲がっている be bent with age ◆人口の高齢化 an aging population ◀少子高齢化社会 aging society with a low birthrate 超高齢社会 super-aged society ▶高齢化社会 aging society 高齢患者 elderly[senior] patient 高齢出産 late childbearing 高齢女性〈男性〉elderly woman〈man〉 高齢人口 the elderly population ☞高齢者

こうれいしゃ 高齢者 elderly person （一般に）older person[adult] （65歳以上）person aged 65[sixty-five] years or older （総称的に）senior citizens, the elderly ☞ライフステージ ◀後期高齢者（75歳以上）(elderly) person aged 75[seventy-five] years and older / senior senior / （総称的に）the old-old 前期高齢者（65〜74歳）(elderly) person aged 65[sixty-five] to 74 [seventy-four] years / junior senior / （総称的に）the young-old 寝たきり高齢者 bedridden older person[patient] ▶高齢

者医療 medical care for elderly[older] people / medical elderly care 高齢者医療制度 the system of medical care for elderly[older] people / the system of medical elderly care 高齢者介護 care of elderly[older] people / elderly care 高齢者虐待 elder abuse / （放置）elder neglect 高齢者差別 ageism / age discrimination 高齢者施設 home[facility] for the elderly

こうレトロウイルスりょうほう 抗レトロウイルス療法 antiretroviral therapy；ART ◀高活性抗レトロウイルス療法 highly active antiretroviral therapy；HAART

こえ 声 voice ◆終わったらスタッフに声をかけて下さい Let one of our staff know when you're finished. ◆ご用のある時は，遠慮しないでスタッフに声をかけて下さい If you need any help, *don't hesitate[feel free] to ask us.
《声の性状の表現》◆声の大きさ voice volume[loudness] / loudness of a voice ◆大きな〈小さな〉声 a loud〈soft〉voice ◆声が大きい speak loudly[in a loud voice] ◆声が響く one's voice vibrates ◆声が太くなる one's voice deepens ◆声が変わる（声変わりする）one's voice breaks ◆声の強さ voice intensity / intensity of a voice ◆声の高さ voice pitch / pitch of a voice ◆高い〈低い〉声 a high〈low〉[high-pitched〈low-pitched〉] voice ◆いつもより高い〈低い〉声で話す speak in a higher〈lower〉voice than usual
《症状の表現》◆声が出ない lose one's voice / be unable to speak ◆使いすぎで声がかれる get hoarse[scratchy] *from using one's voice too much[from excessive use of one's voice] ◆声を出すのがつらい have difficulty speaking ◆声が鼻にかかる speak in a nasal voice / the voice gets[becomes / is] nasal ◆声が震える speak in a quivering voice ◆声がいつもより弱い one's voice gets[becomes / is] weaker than usual
《診察の基本表現》◆私の声が聞こえますか Can you hear me (speaking)? ◆もう少し大きな声で話して下さい Please speak a

little louder. / Please speak up a little.
◆声に何か問題がありますか Do you have any problems with your voice? ◆声がかれますか Does your voice get hoarse? / Do you feel hoarse? ◆最近，声に変化がありましたか Has your voice changed [Have you noticed any changes in your voice] recently? ◆この一節を声に出して〈出さずに〉読んで下さい Please read this passage aloud〈silently〉.
◀歌声 singing voice うぶ声 baby's [newborn's] first cry 金切り声 shrill voice ささやき声 whisper / whispered [whispering] voice しわがれ声 (がらがら声)hoarse voice / (かすれた声)husky voice 鼻声 nasal voice / twang ▶声がれ hoarse voice / hoarseness 声変わり voice change, the change of *one's* voice / (青少年の)adolescent voice change, breaking of *one's* voice

こえる¹ 超える (超過している)**be above** (基準・制限を超える)**exceed** ◆コレステロールが正常値を超えています Your cholesterol level is above normal. ◆カロリー摂取は1日2,000 kcal を超えてはいけません Your caloric intake should not exceed two thousand kilocalories a day.

こえる² 越える be past, pass ◆彼女の容体は峠を越えました She's past[out of] the critical stage. / She has passed the crisis point. / (当座の脅威は去った)She has passed the immediate crisis.

ごえん 誤嚥する aspirate (図aspiration) ☞誤飲 ◆彼女は食事の時に誤嚥してむせやすいですか When she eats, *does she often[does she tend to] breathe in food and choke on it? / Does she easily aspirate food and get choked on it? ◀不顕性誤嚥 silent[asymptomatic / subclinical] aspiration ▶誤嚥性肺炎 aspiration pneumonia

コース course ☞課程 ◆化学療法の全コースを受ける〈終える〉receive〈finish / complete〉the full course of chemotherapy

コーディネーター coordinator ◀移植

コーディネーター transplant coordinator

コーヒー coffee ◆毎日コーヒーを何杯飲みますか How many cups of coffee[How many coffees] do you drink a day? ◆コーヒーを飲むと痛みが悪化しますか Does coffee make the pain worse? ◆この薬と一緒にコーヒーは飲まないで下さい Please don't drink coffee with this medication. ◆コーヒーかす状の液体を吐く vomit liquid *that looks like[with the appearance of] coffee grounds ◀カフェイン抜きのコーヒー decaffeinated coffee / decaf ◀薄い〈濃い〉コーヒー weak〈strong〉coffee ▶コーヒー残渣様吐物 coffee-grounds vomit

コーラ cola (商標名)**Coca-Cola, Coke** ◆コーラにはカフェインが含まれています Coca-Cola contains caffeine.

こおり 氷 ice (小さな角氷)**ice cube** ◆患部を氷で冷やす cool the affected area with ice ▶氷枕 ice pillow / (氷嚢)ice pack[bag]

ゴールドマンしやけい ─視野計 Goldmann perimeter

コールボタン call button ☞呼び出し ◆コールボタンはここにあります Here's the call button. ◆ご用のある時は，遠慮しないでコールボタンを押して下さい If you need any help, please don't hesitate to push[press] the call button. ◀緊急コールボタン emergency call button ナースコールボタン nurse call button

ごおん 語音 speech sound ▶語音聴力検査 speech audiometry 語音弁別検査 speech discrimination test

ごかい 誤解 misunderstanding (動misunderstand) ☞行き違い ◆何か誤解があったようです．お気持ちを傷つけるつもりはありませんでした There must have been some misunderstanding. I didn't mean to hurt your feelings. ◆誤解を招く cause [lead to] a misunderstanding ◆誤解を招きかねない印象を与える give a misleading impression ◆誤解を解く clear up a misunderstanding

コカイン cocaine /koʊkéɪn/ ◆コカイン

を吸う snort[sniff] cocaine　▶コカイン依存 cocaine dependence[(中毒)addiction / poisoning]　コカイン中毒者 cocaine addict　コカイン乱用 cocaine abuse　コカイン離脱 cocaine withdrawal

こがたじょうちゅう　小形条虫　dwarf tapeworm

こかつ　枯渇　depletion

ごがつ　5月　May　☞1月

こかん　股間　(両脚が分かれる部分)crotch (鼠径)groin　★crotch より上の部分.

ごかん　五感　the five senses　★the senses of sight, hearing, smell, taste and touch ともいう.

こかんせつ　股関節　hip joint　◀先天性股関節脱臼 congenital dislocation of the hip；CDH　変形性股関節症 hip osteoarthritis　▶股関節損傷 hip injury　股関節脱臼 hip dislocation　股関節置換術 hip replacement　股関節痛 hip pain

こき　呼気　expiration (↔inspiration) (画expiratory), exhalation (↔inhalation), breath　☞呼吸　▶呼気圧 expiratory pressure　呼気延長 prolonged expiration　呼気終末陽圧換気 *positive end-expiratory pressure[PEEP] ventilation

ごきげん　ご機嫌　☞機嫌

こきざみ　小刻み　◆小刻みに足を引きずって歩く walk with short, quick, and shuffling steps / the steps become short, quick, and shuffling when *a person* walks　◆体が小刻みに震える shake with quick, short movements / tremble　▶小刻み歩行 brachybasia / short-stepped gait

ゴキブリ　cockroach

こきゅう　呼吸　breath /bréθ/ (画breathe /bríːð/), breathing, respiration (画respiratory)　☞息

《診察の基本表現》　◆呼吸に何か問題がありますか Do you have any problems with your breathing?　◆呼吸が苦しいのですか Do you have difficulty breathing?　◆呼吸が苦しくて夜中に目が覚めることがありますか Do you wake up at night because of difficulty with breathing? / Does breath-

ing difficulty cause you to awaken at night?　◆仰向けに寝ると呼吸が苦しくなりますか Do you find breathing more difficult when (you're) lying flat on your back?　◆起き上がると呼吸が楽になりますか Do you find breathing easier when (you're) sitting up (in bed)？　◆家庭や仕事上のストレスが呼吸に影響していますか Does stress at home or work affect your breathing?　◆前より呼吸が楽になりましたか Is it easier to breathe? / Do you find it easier to breathe?　◆手術前に呼吸の練習をして下さい Please do breathing exercises before your surgery.

《呼吸法》　◆鼻〈口〉で呼吸する breathe through *one's* nose〈mouth〉　◆深呼吸する take a deep breath / breathe deeply ◆ゆっくり呼吸する breathe slowly　◆自力で呼吸する breathe *on *one's* own[by oneself]　◆呼吸を止める hold *one's* breath　◆口をすぼめて呼吸をすると楽になります You'll feel better if you breathe *through pursed lips[with your lips pursed].

《呼吸の異常》　◆呼吸が浅い *the breaths are[the breathing is] shallow / (弱い)*the breaths are[the breathing is] weak　◆呼吸が速い *the breaths are[the breathing is] rapid[fast]　◆呼吸が不規則である *the breaths are[the breathing is] irregular　◆彼女の呼吸が荒くなっています She's breathing hard[heavily]. / She's panting for breath.　◆呼吸が苦しそうになる breathing becomes[gets] labored ◆彼の呼吸が止まりました He has stopped breathing. / His breathing has stopped. ◆現在彼女は自発呼吸がない状態です Currently[At present], she's not breathing *on her own[by herself].

◀安静時呼吸 breathing at[during] rest 機械式人工呼吸 mechanical ventilation 急性呼吸窮迫症候群 acute respiratory distress syndrome；ARDS　胸式呼吸 chest [thoracic / costal] breathing[respiration] 強制呼吸 forced breathing[respiration] 口呼吸 mouth breathing / breathing

through *one's* mouth　口すぼめ呼吸 pursed-lip breathing　口対口人工呼吸 mouth-to-mouth resuscitation　呼気終末陽圧呼吸 positive end-expiratory pressure；PEEP　再呼吸法 rebreathing method　持続気道陽圧呼吸 continuous positive airway pressure；CPAP　自発呼吸 spontaneous breathing[respiration] / breathing *on one's own[by oneself]*　人工呼吸 artificial breathing[respiration]　鼻呼吸 nose[nasal] breathing / breathing through *one's* nose　腹式呼吸 abdominal breathing[respiration] / （横隔膜を用いて） breathing using the diaphragm / diaphragm[diaphragmatic] breathing　用手人工呼吸法 manual artificial ventilation
▶呼吸運動 respiratory movement　呼吸管理 respiratory care[management]　呼吸機能［肺機能］検査 respiratory[pulmonary] function test / spirometric test　呼吸筋 respiratory muscle　呼吸筋疲労 respiratory muscle fatigue　呼吸訓練 breathing exercise　呼吸細気管支 respiratory bronchiole　呼吸障害 breathing[respiratory] disorder　呼吸性アシドーシス respiratory acidosis　呼吸性アルカローシス respiratory alkalosis　呼吸性雑音 respiratory murmur　呼吸数 respiratory rate；RR / breathing rate　呼吸中枢 the respiratory center　呼吸抵抗 respiratory resistance　呼吸停止 respiratory arrest / （無呼吸）apnea　呼吸パターン breathing pattern　呼吸バッグ breathing bag　呼吸不全 respiratory failure[insufficiency]　呼吸マスク breathing mask　呼吸麻痺 respiratory paralysis　呼吸抑制 respiratory depression　呼吸リハビリテーション respiratory rehabilitation　☞呼吸音，呼吸器，呼吸困難

呼吸法

■口すぼめ呼吸

●口を閉じて，鼻から息を吸って下さい With your mouth shut, please breathe through your nose.

●口笛を吹くように唇をすぼめて下さい Purse your lips as if you're whistling.

●唇をすぼめたままゆっくり息を吐いて下さい Keeping your lips pursed, breathe out slowly.

●無理に息を強く吐こうとしないで下さい Be careful not to push yourself too hard to force the air out.

●吸う時の2倍くらいの時間をかけてゆっくり吐きます Breathe out twice as slowly as you breathed in.

●慣れたら，息を吐く時間を少しずつ長くして，呼吸回数を減らすようにしてみましょう After some practice try to gradually *increase the time to breathe out[make your breathing out longer] and slow[reduce] your breathing rate.

■腹式呼吸

●まず仰向けに寝て下さい First, please lie on your back.

●リラックスしてお腹に手を当てて下さい Relax, and place your hand(s) on your abdomen.

●鼻からゆっくり息を吸って下さい．息を吸う時お腹が膨らむことを意識するようにして下さい Breathe in slowly through your nose. Try to feel that your abdomen gets larger as you breathe in.

●唇をすぼめてゆっくり息を吐いて下さい．息を吐く時はお腹が引っ込むことを意識するようにして下さい Purse your lips and breathe out slowly. Try to feel that your abdomen falls inward as you breathe out.

（『そのまま使える病院英語表現 5000』第2版，医学書院，2013，pp 408-409 より改変）

異常呼吸の表現

■呼吸様式の異常

●喘ぎ呼吸 gasping[panting] (breathing / respiration)　●下顎呼吸 mandibular breathing[respiration]　●努力呼吸 labored breathing　●起坐呼吸 orthopnea / difficulty breathing when lying down　●奇異呼吸 paradoxical breathing[respiration]　●陥没呼吸 inspiratory retraction / retractive breathing[respiration]

■呼吸数・リズム・パターンの異常
● 頻呼吸 tachypnea / abnormally fast [rapid] breathing　● 緩徐呼吸 bradypnea / abnormally slow breathing　● 過呼吸 hyperventilation / hyperpnea　● 低呼吸 hypopnea / abnormally shallow breathing　● クスマウル大呼吸 Kussmaul breathing[respiration]　● チェーン・ストークス呼吸 Cheyne-Stokes breathing[respiration]　● ビオー呼吸 Biot breathing[respiration]　● 無呼吸 apnea / absence of breathing

こきゅうおん　呼吸音 breath sound, respiratory sound ◀異常〈正常〉呼吸音 abnormal〈normal〉breath sound　肺胞呼吸音 vesicular（breath）sound

こきゅうき　呼吸器 respiratory organs ★通例，複数形で．（[略]肺の pulmonary　胸部の thoracic）▶呼吸器科医 lung specialist / pulmonary specialist / pulmonologist　呼吸器感染 respiratory infection；RI　呼吸器系 the respiratory system　呼吸器外科 the department of thoracic surgery / the thoracic surgery department　呼吸器疾患 respiratory disease　呼吸器内科 the department of respiratory[pulmonary] medicine / the respiratory[pulmonary] medicine department　☞人工呼吸器

こきゅうこんなん　呼吸困難 dyspnea, difficult breathing, breathing difficulty [trouble]（息切れ）**shortness of breath** ◆呼吸困難がありますか Do you have *difficulty breathing[breathing difficulties]? / Do you have difficult and uncomfortable breathing?　◆呼吸困難に陥る start gasping for breath / become unable to breathe ◀安静時呼吸困難 dyspnea [shortness of breath] at[during] rest　吸気性〈呼気性〉呼吸困難 inspiratory〈expiratory〉dyspnea　発作性呼吸困難 paroxysmal dyspnea　労作性呼吸困難 exertional dyspnea / dyspnea on exertion[effort]；

DOE

こきょう　故郷（出身の都市・町など）**hometown, the place** one **grew up in**（出生地）**birthplace**（出身地・実家）**home** ◆あなたの故郷はどちらですか Where are you from? / Where's your hometown?　◆故郷が懐かしいですか Do you miss your home? / Are you homesick?

コキン ◆あごを動かすとコキンという音がしますか Do you notice your jaw clicking?

こくがい　国外(に・で) **abroad**（海外に）**overseas**（日本国外に）**outside Japan, out of Japan** ◆最近，国外に出てどこかへ旅行しましたか Have you recently traveled outside[out of] Japan?　◆国外で治療を受ける get medical treatment outside Japan

こくさい　国際(的な) **international** ▶国際結婚 international marriage　国際疾病分類 International Classification of Diseases；ICD　国際赤十字社 the International Committee of the Red Cross；ICRC　国際単位系 the International System of Units / SI units　☞国際電話

こくさいでんわ　国際電話 international (telephone) call ☞電話 ◆故郷の親類に国際電話をかける make an international (telephone) call to a relative in one's hometown

コクサッキーウイルス coxsackievirus

こくし¹　黒子 ☞黒子(ほくろ)

こくし²　酷使する（使い過ぎる）**use too much, overuse**（過度に使って痛める）**strain** ◆目を酷使する strain one's eyes ◆体を酷使する overwork oneself

ごくしょうみじゅくじ　極小未熟児 ☞極低出生体重児

こくしょく　黒色(の) **black** ◀黒い ▶黒色吐物 black vomit　黒色尿 black urine　黒色表皮腫 acanthosis nigricans　黒色便(tarry) black stool / (下血)melena　☞黒色腫

こくしょくしゅ　黒色腫 melanoma ◀悪性黒色腫 malignant melanoma

こくせき　国籍 nationality ★国籍を表すには，通例，I'm Japanese. She is British. のよう

に形容詞形を用いる. アメリカ人などの場合, He's American. また He's an American. (名詞形) とも言う. ◆国籍はどちらですか What's your nationality? ◆彼女はカナダ国籍です She's (a) Canadian. / She has Canadian nationality. / She is a Canadian citizen. ▶二重国籍 dual citizenship

こくち **告知する** inform, tell ☞巻末付録: 悪い診断結果を伝える時 ◆生検でがんの結果が出たら告知を望みますか Would you like[Do you want] to be told *if the biopsy shows that you have cancer[if the biopsy shows a diagnosis of cancer]? ◆前立腺がんを告知する inform *the patient* that he has prostate cancer

ごくちょうたんぱりょうほう **極超短波療法** microwave therapy

ごくっと ☞ごくんと

ごくていしゅっせいたいじゅうじ **極低出生体重児** very low birth-weight infant; VLBWI (出生体重 1,500 g 未満) infant weighing less than fifteen hundred grams at birth

こくないしょう **黒内障** amaurosis

こくふく **克服する** (乗り切る) overcome, beat (制圧する) conquer (回復する) recover (from) ◆うつ病を克服する overcome[recover from] depression ◆がんを克服する beat[conquer] cancer

こくべつしき **告別式** ☞葬儀

こくみんけんこうほけん **国民健康保険** National Health Insurance (system) ☞健康保険 ▶国民健康保険証 National Health Insurance card[certificate]

こくみんねんきん **国民年金** National Pension (system), government pension ☞年金

こくもうぜつ **黒毛舌** (病) black (hairy) tongue, glossophytia

こくりつ **国立(の)** national ▶国立感染症研究所 the National Institute of Infectious Diseases 国立病院 national hospital

ごくろうさま **ご苦労様** ☞お疲れ様 ◆ご苦労様でした Thank you very much (for your trouble).

ごくんと ☞一気 ◆唾〈この管〉をごくんと飲んで下さい Please swallow *your saliva〈this tube〉*in one gulp[(一度に) in one go].

こけ **苔** (舌の) fur (圏苔が付着した furry) ☞舌苔 ◆舌は苔が生えているような感じですか Does your tongue feel furry?

こけい **固形(の)** solid ◆固形物は食べられますか Can you eat *solid food(s) [solids]? ▶固形腫瘍 solid tumor 固形食 solid food[diet]

ここ

《場所》 ◆ここが痛いのですか Is this where it hurts? ◆ここでしばらく待っていて下さい Can you wait here for a little while? ◆(意識障害の確認) ここはどこですか Where are you now?

《時点》 ◆(訓練の終わりなどで) 今日はここまでにしましょう Let's stop here for today. / So much for today. ◆ここまでのところで何かご質問はありますか Do you have any questions so far? ◆ここが踏ん張りどころですよ This is where you need to be as strong as you can be. / (最善を尽くす) This is where you need to *do your best[(持ちこたえる) hold out].

ごご **午後** afternoon (時刻の後に) pm, p.m. ◆午後 2 時に来て下さい Please come at two in the afternoon. ◆9 月 26 日の午後 3 時に at three on the afternoon of September (the) twenty-sixth ◆今日〈明日〉の午後 this〈tomorrow〉afternoon

こころ **心** (思考・判断・意思決定などをする場所) mind (喜怒哀楽などの感情が宿る場所) heart (精神・意識・霊魂) spirit (圏精神の mental 情動・情緒の emotional 内面の inner 心理の psychological) ◆何か心にかかることがありますか(心配なことがあるか) Do you have any worries? / Is there anything that's worrying you? / Is there anything weighing on your mind? ◆心よりお気の毒に思います I'm truly[so] sorry. / I'm really sad for you. ◆心からお詫び申し上げます I apologize *with all my heart[from the bottom of my heart]. ◆心を閉ざす close one's mind (to / against) / crawl into one's shell ◆心を開く open one's mind (to) / open up to others ◆心を落ち着ける calm down ◆心を決める make up one's mind / decide ◆心と体の関係 relationship between mind and body ◆心の葛藤 emotional conflict[turmoil] / (内面の) inner conflict / (心理的な) psychological conflict ◆心の傷 mental[emotional / psychological] trauma / (傷跡) mental scar ◆心のケア psychological care ◆心の支え emotional support

こころあたり　心当たり ◆不眠の原因に心当たりはありますか What do you think is causing your sleeplessness? / Do you have any idea what's causing your sleeplessness?

こころがける　心がける (努力する)**try** (留意する)**take care** ◆血圧を下げるには減塩を心がけて下さい Please try[take care] to reduce your salt intake *for the sake of[to lower] your blood pressure.

こころぼそい　心細い (途方に暮れる)**feel helpless** (不安に感じる)**feel uneasy** (寂しく感じる)**feel lonesome** ☞寂しい, 心配, 不安 ◆日本での暮らしで心細く感じている点はありますか Is there anything about life in Japan that makes you feel helpless [uneasy / lonesome]?

こころみる　試みる　try, attempt ◆まずこの治療法を試みましょう Let's try this treatment first. ◆減量したければ，まず食事療法と運動療法を試みて下さい If you want to lose weight, you should first try dieting[diet therapy] and exercising[exercise therapy].

ごさ　誤差　error ◀測定誤差 measurement error　標準誤差 standard error ; SE

こし¹　腰 (腰全体)**lower back** (くびれた部分)**waist** (左右に張り出した部分)**hip** 《診察の基本表現》 ◆腰に何か問題がありますか Do you have any problems with your lower back? ◆腰を痛めたのですか Did you hurt your (lower) back? ◆腰が痛みますか Do you have *any pain in your

lower back[any lower back pain]? ◆腰のどのあたりが痛みますか Where in the lower back is the pain? ◆これまでに腰に痛みや不快感がありましたか Have you ever had any pain or discomfort in your lower back? 《基本動作の表現》 ◆腰が曲がっている have a bent[stooped] back / one's (lower) back is bent ◆腰をかがめる bend over[down] / bend one's lower back / stoop (down) ◆腰をさする rub one's (lower) back ◆腰をひねる twist one's (lower) back / twist (one's body) at the waist ◆腰を伸ばす straighten one's (lower) back / stretch one's (lower) back ◆腰をもむ massage one's (lower) back

◀ぎっくり腰(無理をして痛めた腰)strained back / (急性の腰の痛み)acute lower back pain ▶腰骨 hip bone　腰用コルセット back[lumbar] brace[corset] / (腰仙部の装具)lumbosacral brace[corset] ☞腰湯

こし²　固視　(ocular) fixation ◀不安定固視 unstable fixation ▶固視異常 anomalous fixation

こしかける　腰掛ける ☞座る

こしつ¹　個室　private room ◆個室をご希望ですか Would you like to have a private room? ◆個室には１日１万円の差額が必要です An additional ten thousand yen a day will be charged for a private room. / We'll charge you an additional ten thousand yen a day for a private room. ◆今日から個室に移ります You'll be transferred to a private room today.

こしつ²　鼓室　tympanic cavity ▶鼓室形成術 tympanoplasty

こしゆ　腰湯　hip bath (座浴)**sitz bath** ; *a bath in water up to the hips*

ごじゅうかた　五十肩　frozen shoulder, stiff and painful shoulder (due to old age), **fifty-year-old shoulder**

ごじゅうしょうさま　ご愁傷様 ☞愁傷

こしゅく　固縮　rigidity ☞硬直 ◀筋固縮 muscle rigidity

ごしゅじん　ご主人 ☞主人

こじれる　（悪化する）**get worse**　◆風邪がこじれて肺炎を起こしています Your cold has developed into pneumonia. / Your cold got worse and you've developed pneumonia.

こじわ　小皺　fine wrinkles　（特に，目じりの）**crow's feet**

こじん[1]　故人　deceased person, dead person　（特に，最近亡くなった人）**the deceased**　◆故人の遺志を尊重する respect the wishes of the deceased person

こじん[2]　個人　individual　（圏私的な **personal**　個別の **individual**　公的な立場ではない一個人の **private**）　◆私の個人的な意見では in my personal opinion　◆個人的な質問をする ask some personal questions　▶個人差 individual difference　個人識別 personal identification　個人精神療法 individual psychotherapy　（患者の）個人歴 patient profile　☞個人情報

ごしん　誤診　wrong diagnosis, diagnostic error, misdiagnosis　（圏**misdiagnose, wrongly[mistakenly] diagnose**）

こじんじょうほう　個人情報　personal information, private information

こす[1]　越す ☞越える

こす[2]　漉す（濾す）　filter ☞濾過

こすりあらい　擦り洗いする　wash … by rubbing, clean … by rubbing ☞洗う　◆傷口は刺激の少ない石鹸でそっとこすり洗いして下さい please wash[clean] the wound by rubbing it gently with a mild soap.

こする　擦る　rub　（ごしごしこすり落とす）**scrub**　（ひっ搔く）**scratch**　（こそぎ落とす）**scrape**　◆傷口をこすらないで下さい Please avoid rubbing the wound.　◆目を強くこする rub one's eye(s) hard　◆歯垢〈歯石〉をこすり落とす scrape away[off] *dental plaque〈tartar〉

こすれる　擦れる　rubbing　（ギシギシキーキーきしむような）**grating, scraping**　◆こすれるような音〈感じ〉a grating[scraping / rubbing] sound〈sensation〉　◆服にこすれる部分がヒリヒリしますか Does your skin feel irritated *when your clothes rub against it[by the touch of clothes]?

こせい　個性　（個人的特徴・人格）**personality**　（独自性）**individuality**

ごぜん　午前　morning　（時刻の後に）**am, a.m.**　◆午前9時に来て下さい Please come at nine in the morning.　◆3月16日の午前10時に at ten on the morning of March (the) sixteenth　◆今日〈明日〉の午前 this〈tomorrow〉 morning

—こそ　◆今こそリハビリを始める時です It's time to start rehabilitation. / It's time we started rehabilitation.　◆それこそ私が考えていたことです That's exactly what I was thinking about.

こそうねつ　枯草熱 ☞花粉症

こそく　姑息(的な)　palliative ☞緩和　▶姑息医療処置 palliative procedure　姑息手術 palliative surgery　姑息的治療[対症療法] palliative treatment[care]

こそだて　子育てする　（世話する）**take care of one's child〈children〉** ☞育てる　◆彼女は子育てに追われています She's very busy taking care of her child[children].　◆ご主人は子育てに協力的ですか Does your husband help you take care of your child[children]? / Is your husband cooperative when is comes to taking care of your child[children]?　▶子育て相談 counseling for parent(s)

ごぞんじ　ご存知　◆ご存知かもしれませんが As you might[may] already know, …　◆ご存知のとおり，院内は禁煙になっております As you know, smoking is not allowed anywhere inside the hospital.

こたい[1]　固体　solid (body) ☞固形

こたい[2]　個体(の)　individual　▶個体差 individual variation

こだいもうそう　誇大妄想　megalomania, delusion of grandeur　◆誇大妄想の患者 a megalomaniac (patient)

こたえる[1]　応える　（ニーズを満たす）**meet**　（満足させる）**satisfy**　◆残念ながらご要望にはお応えできません I'm sorry that I can't meet[satisfy] your request.　◆ご要望にお応えできるよう努力します We'll try to meet[satisfy] your request. / We'll do our best to respond to your request.

こたえる² 答える （質問に返答する）answer （圏answer）, reply （圏reply） （解答する・解決する）solve （圏solution） （反応する）respond （圏response 圏responsive）
◆ご質問があれば喜んでお答えします I'll be glad[happy] to answer your questions, if you have any. ◆すみませんが，はっきりお答えできません I'm sorry, but I can't give you a definite answer. ◆その難問への答えはまだ出ていません We haven't found the solution to that difficult problem. ◆アンケートに答える answer[（記入する）fill out] a questionnaire ◆（救急電話で）呼びかけには答えますか Does he⟨she⟩ respond to your voice? / Is he⟨she⟩ responsive[responding] to your voice?

こだわり ◆完璧さへのこだわり（強迫観念）an obsession with perfection ◆食べ物へのこだわりがありますか Are you very particular about what you eat?

こちょう 鼓腸 meteorism, tympanism, bloating （of the abdomen）

こちら ◆こちらへどうぞ This way, please. ◆（紹介する時）こちらは清水さんです This is Mr⟨Mrs / Ms / Miss⟩ Shimizu.

こつ¹ knack ◆この器具はこつさえつかめば楽に操作できます Once you get the knack of it, *this instrument is easy to handle[you'll find it easier to handle this instrument].

こつ² 骨 bone （睡頭oste(o)-） ☞骨（ほね）

こついえいようしょう 骨異栄養症 osteodystrophy

こついしゅく 骨萎縮 bone atrophy

こついしょく 骨移植 bone transplant[transplantation / grafting] （骨移植片）bone graft

こつえし 骨壊死 osteonecrosis, bone necrosis

こつえん¹ 骨炎 osteitis, ostitis ◀歯槽骨炎 alveolar osteitis

こつえん² 骨塩 bone mineral

こつか 骨化 ossification ◀異所性骨化

ectopic[heterotopic] ossification 黄色靱帯骨化症 ossification of the ligamentum flavum 後縦靱帯骨化症 ossification of the posterior longitudinal ligament；OPLL

こっかく 骨格 skeleton （睡skeletal） ◀筋骨格系 the musculoskeletal system ▶骨格筋 skeletal muscle 骨格系 the skeletal system

こつがさいぼう 骨芽細胞 osteoblast

こっかっしょく 黒褐色（の） dark brown, blackish brown

こっかん 骨幹 diaphysis ▶骨幹端 metaphysis

こつきゅうしゅう 骨吸収 bone resorption

こつきょく 骨棘 （bone）spur, osteophyte

こつきりじゅつ 骨切り術 osteotomy ◀回旋骨切り術 rotation osteotomy

こつけいせい 骨形成 bone formation （骨発生）osteogenesis （骨化）ossification ▶骨形成術 osteoplasty 骨形成不全症 osteogenesis imperfecta

ごっこあそび ─遊び pretend play, make-believe （play, game） ◆ごっこ遊びをする engage in pretend play ◆お子さんはごっこ遊びが好きですか Does your child like to play make-believe （games）?

こつこうかしょう 骨硬化症 osteosclerosis

こつしゅよう 骨腫瘍 bone tumor

こつシンチグラフィ 骨シンチグラフィ bone scintigraphy

こつずい 骨髄 bone marrow （睡頭myel-(o)-） ◀多発性骨髄腫 multiple myeloma ▶骨髄異形成症候群 myelodysplastic syndrome；MDS 骨髄移植 bone marrow transplant[transplantation]；BMT 骨髄炎 osteomyelitis 骨髄検査 bone marrow examination 骨髄生検 bone marrow biopsy 骨髄線維症 myelofibrosis 骨髄穿刺 bone marrow puncture 骨髄提供者 bone marrow donor 骨髄バンク bone marrow bank 骨髄抑制 myelosuppression

こっせつ 骨折 （bone）fracture （骨折箇所）break　◆これまでに骨折したことがありますか Have you ever broken[fractured] any of your bones?　◆（X線画像を示しながら）ここを見て下さい．骨折しています Here, *the bone is broken[you've got a broken bone].　◆親指が骨折しています You've broken[fractured] your thumb. / You've got a broken[fractured] thumb.　◆骨折を治す fix[repair / set] a broken [fractured] bone / put a broken[fractured] bone right　◆骨折した肋骨 a broken[fractured] rib　◀圧迫骨折 compression fracture　横骨折 transverse fracture　開放〈閉鎖〉骨折 open〈closed〉fracture　陥凹〈嵌入〉骨折 depressed〈impacted〉fracture　亀裂骨折 fissure fracture　線状骨折 linear fracture　脱臼骨折 dislocation fracture　多発骨折 multiple fracture　直達〈介達〉骨折 direct〈indirect〉fracture　剥離骨折 avulsion fracture　病的骨折 pathologic fracture　疲労骨折 stress[fatigue] fracture　不完全骨折 incomplete fracture　吹抜け骨折 blow-out fracture　複雑骨折 compound fracture　不顕性骨折 occult fracture　粉砕骨折 comminuted fracture　分娩骨折 birth fracture　ボクサー骨折 boxer's fracture　らせん骨折 spiral fracture　若木骨折 greenstick fracture　▶骨折固定法 fracture fixation　骨折部位 the site[location] of the fracture

こつそしき 骨組織 bone tissue, osseous tissue

こつそしょうしょう 骨粗鬆症 osteoporosis /ɑ̀stioʊpəróʊsɪs/　◆骨粗鬆症がある have osteoporosis　◆骨粗鬆症になる危険性は更年期後の女性に高くなります The risk of developing osteoporosis is higher in women after menopause. / Postmenopausal women have a higher risk of developing osteoporosis.

こつたいしゃ 骨代謝 bone metabolism

こつたん 骨端 epiphysis, apophysis

こつつう 骨痛 bone pain, bone ache, osteoalgia

こつてんい 骨転移 bone metastasis （㊶

metastases）, metastasis to （the）bone　◆彼の背骨に骨転移がみられます He has bone metastasis in his spine.

ゴットロンちょうこう ―徴候 Gottron sign

こつなんか 骨軟化（の） osteomalacic　▶骨軟化症 osteomalacia

こつなんこつしゅ 骨軟骨腫 osteochondroma　▶骨軟骨腫症 osteochondromatosis

こつにくしゅ 骨肉腫 osteosarcoma

こつねんれい 骨年齢 bone age

こつはっせい 骨発生 osteogenesis

こつばん 骨盤 pelvis （㊶pelvic） （臀部）breech　◆骨盤の手術を受けたことがありますか Have you ever had *pelvic surgery [surgery on your pelvis]?　◆骨盤の診察をする do a pelvic exam　◆広い〈狭い〉骨盤 a broad〈narrow〉pelvis　◀狭骨盤 contracted pelvis　児頭骨盤不均衡 cephalopelvic disproportion；CPD　▶骨盤位 breech presentation　骨盤位分娩 breech delivery[birth]　骨盤腔 pelvic cavity　骨盤牽引 pelvic traction　骨盤骨折 pelvic fracture

コップ （紙製の）（paper）cup　（ガラス製の）glass　（プラスチック製の）（plastic）cup　◆この薬はコップ一杯の水で飲んで下さい Please take this medication with a （full）glass of water.　◆コップの中身を一気に飲んで下さい Please empty the cup in one gulp.　◆このコップに尿を採って下さい Please use this cup to collect your urine.　◆コップ半分 half a cup　◀検尿コップ urinalysis cup / （採尿用の）urine （collection）cup

こつまく 骨膜 periosteum　▶骨膜炎 periostitis

こつみつど 骨密度 bone （mineral）density；BMD　◆骨密度を測る measure *a person's* bone density　▶骨密度検査 bone （mineral）density test

こつりょう 骨量 bone mass

こてい 固定する （支える）brace （図固定具 brace）　（しっかり止める・結ぶ）secure　（取り付ける）fix （図fixation ㊶fixed）, attach

（患部を動かさないようにする）**immobilize**（図 **immobilization**）（包帯を巻く）**dress**（図 **dressing**） ◆頭が動かないように首を固定します I'm going to brace[put a brace on] your neck to prevent your head from moving. ◆捻挫した部位が動かないように固定する secure the sprained area to prevent it from moving ◆ベッドに柵を固定する secure a bed with rails / make a bed safe by fixing[attaching] rails ◀圧迫固定 pressure dressing　頸椎固定具 neck brace / cervical collar　腱固定術 tenodesis　骨折固定法 fracture fixation　髄内釘固定法 intramedullary nailing　脊椎後方固定術 posterior spinal fusion　セメント固定 cement fixation　弾性固定 elastic fixation　内固定 internal fixation　▶固定化 immobilization　固定観念 fixed idea / stereotype　固定具 brace　固定薬疹 fixed drug eruption

こてん **古典（的な）** classic, classical
―ごと ☞―おき

こどう **鼓動** （心拍）**heartbeat** （脈拍）**pulsation** ☞脈 ◆心臓の鼓動に何か問題がありますか Do you have any problems with your heartbeat? ◆鼓動が激しくなる feel *one's* heart pounding[throbbing] ◆鼓動が速くなる the heart beats fast ◆鼓動が不規則になる the heart beats irregularly ◆心臓の鼓動を聞く listen to *the patient's* heartbeat ◆彼の心臓の鼓動は止まりました His heart has stopped beating.

こどく **孤独** **loneliness**（図寂しい **lonely** 単独の **solitary**　独りの **alone**　圖**alone**） ◆孤独に[を]感じる feel lonely[alone] ◆孤独な生活をする live alone / lead a solitary life ☞孤独死

こどくし **孤独死** **lonely death**, **dying alone** ◆孤独死する die a lonely death / die alone

ことし **今年** **this year** ◆今年の夏はニューヨークに帰るご予定ですか Are you planning to go back to New York this summer? ◆（意識障害の確認）今年は何年ですか What year is this?

ことなる **異なる** **differ**（from）, **be different**（from）（様々に変わる）**vary** ☞様々, 違う ◆この病気には3つの異なる治療方法があります There are three different ways to treat this disease. ◆効果や副作用は人によって異なります The effects and side effects differ[vary] from person to person.

ことば **言葉** （話し言葉）**spoken language**, **speech** （書き言葉）**written language** （単語）**word** （表現）**expression** （言語）**language** ☞言語, 語 ◆言葉が出にくいですか Do you have difficulty[trouble] *getting your words out[speaking]? ◆思っていることを言葉で表しにくいですか Do you have difficulty[trouble] putting *what you're thinking[your thoughts] into words? ◆日本に暮らしていて言葉に問題がありませんか While living in Japan, do you have any language problems? ★肯定文で言う. ◆ごめんなさい, 適当な言葉が見つかりません I'm sorry, but I can't find[think of] *the right word[an appropriate expression]. ◆病棟では言葉が通じましたか Were you able to make yourself understood on the ward? ◆ねぎらいの言葉をかける speak[offer / say] words of comfort[thanks] ◆言葉に障害がある have a language disorder ◆言葉につまる stumble over *one's* words / be stuck for words ◆年齢に応じた言葉を話す speak appropriately for *one's* age / speak in an age-appropriate manner ◆言葉が遅れる be slow learning to speak / speech development is delayed[late] ◆平易な言葉 plain language ◆普通の言葉 ordinary language ◆攻撃的な言葉 aggressive words ◆言葉の壁 a language barrier ◆言葉の障害 a speech defect ◀言葉の発達 language development ◀赤ちゃん言葉 baby talk

こども **子供** **child**（圈**children**）（男の子）**boy** （女の子）**girl** ☞子, 児童, 小児, 幼児 ◆子供はいますか Do you have any children? ◆子供は全部で何人ですか How many children do you have? ◆子供のこ

ろ喘息にかかりましたか Did you suffer from asthma *as a child[when you were a child]? ◆4歳の子供 a four-year-old child / a child of four ◆子供への虐待 child abuse ◆子供時代の病気 a childhood illness

ことわる 断る

《前もって知らせる》get permission ◆外出する時は必ず断って下さい Please get permission before going out (of the hospital). ◆お断りしておきますが，当院では看護学生の実習を受け入れております Please be advised that we conduct on-the-job training of nursing students in this hospital.

《拒む》 （申し出などを辞退する）decline （要求・依頼を却下する）turn down （強く断る）refuse ☞拒否 ◆お志はありがたいのですが，贈り物はお断りしております It's very kind of you[We appreciate your kindness], but *we can't accept your gift[we have to decline your present]. ◆申し訳ありませんが，ご依頼はお断りせざるをえません I'm sorry that we *have to turn down [can't accept] your request.

こなぐすり 粉薬 powder, powdered medication, medication in powder form ☞薬 ◆この粉薬が飲み込みにくい時はジュースやアイスクリームに混ぜてお飲み下さい If you can't swallow this powder, you can take it mixed with juice or ice cream. ◆粉薬をぬるま湯で溶かす dissolve the powder in lukewarm water

ゴナドトロピン gonadotropin；Gn ◀ヒト絨毛性ゴナドトロピン human chorionic gonadotropin；hCG ▶ゴナドトロピン欠損症 gonadotropin deficiency ゴナドトロピン産生腫瘍 gonadotropin-producing tumor ゴナドトロピン低下症 hypogonadotropism ゴナドトロピン放出ホルモン gonadotropin-releasing hormone；GnRH / luteinizing hormone-releasing hormone；LH-RH ゴナドトロピン療法 gonadotropin therapy

こなミルク 粉ミルク （乳児用の）formula (milk) （一般に，粉末状の）powdered milk, milk powder

ごねんせいぞんりつ 5年生存率 five-year survival rate ◆胃がんの5年生存率 the five-year survival rate for stomach cancer

このあいだ この間 （先日）the other day （前回）last time （園last） ☞この前 ◆この間はご協力有難うございました Thank you for your cooperation[help] the other day. ◆この間はずいぶん大きい地震でしたが，大丈夫でしたか The last earthquake was a pretty big one—were you all right[okay]?

このさい この際 （状況下で）under the [these] circumstances （現時点で）at this point ◆感染症のため隔離いたしますが，この際やむを得ません We're going to *isolate you from the other patients[put you in quarantine] as you have an infectious disease. There's no help for it under the [these] circumstances. ◆この際ご了解いただきたいことがあります At this point, there's something I need to obtain your approval[consent] for.

このさき この先 ☞今後

このつぎ この次 ☞今度

このば この場 here ◆今この場でお決めになる必要はありません You don't have to decide here and now.

このまえ この前 last time （園last） ☞この間 ◆この前の診察時よりだいぶ良くなっています You're much better than the last time I saw you.

このまま （この状態・現状通り）like this, as it is, as they are （このペースで）at this rate, at this pace ◆このままの調子で食事療法を続けていきましょう Let's keep up the diet therapy *like this[as you've been doing until now]. ◆現状をこのまま放っておくわけにはいきません We cannot leave this matter as it is. ◆このままで行けば来週早々には退院できそうです At this rate[If your recovery keeps up at this pace], you'll probably be able to leave the hospital early next week.

このみ 好み （一般的に）liking （趣味）

taste （好き嫌い）**likes and dislikes** （好物）
one's preference, *one's* favorite （略favorite）　☞好き　◆それは好みの問題です That's a matter of taste[likes and dislikes / preference].　◆好みの料理 *one's* favorite dish[dishes]

このむ　好む　like （…の方を好む）**prefer**
☞好き

このように　like this, (in) **this way**　◆腕をこのように上げて下さい Please raise your arms *like this[in this way].　◆このようにして下さい Please do like this.

ごはん　ご飯 （米飯）**rice** （食事）**meal**
◆ご飯とパンではどちらがいいですか Which would you like, rice or bread?　◀朝ご飯 breakfast　昼ご飯 lunch　夕ご飯 supper / dinner

コピー　copy　◆血液検査のコピーを差し上げます Here's a copy of your blood test results for you. / This copy of your blood test results is for you.　◆この事前指示書をコピーさせていただいてもよろしいですか Would you mind if I[we] make a copy of this advance directive? / If it's all right with you, could I[we] make a copy of this advance directive?

ごピーマイナスしょうこうぐん　5p−症候群　chromosome 5p deletion syndrome, cri-du-chat syndrome, cat-cry syndrome

こびとしょう　小人症　☞小人症（しょうじんしょう）

こぶ　瘤 （打撲傷）**bump** （しこり）**lump** （腫れ）**swelling** （動脈瘤）**aneurysm, bulge in a blood vessel**　◆頭にこぶがある have a bump on the head

ごぶごぶ　五分五分 （半分半分）**fifty-fifty** （均等）**even**　◆彼女が回復する見込みは五分五分です She has *a fifty-fifty[a fifty percent / an even] chance of getting well. / Her chances of recovering are fifty-fifty.

こぶし　fist　◆こぶしを握る make a fist　◆こぶしを握り締める clench *one's* fist

こぶはくせん　股部白癬　ringworm of the groin, tinea cruris （インフォーマルに）**jock**

itch

コプリックはん　─斑　Koplik spot

こべつ　個別(の)　individual （一対一の）**one-on-one, one-to-one** （略単独で）**alone** （内密に）**privately**）　◆お話は個別にうかがいたいのですが Could I talk[have a word] with you alone? / Could we talk one-on-one[(2人だけで)just the two of us / privately]?　▶個別接種 individual vaccination[immunization]

こぼす （液体をこぼす）**spill** （物を落とす）**drop** （涙などを流す）**shed**　◆彼は食事の時によく飲み物や食べ物をこぼしますか Does he often spill drinks or drop food while eating?　◆涙をこぼす shed tears

こまかい　細かい
《小さい》**fine, small, little**　◆細かい字が読みにくいですか Do you have difficulty reading fine print?　◆指の細かい動き fine movements of the fingers / （ピクピクした動き）finger twitching
《細部の》（詳細な）**detailed** （図detail）（些細な）**small, little**　◆細かい注意点などについては看護師にご遠慮なくお尋ね下さい Please don't hesitate to ask the nurses for details[detailed information] on anything.　◆食事療法は，細かいことにこだわらず，まず続けることが肝心です For diet therapy to be successful, it's important not to focus on the small details too much, but to just keep on going with it.　◆細かいことが気にかかるほうですか Do you tend to worry about little[small] things?
《神経が繊細な》**delicate, sensitive**　◆彼は神経がとても細かい He's very sensitive.

ごまかしうんどう　ごまかし運動　trick movement[motion]

こまく　鼓膜　eardrum, tympanic membrane （略頭myring(o)−）　◆鼓膜が破れたことがありますか Have you ever *had a ruptured eardrum[ruptured your eardrum]?　◆鼓膜を切開する make an incision in the eardrum　◀青色鼓膜 blue eardrum[tympanic membrane]　▶鼓膜炎 myringitis　鼓膜切開 myringotomy　鼓膜穿孔 tympanic membrane perforation /

perforation of the eardrum

こまめに often, frequently ◆できるだけこまめに水分補給をして下さい Please drink fluids[water] as often as possible. ◆作業の間にこまめに休息をとってリラックスして下さい Please take *a break and relax frequently[frequent rest] between activities.

こまる 困る 〔苦労する〕have difficulty 〔in〕〔問題を抱えている〕have trouble 〔with〕, have a problem 〔困っている〕be in difficulty[trouble] 《苦労・困難がある》 ◆何かお困りのことがありますか(心配事があるか)Is anything bothering[troubling] you? / (何か問題があるか)Is anything wrong? ◆排尿のコントロールに困っていますか Do you have (any) difficulty (in) controlling your bladder? ◆便秘で困っているのですか Do you have any trouble with constipation? ◆困ることがあれば，相談に来て下さい If you have any problems[If you're ever in trouble], feel free to come and talk with me. ◆それは困りましたねえ That's too bad. / (どうしたものか) What should I do? / (どうしたらよいかわからない) I don't know[I'm not sure] what to do. ◆そうおっしゃられても返事に困ります I don't know[I'm at a loss] how to answer such a question. ◆お金に困っている be in financial difficulties / have money worries 《迷惑だ》 ◆それは困ります．おやめ下さい You can't do that. Please *stop it[don't].

ごみ 〔不用物〕waste 〔ちり・ほこり〕dust 〔古新聞・瓶など〕trash, rubbish ◆目にごみが入る *get some dust[have something] in one's eye(s) ◆ごみを出す take out the trash ◆ごみを捨てる throw out the trash ▶ごみ箱 wastebasket / wastepaper basket

こみいった 込み入った ☞複雑 complicated ◆彼らの別居には込み入った家庭事情があるようです There seem to be some complicated family circumstances behind their separation.

コミュニケーション communication 〔動〕communicate〕 ◆ジェスチャーでコミュニケーションを図る *communicate with [understand] each other by means of gestures ◆周囲と上手くコミュニケーションをとる communicate well with the people around one ◆コミュニケーションに問題がありますか Do you have any difficulty communicating with others? / Do you have any communication problems? ◆彼女のコミュニケーション能力にはやや問題があります There's some question about[as to] her *communication ability [ability to communicate]. ◆彼のコミュニケーション手段は手話です He communicates by (means of) sign language. / He uses sign language to communicate. ◆親子の間には深刻なコミュニケーション断絶があるようです There seems to be a serious *breakdown in communication [communication gap] between parent(s) and child(ren). ◆患者と医療従事者とのコミュニケーション communication between patients and medical personnel ◀言語〈非言語〉コミュニケーション verbal 〈nonverbal〉 communication ▶コミュニケーション技術 communication skills　コミュニケーション障害 communication disorder　コミュニケーション障壁 communication barrier

コミュニティ community ☞地域

こむ 混む ☞混雑

ゴム 〔製品としてのゴム〕rubber 〔材料としてのゴム〕gum ◀ラテックスゴム latex rubber ▶ゴムバンド[輪ゴム] rubber[elastic] band ☞ゴム手袋

こむぎ 小麦 wheat ◆小麦にアレルギーがありますか Are you allergic to wheat? ▶小麦アレルギー wheat allergy / (過敏症) wheat hypersensitivity

ゴムてぶくろ ―手袋 rubber gloves ★通例，複数形で． ◆天然ゴム手袋でアレルギー症状が出る have an allergic reaction to natural rubber gloves

こむらがえり こむら返り leg cramp ◆右足にこむら返りを起こす get a cramp in one's right leg

こめ 米 rice ◆普段，何を食べていますか．お米のご飯ですか，パンですか What do you usually eat, rice or bread? ▶米のとぎ汁様便 rice-water stool[(下痢) diarrhea]

こめかみ temple ◆こめかみに痛みがある have (a) pain in *one's* temple(s) ◆こめかみがずきずきしている *one's* temples are throbbing

ごめん (I'm) sorry （軽い調子で）excuse me ◆遅れてごめんなさい(I'm) sorry I'm late. ◆あ，ごめんなさい．痛かったですか Oh, *excuse me[(I'm) sorry]! Did I hurt you?

こゆび 小指 （手の）little finger （足の）little toe ☞指

こよう 雇用 employment ◀障害者雇用援助 employment support for people with disabilities ▶雇用者 employer 雇用保険 unemployment insurance

ごよう[1] 御用 ☞用

ごよう[2] 誤用 misuse ◆誤用を防ぐために，自己判断で薬の服用を中断し再開しないで下さい To avoid misuse, please do not stop and start taking the medication *on your own[at will].

コラーゲン collagen /kɑ́ləʤən/ （㊕collágenous） ▶コラーゲン線維 collagenous fiber

こらえる ☞抑える，我慢，耐える

ごらん ご覧 ☞見る ◆この写真をご覧下さい Please look at this film. ◆吸入器の使い方をご覧に入れましょう I'll show you how to use the inhaler.

こりごり 懲り懲り ☞うんざりする ◆もう深酒にはこりごりでしょう You've had enough of it with excessive[heavy] drinking, haven't you? / Excessive[Heavy] drinking has already taught you a good lesson, hasn't it?

こりしょう 凝り性（の）（こだわりが強い）particular （気難しい）fastidious ◆ご自分は凝り性なほうだとお考えですか Are you the fastidious type? / Do you tend to be particular in everything you do?

こりつ 孤立 isolation （㊕isolated 単独の

solitary） ◆家族や友人の中で孤立していると感じますか Do you feel isolated from your family and friends? ▶孤立性肺結節 solitary pulmonary nodule

こりる 懲りる ☞懲り懲り

コリン choline （㊕cholinergic） ◀抗コリン薬 anticholinergic (medication / drug / agent) ▶コリンエステラーゼ cholinesterase コリン性蕁麻疹 cholinergic urticaria

こる 凝る get[be, feel] stiff （㊕stiffness） ☞こわばる ◆肩が凝っていますか Are your shoulders stiff? / Do you have stiff shoulders? ◆首が凝る have a stiff neck / feel stiff in the neck ◆肩の凝りをほぐす relieve[lessen] the stiffness in *one's* shoulders

コルサコフしょうこうぐん ―症候群 Korsakoff syndrome

コルセット brace, corset ◆コルセットを着ける put on a brace[corset] ◆コルセットを着けている wear a brace[corset] ▶腰用コルセット back[lumbar] brace[corset] /（腰仙部の装具）lumbosacral brace[corset] 膝用コルセット knee brace

コルチコイド corticoid （副腎皮質ホルモン） adrenal cortex hormone, adrenocortical hormone ▶鉱質コルチコイド mineralocorticoid 糖質コルチコイド glucocorticoid

コルチコステロイド corticosteroid （副腎皮質ホルモン） adrenal cortex hormone, adrenocortical hormone ▶吸入コルチコステロイド薬 inhaled corticosteroid；ICS

コルチコトロピン corticotropin （副腎皮質刺激ホルモン） adrenocorticotropic hormone；ACTH

コルチゾール cortisol

ゴルフひじ ―肘 golfer's elbow

コルポスコピー colposcopy

これから （今すぐに）now （この後で）after this （今後は）from now on ☞今後 ◆これから胸のCT検査をしましょう Let's take [do] a CT scan of your chest now. ◆これから診察があるので失礼します Sorry, but I've got to see my patients after this.

◆これから寒くなりますからお大事に The weather is going to get colder from now on[From now on, the weather will get colder], so please take (good) care of yourself.

コレステロール cholesterol /kəléstəròu/ ◆コレステロールが正常値より高い〈低い〉The cholesterol level is above〈below〉normal. ◆あなたの総コレステロール値は 245 mg/dL で，LDL コレステロールが 175 mg/dL と高値で，HDL コレステロールが 35 mg/dL と低値です Your total cholesterol is two hundred (and) forty-five milligrams (per deciliter)；your LDL cholesterol is high, one[a] hundred (and) seventy-five, and HDL cholesterol is low, thirty-five. ◆LDL コレステロールは 130 に下がり，HDL コレステロールは 40 に上がりました Your LDL cholesterol dropped to one[a] hundred (and) thirty, and your HDL cholesterol rose[climbed] to forty. ◆コレステロールは正常値の範囲内です The cholesterol is in the normal range. ◆この薬は LDL コレステロールを下げます This medication will lower[reduce] the LDL cholesterol (level). ◆上昇したコレステロール値を正常にする normalize an elevated cholesterol level ◆コレステロールをコントロールする control (*one's*) cholesterol ◆コレステロールを多く含む食べ物 food(s) rich in cholesterol / high-cholesterol food(s) ◆動脈にコレステロールが沈着するのを防ぐ prevent cholesterol accumulation[deposits] in the arteries ◀HDL コレステロール HDL[high-density lipoprotein] cholesterol / good cholesterol LDL コレステロール LDL[low-density lipoprotein] cholesterol / bad cholesterol 家族性高コレステロール血症 familial hypercholesterolemia 血中コレステロール増加 increased[elevated] blood cholesterol / (過多) excessive blood cholesterol 高コレステロール high cholesterol 高コレステロール血症 hypercholesterolemia 高コレステロール〈低コレステロール〉食 high-cholesterol〈low-cholesterol〉diet ▶コレステロール管理 cholesterol control[management] コレステロール結石 cholesterol stone コレステロール胆石 cholesterol gallstone コレステロール値 cholesterol level[count] コレステロール低下薬 cholesterol-lowering medication[drug / agent] コレステロールポリープ cholesterol polyp

これだけ 《こればかり（限定）》 ◆これだけは申し上げておきます I'd just like to say this. ◆これだけは忘れないで下さいね I want you not to forget this at least.
《これほどまで》 ◆これだけ早いスピードで回復するとは驚きです I'm really surprised that you recovered so rapidly. ◆これだけ申し上げてもご理解いただけませんか Is it still difficult to understand[Do you still not understand] after I've explained this much?

これで ◆本日はこれですべて終了です It's all over for today. / That's it for today. / You're finished for today.

これまで ◆これまで健康状態はどうでしたか How has your health been up until now? ◆それでは，これまでにかかった病気についてお伺いします Now I'd like to ask you about any illnesses you've had in the past. ◆今日はこれまでにしましょう That's all for today. / So much for today.

コレラ cholera ▶コレラ菌 *Vibrio cholerae* コレラワクチン cholera vaccine

ころがる 転がる （回る）roll ◆ごろんと転がって下さい Please roll over.

ごろごろ ◆お腹がごろごろしますか Does your stomach rumble[make rumbling sounds / make rumbling noises]? ◆目がごろごろしますか Does your eye feel gritty? / Does your eye feel like it has sand[grit] in it? ◆休みの日には家でごろごろしていることが多いですか Do you often *idle the time away[loaf around / lie about] doing nothing at home on your days off?

コロニー colony ▶顆粒球コロニー刺激因子 granulocyte colony-stimulating factor；G-CSF　顆粒球マクロファージコロニー刺激因子 granulocyte-macrophage colony-stimulating factor；GM-CSF

ころぶ 転ぶ　fall（down, over）☞転倒
◆どんなふうに転びましたか How did you fall?　◆よく転びますか Do you often[frequently] fall down?　◆転ばないように注意して下さい Please take care（that）you don't fall. / Please walk carefully so as not to fall down.　◆階段で転ぶ fall down the stairs　◆石につまずいて転ぶ trip[stumble] over a stone and fall down[forward]　◆すべって転ぶ slip and fall　◆うつ伏せに転ぶ fall flat on one's face　◆転んで地面に頭をぶつける fall down and hit one's head on the ground　◆転んで手〈膝〉をつく fall onto one's hands〈knees〉◆前につんのめるように転ぶ fall forward　◆後ろに倒れて転ぶ fall on one's back /（後ろにひっくり返る）tumble down[over]　◆転んで足を折る fall over and break one's leg

コロモジラミ body lice（圖louse）★通例，複数形で.

こわい 怖い
《恐ろしい》scary, frightening（非常に恐ろしい）horrible, dreadful（ぞっとするような）terrifying　◆何か怖い目に遭われたことがありますか Have you ever had any scary[frightening / horrible / terrifying] experiences before?　◆怖い夢を見ることが度々ありますか Do you often have terrifying dreams?
《心配だ》◆今食習慣を変えないと後が怖いですよ（残念に思うだろう）If you don't change your eating habits now, you'll be sorry in the long run.

こわがる 怖がる（おびえる）be scared（of）（心配する）be afraid（of）　◆（MRI検査で）少し大きな音がしますが怖がらなくても大丈夫ですよ This machine makes a slightly loud noise, but there's no need to be scared[afraid].

こわす（身体を）壊す（害を及ぼす）dam-

age（健康を損なう）ruin（傷つける）injure（圖injury）◆過労で体を壊す damage[ruin] one's health by overworking　◆お腹を壊している have *an upset[a bad] stomach / have stomach trouble / one's stomach is upset　◆肩〈肘〉を壊している have *a shoulder〈an elbow〉injury

こわばる（硬直する）have stiffness, get [feel] stiff（こわばっている）be stiff ☞凝る　◆身体のどこかがこわばっていますか Do you have stiffness in any part of your body? / Does any part of your body feel stiff?　◆手がこわばりますか Do your hands get stiff?　◆こわばり始めたのはいつですか When did the stiffness begin?　◆こわばるのはずっとですか，時々ですか Is the stiffness constant[there all the time] or *does it come and go[is it intermittent]?　◆こわばるのはいつですか．早朝〈日中／就眠中／運動後〉ですか When do you have the stiffness? Early in the morning〈During the day / While you're sleeping / After exercise〉?　◆朝のこわばりはどのくらい続きますか How long does your morning stiffness last after you wake up?　◆首筋がこわばる have a stiff neck　◆こわばっている筋肉をほぐす（緩める）loosen one's stiff muscles / relax one's stiff muscles　◆こわばりを和らげる reduce[relieve / relax / ease] stiffness

こわれやすい 壊れやすい ☞もろい

こんいん 婚姻　marriage（圖marital）☞結婚　◆婚姻外で生まれた子（非嫡出子）an illegitimate child ▶婚姻状況 marital status　婚姻届 marriage registration

こんかんちりょう 根管治療　root-canal treatment

こんき 根気（忍耐）patience（圖patient）◆最近根気が続かないと感じますか Do you feel that *you're becoming less and less patient[you have less patience] these days?　◆今回はうまくできなくても根気よく練習していけば大丈夫です Even though you can't do this very well this time, you'll be all right if you keep at it.

こんきょ 根拠（事実としての証拠）evidence

（理由）grounds ★通例，複数形で．（基礎）basis ☞証拠 ◆治療効果についてはっきりした根拠を示す give[provide] clear evidence of the therapeutic effects ◆今のところこのサプリメントの効果を示す十分な根拠はありません At present there isn't enough[sufficient] evidence that this supplement is effective. ◆感染を疑う確かな根拠があります We have reasonable grounds to suspect infection. ◆彼女の不安には根拠がありません Her anxiety has no basis in fact. ◀科学的根拠 scientific evidence ▶根拠に基づく医療 evidence-based medicine；EBM

こんげつ 今月 this month

こんご 今後 （今から）from now （今からずっと）from now on （将来）in the future （このあとで）after this （再び）again （あとで）later ☞これから ◆今後の治療計画についてお話しいたします I'm going to explain[talk about] what the plan of treatment from now on will be. ◆今後どうなさいますか．日本で治療を受けますか What are you going to do (from now on)? Would you like to have the treatment in Japan? ◆今後受診する必要はないでしょう You don't have to come and see me again. ◆今後この症状はしばらく続くかもしれません These symptoms may continue for a while after this. ◆今後の成り行き次第では入院が必要になるかもしれません Depending on how things develop, *you may need to be hospitalized[hospitalization may become necessary]. ◆それは今後の問題です We'll deal with that problem later. /（後回ししてもよい）That's a problem we can deal with later. ◆今後どうなるのか予測がつきません We can't predict *what will happen[how things will develop] in the future. / We'll have to wait and see *what happens[how things develop]. ◆ごめんなさい．今後は遅れないようにします I'm sorry, I'll try not to be late again.

こんごう 混合 mixture, mixing （英mixed,

combined） ▶混合栄養 mixed feeding 混合型インスリン mixed insulin 混合感染 mixed infection 混合診療 treatments partially covered by insurance / mixed treatments 混合性結合組織病 mixed connective tissue disease；MCTD 混合物 mixture / compound ☞混合ワクチン

こんごうワクチン 混合ワクチン combined vaccine ◀ジフテリア・破傷風混合ワクチン diphtheria-tetanus (combined) [DT] vaccine ジフテリア・破傷風・百日咳混合ワクチン diphtheria-tetanus-pertussis (combined)[DTP] vaccine

こんざつ 混雑している be crowded （with） ◆週明けの外来はいつも混雑します Outpatient clinics[departments] are always crowded with patients at the beginning of the week.

コンサルタント consultant

コンサルテーション consultation ▶コンサルテーション精神医学 consultation psychiatry

こんしゅう 今週 this week

コンジローマ condyloma ▶尖圭コンジローマ condyloma acuminatum / genital wart

こんすい 昏睡 coma /kóʊmə/ （英comatose） ◆彼女は深い昏睡状態です She is in a deep coma. ◆まだ半昏睡状態にある be still in a semicoma / be still in a *partially comatose[semicomatose] state ◆回復不能な昏睡状態にある be in an irreversible coma ◆昏睡状態に陥る fall[lapse / go] into a coma ◆昏睡状態から覚める come out of a coma ◆昏睡の深さを測る measure the depth of *a person's* coma ◀外傷後昏睡 coma after (head) injury 肝性昏睡 hepatic coma グラスゴー昏睡尺度 Glasgow coma scale；GCS 子癇性昏睡 eclamptic coma 深昏睡 deep coma 遷延性昏睡 prolonged coma 前昏睡状態 precoma 低血糖昏睡 hypoglycemic coma 糖尿病性昏睡 diabetic coma

こんせき 痕跡 （微量成分の跡）trace （残されたしみ・傷など）mark ☞痕（あと）

こんぜつ　根絶する　eradicate（図eradication）　◆ポリオを根絶する eradicate polio　◆病気を根絶する eradicate a disease

コンセント¹（同意）**consent** /kənsént/　☞同意，同意書

コンセント²（電気の差し込み口）（**electrical**）**outlet, socket**

こんだく　混濁（濁り・曇り）**clouding, cloudiness**（図cloudy, clouded）（不透明・乳白度）**opacity**（主に液体の濁り）**turbidity**（図汚れて濁った **turbid**）（せん妄状態）**delirium**（図**delirious**）　◆彼は意識が混濁しています His consciousness is cloudy[clouded]. / He is delirious[(半ば意識がある) only half conscious].　◆水晶体が混濁しています Your lens has become cloudy.　◀意識混濁 clouded consciousness /（せん妄）delirium　角膜混濁 corneal opacity[clouding]　硝子体混濁 vitreous opacity[clouding]　水晶体混濁 clouding of the lens / lens opacity[clouding]　羊水混濁 meconium staining　▶混濁尿 cloudy[turbid] urine

コンタクトレンズ　contact lens　◆コンタクトレンズを使用していますか Do you wear contact lenses?　◆コンタクトレンズを傷つけたり汚したりしないよう気をつけて下さい Please be careful not to damage or dirty your contact lenses.　◆コンタクトレンズをはめる *put in[insert] one's contact lenses　◆コンタクトレンズを外す *take out[remove] one's contact lenses　◆コンタクトレンズをはめている wear contact lenses　◀ソフト〈ハード〉コンタクトレンズ soft〈hard〉contact lens　連続装用コンタクトレンズ extended-wear contact lens

こんち　根治（完全な回復）**complete cure**（根本的な治癒）**radical cure**　◆手術で根治が望める早期のがんですのでどうぞご安心下さい Your cancer is in its early stages and *can be completely cured[is curable] by surgery, so don't worry.　◆残念ながら現時点ではこの疾患は根治させることができません Unfortunately, at present *there's no complete cure for this disease[we won't be able to cure this illness

completely].　◆彼女は根治が望めない可能性があります She may not be able to achieve a complete cure. / We may not be able to *hope for[expect] a complete cure for her.　◀拡大根治手術 extended radical surgery　▶根治可能性 curability　根治手術 radical surgery　根治切除 radical resection　根治的照射 radical irradiation　根治的治療 radical[curative] treatment

こんちゅう　昆虫　insect　◆ハチなどの昆虫アレルギーがありますか Are you allergic to bees or other insects?　◀有毒昆虫 poisonous[toxic] insect　▶昆虫アレルギー insect allergy　昆虫刺傷 insect bite[sting]　昆虫媒介感染症 insect-borne infection

こんてい　根底(の)　underlying　☞根本　◆根底にある病気を治す cure the underlying disease

こんど　今度

《今回》**this time**（今）**now**　◆今度は上手にできましたね You've done well this time.　◆今度はあなたの番ですよ Now it's your turn.

《次回》**next time**　◆今度来る時に必ず保険証を持ってきて下さい Please be sure to bring your insurance card next time you come.

《別の機会》**some other time**　◆また今度にしていただけますか(婉曲的な断り)Could you come[talk to me] *some other time[next time], maybe?

こんどう　混同する　confuse（図confusion）**, mix up**　◆精神科と神経内科は混同されがちですが，全く違う専門分野です People often confuse (the department of) neurology with (the department of) psychiatry, but they are completely different fields of medicine.

コンドーム　condom /kándəm/　◆コンドームを使う use condoms　◆コンドームを着ける put on a condom　◆コンドームを着けている wear a condom

コントラスト　contrast　◀肝腎エコーコントラスト hepatorenal echo contrast

コントロール ―する （制御する）control （図control） （維持する）maintain （衝動などを抑える）check, restrain ◆排尿〈排便〉をコントロールするのが難しいですか Do you have difficulty controlling your bladder〈bowels〉? ◆あなたは症状のコントロールがうまくできていますね You have your symptoms under control, don't you? / Your symptoms are well controlled, aren't they? ◆血糖値をコントロールする control[maintain] *one's* blood sugar level ◆感情をコントロールする control[check / restrain] *one's* own feelings ◀血糖コントロール sugar control セルフコントロール self-control ペインコントロール pain control マインドコントロール mind control

こんなふうに ☞このように

こんなん 困難 difficulty （図difficult） （問題・トラブル）trouble （苦難）hardship （図hard） （厳しさ）toughness （図tough） ☞困る，難しい ◆歩行に困難がある have some walking difficulties / have some difficulty walking ◆経済的な困難に直面する face financial difficulties ◆困難な問題 a difficult problem ◆困難な仕事 a hard[tough] job / difficult work ◀嚥下困難 dysphagia / difficulty[trouble] (in) swallowing 学習困難 learning difficulty 月経困難（症）dysmenorrhea / painful menstruation[periods] / menstrual[period] pain / menstrual cramps 呼吸困難 dyspnea / difficult breathing / breathing difficulty[trouble] / （息切れ）shortness of breath；SOB 咀嚼困難 difficulty[trouble] (in) chewing / chewing difficulty 入眠困難 difficulty (in) falling asleep 排尿困難 dysuria / urinary difficulty / difficulty (in) urinating / voiding difficulty 排便困難 dyschezia / difficulty (in) moving *one's* bowels 歩行困難 difficulty (in) walking / walking difficulty 哺乳困難 difficulty (in) sucking / sucking difficulty

こんにちは 今日は Hello （子どもの患者やインフォーマルな場面で）Hi （改まった挨拶として）Good afternoon ◆キングさん，こ

んにちは Hello, Mr King! ◆やあスーザン，こんにちは Hi[Hello], Susan!

こんばん 今晩 this evening, tonight

こんばんは 今晩は Hello （子どもの患者やインフォーマルな場面で）Hi （改まった挨拶として）Good evening ◆キムさん，こんばんは Good evening, Ms Kim!

コンピュータ computer ◆コンピュータ使用による眼精疲労はよく起こります Eye strain from[due to] using a computer is very common. ▶コンピュータ支援診断 computer-assisted[computer-aided] diagnosis

コンプライアンス compliance ◆服薬のコンプライアンスが低いと期待される治療効果は得られません Poor drug compliance may result in decreased therapeutic effects.

コンプレックス （劣等感）inferiority complex （↔superiority complex） ◆肥満にコンプレックスを持つ have an inferiority complex about[due to] *one's* *heavy weight [obesity]

こんぽん 根本（的な） （基礎的な）basic, fundamental （根治的な）radical （根底にある）underlying ◆根本的な問題を解決する solve a basic[fundamental] problem ◆残念ですが，現在この病気には根本的な治療法はありません I'm sorry to say, but there's no treatment that can completely cure this disease now. / I'm sorry to say, but there's no radical treatment for this disease at present. ◆ストレスがこの病気の根本的な原因です Stress is the underlying cause of this disease. ▶根本治療 radical treatment 根本的治癒［根治］complete cure / radical cure

こんめい 昏迷 stupor ◆昏迷状態に陥る fall[lapse / go] into a stupor ◆昏迷状態にある be in a stupor

こんや 今夜 this evening, tonight

こんらん 混乱する get[become] confused （図confusion） ☞錯乱 ◆痙攣後どのくらい意識が混乱しますか After a seizure, how long do you stay confused?

さ

さ　差 ☞違い

《相違・差異》difference（動differ）, variation（動vary）　◆この2つの薬は効き目の点で大きな差はありません As regards their effectiveness, there's not much difference between these two medications. / These two medications don't substantially differ in their effectiveness.　◆聞こえ方は左右で差がありますか Is there any difference between the hearing in your left ear and the hearing in your right ear? /（両耳で同じように聞こえるか）Is your hearing the same in both ears?　◆日中の血圧に多少差があるのは正常です Some variation in your blood pressure during the day is normal.　◆成長には個人差があるので，お子さんを焦らずに見守ってあげて下さい Individual differences[variations] in child development are natural, so try not to worry but to enjoy watching how your child grows up.

《隔たり》gap　◆お子さん達の年の差は何歳ですか How far apart in age[How many years apart] are your children?　◆年齢差が大きいのが気になりますか Are you worried about the large[wide] age gap[difference]?

◀人種差 racial difference　性差（男女の違い）sex difference /（社会・文化における男女差）gender difference　世代差 generation gap

サーカディアンリズム　circadian rhythm

サーズ　SARS（重症急性呼吸器症候群）severe acute respiratory syndrome

サービス　service　◆介護サービスを提供する offer[render] a care service　◆訪問介護サービスを利用する use[make use of] a visiting home care service　◀医療サービス medical service　在宅福祉サービス home welfare service　福祉サービス welfare service

サーファクタント　surfactant, surface-active agent

サーベイランス　surveillance

サーモグラフィ　thermography

サーモンパッチ　salmon patch, stork bite

さい¹　際　◆紹介状が必要な際には遠慮なく言って下さい If[In case] you *need a referral letter from me[need me to write a referral letter], please don't hesitate to let me know.　◆この際ゆっくり休養して下さい I hope you'll take this occasion to have a good rest. / Take this opportunity to have a good rest.

さい²　差異 ☞差，違い

さい³　歳 ☞何歳　◆あなたは今何歳ですか May I ask your age? /（子供の患者に）How old are you?　★大人の患者にいきなり"How old are you?"と訊くのは失礼なことがあるので注意．　◆その手術を受けたのは何歳の時でしたか How old were you when you had the surgery?　◆78歳で死ぬ die at the age of seventy-eight　◆8歳の男の子 an eight-year-old boy

ざい　座位・坐位　sitting（position）　◀あぐら座位 sitting crossed-legged / crossed-leg position　半座位 semisitting[Fowler] position　▶座位訓練 sitting exercise　座位バランス sitting balance　座位バランス訓練 exercise to maintain a balanced sitting position / exercise to improve sitting balance　座位分娩 delivery in a sitting position

さいあく　最悪（の）　（the）worst　★the worst のみで「最悪の事態」の意味になる．☞最低　◆起こりうる最悪の事態に備える prepare[be prepared] for the worst（possible thing that can happen）

ざいあくかん　罪悪感 ☞罪責感

ざいいんにっすう　在院日数　the length of one's hospital stay

さいがい　災害　disaster（自然災害）natural disaster　（事故）accident　◀大規模災害 large-scale[mass] disaster　労働災害 work-related[worker / workplace] accident / occupational accident /（産業・工業上の）industrial accident　▶災害派遣医療

チーム disaster medical assistance team；DMAT

さいかんりゅう　再灌流　reperfusion
▶再灌流傷害 reperfusion injury　再灌流療法 reperfusion[（再疎通）recanalization]therapy

さいきかんし　細気管支　bronchiole
◀びまん性汎細気管支炎 diffuse panbronchiolitis；DPB　▶細気管支炎 bronchiolitis

さいきけいせい　催奇形性　teratogenicity
（㊞teratogenic），teratogenic effect　◆この薬は催奇形性があるので，妊婦さんや妊娠している可能性のある女性には使用できません This medication may cause birth defects[This medication carries a teratogenic risk]，so pregnant women or women who may be pregnant should not take it.　◆妊娠 16 週以降は薬による催奇形性のリスクは低くなります The risks of teratogenicity of medications decrease after sixteen weeks of pregnancy.

さいきゅうしゅう　再吸収　reabsorption

さいきょう　最強（の）　（効果的な）(the) most effective　（効き目の強い）(the) most powerful，(the) strongest　◆これが痛み止めとして現在最強の薬効をもつ薬の 1 つです This is currently considered one of *the most effective[the most powerful / the strongest] medications available for pain relief.

さいきょうさく　再狭窄　restenosis
▶冠血管再狭窄 coronary restenosis

さいきん¹　細菌　bacteria（㊞bacterium）
★通例，複数形で．（㊞bacterial　細菌学的な bacteriologic, bacteriological）　（一般的に）germ　☞菌　▶腸内細菌 intestinal bacteria　病原細菌 pathogenic bacteria　▶細菌学 bacteriology　細菌学者 bacteriologist　細菌感染症 bacterial infection　細菌検査 bacterial[bacteriologic] examination　細菌尿 bacteriuria　細菌培養 bacterial culture　☞嫌気性菌，好気性菌，常在細菌

さいきん²　最近
《近い過去》recently, lately　★lately は常に現在完了形で用いる．（このところ）these days　◆最近何か薬を飲みましたか Have you recently taken any medications?　◆彼は最近の事が思い出せないのですか Does he have difficulty remembering *recent events[new things]?　◆最近私はとても忙しい I'm very busy these days. / I've been very busy lately.
《直近の》last　◆最近数か月で体重は変化しましたか Has your weight changed in the last few[several] months?

サイクル　cycle　☞周期，循環
ざいけい　剤形　dosage form
さいげきとうけんびきょうけんさ　細隙灯顕微鏡検査　slit lamp microscopy
さいけつ　採血　blood（specimen）collection　◆明朝 6 時に採血にうかがいます I'll come and take[collect] a blood sample[specimen] at six tomorrow morning.　◆採血しましょう I'm going to[Let me] take a blood sample. / Let's do a blood draw.　▶採血室 phlebotomy room / blood collection room

さいけん　再建　reconstruction（㊞reconstructive）　◀括約筋再建術 sphincter reconstruction　血行再建術 revascularization　肛門再建手術 reconstructive anal surgery　乳房再建術 breast reconstruction surgery　▶再建手術 reconstructive[reconstruction] surgery

さいけんさ　再検査　（再検討のための追加検査）further[additional] test[examination]，another checkup, reexamination　（追跡検査）follow-up test[examination]　◆再検査が必要です You need a *further test[reexamination]. / You need to undergo further testing.　◆診断を確認するため再検査を予定します I'll schedule[You're going to have] an additional test to double-check the diagnosis.　◆再検査のために 3 か月以内にもう一度おいで下さい Please come again in three months for a follow-up test.

さいけんとう　再検討する　（見直す）review（㊞review），reexamine（㊞reexamination）　（考え直す）reconsider（㊞reconsideration）

（確認し直す）double-check, double check（図double check）　（評価し直す）reevaluate（図reevaluation）　（査定し直す）reassess（図reassessment）　◆検査結果が判明したら，治療方針について再検討しましょう When we have the test results, we'll review[reexamine] your treatment plan. ◆CTは放射線診断医が必ず再検討しています Your CT scan will always be double-checked by a diagnostic radiologist. / A diagnostic radiologist will always double-check your CT scan. ◆「心肺蘇生をしない」という決断について再検討した際には，遠慮なくお知らせ下さい If you reconsider your decision that you don't want us to perform CPR[resuscitation], don't hesitate to let us know. / If you change your mind about your DNAR[Do Not Attempt to Resuscitate] order, please don't hesitate to tell us.

さいご¹　**最期**　（臨終）last moments（死の床）deathbed　（最期の日々）last days　☞臨終　◆彼は最期が近いと思われます I'm afraid he is near his last moments. ◆彼女の最期をみとる care for her on her deathbed　◆彼の最期に立ち会う be with him *in his last moments[（亡くなる時）when he passes away] / be present at his deathbed　◆彼女の最期はとても安らかでした She died a very peaceful death. ◆どこで最期を過ごしたいですか，ご自宅ですかそれともホスピスですか Where would you like to spend your last days, at home or in a hospice?

さいご²　**最後**（の）　（一番終わりの）(the) last　（最終段階の）final（図終わり end）☞最終　◆最後に私の診察を受けたのはいつですか When was the last time you came to see me?　◆最後の月経は何歳の時ですか How old were you when you *had your last (menstrual) period [stopped having periods]?　◆排尿の最後に少し痛む have a slight pain at the end of *one's urination　◆膵臓がんの最後の段階 the final stage of pancreatic cancer ◆この薬は症状が良くなっても最後まで飲

み続けて下さい（治療期間ずっと）Please continue taking this medication for the full course of treatment even if your symptoms disappear[clear up].

さいこう¹　**再考する**　☞再検討
さいこう²　**最高**（の）　（最大限の）(the) most　（レベルが一番高い）(the) highest　（一番よい）(the) best　（程度・限度が頂点の）(the) maximum, maximal, peak　最善, 最大, 最長, 最適, ベスト　◆体重は最高でいくらありましたか What is the most you've ever weighed?　◆その施設は最高レベルの医療サービスを提供しています The facility offers the highest level[standards] of medical services.　◆最高の条件[状態] the best conditions　▶最高血圧 maximal [(収縮期の)systolic] blood pressure　最高値 peak value

さいこうかんせんしょう　**再興感染症** reemerging infectious disease

ざいごうぐんじんびょう　**在郷軍人病** ☞レジオネラ

ざいごうもうそう　**罪業妄想**　delusion of guilt

サイコオンコロジー　psychooncology
サイコセラピー　psychotherapy
サイコセラピスト　psychotherapist
さいさん　**再三**　☞何回　many times, over and over again　◆再三の注意にもかかわらず彼は喫煙を止めません He doesn't stop smoking even though I've warned[cautioned] him not to *many times[over and over again]. / He still smokes in spite of my repeated warnings.

さいしゅ　**採取する**　take, collect　◆髄液を採取する take[collect] a spinal fluid sample

さいしゅう　**最終**（の）　（一番後の・前回の）(the) last　（最終段階の）final（図終わり end）☞最後　◆最終決定 *one's final decision　◆最終診断 the final diagnosis　◆最終段階 the end[final] stage[period]　◆最終学歴を教えて下さい Please tell me the last educational institution you attended. / How far did you get in school?　◆最終月経はいつでしたか

When was your last (menstrual) period? ◆最終目標 one's final[(究極的な)ultimate] goal

さいしゅじゅつ **再手術** repeat surgery [operation], resurgery

さいじゅしん **再受診** ☞再診

さいしゅっけつ **再出血** rebleeding
◆この手術は再出血の危険がありますので，追加の処置が必要になるかもしれません This surgery has a risk of subsequent rebleeding, and additional procedures may be necessary.

さいしょ **最初(の)** (一番初めの)first (初期の)initial (図手始めに first, at first) ☞初め，初めて ◆最初の段階 the first[initial] stage ◆最初の月経は何歳の時ですか How old were you when you *had your first (menstrual) period[started your periods]? ◆最初にこのしこりに気づいたのはいつですか When did you first notice this lump? ◆最初に2，3質問いたします First, I'd like to ask you a couple of questions. ◆麻薬性鎮痛薬を使い始めると最初は眠気や吐き気が出ますが，次第に慣れてきます You may feel sleepy and nauseous when you first start taking the narcotic painkillers, but your body will soon get used to them.

さいしょう **最小・最少(の)** (程度・限度が最も低い)(the) minimum, minimal (図minimum 動最小限にする minimize) (数量が最も少ない)(the) least, (the) smallest (レベルが最も低い)(the) lowest ☞最低 ◆1日に必要な最少のカロリーは基礎代謝率に基づいています The minimum[least] number of calories you need each day is calculated based on your basal metabolic rate. ◆薬が最小量で済むように生活習慣を見直して下さい Please change[reexamine] your daily habits or lifestyle so that you can keep the amount of medications you need to a minimum. ◆この薬は最小量から始めて徐々に増量していきます I'll start you on the lowest dose of this medication and gradually increase the dose. ◆化学療法の副作用を最小限に抑

える minimize the side effects of chemotherapy / keep[reduce] the side effects of chemotherapy to a minimum ▶最小血圧 minimal[(拡張期の)diastolic] blood pressure 最小侵襲[低侵襲]手術 minimally invasive surgery 最小値 the[a] minimum value 最小発育阻止濃度 minimum inhibitory concentration；MIC 最小有効量 minimal effective dose；MED

さいしょく **菜食** vegetarian diet (完全菜食)vegan diet ◆彼女は菜食中心の食事をとっています She is on a vegetarian diet. ▶菜食主義 vegetarianism / veganism ☞菜食主義者

さいしょくしゅぎしゃ **菜食主義者** vegetarian /vèdʒətériən/ (完全菜食主義者) vegan /víːgən/ ★卵・牛乳などもとらないのが完全菜食主義者. ◆あなたは厳格な菜食主義者ですか Are you a *strict vegetarian [vegan]?

さいしん¹ **再診** follow-up consultation [examination], reexamination (来院)follow-up[return] visit, revisit ◆6か月後に再(受)診して下さい Please come again in six months for a follow-up consultation [examination]. ★「…後に」の前置詞は after ではなく in を用いる. ◆薬がなくなる前に再(受)診して下さい Please come back again before your medication runs out. ◆お帰りになる前に再診の予約をして下さい Before you leave the hospital, please make a follow-up[return] appointment. ▶再診受付 revisit counter[desk] 再診患者 follow-up patient 再診料 reexamination fee

さいしん² **細心(の)** very careful ◆この器具の取扱いには細心の注意を払って下さい Please be very careful when handling this device. / You have to be very careful when you handle this device. ◆風邪をひかないように細心の注意を払って下さい Please *be very careful[(最大限の注意を払う)take the utmost care] not to catch a cold.

さいしん³ **最新(の)** (最近の)(the) latest, the most recent (最も新しい)(the) new-

est (最先端の) **up-to-date** ☞最先端
◆肺がんについての最新の医療情報 *the latest[the most recent / up-to-date] medical information on lung cancer
◆最新の知識を得る get[obtain] up-to-date knowledge[information]

サイズ **size** ◆最近，ほくろのサイズや形に変化がありましたか Have you noticed any changes in the size or shape of your mole(s)? ◆首周りのサイズが以前より大きくなったのですか Has your collar size become larger? ◆ポリープのサイズは 1 cm 以下です Your polyp is smaller than one centimeter. ◆腫瘍のサイズは 25 mm から 15 mm まで縮小しました The size of the tumor has shrunk from twenty-five (millimeters) to fifteen millimeters. ◆お腹回りのサイズを測る measure *a person's* waist size / measure *a person's* abdominal[waist] circumference ◆傷痕のサイズ scar size / size of a [the] scar

さいせい **再生する** (組織が再生する)**regenerate** (図regeneration 図regenerative) (元の状態に戻る)**grow back** ◆喫煙で傷んだ肺の組織は再生しません Lung tissue damaged by smoking *does not[will not] *grow back[regenerate]. ◆肝臓には再生能力があります The liver has *the capacity to regenerate (itself)[a regenerative capacity]. ◀肝再生 liver regeneration ☞再生医療, 再生不良性貧血

ざいせい **財政** **finance** (圏financial) ☞経済 ◆彼の財政状態は悪い His financial situation[condition] is *not good [bad]. ▶財政援助 financial help[assistance / aid]

さいせいいりょう **再生医療** **regenerative medicine**

さいせいふりょうせいひんけつ **再生不良性貧血** **aplastic anemia**

ざいせきかん **罪責感** **guilty feeling, feeling of guilt** ◆あなたが罪責感をもつ必要は全くありません You don't have to feel guilty at all. ◆無意識のうちに罪責感をもつ have[feel] an unconscious sense of guilt

さいせきじゅつ **砕石術** **lithotripsy**；*a procedure to crush a stone or stones* ◀経尿道的尿管砕石術 transurethral ureterolithotripsy 体外衝撃波砕石術 extracorporeal shockwave lithotripsy；ESWL 膀胱砕石術 cystolithotripsy

さいぜん **最善(の)** **(the) best** (図one's best) ◆最高, 最適, ベスト ◆最善を尽くす do *one's* best / do all *one* can do ◆最善の治療方法を決めなければなりません We have to decide the best option for treating your condition.

さいせんたん **最先端(の)** (最も進んだ) **the most advanced** (技術・装置が最も新しい) **state-of-the-art, cutting-edge, leading-edge** ◆当院は最先端の手術設備を備えています This hospital has the most advanced surgical equipment available. / This hospital is equipped with state-of-the-art surgical equipment. ◆先端技術 state-of-the-art[cutting-edge / leading-edge] technology

さいたい **臍帯** **umbilical cord** ▶臍帯頸部巻絡 umbilical cord around the neck 臍帯血 (umbilical) cord blood 臍帯血幹細胞移植 cord blood stem cell transplant [transplantation] 臍帯結紮 ligature of the umbilical cord 臍帯脱出 umbilical cord prolapse

さいだい **最大(の)** (数量が最も大きい) **(the) biggest, (the) largest** (程度・限度が頂点の) **(the) maximum, maximal** (図maximum 動最大にする maximize), **peak** (最大限の) **(the) utmost** (図utmost) (一番よい) **(the) best** (図best) ☞最高, 最長
◆今, あなたにとって最大の問題は何ですか What's the biggest problem you have in your life right now? ◆治療効果を最大限にあげるには，この薬を指示どおりに飲むことが大切です To get the maximum [maximal] benefit from the treatment, it's important to take this medication exactly as directed. ◆当院は市で最大の医療施設です This hospital is the largest medical facility in the city. ◆感染の拡大

防止に最大限の努力を払います We *do our utmost[do our very best / make the utmost effort] to prevent the spread of infection. ▶最大血圧 maximal[(収縮期の) systolic] blood pressure　最大呼気流量 maximal expiratory flow；MEF / peak expiratory flow；PEF　最大耐容線量 maximum tolerated dose；MTD　最大値 the[a] maximum value

ざいたい　在胎(の) gestational ▶在胎期間 gestational age　在胎週数 gestational week

ざいたく　在宅(の) home, home-based, in-home (圖at home) ◆退院後は在宅介護をお望みですか Do you want *home care[in-home care / care at your home] after your discharge from the hospital? ▶在宅医 home care physician　在宅医療 home-based medical care / medical home care / medical service at *a person's home*　在宅介護サービス in-home (care) service / home care service　在宅介護(支援)センター home care (support) center　在宅看護 home nursing[health] care　在宅患者 homebound patient / patient at home　在宅経腸栄養法 home enteral nutrition；HEN　在宅酸素療法 home oxygen therapy；HOT　在宅静脈栄養法 home parenteral nutrition；HPN　在宅透析 home dialysis　在宅福祉サービス home welfare service　在宅リハビリテーション in-home[home-based] rehabilitation / rehabilitation at home

さいたん　最短(の・で) (時期が最も早い) (the) earliest, (the) soonest　(時間・距離が最も短い) (the) shortest ◆血液検査は最短で1時間後に判明します The results of your blood test will be available in one hour at the earliest.

さいちょう　最長(の・で) (the) longest　(最大限) (the) maximum ◆処方箋の有効期間は(発行した日を含め)最長4日間です The prescription is valid for a maximum of four days from (and including) the date of issue.

さいてい　最低(の) (数量が最も少ない)

(the) least　(レベルが最も低い) (the) lowest　(程度・限度が最も低い) (the) minimum, minimal (圖minimum 圖最小にする minimize)　(最悪の) (the) worst ☞最悪, 最小, 最短 ◆成人になってから最低の体重はいくらですか What is the least you've weighed as an adult? ◆化学療法開始後約2週間で好中球数や血小板数は最低レベルになります Neutrophils and platelets decrease to their lowest levels about two weeks after the start of chemotherapy. ◆最低賃金で働く work on (the) minimum wage ◆リスクを最低限に抑える keep the risk to a minimum / minimize the risk ◆すっかり回復するまでには最低4週間はかかるでしょう It will take at least four weeks to recover completely. ◆あなたが過去最低の状況にあることは理解できます I understand you are in the worst condition ever. ◆最低限度の暮らし the minimum standard of living / the minimum living standard ▶最低血圧 minimal[(拡張期の) diastolic] blood pressure

さいてき　最適(の) (最も適切な) (the) most suitable　(最もよい) (the) best　(条件などが最も望ましい) (the) optimal, (the) optimum ◆最高, 最善, ベスト ◆ストレス解消に最適な方法を選ぶ choose the *most suitable[best / optimal] way to reduce (*one's*) stress ◆薬の最適な量 the optimal[optimum] dose of medication ▶最適温度 the optimal[optimum] temperature　最適条件 the optimal condition

さいど　再度 again ☞もう一度

さいどう　細動 fibrillation ☞除細動, 心室細動, 心房細動

さいどうみゃく　細動脈 arteriole ◀輸出細動脈 efferent arteriole　輸入細動脈 afferent arteriole

サイトカイン cytokine

サイトメガロウイルス cytomegalovirus；CMV ▶サイトメガロウイルス感染症 cytomegalovirus infection　サイトメガロウイルス網膜炎 cytomegalovirus retinitis

さいとやく　催吐薬 emetic /ɪmétɪk/；

medication that induces vomiting ◆催吐薬を投与する give[administer] an emetic

ざいにちがいこくじん 在日外国人 foreign resident of Japan, foreigner residing in Japan

さいにゅういん 再入院 readmission (to the hospital), rehospitalization

さいにゅうこく 再入国 reentry ▶再入国ビザ reentry visa

さいにょう 採尿 urine collection, collection of a urine sample[specimen] ◆こちらのカップに採尿をお願いします Please use this cup to collect your urine. ▶採尿コップ urine (collection) cup

さいねん 再燃する （突然悪化する）flare up again （増悪する）become exacerbated again ☞再発 ◆口唇ヘルペスは免疫力が下がると再燃します Cold sores flare up again when the immune system declines.

さいはつ 再発する （繰り返し起こる）recur /rɪkə́ː/ （図recurrence 図recurrent） （治りかけた病状がぶり返す）relapse /rɪlǽps/ （図relapse 図relapsing） （以前の状態に戻る）return （図return）, come back ◆この病気は再発する恐れがあります There is some possibility of this disease recurring. / You may have a recurrence of this disease. ◆5年以内に再発する可能性は約5%です There is a five percent chance of recurrence within five years. ◆残念ながら，がんの再発が判明しました I'm sorry to tell you this, but I've just found out that your cancer has returned[come back / relapsed]. ◆痛みが再発したら教えて下さい Please let me know when the pain *comes back[starts again]. ◆心臓発作の再発を防ぐ prevent another heart attack ◆うつ病の再発 recurrent depression / （うつ状態の繰り返し）repeated episodes of depression ◀断端再発 stump recurrence ▶再発性潰瘍 recurrent ulcer ☞再発率

さいはつりつ 再発率 recurrence rate ◆この病気は再発率が高い This disease has a high *recurrence rate[rate of recurrence]. / The recurrence rate of this disease is high.

さいはれつ 再破裂 rerupture ◆脳動脈瘤の再破裂は24時間以内に起こるリスクが高い The risk of cerebral aneurysm rerupture is high within the first twenty-four hours.

さいひょうか 再評価 （検討し直す）reevaluation （査定し直す）reassessment ☞再検討

さいふ 財布 wallet, billfold ◆財布などの貴重品は盗難防止のため部屋のセーフティボックスで保管して下さい To prevent theft[For theft prevention], please keep valuables, such as your wallet, in the safety box in your room.

さいぶ 臍部 umbilical region

さいヘルニア 臍ヘルニア umbilical hernia

さいべん 採便 stool collection, collection of a stool sample[specimen], feces collection ◆ご自宅でこの容器に採便して，次回受診時にお持ち下さい Please collect your stool sample in this container and bring it with you when you come *for your next visit[to see me next time]. ▶採便袋 colostomy bag

さいぼう 細胞 cell （図cellular 接頭 cyt(o)-） ◆正常な細胞 a normal cell ◆異常な細胞 an abnormal cell ◀悪性細胞 malignant cell 異型細胞 atypical cell 角化細胞 keratinocyte 幹細胞 stem cell がん細胞 cancer cell 腫瘍細胞 tumor cell 上皮細胞 epithelial cell 生殖細胞 reproductive cell 造血幹細胞 hematopoietic [blood-forming] stem cell 標的細胞 target cell 分化細胞 differentiated cell 未分化細胞 undifferentiated cell 免疫担当細胞 immunologically competent cell ▶細胞異型 cellular atypia 細胞学 cytology 細胞学者 cytologist 細胞検査士 cytotechnologist 細胞死 cell death 細胞質 cytoplasm 細胞周期 cell cycle 細胞性免疫 cellular immunity 細胞増殖 cell growth 細胞毒性 cytotoxicity 細胞培養 cell culture 細胞分化 cell differentiation

細胞分裂 cell division　細胞壁 cell wall
細胞膜 cell membrane　☞細胞診

さいぼうしん　**細胞診**　**cytology** /saɪtálə-
ʤi/, **cytodiagnosis**　(塗抹検査法) **smear**
/smíə/　(子宮頸がんの検査法) **Pap smear**
[**test**]　◆鼻汁の細胞診をしましょう Let's
do[get] a nasal smear.　◆細胞診の結果は
陽性〈陰性〉です The cytology results are
positive〈negative〉.　◆正常な〈異常な〉細
胞診結果 *a normal〈an abnormal〉cytol-
ogy result　◀喀痰の細胞診 sputum cytology[smear]　◀擦過細胞診 scraping cytology　穿刺吸引細胞診 fine needle aspiration cytology；FNAC　尿細胞診 urine
[urinary] cytology　ブラシ細胞診 brush
cytology

さいほつさ　**再発作**　(繰り返し起こる発作)
recurrent attack　(2回目の発作) **second**
[**another**] **attack**　◆一過性虚血の再発作
を起こす have recurrent transient ischemic attacks　◆この病気は再発作を起こす
と非常に危険です A second attack of this
disease is very serious[critical].

さいみん　**催眠**　**hypnosis** (㊀**hypnotic**)
◀自己催眠 self-hypnosis　◀催眠薬 hyp-
notic (medication / drug / agent) / (睡眠
導入薬) sleep-inducing medication　催眠
療法 hypnotherapy / hypnotic　therapy
催眠療法士 hypnotherapist　☞催眠術

さいみんじゅつ　**催眠術**　**hypnotism** (㊀**催
眠術をかける hypnotize**)　◆催眠術がか
かっている be under hypnosis

さいらい　**再来**　☞再診
さいらん　**採卵**　**oocyte retrieval**
ざいりゅう　**在留**　**residence** (㊀**reside**)
▶在留カード residence card　在留外国人
foreign resident of Japan / foreigner residing in Japan　在留期間 period of residence in Japan　在留許可 residence permit　在留資格 visa[residence] status
さいりょう　**最良**　☞最高, 最善
さいるいやく　**催涙薬**　**lacrimator**
サイロキシン　**thyroxine**；**T₄**　◀遊離サイ
ロキシン free thyroxine[T₄]
サイログロブリン　**thyroglobulin**
サイロニン　**thyronine**　◀トリヨードサイ

ロニン triiodothyronine；T₃

さいわい　**幸い(な)**　**lucky, fortunate** (㊀
luckily, fortunately)　◆その事故で大怪我
をしなくてすんだのは幸いでしたね You're
lucky not to have suffered any serious
injuries in the accident. / Luckily[Fortu-
nately], you were not seriously injured in
the accident.　◆幸いにも，ポリープは良性
でした Luckily[Fortunately], the polyp
was benign.

サイン　(署名) **signature** /sígnətʃʊ/ (㊀
sign)　◆この同意書をよく読んでサインし
て下さい Please read this (informed)
consent form carefully and sign it.　◆こ
こにサインをお願いします Sign here,
please. / Could I have your signature
here?　◆所定の欄にサインする sign in
the space provided

サウジアラビア　**Saudi Arabia** (㊀**Saudi
Arabian**)　☞国籍　▶サウジアラビア人
(の) Saudi Arabian

さえる　**冴える**　(目覚めている) **be wide
awake**　(頭の働きがよい) **be alert**[**sharp**,
clear-headed]　◆目が冴えて眠れません
か Are you wide awake and unable to fall
asleep?　◆今日，彼は頭が冴えています
His mind is alert[sharp] today. / He's
really clear-headed today.　◆顔色が冴え
ないようですね，大丈夫ですか(落ち込んでい
る) You look down[depressed]. Are you
*all right[okay]?　◆気分が冴えない日が
ずっと続いているのですか Have you been
feeling down[depressed / blue] for a long
time?

さか　**坂**　(斜面) **slope**　(坂道・丘) **hill**　◆坂
や階段を上がったりする時，胸が痛みますか
Do you have chest pain when you go up
slopes or stairs?

さかい　**境**　**border**　(境界線) **borderline**
☞境界

さがく　**差額**　(差し引き残高) **difference**,
balance　(追加の料金) **additional charge**
(余分の料金) **extra charge**　◆会計窓口で差
額を払って下さい Please pay the difference[balance] at the cashier's window.
▶差額病室 special (charge) room；*room*

that is only partially covered by health insurance 差額料金(保険適応外の料金) charge not covered by health insurance / (差額室料) special room charge ☞差額ベッド

さがくベッド **差額ベッド** (特別提供の部屋)special (charge) room (有料のベッド) extra-charge bed, pay bed ◆差額ベッド代は保険の適用外です Additional fees for special rooms are not covered by health insurance. ◆差額ベッド代として1日当たり1万円かかります We'll charge you an additional ten thousand yen a day for a special room.

さかご **逆子** **breech baby** (骨盤位分娩) breech delivery ◆赤ちゃんは逆子になっています The baby is in the *breech position[(臀部が先)bottom-first position / (足が先)feet-first position].

さかさまつげ **逆さまつげ** **ingrown eye-lashes** (睫毛乱生)trichiasis

さがす **探す・捜す** **look for, search** (for) (見つける)find out ◆彼は失業して仕事を探しています He has lost his job and is looking for work. ◆アレルギーの原因を探しましょう Let's find out what's causing your allergies.

さかな **魚** **fish** (圏fishy) ◆生の魚を食べる eat raw fish ◆魚くさいおりもの fishy vaginal discharge

さかみち **坂道** **hill** ☞坂

さがる **下がる** (数値・水準などが低下する) **come[go] down, fall, drop** (減少・下落する)decline, decrease ◆熱が下がりましたか Did your fever come[go] down? ◆血圧が正常値まで下がっています Your blood pressure has fallen[dropped] to within normal. ◆近年、乳児死亡率が下がっています The infant mortality rate has declined[fallen / decreased] in recent years. ◆2, 3歩だけ後ろへ下がって下さい Just a few steps backward(s), please.

さき **先** 《先端》(舌・指などの先端)tip (尖った部分)point (端の部分)end ◆舌の先 the tip of one's tongue ◆手の指先 a fingertip / the

tip of a finger ◆足の指先 the tip of a toe 《前方に》ahead ◆お手洗いはこの先少し行ったところにあります There is a restroom just a little ahead. 《順番》ahead ◆どうぞお先に Go ahead, please. / After you. 《今後・将来》from now on, in the future ◆これから先はどうなさいますか What are you going to do from now on? ◆この治療は先が長い There's still a long way to go with this treatment.

さきほど **先程** (つい今しがた) **just now** (少し前)a little while ago ◆先程は失礼しました〈行為に対して〉I'm sorry about *what I did〈発言に対して〉what I said〉to you *just now[a little while ago]. ◆お友達が先程からラウンジでお待ちかねです Your friend has been waiting for you in the lounge *for a while[for some time].

さきゃくブロック **左脚ブロック** **left bundle branch block；LBBB** ◆完全左脚ブロック complete left bundle branch block；CLBBB 不完全左脚ブロック incomplete left bundle branch block；ILBBB

さぎょう **作業** (仕事一般)work (任務・職務)task ☞仕事, 労働 ◆作業中に事故に遭う have an accident while at work ◆日常生活に必要な作業を行うのが難しい have difficulty *carrying out[performing] tasks necessary for one's everyday life ◀共同作業 group[collaborative] work 単純作業 simple work 日常的作業 everyday task ▶作業環境 working [work] environment 作業関連疾患 work-related disease 作業効率 work efficiency 作業時間 working hours 作業所 workshop 作業能力 working[work] capacity[ability] 作業量 workload ☞作業員, 作業療法

さぎょういん **作業員** **worker** ◀工事作業員 construction worker

さぎょうりょうほう **作業療法** **occupational therapy；OT** ◀機能的作業療法 functional occupational therapy ▶作業療法士 occupational therapist；OT 作業

療法室 occupational therapy room

さく¹ 柵 rail （ベッドの）bedside rail
◆このベッドの柵は転落防止のためのものです This bedside rail is to keep you from falling out of the bed. / This bedside rail is for your safety so that you won't fall out of the bed. ◆ベッドの柵を上げる〈下げる〉raise〈lower〉the bedside rail

さく² 策 measure ☞手段, 対策 ◆感染防止の策を講じる必要があります We must [need to / have to] take measures to prevent the spread of infection.

さく³ 割く （時間を都合する）spare ◆検査結果についてお話ししたいので10分ほど時間を割いていただけますか I'd like to talk about the test results, so could you spare me ten minutes or so? ◆貴重なお時間を割いていただきありがとうございます Thank you very much for giving me your valuable time.

さくかんかく 錯感覚 paresthesia, dysesthesia ; *an abnormal feeling in the body such as tingling or burning*

さくご 錯語 paraphasia

さくさん 酢酸 acetic acid

さくし 錯視 optical illusion

さくじつ 昨日 yesterday

さくせい 作成する （作る・準備する）make, prepare, draw up （手配する）set up, arrange ◆同意書を作成する prepare a consent form ◆介護計画を作成する make[set up] a person's care plan

さくにゅう 搾乳する pump *one's* breast milk ▶搾乳器 breast pump

さくねん 昨年 last year

さくや 昨夜 last night, yesterday evening

さくらん 錯乱 （意識の混乱）(mental) confusion （形confused）, derangement （形deranged）◆彼は錯乱することがありましたか Has he ever had any (bouts of) confusion? ◆錯乱状態に陥る become [be] confused[deranged] / fall into a state of confusion

さくわ 作話 confabulation

さけ 酒 alcohol /ǽlkəhɔːl/, alcoholic drink[beverage] （日本酒）sake ☞アルコール, 飲酒, 酒量
《飲酒習慣の質問》◆お酒を飲みますか Do you drink alcohol? ◆いつもはどんなお酒を飲みますか What kind of alcohol do you usually drink? ◆お酒はどのくらいの頻度で飲みますか How often do you drink alcohol? ◆お酒は1日にどのくらい飲みますか How much (alcohol) do you drink a day?
《節酒・断酒の指導》◆お酒を飲まないように努力して下さい Please try to stop drinking alcohol. ◆24時間はお酒を飲まないで下さい You should not drink alcohol for twenty-four hours. ◆お酒は適量であればかまいません You can drink alcohol in moderation. ◆この薬を飲んでいる間はお酒を控えて下さい Please do not drink alcohol while taking this medication.
◆酒をやめる *give up[quit] drinking ◆適量の酒 a moderate amount of alcohol ◆大量の酒 a large amount of alcohol ◆酒の消費量 alcohol consumption
▶酒飲み drinker /（大酒家）heavy drinker /（適度に飲む人）moderate drinker /（付き合いで飲む人）social drinker /（たまに飲む人）occasional drinker /（問題のある酒飲み）problem drinker ☞寝酒

さけぶ 叫ぶ （悲鳴を上げる）cry out （大声を出す）shout ◆痛いと叫ぶ *cry out [shout] in pain

さけめ 裂け目 （割れ目・亀裂）crack （動crack）（縦長の細い割れ目）split （動split）（細長い割れ目・細隙）slit （動slit）（深い割れ目・裂溝）fissure （破れ目・裂孔）tear /téə/ （唇・口などの割れ目）cleft （形cleft）◆錠剤の裂け目で(半分に)割る split the tablets (in half) ◆細い裂け目のあるランプ a slit lamp ◆踵の裂け目 a heel crack ◆肛門の裂け目 an anal fissure ◆網膜の裂け目 a retinal tear ◆裂け目のある口唇 a cleft lip

さける¹ 裂ける ☞破裂, 破れる

さける² 避ける avoid, stay away （from）, keep away （from）◆過労を避ける try not to overwork *oneself* / try to avoid overworking　◆塩分の強い食品を避ける avoid[stay away from] eating salty foods　◆今となっては透析が避けられないようです Dialysis now seems inevitable. / It looks like you'll have to go on dialysis. / I'm afraid you cannot avoid going on dialysis.

さげる　下げる

《低くする》**bring down, lower**　（減少させる）**reduce**　◆熱を下げるためのお薬を出しましょう I'm going to[Let me] give you something to *bring down[lower / reduce] your fever.　◆血圧を下げる *bring down[lower] *one's* blood pressure　◆（診察時に）スカートを下げてお腹を見せて下さい Please lower your skirt and show me your abdomen.　◆ベッドを下げる lower *one's* bed

《片づける》**take away, remove**　◆（食後に）トレイを下げましょうか Shall I take away *your tray[the dishes]?

《音量を絞る》**turn down**　◆ラジオの音量を少し下げていただけますか Could you please turn the radio down（a little）?

さこう　鎖肛　anal atresia

ざこう　座高　sitting height

さこつ　鎖骨　collarbone, clavicle（屬clavian, clavicular）　◆骨折した鎖骨 a broken collarbone　▶鎖骨下静脈 subclavian vein　鎖骨下動脈 subclavian artery　鎖骨下動脈盗血症候群 subclavian steal syndrome　鎖骨骨折 clavicle fracture　鎖骨上窩リンパ節 supraclavicular lymph node

ざこつ　坐骨　ischium, ischial bone（屬ischial, sciatic）　（一般的に）**sit bone**　▶坐骨支持装具 ischial weight-bearing brace　坐骨神経 sciatic nerve　坐骨神経痛 sciatic neuralgia / sciatica

ざざい　坐剤　☞坐薬

ささえる　支える　support（図support、supportive）　☞援助，サポート，支援，助ける　◆杖で体を支える support *oneself* with a cane　◆友人〈家族〉が彼女にとって大きな心の支えになっています Her friends give〈Her family gives〉her a lot of emotional support.　◆認知症の患者とその家族〈介護者〉を支える support[give support to] patients with dementia and their *family members〈carers〉

ささくれる　become split　◆冬は乾燥して水分が失われるので指にささくれができやすくなります In winter, when the skin becomes dry and dehydrated, *it's easy for the fingers to become split[it's easy to get split fingers].

ささやく　whisper　◆ささやき声が聞こえる hear whispering in *one's* ears　◆誰かが自分に何かするようささやくのが聞こえたりしますか Do you ever hear someone whispering and telling you to do something?　◆ささやき声で話す speak in a whisper / speak in a low[soft] voice

ささる　刺さる　stick（in）, get[become] stuck　◆小さな魚の骨が彼の喉に刺さっています A little fish bone has got stuck in his throat. / He has got a little fish bone stuck in his throat.　◆指にとげが刺さっています You've got a splinter in your finger.

さされる　刺される　（蚊・のみなどに）be bitten（by）, get bitten（by）　（針でハチなどに）be stung（by）, get stung（by）　◆蚊に刺される be bitten by *a mosquito[mosquitoes]　◆腕をスズメバチに刺される be stung on the arm by a hornet[wasp]

さしあげる　差し上げる　give　◆睡眠薬を差し上げましょう Let me give[（処方する）prescribe] you some sleeping pills.　◆よろしければこの乳房自己触診のパンフレットを差し上げます If you like, *you can have this pamphlet on breast self-exam[I'll give you this pamphlet on breast self-exam].

さしきず　刺し傷　（刺されて穴のあいた傷）**puncture wound**　（ナイフなどによる傷）**stab wound**　（ハチ・とげなどの刺し傷）**sting**　（虫による刺し傷・かみ傷）**bite**

さじくへんい　左軸偏位　left axis deviation

さしこむ　差し込む

《コンセントに差し込む》**plug in**　◆プラグをコンセントに差し込む plug *in to[into] *a socket[an outlet] / put the plug into *a socket[an outlet]

《痛み》（腹などがきりきり痛む）**griping**[**colicky**] **pain** ★激しい腹痛・月経痛は cramps という.

さしさわる　差し障る　☞差し支えない，障る ◆もし差し障りがなければ，結婚生活についてもう少し詳しくお聞かせいただけますか If you don't mind me[my] asking, could you tell me about your married life in more detail?　◆仕事に差し障る interfere with *one's* work　◆傷に差し障りますので，24 時間はベッドで安静にしていて下さい（傷へのダメージを防ぐために）Please stay in bed for at least twenty-four hours to avoid harming the wound[injury].

さししめす　指し示す　☞指す

さじじょうづめ　匙状爪　**spoon nail**

さしず　指図　☞指示

さしせまる　差し迫る　draw near, approach　◆ビザの有効期日が差し迫っているのですぐ更新するといいでしょう The expiration date on your visa is *drawing near[approaching], so you should renew it soon.　◆手術を行う差し迫った必要性はないでしょう I don't think you're in urgent need of surgery.

さしつ　左室　left ventricle；LV（形left ventricular）　▶左室肥大 left ventricular hypertrophy　左室不全 left ventricular failure

さしつかえない　差し支えない　◆シャワーは差し支えありません You can take a shower. / It's all right to take a shower.　◆日常生活に差し支えなければ，しばらく様子を見ることにしましょう As long as you're physically fit enough for everyday life, let's wait a while and see if anything develops.　◆差し支えなければ，詳細をお聞かせ下さい If you don't mind me[my] asking, could you tell me about that in more detail?　◆差し支えなければ，明日の朝おいで下さい If it's not inconvenient for you[If it's not too much trouble (for you)], please come tomorrow morning.

さしば　差し歯　post crown　☞継ぎ歯

さしひかえる　差し控える　（見合わせる）　**hold back　（遠慮する）reserve　（慎む）refrain（from）**　☞遠慮，控える　◆その問題についての判断を差し控える *hold back[reserve]（*one's*）judgment on that issue / refrain from making a judgment on that issue　◆患者さんの書面による同意のない場合，個人情報の開示は差し控えさせていただきます（公表しない）We do not disclose [release] patients' personal health information *without receiving their written consent first[without their prior written consent].

さしょう　査証　visa　☞ビザ

ざしょう　挫傷　（打撲傷）contusion, bruise （筋肉などを痛めること）strain　☞挫創　▶脳挫傷 brain contusion　肺挫傷 pulmonary contusion　腰仙部挫傷 lumbosacral strain

さしん　左心　left heart　▶左心負荷 left heart overload　左心不全 left-sided[left] heart failure

さしんしつ　左心室　☞左室

さしんぼう　左心房　☞左房

さす¹　刺す　（刃物でぐさりと刺す）stab　（針などでちくっと刺す）prick　（尖った物で穴を開ける）pierce, puncture　☞刺さる，刺される ◆刺すような痛みがある have a stabbing pain　◆これは痛み止めの注射です。さあ刺しますよ This shot will help stop the pain. Here we go.

さす²　指す　point（to）　◆痛む所を指して下さい Please point to the place where it hurts.　◆私が指し示した物の名前を言って下さい Please tell me the names of the objects I point to.

さす³　差す　◆目薬をさす *put in[apply] eye drops / apply eye lotion　◆1，2 滴ずつそれぞれの目にさす put one to two drops into each eye

さする　rub（gently）　（マッサージする）massage　◆脚をさすりましょうか Shall I rub your leg(s)?

させい　嗄声　hoarse voice, hoarseness

させつ　左折する　turn left, make a left turn　◆3 つめの角を左折して下さい

Please *turn left[make a left turn] at the third corner.

ざそう¹ 挫創 contused wound ☞挫傷 ◀圧挫創 crush wound

ざそう² 痤瘡 acne /ǽkni/ ☞にきび ◀酒皶性痤瘡(acne) rosacea 尋常性痤瘡 acne vulgaris / common[simple] acne 嚢胞性痤瘡 cystic acne ▶痤瘡様発疹 acneiform[acnelike] eruption

さだめる 定める (規則などを明記する)stipulate (基準・目標などを決める)set, establish (決定する)decide (on) ☞決める, 決定 ◆結核の症例は保健所に届け出ることが法律で定められています It is stipulated by law that *we report cases of tuberculosis to the health center[cases of tuberculosis must be reported to the health center]. ◆例えば、毎週水曜日を休肝日と定めてみてはいかがですか For example, how about *setting Wednesday [deciding on Wednesday] as your alcohol-free day each week? ◆リハビリの具体的な目標を定める set[establish] specific rehabilitation goals

さつえい 撮影する (写真を撮る)take ◆胸部 CT を撮影しましょう I'm going to [Let me] take a CT scan of your chest. ◀冠動脈動画撮影 cinecoronary angiography 胸部単純撮影 plain chest radiography デジタル X 線撮影 digital radiography；DR 動脈撮影 arteriography ポジトロン断層撮影 positron emission tomography；PET

ざつおん 雑音 (かすかな音)murmur (不快な音)noise (一般的に音)sound ◆心雑音を指摘されたことがありますか Have you ever been told by a doctor that you have a heart murmur? ◆雑音が気になりますか Does noise bother you? ◆耳の中で雑音がする hear noises in *one's* ears ◀拡張期雑音 diastolic murmur 逆流性雑音 regurgitant murmur 駆出雑音 ejection murmur 血管雑音 vascular murmur 収縮期雑音 systolic murmur 副雑音(呼吸音の) adventitious sound

さっか 擦過 scratch (🖻scratchy) ▶擦

過音 scratchy sound ▶擦過細胞診, 擦過傷

さっかく 錯覚 illusion ◆喫煙者はタバコを吸うことでストレスが軽減されると錯覚しています Smokers are under the illusion that smoking relieves stress. ◆目の錯覚 *an optical[a visual] illusion

さっかさいぼうしん 擦過細胞診 scraping cytology, scrape cytology

さっかしょう 擦過傷 (すり傷)scrape, abrasion (引っ掻き傷)scratch

サッカリン saccharin

さっき ☞先程

さっきん 殺菌する (滅菌する)sterilize /stérəlàɪz/ (🖻sterilization) (特に感染予防のために消毒する)disinfect (🖻disinfection) (食品などを低温殺菌する)pasteurize (🖻pasteurization) ☞消毒, 滅菌 ◆医療器具を高温で殺菌する sterilize medical instruments at a high temperature ◀最小殺菌濃度 minimum bactericidal concentration；MBC 低温殺菌(low-temperature) pasteurization ▶殺菌作用 germicidal[bactericidal] effect 殺菌消毒器 sterilizer 殺菌薬 bactericide, germicide, bactericidal[germicidal] sterilization [agent] / (殺菌用の)antiseptic / (感染予防用の) (germicidal) disinfectant 殺菌力 bactericidal activity

ざっくばらん ☞率直

さっしょう 擦傷 ☞擦過傷

さっする 察する ◆お子さんのことでご心配のこととお察しいたします I know you must be very worried[concerned] about your child. / I understand how worried [concerned] you are about your child. ◆お気持ちをお察しいたします(適当な言葉が見つかりませんが、あなたのお力になるためにここにおります)I don't know what to say, but I'm here to help you. ★I know how you feel. という表現は患者の感情を害することもあるので避けたい.

さつせいしやく 殺精子薬 spermatocide, spermatocidal agent

さっちゅうやく 殺虫薬 insecticide

さっぱり
《すっきりした》**refreshed** ◆シャワーを浴びてさっぱりしましたか Did you feel refreshed after the shower?
《あっさりした》 ◆さっぱりした食べ物（あっさりした味の）**plain[simple] food** / （味付けの薄い）**lightly-seasoned food** ◆さっぱりした味付け **plain[simple] seasoning** ◆さっぱりした人（性格が淡白な）**a frank person**
《全然…ない》 ◆どうしたらいいのかさっぱり分かりません I just don't know[I have no idea] what to do. / I don't know what to do at all.

サディスト **sadist**
サディズム **sadism**（形**sadistic**）
さとう 砂糖 **sugar** ☞糖分 ◆人工甘味料を使うことで砂糖の摂取を抑えることができます You can cut down on sugar by using artificial sweeteners. ◆低血糖の症状を感じたら、すぐに砂糖を約 20 g 摂取してください If you have any of the symptoms of *low blood sugar[hypoglycemia], eat about twenty grams of sugar right away.

さどうやく 作動薬 **agonist** ◀ドパミン作動薬 **dopamine[dopaminergic] agonist** ニコチン作動薬 **nicotinic agonist** 副交感神経作動薬 **parasympathomimetic（medication / drug / agent）**

さとおや 里親 **foster parent(s)**

さとがえり 里帰り ◆里帰りされるご予定はありますか Are you planning to go back to your country to see your family? / （出産のために）Are you planning to return[go back] to your parents' home to have the baby?

さとご 里子 **foster child**

サドルブロックますい ―麻酔 **saddle block anesthesia**

さねつ 詐熱 **factitious fever**

さのう 左脳 **the left brain, the left hemisphere（of the brain）**

さびしい 寂しい **lonely**（動**寂しく思う miss**）◆故郷のご家族やお友達がいなくて寂しいですか Do you miss your family

and friends (from) back home? ◆ご主人が亡くなられてお寂しいでしょう Since your husband passed away, you must be lonely without him.

さびょう 詐病 **malingering** ☞仮病

サプリメント （dietary）**supplement** ◆サプリメントを飲んでいますか Are you taking any supplements? ◀カルシウムサプリメント **calcium supplement**

さべつ 差別 **discrimination**（動**discriminate**）☞偏見 ◆当院では患者差別はいたしません（平等に扱う）We treat all patients equally in this hospital. ◀人種差別 **racial discrimination / racism** 性差別 **sex[sexual] discrimination / sexism** 年齢差別 **age discrimination** / （特に高齢者に対する）**ageism**

さぼう 左房 **left atrium；LA**（形**left atrial**）▶左房圧 **left atrial pressure** 左房径 **left atrial diameter[dimension]；LAD**

さほういどう 左方移動 **shift to the left, left shift**

サポーター **support, supporter** ▶足首〈膝〉用サポーター **ankle〈knee〉support** スポーツ用[局部]サポーター **jockstrap / athletic supporter**

サポート **support** ☞援助，支える，支援，助ける ◆彼には精神的なサポートが必要です He needs moral[emotional / psychological] support. ◆家族のサポートがありますか Do you have family support? ◆家族のサポートがない **have no family support** / **have no support from** *one's* **family** ▶サポートグループ **support group** サポートストッキング **support hose[stockings]** サポート用包帯 **support bandage**

さまざま 様々（な） （種々の）**various, a variety of, many kinds[sorts] of, all kinds[sorts] of** （異なる）**different, diverse** ☞いろいろ，種々 ◆この問題の解決には様々なやり方があります There are various ways to solve this problem. ◆彼は様々なストレスを受けています He is under many[all] kinds of stress. ◆その薬による影響は人によって様々です The medica-

tion affects different people in different ways.

さます¹ 冷ます （冷やす）**cool down** （下げる）**bring down, lower** ☞冷やす ◆食事は冷まして召し上がって下さい Please let your meals cool down before you eat them. ◆熱を冷ますのに何か市販の薬を飲みましたか Did you take any over-the-counter drugs to *bring down[lower] the fever? ◀熱冷まし antipyretic （medication / drug / agent）

さます² 覚ます ☞覚める

さまたげる 妨げる （妨害する）**disturb** （支障をきたす）**interfere with** （阻止する）**prevent ... from** ◆寝る前のパソコンや携帯電話は良質な睡眠の妨げになることがあります Using computers or mobile phones before bedtime can sometimes *disturb you from[interfere with] getting a good sleep. ◆栄養不良は子供の正常な発育を妨げます Malnutrition[Malnourishment] prevents children from attaining *normal growth[their full growth potential].

さむい 寒い cold （ひんやりした）**chilly** ◆寒い時に痛みますか Do you have pain when it's cold? ◆寒がりですか Are you sensitive to (the) cold? ◆以前と比べて寒がりになっていますか Do you feel the cold more than you used to? ◆この部屋は少し寒いですか Is it a little chilly in this room?

さむけ 寒気 chill （寒さによる震え）**shiver** ◆寒気がしますか Do you have the chills[shivers]?

さめはだ 鮫肌 （荒れた皮膚）**rough skin** （魚鱗癬）**ichthyosis, fish skin**

さめる 覚める （目が覚める）**wake up** （🈩awake） （麻酔などから脱する）**come out** ◆夜中に目が覚めますか Do you wake up during the night? ◆早朝目が覚めてその後なかなか眠れないのですか Do you wake up early in the morning and then can't get back to sleep? ◆目が覚めていますか Are you awake? ◆手術中目が覚めているでしょう You'll be awake during the surgery. ◆彼女はあと1時間ほどで麻酔が覚

めるでしょう She'll come out of the anesthesia in about an hour. / The effects of her anesthetic will wear off in an hour or so.

ざやく 坐薬 suppository /səpázətòːri/ ◆坐薬をお出ししましょう I'm going to [Let you] give you a suppository. ◆この坐薬は肛門に入れて下さい Please insert this suppository into your bottom[（直腸）rectum / back passage]. ★anus（肛門）という語は患者に不快な思いを抱かせることがある. ◀肛門坐薬 rectal suppository 膣坐薬 vaginal suppository

さゆ 白湯 （plain）**hot water,** （plain）**warm water** ◆この薬は白湯でお飲み下さい Please take this medication with hot [warm] water.

さゆう 左右 left and right ★right and left ともいう. （横に）**from side to side** ◆感触に左右差はありますか Do you feel any difference between your left and right sides? / （左右同じか）Do you feel the same *on both sides[on the left and right]? ◆舌を左右に動かして下さい Please move your tongue *from side to side[from left to right]. ◆体を左右に曲げて下さい Please bend from side to side. ◆左右のバランス the balance between left and right ☞左右対称，左右不同

さゆうする 左右する influence ◆環境に左右される be influenced by one's environment

さゆうたいしょう 左右対称 symmetry （🈩symmetric, symmetrical） ◆乳房の形や大きさは左右対称ですか Are your breasts symmetrical in appearance and size?

さゆうふどう 左右不同 asymmetry （🈩asymmetric, asymmetrical） ◀瞳孔左右不同 asymmetric pupils / anisocoria

さよう 作用する act （🈩action, 影響・効果 effect）**, work** （相互作用する）**interact** （🈩interaction） （機能する）**function** （🈩function） ◆この薬は血小板に作用して血栓を予防します This medication acts on platelets to prevent the blood from clotting.

◆この 2 つの薬は相互に作用し合います These two medications will interact with each other. ◆胃に対するこの薬の作用 the action[effect] of this medication on the stomach ◀抗菌作用 antibacterial [antimicrobial] effect[action] 相互作用 interaction 相乗作用 synergism / potentiation 鎮静作用 sedative effect[action] 副作用(一般的に)side effect /(有害の)adverse effect[reaction] /(逆の)contrary effect[reaction] 薬理作用 pharmacologic action ▶作用機序 mechanism of action；MOA / action mechanism 作用時間 reaction time 作用点 working point 作用薬 agonist

さようなら Goodbye! ◆(また明日)See you tomorrow. ◆(お大事に)Take care (of yourself). ◆(夜別れる時)Good night.

ざよく 座浴 sitz bath （腰湯）hip bath；*a bath in water up to the hips*

さらさら(の) thin (↔thick) （漿液性の）serous ◆さらさらした分泌物 thin[serous] discharge ◆血液をさらさらにする薬を処方する(血液の凝固を防ぐ)prescribe a medication *to prevent the clotting of blood[to stop the blood from clotting]

ざらざら(の) （荒れてかさかさの）rough, coarse (↔smooth) （砂利っぽい）sandy, gritty ◆皮膚にざらざら感がありますか Does your skin feel rough? ◆舌がざらざらする The tongue gets[becomes] rough [sandy / gritty]

さらす 曝す expose (to) ◆騒音に曝された経験がありますか Have you ever been exposed to loud noise? ◆仕事場で何か刺激物に曝されていますか Are you exposed to any irritants at work? ◆強い直射日光や高温に曝される be exposed to strong direct sunlight or high temperatures

サラセミア thalassemia

サリチルさん 一酸 salicylic acid

サリドマイド thalidomide ▶サリドマイド児 thalidomide baby[child]

サリン sarin ▶サリン中毒 sarin poisoning

サルコイドーシス sarcoidosis ◀眼〈心 / 肺〉サルコイドーシス ocular〈cardiac / pulmonary〉sarcoidosis

さるて 猿手 ape hand

サルファざい 一剤 sulfa drug

サルモネラ salmonella （学名）*Salmonella* ▶サルモネラ食中毒 salmonella food poisoning

さわやかな ◆さわやかな気分になる feel refreshed ◆さわやかな飲み物 a refreshing drink

さわる¹ 触る （手や指で）touch （刷毛などで）brush （触って感じる）feel ☞触れる ◆皮膚をピンで触ります I'm going to touch you with a pin. ◆(刷毛で)額に触ります Let me brush your forehead. ◆触った感覚が過敏になって〈鈍くなって / しびれて〉いますか Are your touch sensations sharp〈dull / numb〉? ◆この辺を触ると痛みますか Is this area tender? ★tender は体の一部を触った時に感じる痛みをいう.

さわる² 障る （害する）be bad (for), be harmful (to) （影響を及ぼす）affect （支障をきたす）interfere (with) ◆カフェインの摂り過ぎは体に障ります Too much caffeine is *bad for you[bad for (your) health]. / Too much caffeine affects your health. ◆お気に障ったとしたらごめんなさい(気持ちを傷つけたとしたら)I'm sorry if I've hurt your feelings. ◆仕事に障る interfere with *one's* work ◆神経に障る get [grate] on *one's* nerves

さん 酸 acid （医acid）◀胃酸 stomach [gastric] acid 脂肪酸 fatty acid 制酸薬 antacid 胆汁酸 bile acid 乳酸 lactic acid 尿酸 uric acid；UA ▶酸塩基平衡 acid-base balance 酸塩基平衡異常 acid-base imbalance 酸逆流 acid reflux 酸損傷 acid injury 酸熱傷 acid burn ☞酸化，酸性，酸味

ざんい 残胃 residual stomach ▶残胃炎 gastritis of the residual stomach

さんいん 産院 （病院）maternity hospital （診療所）maternity clinic

さんか¹ 参加する participate (in), take part (in), join (in) （出席する）attend

さんか¹

◆治験に参加する participate[take part] in a clinical trial ◆（妊婦のための）両親学級に参加する attend[take part in] parenting classes

さんか² 産科 obstetrics /əbstétrɪks/ ; OB （略obstetric）（診療科）the department of obstetrics, the obstetric(s) department ☞産婦人科 ▶産(科医)院 maternity clinic 産科医 obstetrician 産科診察 obstetric examination 産科病棟 maternity ward[unit / floor] 産科病院 maternity hospital 産(科)婦人科 obstetrics and gynecology ; OB/GYN

さんか³ 酸化 oxidation （略oxidative 酸化体の oxidant）◀抗酸化作用 antioxidant effect[action] / antioxidation ▶酸化酵素 oxidase 酸化ストレス oxidative stress ☞酸化物

さんかくきん¹ 三角巾 triangular bandage （吊り包帯）sling ◆三角巾を結ぶ tie a triangular bandage ◆三角巾で腕を吊る have *one's* arm in a sling

さんかくきん² 三角筋 deltoid muscle

さんがた 3型・Ⅲ型 type 3, type Ⅲ ▶Ⅲ型アレルギー反応 type Ⅲ allergic reaction

さんがつ 3月 March ; Mar. ☞1月

さんかぶつ 酸化物 oxide （compound）◀窒素酸化物 nitrogen oxide

さんき 3期 （第3の段階）third stage, stage three （3つの期間・時期）three periods[terms] ☞期 ◆胃がんのⅢ期 the third stage of stomach cancer ◆Ⅲ期の肺がん stage three lung cancer / third stage lung cancer

さんきゃくづえ 三脚杖 tripod cane, three-legged cane

さんきゅう 産休 （母親の）maternity leave （父親の）paternity leave ◆産休をとる take maternity leave ◆14週間の産休をとる take fourteen weeks' maternity leave / take maternity leave of fourteen weeks ◆産休中である be on maternity leave

さんぎょう 産業(の) （職業上の）occupational （工業の・職場の）industrial ▶産業医 *occupational health[industrial] physician 産業医学 occupational[industrial] medicine 産業衛生 industrial sanitation[hygiene] 産業看護師 occupational health nurse ; OHN / industrial nurse 産業廃棄物 industrial waste

ざんぎょう 残業 overtime work （略work overtime）, extra work ◆よく残業しますか Do you often work overtime?

サングラス sunglasses ◆サングラスをかけている wear sunglasses

さんけ 産気づく （陣痛がある）have labor pains （分娩が始まる）go into labor

さんけつ 酸欠 oxygen deficiency, lack of oxygen （supply）（低酸素症）hypoxia ◆彼女は酸欠状態です Her body isn't receiving enough oxygen. / She doesn't have an adequate oxygen supply.

さんけつしょう 酸血症 ☞アシドーシス

さんご 産後(の) postpartum ▶産褥 ◆産後はゆっくり休まないといけません You need to get some good rest after *you give birth[the delivery]. ◆産後元の体に戻るには通常1, 2か月かかります After the delivery, it usually takes one to two months for the body to return to its prepregnant state. ▶産後うつ病 postpartum depression

さんこう 参考 （情報）information （参照）reference （略refer）◆ご参考までに、これは英語を話すスタッフのいるクリニックに関するパンフレットです For your information[reference], here's a leaflet about the clinics that have English-speaking staff. ◆食事療法についてはこのパンフレットを参考にして下さい Please refer to this leaflet for information on your diet therapy. ◆痛風について，また痛風とどう向き合うかについて参考になる資料を差し上げます I'll give you a booklet which will help you understand what gout is and how to cope with it. ▶参考資料 reference data[material] 参考図書 reference book

サンゴじょう ―状 coralliform （鹿角状の）staghorn ▶サンゴ状結石 coralliform [staghorn] stone

ざんさ 残渣 **residue** ◀コーヒー残渣様吐物 coffee-grounds vomit 食物残渣 food residue 低残渣食 low-residue diet；LRD／low-fiber diet；LFD

さんざい¹ 散剤 **powder, powdered medication**［**drug**］ ☞粉薬

さんざい² 散在(性の) (びまん性・広汎性の)**diffuse** (播種性の)**disseminated** (散発的な)**sporadic**

さんさしんけい 三叉神経 **trigeminal nerve** ▶三叉神経痛 trigeminal neuralgia／tic douloureux 三叉神経麻痺 trigeminal nerve palsy［paralysis］

さんじ¹ 産児 (赤ん坊)**baby** (乳児)**infant** ◀正期産児 full-term baby［infant］／baby born at term ☞産児制限

さんじ² 三次(の) **tertiary**, (the) **third** ▶三次救急 tertiary emergency care 三次元イメージング three-dimensional imaging 三次予防 tertiary prevention

さんしきかく 3色覚 **normal trichromatism**

さんじせいげん 産児制限 **birth control**

さんしまひ 三肢麻痺 **triplegia**

さんしゅこんごうワクチン 三種混合ワクチン (ジフテリア・破傷風・百日咳混合ワクチン)**diphtheria, tetanus, and pertussis**［**DTP**］**vaccine**

さんしょう 参照 ☞参考

さんじょく 産褥 **puerperium** (圏**puerperal, postpartum**) ☞産後 ▶産褥感染症 puerperal infection 産褥期 the postpartum［puerperal］period 産褥精神病 puerperal psychosis 産褥体操 puerperal exercise 産褥乳腺炎 puerperal mastitis 産褥熱 puerperal［childbed］fever 産褥無月経 puerperal amenorrhea

サンスクリーン **sunscreen, sunblock**

さんせい¹ 酸性(度) **acidity** (圏**acid, acidic**) ◀強酸性 strong acidity 弱酸性 weak acidity ▶酸性尿 acidic urine／aciduria 酸性ホスファターゼ acid phosphatase；ACP

さんせい² 産生する **produce** (圏**production**) ◆インスリンは膵臓で産生されます

Insulin is produced in the pancreas. ◆クッシング症候群は副腎皮質ホルモンが過剰に産生されることで起こります Cushing syndrome can result from overproduction of adrenocortical hormones. ◀アルドステロン産生腺腫 aldosteronoma／aldosterone-producing［aldosterone-secreting］adenoma ゴナドトロピン産生腫瘍 gonadotropin-producing tumor ホルモン産生腫瘍 hormone-producing tumor

さんせい³ 賛成する (同意する)**agree** (**with, to**) (認める)**approve** (**of**) ◆全面的に賛成いたします I completely agree. ◆その点についてはあなたの考えに賛成です I agree with you on that point. ◆喫煙には賛成しません I don't approve of your smoking.

さんぜんさんご 産前産後 **before and after childbirth** ▶産前産後休暇 maternity leave

さんせんべん 三尖弁 **tricuspid valve** ▶三尖弁逆流症 tricuspid (valve) regurgitation；TR 三尖弁狭窄症 tricuspid (valve) stenosis；TS 三尖弁膜症 tricuspid valve disease

さんそ 酸素 **oxygen** /ɑ́ksɪdʒən/ ◆家で酸素を使っていますか Do you use oxygen at home? ◆血液中に酸素が不足しているので、在宅酸素療法をお勧めします Since your blood oxygen levels are low［Since there is a shortage of oxygen in your blood］, I recommend home oxygen therapy. ◆酸素を使う時は禁煙し、酸素濃縮器を少なくとも2 m 火気から離して下さい When using oxygen, do not smoke and be sure to keep the oxygen concentrator at least two meters away from any source of heat. ◆酸素を吸う breathe oxygen ◆酸素を吸入する inhale oxygen ◆血液中に酸素を取り込む supply oxygen to the blood ◆血液中の酸素量を増やす increase the amount of oxygen in the blood ◆患者の酸素レベルを測る〈モニターする〉measure〈monitor〉a patient's oxygen levels ◀液化酸素 liquid oxygen

活性酸素 active oxygen / oxygen (free) radical / reactive oxygen species；ROS 携帯用液化酸素型タンク portable liquid oxygen tank 携帯用酸素ボンベ portable oxygen cylinder 低酸素症 hypoxia 低酸素脳症 brain hypoxia 無酸素症 anoxia 無酸素性脳障害 anoxic brain damage ▶酸素供給装置 oxygen supply equipment 酸素消費量 oxygen consumption 酸素摂取量 oxygen intake 酸素タンク oxygen tank 酸素中毒 oxygen poisoning 酸素テント oxygen tent 酸素投与 oxygen administration 酸素毒性 oxygen toxicity 酸素濃縮装置 oxygen concentrator ☞酸(素)欠(乏), 酸素カニューラ, 酸素吸入, 酸素濃度, 酸素分圧, 酸素飽和度, 酸素マスク, 酸素療法

ざんぞう 残像 afterimage

さんそカニューラ 酸素カニューラ oxygen cannula ◀鼻腔酸素カニューラ nasal oxygen cannula

さんそきゅうにゅう 酸素吸入 oxygen inhalation ◆手術中患者に酸素吸入を行う give the patient oxygen during surgery /（患者に吸わせる）have the patient inhale oxygen during surgery ▶酸素吸入器 oxygen inhaler 酸素吸入療法 oxygen (inhalation) therapy

さんそけつぼう 酸素欠乏 ☞酸欠

さんそのうど 酸素濃度 oxygen concentration ◀吸入酸素濃度 fraction of inspired oxygen；FiO₂

さんそぶんあつ 酸素分圧 partial pressure of oxygen, oxygen partial pressure ◀動脈血酸素分圧 partial pressure of oxygen in arterial blood；PaO₂ / arterial partial pressure of oxygen

さんそほうわど 酸素飽和度 oxygen saturation ◀経皮的酸素飽和度 percutaneous oxygen saturation 動脈血酸素飽和度 arterial (blood) oxygen saturation；SaO₂ 夜間酸素飽和度低下 nocturnal oxygen desaturation

さんそマスク 酸素マスク oxygen mask ◆この酸素マスクをお口に掛けますね I'm going to[Let me] slip this oxygen

mask over your mouth. ◆酸素マスクをつける put on an oxygen mask ◆酸素マスクをしている wear an oxygen mask ◆酸素マスクを取る *take off[remove] an oxygen mask

さんそりょうほう 酸素療法 oxygen therapy ◀高圧酸素療法 hyperbaric oxygen therapy 在宅酸素療法 home oxygen therapy；HOT

ざんぞんきのう 残存機能 residual function ◆術後の残存肺機能が十分でないと肺葉切除術はできません Unless we can be sure that the lungs will retain enough ability to keep functioning after surgery, we can't do[perform] a lung resection. ◆残存機能を最大限に生かす make the best use of *one's* residual function capacity

さんだい 散大する dilate /dáɪleɪt/ (図dilation, dilatation) ☞散瞳 ◆散大した瞳孔 dilated pupils ◆瞳孔を散大する dilate *a person's* pupils ◆瞳孔散大 pupil dilation / mydriasis

さんちょう 産徴 bloody show, sign of the onset of labor ◆産徴がありましたか Have you noticed a bloody show?

ざんてい 暫定 ☞仮

さんてんほこう 三点歩行 three-point gait

さんど 3度・Ⅲ度 (the) third degree ▶Ⅲ度熱傷 third-degree[full-thickness] burn 3度房室ブロック third-degree atrioventricular[AV] block

さんどう¹ 産道 birth canal ▶産道感染 birth canal infection 産道損傷 birth canal injury[tear]

さんどう² 散瞳 pupil dilation, dilation of the pupil (of the eye) (動dilate), mydriasis (形mydriatic) ☞散大 ◆散瞳するために点眼薬を入れます I'm going to[Let me] put eye drops in your eye(s) to dilate your pupil(s). ◆散瞳するまでここでお待ち下さい Please wait here *for your pupils to dilate[while your pupils dilate]. ▶散瞳薬 mydriatic (medication / drug / agent / eye drop)

さんとうきん 三頭筋 triceps（muscle），three-headed muscle ◀上腕三頭筋 triceps muscle of the arm／triceps brachii muscle 上腕三頭筋反射 triceps（brachii）reflex[jerk]

ざんにょう 残尿 residual urine ◆残尿感がありますか After you *pass water[urinate]，do you feel that *your bladder is not completely empty[you haven't completely emptied your bladder]? ▶残尿感 constant urge to urinate

ざんねん 残念 （気の毒に思う）I'm sorry, I'm afraid （圏残念ながら unfortunately） ◆（大変）残念です I'm（very）sorry. ◆残念ですが，私にはできません I'm sorry, but I can't.／I'm afraid that I can't. ◆残念ながら，よくないお知らせです I'm afraid the news isn't good.／I'm sorry to have to tell you that the news isn't good. ◆残念ながら，悪性です Unfortunately, it's malignant. ◆残念ですが，彼女に手術はできません I'm afraid that we can't give her surgery. ◆残念ですが，この病気には治療法がないのです Unfortunately, there's no cure for this disease.

さんぱつ 散発（性の） sporadic

さんはんきかん 三半規管 three semicircular canals[ducts]

さんぴ 賛否 ◆その治療が妥当かどうかについては医師の間でも賛否が分かれていますOpinionsamongdoctorsaredividedastowhetherthetreatmentisappropriate（or not）.／There are arguments both for and against the treatment among doctors as to whether it is appropriate（or not）.

さんぷ 産婦 women who have recently given birth ★複数形で.

さんふじんか 産婦人科 obstetrics and gynecology /əbstétrɪks ən gàɪnəkáləʤi/ （診療科）the department of obstetrics and gynecology, the obstetrics and gynecology department；OB/GYN department ☞産科, 婦人科 ▶産婦人科医 obstetrician-gynecologist；OB/GYN

さんぶそう 散布巣 satellite lesion

さんぶつ 産物 product ◀代謝産物 metabolic product 副産物 by-product[byproduct]／（派生物）outgrowth

サンプリング sampling ◀副腎静脈サンプリング adrenal venous sampling；AVS

サンプル （見本）sample （検体・試料）specimen ☞検体, 標本 ◆血液のサンプルを採ります I'm going to[Let me] get a blood sample from you. ◆2 日にわたって便のサンプルを採る collect a stool sample on two different days ◆無作為にサンプルを抽出する draw samples at random ◀尿サンプル urine sample[specimen]

さんぽ 散歩 walk （圏take a walk, go for a walk） ◆できるだけ散歩なさることをお勧めします I recommend that you take a walk whenever you can. ◆散歩に行きましょう Let's go out for a walk. ◆気晴らしに散歩はいかがですか How about[What about] taking a walk to relax?

さんみ 酸味 sourness /sáʊə-nəs/ （酸っぱい味）tart flavor[taste], zesty flavor[taste] （酸味度）acidity ☞酸っぱい ◆減塩で酸味が足りないと感じるようでしたら酢やレモン汁などの酸味を入れるといいですよ If you cut down on salt and feel your food isn't salty enough, you could add[season it with] tart flavors[tastes] such as vinegar or lemon juice.

さんやく 散薬 powder, powdered medication[drug] ☞粉薬

さんりゅう 産瘤 cephalhematoma

ざんりゅう 残留（の） （残って溜まっている）residual （図residue） （保持している）retained ◀胎盤残留 retained placenta ▶残留塩素 residual chlorine 残留毒性 residual toxicity 残留農薬 pesticide residue

さんりゅうしゅ 霰粒腫 chalazion

さんれつ 参列する attend ◆明日の葬儀に参列いたします I'm going to attend the funeral tomorrow.

し

し 死 death ☞死ぬ, 死亡, 亡くなる
◆非常にまれですが, 死を含めた重い合併症が生じることがあります Very rarely, serious complications can occur, including death. ◆死が迫っている death is imminent / not have long to live ◆彼女の死を悲しむ mourn[grieve] over her death ◆肝臓がんによる死 death from liver cancer ◆原因不明の死 *an unknown[an unexplained / an undetermined / a suspicious] (cause of) death ◆苦しまない死 a painfree[painless] death ◆安らかな死を迎える die a peaceful[quiet] death / die peacefully ◆死に備える prepare for death ◆死を受け入れる accept death ◆患者が死と向き合うよう援助する help the patient face[cope with / confront] death ◆死に至る過程を支える support the dying process ◆患者の死を看取る care for a dying patient

◁縊死 death by hanging 異状死 unnatural death / death from[by] unnatural cause 餓死 death from starvation / (食事を与えられないことによる死)death by starvation 過労死 death from overwork 感電死 death by electric shock / electrical death 交通事故死 traffic death 孤独死 lonely death / dying alone 事故死 accidental death 失血死 death from loss of blood 焼死 fire death / death from fire 喘息死 asthma death 即死(瞬間の死)instant[instantaneous] death / (その場での死)death on the spot 窒息死 death from suffocation 中毒死 death by[from] poisoning 電撃死 lightning death 転落死 fall[falling] death 凍死 death from[by] freezing 突然死 sudden death / (予期せぬ死)unexpected death / (早すぎる死)untimely death 熱傷死 death due to burns[burn injuries] 脳死 brain[cerebral] death 病死 death from disease[sickness / illness] 不審死 suspicious death

▶死の徴候 sign of death 死への準備教育 death education ☞安楽死, 検死, 死因, 死期, 死後, 死産, 死者, 死生観, 自然死, 死体, 死胎児, 死に目, 死斑, 死別, 尊厳死

― し ― 歯 tooth (圏teeth) ☞歯 (は)
◁う歯 tooth decay / tooth[dental] caries 永久歯 permanent tooth 過剰歯 supernumerary tooth 義歯 dentures / (各々の歯)false[artificial] tooth 欠損歯 missing tooth 犬歯 canine (tooth) 充填歯 filled tooth 小臼歯 premolar (tooth) 切歯 incisor (tooth) 大臼歯 molar (tooth) 智歯 wisdom tooth 転位歯 displaced[malposed] tooth 乳歯 milk[baby] tooth 抜歯 tooth extraction 浮遊歯 floating tooth 埋伏歯 impacted tooth ☞歯科, 歯学, 歯牙欠損, 歯冠, 歯間ブラシ, 歯垢, 歯根, 歯周, 歯髄, 歯石, 歯槽, 歯痛, 歯肉

じ[1] 字 (漢字などの文字)**character** (かな・アルファベットなどの文字)**letter** (筆跡)**handwriting** ◆字が下手になったと感じますか Do you feel that your handwriting has become poorer? ◆字が読みにくいですか Do you have difficulty reading? ◆私が指示した字を読んで下さい Please read the letters I point at.

じ[2] 痔 hemorrhoids /héməridz/ (圏hemorrhóidal), **piles** /páilz/ ★いずれも通例, 複数形で. ◆痔がありますか Do you have hemorrhoids? ◁切れ痔(裂肛)anal fissure / (出血性痔核)bleeding hemorrhoids[piles] ▶痔出血 hemorrhoidal bleeding ☞痔核

じ[3] 時 o'clock ☞時間 ◆診察は9時に始まります The examination starts at nine (o'clock). ◆今, 何時ですか What time is it (now)? / Do you have the time? ◆今2時半です It's two-thirty. / It's half past two. ★毎時ちょうどの場合以外は通例 o'clock を付けない. ◆ご希望の予約時間は何時ですか What time is good[best] for your appointment? / When's a good time for your appointment?

じあえんそさんナトリウム 次亜塩素酸ナトリウム **sodium hypochlorite**

しあつ 指圧 shiatsu（massage）, acupressure, finger-pressure ▶指圧師 shiatsu practitioner[therapist] 指圧点[つぼ] acupressure[finger-pressure] point 指圧療法 shiatsu[acupressure / finger-pressure] therapy

しあわせ 幸せ（な） happy（图happiness）（運が良い）fortunate, lucky ☞幸運, 幸福 ◆今，幸せなご気分ですか Do you feel happy now? ◆良いご主人でお幸せですね You are fortunate to have such a good husband.

シアンかぶつ 一化物 cyanide ▶シアン化物中毒 cyanide poisoning

しい 肢位 position ◀蛙型肢位 frog-leg position 機能肢位 functional position 不良肢位 malposition

じい 自慰（行為） masturbation（動masturbate）☞巻末付録：訊きにくい質問のコツ ◆自慰行為をしますか Do you masturbate? ◆お子さんは自慰行為をしますか Does your child play with his〈her〉 private parts[genitals]?

シーアールピー CRP（C 反応性蛋白質）C-reactive protein ◆CRP は体内での炎症の指標です CRP is a marker of inflammation in the body. ◆体内の炎症に応じて CRP の数値が上がります CRP levels rise in response to inflammation in the body. ◆今日の検査結果では CRP は 3 まで下がっています〈上がっています〉The test results today show that your CRP levels have fallen〈risen〉to three.

シーオーピーディー COPD（慢性閉塞性肺疾患）chronic obstructive pulmonary disease ◆COPD は気道が炎症を起こして狭くなり，呼吸困難をきたす進行性の病気です COPD is a progressive disease that results in inflamed and narrowed airways that make it hard to breathe.

シーがたかんえん C 型肝炎 hepatitis C, type C hepatitis ▶C 型肝炎ウイルス hepatitis C virus；HCV C 型肝炎ウイルスキャリア *hepatitis C virus[HCV] carrier C 型肝炎ウイルスマーカー *hepatitis C virus[HCV] marker

シークきょう 一教 Sikhism ▶シーク教徒 Sikh

シーシーユー CCU（冠疾患集中治療室）coronary care unit

じいしき 自意識 self-consciousness（圏自意識の・自意識過剰の self-conscious）◆…について自意識過剰である feel[be] self-conscious about …

シーツ sheets ★複数形で. ◆清潔なシーツをベッドに敷く put clean sheets on the[a] bed ◆シーツを交換する change the sheets ◆シーツを直す straighten the sheets

しいて 強いて ◆強いてとおっしゃるなら外泊を許可しましょう If you insist, I'll allow you to go home for the night.

シーティー CT（コンピュータ断層撮影）computed tomography ◆頭の CT が必要です You need to have a CT scan of your head. ◆胸の CT を撮りましょう Let's take[do] a CT scan of your chest. / I'm going to take a CT of your chest. ◀高分解能 CT high-resolution CT；HRCT 動画 CT cine CT マルチスライスヘリカル CT multislice helical CT

シーディーシー CDC（米国疾病予防管理センター）Centers for Disease Control and Prevention

シートベルト seat belt, safety belt ◆（車椅子用の）シートベルトを膝と胸にかけて締めて下さい Please put the（wheelchair）seat belt across your lap and chest and fasten it. ◆シートベルトをつける wear[use] *one's* seat belt

シーピーアール CPR（心肺蘇生法）cardiopulmonary resuscitation ☞心肺蘇生 ◆CPR を施す do[perform / administer] CPR on *a person*

しいん¹ 子音 consonant

しいん² 死因 the cause of death ◆彼女の死因は心不全でした The cause of her death was heart failure. / She died of heart failure. ◆直接の死因 immediate cause of death / the direct cause of death / the cause directly leading to death ◆死因不明で亡くなる die[pass away] of unknown causes ▶死因別死亡率 cause-specific death rate

ジーン gene ☞遺伝子

じえいぎょう 自営業 *one's* own business ◆自営業である be self-employed / have[run] *one's* own business

シェーグレンしょうこうぐん —症候群 Sjögren syndrome

ジェットラグ (時差ボケ)jet lag ☞時差

ジェネリックいやくひん —医薬品 generic drug[medication] (↔brand-name drug[medication]) ◆ジェネリック医薬品をお使いになりたいですか Would you like to use generic drugs? ◆この薬はジェネリック(医薬品)のタイプを購入できます Generic forms of this medication are available.

ジェル gel ☞ゼリー ◀消毒ジェル(手の) hand sanitizer gel

しえん 支援 (支え)support (サービス)service (援助)assistance ☞援助, 支える, サポート, 助ける ◀医療支援 medical support[assistance] 介護支援サービス care (support) service 在宅介護支援センター home care (support) center[agency] 社会的支援 social support 情緒的支援 emotional support 要支援(long-term) support needs / (long-term) support required[needed] ▶支援グループ support group 支援センター support center 支援組織 support organization

しお 塩 salt (塩塩辛い salty) ☞塩分 ◆塩気の強い食品を避ける avoid eating salty foods ▶塩味 salty taste / saltiness 塩水 salt water

しか 歯科 dentistry (塩dental) (診療科)the department of dentistry, the dentistry department ◀学校歯科医 school dentist 矯正歯科(診療所)orthodontics clinic / (病院の) the orthodontics department ▶歯科医 dentist 歯科医院 dental clinic 歯科衛生士 dental hygienist 歯科技工士 dental technician 歯科矯正医 orthodontist 歯科矯正学 orthodontics 歯科矯正装置 orthodontic appliance 歯科治療 dental treatment / (歯列矯正の)orthodontic treatment 歯科麻酔 dental anesthesia 歯科用ドリル dental drill ☞歯(科)学

じか 自家(の) auto- ▶自家移植 autotransplant / autotransplantation / autologous transplant[transplantation] / (移植片)autograft 自家骨髄移植 autologous bone marrow transplant[transplantation] 自家中毒 autointoxication ☞自家用車

じが 自我 (自己認識)sense of identity, sense of self (哲学的な意味での我)ego ◆自我を確立する establish a sense of identity[self] ◀超自我 superego ▶自我同一性危機 identity crisis

しかい 視界 visual field, field of vision ☞視野

じかい¹ 耳介 auricle (塩auricular), pinna ▶耳介軟骨 auricular cartilage

じかい² 次回(の) next (塩next time) ◆受付で次回の予約をして下さい Please make an appointment for your next visit at the reception desk. ◆次回の予約をする make the[*one's*] next appointment ◆検査結果は次回お話しましょう Let's talk about the result of the tests next time. ◆保険証は次回に必ず持ってきて下さい Please be sure to bring your insurance card next time you come.

しがいせん 紫外線 ultraviolet rays[light], UV rays[light] ★rays は複数形で。(塩ultraviolet, UV) ◆日焼け止めで紫外線対策を行う protect *oneself* from UV rays by using sunscreen ▶紫外線照射 ultraviolet irradiation 紫外線ランプ ultraviolet lamp 紫外線療法 ultraviolet therapy

ジカウイルス Zika virus ▶ジカウイルス感染症 Zika virus infection / (ジカ熱)Zika fever

しかく¹ 視覚 vision (塩視力の visual 眼の optic, optical, ocular) ☞視野, 視力 ◆視覚に変化がありましたか Have you noticed any changes in your vision[ability to see]? ▶視覚検査 vision[eye] test 視覚失認 visual agnosia 視覚障害 vision

しかく¹

[visual] disorder / vision[visual] impairment　視覚障害者 visually impaired [challenged] person / blind person ★the blind には差別的なニュアンスがあるので，総称的には blind people を用いる．　視覚性めまい visual[ocular] vertigo　視覚野 field of vision / visual area　視(覚)中枢 the visual[optical] center

しかく²　資格　qualification（圏qualified）（身分）status　◆ストーマケアの資格がある be qualified for stoma care　◆資格のある助産師 a qualified midwife　◀在留資格 visa[residence] status

しがく　歯学　dentistry, dental medicine　▶歯学部 dental school / the school of dentistry　歯学部生 dental student

じかく¹　痔核　hemorrhoids, piles　★通例，複数形で．　◀外痔核 external hemorrhoids　嵌頓内痔核 strangulated[incarcerated] internal hemorrhoids　出血性痔核 bleeding hemorrhoids　脱出痔核 prolapsed hemorrhoids　内痔核 internal hemorrhoids　▶痔核切除術 hemorrhoidectomy

じかく²　自覚する（気づく）notice（気づいている）be aware[conscious] (of)（悟る）realize（圏主観的な subjective）◆自覚症状 a subjective symptom /（自覚的徴候）a subjective sign　◆軽い胃炎がありますが，自覚症状はありましたか You have mild gastritis. Have you noticed any symptoms yourself?　◆初めて症状を自覚したのはいつですか When did you first notice the symptom?　◆彼女は忘れっぽいことを自覚していますか Is she aware of being forgetful (about things)?　◆彼女は親としての自覚が足りない She should be more aware[conscious] of her responsibility as a parent. / She lacks a sense of *parental responsibility[her duties as a parent].

しがけっそん　歯牙欠損　tooth loss

じかせん　耳下腺　parotid gland　◀耳下腺腫瘍 parotid gland tumor　☞耳下腺炎

じかせんえん　耳下腺炎　parotitis　◀反復性耳下腺炎 recurrent parotitis　流行性

耳下腺炎 epidemic parotitis /（ムンプス）mumps

しかたない　仕方ない（どうしようもない）can't help but …（選択の余地がない）have no choice but …　◆がんが腹腔に広がっていたので，仕方なく閉腹しました Since the cancer had spread to the peritoneal cavity, we had no choice but to close the abdomen.　◆当院の規則に従わないのでしたら，仕方ありません．退院していただかざるを得ません If you don't follow our hospital regulations, we have no other choice but to ask you to leave the hospital.　◆喉が渇いて仕方ないようでしたら，うがいしてみて下さい If you become really thirsty[If you're dying for some water], try to gargle.　◆ご主人の日本への転勤で，仕方なくキャリアを諦めたのですね Because of your husband's transfer to Japan, you quit your career against your will, didn't you?

じがためりょうほう　地固め療法（白血病の）consolidation chemotherapy

しがつ　4 月　April ; Apr.　☞1 月

ジカねつ　―熱　Zika fever

しかめる（苦痛で）grimace /grímǝs/（不快感で）frown /fráun/（顔・口をゆがめる）twist　◆彼は痛みで顔をしかめた He grimaced with pain. / His face twisted with pain.

じかようしゃ　自家用車　*one's* own car　▶自家用車通勤 commuting to work *by car[in *one's* own car] / driving to work

しかる　叱る　scold　☞怒る　◆子供を叱る時には，深呼吸して気持ちを落ち着けるとよいでしょう Before you scold your child, you should take a deep[big] breath and calm yourself.　★英語では子供を叱る前に You should first count to ten.（10 数えてから）などという．

しかるべき　然るべき　☞適切

しかん¹　子癇　eclampsia（圏eclamptic）▶子癇性昏睡 eclamptic coma

しかん²　弛緩（筋肉などのほぐれ）relaxation（圏relax）（無緊張）atony（圏atonic）（筋肉などのたるみ）flaccidity（圏flaccid）

しかん²　《胃噴門などの弛緩》chalasia　◆筋肉が弛緩する muscles relax　◆筋肉が硬直と弛緩を交互に繰り返す The muscles contract and relax *by turns[alternately]. ◀横隔膜弛緩症 diaphragmatic relaxation　筋弛緩 muscle relaxation　筋弛緩薬 muscle relaxant　無弛緩症 achalasia ▶弛緩期 relaxation period　弛緩出血 atonic bleeding　弛緩性便秘 atonic constipation　弛緩性麻痺 flaccid paralysis

しかん³　歯冠　tooth crown, dental crown

しがん　志願する　《申し込む》apply（for）《進んで申し出る》volunteer（for）　◆治験に志願する volunteer for a clinical trial ▶志願者 applicant / volunteer

じかん¹　耳管　eustachian tube, auditory tube, pharyngotympanic tube（㊑tubal）▶耳管咽頭口 pharyngeal opening of the eustachian tube　耳管炎（eustachian）salpingitis / eustachitis　耳管カテーテル tubal catheter　耳管機能検査 tubal[eustachian tube] function test　耳管狭窄症 tubal stenosis / stenosis of the eustachian tube　耳管通気法（鼓室の）tympanic inflation[insufflation]　耳管扁桃 tubal tonsil

じかん²　時間　《時の長さ》《一般的に》time　《1時間》hour；h, hr　◆来院にどのくらい時間がかかりますか How long does it take（for）you to come to the hospital?　◆診察にはまだ少し時間がかかりそうです（I'm afraid）it will take some time before the doctor sees you.　◆今は時間がないので後でお話ししましょう（予定が詰まっているので）I'm tied up at the moment, so let's talk about it later.　◆時間は十分にある have enough [plenty] of time　◆期限までに完成させるのは時間的に厳しい Timewise, it's difficult to finish it by the deadline.　◆2, 3時間 a few hours　◆5, 6時間 several hours　◆毎時間 every[each] hour　◆6時間ごとに every six hours　◆4時間に1回 once every four hours　《時刻・時間帯》time　《期間》period　（…時間）hour　☞時刻　◆検温の時間です It's time to take your temperature.　◆時間厳守で

お願いします Please don't be late. / Please be punctual.　◆約束の時間に遅れる be late for *one's* appointment　◆朝食の時間は6時から7時までとなります Breakfast（time）is from six to seven. / Breakfast is served between six and seven.　◆熱は決まった時間帯に出ますか Do you have the fever[Does the fever come on] at a specific time of day?　◀空き時間 free[spare] time　遊び時間 playtime　凝固時間 coagulation time　虚血[阻血]時間 ischemic time　勤務時間 working hours[time]　作業時間 working hours　作用時間 reaction time　就寝時間 bedtime / time to go to bed　出血時間 bleeding time　授乳時間 time to feed the baby　消灯時間 lights-out　食事時間 mealtimes　所要時間 the time required [needed]　診察時間 office[consultation] hours　睡眠時間 hours of sleep / sleeping hours　通勤時間 commuting time　トロンビン時間 thrombin time；TT　排尿時間 voiding time　プロトロンビン時間 prothrombin time；PT　待ち時間 waiting time[period]　面会時間 visiting hours　予約時間 appointment time ▶時間感覚 time sense[perception / sensation] ☞時間外

じかんがい　時間外（の・に）　after-hours, out-of-hours, off-hour（㊑out of hours）◆当院は時間外の救急対応をしています We provide emergency services out of hours in this hospital. / After-hours[Off-hour] emergency services are available in this hospital. ▶時間外勤務 overtime work　時間外診療 after-hours outpatient services　時間外窓口 after-hours counter [window]

しかんブラシ　歯間ブラシ　interdental brush　◆歯間ブラシを使って歯の隙間から歯垢を取り除いて下さい Please use an interdental brush to remove the plaque from between your teeth.

しき¹　死期　*one's* end, the time[hour] of death　◆死期が迫っている be near *one's* end / be close to death / death is imminent

しき² **式** （公式・化学式）**formula** ◆構造式 structural formula

しき³ **式** （儀式）**ceremony, service** ◆式は土曜日に執り行われます The ceremony will be held on Saturday. ◆式に参列する attend the ceremony　告別式 funeral （ceremony / service）

—しき **—式** （やり方）**way, style** ◆日本式の方法 the Japanese way of doing things ◆洋式トイレ a Western-style toilet

じき¹ **時期** （一般的に）**time** （期間）**period** （of time） （ある特定の日付）**date** （季節）**season**

《期間》 ◆楽しい〈苦しい〉時期 a good 〈bad / hard〉time ◆喫煙していた時期はありますか Was there any time when you smoked?

《タイミング》 ◆時期が来れば楽になります In time, you'll feel better. ◆ご帰国の時期はもう決めましたか Have you set a date for returning to your country? ◆この薬が効かないと結論づけるのは時期尚早です It would be *too early[premature] to conclude that this medication isn't working. ◆おまるの便座に興味を持つようになった時が，トイレトレーニングを始めるのにベストな時期です The best time for starting your baby on potty training is when he〈she〉shows an interest in the potty. ◆この件については時機を見てお子さんに話されたほうがよいでしょう You should find a good time to tell your child about this （matter）.

じき² **磁気（の）** **magnetic** ▶磁気共鳴画像 magnetic resonance imaging；MRI　磁気共鳴血管撮影 magnetic resonance angiography；MRA

じき³ **直（に）** （はやく）**quickly** （まもなく）**soon** ☞すぐ

じきあつしょうがい **耳気圧障害** **otic barotrauma, ear barotrauma**

しきいしぞう **敷石像** **cobblestone appearance**

しきかく **色覚** **color vision[sense]**

◀1 色覚 achromatopsia / total color blindness　2 色覚 dichromatism / color blindness　3 色覚 （normal） trichromatism 異常 3 色覚 anomalous trichromatism 正常色覚 normal color vision

▶色覚検査 color vision test ☞色覚異常

しきかくいじょう **色覚異常** **color blindness, color vision defect[anomaly]** ◀1型色覚異常 protan defect / red color blindness　2型色覚異常 deutan defect / green color blindness　3型色覚異常 tritan defect / blue color blindness　赤緑色覚異常 red-green （color） blindness / red-green color vision defect　先天性〈後天性〉色覚異常 congenital〈acquired〉 *color blindness[vision defect]

しきそ **色素** **pigment, pigmentation** （色素性の **pigmentary** 色素が沈着した **pigmented**） ◆皮膚の色素沈着 pigmentation[（黒ずみ）darkening] of one's[the] skin ◀正色素性〈低色素性〉貧血 normochromic〈hypochromic〉anemia　メラニン色素 melanin pigment　▶色素細胞 pigment cell　色素性母斑 pigmented nevus　色素沈着（skin） pigmentation / accumulation[deposit] of pigments　色素内視鏡検査 dye endoscopy

ジギタリス **digitalis, foxglove** ▶ジギタリス中毒 digitalis poisoning[intoxication] / digitalism

しきち **敷地** **premises** ★複数形で. ◆病院の敷地内は禁煙です Please do not smoke[Smoking is not allowed] anywhere on the hospital premises.

しきのう **視機能** **visual function** ☞視覚，視野，視力

しきべつ **識別** （相違）**distinction** （身元などの確認）**identification** ☞区別 ◀個人識別 personal identification

しきもう **色盲** ☞色覚異常

じぎゃく **自虐（的な）** **masochistic** （masochism）

しきゅう¹ **子宮** **uterus** /júːtərəs/ （uterine /júːtəràin/）, **womb** /wúːm/ （hyster(o)-, metr(o)-） ◀後屈子宮 retroflexed uterus　▶子宮外妊娠 ectopic pregnancy 子宮下垂 descent of the uterus／hysteroptosis 子宮がん uterine cancer 子宮鏡検査 hysteroscopy 子宮筋腫 uterine myoma 子宮筋腫摘出術 myomectomy 子宮腔 uterine cavity 子宮後屈症 uterine retroflexion／retroflexion of the uterus 子宮収縮 uterine contraction 子宮収縮ホルモン oxytocin；OXT 子宮収縮薬 oxytocic (medication／drug／agent) 子宮腺筋症 uterine adenomyosis 子宮前屈 anteflexion of the uterus 子宮体がん uterine corpus cancer 子宮体部 uterine body／body of the uterus 子宮脱 uterine prolapse 子宮底 fundus of the uterus 子宮内胎児死亡 intrauterine fetal death；IUFD 子宮内避妊器具 intrauterine (contraceptive) device；IUD／(リング状のもの)intrauterine contraceptive ring 子宮発育不全 uterine hypoplasia 子宮破裂 uterine rupture 子宮復古 uterine involution 子宮壁 uterine wall 子宮卵管造影 hysterosalpingography；HSG／X-ray recording of the uterus and fallopian tubes ☞子宮頸管, 子宮頸がん, 子宮口, 子宮摘出術, 子宮内膜

しきゅう² 支給する （与える）**give** （用意・供給する）**supply, provide** （配る）**distribute** （発行する）**issue** ◆赤ちゃんのおむつは支給します We provide diapers for babies. ◆生活保護費を支給する distribute[issue] welfare payments

しきゅう³ 至急 （直ちに）**immediately**／ɪmíːdiətli/, **right away, at once**, 《英》**straightaway** （緊急に）**urgently** ☞緊急, すぐ ◆至急連絡して下さい Please contact[call] us immediately[at once]. ◆この傷は至急手当てが必要です This wound should be treated *right away[immediately]. ／ This wound is in urgent need of treatment.

しきゅうけいかん 子宮頸管 **cervical canal of the uterus, uterocervical canal** （子宮頸部）**uterine cervix** ◀クラミジア子宮頸管炎 chlamydial cervicitis ▶子宮頸管炎 cervicitis 子宮頸管拡張術 cervical dila-

tion[dilatation] 子宮頸管熟化薬 cervical ripening agent 子宮頸管妊娠 cervical pregnancy 子宮頸管粘液 cervical mucus 子宮頸管縫縮術 cervical cerclage／circumferential suture of the cervix 子宮頸管ポリープ(uterine) cervical polyp 子宮頸管無力症 cervical incompetence[atony] 子宮頸管裂傷 cervical tear[laceration]

しきゅうけいがん 子宮頸がん （uterine）**cervical cancer** ▶子宮頸がん検査 Papanicolaou[Pap] smear (test)

しきゅうけいぶ 子宮頸部 ☞子宮頸管

しきゅうこう 子宮口 **uterine os, opening of the uterus** ◆子宮口がまだ開いていません Your cervix hasn't dilated yet. ◆子宮口は6 cm開いています Your cervix has dilated to six centimeters.

じきゅうせい 持久性 ☞持久力

しきゅうたい 糸球体 **glomerulus** ☞糸球体硬化症, 糸球体腎炎

しきゅうたいこうかしょう 糸球体硬化症 **glomerulosclerosis** ◀巣状糸球体硬化症 focal glomerulosclerosis；FGS

しきゅうたいじんえん 糸球体腎炎 **glomerulonephritis** ◀血尿や蛋白尿は, 糸球体腎炎が原因のようです The blood and protein in your urine seem to be due to glomerulonephritis. ◀急速進行性糸球体腎炎 rapidly progressive glomerulonephritis；RPGN 巣状糸球体腎炎 focal glomerulonephritis 膜性増殖性糸球体腎炎 membranoproliferative glomerulonephritis；MPGN 慢性糸球体腎炎 chronic glomerulonephritis；CGN メサンギウム増殖性糸球体腎炎 mesangial proliferative glomerulonephritis 連鎖球菌感染後糸球体腎炎 poststreptococcal glomerulonephritis

しきゅうてきしゅつじゅつ 子宮摘出術 **hysterectomy** ◀広汎性子宮全摘出術 radical hysterectomy 超広汎性子宮全摘出術 extended radical hysterectomy

しきゅうないまく 子宮内膜 **endometrium** (形endometrial) ◀異所性子宮内膜症 ectopic endometriosis ▶子宮内膜が

ん endometrial cancer　子宮内膜症 endometriosis　子宮内膜増殖症 endometrial hyperplasia　子宮内膜生検 endometrial biopsy

じきゅうりょく　持久力　(耐える力) endurance　(スタミナ) stamina　◀身体的持久力 physical endurance　▶精神的持久力 mental endurance　▶持久力訓練 endurance training[exercise]

しきょ　死去　☞死, 死ぬ, 死亡, 亡くなる

じきょう　耳鏡　otoscope　(形otoscopic)　▶耳鏡検査 otoscopic exam[examination] / otoscopy

しきり　仕切り　partition　(形partition)　(衝立) screen　(形screen)　◆仕切りのカーテン a partitioning curtain / a partition curtain　◆プライバシー保護のため病室の一部を仕切る partition[screen] off part of the room for privacy

じく　軸　(回転体の) axis　(複axes)　(骨幹など棒状の) shaft　◀縦軸 longitudinal axis　横軸 horizontal axis

しくうかんしつにん　視空間失認　visual-spatial agnosia

じくさく　軸索　axon　(形axonal)　▶軸索断裂 axonotmesis　軸索変性 axonal degeneration

しくしく　◆胃がしくしく痛む have *a nagging[an incessantly dull] pain in the stomach　◆しくしくする痛み a gnawing [nagging] pain　☞痛み

じくじく　◆傷口がじくじくしている The cut[wound] is oozing[wet and sticky].

しくみ　仕組み
《構造》structure　◆からだの仕組み the structure of the body / body structure
《メカニズム》mechanism　◆がんが発症する仕組みはまだよく分かっていません We still don't fully understand how cancer develops. / The mechanism of cancer development has not yet been fully clarified.
《方式》system　◆ベッドサイドのテレビはプリペイドカードで視聴する仕組みです The bedside TV works on a prepaid card system.

しげき　刺激　(一般的に) stimulation　(動stimulate　形stimulating, stimulant)　(生理・心理的な刺激) stimulus　(複stimuli)　(炎症性の刺激) irritation　(動irritate　形irritating, irritable)　◆咳や喘鳴の原因となるアレルゲンや刺激物に曝されないようして下さい You should avoid exposure to allergens or irritants that cause coughing or wheezing.　◆筋肉を刺激する stimulate *one's muscles　◆胃に刺激のある食べ物を避ける avoid foods that stimulate the stomach　◆胃を刺激する irritate *one's stomach　◆刺激の少ない石鹸 mild[hypoirritant] soap　◀易刺激性 irritability　温度刺激 caloric stimulation　寒冷刺激 low temperature stimulus　条件〈無条件〉刺激 conditioned〈unconditioned〉stimulus　性的刺激 sexual stimulation　単一刺激 single stimulus　聴覚刺激 acoustic stimulation　電気刺激 electric stimulation　反復刺激 repetitive stimulation　光刺激 photic stimulation　▶刺激症状 irritation[irritable] symptom　刺激伝導系(心臓の) the (heart) conduction system　刺激伝導障害 conduction defect　刺激物 stimulant / stimulator　(炎症などを引き起こす物) irritant　☞刺激薬

しげきやく　刺激薬　stimulant, stimulator　◀精神刺激薬 psychostimulant / psychic energizer　ドパミン受容体刺激薬 dopamine receptor stimulant　β(受容体)刺激薬 β(-receptor) stimulant

しけつ　止血する　stop (the) bleeding[hemorrhage]　(形hemostasis　形hemostatic)　◆傷口を圧迫して止血する stop the bleeding[hemorrhage] by applying pressure to the wound　◆止血帯を使って止血する use the tourniquet to stem[staunch] the bleeding　◀圧迫止血法 arrest of bleeding[hemorrhage] by *application of pressure[compression]　内視鏡的止血法 endoscopic hemostasis　▶止血ガーゼ hemostatic gauze　止血機能 hemostatic function　止血点 blood pressure point / hemostasis site　止血綿 styptic cotton　止血薬 hemostatic

(medication / drug / agent)

しけん 試験 （一般的に）examination, exam （検査）test （安全性などの試験）trial （圏実験的な experimental 予備的な・検査目的の exploratory）☞検査 ◆その薬はまだ試験的な段階です The medication is still in the experimental[test] stage. ◀かかと膝試験 heel-knee test クームス試験 Coombs test 血液交差適合試験 blood crossmatching (procedure) 第Ⅲ相試験 phase III trial 貼付試験 patch test トレッドミル運動負荷試験 treadmill exercise test ブドウ糖負荷試験 glucose tolerance test；GTT マスター二段階（昇降）試験 Master two-step (exercise) test 無作為化比較試験 randomized controlled trial；RCT 無作為化臨床試験 randomized clinical trial；RCT 薬剤感受性試験 drug susceptibility[sensitivity] test 誘発試験 provocative[provocation] test 指鼻試験 finger-to-nose test 臨床試験 clinical trial[test] リンパ球刺激試験 lymphocyte stimulation test；LST ▶試験開腹 exploratory laparotomy 試験管 test tube 試験穿刺 exploratory puncture 試験投与 test dosing

しげん 資源 resources ★通例，複数形で．◀社会資源 social[community] resources 人的資源 human resources / manpower

しご 死後（の）postmortem （圏after death）◆死後の処置を行う provide postmortem care ☞死後解剖，死後硬直

じこ¹ 事故 accident /ǽksədənt/ （圏accidéntal）◆大きな事故や怪我をしたことがありますか Have you ever had any serious accidents or injuries? ◆事故を起こす〈事故に遭う〉have an accident ★同じ表現を使うことができる．◆事故が起こった時の状況を教えて下さい Please describe how the accident happened[occurred]. ◆事故を避ける avoid an accident ◆通勤中に〈作業中に〉起こった事故 an accident that occurred *on the way to work〈at work〉◀医療事故 medical accident 交通事故 traffic accident 自動車

事故 car[automobile] accident 死亡事故 fatal accident 転落[転倒]事故 fall[falling] accident / accident from a fall 針刺し事故 needlestick accident ▶事故死 accidental death 事故報告（医療事故の報告）accident[occurrence] report / （ニアミス・軽微な事故の報告）incident report

じこ² 自己 self （腰頭self-, auto-）☞自家，自分 ◆自己紹介をさせていただきます．医師の加藤です Let me introduce myself. I'm Dr Kato. ◆インスリンの自己注射をする give *oneself* an insulin injection / self-inject insulin ◆自己評価が低い The self-evaluation[self-assessment] score is low. ▶自己愛 narcissism / self-love 自己暗示 autosuggestion 自己概念 self-concept 自己管理 self-monitoring / self-management 自己血輸血 autologous blood transfusion / transfusion of *one's* own blood 自己抗体 autoantibody 自己催眠 self-hypnosis 自己実現 self-realization / self-actualization 自己主張 self-assertion / self-assertiveness 自己像 self-image 自己注射 self-injection 自己中心 self-centeredness 自己貯血 autologous blood donation / donation of *one's* own blood 自己導尿 self-catheterization / self-urethral catheterization 自己投薬 self-medication / self-administration 自己認識 self-understanding / self-awareness / self-recognition 自己分析 self-analysis 自己防衛本能 instinct for self-defense[self-protection] ☞自己触診，自己同一性，自己負担，自己免疫

しこう¹ 志向 （方向性・関心）orientation （圏oriented）（好み）preference ◆仕事志向の人 a work-oriented person ◀性的志向 sexual orientation[preference] 問題志向型システム problem-oriented system；POS 問題志向型診療録 problem-oriented medical record；POMR

しこう² 思考 thought, thinking ☞考え ◆このタイプの認知症は思考に影響を与えます This type of dementia affects thinking. ◆軽い思考障害の兆候が認められます The patient shows[is showing]

signs of mild thought[thinking] disorder [disturbance]. ◀分裂思考 schizophrenic thinking ▶思考化声 thought hearing / audible thoughts / thought echo 思考吹入 thought insertion 思考伝播 thought broadcasting 思考途絶 thought blocking 思考滅裂 thought incoherence / incoherent thinking [thought]

しこう³ 歯垢 (dental) plaque ☞歯石
◆歯垢が溜まっています You have plaque buildup on your teeth. ◆歯垢を取る remove the plaque from[on] the teeth / (こすり落とす) scrape away[off] dental plaque ◆歯垢のスケーリングを行う deepscale the plaques ▶歯垢形成 plaque formation 歯垢コントロール plaque control

しこう⁴ 嗜好 (味覚) taste (好み) preference ☞好き嫌い ◆最近食べ物の嗜好が変化しましたか Has your taste in food changed recently?

じこう¹ 耳垢 earwax, ear wax, cerumen (形 ceruminal) ☞耳垢(みみあか) ▶耳垢除去 earwax removal 耳垢栓 earwax[ceruminal] impaction / earwax buildup and blockage

じこう² 事項 (検討を要する事柄) matter (項目) item (主題) subject ◆注意事項をよくお読み下さい Please read the directions[instructions] carefully. ◀関連事項 related matters[items / subjects] 引継ぎ事項 matter to be handed over

じこう³ 持効(型の) long-acting ▶持効型インスリン long-acting insulin 持効薬 long-acting medication[drug / agent]

じこうかしょう 耳硬化症 otosclerosis

しこうさ 視交叉 optic chiasm, chiasm of the optic nerve

しこうさくご 試行錯誤 trial and error
◆試行錯誤で by[through] trial and error

しごかいぼう 死後解剖 postmortem examination ☞検死

じこく 時刻 time ☞時間 ◆予約の時刻 the appointed time ◆終了予定の時刻 the estimated time of completion ◀死亡時刻 the time of death

しごうこうちょく 死後硬直 rigor mortis, postmortem rigidity (死体硬直) cadaveric rigidity ◆死後硬直がすでに起きています The stiffness[rigor mortis] has already set in.

じこしょくしん 自己触診 (乳房の) breast self-examination;BSE, breast self-exam
◆乳房の自己触診を定期的にやっていますか Have you been doing regular breast self-exams?

しこつ¹ 指骨 bone of the finger ▶指骨骨折 finger fracture

しこつ² 趾骨 bone of the toe

しこつ³ 篩骨 ethmoid bone, ethmoidal bone ▶篩骨洞 ethmoid[ethmoidal] sinus 篩骨洞炎 ethmoidal sinusitis

しごと 仕事 (一般的に) work (収入を得る仕事) job (職業) occupation (職務) duties (and responsibilities) ★複数形で. ☞作業,働く,労働 ◆仕事に行く go to work / go to the office ◆仕事を得る get a job ◆仕事に就く take a job ◆仕事を失う lose a job ◆仕事を辞める quit a job / resign from a job ◆仕事に復帰する return[go back / get back] to work[one's job]
《職種・職務を尋ねる》 ◆現在,仕事をしていますか Are you working at present? / Are you currently employed? ◆どんな仕事をしていますか What kind[type] of work do you do? / What do you do for a living? / What's your occupation? ◆今までどんなお仕事に就かれたかをお話し下さい Please tell me about the jobs you've had in the past. ◆どんな仕事内容ですか What are your duties and responsibilities? ◆体を使う仕事 physical work[labor] ◆事務の仕事 office[clerical] work ◆人と会うことの多い仕事 work[a job] that requires you to meet people / a people-based job ◆ボランティアの仕事 volunteer work ◆仕事場の住所はどちらですか Where's your *place of work [workplace]? / Could you tell me your work address?
《仕事量を尋ねる》 ◆仕事はお忙しいですか

Are you busy at work? ◆いつも遅くまで仕事をしますか Do you usually work late? ◆どのくらい体を使うお仕事ですか How much physical labor does your work require? ◆フルタイムの仕事 full-time work / a full-time job ◆パートの仕事 part-time work / a part-time job

《心身への影響を尋ねる》 ◆仕事は気に入っていますか How do you like your work [job]? ◆仕事の面で何か問題がありますか Do you have any problems at work? ◆仕事にストレスを感じていますか Do you feel stressed in your work? / Are you stressed at work? ◆ストレスの多い仕事 a stressful[stress-filled] job ◆目の疲れは仕事に関係していると思いますか Do you think your eye strain may be related to your work?

《アドバイスの表現》 ◆仕事量を減らして下さい Please cut back on your work. ◆仕事は休んで，少し休養して下さい You should not go to work. Please rest for a while. ◆仕事を休む take some time off work / (病気休暇を取る) take sick leave from work ◆仕事は続けても構いません You can[may] go on with your work.

▶仕事環境 working environment 仕事(上の)関係 working relationship 仕事中毒(人) workaholic, work addict / (状態) workaholism, work addiction 仕事量 the amount of work

じこどういつせい 自己同一性 identity
◆自己同一性の危機を経験する experience an identity crisis

じこふたん 自己負担 self payment, out-of-pocket payment ◆医療費の3割は自己負担です You'll have to pay thirty percent of your (medical) expenses. ◆美容整形の医療費は全額自己負担です You'll have to pay the full cost of your medical expenses for cosmetic surgery. / (保険の適用外) The medical expenses of cosmetic surgery are not covered by your health insurance.

じこめんえき 自己免疫 autoimmunity (形autoimmune) ▶自己免疫疾患 auto-immune disease 自己免疫性肝炎 auto-immune hepatitis 自己免疫性甲状腺疾患 autoimmune thyroid disease；AITD 自己免疫性溶血性貧血 autoimmune hemolytic anemia；AIHA

しこり lump, mass (腫瘤)tumor ◆しこりに気づいたのはいつですか When did you first notice the lump? ◆しこりはどこにありますか Where is the lump (located)? / Could you show me where the lump is? ◆しこりは大きくなっていますか Is the lump getting bigger? ◆しこりは痛みますか Is the lump painful? ◆乳房にしこりがないかをチェックします I'm going to [Let me] feel for any lumps in your breast. / I'm going to[Let me] do a thorough breast exam to check for any lumps. ◆首にしこりがある have a lump on *one's* neck ◆乳房〈鼠径部〉にしこりを発見する find a lump in *one's* breast 〈groin〉 ◆皮下〈わきの下〉に硬いしこりがある have a firm[hard] lump *under the skin〈under *one's* arm〉

しこん 歯根 tooth root, dental root
◀人工歯根 artificial tooth[dental] root
▶歯根う蝕 root caries

しさ 示唆する suggest (図suggestion 形示唆に富む suggestive) ☞示す ◆これらの検査結果は化学療法が有効であったことを示唆しています These test results suggest that the chemotherapy was effective.

じさ 時差 (時間のずれ)time lag (時間の差) time difference ◆時差ぼけする have jet lag / suffer from jet lag / be jet-lagged ▶時差症候群 jet lag syndrome

じさつ 自殺 suicide /súːəsàːd/ (形自殺願望の suicídal) ◆自殺する kill *oneself* (by) / take *one's* own life (by) / commit suicide (by) ◆睡眠薬自殺する kill *oneself* by taking sleeping pills / commit suicide with sleeping pills ◆飛び降り自殺する kill *oneself* by jumping (from) ◆首吊り自殺する hang oneself / kill oneself by hanging ◆リストカットで自殺を試みる attempt (to commit) suicide by cutting one's wrist(s) ◆自殺願望がある

feel[be] suicidal / want to kill oneself / have suicidal thoughts ◆自殺したいと言う express *thoughts about committing suicide[suicidal thoughts] ◆自殺を予防する prevent suicide ◀ガス自殺 gas suicide / suicide by gas (inhalation) 集団自殺 group suicide 入水自殺 suicide by drowning (oneself) 飛び降り自殺 jumping suicide 服毒自殺 suicide[killing oneself] by taking poison 硫化水素自殺 hydrogen sulfide suicide ▶自殺企図 suicide attempt 自殺傾向 suicidal[suicide] tendency 自殺行為 suicidal behavior / (1回の行為) suicidal act 自殺者 suicide 自殺未遂 attempted suicide / attempt to kill oneself / (行為) suicide attempt

しさん 死産 **stillbirth** (形stillborn) ◆死産したことがありますか Have you ever *had a stillbirth[given birth to a baby who was stillborn]? ◆死産の子供 a stillborn baby / a baby that died shortly after birth ▶死産証書 certificate of stillbirth 死産届 notice[registration] of stillbirth

じさん 持参する (持ってくる)**bring** (持って行く)**take** ◆入院の際には常用している薬を持参して下さい Please bring your medications with you on the day of your admission to the hospital. ◆心臓の専門医を受診する時には、この紹介状を持参して下さい Please take this referral letter with you when you *see the heart specialist[go for your appointment with the heart specialist].

しし 四肢 **limbs** /límz/, **arms and legs** (特に先端部分)**extremities** ★いずれも通例, 複数形で. ☞四肢麻痺, (四)肢誘導

しじ[1] 支持 **support** (形supportive) ☞援助, 支える, サポート, 助ける ▶支持器具 (足首の) (ankle) support 支持的ケア supportive care 支持療法 supportive therapy

しじ[2] 指示 (やり方に関する指図)**instructions** (動instruct) (口頭による指図)**directions** (動direct) ★いずれも通例, 複数形で. (正式な指示・命令)**order** (動order) ◆私の指示がわかりますか Do you understand my instructions? ◆この薬は指示通りに飲んで下さい Please take this medication exactly as directed[instructed]. ◆看護師の指示に従って下さい Please follow the nurse's instructions[directions]. ◆痛み止めの注射は必要に応じて4時間ごとに打つようにと担当医から指示されています Your doctor has instructed[ordered] a shot of pain medication every four hours *if you need it[as needed]. ◆指示するまで動かないで下さい Please don't move till *I say "OK"[I give you the signal]. ◆指示があったら深く息を吸って止めて下さい Please breathe deeply and hold when I tell you to. ◆鈴木先生からの指示ではタバコは控えるようにとのことです Dr Suzuki wants you to refrain from smoking. ◆具体的な指示を与える give specific instructions[directions] ◆明確な指示 clear[specific] instructions[directions] ◆口頭の指示 verbal instructions[directions] ◆書面の指示 written instructions ◀退院指示 discharge instructions ☞事前指示書

じし[1] 示指 **index (finger)**, **forefinger**

じし[2] 自死 ☞自殺

ししつ 脂質 **lipid** ◀過酸化脂質 lipid peroxide 糖脂質 glycolipid リン脂質 phospholipid 類脂質 lipoid ▶脂質代謝 lipid metabolism 脂質低下薬 lipid-lowering medication[drug / agent] ☞脂質異常症

じじつ 事実 **fact** (真実)**truth** ◆事実をありのままに話して下さい Please tell me the facts[truth] frankly. ◆事実を確認する confirm a fact ◆事実を調べる check a fact ◆事実関係を調べる check[investigate] what actually[really] happened ◆がんであるという事実を受け入れる accept the fact that one has cancer ◆統計上の事実 a statistical fact ◆明白な事実 *an obvious[a clear] fact

ししついじょうしょう 脂質異常症 **dyslipidemia**

ししまひ 四肢麻痺 **quadriplegia** ◀周期性四肢麻痺 periodic paralysis

ししゃ 死者 dead person （故人）the deceased /dɪsíːst/

ししゃやく 止瀉薬 antidiarrheal（medication, drug, agent）

ししゅう 歯周（の） periodontal ▶歯周炎 periodontitis　歯周病 gum[periodontal] disease　歯周ポケット periodontal pocket

しじゅう 始終 （しょっちゅう）all the time （必ず）always ☞いつも

ししゆうどう 四肢誘導 ☞肢誘導

じしゅっけつ 耳出血 bleeding from the ear, ear bleeding

じしゅてき 自主的 ☞主体的

ししゅんき 思春期 puberty /pjúːbəti/, adolescence /æ̀dəlésəns/（㊣adolescent） ☞ライフステージ ◆思春期に入る reach (the age of) puberty ◀児童思春期精神保健 child and adolescent mental health　早発思春期 premature puberty ▶思春期医学 adolescent medicine　思春期早発 precocious puberty　思春期遅発 delayed puberty

じしょ 自書 ◆この欄にお名前を自書して下さい Please write your name in your own handwriting in this column.

じじょ 自助 self-help ▶自助グループ self-help[peer support] group ☞自助具

ししょう¹ 支障 （問題点・トラブル）trouble （妨げ）obstacle, hindrance（㊣妨害する interfere with　影響を及ぼす affect） ◆すべて支障なくいきました Everything went off without any trouble. / Everything went well[smoothly]. ◆腰痛は日常生活に支障を来していますか Is your lower back pain interfering with your daily activities? / Does your lower back pain affect your *daily routine[everyday life]?

ししょう² 視床 thalamus（㊣thalamic） ▶視床核 thalamic nuclei　視床出血 thalamic hemorrhage　視床痛 thalamic pain ☞視床下部

ししょう³ 刺傷 （ハチの針・とげなどの刺し傷）sting

しじょう 矢状（の） sagittal ▶矢状断 sagittal section　矢状面 sagittal plane

じしょう 自傷 self-inflicted injury [wound] ◀手首自傷症候群 wrist-cutting syndrome ▶自傷行為 self-inflicted [self-injurious] behavior

じじょう 事情 （周囲の状況）circumstances （特に生活・仕事面での状態）conditions ★いずれも通例，複数形で．（事態）situation （理由）reason ☞状況，理由 ◆事情により under the circumstances / because of the circumstances ◆やむを得ない事情によって by[through] force of circumstances ◆そういう事情で手術を延期せざるを得ません Under the circumstances[Because of the circumstances], we'll have to postpone the surgery. ◆事情の許す限り喜んでお手伝いいたします As far as circumstances permit, I'll be glad to help you. ◆家庭の事情で帰国する return home for family reasons ◀住宅事情 housing conditions[situation]　経済事情 financial conditions[situation]

ししょうかぶ 視床下部 hypothalamus （㊣hypothalamic） ▶視床下部疾患 hypothalamic disease

しじょうきん 糸状菌 mold ▶糸状菌症 hyphomycosis

ししょうこつ 耳小骨 auditory ossicles, ear ossicles

しじょうちゅう 糸状虫 filaria ▶糸状虫症 filariasis

じじょぐ 自助具 （食事用の）self-help device

ししょくしん 視触診 inspection and palpation

ししん¹ 指針 guidelines ★通例，複数形で．☞ガイドライン

ししん² 指診 digital examination ◀肛門指診 digital anal examination / digital examination of the anus　直腸指診 digital rectal examination；DRE / digital examination of the rectum

じしん 自信 confidence, self-confidence, confidence in *oneself*（㊣confident） ◆自信がある have confidence in *oneself* ◆自信をつける develop[build] confidence in *oneself* ◆自信を喪失する

lose *one's self-confidence[confidence in oneself] ◆自分に自信が持てない(精神的に不安定な)feel insecure about oneself ◆自信を取り戻す recover[regain](one's) confidence ◆禁煙できるという自信を持ちましょう You should have confidence in your ability to quit smoking. / Have confidence[Be confident] in yourself that you can give up smoking.

じしんおん 児心音 **fetal heart sound [tone]** ◆児心音を聴く listen to the fetal heart sounds

じしんき 持針器 **needle holder**

ししんけい 視神経 **optic nerve** ▶視神経萎縮 optic nerve atrophy 視神経腫瘍 optic nerve tumor 視神経脊髄炎 optic neuromyelitis 視神経損傷 optic nerve injury 視神経乳頭 optic disc 視神経乳頭陥凹 excavation of the optic nerve head ☞視神経炎

ししんけいえん 視神経炎 **optic neuritis** ◀球後視神経炎 retrobulbar optic neuritis

しずい 歯髄 **dental pulp** ◀露出歯髄 exposed pulp ▶歯髄炎 pulpitis 歯髄処置 pulp treatment

しすう 指数 (指標)**index** (比率)**quotient** (数値)**score** ◀知能指数 intelligence quotient；IQ 熱傷指数 burn index；BI 発達指数 developmental quotient；DQ 不快指数 discomfort index；DI / (天候の)temperature-humidity index

しずか 静か(な・に) (物音をたてない)**quiet, silent** (穏やかな)**peaceful, calm** (動かない)**still** ◆静かにして下さい Please be quiet. / Be quiet, please. ◆少しの間静かにしていただけませんか May I ask you to keep quiet for a while? ◆お子さんは静かに眠っています Your child is sleeping peacefully[quietly]. ◆検査が済むまで静かにしていて下さい Please keep still until the test is finished.

ジスキネジア **dyskinesia** ◀口部ジスキネジア oral dyskinesia 胆道ジスキネジア biliary dyskinesia

しすぎる し過ぎる ☞―過ぎる ◆パソコ

ン作業のし過ぎで目が疲れる have eye strain from using one's computer too much ◆痛いからといってあまり安静にし過ぎると，かえってよくありません Even if you're in pain, it's no good staying in bed all the time.

シスチン **cystine** ▶シスチン結石 cystine stone[calculus] シスチン尿 cystinuria

システム **system** (㋫systematic) ▶システム分析 systems analysis システムレビュー systems[systematic] review / review of systems；ROS

ジストニア **dystonia** (㋫dystonic) ▶ジストニア運動 dystonic movement

ジストロフィー **dystrophy** /dístrəfi/ ◀異染性白質ジストロフィー metachromatic leukodystrophy 外陰ジストロフィー vulvar dystrophy 筋緊張性ジストロフィー myotonic dystrophy；MD / dystrophia myotonica；DM 反射性交感神経性ジストロフィー reflex sympathetic dystrophy 副腎白質ジストロフィー adrenoleukodystrophy ☞筋ジストロフィー

しずまる 静まる・鎮まる (落ち着く)**calm (down)** (痛み・苦しみが徐々に和らぐ)**subside** ◆動悸は鎮まりましたか Have the palpitations subsided?

しずむ 沈む (気分が)**feel[get, become] depressed, feel down** ☞落ち込む

しずめる 静める・鎮める (落ち着かせる)**calm (down), soothe** (和らげる・安心させる)**relieve** ◆気を静める calm down / calm oneself / (神経を)calm[soothe] one's nerves / (不安を)calm one's fear ◆痛みを鎮める relieve[soothe] the pain

しせい¹ 刺青 **tattoo** ▶刺青除去 tattoo removal

しせい² 姿勢 (体の構え)**posture** (㋫postural) (体の置き方)**position** ☞体位 ◆姿勢が良い have good posture ◆姿勢が悪い have poor[bad] posture ◆姿勢を変える change one's position ◆真っ直ぐな姿勢をとる assume a straight posture ◆いつも同じ姿勢でいますか Do you always hold[adopt] the same posture?

◆その姿勢を10秒間保てますか Can you hold that posture for ten seconds? ◀異常姿勢 abnormal posture　屈曲姿勢 crouched[crouch] posture　除脳姿勢 decerebrate posture　除皮質姿勢 decorticate posture　静的姿勢 static posture　前傾[前屈]姿勢 stooped[forward-bent] posture　胎児姿勢 fetal position　はさみ姿勢 scissoring posture　不良姿勢 malposture　▶姿勢訓練 postural exercise　姿勢時振戦 postural tremor　姿勢反射 postural reflex

しせい³　脂性(の)　oily, greasy　▶脂性皮膚 oily[greasy] skin

しせい⁴　視性(の)　(視覚・視力の)visual　(眼球の)ocular　(光・視覚上の)optical　▶視性眼振 visual[ocular] nystagmus　視性めまい visual[ocular] vertigo

じせい¹　耳性(の)　aural, auditory　(耳原性の)otogenic　(耳の)otic　▶耳性眼振 aural nystagmus　耳性めまい aural[auditory] vertigo　耳性斜頸 otogenic torticollis

じせい²　自制する　control *oneself* (図 self-control)　◆食べ過ぎ〈飲み過ぎ〉ないように，よく自制されていますね You're good at controlling yourself from eating〈drinking〉too much.　◆彼女には自制心がない She has no self-control.　◆自制心を失う lose *one's* self-control

しせいかつ　私生活　(公的な立場を離れた生活)private life　(個人としての生活)personal life　◆私生活に立ち入った質問かと思いますが，この情報はあなたの診療に役立てるためのものです I know I'm asking questions that concern your private[personal] life, but this information will help me take better care of you.

しせいかん　死生観　view of life and death

じせいきょうちょう　自声強聴　autophony

しせき　歯石　tartar, dental calculus　☞歯垢　◆歯石を取り除く remove tartar from[on] the teeth / get rid of tartar / (こすり落とす)scrape away[off] tartar　▶歯石形成 tartar formation　歯石沈着 tartar deposi-tion

しせつ　施設　home, facility　(公共的な機関)institution　(圏institutional)　☞ホーム　◆知的障害者のための施設 *an institution [a facility] for people with intellectual disabilities　◆高齢者のための施設 a home[facility] for the elderly　◆施設に入所する enter[be admitted to] a facility [home]　◆彼女を施設に入れる *put her in[have her admitted to] a home[facility]　◀医療施設 medical facility[institution]　介護施設 (residential) care home / nursing facility[home]　児童福祉施設 child welfare facility　社会福祉施設 social welfare facility　授産施設 sheltered *work institution[workshop]　生活支援施設 assisted living facility　通所介護施設 day care facility　保健医療施設 health care facility　保護施設 public assistance institution　養護施設 (児童の)children's home / residential facility for children　▶施設内審査委員会 institutional review board；IRB

しせつうんどうしっこう　肢節運動失行　limb-kinetic apraxia

しせつかんかんせつ　指節間〈趾節間〉関節　finger〈toe〉joint, interphalangeal joint of the hand〈foot〉　◀遠位指節間〈趾節間〉関節 *distal interphalangeal[DIP] joint of the hand〈foot〉　近位指節間〈趾節間〉関節 *proximal interphalangeal[PIP] joint of the hand〈foot〉

しせつこつ　指〈趾〉節骨　finger〈toe〉, phalanx of the hand〈foot〉　(圏phalangeal)　▶指〈趾〉節骨骨折 phalangeal fracture of the hand〈foot〉

しせん¹　脂腺　sebaceous gland, oil-producing gland of the skin

しせん²　視線　eye(s)　(凝視)stare　(圏stare)　◆視線を合わせる make eye contact (with)　◆視線を避ける avoid eye contact / avert *one's* eyes away (from)　◆常に周囲の人の視線が気になりますか Do you always feel uncomfortable and bothered by being seen or stared at by the people around you?　▶視線恐怖 scopophobia；*abnormal fear of being seen by others*／（自己視線恐怖を含めて）fear of eye-to-eye contact[confrontation]

しぜん **自然（の）** （自然による・自然に関する）**natural** （自然発生的な）**spontaneous** （圖ひとりでに **by** *oneself*） ◆分泌物は自然に出ますか，押すと出ますか Do the discharge come out by itself or by squeezing? ▶自然回復 spontaneous recovery 自然科学 natural science 自然寛解 spontaneous remission 自然気胸 spontaneous pneumothorax 自然受精 natural insemination 自然食品 natural food(s) 自然治癒 spontaneous cure／natural healing 自然分娩 natural childbirth[delivery] 自然免疫 natural immunity 自然流産 spontaneous abortion ☞自然死

じぜん **事前（の）** **advance** （圖**in advance**, **beforehand**） ◆事前に予約をとって下さい Please make *an advance appointment [your appointment in advance]. ▶事前予約 advance appointment ☞事前指示書

しぜんし **自然死** **natural death** ◆自然死する die of natural causes

じぜんしじしょ **事前指示書** **advance** **(medical, health care) directive** （リビングウィル）**living will**

しそう¹ **刺創** **stab wound**

しそう² **歯槽** **tooth socket**, **(dental) alveolus** （圈**alveolar**） ▶歯槽骨 alveolar bone 歯槽骨炎 alveolitis 歯槽膿瘍 alveolar abscess 歯槽膿漏 alveolar pyorrhea ★alveolar は肺胞という意味もあるので注意.

じぞく **持続する** （一般的に）**continue** （効果などが続く）**work** （特定の期間続く）**last** （維持する）**maintain**, **keep up** （圈連続した**constant**, **continuous** 慢性的でしつこい**persistent** 効き目の長い**long-acting** 長期に及ぶ**prolonged**） ☞続く，連続 ◆鎮痛薬の効果がまだ持続しています The painkiller is still working.／The analgesic effect is still continuing[working]. ◆集中力を持続させるのは難しいですか Do you have trouble *maintaining attention[concentrating]? ◆持続的に痛みますか Do

you have the pain[Does it hurt] all the time? / Is the pain constant[persistent]? / Are you constantly in pain? ◆その痛みは一過性ですか，持続性ですか Does the pain come and go, or *does it stay[is it there all the time]? ◆持続的な咳 a constant[continuous] cough ▶持続型インスリン long-acting insulin 持続感染 persistent infection 持続気道陽圧呼吸 continuous positive airway pressure；CPAP 持続吸引 continuous suction 持続携行式腹膜透析 continuous ambulatory peritoneal dialysis；CAPD 持続血糖測定 continuous glucose monitoring；CGM 持続痛 continuous[persistent] pain 持続的血液濾過 continuous hemofiltration；CHF 持続点滴 continuous drip infusion 持続陽圧換気 continuous positive pressure ventilation；CPPV

じそんしん **自尊心** **self-respect** （誇り）**pride** ◆自尊心を失う lose *one's* self-respect ◆自尊心を傷つける hurt[wound] a *person's* pride

した¹ **下** （方向が下の方）**down** （↔up） （位置がすぐ真下）**under** （↔on top of） （位置が下方）**below** （↔above） ◆下を見て下さい Please look down. ◆ずっと下まで見て下さい Please look all the way down. ◆左の目の下に大きなほくろがある have a big mole under *one's* left eye ◆心電図室は下の階にあります The EKG[electrocardiography] room is on the floor below (this one). ◆右〈左〉を下にして寝る sleep on *one's* right〈left〉side ◆血圧は上が135，下が90です Your blood pressure is a[one] hundred (and) thirty-five over ninety.

した² **舌** **tongue** /táŋ/ ☞舌（ぜつ） ◆舌に何か問題がありますか Do you have any problems with your tongue? ◆舌を診せて下さい Let me examine your tongue. ◆舌の先 the tip of *one's* tongue 《症状・所見の表現》 ◆舌が痛みますか Do you have (a) pain in your tongue? / Is your tongue sore[painful]? ◆舌がよく

荒れますか Does your tongue often get [become] rough? / (舌苔が付着するか) Does your tongue often get[become] coated[furred]? ◆舌に潰瘍がよくできますか Do you often have ulcers on your tongue? ◆舌が乾燥する the tongue gets [becomes] dry ◆舌が利かない(味覚障害がある)lose *one's* sense of taste ◆舌が黒ずむ the tongue gets[becomes] dark ◆舌がざらざらする the tongue gets[becomes] rough[sandy / gritty] ◆舌がしびれる the tongue gets[becomes] numb ◆舌が腫れている have a swollen tongue / the tongue is swelling up ◆舌がひりひりする the tongue burns[tingles] ◆舌がもつれる(話し方が不明瞭) *one's* speech becomes slurred / have slurred speech / have trouble speaking ◆舌を噛む bite *one's* tongue

《指示》◆舌を突き出して下さい Please stick out your tongue. ◆舌を上にあげる lift up *one's* tongue ◆舌を左右に動かす move *one's* tongue from left to right ◆この錠剤は舌の下に入れたままゆっくり溶かして下さい Please place this tablet under your tongue and let it dissolve slowly.

したあご 下顎 lower jaw ☞顎(あご, がく), 下顎(かがく)

したい¹ 死体 (dead) body, corpse (解剖用の)cadaver (⊞cadaveric) ▶死体安置所(hospital) morgue 死体解剖 autopsy / postmortem examination 死体検案書 death certificate 死体硬直 cadaveric rigidity 死体腎移植 kidney transplant [transplantation] from a dead donor / cadaver kidney transplant[transplantation] 死体防腐処置 embalming

したい² 肢体 limbs /límz/, arms and legs (特に先端部分)extremities ★いずれも通例, 複数形で. ☞肢体不自由

じたい¹ 事態 (状況)situation (物事) things ★複数形で. ☞状況 ◆事態はかなり深刻です I'm afraid that *the situation is[things are] rather serious[critical]. ◆最悪の事態に備える prepare for the worst (situation) ◆事態を見守る keep

an eye on the situation ◀緊急事態 emergency

じたい² 辞退する decline ☞拒否, 断る ◆贈り物は辞退させていただきます I'm sorry, but *we have to decline your gift [we cannot accept your gift].

したいじ 死胎児 dead fetus

したいふじゆう 肢体不自由(の) physically disabled[challenged] ▶肢体不自由者〈児〉physically disabled[challenged] person〈child〉/ person〈child〉with physical disabilities[challenges]

したがう 従う (指示に)follow (規則などに)observe (命令などに)obey ☞順守 ◆担当医の指示に従う follow the attending doctor's instructions ◆病院の規則に従う follow[observe] the hospital (rules and) regulations

したぎ 下着 underwear, underclothes ★複数形で. (下着のシャツ)undershirt (下着のパンツ)underpants ★複数形で. ◆下着のシャツを脱いで下さい Please *take off [slip off] your undershirt. ◆下着のパンツ以外全部脱いで下さい Please *take off [remove] all your clothes except (for) your underpants. ◆下着を引き上げて下さい Please pull up your underwear. ◆木綿の下着を着て下さい Please wear cotton underwear. ◆ウールや化繊の下着を避ける avoid wearing underwear made from wool or synthetic fibers

じたく 自宅 *one's* home, *one's* house ◆自宅のお電話は何番ですか What's your (home) phone number? ◆自宅療養をご希望ですか Would you like to recuperate [convalesce] at home? ◆自宅で介護してくださる方はいますか Do you have someone who can *take care of you[care for you] at home? ◆手術前1, 2週間自宅で待機して下さい Please *spend a couple (of) weeks at home[stay at home a couple (of) weeks] before the surgery. ◆自宅近くの病院で治療を受ける have (the) treatment at a hospital near *one's* home ◆自宅に帰る go home ▶自宅住所 home address 自宅分娩 home childbirth[delivery]

したくちびる 下唇　lower lip

したしい 親しい　(仲がいい)close　(友好的な)friendly　(気さくな)easy　(圏easily)　◆日本に親しい友人はいますか Do you have any close friends in Japan?　◆見知らぬ人とでも親しく話せるほうですか Can you speak easily[in a friendly way] with strangers?

したたる 滴る　(ポタポタ落ちる)drip　(尿などが垂れる)dribble　(尿などが漏れる)leak　◆排尿後も尿がしたたることがありますか Do you have any dribbling[leaking] after you urinate[pass water]?

したばら 下腹　☞下腹部

したみ 下見　preliminary look[inspection]　◆手術前に集中治療室の下見に行きましょう Let's go and take a (preliminary) look at the intensive care unit before your surgery.

しちがつ 7月　July；Jul.　☞1月

しちゅう[1] 市中　(地域社会)community　(地方自治体)municipality　(圏municipal)　◆市中でインフルエンザが流行っています Flu is going around this community.　▶市中肺炎 community-acquired pneumonia；CAP　市中病院 community[municipal] hospital

しちゅう[2] 支柱　upright bar

しちょう 師長　supervisor, manager　▶看護師長 nursing[nurse] supervisor　病棟師長 ward[floor／unit] nursing supervisor

しちょうねつ 弛張熱　remittent fever

しつ 質　quality　(↔quantity)　(圏qualitative)　◆医療の質が高い〈低い〉The quality of medical care is high〈low〉.　◆患者ケアの質を改善する improve the quality of care for patients　◆生活の質を向上させる improve the *quality of life[QOL]　▶質的研究 qualitative research　質的相違 qualitative difference　質的分析 qualitative analysis

じつ 実　☞実に，実の，実は

しつう 歯痛　toothache, tooth pain, dentalgia

じつう 耳痛　earache, ear pain, otalgia

しつおん 室温　room temperature　◆この薬は室温で保管して下さい Please keep this medication at room temperature.

しつか 膝窩　popliteal space, posterior part of the knee

しつがい 膝蓋　patella　(圏patellar)　▶膝蓋腱反射 patellar tendon reflex；PTR／knee jerk[reflex]　膝蓋骨 kneecap／patella　膝蓋靱帯 patellar ligament　膝蓋軟骨軟化症 chondromalacia patellae

しっかり firmly, tightly　◆赤ちゃんをしっかり抱っこする hold *one's* baby firmly[tightly]　◆(電話相談で)彼の意識はしっかりしていますか Is he conscious?　◆(意識レベルの低い患者に)大丈夫ですか，しっかりして下さい！救急車がすぐに来ますから Are you OK? Hold on! The ambulance will be right here.　★hold on は「ちょっと辛抱する・頑張る」という意味。　◆朝食をしっかり摂ると1日のスタートがよくなります Eating[Having] a good breakfast will give you a good start to the day.

しっかん 疾患　(具体的な病名のつく病気)disease　(障害)disorder　(一般的に病気)sickness, illness　☞疾病, 病気　◀胃腸疾患 gastrointestinal disease／GI tract disorder　遺伝疾患 genetic disease　肝疾患 liver disease　冠(動脈)疾患 coronary artery disease；CAD　基礎疾患 underlying disease　血液疾患 hematologic[blood] disease　呼吸器疾患 respiratory disease　心因性疾患 psychogenic disease　心疾患 heart disease　腎疾患 kidney disease　心臓血管疾患 cardiovascular disease　精神疾患 psychiatric[mental] disease　染色体疾患 chromosome disorder　全身性疾患 systemic disease　先天性疾患 congenital disease[disorder]　代謝性疾患 metabolic disease　特定疾患 specified disease／(指定難病)designated intractable disease　内分泌系疾患 endocrine (system) disease　脳血管疾患 cerebrovascular disease；CVD　泌尿器疾患 urologic disease　婦人科疾患 gynecologic[women's] disease

しつかんじょうしょう 失感情症 alexithymia

しつかんせつ 膝関節 knee joint ▶変形性膝関節症 knee osteoarthritis ▶膝関節痛 knee pain

しつぎょう 失業する lose *one's* job ◆失業中である be out of work ◆失業後はどのように過ごしていますか How have you been spending your time[days] since losing your job? ▶失業保険 unemployment insurance

しつきょうい 膝胸位 knee-chest position

しっきん 失禁 incontinence (形incontinent) ◆この手術に伴う合併症として尿の失禁が起こるかもしれません Loss of bladder control[Urinary incontinence] is a possible complication after this surgery. / A possible complication of this surgery is that you may have trouble *controlling your bladder[holding your water]. / You may have toilet[bathroom] accidents as a complication of this surgery ◆尿失禁はどのような時によく起こりますか When do you usually *have this bladder incontinence[leak urine]? ◀溢流性失禁 overflow (urinary) incontinence 感情失禁 emotional incontinence 腹圧性尿失禁 stress urinary incontinence；SUI 便失禁 fecal[bowel] incontinence / loss of bowel control / (小児語) fecal soiling 夜間失禁 nocturnal incontinence ▶失禁ケア incontinence care 失禁用パッド incontinence pad

シックハウスしょうこうぐん —症候群 sick house syndrome

しつけ (訓練) training (動train) (規律などのしつけ) discipline (動discipline) /dísə-plɪn/ (礼儀) manners ★複数形で. ◆お子さんはトイレのしつけが済んでいますか Is your child toilet-trained? ◆トイレのしつけを急ぐ必要はありません There's no hurry to toilet-train your child. ◆その子はとてもよくしつけられています The child has very good manners. / The child is well disciplined. ◆お子さんのしつけは根

気強くすることが大切です Patience is very important[It's important to be patient] when disciplining your child.

しっけ 湿気 (湿度) humidity (形humid) (湿り気) moisture (形moist) (じめじめした状態) dampness (形damp) ☞湿度 ◆日本の夏は湿気が多いので，かび対策をしたほうがよいでしょう Japanese summers are humid, so you should take some steps against mold.

しつけいさん 失計算 ☞失書

しっけつ 失血 blood loss (動lose blood) ☞出血 ◆怪我で失血する lose blood from *an injury[a wound] ◆失血死する die from loss of blood

じっけん 実験 experiment (形experimental), test ◆この薬の効果は多くの実験によって確かめられています The efficacy of this medication has been confirmed by many experiments. ◆ヒトでの臨床試験は，必ず前もって動物で実験し，安全性や有効性を確認してから行います Before clinical trials on human beings, a drug's safety and effectiveness are first confirmed in *animal experiments[experiments using animals]. ◀対照実験 control experiment[test] ▶実験計画 experimental design 実験動物 laboratory[experimental] animal

しつけんとうしき 失見当識 disorientation ☞見当識

しつご 失語(症) aphasia；*partial or total loss of the ability to communicate in speech or in writing* (形aphasic) ◆失語症の人 an aphasic person / a person with aphasia ◀ウェルニッケ失語 Wernicke aphasia 運動性〈感覚性〉失語 motor〈sensory〉 aphasia 健忘性失語 amnestic aphasia 全失語 total[global] aphasia 伝導性失語 conduction aphasia ブローカ失語 Broca aphasia

しつこい 《不快な感覚・症状が》 (慢性的に続く) persistent (しくしくする) gnawing /nɔ́:ɪŋ/, nagging ◆しつこい咳〈かゆみ〉 a persistent cough〈itch〉 ◆しつこい痛みa

gnawing[nagging] pain
《食べ物が》（腹にもたれる）**heavy** （脂っこい）**greasy** ◆しつこい食べ物 heavy[greasy] food

しっこう 失行 **apraxia** ◀観念運動失行 ideomotor apraxia 構成失行 constructional apraxia 肢節運動失行 limb-kinetic apraxia 発語失行 speech[verbal] apraxia 歩行失行 gait apraxia

じっこう 実行する （行う）**carry out** （行動する）**act on** （実行に移す）**put … into practice** ☞実践 ◆その治療計画を実行する carry out the treatment plan ◆それはいい考えですね．すぐに実行なさってはいかがですか That's a good idea. I suggest you *act on that[put it into practice] right away. ◆その計画は実行不可能です The plan is impractical.

じっさい 実際（に） （現に）**actually** （本当に）**really** （実は）**as it is** （ほとんど・事実上）**practically** （圏**practical**） ☞現実, 実は ◆実際に手術してみなければ何とも言えません I can't say anything definite until we actually perform the surgery. ◆その方法は実際には応用できません We can't actually put that method into practice. ◆実際のところ, ご自分の病気についてどのようにお考えですか What are you really thinking about your illness? / How do you really think about your illness? ◆彼女の病状はよくなると期待したのですが, 残念ながら実際のところ悪化しています I had hoped her condition would get better, but as it is, I'm afraid it's getting worse. ◆あなたと私の考えには実際的な相違はありません There is no practical difference between your opinion and mine.

しっさん 失算 **acalculia**

じっしつ 実質（的な） （中身のある）**substantial** （圏**substantially**） （本質的な）**essential** （圏**essentially**） ◆ジェネリック医薬品は先発医薬品と実質的には変わりありません Generic drugs and brand-name drugs are essentially the same. / There is no substantial difference between generic drugs and brand-name drugs. ▶実

質臓器 parenchymal organ

じっしゅう 実習 （practical） **training** （大学などの実習科目）**practicum** （職場での実地訓練）**on-the-job training** ◆看護技術の実習をする have (practical) training in nursing skills ◆当院は大学病院なので, 医学生や看護学生が臨床実習をさせていただくことがあります．ご理解とご協力をお願いします This is a university-affiliated hospital, in which medical and nursing students sometimes undergo clinical training. Your understanding and cooperation are appreciated. ◀看護実習 nursing practicum 臨床実習 clinical training ▶実習生 trainee

しつじゅうじじんたい 膝十字靱帯 **cruciate ligament of the knee**

しつじゅん 湿潤（性の） **moist, wet** ▶湿潤性湿疹 moist eczema

しっしょ 失書 **agraphia** ◀失読失書 alexia with agraphia

じっしょう 実証する （証明する）**prove** （確認する）**confirm** （実物を見せながら説明する）**demonstrate** （根拠を示す）**give evidence** ◆この新薬は有効であると海外ですでに実証されています The effectiveness of this new medication has already been proved[confirmed] overseas.

じつじょう 実情 （実際の状態）**the actual condition[state of affairs], the real condition[state of affairs]** ☞状況 ◆職場環境の実情をお聞かせ下さい What are your working conditions really like? / Please tell me the actual[real] state of affairs in your work environment. ◆脳死については日本では国民の中でまだ十分な了解が得られていないのが実情です（実は…）The fact is that people in Japan *have not yet fully come to terms with[have yet to fully agree with] brain death.

しっしん[1] 湿疹 （皮膚病の）**eczema** / ékzəmə/ （圏**eczématous**） （発疹）**rash** ☞発疹 ◆顔に湿疹ができる get eczema on the face ◆湿疹が出る break out in a rash / have a rash ◆お腹に湿疹が出ていますか Do you have a rash on your abdomen? ◆この軟膏を塗れば湿疹が治まります This ointment will cure[clear up] your rash. ◀アトピー性湿疹 atopic eczema 陰部湿疹 genital eczema 外因性湿疹 exogenous[exogenic] eczema 貨幣状湿疹 nummular[coin-shaped] eczema 間擦性湿疹 intertriginous eczema 乾性湿疹 dry eczema 汗疱状湿疹 dyshidrotic eczema 紅斑性湿疹 erythematous eczema 湿潤湿疹 moist eczema 脂漏性湿疹 seborrheic eczema 手湿疹 hand eczema 乳児湿疹 infantile eczema

しっしん² 　**失神する**　(一時的に気を失う) **faint, pass out, black out** (図**faint** 専門用語 **syncope** 図**syncopal**) 　(倒れる) **collapse** ☞意識 ◆失神したことがありますか Have you ever fainted[passed out]? ◆過呼吸で失神する faint from[due to] hyperventilation ◆失神して倒れる *fall down*[collapse] in a faint ◀起立性失神 orthostatic syncope 頸動脈洞性失神 carotid sinus syncope 血管迷走神経性失神 vasovagal syncope 心原性失神 cardiogenic syncope 咳失神 cough[tussive] syncope 体位性失神 postural syncope 排尿失神 micturition syncope 排便失神 defecation syncope ヒステリー性失神 hysterical syncope ▶失神感 fainting feeling 失神発作 fainting[syncopal] attack

しっせい¹ 　**失声**(症) **voice loss, loss of the voice, aphonia** (発声障害) **dysphonia** ☞発声障害

しっせい² 　**湿性**(の) **wet, moist** (痰を伴う) **productive** ▶湿性咳 wet[productive] cough 湿性ラ音 moist rale

じっせき 　**実績** (業績) **achievement** (動**achieve**) (よい結果) **good result** (成功経験) **successful experience** ◆実績を上げる achieve[get] a good[(満足のいく)satisfactory] result ◆彼にはこの手術に関して十分な実績があります He has plenty of successful experience with performing this surgery.

じっせん 　**実践する** (行う) **do, carry out** ☞実行 ◆健康の維持増進のために何を実

践していますか What do you do exactly to get and stay healthy? ◆運動療法は無理なく実践できるような内容にすると, 長続きします If your exercise therapy is *a doable[an easy / a reasonable] one, you'll be able to keep it up for a long time.

しつそうぐ 　**膝装具** **knee brace**

しっちょう 　**失調** **ataxia** (図**ataxic**) ◀栄養失調 malnutrition / malnourishment / lack of nourishment 自律神経失調症 autonomic imbalance / dysautonomia 心因性失調 psychogenic ataxia 体幹運動失調 truncal ataxia 片側運動失調 hemiataxia ▶失調性眼振 ataxic nystagmus 失調性歩行 ataxic gait / gait ataxia

しっと 　**嫉妬** **jealousy** (図**jealous**) ◆嫉妬深い夫 a jealous husband ▶嫉妬妄想 delusion of jealousy

しつど 　**湿度** **humidity** (図湿度の高い **humid**) ◆日本の夏は湿度が高いので, 体調管理に注意が必要です Japanese summers are very humid, so you should take care to look after your health[physical condition]. ◀相対湿度 relative humidity

じっと 　(動かずに) **still, fixedly** (図**fixed**) (辛抱強く) **patiently** ◆目を閉じてじっとしていて下さい Please close your eyes and keep still. ◆緑の点をじっと見て下さい Please keep your eyes fixed on the green point. / Please keep[continue] looking at the green point. ◆少しの間じっとしていて下さい Please don't move for a while. ◆じっと立っている時ふらつきますか Do you feel unsteady when you're standing still? ◆じっと待つ wait patiently

しっとう 　**執刀する** **perform surgery, operate** ◆あなたの脊椎手術を執刀するのは佐々木先生です Dr Sasaki will perform your spinal surgery. / Dr Sasaki will be in charge of your spinal surgery. ▶執刀医 operating surgeon

しつどく 　**失読** (読字困難)**alexia, acquired dyslexia, text[word] blindness** ▶失読失書 alexia with agraphia

しつない 　**室内**(の) **indoor** (図室内で **indoors**) ◆室内に閉じこもる shut *oneself*

しつない 311 **しっぺい**

up[stay] in *one's* room / stay indoors ▶室内運動 indoor exercise　室内空気汚染 indoor air pollution　室内塵アレルギー house dust allergy　室内塵ダニ house dust mite

じつに 実に　(とても・非常に)very, extremely　(本当に)really　(実際に)actually　(ひどく)terribly, awfully　(極めて)quite　◆実によく頑張りましたね You did very [extremely] well. /(やり遂げた)You've really made it.　◆この病気の症状は実に様々で複雑です The symptoms of this disease are really numerous and quite complex.　◆この問題を解決するのは実に難しい This problem is terribly[very / really] difficult to solve.　◆この吸入器を使うのは実に簡単です It's really[actually] quite simple to use this inhaler.

しつにん 失認　agnosia；*loss of the ability to recognize people and objects*　◀視覚失認 visual agnosia　視空間失認 visual-spatial agnosia　手指失認 finger agnosia　身体失認 asomatognosia　相貌失認 prosopagnosia　聴覚失認 auditory agnosia　病態失認 anosognosia　物体失認 object agnosia　立体失認 astereognosia

じつの 実の　(本当の)real, true　(実際の)actual　(生物学上の)biological, biologic　◆実の母親〈父親〉a biological[birth] mother〈father〉　▶実年齢 *one's* real age

じつは 実は　(実際のところ)actually, in fact, the fact is(that …)　(本当を言うと)To tell(you)the truth, The truth is(that …)　(残念なことに)unfortunately　☞実際　◆総コレステロールのことを気にしておられますが，実は LDL コレステロールの高い数値のほうがずっと危険です You're concerned about your total cholesterol levels, but, in fact, high LDL levels are considered more dangerous.　◆実はしびれの診断と治療は大変難しいのです The fact is that it is very difficult to diagnose the cause of numbness and to treat it.　◆実はあなたの回復が早いので驚いています To tell the truth, I'm surprised by your speedy recovery.　◆実はあまりよいお話ではありません Ac-tually[Well], I'm afraid I have some bad news for you.　◆実は，CT 検査は 1 か月先まで予約がいっぱいです Actually[Unfortunately], the next available CT appointment is not until next month.

しっぱい 失敗する　(しくじる)fail (図failure ↔success)　(ミスをする)make a mistake (図mistake)　◆その実験は失敗でした The experiment failed. / The experiment ended in failure.　◆失敗したからといってがっかりしないで，もう一度やってみて下さい Don't be discouraged just because you failed. Please try again.　◆失敗から学ぶ learn from *one's* mistakes　◆不注意により失敗する make a careless mistake　◆大失敗 a big[terrible / serious] mistake　◆ちょっとした失敗 a slight [minor] mistake

じっぴ 実費　actual expense　◆おむつは実費をご負担いただきますのでご了承下さい Please be advised that *patients* will pay for diapers[(成人用の)incontinence underwear] at their own expense.

しっぷ 湿布　compress /kámpres/, poultice, medicated(skin)patch　◆肩に湿布をする *put a compress on[apply a compress to] *one's* shoulder　◆1 日に 2 回この湿布を腰に貼って下さい Please apply this compress to your lower back twice a day.　◆温湿布 hot compress /(温パック)hot[heat] pack / hot[heat / heating] pad　冷湿布 cold compress[pack / pad] /(氷の)ice pack[pad]

じつぶつ 実物(大の)　(本物そっくりの)life-like　◆母親学級では，実物大の人形を使って沐浴の練習をします In *the antenatal class[the class for expectant mothers], participants practice bathing a baby using lifelike demonstration dolls.

しっぺい 疾病　(具体的な病名のつく病気)disease　(一般的に病気)sickness, illness　☞病気　◀国際疾病分類 International Classification of Diseases；ICD　▶疾病恐怖 nosophobia / pathophobia　疾病否認 denial of illness　疾病利得 gain from illness

しつぼう 失望する be disappointed (at, with, in) (落胆する) be discouraged (by) (望みを失う) lose hope ☞がっかりする
◆1回ぐらい検査結果が悪いからといって失望しないで下さい Please don't be *disappointed at[discouraged by] one bad test result.

しつめい 失明する lose one's eyesight, become[go] blind ◆治療しないと失明する恐れがあります Without treatment, I fear that you'll lose your eyesight.

しつもん 質問 question (問い合わせ) inquiry ◆よくある質問 frequently asked question(s)；FAQ(s) ◆重要な質問 *a key[an important] question ◆次の質問にお答え下さい Please answer the following questions. ◆質問を言い換えましょう Let me rephrase my question. ◆何か質問はありますか(Do you have) any questions? ◆何か質問があったら遠慮せずに訊いて下さい If you have any questions, feel free to ask me. ◆いくつか質問いたします I'd like to ask you some questions. / I'd like to get some information from you. ◆結婚生活について質問してもいいですか May I ask you some questions about your married life? ◆個人的なことを質問してもいいですか Would you mind *my asking[if I ask] some personal[private] questions? ☞質問票

しつもんひょう 質問票 questionnaire (sheet) /kwèstʃənéə-/ ◆この質問票に記入して下さい Please fill out[in] this questionnaire. ◆この質問票にお答え下さい Please answer the questions on this form.

しつよう 執拗(な) ☞しつこい

じつよう 実用(的な) practical (↔impractical) ◆このガイドブック〈小冊子〉は食事療法を理解するうえで実用的な情報を与えてくれます This guide〈brochure〉gives practical information to help you understand diet therapy.

しつりつ 失立 astasia (彨astatic) ▶失立失歩 astasia-abasia 失立発作 astatic seizure

しつれい 失礼
《挨拶》 ◆失礼します(席を立つ時) Excuse me. / (病室に入る時) May I come in? ★Good morning[Hello], Mrs Brown. などとも言う. ◆それではこれで失礼します(別れる時) Well, I must be going. / Goodbye (for now). / See you. ★文末に tomorrow や next Monday など, 次に再会する日時に言及することも多い.
《謝罪》 ◆お待たせして失礼しました I'm sorry I've kept you waiting. / I'm sorry to have kept you waiting. ◆失礼します. 浣腸しますよ I'm sorry, I'm just going to give you an enema.

じつれい 実例 (代表的な例) example (個別の例) instance (事例) case (サンプル・見本) sample ☞例

しつれん 失恋する break up with one's boyfriend〈girlfriend〉, suffer a broken heart ◆彼女は失恋の痛手がきっかけで過食症に陥った Breaking up with her boyfriend[Suffering a broken heart] triggered her bulimia[binge eating disorder].

してい 指定(の) designated /dézɪɡnèɪtɪd/ (日時を約束した) appointed ◆指定の喫煙所は救急外来待合室の入口の外にあります There is a designated smoking area outside the emergency waiting room entrance. ◆この病気は難病に指定されています This disease is designated as an intractable disease. ◆特にご指定の日時〈銘柄〉はありますか Do you have any particular date〈brand / product〉in mind?
▶指定医薬品 designated drug 指定医療機関 designated medical institute[institution] 指定感染症 designated infectious [communicable] disease

してき¹ 私的(な) (公的な立場を離れた個人の) private (一般的に個人の) personal
◆すみませんが, 私的な事柄についてはお話しできません I'm sorry, but I can't tell you about my private[personal] matters. ◆私的なお誘いには応じられません I'm afraid that I can't accept private [personal] invitations.

してき² 至適(な) optimal, optimum

してき² ☞最適 ▶至適温度 optimal[optimum] temperature

してき³ 指摘する tell, point out ◆健診で蛋白尿〈高血圧〉を指摘されたことがありますか Have you ever been told[Has it ever been pointed out to you] by a doctor that *protein was found in your urine 〈your blood pressure was high〉at your checkup? ◆加藤先生が指摘したように，喫煙は体に有害です As Dr Kato *told you [pointed out], smoking is harmful to health.

してん 視点 point of view, viewpoint ◆違う視点からその問題を考えてみましょう Let's think of the problem from another[a different] point of view.

じてんしゃ 自転車 bicycle, bike ◆自転車に乗る ride a bicycle ◆自転車で通勤する *go to work[commute] by bicycle ◆自転車で通学する go to school by bicycle ◆自転車をこいで下さい Please push the pedals. ▶自転車エルゴメーター bicycle ergometer

しどう 指導 （指示・指図）instructions ★通例，複数形で．（勧告）recommendation （ガイダンス）guidance （教育）education, teaching （相談・カウンセリング）counseling （助言）advice ◆専門医〈前の医師〉からどのような指導を受けましたか What instructions[recommendations] did you get[have] from *the specialist〈your previous physician〉? ◆助産師が母乳指導を行います The midwife will *show you how to breastfeed your baby[give you guidance on breastfeeding]. ◆この後，栄養指導〈禁煙指導〉の講座を受けて下さい After this, I'd like you to take the nutrition 〈quit-smoking〉class. ◆アルコール問題を抱える患者を指導する provide guidance to a patient with an alcohol problem ◀家族指導 family guidance 患者指導 patient education[instructions] 食事指導 dietary guidance[instructions] 生活指導 life counseling[guidance] 退院指導 discharge guidance 服薬指導 medication counseling[teaching] 訪問指導 guidance by a visiting health worker / visiting[home-visit] guidance 保健指導 health guidance ▶指導医 medical supervisor 指導員 instructor / adviser / （集団の）leader

じとう 児頭 fetal head ▶児頭下降 descent of the fetal head 児頭嵌入 engagement of the fetal head 児頭骨盤不均衡 cephalopelvic disproportion；CPD 児頭浮動 floating fetal head

じどう¹ 自動（の）automatic （オートメーション化された）automated （能動の）active （↔passive） ◆このエアコンは自動的に室温を調節します This air conditioner automatically regulates room temperature. ◆ドアは自動的に開きます The door opens automatically[by itself]. ▶自動血圧計 automatic blood pressure measuring device / automated sphygmomanometer 自動制御 automatic control 自動精算機 automatic bill payment machine 自動体外式除細動器 automated external defibrillator；AED 自動販売機 vending machine 自動腹膜透析 automated peritoneal dialysis；APD 自動分析装置 automatic analyzer / autoanalyzer

じどう² 児童 child （㣎children） ☞子供，小児 ▶児童虐待 child abuse 児童相談所 child guidance center / counseling clinic for children 児童手当 child benefit [allowance] 児童福祉 child welfare 児童福祉施設 child welfare facility 児童扶養手当 child care benefit / child-rearing allowance 児童養護施設 residential facility for children / children's home / （孤児院）orphanage

じどうしゃ 自動車 car, automobile ☞車 ◆自動車を運転する drive a car ◆自動車事故に遭う have *a car[an automobile] accident ◆自動車事故で死ぬ die[be killed] in *a car[an automobile] accident ▶自動車排気ガス automobile exhaust gas

じどうしょう 自動症 automatism

シトルリン citrulline ▶シトルリン血症 citrullinemia

しにく 歯肉 gum, gingiva /ʤɪndʒáɪvə/ (形gingival) ☞歯茎 ◆歯肉が腫れて赤黒くなっています The gums are swollen and dusky red. ◆歯肉が炎症を起こしています You have inflamed gums. ◆歯肉は触ると痛みますか Do your gums feel tender to the touch? ◆歯磨きをすると歯肉から出血がありますか Do your gums bleed when you brush your teeth? ◆歯肉が後退して歯を失う危険があります You have receding gums[Your gums have receded] and you're in danger of losing your teeth. ◆歯と歯肉の間から膿が出る have pus between *one's* teeth and gums ◆歯肉が変色する the gums change color / have discolored gums ▶歯肉炎 gingivitis / inflammation of the gum(s) 歯肉口内炎 gingivostomatitis 歯肉出血 gingival bleeding[hemorrhage] / bleeding (of the) gums 歯肉増殖症 gingival hyperplasia 歯肉膿瘍 gingival abscess

しにめ 死に目 ◆父親の死に目に会う be at *one's* father's bedside when he dies / be with *one's* father when he dies

しにゅうぶ 刺入部 (注射の)injection site (穿刺の)puncture site

しぬ 死ぬ die (of, from) (事故などで)be killed (婉曲的に)pass away (死に瀕している)be dying ▶死，死亡，亡くなる ◆彼女は肺炎で死にました She died of[from] pneumonia. ★病気による死因を指す場合には by や with を用いない。by や with の例としては，「毒で死ぬ die by[from] poison」「尊厳死する die with dignity」などという。 ◆彼は怪我で死にました He died from his injuries. ◆出血多量で死ぬ(失血により死ぬ) die from loss of blood / (死に至るまで出血する)bleed to death ◆自動車事故で死ぬ die[be killed] in a car accident ◆死ぬのではないかと恐怖を覚えることがありますか Do you ever fear that you may be dying? ◆安らかに死ぬ die peacefully ◆死にゆくプロセス the dying process

しのうくんれん 視能訓練 orthoptic exercise, orthoptics ▶視能訓練士 orthoptist：ORT

しはい 支配する control ◆右脳は左半身の運動や感覚を支配し，左脳は右半身を支配しています The right half of the brain controls the movement and sensation of the left side of the body, while the left half of the brain controls the right side of the body.

しばしば often, frequently (何回も)many times ☞頻繁

じはつ 自発(的な) (自然発生的な)spontaneous (随意の・自由意思による)voluntary (↔involuntary) ▶自発痛 spontaneous pain 自発的臓器提供 voluntary organ donation ☞自発呼吸

じはつこきゅう 自発呼吸 spontaneous breathing[respiration], breathing *on one's* own[by *oneself*] ◆彼女は血圧が低下し，自発呼吸が無くなっています Her blood pressure has dropped and she is not breathing *on her own*[spontaneously].

しはらう 支払う pay (図payment), make (a) payment (保険対象とする)cover ◆病院の費用は何で支払いますか How will you pay your hospital fees? ◆お支払いは現金でお願いします Please pay by cash. / You are requested to make payments in cash. ◆当病院ではクレジットカードによる支払いに応じます We accept [Our hospital accepts] payment by credit card. / You can pay by credit card. ◆自費で支払う pay at *one's* own expense ◆その医療費は労災保険から支払われます The medical expenses will be covered by *worker compensation insurance[the Workers' Accident Compensation Insurance]. ◆定額の支払い flat[fixed] sum payment ◆出来高による支払い料金 fees for services

しばらく (少しの間)for a (little) while (ほんのちょっと)a moment (やや長めの間)for a long time (少ししたら)in a little while ◆しばらくお待ち下さい Please wait *for a while[a moment]. ◆先生はしばらくしたら戻って来ます The doctor will be back in a little while. ◆しばらくおそばについてい

ましょう I'll just sit with you for a while.
◆しばらく麻酔が残っていますので飲食は控えて下さい The (effects of the) anesthesia won't wear off for a while, so please don't eat or drink anything. ◆しばらくぶりですね。具合はどうでしたか It's been such a long time (since I saw you last)〔I haven't seen you for a long time〕. How have you been?

しばられる **縛られる** (固執する)stick to (閉じ込められる)be trapped ◆固定観念に縛られず，もう少し自由に考えてみませんか Instead of sticking to stereotypes, how about thinking more freely[flexibly]? ◆彼は自分なしでは仕事が回らないという思いに縛られています He is trapped in the idea that things can't go on without him at work.

しはん¹ **死斑** livor mortis, postmortem lividity[staining]

しはん² **紫斑** purpura, purplish-red spot ◆紫斑が足に出ました The purpura appeared on the legs. ◀触知可能紫斑 palpable purpura 単純性紫斑 purpura simplex ☞紫斑病

しはん³ **市販する** sell ... in the stores, sell ... over the counter ◆市販されている血圧計を購入し，血圧を毎日測って下さい Please buy a blood pressure machine that *they sell[you can buy] in the stores and take your blood pressure every day. ◆この薬は市販されているので，処方箋なしでも薬局で購入できます This medication is sold over the counter, so you can buy it at a *drug store[pharmacy]. ☞市販後調査，市販薬

しはんごちょうさ **市販後調査** postmarketing surveillance；PMS

しはんびょう **紫斑病** purpura ◀アナフィラクトイド紫斑病 anaphylactoid purpura アレルギー性紫斑病 allergic purpura 血栓性血小板減少性紫斑病 thrombotic thrombocytopenic purpura；TTP 特発性血小板減少性紫斑病 idiopathic thrombocytopenic purpura；ITP ヘノッホ・シェーンライン紫斑病 Henoch–

Schönlein purpura；HSP

しはんやく **市販薬** over-the-counter drug[medication], OTC drug[medication] ◆その薬は医師の処方によるものですか，それとも市販薬ですか Did your doctor prescribe the medication or did you buy it over the counter? ◆市販薬を飲む take an over-the-counter drug

じひ **自費** *one's* own expense ☞自費診療

じびいんこうか **耳鼻咽喉科** the department of otorhinolaryngology, the ENT[Ear(s), Nose, and Throat] department, the department of ENT ▶耳鼻咽喉科医 ENT doctor[specialist] / otorhinolaryngologist 耳鼻咽喉科学 otolaryngology / otorhinolaryngology

じひしんりょう **自費診療** medical services not covered by insurance, out-of-pocket medical services ◆健康保険がないと自費診療になります(医療費全額を支払う必要がある) If you do not have health insurance, you will have to pay all your medical expenses.

じひつ **自筆** ☞自書

しひょう **指標** (ある事の徴候)indicator (目印)index, marker (発達段階などにおける道標)milestone ◆血圧の数値は健康の指標の1つです Your blood pressure level is one of the indicators of your overall health. ◆HbA1c は過去1〜2か月間の血糖値レベルを示す指標です HbA1c is *an index[a marker] of *a person's* average blood sugar level over the previous one to two months. ◀発達指標(目安)developmental milestone / (数標)developmental index

じびょう **持病** (慢性の健康問題)chronic *health problem[illness] (慢性疾患)chronic disease (長い間の病気)old complaint ◆何か持病はありますか Do you have any chronic *health problems[illnesses]? ◆リウマチは彼女の持病です She's had rheumatism for a long time.

しびれ **痺れ** (無感覚)numbness /nʌ́mnəs/ (🔈numb, asleep 🔈go[become,

get] **numb**）（麻痺）**paralysis, palsy**
☞麻痺 ◆どんなしびれか話して下さい Tell me more about the numbness. ◆右腕〈手〉がしびれていますか Is your right arm〈hand〉numb? / Do you have any numbness in your right arm〈hand〉? ◆手がしびれるのはどんな状況の時ですか In what situations does your hand usually go numb[asleep]? ◆彼は左腕にしびれがある He has numbness in his left arm. / His left arm feels[has gone] numb. ◆舌がしびれる the tongue goes[becomes] numb

しびん 尿瓶 ☞尿器, 便器

しぶつ 私物 *one's*（**personal**）**belongings** ★複数形で．☞持ち物

ジフテリア **diphtheria**／dɪfθíriə／ ◀咽頭〈喉頭〉ジフテリア **pharyngeal〈laryngeal〉diphtheria** ▶ジフテリア菌 *Corynebacterium diphtheriae* ジフテリア抗毒素 **diphtheria antitoxin** ジフテリア破傷風無細胞百日咳ワクチン *diphtheria, tetanus, and acellular pertussis[DTaP] vaccine ジフテリア破傷風ワクチン *diphtheria and tetanus[DT] vaccine

シフト （勤務体制）（**work**）**shift**

しぶり 渋り **tenesmus**；*straining to pass stools or to urinate* ◀尿しぶり **urinary tenesmus** ▶しぶり腹 **tenesmus**

じぶん 自分 **oneself**（図自分自身の **one's own**）☞自己 ◆ご自分を大切にして下さい Please take care of yourself. ◆ご自分のことについて話して下さい Please tell me about yourself. ◆自分のことは自分でやる do things for *oneself* / do what *one* can do *by oneself*[on *one's* own] ◆自分をコントロールする control *oneself* ◆自分から進んで治療を受ける have the treatment of *one's* own（free）will ◆自分自身の病気について正しく認識する have an accurate understanding of *one's* own disease ◆しびれていて自分の腕ではないような感じですか Does your arm feel numb and as if it's not part of your body? ◆自分自身がぐるぐる回る感じですか Do you feel as if you're spinning round and

round?

じへい 自閉 **autism**（図**autistic**）▶自閉スペクトラム症 **autism spectrum disorder**；**ASD** /（アスペルガー症候群）**Asperger syndrome**；**AS** 自閉スペクトラム症児 **autistic child** 自閉的態度 **autistic attitude**

じへいそくかん 耳閉塞感（耳が塞がっている感じ）**aural fullness, ear fullness, sensation of fullness and〈or〉pressure in** *one's* **ear(s)**（うっ血している感じ）**congested feeling in** *one's* **ear(s)**（詰まった感じ）**plugged-up feeling in** *one's* **ear(s)**

しへき 嗜癖 **addiction**（図**addictive**）◀アルコール嗜癖 **alcohol addiction** 麻薬嗜癖 **narcotic addiction** 薬物嗜癖 **drug addiction** ▶嗜癖行動 **addictive behavior**

しべつ 死別 ◆何歳の時にご主人と死別なさいましたか How old were you when you lost your husband? ◆配偶者と死別している be widowed

しぼう¹ 死亡する **die**（図**death**, 図**dead**）（事故などで）**be killed**（婉曲的に）**pass away** ☞死, 死ぬ, 亡くなる ◆肝臓がんで死亡する die of[from] liver cancer ◆患者の死亡を確認する confirm the death of the patient ◆患者の死亡を宣告する pronounce the patient dead ◆お父様の死亡原因は何でしたか What was the cause of your father's death? ◆心臓手術中に死亡する die during heart surgery ◆入院中に死亡する die *in the hospital[during a hospital stay / during hospitalization] ◀子宮内胎児死亡 **intrauterine fetal death**；**IUFD** 周産期死亡 **perinatal death** 来院時死亡 **death on arrival**；**DOA** ▶死亡事故 **fatal accident** 死亡時刻 the time of death 死亡診断書 **death certificate** 死亡統計 **mortality statistics** 死亡届 **notification of death** / **death registration** ☞死亡率

しぼう² 脂肪 **fat**（図脂肪分の多い **fatty, fat-filled** 脂肪の **adipose**）◆脂肪の摂取量を減らす reduce[cut down on] *one's* fat intake ◆脂肪と糖分を多く含む食べ物を

減らして下さい You should cut down on foods that contain a lot of fat and sugar. ◆脂肪分の多い食べ物を避ける avoid fatty [fat-filled] foods / avoid high-fat foods / avoid foods high in fat ◆お腹と内臓周辺に脂肪が溜まっている have a lot of fat in the abdomen and surrounding internal organs ◆低脂肪の食べ物 low-fat foods [diet] / foods low in fat / (脂肪制限食)fat-restricted diet ◆無脂肪の牛乳 fat-free milk ◀植物性脂肪 vegetable fat　体脂肪 body fat　体脂肪率 body fat percentage / percent body fat　中性脂肪 neutral fat / triglyceride　貯蔵脂肪 depot fat　動物性脂肪 animal fat　内臓脂肪 visceral fat　皮下脂肪 subcutaneous fat / fat just under the skin　飽和脂肪 saturated fat ▶脂(肪)質 lipid　脂肪過多 excess[excessive] fat / adiposity / adiposis　脂肪含有量 fat content　脂肪吸収試験 fat absorption test[study]　脂肪摂取量 fat intake　脂肪塞栓(症) fat embolism　脂肪組織 fatty[adipose] tissue　脂肪分解 lipolysis　脂肪便 fatty stool　脂肪変性 fatty degeneration ☞脂肪肝, 脂肪酸, 脂肪腫

しほうかいぼう　司法解剖　forensic autopsy, judicial autopsy

しぼうかん　脂肪肝　fatty liver

しぼうさん　脂肪酸　fatty acid ◀一価不飽和脂肪酸 monounsaturated fatty acid　多価不飽和脂肪酸 polyunsaturated fatty acid；PUFA　必須脂肪酸 essential fatty acid　不飽和脂肪酸 unsaturated fatty acid；UFA　飽和脂肪酸 saturated fatty acid；SFA　遊離脂肪酸 free fatty acid

しぼうしゅ　脂肪腫　lipoma

しぼうりつ　死亡率　death rate, mortality (rate) ◆術後合併症による死亡率は約2％です The death rate from *postoperative complications[complications following surgery] is around two percent. ◀累積死亡率 cumulative mortality[death] rate

しぼる　絞る・搾る
《力を加えて内容物を出す》 (布などをねじって水分を出す)wring (out)　(ぎゅっと締めつけ

る)squeeze　(液体や気体を吸い上げる・送る) pump ◆タオルを絞る wring (out) a towel ◆レモンを搾る squeeze a lemon ◆母乳を搾る pump (breast) milk 《対象を限定する》narrow (down), pinpoint, focus (on) ◆頭痛の原因を2つの可能性に絞る narrow the cause of *a person's* headache down to two possibilities

しまい　姉妹　sister ☞兄弟

しみ　染み　(皮膚・顔などのしみ) (skin) blemish, blotch　(皮膚の変色)skin discoloration　(小さな斑点)speck　(汚れ) stain ☞色素 ◆日焼けはしみの原因になります Too much suntan causes skin blemishes. ◆顔のしみをとるクリーム a cream to remove blemishes from the face ◆加齢によるしみ age-related blotches / skin discoloration due to old age ◆しみのある皮膚 blotched skin ◆血のしみ a blood stain

しみでる　染み出る　(粘性の液体が)ooze (out)　(水などが)seep (out) ☞滲む

しみる　染みる　(鋭い痛みがある)have a sharp pain　(ヒリヒリ・チクチク痛む)sting (うずくように痛む)smart　(皮膚に炎症を起こす)irritate ◆冷たい水が歯にしみますか Do your teeth hurt when you drink cold water? / Do you have a sharp pain in the teeth after drinking cold water? ◆この塗り薬は傷口にはしみません This ointment won't make the cut sting[smart]. ◆目がしみる The eyes sting. ◆タバコの煙が目にしみる Cigarette smoke irritates the eyes.

しみん　嗜眠　☞傾眠

しみんびょういん　市民病院　(市の)city hospital　(地方自治体の)municipal hospital　(地域の)community hospital

じむ　事務　office work, clerical work　(事務部)department of hospital administration (㊟事務的な businesslike　書類などを処理する clerical) ◆手続きを事務的に進める go through the procedure[formalities] in a businesslike manner ◆申し訳ございません，当方の事務的ミスでご迷惑をおかけしました We are very sorry[We apologize] for the inconvenience caused by our clerical mistake. ◀一般事務職員（general office）clerk　医療事務職員 medical clerk　受付事務職員 receptionist　入院事務室 hospital admissions office　福祉事務所（public / social）welfare office　▶事務室（hospital business）office　事務職員（職員全体）clerical staff /（一人ひとりの職員）clerk, clerical worker　事務長 director of administration / business manager

シムスたいい　一体位　Sims position
しめい　氏名　(full) name　☞名前
じめじめ　☞湿気
しめす　示す　（表す）show, indicate　（指し示す）point（to, out）（意味する）mean　☞示唆，見せる　◆生検結果はポリープが良性であることを示しています The biopsy result shows that the polyp is benign.　◆痛む場所を指で示して下さい Please point to where it hurts.　◆この血液検査所見は体のどこかに炎症があることを示しています This result of the blood test indicates[means] that you have inflammation somewhere in your body.
しめつける　締め付ける　tighten /táitn/（图tightness 图tight）（ぎゅっと搾るように）squeeze　（押しつぶすように）crush　◆胸が締め付けられるように痛む have a tightening[squeezing / crushing / tight] pain in one's chest / have pressure or tightness in the chest　◆バンドで頭を締め付けられるように痛む have a pain that feels like a *tight band around the head[band squeezing the head] / have a tightening band-like headache　◆胃が締め付けられる have knots in the stomach
しめっぽい　湿っぽい　☞湿気
しめらす　湿らす　（軽く水気を含ませる）moisten, dampen　（水などで濡らす）wet　◆唇を湿らせる moisten one's lips　◆アルコールを湿らせた綿 cotton dampened with alcohol
しめる¹　湿る　（濡れる）get wet　（じめじめする）get damp　◆湿った咳 a wet cough
しめる²　閉める　close（↔open），shut

◆カーテンを閉めましょうか Shall I close the curtains?
しも　下　（陰部）private parts　★複数形で.　◆お下の清拭はご自分でなさいますか Would you rather wash your private parts by yourself?
しもやけ　霜焼け　（凍瘡・軽度の凍傷）chilblains　★複数形で.　（凍傷）frostbite　◆霜焼けがある have chilblains　◆足の指に霜焼けができやすいですか Do you tend to get chilblains on your toes?
しもん　指紋　fingerprint
しや　視野
《眼で見える範囲》visual field, field of vision　◆視野が狭くなっていますか Has your visual field become narrower?　◆視野に障害がある be visually impaired / have visual impairment / have *disturbed vision[visual disabilities]　◆周辺の視野が欠ける have peripheral vision loss / have loss of side vision　◆視野の中に黒い点が浮かぶ black specks float in the field of vision
《見方》perspective, point of view　◆もう少し広い視野から今後の治療方針を検討しましょう Let's examine[review] your future treatment plan from a broader perspective[point of view].　◆切断も視野に入れつつ，当面は保存的治療に努めます Considering the possibility of amputation, for the time being, we'll do our best to give you conservative treatment.
◀周辺視野 peripheral visual field　対面視野検査 confrontation（visual field）test[method]　中心視野 central visual field / field of central vision　明視野 bright field　らせん状視野 spiral visual field　両眼視野 binocular visual field　▶視野異常 visual field abnormality　視野狭窄 visual field constriction / narrowing of the visual field　視野計 perimeter　視野欠損 visual field defect　視野検査 visual field test / perimetry
シャイ・ドレーガーしょうこうぐん　一症候群　Shy-Drager syndrome；SDS
しゃかい　社会　society（图social）（地域

社会〕community ◀高齢〈超高齢〉社会 aged〈super-aged〉society　少子高齢化社会 aging society with a low birthrate　地域社会 local community　▶社会階層 social class　社会環境 social environment　社会[社交]恐怖 social phobia　社会資源 social[community] resources　社会生活技能訓練 social skills training；SST　社会組織(構造) social structure／(集団・機構) social organization　社会適応 social adaptation[adjustment]　社会的孤立 social isolation　社会的支援 social support　社会的疎外 social alienation　社会的入院 non-medical hospitalization　社会的不適応 social maladjustment　社会的不利 social disadvantage[handicap]　社会[社交]不安症 social anxiety disorder；SAD　社会福祉 social welfare　社会福祉協議会 council of social welfare　社会福祉士 social worker；SW　社会福祉施設 social welfare facility　社会負担 burden on society　社会保険 social insurance　社会保障給付 social security benefits　社会問題 social problem　社会リハビリテーション social rehabilitation

しゃかいふっき　社会復帰 returning to work　◆社会復帰する(病気から) return to work after *one's* illness[(怪我から) injury]／(普通の生活に戻る)*get back[return] to normal life　◆職場への社会復帰をご希望ですか Would you like to *return to work[go back to your job]?　◆元通りの状態での社会復帰は難しいかもしれません It might be difficult for you to return to life as it was before.　◆回復の期間はそれぞれ異なりますが，ほとんどの患者さんは2，3か月で社会復帰できます The time to recovery varies from person to person, but most patients are able to *get back[return] to normal life in a few months.　▶社会復帰プログラム return-to-work program

しゃがむ　squat (down) /skwάt-/, **crouch (down)** /krάʊʧ-/　◆しゃがみ込んだ姿勢になる crouch down (in a squatting posi-

tion)／ sit in a squatting position　◆ゆっくりしゃがんでみて下さい Try to squat down slowly.　◆しゃがんだ姿勢から支えなしで立ち上がれますか Can you stand up from a squatting position without any support?

しゃがれごえ　しゃがれ声　☞しわがれ声

しゃがんし　遮眼子 occluder　◆この遮眼子で右目を隠して下さい Please cover your right eye with this occluder.

しやく　試薬 reagent, experimental medication[drug]

じゃくかくだい　弱拡大 (顕微鏡の)**low-power field**

じゃくさん　弱酸 weak acid　▶弱酸性 weak acidity

じゃくし　弱視 amblyopia, weak eyesight, poor vision, lazy eye　◀不同視性弱視 anisometropic amblyopia

しやくしょ　市役所 (市の)**city hall, city office** (地方自治体の)**municipal office**

しゃくそくへんい　尺側偏位 ulnar drift[deviation]

ジャクソンけいれん　―痙攣 jacksonian seizure[convulsion]

ジャクソンてんかん　jacksonian epilepsy

じゃぐち　蛇口 faucet, tap

じゃくてん　弱点 (弱い点)**weak point** (不都合な点)**drawback** (短所・不十分な点)**shortcomings**　★通例，複数形で．(欠陥)**defect**　◆欠点　◆誰にでも弱点はあります Everyone has their weak points.　◆この薬は高い効果を発揮しますが，副作用が出やすいことが弱点です This is a very effective medication, but its drawback is that it tends to have some side effects.　◆これを機会にご自分の弱点を克服してみませんか How about taking this opportunity[chance] to overcome your shortcomings?

しゃくど　尺度 (目盛)**scale** (計量の単位)**measure**　◀痛みの数値評価尺度 *Numerical Rating Scale[NRS] for pain measurement　グラスゴー昏睡尺度 Glasgow coma scale；GCS

じゃくどく　弱毒(性の) (弱めた)**attenu-**

ated （毒性の弱い）low-virulent （低病原性の）low-pathogenic ▶弱毒化ウイルス attenuated virus 弱毒菌 low-virulent bacilli 弱毒生ワクチン attenuated live vaccine

しゃくねつ　灼熱　burn ◀排尿時灼熱感 urinary burning / urine ardor ▶灼熱感 burning sensation 灼熱痛 burning pain

じゃくねん　若年(性・型の) （未成年者の・未成熟の）juvenile /ʤúːvənaɪl/ （若年発症の）early-onset （時期尚早の）premature ▶若年型糖尿病 juvenile diabetes 若年性アルツハイマー病 early-onset Alzheimer disease 若年性関節リウマチ juvenile rheumatoid arthritis；JRA 若年性白髪 premature gray hair

じゃくようせい　弱陽性(の)　weak positive, weakly positive

しゃけい　斜頸　wryneck, torticollis ◀眼性斜頸 ocular torticollis 筋性斜頸 muscular torticollis 痙性斜頸 spasmodic torticollis 耳性斜頸 otogenic torticollis

しゃけつ　瀉血　phlebotomy

しゃこう　社交(の) （人付き合いの良い）social, sociable （外向的な）outgoing ◆彼には社交性がある He is quite a social[sociable] person. / He mixes well with other people. ◆彼女はあまり社交的なタイプではない She is not the social[sociable] type. ◆社交的な性格 an outgoing personality ▶社交恐怖 social phobia 社交不安症 social anxiety disorder；SAD

しゃざい　謝罪　apology（動apologize）☞謝る，すみません，申し訳，詫びる

しゃし　斜視　strabismus, squint （寄り目）crossed eyes ◆斜視がある have a squint / （内斜視）have crossed eyes ◀外斜視 external[divergent] strabismus / exotropia；XT 仮性斜視[偽斜視] false strabismus / pseudostrabismus 顕性斜視 manifest strabismus 交代性斜視 alternating strabismus 上下斜視 vertical strabismus 内斜視 internal[convergent] strabismus / esotropia；ET / crossed eyes 非共同性斜視 incomitant strabismus

しゃしん　写真 （一般的に）picture, photograph, photo （フィルム）film ◆それでは今から胸のＸ線写真を撮ります Well now, I'm going to take an X-ray of your chest. ◆この CT 写真を見て下さい Please look at this CT film. ◆病変部の写真を撮らせていただいてもよろしいですか May I take a picture of the lesion? ◀超音波写真 ultrasound film Ｘ線写真 X-ray[x-ray] film

しゃせい　射精　ejaculation（動ejaculate）☞巻末付録：訊きにくい質問のコツ ◆射精に問題がありますか Do you have any problems[trouble] ejaculating? / Do you have any ejaculation problems? ◆射精時に痛みがありますか Do you experience any pain during ejaculation? ◆射精が早すぎる have premature ejaculation ◆射精に時間がかかる have delayed ejaculation ◆射精をコントロールする control ejaculation ◀逆行性射精 retrograde ejaculation

しゃだん　遮断する （遮る・阻止する）block （止める）stop （切り離す）cut off ◆負の連鎖反応を遮断する block[cut off] a negative chain reaction ◀遮断薬

しゃだんやく　遮断薬　blocker, blocking medication[drug, agent] ◀アドレナリン遮断薬 adrenergic blocker カルシウムチャネル遮断薬 calcium channel blocker 競合的遮断薬 competitive blocker 副交感神経遮断薬 parasympatholytics / parasympathetic blocking medication[drug / agent]

シャツ　shirt （下着）undershirt ☞下着

じゃっかん　若干(の) （いくらか）some （ちょっと）a little ☞少し

しゃっくり　hiccups ★通例，複数形で。 ◆しゃっくりがよく出ますか Do you often have[get] (the) hiccups? ◆しゃっくりが止まらない can't get rid of (the) hiccups

しゃっこつ　尺骨　ulna（形ulnar） ▶尺骨管症候群 ulnar tunnel syndrome 尺骨神経 ulnar nerve

しゃび　斜鼻　crooked nose, twisted nose

しゃふつしょうどく　煮沸消毒する　steri-

lize … by boiling（図sterilization[disinfection] by boiling）　◆哺乳瓶を煮沸消毒する sterilize a baby's bottle by boiling

しゃぶりだこ　◆指を吸い過ぎてしゃぶりだこができる have a callus from sucking *one's* thumb too much　★callus は皮膚肥厚・たこをさす．

しゃぶる　suck /sʌ́k/　◆親指をしゃぶる suck *one's* thumb　◆おしゃぶりをしゃぶる suck on a pacifier　◆おしゃぶり（形が乳首をした）pacifier / dummy /（リング状の）teething ring　指しゃぶり（親指の）thumb-sucking /（手指の）finger-sucking

しゃべる　talk　（雑談する）chat, have a chat　☞話す　◆少しおしゃべりしませんか Can we have a little chat? / How about talking with me for a while?

じゃま　邪魔する
《妨害する》disturb　（行く手をふさいでいる）be in the way　◆通行の邪魔になりますので，お荷物は窓際にお寄せ下さい Your things are in the way. Please move them closer to the window.
《挨拶として》　◆お邪魔ではないでしょうか I hope I'm not disturbing you.　◆ちょっとお邪魔してよろしいですか May I come in for a moment? / Do you mind if I come in for a moment?　◆お邪魔しました Thank you for your time.　★I've enjoyed talking with you. / It was good talking with you. / I must be going now. などともいう．

シャルコーかんせつ　―関節　Charcot joint

しゃれい　謝礼　（専門職への礼金）fee　（お礼）reward　（贈り物）thank-you gift　◆謝礼を支払う pay a fee　◆謝礼として（感謝のしるしとして）as a gesture of thanks / as a thank-you gift　◆謝礼はお受けできません．お気持ちだけいただきます I'm not allowed to accept（thank-you）gifts, but I do appreciate the thought[gesture].

シャワー　shower　◆シャワーは結構ですが，お風呂には入らないで下さい You can take a shower, but avoid taking a bath.　◆シャワーやお風呂はぬるま湯にして下さい Please take a shower or bathe in

lukewarm water.　◆シャワーを浴びてはいかがですか．さっぱりしますよ How about taking a shower. It'll help you feel refreshed.　▶シャワー室 shower room

シャント　shunt　◆透析のためのシャントを造設する create a shunt for use in dialysis　◀髄液シャント cerebrospinal fluid shunt　動静脈シャント arteriovenous shunt

ジャンパーひざ　―膝　jumper's knee

シャンプー　shampoo /ʃæmpúː/　◆どんなシャンプーを使っていますか What type of shampoo do you use?　◆シャンプーをいたしましょうか Would you like（to have）a shampoo?　◆シャンプーをしましょう Let me give you a shampoo.

しゅ　主（たる）　main, chief, primary　☞主な

しゅいん　主因　（最重要の原因）the primary cause　（主な要因）the main factor

しゅう　週　week；w, wk　（図weekly）
◆週に何回くらいお酒を飲みますか How often *in a week[per week]* do you drink alcohol? / On average, how many times in the[a] week do you drink alcohol?
◆その時妊娠は何週でしたか How many weeks pregnant were you then?　◆週に1回〈2回 / 3回〉once〈twice / three times〉a week　◆週の前半 the first half of the week　◆週の後半 the latter[second] half of the week　◀隔週 every other week　今週〈先週 / 来週〉this〈last / next〉week　★week の前に this, last, next が来る時には前置詞 in は付けない．　妊娠週数 week of pregnancy[gestation] / gestational week　毎週 every[each] week
▶週末に on weekends

―しゅう　―臭　（一般的に）smell　（嫌なにおい）odor　◆アルコール臭 alcohol（breath）odor

じゆう　自由　（他の影響を受けず意のままになる状態）freedom（図free）　（公権力から思想・行動を抑圧されない状態・権利）liberty　◆病院内はどうぞ自由に歩いて下さい Please feel free to walk about inside the hospital.　◆どうぞ自由に質問して下さい Please feel free to ask questions. ◆動作の自由を制限する restrict *a person's* freedom of movement ◆彼は脳血栓で右半身の自由がききません He can't move the right side of his body as a result of a cerebral thrombosis. ◆行動の自由 freedom of movement[action] ▶自由意志[意思] freedom of will / free will　自由時間 free time　自由連想法 free association

じゅうあつ　**重圧**　**burden**　☞プレッシャー　◆精神的な重圧がある carry a psychological burden　▶重圧感(胃の)feeling of heaviness (in the stomach)

しゅうい　**周囲**　(周辺)**circumference**, **periphery** (回り)**around** (付近の)**surrounding** (頭peri-)　☞周辺, 周り　◆周囲に同じような症状の人がいますか Does anyone around you have similar symptoms? ◆口の周囲がしびれる feel numb around *one's* mouth ◆周囲の環境 the surrounding environment ◀ウエスト周囲長 waist circumference　肛門周囲膿瘍 perianal abscess　扁桃周囲膿瘍 peritonsillar abscess　▶周囲浸潤麻酔 field block (anesthesia) ☞周囲炎

じゅうい　**獣医(師)**　**veterinarian**; **vet**, **animal doctor** ▶獣医学 veterinary medicine

しゅういえん　**周囲炎**　◀肩関節周囲炎 periarthritis of the shoulder / scapulohumeral periarthritis / stiff shoulder　智歯周囲炎 pericoronitis of a wisdom tooth　扁桃周囲炎 peritonsillitis　毛包周囲炎 perifolliculitis

じゅういちがつ　**11月**　**November**; **Nov.** ☞1月

じゅうおうひ　**縦横比**　**depth-width ratio**

じゅうかく　**縦隔**　**mediastinum** (mediastinal) ▶縦隔炎 mediastinitis　縦隔気腫 mediastinal emphysema　縦隔鏡検査 mediastinoscopy　縦隔腫瘍 mediastinal tumor　縦隔リンパ節 mediastinal lymph node

しゅうがくじけんしん　**就学児健診**　**school entry health checkup**

しゅうがくてきちりょう　**集学的治療**　multidisciplinary treatment

じゅうがつ　**10月**　**October**; **Oct.**　☞1月

じゅうかぶつ　**臭化物**　**bromide**

しゅうかん[1]　**習慣**　(個人の習慣・癖)**habit** (habitual) (意識的に実践する習慣)**practice** (日常の仕事・雑事)**routine** (社会のしきたり)**custom** ◆慣習, 癖 ◆飲酒は習慣になっていますか Is your drinking a habit? / Are you a habitual drinker? ◆よい習慣を身につけて下さい You should develop good habits in your daily life. ◆あなたは生活習慣を変える必要があります You need to make *some changes to your lifestyle[some lifestyle changes]. ◆生活習慣を改める modify *one's* daily habits ◆散歩を習慣づける make a habit of taking a walk ◆長年の習慣を直す break a long-standing habit ◆この薬には習慣性があります This medication *may become [is] habit-forming[addictive]. ▶習慣性嘔吐 habitual vomiting　習慣性脱臼 habitual dislocation　習慣性チック habit[habitual] tic　習慣性便秘 habitual constipation　習慣性薬物 habit-forming drug[substance]　習慣流産 habitual abortion ☞食習慣, 生活習慣

しゅうかん[2]　**週間**　**week**　☞週　◆2, 3週間 a few weeks / a couple of weeks

じゅうかんきょう　**住環境**　(住宅事情)**housing conditions[situation]** (生活環境)**living conditions**　★condition は通例, 複数形で.

しゅうかんしょう　**臭汗症**　**bromidrosis**

しゅうき[1]　**周期**　(循環する過程)**cycle** (cyclic) (一定の期間)**period** /píriəd/ (定期的な)**periodic**, **periodical**) ◆その痛みは周期性ですか Does the pain come on at regular intervals? / Is the pain periodic? ◆周期的に起こる occur[come on] periodically ◆短い周期で in short cycles ◆周期性の痛み (a) periodic pain ◀月経周期 menstrual cycle　睡眠周期 sleep cycle　排卵周期 ovulation cycle　毛周期 hair cycle ▶周期性アルブミン尿 cyclic albuminuria　周期性嘔吐 periodic vomiting　周期性過眠 periodic hypersomnia 周期性呼吸 periodic respiration 周期性麻痺 periodic paralysis 周期熱 periodic fever

しゅうき² 臭気 bad smell, offensive odor, unpleasant odor ☞におい

しゅうきゅう 週休 ◆お勤め先は週休2日制ですか Are you on a five-day (work) week in your company? / Does you company have a five-day week?

じゅうきょ 住居 house, residence ☞住宅, 住まい

しゅうきょう 宗教 religion (麗religious) ◆あなたの宗教は何ですか What's your religious background? / Could you tell me your religion? ★この質問は唐突にならないように，前もって"Are you religious?"などと訊いてからにするとよい.
◆宗教上の理由で食べられないものはありますか Are there any kinds of food that you can't eat for religious reasons? ◆宗教上，何かご要望や食事の制限はありますか Do you have any religious needs or dietary restrictions? ◆彼は宗教上の理由で肉〈豚肉〉を食べません He doesn't eat meat〈pork〉for religious reasons.

宗教の確認

外国人患者を受け入れる場合には宗教に関する情報を得る必要がある．病気とは無関係のように思われるが，宗教上の理由で，ある種の診療拒否や輸血などの治療拒否もありうるし，イスラム教徒は豚肉を食べない，あるいは1日に5回メッカの方向に向かってお祈りをするなど，食事や生活面などにも配慮が必要な場合が出てくるかもしれない．また危篤状態になったとき宗旨によっては特別な儀式を行うので，前もって訊いておきたい．

● キリスト教 Christianity / キリスト教徒 Christian
● カトリック教 Catholicism / カトリック教徒 Catholic
● プロテスタント(新教)Protestantism / プロテスタント Protestant
● ギリシャ正教 Orthodox Christianity / ギリシャ正教徒 Orthodox Christian
● ユダヤ教 Judaism / ユダヤ教徒 Jewish ★Jew は差別的な響きがあるので避ける.
● イスラム教 Islam / イスラム教徒 Muslim
● ヒンズー教 Hinduism / ヒンズー教徒 Hindu
● シーク教 Sikhism / シーク教徒 Sikh
● 仏教 Buddhism / 仏教徒 Buddhist
● エホバの証人 Jehovah's Witnesses / エホバの証人の信徒 Jehovah's Witness
● 無神論 atheism / 無神論者 atheist
★カルテに記載する場合，宗教を書く欄があれば，その他の宗教という意味で"other"としたり，特定の宗教を持たないことを示すために"none"と書いてもよい.

じゅうきんぞく 重金属 heavy metal
▶重金属中毒 heavy metal poisoning

しゅうけいきょうふ 醜形恐怖 dysmorphophobia (醜形恐怖症)body dysmorpric disorder

じゅうけつ 充血 congestion (麗congested), injection, hyperemia (怒張)engorgement (麗目が血走った bloodshot)
◆充血した目をしている have bloodshot eyes /（炎症を起こしている）have inflamed eyes ◀結膜充血 conjunctival injection / congestion of the conjunctiva

じゅうけつきゅうちゅう 住血吸虫 schistosome, blood fluke ▶住血吸虫症 schistosomiasis

しゅうさんき 周産期 the perinatal period ▶周産期医学 perinatal medicine / perinatology 周産期医療センター perinatal medical center 周産期ケア perinatal care 周産期死亡 perinatal death

しゅうし 修士 （修士号）master's degree ▶修士課程 master's (degree) program

じゅうじ 従事する （活動・仕事をする）be engaged (in) （職業などに携わる）be employed (in) （関与している）be involved (in) ◆現在彼女は膵臓がんの研究に従事しています She is currently engaged in pancreatic cancer research. ◆建設業に

従事したことがありますか Have you ever been (employed) in the construction business? ◀医療従事者 the medical staff[personnel]

じゅうじじんたい 十字靱帯 cruciate ligament ◀後十字靱帯 posterior cruciate ligament；PCL 膝十字靱帯 cruciate ligament of the knee 前十字靱帯 anterior cruciate ligament；ACL

じゅうじつ 充実(した) (中身の詰まった)solid (生活・仕事に満足できる)fulfilling (図fulfillment) ◆毎日の生活は充実していますか Is your everyday life fulfilling? ◆仕事は充実していますか Is your work fulfilling? / Does your work give you a sense of fulfillment? ◆充実性腫瘤 solid tumor

しゅうしゅう¹ 収拾する (決着をつける)settle (解決する)solve ◆事態を収拾する settle the situation ◆問題を収拾する solve the problem

しゅうしゅう² 収集する gather (目的をもって集める)collect (図collection) ◆前立腺がんの情報を収集する gather[collect] information about[on] prostate cancer ◆データ収集 data collection

しゅうしゅく 収縮 (筋肉などの収縮)contraction (↔dilation)(形contractile) (血管などの収縮や狭窄)constriction (形constrictive) (萎縮)shrinkage (形心収縮の)systolic ◆気管支収縮 bronchoconstriction 筋収縮 muscle contraction 血管収縮 vasoconstriction / constriction of the blood vessels 子宮収縮 uterine contraction 随意〈不随意〉収縮 voluntary〈involuntary〉contraction 線維性収縮 fibrillation 線維束性収縮 fasciculation 等尺性〈等張性〉収縮 isometric〈isotonic〉contraction 律動性収縮 rhythmic contraction ▶収縮期(心臓の)systolic period / (筋肉の)contractile period 収縮期血圧 systolic blood pressure 収縮期雑音 systolic murmur 収縮筋 contractile muscle 収縮性心膜炎 constrictive pericarditis

しゅうじゅつき 周術期(の) perioperative ▶周術期看護 perioperative nursing 周術期管理 perioperative management 周術期ケア perioperative care

じゅうしょ 住所 address /ǽdres/ ◆ご住所はどちらですか What's your (home) address? ◆この欄に住所と名前を書いて下さい Please write down your name and address in this space. ★日本語は住所，氏名の順で言うが，英語では順序が逆で名前が先に来る. ◆自宅の住所 one's home address ◆仕事場の住所 one's work address ◆現住所 one's present[current] address

しゅうしょう 愁傷 ◆ご愁傷さまです I'm very sorry for your loss. / Please accept my sincere condolences[sympathy] (for the loss of someone).

じゅうしょう¹ 重症(の) (病状が深刻な)serious, seriously ill[sick] (図serious illness) (危篤の)critical, critically ill[sick] (命に関わる)life-threatening (病気・怪我が重い)severe (図重症度 severity) ▶重度，重篤 ◆お気の毒ですが，彼は重症です I'm sorry but he is very[critically] ill. / I'm afraid that he is in (a) serious[critical] condition. ◆重症の患者 a seriously ill patient / (ハイリスクの)a high-risk patient ◆重症化する become seriously[critically] ill ▶重症急性呼吸器症候群 severe acute respiratory syndrome；SARS 重症筋無力症 myasthenia gravis；MG 重症度指数 severity score 重症度分類 classification of severity 重症複合免疫不全症 severe combined immunodeficiency；SCID

じゅうしょう² 重傷 (重い怪我)serious injury[wound] (致命的な怪我)fatal injury[wound] ◆交通事故で重傷を負う be seriously injured in a traffic accident ◆彼女の怪我は重傷ですが，命に関わることはありません Her injury is serious, but not life-threatening. ◆頭に重傷を負う have a serious head injury / have a serious injury to the head

しゅうしん¹ 終身(の) (生涯続く)lifelong (図for life, all through one's life) ▶終身介護 lifelong care

しゅうしん² 就寝する go to bed (寝入

る)fall asleep ☞眠る，寝る ◆この薬は就寝時に〈就寝直前に〉服用して下さい Please take this medication *at bedtime〈right before bedtime〉. ◆就寝中に during *one's* sleep / while sleeping ▶就寝時間 bedtime / time to go to bed

じゅうしん 重心 （体のバランス）balance （圖balance）（重力の中心）the center of gravity ☞バランス ◆重心を失う lose *one's* balance ◆重心をとる balance *oneself*

ジュース （果汁）juice （清涼飲料）soft drink (s) ◆りんごジュースはいかがですか Would you like[care for] some apple juice? ◆ジュースに薬を混ぜて飲む take the medication mixed with juice ◆野菜ジュースは糖分が少ない Vegetable juices are low in sugar.

しゅうせい 修正する （改訂）revise （圖revision）（全面変更）change（圖change）（部分変更）alter（圖alteration）（一部修正）modify（圖modification）☞変える，変更

しゅうせいだいけっかんてんい 修正大血管転位 corrected transposition of the great arteries

しゅうせいめんえき 終生免疫 lifelong immunity

しゅうせき 集積 （蓄積）accumulation （同種のものが集まること）clustering, cluster （統合）integration（圖integrated）◆家族集積性 familial[family] clustering ◆集積回路 integrated circuit

じゅうせき 重積 overlapping ◀頭蓋骨重積 overlapping of the cranial bones 喘息発作重積状態 status asthmaticus 腸重積 intussusception（of the intestine）てんかん重積状態 status epilepticus

しゅうそ¹ 臭素 bromine

しゅうそ² 愁訴 complaint ◀更年期愁訴 menopausal[climacteric] complaint ☞不定愁訴

じゅうそう¹ 重曹 sodium bicarbonate, bicarbonate of soda, baking soda

じゅうそう² 銃創 gunshot wound

じゅうそう³ 縦走（の） longitudinal ▶縦走潰瘍 longitudinal ulcer

じゅうたい 重体（の）（危篤の）critical （病状が深刻な）serious （命に関わる）life-threatening ▶重症

じゅうだい 重大（な）（重要な）important （意義深い）significant （深刻な）serious, grave ◆これは重大な問題です This is *an important[a serious] problem. / This is a matter of grave concern. ◆重大な過ち a serious mistake[error]

じゅうたく 住宅 house, residence （住環境）housing ☞住まい ▶住宅事情 housing conditions[situation] /（生活環境）living conditions ★condition は通例，複数形で. 住宅手当 housing benefit 住宅問題 housing problem

しゅうだん 集団 group （圖大規模な mass, large-scale）☞グループ ◀母集団 population ▶集団感染 mass infection 集団検診 mass screening 集団食中毒 mass[large-scale outbreak of] food poisoning 集団心理学 group psychology 集団精神療法 group psychotherapy 集団発生 *mass outbreak[epidemic] 集団保育 group *day care[nursery] 集団療法 group therapy

じゅうたんさん 重炭酸 bicarbonate ▶重炭酸緩衝系 the bicarbonate buffer system 重炭酸透析 bicarbonate dialysis

しゅうちゅう 集中する concentrate (on)（圖concentration）（重点を置く）focus (on)（圖intensive）◆集中力に変化がありましたか Have you noticed any changes in your ability to concentrate? ◆以前楽しんでやっていた活動に集中するのが難しいですか Do you have difficulty concentrating on activities that you once enjoyed? ◆集中力に欠ける lack concentration / lack the ability to concentrate ◆当面は疼痛管理に集中して治療にあたる treat *the patient*, focusing for the time being on pain management ◆抗がん剤を集中的に投与する administer dose-intensive[dose-intense] chemotherapy ☞集中治療室

しゅうちゅうちりょうしつ 集中治療室 intensive care unit；ICU, intensive care

room ◆手術後は集中治療室で麻酔から覚めることになるでしょう After the surgery, you'll wake up in the ICU[intensive care unit] after the anesthesia wears off. ◆集中治療室に入っている be in the intensive care room ◀冠疾患集中治療室 coronary care unit；CCU　新生児集中治療室 neonatal[newborn] intensive care unit；NICU　母体胎児集中治療室 maternal fetal intensive care unit；MFICU

じゅうてん[1]　**充塡 filling**（略fill）　▶充塡剤 filling material / filler　充塡歯 filled tooth

じゅうてん[2]　**重点**（強調）**emphasis**（優先）**priority**（焦点）**focus**（略focus）（重視・力点）**stress** ◆この治療は痛みの緩和に重点を置いています The emphasis[priority] in this treatment is on pain relief. / This treatment focuses on pain relief. ◆けがを予防するための機能訓練を重点的に行う treat *patients* with an emphasis on functional training to prevent injury

じゅうど　**重度（の）**（病気・怪我が重い）**severe**（⟷mild）（状態が深刻な）**serious**（重大な）**major**（⟷minor）☞重症, 重篤 ◆重度の障害がある be severely[seriously] disabled[challenged] ◆重度のやけど a severe[serious / major] burn　▶重度障害者 severely disabled[challenged] person / person with *severe disabilities[a serious disability]　重度精神遅滞 severe mental retardation

しゅうどう　**肢誘導 limb lead** ◀標準肢誘導 standard limb lead

じゅうどうせいふくし　**柔道整復師 judo therapist, bonesetter**；BS

じゅうとく　**重篤（な）**（病状が非常に深刻な）**very serious**（危篤の）**critical**（命に関わる）**life-threatening** ☞重症, 重度 ◆重篤な合併症 very serious complications ◆重篤な副作用 a very serious adverse effect[reaction]

じゅうなん　**柔軟（な）**（弾力性に富んだ）**flexible**（略flexibility）（伸縮性の）**stretching** ◆仕事のスケジュールに柔軟性はありますか Do you have a flexible work

schedule? / Is there any flexibility with your work schedule? ◆柔軟性のある勤務時間 flexible working hours ◆柔軟体操をすると関節の可動域が拡がります Stretching exercises will improve the range of motion in your joints.

じゅうにがつ　**12月 December; Dec.** ☞1月

じゅうにしちょう　**十二指腸 duodenum** /djùːoʊdíːnəm/（略duodenal）　▶胃十二指腸潰瘍 gastroduodenal ulcer　膵頭十二指腸切除術 pancreaticoduodenectomy　▶十二指腸潰瘍 duodenal ulcer　十二指腸穿孔 duodenal perforation

しゅうにゅう　**収入 income** ☞所得 ◆安定した収入がある have a steady income ◆収入が不安定である the income is not steady / the income is precarious

じゅうびょう　**重病 serious illness** ☞重症 ◆彼女は重病です She is seriously [critically] ill. ▶重病患者 seriously ill patient

じゅうひようぼはん　**獣皮様母斑 giant hairy nevus**

しゅうふく　**修復する repair**（図repair），**perform a repair**（復元する）**restore**（図restoration） ◆外科的修復を行う repair surgically / perform a surgical repair ◆夫婦関係を修復する restore a marriage (relationship)

じゅうふく　**重複（の）** ☞ダブる, 重複（ちょうふく）

じゅうぶん　**十分（な）**（量が必要を満たす）**enough, sufficient**（沢山の）**plenty of**（満足できる）**satisfactory, good enough**（最大の）**full** ☞たっぷり ◆時間は十分にあります We have enough[plenty of] time. ◆休息と睡眠を十分にとって下さい Please get plenty of rest and sleep. ◆その説明は十分ではありませんでした The explanation wasn't *good enough[satisfactory]. ◆十分な証拠を集める collect enough[sufficient] evidence ◆患者のプライバシーに十分配慮する pay sufficient attention to a patient's privacy

しゅうへき　**習癖 habit** ☞癖, 習慣

しゅうへん 周辺 periphery (📖peripheral), circumference (副📖周りに around) ◆周囲, 周り ◆目の周辺部 the area around *one's* eyes ▶周辺視 peripheral[side] vision 周辺視野 peripheral visual field

しゅうまつ 終末 end (📖terminal, final) ▶終末回腸 terminal ileum 終末細気管支 terminal bronchiole ☞終末期

しゅうまつき 終末期 the terminal stage, the last stage, the final stage ☞末期 ▶終末期医療 terminal (medical) care / end-of-life care 終末期がん患者 terminal cancer patient 終末期緩和ケア terminal palliative care

じゅうまん 充満する be filled with, be full of ◆副鼻腔内に膿が充満しています Your (paranasal) sinus is filled with pus.

しゅうみん 就眠する ☞就寝

じゅうみん 住民 resident ◆市〈町／村〉で行う住民健診を受ける have a health checkup for city〈town／village〉 residents ◀地域住民 local[community] resident

しゅうめい 羞明 (光線過敏) photophobia, photosensitivity, light sensitivity

じゅうもう 絨毛 villus (📖villous) (絨毛膜) chorion, chorionic membrane (📖chorionic) ▶絨毛運動 villous movement 絨毛癌 choriocarcinoma 絨毛採取 chorionic villus sampling；CVS

じゅうよう 重要(な) (大切な) important (極めて重要な) vital (鍵となる) key (意義深い) significant (不可欠な) essential ☞大事 ◆規則正しい運動は健康にとって重要です Regular exercise is important[vital] for your health. ◆ここに重要事項が書かれていますので, よくお読み下さい This contains some important information that you should know, so please read it carefully. ◆そのことはさほど重要ではありません That's not so important. ◆緩和ケアにはご家族が重要な役割を果たします The family plays *an important[a key] role in a patient's* palliative care. ◆重要な問題について話し合う discuss *an im-portant[a significant] matter* ▶重要臓器 vital organs ★通例, 複数形で.

しゅうり 修理 repair (📖repair) ☞修復

じゅうりゅうしせんちりょう 重粒子線治療 heavy particle radiotherapy

しゅうりょう 終了する (一般的に) be over, end (完了する) finish, be finished (閉じる) close ☞終わる ◆手術は1時頃に終了する予定です The surgery will *be over[end] at approximately one o'clock.*

じゅうりょう 重量 weight ▶重量感覚 sense of weight / weight perception

じゅうりょく 重力 gravity ◀抗重力筋 antigravity muscle 無重力状態 weight-lessness / zero gravity

しゅうれんやく 収斂薬 astringent

しゅうろう 就労する (働く) work (雇用される) be employed ☞仕事, 働く ◀不法就労者 illegal[illegally-employed] worker ▶就労時間〈日数〉 working hours〈days〉 就労ビザ work[working] visa

しゅえい 守衛 (警備員)(security) guard (用務員) janitor ◆守衛を呼ぶ call a guard

しゅかん 主観(的な) subjective (↔objective) ◆主観的な症状 a subjective symptom ◆主観的な見かた a subjective view

しゅかんせつ 手関節 wrist joint

しゅぎ 主義 (行動規範) principle (決まり事・習慣) rule ◆今提案しているように生活を変更するのはあなたの主義に反していますか Is it against your principles to change your way of living in the way that I'm suggesting? ◆晩酌は欠かさない主義ですか Is it a rule of yours to always have a drink with dinner?

じゅくこう 熟考する ☞熟慮

しゅくしゅ 宿主 host ◀易感染性宿主 compromised host / (免疫不全の) immunocompromised host ▶宿主寄生体関係 host-parasite relationship 宿主適応 host adaptation

じゅくしゅ 粥腫 ☞アテローム

しゅくしょう 縮小する (縮む) shrink (小さくなる) become smaller (収縮する) constrict (📖constriction) (減らす) reduce

しゅくしょう　328　しゅじゅつ

（図reduction）　◆（がんの）原発巣の大きさが縮小しました The primary lesion has shrunk[become smaller].　◀瞳孔縮小 pupil[pupillary] constriction / miosis　▶縮小手術 limited surgery

じゅくじょうこうか　粥状硬化（症） atherosclerosis

しゅくすい　宿酔　☞二日酔い　◀放射線宿酔 radiation sickness

じゅくすい　熟睡する have a sound sleep, sleep soundly[well]　☞眠る　◆熟睡している be fast[sound] asleep　◆熟睡できないのですか Are you not able to have a sound sleep? / Can you not get a good sleep?　◆熟睡感がないのですか Do you feel unable to have a sound sleep?　◆昨晩は熟睡できましたか Did you sleep well last night?

しゅくだい　宿題 homework　（研究課題）assignment　（解決すべき問題）subject, problem

しゅくどう　縮瞳 pupil constriction, pupillary constriction, miosis　▶縮瞳薬 miotic (medication / drug / eye drop)

しゅくはく　宿泊する stay overnight　◆個室では，ご家族も患者さんと一緒に宿泊することが可能です Family members can[may] stay overnight with patients in private rooms.

しゅくべん　宿便 stool impaction, fecal impaction : *mass of hardened stool that becomes stuck in the intestine*　☞便秘　▶宿便性潰瘍 stercoral ulcer

じゅくみん　熟眠　☞熟睡

じゅくりょ　熟慮する think over, consider　◆熟慮なさってから最終的な結論を出して下さい Please *think it over[think about it very carefully] before you make a final decision.

しゅこん　手根 wrist, carpus（図carpal）　▶手根管 carpal tunnel　手根間関節 intercarpal joint　手根管症候群 carpal tunnel syndrome　手根骨 carpal[wrist] bone

しゅさ　酒皶 rosacea　▶酒皶性痤瘡 acne rosacea

じゅさんしせつ　授産施設 sheltered workshop[work institution]

しゅし[1]　手指 finger　（親指）thumb（図digital）　◆手，指　◆手指の間まで石鹸で丁寧に洗って下さい Please wash your hands properly with soap, including between the fingers.　▶手指失認 finger agnosia　手指切断 digital amputation　手指変形 digital deformity

しゅし[2]　主旨 main point　（根本となる原理）main principle　（物事のかなめ）keystone　◆この治療の主旨をご説明いたします Let me explain the main point[principle] of this treatment.

しゅし[3]　趣旨　（目的）purpose, aim　（意図）point　◆ご提案の趣旨をお聞かせいただけますか Could you tell me the purpose[aim] of your proposal? / What's the main point of your proposal?　◆お話の趣旨はよくわかります I understand *what you meant[what you're saying]. / I [understand] your point.

じゅし　樹脂 resin　◀合成樹脂 synthetic resin / plastic

しゅじい　主治医　（病院の担当医）attending physician, doctor in charge　☞担当医　（かかりつけ医）regular doctor[physician]　（家庭医）family doctor[physician]

しゅじゅ　種々（の）　（多種類の）many kinds[sorts] of　（いろいろの）various, a variety of　（いくつかの）a number of　☞いろいろ，様々　◆治療には種々の選択肢があります There are *many kinds of[various] treatment options available.　◆種々の理由で手術は延期されました Surgery was put off for a number of reasons.

しゅじゅつ　手術 surgery（図surgical）, operation（図operative）　（外科的処置）(surgical) procedure　◆（医師が）胆嚢の手術をする perform[do] surgery[an operation] on *the patient's gallbladder　◆（患者が）手術を受ける have[undergo] surgery[an operation]　◆手術前 before surgery / preoperatively　◆手術後 after surgery / postoperatively　◆手術当日 the day of surgery　◆手術中に during (the) surgery

《手術歴》 ◆手術を受けたことがありますか Have you ever had (any) surgery before? ◆何の手術でしたか What surgery did you have? ◆手術はいつでしたか When was the surgery? ◆どこの病院で手術を受けましたか In what hospital did you have the surgery?

《手術時期》 ◆虫垂が炎症を起こして破れる寸前なので，すぐに手術をする必要があります You need to have surgery on your appendix immediately because it is inflamed and about to rupture. ◆手術を急ぐ必要はありません You don't have to rush into having the surgery. / There's no hurry to have the surgery. ◆この手術に緊急性はないので，いつするかはあなた次第です This surgery is not an emergency, so *you can wait until you feel it's necessary [when to have it is up to you].

《手術の説明》 ◆あとで外科医が手術についてあなたとご家族に説明いたします The surgeon will *explain the surgery to[discuss the surgery with] you and your family later. ◆麻酔医が麻酔について説明します Your anesthesiologist will explain[talk to you about] your anesthesia. ◆手術は乳房温存術を予定しています The surgery you're going to have is breast-conserving surgery. ◆ポリープをとる手術をお勧めします I recommend surgery to remove the polyp(s). ◆この手術は外来で行います This is an outpatient procedure. / This surgery will be performed on an outpatient basis. ◆これは日常的によく行う手術で，手術成績も非常に良好です This is routine surgery, with very good (surgical) outcomes. ◆残念ですが，この手術が成功する確率は50％未満です I'm afraid to say that the chances of success with this surgery are not more than fifty percent. ◆手術中あるいは術後に輸血が必要になるかもしれません You may need (to have) a blood transfusion during or after the surgery.

《手術までの流れ》 ◆水曜日の午前に手術の予定です Your surgery is scheduled for Wednesday morning. ◆手術は朝9時から行います The surgery will start at nine in the morning. ◆手術はおよそ3時間かかります The surgery will take about three hours. ◆全身麻酔なので手術中は眠っていて痛みはありません You'll be under general anesthesia for this surgery, so it'll put you to sleep and you won't feel[have] any pain during the surgery. ◆局所麻酔ですから手術中目が覚めているでしょう You'll have a local anesthetic[You'll be under local anesthesia], so you'll be awake during the surgery. ◆手術当日の朝，装身具，入れ歯，コンタクトレンズなどをすべてとって，このガウンに着替えます On the day of the surgery, we will ask you to remove all jewelry, dentures, and contact lenses, and to change into this gown. ◆朝7時に手術室にお連れします We're going to take you to the operating room at seven in the morning. ◆手術前日の晩よく眠れるように睡眠薬を差し上げます The night before the surgery, I'm going to give you a sleeping pill so that you can have a good night's sleep. ◆手術準備のために胸の部分の毛を剃ります To prepare for your surgery, I'm going to shave your chest.

《手術後の声かけ》 ◆手術は終わりました Your surgery is over. ◆手術は無事に終わりました The surgery went well[successfully]. /（うまくいった）Your surgery was successful. ◆あなたは今ICUにいます You're now in the ICU[intensive care unit]. ◆明日の朝までここで過ごします You'll stay here until tomorrow morning. ◆痛みがありますか Are you having any pain? / Do you have any pain? ◆吐き気がありますか Do you have nausea? / Do you feel nauseous? ◆お水はまだ飲めませんが，唇を湿らせてあげましょう You can't drink water yet, but I'm going to moisten your lips. ◆ガスが出たら知らせて下さい Please let us know when you've passed gas.

◀移植手術 transplant surgery[operation] 開胸手術 thoracotomy / （心臓の）open heart surgery 開腹手術 abdominal surgery / laparotomy 機能温存手術 function-preserving surgery 緊急手術 emergency[urgent] surgery 顕微鏡手術 microsurgery 姑息手術 palliative surgery [procedure] 根治手術 radical surgery 再建手術 reconstructive[reconstruction] surgery 再手術 repeat surgery / resurgery 縮小手術 limited surgery 早期手術 early surgery 待機手術 elective [planned / nonemergency] surgery 大〈小〉手術 major〈minor〉surgery 治癒手術 curative surgery 低侵襲手術 minimally invasive surgery 凍結手術 cryosurgery 内視鏡手術 endoscopic surgery [surgical procedure] 二期的手術 two-stage surgery 日帰り手術 day[same-day] surgery / （外来手術）outpatient[ambulatory] surgery 腹腔鏡下手術 laparoscopic[keyhole] surgery 無輸血手術 surgery without blood transfusion ▶手術器具 surgical instrument[tool] 手術危険度 surgical risk 手術室 operating room；OR 手術侵襲 stress under surgery / surgery stress 手術成績 surgical [surgery] outcome 手術創 surgical wound 手術台 operating[surgical] table 手術体位 surgical position 手術適応 indication for surgery 手術部位 surgical site[area] 手術帽子 surgical cap 手術用手袋 surgical gloves 手術用マスク surgical mask ☞手術同意書，(手)術衣，(手)術後，(手)術前，(手)術中

しゅじゅつどういしょ　手術同意書　(informed) consent form for surgery, surgery consent form ◆手術には手術同意書に署名が必要です You'll need to sign a consent form for the surgery. ◆これは手術同意書です．よく読んで署名と日付を入れて下さい Here is the consent form for your surgery. Please read it carefully, and sign and date[put the date on] it.

しゅしょう　手掌　palm　(㊣palmar) ▶手掌紅斑 palmar erythema / red palm

じゅしょう　受傷する　get[become] injured　(受傷している)be injured, have an injury ☞怪我

じゅじょうさいぼう　樹状細胞　dendritic cell；DC

しゅじん　主人　one's husband ◆（ブラウン夫人に）ご主人にもこの同意書にサインをしていただきたいのですが(Mrs Brown,) may I ask *your husband[Mr Brown] to sign this consent form, too?

じゅしん　受診する　consult　(㊣consultation)　(医師の診察を受ける)see a doctor ★実際の会話では see a dentist, see a dermatologist などと具体的に言う． (来院する)come [go] to the hospital (㊣visit) ◆今日受診された主な理由を話して下さい What's brought you here today? / How can I help you today? ◆当院を以前受診されたことはありますか Have you ever been to our hospital before? / Is this your first visit to our hospital? ◆めまいの原因を調べるために神経内科医を受診することをお勧めします I would recommend that you consult a neurologist to find out what's causing your dizziness. ◆激しい痛みが続くようでしたら当院の救急外来を受診して下さい If the severe pain persists, please come to the emergency room of the hospital. ◆薬が切れたら再度受診して下さい Please *come and see me again [come back again] when your medication runs out. ◆緊急に受診する see a [the] doctor urgently ◀再受診 follow-up consultation[examination] / re-examination / (来院)*follow-up visit[revisit] / (予約)follow-up[return] appointment ▶受診着 hospital gown 受診票 consultation form / registration card 受診料 consultation fee

じゅせい　授精・受精　(精子注入による授精) insemination　(㊣inseminate)　(精子と卵子の融合)fertilization　(㊣fertilize) ◆人工授精する artificially inseminate ◀人工授精 microinsemination / microfertilization 自然受精 natural insemination 人工授精 artificial insemination 体外受精 in vitro fertilization；IVF

じゅせいらん 受精卵 **fertilized egg** （胚）**embryo** ▶受精卵診断 preimplantation assessment[diagnosis]

しゅそ 主訴 **chief complaint**；**CC** ◆主訴を訊く inquire about the chief complaint

しゅたい 主体 ◆糖尿病の治療は食事療法が主体となります Diabetes treatment mainly involves diet therapy. ☞主体的

しゅだい 腫大 ◀腫脹，腫れ ◀肝腫大 hepatomegaly

じゅたいちょうせつ 受胎調節 ☞避妊

しゅたいてき 主体的(に) （ひとりで・独力で）**on** *one's* **own, by** *oneself* （自分で・自分のために）**for** *oneself* （自主的に）**independently** （自発的に）**voluntarily** ◆可能な治療法をいくつか説明しますので，どれにするかはご自身で主体的にご判断下さい I'm going to explain the treatment options available, so please *make your own judgment about[judge for yourself] which one to choose. ◆主体的に行動する act independently[on *one's* own initiative] ◆主体的に治験に参加する voluntarily participate in a clinical trial

しゅだん 手段 （方法）**means** ★単複同形．（やり方）**way** （対策）**measure** （やむをえない手段）**resort** ◆方法 ◆あらゆる手段を尽くします We'll try all possible means. / We'll try every means available. ◆他に手段はなさそうです I'm afraid there's no other way. ◆院内感染を予防する手段を講じる take measures to prevent hospital-acquired infections ◆手術は最後の手段になります We'll do surgery as a last resort. ◆コミュニケーション手段 means of communication

しゅちょう¹ 主張する （言い張る）**insist (on)** （図**insistence**） （事実として言い張る）**claim** （図**claim**） （確信をもって言う）**assert** （図**assertion**） ◆彼は症状が改善していないのに退院すると主張しています He insists on leaving the hospital even though his symptoms have not improved. ◆彼女は父親の死がうつ病の引き金になったと

主張しています She claims that her father's death triggered her depression. ◆権利を主張する assert *one's* right ◀自己主張 self-assertion / self-assertiveness

しゅちょう² 腫脹 （腫れもの）**swelling** （肥大）**enlargement** ☞腫れ ◀陰嚢腫脹 scrotal swelling / swelling of the scrotum 乳頭腫脹（視神経乳頭の）optic disc swelling 脳腫脹 brain[cerebral] swelling 両側肺門リンパ節腫脹 bilateral hilar lymphadenopathy；BHL リンパ節腫脹 lymph node swelling[enlargement]

じゅつい 術衣 （患者用）**hospital gown** （医師用）**surgical gown[wear], scrubs** ★通例，複数形で．

しゅっきん 出勤する **go to work, go to the office** ◆熱が下がっても3日間は出勤を控えて下さい Even if your fever comes [goes] down, please refrain from going to work for three days. ◆出勤は可能ですが，あまり無理をなさらないように You can go to work, but don't *overdo things[work too hard]. ▶出勤拒否 refusal to go to work 出勤日数 the number of days worked 出勤日 working day / workday

しゅっけつ 出血 **bleeding** （颾**bleed**） （専門的に）**hemorrhage** /hémərɪʤ/ （颾**hemorrhage** 颾**hemorrhágic**） ◆出血し始めたのはいつですか When did the bleeding start? ◆出血の場所はどこですか Where is the bleeding? ◆出血の量はどのくらいでしたか How much did you bleed? ◆多量の出血（膨大な）massive [excessive / a lot of / heavy / abundant] bleeding / （激しい）severe bleeding ◆少量の出血 slight[a little bit of / light / a small amount of] bleeding ◆CTの結果では少し出血がみられます The CT shows that there's some slight bleeding. ◆後で少し出血するかもしれませんが，心配はありません You may notice some slight bleeding later, but there's nothing to worry about. ◆（月経時の）通常の出血量はどのくらいですか What is your usual flow? ◆（月経時の）彼女の出血量は通常多め〈普通 / 少なめ〉だ Her menstrual flow is usually heavy〈normal / light〉. / She has heavy〈normal / light〉 periods. ◆腔からの出血がある have some vaginal bleeding ◆歯を磨く時歯肉からの出血がある the gums bleed when *one* brushes *one's* teeth ◆出血が止まらない the bleeding doesn't stop ◆出血を止める stop the bleeding ◆出血多量で死ぬ die from *loss of blood[excessive bleeding] / bleed to death ◀再出血 rebleeding 術後出血 postoperative bleeding[hemorrhage] 潜在出血 occult bleeding 点状出血 petechia / petechial hemorrhage 動脈性出血 arterial bleeding[hemorrhage] 内出血 internal bleeding[hemorrhage] 皮下出血 subcutaneous bleeding [hemorrhage] / bleeding under the skin / (打ち身)bruise 毛細管出血 capillary bleeding ▶出血時間 bleeding time 出血性ショック hemorrhagic shock 出血性素因 hemorrhagic diathesis ☞出血傾向

しゅっけつけいこう 出血傾向 bleeding tendency, tendency to bleed ◆出血傾向がありますか Do you bleed easily? / (皮下出血を起こしやすいか)Do you bruise easily? ◆出血傾向は生まれつきですか Were you born with a bleeding tendency?

しゅつげん 出現する appear (图appearance) (発生する)occur /əkə́ː/ (图occurrence) ◆現れる ◆薬を飲み始めて数日のうちに副作用が出現しました The side effects appeared[occurred] within a few days of starting the medication. ◆新しい症状が後から出現するかもしれません New symptoms may appear later. ◆黄疸が出現している have jaundice / be jaundiced

じゅつご 術後(の) postoperative (圖after surgery, postoperatively) ◆術後の経過は良好です You're making good progress[You're doing well] after the surgery. ◆患者の術後の経過は良好でした (合併症はなかった)The patient's postoperative progress was uncomplicated. ◆術

後6日目に on the sixth postoperative day ▶術後化学療法 postoperative chemotherapy 術後合併症 complication(s) after surgery / postoperative complication(s) 術後感染 postoperative infection 術後管理 postoperative management 術後ケア postoperative care 術後出血 postoperative bleeding[hemorrhage] 術後照射 postoperative irradiation 術後せん妄 postoperative delirium 術後疼痛 postoperative pain 術後肺炎 postoperative pneumonia

しゅっこく 出国する leave a country ◆日本を出国なさる予定はありますか Are you planning on leaving Japan?

しゅっさん 出産 birth (圖give birth, have a baby), childbirth, childbearing (分娩)delivery ☞お産, 分娩 ◆出産したことがありますか Have you ever given birth? ◆最近, 出産しましたか Have you recently had a baby? ◆これまでに何回出産しましたか How many babies[deliveries] have you had? ◆自然分娩, 計画分娩, 無痛分娩など, どのような出産を希望しますか Which childbirth method do you prefer? Natural, planned, or painless delivery? ◆立会い出産をご希望ですか Would you like to have your husband 〈partner〉 in the delivery room? ★partner は夫婦あるいは同棲相手を指す. ◆出産が間近です It's almost time for your baby to be born. / Your baby is due soon. ◀計画出産 planned childbirth 高齢出産 late childbearing 代理出産 surrogate birth 多胎出産 multiple birth ▶出産育児一時金 lump-sum birth allowance / childbirth and nursing allowance 出産可能年齢 childbearing age 出産休暇(母親の)maternity leave / (父親の)paternity leave 出産給付金 childbirth[maternity] benefits 出産手当 maternity allowance 出産方法 childbirth method ☞出産予定日

しゅっさんよていび 出産予定日 due date, expected[estimated] date of delivery ; EDD, expected date of confinement ; EDC, probable date of confinement ; PDC

☞予定日　◆出産予定日はいつですか When is your baby due? / When is your [your baby's] due date?

しゅっしゃ　出社する　☞出勤

しゅっしょう　出生　☞出生（しゅっせい）

しゅっしん　出身　◆ご出身はどちらですか Where are you from?　◆アメリカはどちらのご出身ですか What part of the United States are you from?　▶出身国 one's country / country of origin　出身地 one's hometown

しゅっせい　出生　birth, childbirth　◆出生時の体重はいくらでしたか How much did your baby weigh at birth? / What was your baby's weight at birth?　◆出生地はどこですか What's your place of birth? / Where were you born?　▶出生証明書 birth certificate　☞出生前，出生届，出生率

しゅっせいぜん　出生前（の）　prenatal （胎児の）**fetal**　◆出生前の時期に何か問題がありましたか（妊娠中に）Did you have any problems during pregnancy?　▶出生前ケア prenatal care　出生前診断 prenatal [fetal] diagnosis　出生前治療 prenatal treatment

しゅっせいとどけ　出生届　（通知）**notice of birth, notification of birth**　（登記）**registration of birth**　◆出生届を忘れずに出して下さい Please don't forget to register the birth of your baby. / Please don't forget to have your baby's birth registered.　◆出生届書は（出生日を含めて）14日以内に市役所〈区役所／町役場〉に提出する必要があります You need to submit a notice[notification / report] of birth form to your local city〈ward / town〉office within fourteen days of the birth（including the date of the birth）.

しゅっせいりつ　出生率　birthrate, birth rate　◆出生率の低下 declining birthrate / decrease in the number of children

じゅつぜん　術前（の）　preoperative （圏 **before surgery, preoperatively**）　▶術前オリエンテーション preoperative orientation　術前化学療法 preoperative chemotherapy　術前カンファレンス preoperative confer-

ence　術前管理 preoperative management　術前ケア preoperative care　術前検査 preoperative test[examination]　術前照射 preoperative irradiation

じゅつちゅう　術中（の）　intraoperative （圏 **during surgery, intraoperatively**）　▶術中迅速診断 intraoperative rapid diagnosis　術中モニタリング intraoperative monitoring

しゅっぱつ　出発する　leave, depart （圏 **departure**）　◆日本をいつご出発ですか When are you leaving Japan?　◆ご出発前に一度診察を受けて下さい Please come and see me before your departure.

しゅどう　手動（の）　manual, hand-operated　（自力推進式の）**self-propelled**　▶手動車椅子 manual[self-propelled] wheelchair

じゅどう　受動（的な）　passive （↔active）　◆受動的な動作 a passive movement　▶受動運動 passive exercise [movement]　受動喫煙 passive[（間接的な）indirect / secondhand] smoking　受動状態 passive state　受動免疫 passive immunity[immunization]

しゅとして　主として　mainly, chiefly, mostly　☞主に，主体，中心

じゅにゅう　授乳する　feed （圏 **feeding**）（母乳を与える）**breastfeed** （圏 **breastfeeding**），**nurse** （圏 **nursing**）　☞哺乳　◆現在，授乳していますか Are you breastfeeding now?　◆授乳は何で行っていますか，母乳，ミルク，あるいは混合ですか What are you feeding your baby? Breast milk, formula, or a combination of the two?
◆この薬を飲んでいる間は授乳を控えて下さい While taking this medication, please refrain from breastfeeding.　◆ホプキンズさん，新生児室に行って下さい。授乳のお時間です Mrs Hopkins, please go to the nursery. It's time to feed your baby.　▶授乳間隔 feeding interval　授乳期（乳汁分泌の）lactation period　授乳室 breastfeeding room　授乳性無月経 lactation amenorrhea　授乳不足 underfeeding　授乳用ブラジャー nursing[breastfeeding] bra

しゅにん　主任　（責任者）person in charge　（組織などの長）charge, head　▶主任看護師 charge[head] nurse

しゅひぎむ　守秘義務　(duty of) confidentiality　（医師・患者間の）doctor-patient confidentiality　（医療記録の）duty to keep patient records confidential, duty to protect patient confidentiality　▶守秘義務違反 breach of confidentiality

しゅふ　主婦・主夫　homemaker　（主婦）housewife　（主夫）househusband

しゅみ　趣味　hobby　（気晴らし）pastime　◆どんな趣味をお持ちですか What are your hobbies? / What do you do in your free time?

じゅみょう　寿命　（命の長さ）life span, lifespan　（生命）life　☞命　◆寿命を縮める shorten *one's* life　◆この手術で彼の寿命は延びるでしょう This surgery will prolong his life.　◀平均寿命 average life span

しゅやく　主役　（鍵となる）key role[part]　（第一の）leading role[part]　◆治療の主役はあなたご自身なのですから，もっと積極的に取り組んで下さい You have[play] a key [leading] role in the treatment, so try to be more positive about it.

しゅよう¹　主要（な）　（最も重要な）main, chief　（他と比較して大きな）major　（鍵となる）key　（第一の）leading　◆主な，重要 ◆パーキンソン病の主要な症状 the main [major / key] symptoms of Parkinson disease　◆心不全の主要な原因 the major [leading] cause of heart failure　▶主要組織適合遺伝子複合体 major histocompatibility complex；MHC

しゅよう²　腫瘍　tumor　（新生物）neoplasm　（腰頭onco-）☞がん　◆悪性〈良性〉腫瘍 a malignant〈benign〉tumor　◆胃に腫瘍がありますが，悪性の所見は認められません You have a tumor in your stomach, but the test findings don't show any signs of malignancy.　◆腫瘍は小さいので内視鏡で切除できます The tumor is still small enough that we can *remove it[take it out] using an endoscope.　◆腫瘍が神経

を圧迫しているために痛みや麻痺が起こっているのです The tumor puts pressure on the nerves and causes pain and paralysis.　◆恐らくこの薬で腫瘍は小さくなるでしょう This medication will probably *shrink the tumor[make the tumor smaller].　◆まず放射線治療でできるだけ腫瘍を縮小させましょう First, let's shrink the tumor as much as possible with radiation therapy.　◀原発腫瘍 primary tumor　抗腫瘍薬 antineoplastic （medication / drug / agent)　充実性腫瘍 solid tumor　神経内分泌腫瘍 neuroendocrine tumor　ホルモン産生腫瘍 hormone-producing tumor　▶腫瘍陰影 tumor shadow　腫瘍壊死因子 tumor necrosis factor；TNF　腫瘍学 oncology　腫瘍細胞 tumor cell　腫瘍生検 tumor biopsy　腫瘍切除 tumor resection　腫瘍専門医 oncologist / tumor specialist　腫瘍摘出 tumor excision　腫瘍部位 the site of the tumor　腫瘍免疫 tumor immunity　☞腫瘍マーカー

じゅよう　受容　acceptance （動accept）◆障害の受容 acceptance of disability ◆死を受容する accept death

じゅようたい　受容体　receptor　◀エストロゲン受容体 estrogen receptor　ドパミン受容体刺激薬 dopamine receptor stimulant　ヒスタミン受容体拮抗薬 histamine receptor antagonist　ロイコトリエン受容体拮抗薬 leukotriene receptor antagonist；LTRA

しゅようマーカー　腫瘍マーカー　tumor marker　◆治療で腫瘍マーカー値が下がりました Your tumor marker level has *gone down[decreased] with treatment.　◆腫瘍マーカー値が上がる the tumor marker level *goes up[rises / increases]　◆腫瘍マーカーを測って治療を評価する measure tumor markers for evaluation of the treatment

しゅりゅう　腫瘤　tumor, mass　☞腫瘍 ◀カリフラワー状腫瘤 cauliflower-like tumor　腹部腫瘤 abdominal tumor

しゅりょう　酒量　alcohol consumption ◆1日あたりの酒量はどの程度ですか How

much do you drink a day? ◆酒量がちょっと多いようですね It seems to me that you drink a little too much. ◆酒量を減らす reduce *one's* alcohol consumption ◆酒量が増える〈減る〉drink more〈less〉alcohol than before

しゅるい 種類 kind, sort （タイプ・型）type （同類の中の異種）variety ◆2種類のお薬を飲んでいただきます You'll take two kinds of medication. ◆この種類の病気はごく一般的です This type of illness is quite common. ◆どんな種類の運動をしていますか What kind of exercise[sports] do you do? ◆色々な種類のウイルス a variety of viruses

しゅわ 手話 sign language, manual language[communication] ◆手話で話をする talk by sign language / use sign language

シュワンさいぼう ―細胞 Schwann cell ▶シュワン細胞腫 schwannoma

じゅん 順 ☞順番 ◆初めから順を追ってその出来事についてお話し下さい Please tell me what happened in order, from the beginning. ◆先着順にお名前をお呼びします We'll call your names *in order of arrival[on a first-come, first-served basis]. ◆語をABC順に並べる list[arrange] words *in alphabetical order[alphabetically] ◆アイウエオ順に in a-i-u-e-o order ◆年齢の順に in order of age ◆頻度の順に in order of frequency ◆順不同に in random order

じゅんおんちょうりょくけんさ 純音聴力検査 pure tone audiometry

じゅんかい 巡回する make *one's* rounds, go on *one's* rounds

しゅんかん 瞬間 moment (㋰momentary), instant ☞瞬時 ◆急に立ち上がった瞬間に目がくらみますか Do you get dizzy *the moment[when] you get up suddenly from a sitting position? ◆瞬間的な鋭い痛み sharp momentary pain

じゅんかん 循環 （血液などの巡り）circulation (㋰circulate ㋰circulatory) （サイクル・周期）cycle ◆血液の循環が良い〈悪い〉

have good〈bad / poor〉(blood) circulation ◆この薬は血液の循環を良くします This medication will improve your circulation. ◀悪循環 vicious cycle 　血液循環 blood circulation 　側副循環 collateral circulation 　体外循環 extracorporeal circulation 　体循環 systemic circulation 　脳循環 brain[cerebral] circulation 　肺循環 pulmonary circulation 　微小循環 microcirculation 　末梢循環障害 peripheral circulatory disturbance 　門脈循環 portal circulation ▶循環管理 hemodynamic control / circulatory care 　循環気質 cyclothymic personality / cyclothymia 　循環血液〈血漿〉量 circulating blood〈plasma〉volume 　循環血液量減少性ショック hypovolemic shock 　循環障害 circulatory disturbance 　循環不全 circulatory failure ☞循環器

じゅんかんき 循環器 circulatory organ ▶循環器科医 heart specialist / cardiologist 　循環器系 the circulatory system 　循環器疾患 circulatory disease 　循環器障害 circulatory disorder 　循環器内科 the department of cardiology / the cardiology department ☞心臓

じゅんかんごし 准看護師 associate nurse, assistant nurse ★米国の licensed practical nurse；LPN に相当する.

しゅんきカタル 春季カタル spring catarrh （春季角結膜炎）vernal keratoconjunctivitis （春季結膜炎）vernal conjunctivitis

じゅんきょうじゅ 准教授 associate professor

しゅんじ 瞬時（の）momentary (㋰moment, instant), fleeting ☞瞬間 ◆瞬時の痛み a momentary[fleeting] pain ◆刺激に瞬時に反応する respond to the stimulus instantly[in just a moment / momentarily] ◆それは瞬時の出来事でした It all happened in *a moment[an instant].

じゅんしゅ 順守する・遵守する observe, obey, abide (by), comply (with) (㋰in compliance with 　従って in accordance with) ☞従う ◆病院内の規則を順守して

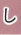

下さい Please observe[obey / abide by] the hospital regulations. ◆この臨床試験は国の倫理指針を順守して行っています We are conducting this clinical trial in compliance[accordance] with the Japanese ethical guidelines for clinical studies. ◀服薬順守 medication[drug] compliance

じゅんじょ 順序 order ☞順, 順番

じゅんじる 準じる (基づいて)based on (従って)in accordance with ◆この治療は学会が取り決めたガイドラインに準じて行います We give this treatment *based on [in accordance with] the guidelines of the medical society.

じゅんちょう 順調(な) (よい)fine, good (正常な)normal (規則的な)regular (圏well, all right) ◆万事順調です Everything is fine. / Everything is *going well[all right]. ◆(患者の行為に対して)順調ですよ You're doing fine. ◆月経は順調ですか Are your (menstrual) periods normal [regular]? / Do you have regular periods? ◆赤ちゃんは順調に発達しています Your baby is growing well. / (期待通りに)Your baby is developing *as expected[(申し分なく)satisfactorily]. ◆順調にいけば1週間で退院できます If things go well, you'll be able to leave the hospital in a week. ◆手術後順調に回復する make good progress after the surgery

じゅんど 純度 purity (↔impurity) ◆このインプラントは高純度のチタンで作られています This implant is made of high-purity titanium.

じゅんのう 順応 adaptation (動adapt) ☞適応 ◆新しい環境に早く順応なさいましたね You quickly adapted yourself to your new environment, didn't you? ◀暗順応 dark adaptation 明順応 light adaptation ▶順応性 adaptability

じゅんばん 順番 turn (順序)order, sequence ☞順 ◆順番が来たらお名前をお呼びします We'll call your name when your turn comes. / Patients are seen on a first-come, first-served basis. ◆どうぞ

順番にお入り下さい Come in in turn, please. / (1人ずつ)Please come in one at a time. ◆病状によって順番が変わることがあります Some patients may be seen out of order of arrival *owing to[because of] the severity of their condition. ◆100から7を順番に引いて下さい Please count down from one hundred *by subtracting seven each time[by sevens]. ◆順番を待つ wait for *one's* turn / wait until it's *one's* turn

じゅんび 準備する prepare (図preparation), get ready ☞手配, 用意 ◆この説明書に入院に際しご準備いただく物についての情報が載っています You'll find information about *what to prepare for admission to the hospital[what to pack in your hospital bag] in this brochure. ◆この検査には特別な準備は必要ありません No preparation is necessary for this test. ◆手術の準備のためにお腹の部分の毛を剃りましょう To prepare[get ready] for your surgery, I'm going to shave your abdomen. ◆準備完了です Everything is *ready now[set]. / We're all set. ▶準備運動 warm-up

しゅんもくはんしゃ 瞬目反射 blink reflex, blinking reflex

じゅんやきん 準夜勤 evening shift ◆準夜勤で働く work the evening shift / work on the evening shift

しよう¹ 試用 trial ◆1か月薬を試用する have the medication on trial for one month / take the medication on a[a one] month's trial basis ▶試用期間 trial period

しよう² 使用する use, make use (of) ☞使う, 利用 ◆吸入器は定期的に使用して下さい Please use the inhaler regularly. ◆自己判断で薬の使用を中止しないで下さい Don't stop taking[using] the medication *on your own[without consulting me first]. ◆トイレは現在使用中です The restroom[toilet] is occupied right now. ◆使用済みの針を処分する dispose of used needles ◆未使用の吸入器 an unused

inhaler ☞使用期限, 使用法

しょう¹ 小(の) small (↔large, big) (事柄が容易な・重要でない) minor (↔major)
◆検査着には大, 中, 小と3つのサイズがあります Exam gowns are available in three sizes: small, medium, and large. ★この場合は, 通例, small を先にする. ▶小手術 minor surgery

しょう² 性 ◆今の仕事は性に合わないのですか Do you think[feel] that your current job *doesn't suit you[isn't right for you]?

—しょう¹ —性 ◆肌は荒れ性ですか(かさかさになるか)Does your skin chap easily? / (乾燥肌か)Do you have dry skin? ◆脂性の皮膚 greasy[oily] skin ◆あなたは心配性のほうですか Do you tend to be an anxious or nervous person? / Do you worry a lot?

—しょう² —床 -bed ◆300床の病院 a three hundred-bed hospital

じょう 滋養 ☞栄養

—じょう —錠 (錠剤)tablet (丸剤)pill (カプセル)capsule ☞薬 ◆この薬は1回2錠飲んで下さい Please take two of these tablets[pills] at a time.

しょうあつやく 昇圧薬 pressor, vasopressor

じょういうんどうニューロン 上位運動ニューロン upper motor neuron; UMN

じょういたいばんそうきはくり 常位胎盤早期剥離 abruptio placentae; *premature separation of the placenta from the inner wall of the uterus*

しょういんしん 小陰唇 labium minus (🔠labia minora)

じょういんとう 上咽頭 epipharynx (🔠epipharyngeal) ▶上咽頭炎 epipharyngitis 上咽頭がん epipharyngeal cancer

しょうえき 漿液 serum, serous fluid
▶漿液性滲出液 serous effusion 漿液性分泌物 serous[thin] discharge

しょうえんやく 消炎薬 antiinflammatory (medication, drug, agent) ▶非ステロイド系消炎薬 nonsteroidal antiinflammatory drugs; NSAIDs

じょうおん 常温 room temperature
◆薬を常温で保管する keep the medication at room temperature

しょうか 消化 digestion /daɪdʒéstʃən/ (🔠digest 🔠digestive, digestible 消化促進性の peptic) ◆消化の具合が悪いのですか Do you have problems with your digestion? ◆この薬は消化を良くしてくれます This medication aids[stimulates] digestion. ◆消化に良い軽い食事にして下さい Please eat light meals that are easy to digest. ◆消化に良い食べ物(an) easily digestible food / (a) food that is easy to digest ▶消化液 digestive[peptic] juice 消化機能 digestive function 消化吸収試験 digestion-absorption test 消化酵素 digestive enzyme 消化性潰瘍 peptic ulcer 消化薬 digestant / digestive (medication / drug / agent) ☞消化管, 消化器, 消化不良

じょうか 浄化 purification (🔠purify)
◀血液浄化 blood purification

しょうかい¹ 紹介する (一般的な紹介)introduce (🔠introduction) (専門医などへの紹介)refer /rɪfə́ːr/ (🔠referral /rɪfə́ːrəl/) ◆同室の方をご紹介しましょう. こちらは金子さんです Let me introduce you to your roommate. This is Ms Kaneko. ◆自己紹介させて下さい. 麻酔医の佐々木です Let me introduce myself. I'm Dr Sasaki, your anesthesiologist. ◆肺の専門医をご紹介します I'm going to *refer you[give you a referral] to a lung specialist (for consultation). ◆どなたの紹介で来院なさいましたか Who referred you here[to this hospital]? ▶紹介と相談 referral and consultation ☞紹介状

しょうかい² 照会する (問い合わせる)ask, inquire (🔠inquiry) (専門医などに問い合わせる)refer (🔠reference) ◆係に照会しますのでしばらくここでお待ち下さい I'm going to ask the person in charge about this, so please wait here for a while. ▶照会状 letter of inquiry[reference] / reference letter

しょうがい¹ 障害・障がい disability (心

しょうがい[1]

(身の疾患)disorder （心身機能の乱れ)disturbance （心身機能の低下)impairment (身体の機能不全)dysfunction （問題)problem, trouble （妨げ・邪魔もの)obstacle （欠陥)defect ★handicapには差別的なニュアンスがある. ◆身体に〈知的に〉障害がある have *a physical〈an intellectual〉disability / be physically〈intellectually〉disabled ◆腎臓に障害がある have a kidney disorder[problem] ◆脳に障害がある(損傷がある)be brain-damaged ◆彼女は脳出血で倒れてから左半身に障害が残っています(麻痺がある)The left side of her body has been paralyzed since she had a brain hemorrhage./The stroke has left her paralyzed on the left side of her body. ◆軽度〈中程度／重度／最重度〉の障害 a mild〈moderate / severe / profound〉disability ◀意識障害 consciousness disturbance / disturbance of consciousness /（錯乱状態）confusional state　胃腸障害 stomach[gastrointestinal] trouble　運動障害 movement[motor] disorder[disturbance]　栄養障害 nutritional[nutrition] disorder　感覚障害 sensory disorder[disturbance / impairment]　肝機能障害 liver[hepatic] dysfunction　記憶障害 memory disorder[disturbance]　機能障害 functional disorder[impairment / dysfunction]　血行障害 disturbance of blood circulation / disturbed blood flow　言語障害 verbal[language / speech] disorder[impairment]　更年期障害 menopausal[climacteric] disturbance　視覚障害 vision[visual] disorder[impairment]　循環障害 circulatory disturbance　睡眠障害 sleep disorder[disturbance]　精神障害 mental disorder[disability] /（精神病的な）psychiatric disorder　摂食障害 eating disorder　先天性障害 congenital disorder　知的障害 intellectual disability[impairment]　聴覚障害 *hearing impairment[auditory disorder]　脳血管障害 cerebrovascular disorder　排尿障害 urinary[urination] disorder[disturbance / problem]　発育障害 growth disorder　歩行障害 walking difficulty / gait disorder[disturbance]　▶障害(補償)給付 disability (compensation) benefit　障害手当金 disability allowance　障害等級 degree of disability[invalidity]　障害(基礎)年金 disability (basic) pension　障害(厚生)年金 disability (employees') pension　☞障害児, 障害者

しょうがい[2]　傷害 injury ☞怪我 ▶傷害保険 accident insurance

しょうがい[3]　生涯 one's life, one's lifetime ◆幸せな生涯を送る live a happy life ◆生涯にわたる病気 a lifelong disease ◆この治療はたいていの場合生涯にわたって続けなければなりません This treatment usually has to be continued indefinitely./This illness usually requires lifelong treatment.

しょうがいじ　障害児・障がい児　child with special（health, care）needs, child with *a disability[disabilities], disabled child, challenged child　☞障害者 ◀学習障害児 child with a learning disability　情緒障害児 child with emotional problems / emotionally disturbed child　身体障害児 child with a physical disability / physically disabled[challenged] child　知的障害児 child with an intellectual disability / intellectually disabled[challenged] child

しょうがいしゃ　障害者・障がい者　person with *a disability[disabilities], disabled person, challenged person　☞障害児 ◀視覚障害者 visually impaired[challenged] person　身体障害者 person with a physical disability / physically disabled[challenged] person　精神障害者 person with a mental disability / mentally disabled[challenged] person　知的障害者 person with an intellectual disability / intellectually disabled[challenged] person　聴覚障害者 person with a hearing impairment[disorder] / deaf[hard-of-hearing] person　▶障害者施設 facility for people with disabilities　（身体）障害者手帳（physical）disability handbook / handbook for the（physically）disabled

しょうかいじょう　紹介状（専門医などへ）referral letter /rɪfə́ːrəl-/（一般的に）letter of introduction　◆乳腺外科医に紹介状を書きましょう I'd be happy to write a referral letter to a breast surgeon.　◆かかりつけ医の紹介状をお持ちですか Do you have a referral letter from your family doctor?　◆紹介状をお持ちでないと5,000円の追加料金が必要となりますがよろしいですか If you don't have a referral letter, *you'll be required[you'll have] to pay an extra charge of five thousand yen. Is that all right with you?

しょうかかん　消化管　digestive tract, gastrointestinal[GI] tract, alimentary canal[tract]　☞胃腸　◆消化管を拡げるために空気を入れますのでゲップを我慢して下さい I'm going to insert air to expand your digestive tract, so please don't belch.　◆上部〈下部〉消化管 the upper〈lower〉gastrointestinal[GI] tract　▶消化管間質腫瘍 gastrointestinal stromal tumor；GIST　消化管出血 gastrointestinal bleeding[hemorrhage]　消化管穿孔 perforation of the digestive tract　消化管ホルモン gastrointestinal hormone

しょうかき　消化器　digestive organ　▶消化器科医 gastroenterologist　消化器系 the digestive system　消化器外科（診療科）the department of gastroenterological surgery / the gastroenterological surgery department　消化器内科 the department of gastroenterology / the gastroenterology department　消化器病学 gastroenterology

じょうがく　上顎　upper jaw, maxilla（形 maxillary）☞顎（あご，がく）▶上顎がん maxillary cancer　上顎骨 upper jawbone / maxillary bone　上顎骨骨折 maxillary bone fracture　上顎前突 maxillary protrusion　上顎洞 maxillary sinus

しょうかたい　松果体　pineal gland[body]

しょうかふりょう　消化不良　indigestion, dyspepsia（形 dyspeptic）◆消化不良を起こす get[have] indigestion　◆どんな物を食べたり飲んだりした時に消化不良が起こりますか What kind of food or drinks cause your indigestion?　▶消化不良便 dyspeptic[undigested] stool

しょうき　笑気　laughing gas（亜酸化窒素）nitrous oxide

しようきげん　使用期限　use-by-date, expiration date,《英》expiry date　◆使用期限が切れた薬は使わないで下さい Please don't use the medication after its use-by-date[expiration date] has passed.　◆その薬については，未開封の状態で使用期限内であれば使っていただいて結構です You can use the medication if it is sealed[unopened] and within its use-by-date.

じょうきどう　上気道　upper airway[respiratory tract]　▶上気道感染症 upper respiratory infection；URI / upper airway infection　上気道閉塞 upper airway obstruction

しょうきゅうし　小臼歯　premolar (tooth)

じょうきょう　状況（事態）situation（人が置かれた状態）condition（周囲の環境）circumstances ★通例，複数形で.（形 circumstantial）（人・物の様子・状態）state, status　☞現状，事情，事態，状態　◆動脈瘤はまだ非常に小さいので，今は何もせず状況を見守りましょう The aneurysm is still very small, so let's leave it for now and keep an eye on the situation.　◆ストレスを感じるのはどんな状況の時ですか In what situations do you feel stressed?　◆現在の状況では，まだ退院しないほうがいいでしょう Judging from your present condition, it would be better for you not to leave the hospital yet.　◆事故の状況を教えて下さい Please describe how the accident happened. / Please tell me the circumstances of the accident.　◆彼女は自分の状況を理解できない様子です It seems that she doesn't understand *her situation[how matters stand with her].　◆状況はだんだん好転〈悪化〉しています Things are gradually getting better〈worse〉.　◆深刻な状況 a serious[critical] situation ◆望ましくない状況 unfavorable circumstances ◀経済状況 financial[economic] situation 婚姻状況 marital status ▶状況証拠 circumstantial evidence

しょうきょうきん 小胸筋 pectoralis minor (muscle), smaller pectoral muscle

しょうきょく 消極的(な) (否定的な)negative (↔positive) (受動的な)passive (↔active) ◆治療に消極的になっておられますね。お気持ちはよくわかります You have negative feelings toward[You feel negative about] the treatment, don't you? I can understand why you feel that way. ◆消極的な意見 a negative opinion ◆消極的な性格 a passive personality ▶消極的安楽死 passive euthanasia

じょうきん 常勤(の) full-time (↔part-time) ☞フルタイム ▶常勤医 full-time hospital-employed[hospital-based] physician 常勤スタッフ full-time staff

じょうげ 上下(の) up and down (垂直方向の)vertical (圏rise and fall, go up and down) ☞変動 ◆熱は1日のうちで上下しますか Does the fever rise and fall within a day? ▶上下運動 up-and-down movement[motion] 上下斜視 vertical strabismus 上下注視麻痺 vertical gaze palsy

しょうげき 衝撃 shock (影響)impact ☞ショック ▶衝撃波 shock wave

しょうけっせつ 小結節 nodule, small knot

じょうけん 条件 condition (条件づけ) conditioning (圏条件づけられた condi-tioned) (必要条件)requirement ◆血圧はいつも同じ条件で測って下さい Please take your blood pressure under the same conditions as usual. ◆最高の条件でも手術は時に危険を伴います Even under the best conditions, *surgery can sometimes be risky[there is some risk involved in surgery]. ◆明日の朝8時までに戻るという条件で外泊を許可しましょう We'll allow you to stay home overnight on condition that you return by eight o'clock tomorrow

morning. ◆悪条件 bad[unfavorable] condition 最適条件 the optimal condition 前提条件 precondition / prerequisite condition 必要条件 necessary requirement[condition] ▶条件刺激 conditioned stimulus 条件反射 conditioned reflex；CR 条件反応 conditioned response

じょうげん 上限 the upper limit (最大・最高)the maximum (圏maximal) ◆最高血圧の正常上限値は…です The upper limit for normal maximal[systolic] blood pressure is …. ◆正常上限値を超えている be above the upper limit of normal ◆医療負担額の上限 the maximum charge for the medical treatment

しょうこ 証拠 (事実としての証拠)evidence (徴候)sign (証明)proof ☞根拠 ◆ウォーキングが減量に効果的だという十分な証拠があります There's[We have] enough[sufficient] evidence on the effectiveness of walking (exercise) for losing weight. ◆手術後ガスが出るのは腸の動きが回復している証拠です Passing gas after surgery is a sign that the intestines are returning to normal. ◆説明内容を了解していただいた証拠として、こちらにご署名をお願いします Please sign this form as proof that you have understood my explanation. ◆確かな証拠を出す provide[give] good[strong] evidence ◆具体的な証拠 concrete evidence ◆はっきりした証拠 clear evidence ◆説得力のある証拠 persuasive[convincing] evidence ◀状況証拠 circumstantial evidence

しょうこう¹ 小康 (寛解)remission (中休み)respite ◆彼女は現在小康状態にあります Her disease is now in remission. / (病状が安定している)Her condition is now stable.

しょうこう² 症候 symptom /símptəm/ (圏symptomátic) ☞症状 ◆彼女に髄膜炎を示す症候が現れています She has symptoms that suggest meningitis. / She has the typical symptoms of meningitis.

▶症候性てんかん symptomatic epilepsy ☞症候群, 無症候性

じょうこう 上行(性の) ascending (↔descending) ◀脊髄上行路 spinal ascending tract ▶上行結腸 ascending colon 上行大動脈 ascending aorta

しょうこうぐん 症候群 syndrome ▶後天性免疫不全症候群 acquired immunodeficiency syndrome；AIDS 上大静脈症候群 *superior vena cava[SVC] syndrome

しょうこうねつ 猩紅熱 scarlet fever, scarlatina

しょうこつ 踵骨 heel bone, calcaneus

しょうさい 詳細 detail (⊞detailed ▥in detail) ☞詳しい ◆なお詳細は担当医に訊いて下さい Please ask your doctor for further details. ◆詳細は明日お話しします I'll *give you[go over] the details tomorrow. ◆詳細な説明 a detailed explanation[description]

しようざい 止痒剤 ☞痒み止め

じょうざい 錠剤 tablet ☞薬, 一錠 ◆薬は錠剤でお出しします I'm going to give you some tablets. ◆この錠剤は1回2錠飲んで下さい Please take two tablets each time. ◆錠剤を舌の下に入れてゆっくり溶かして下さい Place the tablet under your tongue and let it melt[dissolve] slowly.

じょうざいさいきん 常在細菌 indigenous bacteria (⊞bacterium) ▶常在細菌叢 normal microbial flora

しょうさいぼうがん 小細胞癌 small cell carcinoma ◀非小細胞肺癌 non-small cell lung cancer[carcinoma]；NSCLC ▶小細胞肺癌 small cell lung cancer[carcinoma]；SCLC

しょうさっし 小冊子 ☞パンフレット

しょうさん[1] 硝酸 nitric acid ◀亜硝酸 nitrous acid ▶硝酸銀 silver nitrate

しょうさん[2] 称賛する admire (图admiration) (ほめる) praise (图ほめ言葉 praise) ◆これまで治療に頑張ってこられたことは称賛に値します I admire you for all the effort you've put into your treat-

ment. / The effort you've put into your treatment deserves a lot of praise.

しょうし[1] 小指・小趾 (手の) little finger (足の) little toe ☞指 ▶小指球 hypothenar eminence

しょうし[2] 焼死 fire death, death from fire ◆火災で2人が焼死した Two people *were burned to death[died] in the fire.

しょうし[3] 硝子(様の) hyaline ▶硝子円柱 hyaline cast 硝子軟骨 hyaline cartilage 硝子変性 hyaline degeneration 硝子膜 hyaline membrane

じょうし 上肢 arms, upper limbs[extremities] ★通例, 複数形で. ▶上肢筋 upper limb muscle / muscle of the upper limbs

しょうしか 少子化 (出生率低下)declining birthrate (子供の数の減少)decrease in the number of children ☞少子高齢化

しょうじき 正直(な) (誠実な)honest (率直な)frank ◆正直に申し上げて彼女の回復はあまり芳しくありません Honestly speaking[To be honest / To be frank], she's not recovering as quickly as she should. / To tell the truth, the pace of her recovery is *rather unsatisfactory[not very good]. ◆正直に答える answer honestly

じょうしき 常識 (良識)common sense (一般的知識)common knowledge ◆彼は常識的な人です He has (good) common sense. / He is a sensible man. ◆常識的な判断をすれば, 治療の選択肢としてこれがベストです Judging by common sense, [Common sense tells me that] this treatment option is the best of all. ◆塩分を摂り過ぎると高血圧になるのは常識です It's common knowledge[Everyone knows] that too much salt causes high blood pressure.

しょうしこうれいか 少子高齢化 low [declining] birthrate and aging population ▶少子高齢化社会 aging society with a low birthrate

しょうしたい 硝子体 vitreous body ▶硝子体混濁 vitreous opacity[clouding]

しょうしたい 342 **しょうじょう**¹

硝子体出血 vitreous bleeding[hemor-rhage] 硝子体剝離 vitreous detachment 硝子体浮遊物 vitreous floater

しょうしつ **消失する** **disappear, lose** （図 **loss**） ☞消える ◆吐き気は一時的なもので通常 2〜3 日で消失します Nausea is temporary and will usually disappear in a couple of days. ▶意識消失 loss of consciousness；LOC / unconsciousness 感覚消失 sensory loss / loss of sensation

じょうしつきがいしゅうしゅく **上室期外収縮** **supraventricular extrasystole[ectopic complex], supraventricular premature contraction[beat / complex / systole]**；**SVPC**

じょうしつせいひんぱく **上室性頻拍** **supraventricular tachycardia**；**SVT**

しょうしゃ **照射** **irradiation** （動**irradiate**）, **radiation** （動**radiate**） ◆患者に γ 線を照射する irradiate the patient with gamma rays ◆患部に放射線を照射する apply radiation to the affected area ◀X 線照射 X-ray irradiation 外部〈内部〉照射 external〈internal〉 irradiation[radiation] 腔内照射 intracavitary irradiation 紫外線照射 ultraviolet irradiation 術前〈術後〉照射 preoperative〈postoperative〉 irradiation 分割照射 fractionated irradiation 放射線照射血液 irradiated blood 予防照射 prophylactic irradiation ▶照射時間 exposure time 照射線量 exposure dose 照射野 irradiation field

しょうしゃく **焼灼** （焼き切ること）**ablation** （傷などを焼くこと）**cauterization** ◀カテーテル焼灼術 catheter ablation 電気焼灼術 electric cauterization / electrocauterization ラジオ波焼灼療法 radiofrequency ablation；RFA

しょうしゅう **召集** **call** （動**call a code**） ◀緊急召集 emergency call[code] /《米》 code blue, stat call

じょうしゅう **常習（の）** **habitual** （習慣性の）**habit-forming, addictive** ◆この薬は常習性がありますので，本当に必要な時だけお飲み下さい Please take this medication only when you really need it, because

it *may become[is] habit-forming[addictive]. ◆彼は遅刻の常習者です He is habitually[always] late for work〈school〉. ◆麻薬の常習者である be a drug addict / have a drug habit ▶常習飲酒家 habitual drinker

しょうしゅうざい **消臭剤** **deodorant, deodorizer, odor remover**

しょうしょ **証書** ☞証明書

しょうじょ **少女** **girl** （図少女[少年]の ju-venile /dʒúːvənàil/） ◀非行少女 female juvenile delinquent ▶少女期[時代] girl-hood 少女犯罪 juvenile[youth] crime 少女非行 juvenile delinquency

しょうしょう **少々** ☞少し ◀少々お待ち下さい Please wait a moment[minute]. /（電話で）Please hold on. ◆運動は，少々であれば差支えありません It's all right to do some light exercise. / You can do some light exercise. ◆少々の痛みであればこの鎮痛薬で治まります If you have only a little pain, it will disappear[go away] with this painkiller.

しょうじょう¹ **症状** （病気の徴候）**symptom** /símptəm/ （健康上の問題）**problem** （体の状態）**condition** ☞病歴 ◆どんな症状ですか What kind of symptoms do you have? ◆最初にこの〈これらの〉症状に気づいたのはいつですか When did you first notice *this symptom〈these symptoms〉? ◆このような症状を経験したことがありますか Have you ever had *anything like this[this kind of symptom] before? ◆この症状はどのくらい続いていますか How long have you had these symptoms? ◆あなたの症状はおそらく風邪によるものでしょう Your symptoms probably come from a cold. ◆めまいの症状が再発したら再度受診して下さい Please come back again if your dizziness returns. ★この場合は symptom を使わず具体的な症状（頭痛・腹痛など）を言うことが多い. ◆熱や痛みなどの症状が現れた時にこの薬を服用して下さい Please take this medication when *you get symptoms such as fever or pain[symptoms, such as fever or

しょうじょう¹ pain, come on]. ◆症状がなくなっても最後まで飲み続けて下さい Please continue taking this medication even if your symptoms have disappeared[gone away / cleared up]. ◆彼女の症状は安定しています She is in (a) stable condition. / Her condition is stable. ◆症状が改善する one's symptoms[conditions] improve ◆風邪のような症状がある have cold-like[flu-like] symptoms ◆痒い〈息苦しい〉ような症状がある have a symptom like itchiness〈breathlessness〉 ◆パーキンソン病の症状がある have symptoms of Parkinson disease ◆心不全の主要な症状 the main[major / key] symptoms of heart failure ◀アレルギー症状 allergic symptom[condition] 胃腸症状 gastrointestinal symptom 局所症状 local symptom 禁断[離脱]症状 withdrawal symptom 更年期症状 menopausal[climacteric] symptom 自覚〈他覚〉症状 subjective〈objective〉symptom 初期症状 early[initial] symptom 前駆症状 premonitory symptom / symptom indicative of an approaching disease / prodrome 脱水症状 dehydration 中毒症状 poisoning[toxic] symptom

しょうじょう² 床上 ▶床上安静 bedrest / bed rest 床上運動 bed exercise / exercise in bed 床上動作 bed activity 床上排泄 using a bedpan

じょうしょう 上昇する rise, go up, elevate （増大する）increase /ɪnkríːs/, （図rise, elevation, íncrease 急騰 surge） ☞上がる ◆彼女の血圧が急に上昇しました Her blood pressure has risen[gone up / elevated / increased] suddenly. ◆体温の上昇 elevation of body temperature ◀ST上昇 ST elevation 早朝血圧上昇 morning blood pressure rise[surge]

しょうしょく 少食・小食 ◆今日は少食ですね You haven't eaten much today, have you? / （食欲がない）You don't have much (of an) appetite today, do you? ◆いつも少食のほうですか Are you usually a light eater? / Do you usually not eat much?

じょうしょく 常食 regular diet, normal diet, ordinary meal ☞食事

しょうじる 生じる come on, occur /əkɚː/, happen （原因となる）cause, lead to （引き起こす）bring about （結果として起こる）result from ☞起こる ◆痛みが生じるのは突然ですか, ゆっくりですか Does the pain *come on[occur] suddenly or gradually? ◆糖尿病により網膜症, 心臓病, 腎不全など深刻な合併症が生じることがあります Diabetes can cause[have] serious complications including retinopathy, heart disease, and kidney failure. ◆コミュニケーション不足により誤解が生じたようです I'm afraid that a lack of communication has caused[led to] this misunderstanding. ◆この病気は時にストレスから生じることがあります This illness sometimes results from stress.

しょうじんしょう 小人症 （低身長）short stature ◀下垂体小人症 pituitary dwarfism

じょうず 上手（な） good （圖well） ☞うまい ◆箸を使うのがお上手ですね You're good at using chopsticks, aren't you? / You can use chopsticks well, can't you? ◆娘さんは日本語がお上手です Your daughter speaks good Japanese. / Your daughter is good at speaking Japanese. ◆お酒とは上手に付き合って下さい（適度に飲む）Please try to moderate your drinking. / You should drink sensibly and in moderation.

しょうすい¹ 小水 urine ☞尿

しょうすい² 憔悴する ◆彼は憔悴しきった様子でした（疲れ果ててた）He looked exhausted[worn out]. ◆憔悴しきった顔をしている（やつれた）look haggard / have a haggard look

しようせいビタミン 脂溶性ビタミン fat-soluble vitamin

しょうせきかくひしょう 掌蹠角皮症 palmoplantar keratoderma

しょうせきのうほうしょう 掌蹠膿疱症 palmoplantar pustulosis

しょうせっかい 小切開 minimal incision

じょうせんしょくたい 常染色体 auto-some（⌐autosomal）　◆常染色体異常 autosomal[autosome] abnormality[aberration]　常染色体性遺伝病 autosomal genetic disease　常染色体優性遺伝 autosomal dominant (inheritance)；AD　常染色体性劣性遺伝 autosomal recessive (inheritance)；AR

じょうたい¹ 状態　（特に健康状態・容態）condition　（周囲の状況・情勢）situation　（人・物の状態）state　☞状況，症状　◆この状態はどのくらい続いていますか How long have you felt this way?　◆今の状態はどうですか How are you now?　◆あなたはまだ通勤できるような状態ではありません You're in no condition to go to work yet.　◆状態が良い〈悪い〉be in good〈bad〉condition　◆健康状態がよい〈あまり良くない〉be in good〈poor〉health　◆危篤状態である be in critical condition　◆危篤状態を脱する come out of critical condition　◆危篤状態を脱している be no longer in critical condition　◆寝たきりの状態である be bedridden　◆ショック状態にある be in (a state of) shock　◆錯乱状態に陥る fall into a state of confusion /（精神的な疾病によって）become deranged　◆正常な状態に戻る return[get back] to normal　◆安定した状態 (a) stable condition　◆意識の状態 a state of consciousness　◆意識不明の状態 a state of unconsciousness　◀うつ状態 depressive state / state of depression　衛生状態 sanitary[hygienic] conditions　栄養状態 nutritional state　覚醒状態 arousal state / state of arousal / vigilance　仮死状態 state of *apparent death[suspended animation]　経済状態 financial[economic] situation　健康状態 state of health / physical[health] condition　心停止状態 state of cardiac[heart] arrest　生活状態 living conditions　精神状態 mental[（心理的な）psychological /（情動的な）emotional] condition[state]

じょうたい² 上体 the upper part of *one's* body, upper body　◆ベッドから上

体を起こす sit up in bed　◆上体を前に傾ける lean[bend] forward　◆上体を後ろに反らす lean[bend] backward

しょうたいしゅっけつ 消退出血 withdrawal bleeding

じょうだいじょうみゃく 上大静脈 superior vena cava；SVC　▶上大静脈症候群 *superior vena cava[SVC] syndrome

しょうだく 承諾　（同意）consent　（賛同）approval　（許可）permission　◆この検査に対する承諾をいただけますか Could I have your consent to do this test?　◆この手術承諾書をよく読んでサインをお願いします Please read this consent form for surgery carefully and sign it.　◆退院するには担当医の承諾が必要です You must have your doctor's consent[permission] to leave the hospital.　◆担当医の承諾なく外出しないで下さい Don't go out of the hospital without your doctor's permission.　▶承諾書 written consent

しょうち 承知　◆承知しました Certainly. / All right.　／（インフォーマルに）OK.

じょうちゅう¹ 条虫 tapeworm　◀広節裂頭条虫 broad[fish] tapeworm　小形条虫 dwarf tapeworm　無鉤条虫 beef tapeworm / *Taenia saginata*　有鉤条虫 pork tapeworm / *Taenia solium*　裂頭条虫症 diphyllobothriasis　▶条虫症 tapeworm infection

じょうちゅう² 静注 intravenous injection, IV injection　☞注射　◀点滴静注 IV [intravenous] drip

じょうちょ 情緒 emotion（⌐emotional）　☞感情，情動　◆息子さんは新しい日本の環境になじめなくて情緒不安定になったのですか Did your son become emotionally unstable because he couldn't adapt to his new surroundings in Japan?　▶情緒安定〈不安定〉emotional stability〈instability / lability〉　情緒障害 emotional disorder [disturbance]　情緒障害児 emotionally disturbed child / child with emotional problems　情緒的支援 emotional support　情緒反応 emotional response

しょうちょう 小腸 small intestine[bowel] ★intestine は /ɪntéstɪn/, bowel は /báʊəl/ と発音する.

じょうちょうかんまくどうみゃく 上腸間膜動脈 superior mesenteric artery

しょうてん 焦点 focus (圖焦点が合う・焦点を合わせる focus), focal point ◆焦点が合っている in focus ◆焦点がずれている out of focus ◀てんかん焦点 epileptic focus 二重焦点眼鏡 bifocal glasses 二重焦点レンズ bifocal lens ▶焦点発作〈てんかん〉focal seizure〈epilepsy〉

しょうとう 消灯する turn off the light ◆消灯時間は午後9時です Lights are turned off at nine pm. ▶消灯時間 lights-out

しょうどう 衝動 (本能的な心の動き)impulse /ímpʌls/ (圖impúlsive) (行動を駆り立てる欲求)urge, drive ◆タバコを吸いたいという衝動に駆られることがよくありますか Do you often feel an impulse[urge] to smoke? ◆衝動を抑える方法として何かアイディアがありますか Do you have any ideas about how you can control[resist] your impulses? ◆衝動的に行動する behave on impulse ◆衝動的な行動 impulsive behavior ◀性衝動 sexual impulse[urge] / sex drive

じょうどう 情動 (強い感情)emotion (圖emotional, affective) ☞感情, 情緒 ▶情動障害 affective disorder[disturbance] 情動ストレス emotional stress 情動脱力発作 cataplexy 情動不安(落着きのなさ) restlessness

しょうとうしょう 小頭症 microcephaly

じょうどうしょう 常同症 stereotypy

しょうとうだい 床頭台 bedside cabinet[table]

じょうどうみゃくバイパス 静動脈バイパス venoarterial bypass

しょうどく 消毒する (滅菌・殺菌する) sterilize (圖sterilization) (感染予防として消毒する)disinfect (圖disinfection) (消毒綿などで傷口を拭く)swab (圖swab) ☞殺菌, 滅菌 ◆ご家族への感染を防ぐために, 患者さんが触ったドアノブや便器などを拭いて消毒して下さい To prevent the spread of infection to family members, clean and disinfect items that are touched by patients such as door knobs or toilets (with a disinfectant). ◆消毒液で傷口をきれいにします I'm going to cleanse the wound with an antiseptic solution. ◆傷口をアルコールで消毒する swab the wound with alcohol ◆(採血の前などで)アルコール消毒でかぶれたことがありますか Do you ever get a skin rash from using alcohol wipes[swabs]? ◆哺乳瓶を熱湯で消毒する sterilize baby[milk] bottles in boiling water ◀アルコール消毒 alcohol-based antisepsis アルコール消毒綿 alcohol wipe[swab] 皮膚消毒 skin antisepsis[disinfection] ▶消毒液 antiseptic solution 消毒器具 sterilizer 消毒ジェル(手の)hand sanitizer gel 消毒綿 antiseptic wipe / (cotton) swab 消毒用アルコール(傷口・皮膚用) rubbing alcohol ☞煮沸消毒, 消毒薬

しょうどくやく 消毒薬 (殺菌用)antiseptic (感染予防用)disinfectant (手消毒用) hand sanitizer, antiseptic wash ◆病室にお入りになる時には消毒薬で手をきれいにして下さい〈拭いて下さい〉Please clean〈wipe〉your hands with the hand sanitizer when entering the room. ◆病棟に入る前と後には備え付けの手指消毒薬を使って下さい(消毒ジェルを使う)Please use the hand hygiene gel provided before and after visiting the ward.

しょうに 小児 (小さい子供)small[little] child (乳児)infant ◆子供, 児童, 幼児, ライフステージ ◆小児が罹りやすい病気 common diseases in small children / usual childhood diseases ; UCHD ◆この薬は小児の手の届かない所に保管して下さい Please keep this medication out of the reach of (small) children. ▶小児がん childhood cancer 小児期 childhood 小児虐待 child abuse[(放置)neglect] 小児ケア child care 小児語 child language 小児喘息 childhood asthma 小児病院 children's hospital 小児麻痺 polio /

しょうに 346 じょうぶ[1]

infantile paralysis／(急性灰白髄炎) polio-myelitis　☞小児科, 小児外科

しょうにか 小児科 pediatrics／pìːdiǽtrɪks/ (診療科) the department of pediatrics, the pediatrics department ▶小児科医 pediatrician／children's doctor 小児科医院 children's clinic 小児(科)病棟 children's ward[floor／unit]／pediatric(s) ward[floor／unit]

しょうにげか 小児外科 pediatric surgery (診療科) the department of pediatric surgery, the pediatric surgery department ▶小児外科医 pediatric surgeon

しょうにん[1] 証人 witness

しょうにん[2] 承認する (認可する) approve (図 approval) ▶許可, 承諾, 同意 ◆この薬は現在乳がんの治療薬として承認されています This medication is currently approved for the treatment of breast cancer. ◆日本ではこの薬は承認されていないので処方できません This medication has not been approved for use in Japan, so I can't prescribe it for you. ▶未承認薬 unapproved medication[drug] ▶承認薬 approved medication[drug]

しょうねん 少年 boy (図 少年[少女]の juvenile／dʒúːvənàɪl/) ◀青少年 youth／young adult 非行少年 juvenile delinquent ▶少年期[時代] boyhood 少年犯罪 juvenile[youth] crime 少年非行 juvenile delinquency

しょうのう[1] 小脳 cerebellum／sèrəbéləm/ (図 cerebellar) ▶小脳出血 cerebellar bleeding[hemorrhage] 小脳半球 cerebellar hemisphere 小脳皮質 cerebellar cortex

しょうのう[2] 樟脳 camphor

じょうはつ 蒸発 evaporation ▶蒸発器 evaporator 蒸発熱 evaporation heat

じょうはんしん 上半身 the upper half [part] of the body, upper body ☞上体 ◆服は上半身脱いで下さい Please take off your clothes from the waist up.

しょうひ 消費 consumption (図 consume) (時間・エネルギーなどの) expenditure ◆お酒の消費量が徐々に増えましたか Has your alcohol consumption increased steadily? ◆運動してカロリーを消費する (燃焼させる) burn off calories by exercising [doing exercises] ◆差額ベッド代や各種診断書には消費税が課税されます Additional fees for special rooms and various certificates are subject to consumption tax. ◀アルコール消費量 alcohol consumption エネルギー消費量 energy expenditure／the amount of energy consumed 酸素消費量 oxygen consumption ▶消費者 consumer 消費性凝固障害 consumption coagulopathy ☞消費期限

じょうひ 上皮 epithelium (図 epithelial, epidermal) ◀異型上皮 atypical epithelium 非上皮性腫瘍 nonepithelial tumor ▶上皮化 epithelialization 上皮細胞 epithelial cell 上皮性腫瘍 epithelial tumor 上皮成長因子 epidermal growth factor；EGF 上皮組織 epithelial tissue 上皮内癌 carcinoma in situ；CIS

しょうひきげん 消費期限 use-by-date, expiration date,《英》expiry date ◆食品はなるべく早く消費期限内に食べて下さい Please eat all foods quickly and before the use-by-date.

じょうびやく 常備薬 (家庭に置く薬) household medication (家庭用救急箱) home first aid kit

しょうびょう 傷病 sickness and injury, trauma and disease ▶傷病者 sick and injured[wounded] person／invalid 傷病手当金 injury and disease allowance 傷病補償年金 injury and disease compensation pension 傷病名 name of disability／name of sickness and injury

じょうぶ[1] 上部 upper part ▶上部消化管 *upper gastrointestinal[GI] tract 上部消化管出血 upper gastrointestinal bleeding 上部消化管造影 *upper gastrointestinal[GI] series[radiography]／barium swallow 上部消化管内視鏡検査 *upper gastrointestinal[GI] endoscopy／upper endoscopy 上部食道 (上 1／3) upper third of the esophagus

じょうぶ² 丈夫（な）（strong and）healthy （頑健な）robust ☞健康

じょうふくぶ 上腹部 the upper abdomen, the epigastric region, the epigastrium ▶上腹部［心窩部］痛 upper abdominal［epigastric］pain / epigastralgia

しょうへき 障壁 barrier ◆2人の間には言葉の障壁がありました There was a language barrier between the two. ◀コミュニケーション障壁 communication barrier 文化障壁 cultural barrier

しょうべん 小便 ☞尿

しようほう 使用法 how to use （薬などの指示）directions （for use）★通例，複数形で．◆吸入器の使用法がわかりますか Do you know how to use an inhaler? ◆この薬は使用法に従ってお飲み下さい Please take this medication according to the directions.

じょうほう 情報 information ★information は数えられない名詞なので，1件の情報は a piece of information という．◆受傷状況についてもっと情報をいただけますか Would you please give me more information about how you injured yourself? ◆前立腺がんについての最新情報を与える provide the latest information about［on］prostate cancer ◆インターネットは最新の医療情報を入手できる利点がありますが，信頼できる情報かを見極めることが重要です The *good points［advantages］of the internet are that you can get［obtain］up-to-date *health care［medical］information, but it's important to make sure that the information is reliable. ◆あなたからの情報は守秘し，許可なく開示することはいたしません The information you provide is confidential and will not be disclosed without your permission. ◆患者同士で情報を交換する exchange information with［among］other patients ◆正確な情報を得る have［get / obtain / collect］accurate［precise］information ◆実用的な〈信頼できる〉情報 practical〈reliable〉information ◆不十分な〈不正確な〉情報 insufficient〈incorrect〉information ◆診

療記録を情報開示する disclose *a person's medical record* ◀医薬品等安全情報 drug safety information 花粉情報 pollen forecast［information］ 基礎情報 basic［fundamental］information /（データベース）database 個人情報 personal［private］information 中毒情報センター poison information center 副作用情報 side effects information ▶情報開示（information）disclosure

じょうほうちゅうししまひ 上方注視麻痺 upward gaze palsy

しょうほっさ 小発作 minor attack （痙攣性の）minor seizure

しょうまく 漿膜 serous membrane, serosa ▶漿膜炎 serositis

じょうみゃく 静脈 vein /véin/（↔artery）（圏静脈（性）の venous /víːnəs/ 腰頭 phleb(o)-）◆静脈注射をする give an IV［intravenous］injection ◀下大静脈 inferior vena cava；IVC 頸静脈 jugular vein 鎖骨下静脈 subclavian vein 上大静脈 superior vena cava；SVC 大腿静脈 femoral vein ▶静脈確保 venous access / establishment of a venous route 静脈カテーテル法 venous catheterization 静脈系 the venous system 静脈血 venous blood 静脈性腎盂造影 intravenous pyelography；IVP / X-ray recording of the kidneys and urinary tract 静脈造影（下肢の）phlebography［venography］（of the lower limbs）▷静脈栄養, 静脈炎, 静脈血栓症, 静脈瘤

じょうみゃくえいよう 静脈栄養 intravenous nutrition［feeding］◀完全静脈栄養 total parenteral nutrition；TPN 在宅静脈栄養法 home parenteral nutrition；HPN

じょうみゃくえん 静脈炎 phlebitis ◀血栓性静脈炎 thrombophlebitis

じょうみゃくけっせんしょう 静脈血栓症 venous thrombosis ◀深部静脈血栓症 deep vein thrombosis；DVT

じょうみゃくりゅう 静脈瘤 varices （圏 varix），varicose veins ★通例，複数形で．◀胃静脈瘤 gastric varix 下肢静脈瘤

varicose veins of the lower limbs[extremities] / lower limb varicose veins ☞食道静脈瘤

しょうめい¹　照明　illumination, lighting　(電灯)light　◆照明をつける〈消す〉turn on〈off〉the lights　◆照明を落とす turn[dim] the lights down　◀間接照明 indirect illumination

しょうめい²　証明する　prove (図proof)　◆身元を証明するものを何か持っていますか Do you have anything to prove your identity?　◆検査でポリープは良性であることが証明されました The tests have proved that your polyp is benign.　☞証明書

しょうめいしょ　証明書　certificate /sə-tíf ı kət/　◀証明書を発行する issue a certificate　◀外国人登録証明書 alien registration card　死産証書 certificate of stillbirth　死亡証明書 death certificate　出生証明書 birth certificate　接種証明書 certificate of immunization　卒業証明書 diploma / graduation certificate　妊娠証明書 certificate of pregnancy　年金証明書 pension certificate　身分証明書 identification[ID] card

しょうめん　正面　front (図front 図ahead, forward(s))　◆こちらに〈あちらに〉真っ直ぐ向いて下さい Please look straight ahead *this way〈that way〉. / Please face forward *this way〈that way〉.　▶正面玄関 the main entrance / the front door　正面像 anterior view

しょうもう¹　消耗する　(疲れ果てる)exhaust /ıgzɔ́ːst/ (図exhaustion)　(痩せ衰える)waste away　◆咳で体力が消耗している be exhausted from coughing　◆消耗させる病気 a disease that causes *a person to waste away*

しょうもう²　睫毛　eyelash　☞まつげ

しょうやく　止痒薬　☞痒み止め

しょうやく　生薬　crude drug, galenical preparation

しょうゆ　醤油　soy sauce　◆醤油をかける add soy sauce / flavor with soy sauce　◀減塩醤油 low-salt[low-sodi-um] soy sauce

しょうよう　小葉　lobule (図lobular)

じょうよう　常用する　(いつも使う)take[use] … regularly　(常習的になっている)take[use] … habitually　◆薬を何か常用していますか Are you taking any regular[Are you on any] drugs or medications?　◆この薬は常用してはいけません You should not take this medication habitually. / Avoid habitual use of this medication.　◆睡眠薬を常用している be on sleeping pills / use sleeping pills regularly[habitually]　◀麻薬常用[乱用](narcotic) drug abuse　麻薬常用者[中毒者](narcotic) drug addict[user]　▶常用癖 addiction　常用量 usual dose

しょうようきん　小腰筋　psoas minor muscle

しょうらい　将来　the future　☞今後　◆近い将来に in the near[immediate] future　◆このまま放置すると将来的に失明する可能性があります If you leave this untreated, you may go blind in the future.　◆この研究には将来性があります(有望である)This research *is very promising[(可能性がある)has great potential].　◆(子供の患者に)将来何になりたいの What do you want to be when you grow up?

じょうりゅうすい　蒸留水　distilled water　◀滅菌蒸留水 sterile distilled water

しょうりょう　少量(の)　a small amount of (↔a large amount of), a small quantity of, a little (↔much)　(わずかな)slight　☞少ない, 大量, 多量　◆ごく少量の痰 *a small amount[a little bit] of phlegm　◆少量の出血〈おりもの〉slight bleeding〈discharge〉　◆少量のアスピリンを毎日飲む take a small dose of aspirin each day

しょうれい　症例　case　▶症例研究 case study　症例検討会 case conference　症例対照研究 case-control study　症例報告 case report

しょうわん　小彎　lesser curvature of the stomach

じょうわん　上腕　upper arm, brachium

（圏above-elbow；AE, brachial）　▶上腕義手 above-the-elbow[AE] prosthesis　上腕筋 brachial muscle　上腕骨 arm bone / humerus　上腕骨外側上顆炎（テニス肘）tennis elbow / lateral humeral epicondylitis　上腕三頭筋 triceps muscle of the arm / triceps brachii muscle　上腕三頭筋反射 triceps (brachii) reflex[jerk]　上腕切断 above-the-elbow[AE] amputation　上腕二頭筋 biceps muscle of the arm / biceps brachii muscle　上腕二頭筋反射 biceps (brachii) reflex[jerk]

ショートステイ　short stay, short-term stay　▶ショートステイ施設 short[short-term] stay facility /（介護の一時的な代行施設）respite care facility

しょかい　初回　first time（圏first, at first）　☞最初, 初め

じょがい　除外する　rule out, exclude（圏exclusion）　☞除く　◆この検査結果で他の病気の可能性を除外できます With the results of this test, we can *rule out [exclude] the possibility of other diseases.　▶除外診断 diagnosis by exclusion

しょかんせん　初感染　primary infection　▶初感染結核 primary tuberculosis

しょき　初期（の）（時間的に早い）early（初期段階の）initial　（一次の・原発の）primary（第一の）first　☞早期　◆がんは初期です Your cancer is in its early stage.　◆初期の前立腺がんです You have early-stage prostate cancer.　◆初期のうちに治療する treat the disease in its early stages　◆中年の初期 early middle age　◀妊娠初期 the early[first] stage of pregnancy / the first trimester　▶初期医療 primary care　初期救急 primary emergency care　初期症状 early[initial] symptom　初期段階 the first[initial] stage[period]　初期治療 early[initial] treatment　初期尿 initial urine　初期病巣 primary[initial] lesion

じょきょ　除去する　remove（圏removal）, take out, get rid of　（特に身体に有害なものを排除する）eliminate（圏elimination）（減少させる）deplete（圏depletion）　☞除く

◆皮膚がんを除去するには手術が必要です You need to have surgery to remove[get rid of] the skin cancer.　◆外耳道から異物を除去する remove[take out] a foreign body from the ear canal　◆手術によるほくろの除去 surgical removal of a mole　◀アレルゲン除去製品 allergen-free product(s)　耳垢除去 earwax[cerumen] removal　刺青除去 tattoo removal　白血球除去フィルター leukocyte depletion filter　▶除去食 elimination diet

じょきん　除菌（消毒）disinfection（根絶）eradication　◆殺菌, 消毒, 滅菌　◆ピロリ菌の除菌治療 Helicobacter pylori eradication treatment[therapy]

ジョギング　jogging（圏jog）　◆ジョギングをしますか Do you enjoy jogging? / Do you jog?

しょく¹　食（食事）meal　（食べ物）food（食欲）appetite /ǽpətàɪt/（治療食）diet　☞食事, 食べ物　◆1 日に 3 食食べる eat three meals a day　◆食が進む have a good appetite　◆食が進まない have a poor appetite / not have much appetite　◆最近食が落ちていますか Have you recently lost your appetite?　◆食が細い eat only a small amount of food　◆食前〈食後 / 食間〉服用 To be taken before〈after / between〉meals　◀検査食 special[prescribed] diet before the test[examination]　高脂肪食 high-fat diet　高繊維食 high-fiber diet　常食 regular[normal] diet / ordinary meal　調整食（既定食・処方食）formula diet / formulated food /（均衡食）balanced diet　日本食 Japanese dish [food]　乳児食 baby[infant] food　病院食 hospital food[meal]　病人食 diet [food] for sick people /（患者用の）diet [food] for patients /（調理法）special recipe for sick people　ベジタリアン食 vegetarian food[meal]　▶食材 food item　☞食後, 食行動, 食事, 食習慣, 食生活, 食前, 食中毒, 食直後, 食直前, 食堂, 食品, 食物（しょくもつ）, 食欲, 食間, 食べ物

しょく²　職　job　☞仕事, 職業　◆病気で職を失うことにならないか心配なのですね

You're worried[concerned] about losing your job because of your[this] illness, aren't you? ☞職員，職種，職場

しょくあたり　食あたり　☞食中毒

しょくいん　職員　(職員1人)staff member, member of staff　(職員全体)the staff, the personnel　(事務員)clerk　☞スタッフ　◆ご不明な点は職員に尋ねて下さい If you're unsure about anything, please ask one of the staff. /(追加情報が必要な場合には)Please ask one of the staff if you need additional information.　◀医療事務職員 medical clerk　医療職員 the medical staff [personnel]　受付事務職員 receptionist　看護職員 the nursing staff[personnel]　事務職員 clerk / clerical worker /(職員全体)the clerical staff

しょくえん　食塩　salt　(㊟salt, salty)　(含塩物)saline　(㊟saline)　(ナトリウム)sodium　☞塩分，塩　◆食塩抜きの食事 *a salt-free[no-salt] diet　◀生理食塩水 physiologic saline[salt] solution　▶食塩水 saline[salt] solution　食塩制限食 low-salt[low-sodium] diet / sodium-restricted diet

しょくかんかく　触感覚　sense of touch, touch sensation　☞触覚

しょくぎょう　職業　(一般的に)occupation　(㊟occupational, vocational)　(仕事)work　(勤め口)job　(専門職)profession　(㊟professional)　☞仕事，職　◆ご職業は何ですか What's your occupation? / What type of work do you do? / What do you do for a living?　◆ストレスの多い職業 a stressful occupation[job]　▶職業訓練 vocational training　職業ストレス occupational stress　職業性喘息 occupational asthma　職業性難聴 occupational hearing loss　職業病 occupational disease　職業復帰 return to work[one's job]　職業リハビリテーション occupational rehabilitation　職業倫理 professional ethics　職業歴 occupational history

しょくご　食後(に)　after meals　◆この薬は食後に飲んで下さい Please take this medication after meals.　◆食後2時間く

らいは横にならないようにして下さい Please try to wait at least two hours before lying down after eating. / Please avoid going to bed within two hours of eating.　◆毎食後に after every[each] meal　◆食後高血糖 after-meal hyperglycemia　食後服用(服薬指示)To be taken after meals

しょくこうどう　食行動　eating behavior, dietary behavior　(授乳の)feeding behavior　▶食行動異常 eating disorder　食行動パターン eating behavior pattern

しょくじ　食事　(一般的に)meal　(治療などのための規定食)diet　(㊟dietary)　☞食，食習慣，食生活，食べ物，食べる
《食習慣の基本表現》　◆食事は規則的にとっていますか Do you eat *at regular times [regularly]? / Are you eating regularly?　◆食事は不規則なほうですか Do you eat at irregular times? / Do you tend to eat irregularly?　◆食事は1日何回食べますか How many times a day do you eat?　◆食事を抜く skip meals　◆食事制限をしている be on a restricted diet
《食事に関する指示》　◆検査の前夜は軽い食事にして，0時以後は飲食を控えて下さい On the night before the day of the test, please eat a light meal, and don't eat or drink after midnight.　◆食事と生活習慣を変える change one's diet and daily habits　◆食事の調節で体重増加を抑える control weight increase by dietary regulation　◆食事を減らす eat less
《食事の内容》　◆脂っこい食事 a fatty [greasy] meal　◆脂肪分を抑えた食事 a diet that is low in fat　◆塩分の多い食事 a salty meal　◆バランスのとれた食事 a well-balanced meal　◆果物や野菜の多い食事 a diet that is rich in fruits and vegetables　◆繊維の多い食事 a diet rich in fibers / a high-fiber diet　◆菜食主義者の食事 a vegetarian diet /(卵・牛乳も摂らない厳格な食事)a vegan diet　◆軽い食事 a light meal　◆温かい食事 a hot meal
《配膳・下膳》　◆お食事をお持ちしました(朝食)Here's your breakfast〈(昼食)lunch /

（夕食）dinner．　◆食事はお済みになりましたか Have you finished eating? / Are you through with your meal?

▶食事記録 diet record　食事時間 meal times　食事指導 dietary guidance[instruction]　食事摂取量 dietary intake　食事箋 dietary recipe[slip]　☞食事制限，食事療法

食事の種類

★diet のかわりに food を用いてもよい．

■一般食 general diet
●普通食 regular[normal] diet / ordinary meal　●固形食 solid diet　●軟食 soft diet　●半流動食 semiliquid [semisoft] diet　●流動食 liquid diet　●粥食 semisolid diet / rice porridge (diet)

■特別食 special diet・治療食 therapeutic diet
●嚥下食 dysphagia diet / diet for patients with a swallowing disorder　●減量食 reduction[reducing] diet / (体重の) weight-reduction[weight-reducing] diet　●除去食 elimination diet　●心臓病食 cardiac[heart-healthy] diet　●腎臓病食 renal[kidney-healthy] diet　●痛風食 gout diet　●糖尿病食 diabetic diet　●減塩食 low-salt[low-sodium] diet / sodium-restricted diet　●低カリウム食 low-potassium diet　●低カロリー食 low-calorie diet；LCD / calorie-restricted diet　●高カロリー食 high-calorie diet；HCD　●低コレステロール食 low-cholesterol diet　●低残渣食 low-residue diet；LRD　●低脂肪食 low-fat [fat-restricted] diet　●低繊維食 low-fiber diet；LFD　●高繊維食 high-fiber diet　●低炭水化物食 low-carbohydrate diet　●低蛋白食 low protein[protein-restricted] diet　●高蛋白食 high-protein diet　●低プリン食 low-purine diet　●低ヨード食 low-iodine diet　●低リン食 low-phosphorus diet　●無グルテン食 gluten-free diet　●無乳糖食 lactose-free diet

しょくじせいげん　**食事制限**　dietary restriction（🈺restrict *one's* diet）　☞食事，食事療法，ダイエット　◆食事制限はありますか Do you have any restrictions in your diet?　◆血糖値が高いので食事制限が必要です Your blood sugar level is high, so you need to restrict your diet.　◆食事制限はきちんと守っていますか Are you keeping [sticking] to your diet?　◆明日から彼女は流動食に食事制限されます She'll be put on a liquid diet starting tomorrow. / We're going to restrict her to a liquid diet from tomorrow.

しょくしふしん　**食思不振**　☞食欲不振

しょくじりょうほう　**食事療法**　diet therapy, dietary therapy　☞食事，食事制限，ダイエット　◆特別な食事療法をしていますか Are you on a special diet?　◆厳しい食事療法をしている be on a strict diet　◆慢性腎不全の食事療法 a diet therapy for chronic kidney failure / a renal failure diet

しょくしゅ　**職種**　type of work, kind of work　☞仕事，職業　◆現在の仕事はどのような職種ですか What type of work do you do?

しょくしゅうかん　**食習慣**　eating habits　★通例，複数形で．　☞食事，食生活　◆食習慣についてお話し下さい Please tell me about your eating habits.　◆食習慣を変える〈改める〉必要があります You need to change〈modify〉your eating habits.　◆食習慣を改善する improve *one's* eating habits

しょくしん　**触診**　palpation　◆お腹を触診しましょう Let me feel[examine] your abdomen.　◆定期的に乳房の自己触診をしていますか Have you been doing regular breast self-exams?　◆視触診 inspection and palpation　直腸触診 digital rectal examination；DRE

しょくせいかつ　**食生活**　eating habits　★通例，複数形で．　☞食事，食習慣　◆規則正しい食生活をして下さい（決まった時間に食べる）Please eat regularly[at regular times]. /（1 日に 3 度きちんと食べる）Please have three regular meals a day. ◆不規則な食生活 irregular eating habits

しょくぜん 食前(に) **before meals, before food** ◆この薬は食前に飲んで下さい Please take this medication before meals. ▶食前服用(服薬指示) To be taken before meals

じょくそう 褥瘡 **bedsore, pressure sore, decubitus** ◆床擦れ ▶褥瘡ケア bedsore [pressure sore] care 褥瘡性潰瘍 pressure[decubitus] ulcer

しょくち 触知(可能な) **palpable** ◆触知可能な紫斑 palpable purpura ◆非触知乳がん nonpalpable[impalpable] breast cancer

しょくちゅうどく 食中毒 **food poisoning** (食物による疾病〈感染症〉)**foodborne disease〈infection〉** (飲料水による疾病〈感染症〉)**waterborne disease〈infection〉** ◆症状からはどうも食中毒のようです From your symptoms, I think you probably have food poisoning. ◆最近ノロウイルス食中毒が保育園で発生しました Foodborne norovirus illness[infection] recently broke out at a day care center. / There was a recent outbreak of foodborne norovirus illness[infection] at a day care center. ◆食中毒の予防 prevention of food poisoning ◀細菌性食中毒 bacterial food poisoning サルモネラ食中毒 salmonella food poisoning 集団食中毒 mass food poisoning / large scale outbreak of food poisoning ブドウ球菌食中毒 staphylococcal food poisoning

しょくちょくご 食直後(に) **immediately after meals[eating], right after meals[eating]**

しょくちょくぜん 食直前(に) **immediately before meals[eating], right before meals[eating]**

しょくどう¹ 食堂 **dining room** (カフェテリア)**cafeteria** ◆食事はお部屋でも食堂でも召しあがることができます Your meals can be served to you in your room or in the dining room.

しょくどう² 食道 **esophagus** /ɪsɑ́fəgəs/ (圏**esophagéal**), **gullet** ◆胃酸の逆流により食道が炎症を起こしています Your esophagus is inflamed because of *backflow of acid[acid backing up] from the stomach. ◀胃食道逆流症 gastroesophageal reflux disease；GERD 気管食道瘻 tracheoesophageal fistula 頸部〈胸部／腹部〉食道 cervical〈thoracic / abdominal〉esophagus 上部〈中部／下部〉食道 upper〈middle / lower〉third of the esophagus バレット食道 Barrett esophagus ◆食道アカラシア esophageal achalasia 食道がん esophageal cancer / cancer of the esophagus 食道カンジダ症 *Candida* esophagitis / esophageal candidiasis 食道狭窄 esophageal stenosis[stricture] 食道ステント esophageal stent 食道造影 esophagography / barium swallow 食道発声 esophageal speech 食道裂孔ヘルニア esophageal hiatal hernia ☞食道炎, 食道静脈瘤

しょくどうえん 食道炎 **esophagitis** ◀逆流性食道炎 reflux esophagitis 放射線食道炎 radiation esophagitis

しょくどうじょうみゃくりゅう 食道静脈瘤 **esophageal varices** (圏**varix**) ▶食道静脈瘤硬化療法 sclerotherapy for esophageal varices 食道静脈瘤破裂 rupture of the esophageal varices

しょくば 職場 **place of work, workplace** ◆職場に同じような症状の人がいますか Does anyone around you at work have similar symptoms? ◆職場まで歩いて通う walk to work ◆職場までバスで〈電車で〉通う take the bus〈train〉to work ◆職場復帰する return to work[*one's job*] ◆職場の人間関係に悩んでいる have trouble with people at work / worry about relationships with colleagues ▶職場環境 working conditions / work environment 職場ストレス job[work-related] stress

しょくひ¹ 食費 **food expenses**

しょくひ² 植皮(術) ☞皮膚移植

しょくひん 食品 **food** ☞食物(しょくもつ), 食べ物 ◆塩分の強い食品は避けるよ

うお勧めします I recommend that you avoid[stay away from] eating salty foods. ◆体に悪い食品 unhealthy[unwholesome] food(s) ◀アレルゲン除去食品 allergen-free food　遺伝子組み換え食品 *genetically modified[GM] food　栄養補助食品 dietary[nutritional] supplement　減塩食品 low-salt[low-sodium] food / sodium-restricted food　健康食品 health food　自然食品 natural food　生鮮食品 fresh food　ダイエット食品 diet[dietetic] food　凍結乾燥食品 freeze-dried food　特定保健用食品 food for specified health use(s)　病人用食品 food for sick people[patients]　補強食品 supplementary[supplemental] food　保存食品 preserved food / (腐りにくい食品) nonperishable food　冷凍食品 frozen food　▶食品アレルギー food allergy　食品衛生 food hygiene[sanitation]　食品衛生法 Food Sanitation Law　食品添加物 food additives

しょくぶつ　植物　plant (㊎植物性の vegetable　植物状態の vegetative) ◆植物にアレルギーがありますか Are you allergic to any plants? ◀遷延性植物状態 persistent vegetative state；PVS　薬用植物 medicinal plant[(薬草) herb]　有毒植物 toxic [poisonous] plant　▶植物性脂肪 vegetable fat　植物性蛋白 vegetable protein　植物繊維 vegetable fiber　植物油 vegetable oil

しょくもう　植毛　hair transplant[transplantation] (㊎transplant hair), hair implant[implantation] ◆後頭部と側頭部の毛を脱毛部へ植毛する transplant hair from the back and side of the scalp into [to] the bald areas　▶人工植毛 synthetic [artificial] hair implant

しょくもつ　食物　food ☞食品, 食べ物　▶食物アレルギー food allergy　食物アレルゲン food allergen　食物残渣 food residue　食物消化 food digestion ☞食物繊維

しょくもつせんい　食物繊維　dietary fiber ◆食物繊維は便通を調節してくれます

Dietary fiber helps promote[regulate] bowel function. ◆便秘はたいてい食物繊維の不足が原因で起こります Constipation usually results from a lack of dietary fiber. ◆食物繊維が豊富な果物や野菜を食べる必要があります You need to eat fruit or vegetables rich[high] in (dietary) fiber.

しょくよく　食欲　appetite /ǽpətàit/ ◆食欲はどうですか How is your appetite? ◆食欲はありますか Do you have a good appetite? / Are you eating all right? ◆食欲がある〈まあまあ / ほとんどない〉have a good〈fair / poor〉appetite ◆食欲がまったくない have no appetite (at all) ◆最近食欲に変化がありましたか Has there been any change in your appetite? ◆食欲が増した〈減った / ほぼ同じ〉the appetite has increased〈decreased / stayed about the same〉 ◆食欲が低下したのはつい最近ですか, それともかなり前ですか Did you lose your appetite just recently or some time ago? ◆食欲を満足させる satisfy *one's* appetite　▶食欲異常 appetite disturbance / disturbance of appetite　食欲障害 appetite disorder ☞食欲不振

しょくよくふしん　食欲不振　appetite loss, lack[loss] of appetite, anorexia ◆食欲不振である have a poor appetite ◆食欲不振に陥る lose *one's* appetite ◀神経性食欲不振症 anorexia nervosa；AN　★一般的には anorexia のみ.

しょけい¹　初経　the first (menstrual) period, initial (menstrual) period, menarche ◆初経年齢は何歳の時ですか How old were you when you had your first (menstrual) period?

しょけい²　書痙　writer's cramp

しょけん　所見 (検査などの結果)**findings** ★通例, 複数形で. (観察に基づく意見)**observation** ◆心電図所見は正常です The EKG findings[observations] are normal. ◆検査でがんの所見がみられました The test findings show signs of cancer. / The tests show signs of cancer.

◆大腸内視鏡の所見では according to your colonoscopy ◀入院時の所見 findings on admission ◀X線所見 radiologic findings 検査所見 examination[laboratory] findings 身体所見 physical findings 他覚的所見 objective findings[(徴候) signs] 病理所見 pathologic findings 剖検所見 autopsy findings 臨床所見 clinical findings

じょげん **助言** advice (動advise) ☞勧める，忠告 ◆精神科医の助言を受ける〈助言に従う〉take〈follow〉the psychiatrist's advice ◆腫瘍専門医の助言を求める ask (for) an oncologist's advice / go to an oncologist for advice ◆感染を防ぐために適切な助言を与える *give proper advice [advise appropriately] on how to prevent infection

じょさいどう **除細動** defibrillation ◀電気的除細動 electric defibrillation / cardioversion ☞除細動器

じょさいどうき **除細動器** defibrillator, **cardioverter** ◀植込み型除細動器 implantable (cardioverter) defibrillator；ICD 自動体外式除細動器 automated external defibrillator；AED 直流除細動器 *direct current[DC] defibrillator

しょさん **初産** one's first childbirth, the **delivery of** one's **first baby** ◀高年初産婦 elderly woman in her first pregnancy / elderly primipara ▶初産婦 (出産予定の) woman in her first pregnancy / woman expecting a baby for the first time / primipara / (出産後の) woman who has had her first baby

じょさん **助産** ▶助産院 maternity[midwife] clinic 助産師(nurse) midwife

しょじ **所持する** (所有する)**have**, **possess** (持ち歩く)**carry** ◆必ずこの糖尿病 ID カードを所持して下さい Please always carry this diabetic ID[identification / identity] card with you. ☞所持品

じょし **女子** girl (女性)woman (動women 形female) ☞女性 ◆女子学生 a female student

しょじしょうがい **書字障害** dysgraphia

じょしつき **除湿器** dehumidifier ◆除湿器をかける turn on a dehumidifier

しょじひん **所持品** one's (personal) belongings[things] ★通例，複数形で. ☞持ち物

じょしゅ **助手** assistant ◀看護助手 nursing assistant / nurses' aide 外科助手 surgical assistant 病棟助手 ward [floor / unit] assistant

じょしゅう **除臭** (消臭)deodorization, **odor removal**

じょじょ **徐々(に)** (次第に)gradually (ゆっくりと)slowly (少しずつ)little by little ◆痛みは徐々に起こったのですか，それとも突然でしたか Did the pain come on gradually or suddenly? ◆抑うつ気分は徐々に軽く〈ひどく〉なっていますか Is your depressed mood getting better 〈worse〉? ◆軽い運動をして徐々に体力をつけて下さい Please build up your strength little by little by doing light exercise. ◆彼は手術から徐々に回復しています He is slowly recovering from his surgery. ◆血糖値が徐々に上がって〈下がって〉います Your blood sugar level is going up〈down〉slowly[gradually].

しょじょまく **処女膜** hymen

しょしん **初診** first visit (to the hospital 〈clinic〉) ◆初診ですか Is this your first visit? / Are you a new patient? / Have you visited this hospital before? ▶初診受付 new patient registration counter [desk] 初診料 initial fee[charge]

じょせい¹ **女性** woman (複women 形 **female**) ◆高齢女性 an elderly woman ▶女性仮性半陰陽 female pseudohermaphroditism 女性看護師 female nurse 女性性器 female genitals[genitalia / genital organs] 女性生殖器系 the female reproductive system 女性専門外来 the women-only outpatient department [clinic] 女性ホルモン female (sex) hormone 女性用トイレ (the) women's [ladies'] room ☞女性化

じょせい² **助成** (支援)support, assistance (政府などからの金銭援助)subsidization（圏subsidize）　◆難病には政府からの助成があります Patients with intractable diseases can receive government support [assistance]. / Medical costs for intractable diseases are subsidized by the government.　◀難病医療費助成制度 financial assistance for intractable diseases　▶助成金 subsidy /（研究などに与えられる奨励金）grant

じょせいか　**女性化**　feminization　◀精巣性女性化症候群 testicular feminization syndrome　副腎性女性化 adrenal feminism　▶女性化乳房 gynecomastia

しょせつ　**諸説**　various opinions [views]　◆その原因については諸説ありますが，どれも決め手に欠けています There are various opinions[views] about what causes it, but no conclusive evidence exists for any of them.

じょそうざい　**除草剤**　weedkiller, herbicide　◆除草剤を飲んで自殺する kill *oneself* by drinking[swallowing] weedkiller [herbicide]　▶除草剤中毒 herbicide poisoning

しょち　**処置**　（治療）treatment　（圏treat）（ケア）care（圏care）　（治療の手順）procedure　（対策）measure　☞治療　◆傷口の処置をしましょう Let me treat your wound.　◆一時的な処置をしておきます I'm going to give you a temporary treatment.　◆この処置で一時的に症状は和らぐでしょう This treatment will relieve your symptoms for the time being.　◆必要とされる適切な処置を施す give *a person* appropriate treatment as required[necessary]　◆彼が病院に到着した時にはすでに処置の施しようがありませんでした When he arrived at the hospital, there was nothing we could do for him.　◆未処置の虫歯 untreated tooth decay　◀一次救命処置 basic life support；BLS　応急処置 first aid / emergency treatment[care]　外科的〈内科的〉処置 surgical〈nonsurgical / medical〉treatment　追加処置 additional procedure　二次救命処置 advanced cardiac[cardiovascular] life sup-

port；ACLS　入院処置 hospital treatment　予防処置 preventive treatment /（予防策）preventive[precautionary] measure　▶処置室 treatment room

しょちょう　**初潮**　☞初経

じょちょう　**助長する**　（増す）increase（促進する）encourage, promote　◆薬によっては手術後に出血の危険を助長する恐れがありますので，常用している薬があれば教えて下さい Could you tell me if you are on any medications because some of them may increase your risk of bleeding after surgery.　◆この病名は患者さんへの偏見を助長するので，今は使われません This term for the illness encourages [promotes] prejudice against patients, so it isn't used any longer.

しょっかく　**触覚**　sense of touch, touch sensation（圏tactile）　◆触覚は過敏ですか Do you have an acute sense of touch?　◆触覚が鈍くなったような感じはありますか Do you feel that your sense of touch has become less sharp[acute]?　◆触覚に左右差がある the sense of touch is different *between the left and the right sides [between the two sides]　▶触覚過敏 tactile hyperesthesia　触覚減退 tactile hypesthesia　触覚麻痺 tactile paralysis

しょっかん¹　**触感**　（物の質感）texture（触った感触）the feel, the touch　☞肌触り

しょっかん²　**食間（に）**　between meals　▶食間服用（服薬指示）To be taken between meals

ショック　**shock**
《精神的な衝撃》　◆ショックを与える shock / give a shock　◆精神的ショックを受けている be in（a state of）emotional [psychological] shock / be in shock　◆この検査結果はさぞショックなことと思います I understand[I can see] that this test result must be a shock for you.
《循環障害による症候》　◆ショック症状を起こす get a shock　◆ショック死する die of [from] shock
《通電ショック》　◆直流通電ショック *direct current[DC] shock　◆電気ショック療法

*electric shock[electroshock] therapy；EST / electroconvulsive therapy；ECT

◀アナフィラキシーショック anaphylactic shock 外傷性ショック traumatic shock 出血性ショック hemorrhagic shock 循環血液量減少性ショック hypovolemic shock 神経原性ショック neurogenic shock 心原性ショック cardiogenic shock 毒素性ショック症候群 toxic shock syndrome；TSS 敗血症性ショック septic shock

▶ショック体位 shock position

しょてい 所定(の) (必要な)necessary (規定の)prescribed ◆入院される方は所定の手続きを済ませて下さい Upon admission to the hospital please complete the necessary admission procedures [forms]. ◆所定の用紙がありますのでご記入の上提出して下さい Here is the prescribed form, so please fill it out and hand it in to us.

しょとう ショ糖 sucrose

しょとく 所得 income ☞収入 ◆彼には年間300万円の所得があります He has *an annual[a yearly] income of three million yen. ◆所得が多い〈少ない〉have a large〈small〉income / 低所得の家庭 a low-income family / a family with a low income ◀世帯所得 family income ▶所得税 income tax

しょにち 初日 the first day ◆最終月経の初日はいつでしたか When was the first day of your last (menstrual) period?

しょにゅう 初乳 colostrum, the first breast milk

じょのう 除脳 decerebration (形decerebrate) ▶除脳硬直 decerebrate rigidity 除脳姿勢 decerebrate posture

じょはすいみん 徐波睡眠 slow-wave sleep

じょひしつ 除皮質 decortication (形decorticate) ▶除皮質硬直 decorticate rigidity 除皮質姿勢 decorticate posture

しょひよう 諸費用 miscellaneous (small) expenses, sundry expenses ◆諸費用と合わせて会計は1万円になります Including *miscellaneous small[sun-

dry] expenses, the cost is[comes to] ten thousand yen.

しょほう 処方する prescribe (图prescription) ◆抗菌薬を処方します I'm going to *prescribe an antibiotic[give you a prescription for an antibiotic]. ◆7日分の薬を処方しましょう I'll prescribe the medication for seven days. ◆処方された薬以外は飲まないで下さい Please don't take any medication unless prescribed by me. / Please don't take any medication other than the prescription one. ◆電話による処方はできません I'm sorry, but we can't give you a telephone prescription.

▶処方食 prescribed diet ☞処方箋, 処方薬

しょほうせん 処方箋 prescription ◆これが薬の処方箋です This is a prescription for your medication. / Here's your prescription. ◆この処方箋を薬局へ持参して下さい Please take this prescription to the pharmacy. ◆処方箋は今日〈発行日〉を含め4日間有効です The prescription is valid for four days from and including today〈the date of issue〉. ◆その薬は処方箋によってのみ入手できます That medication is available by prescription only. ◆睡眠薬の処方箋を書く write a prescription for sleeping pills ◆処方箋の薬を調合する fill the prescription ◀院外処方箋 prescription to be filled at an outside pharmacy 麻薬処方箋 narcotic prescription ▶処方箋料 prescription fee [charge]

しょほうやく 処方薬 prescription medication[drug], prescribed medication [drug] ◆今飲んでいるのは医師からの処方薬ですか, それとも市販薬ですか Are you taking a prescription medication or an over-the-counter[OTC] drug? / Is the medication you're taking a prescription or an over-the-counter[OTC] drug? ◆処方薬は今日〈処方箋の発行日〉から4日以内に受け取って下さい Please get your prescription medication within four days *including today〈of the date of issue）．

しょぼしょぼ ◆目がしょぼしょぼする get bleary eyes / the eyes go[become] bleary

じょみゃく 徐脈 bradycardia （↔tachycardia）, infrequent pulse ◀洞徐脈 sinus bradycardia ▶徐脈性不整脈 bradyarrhythmia

しょめい 署名 signature （動sign）☞サイン ◆この同意書に署名して下さい Please sign this consent form. / Could you please sign this consent form?

しょめん 書面 （文書）writing （過written） （手紙）letter ◆文書 ◆担当医の書面による許可を必要とする need one's doctor's written permission ◆書面で返事をする reply *in writing[by letter]

しょよう 所要（の） required （図requirement）, needed （図need） ◆カロリー所要量は，年齢，性別，身体活動レベルから推計されます A person's daily calorie *requirement is[needs are] estimated by his〈her〉age, gender, and physical activity level. ◆この検査の所要時間は約30分です This test takes approximately thirty minutes. ◆通勤の所要時間はどのくらいですか How long does it take to commute [get] to your office? ◀エネルギー所要量 energy requirement[（許容量）allowance] ▶所要時間 the time required [needed]

しょり 処理する 《物事をさばく》（取り扱う）handle, deal （with） （うまく対処する）manage, cope （with） ☞対応, 対処 ◆問題を処理する handle[deal with / manage] a problem ◆どうやってストレスを処理していますか What do you do to *cope with[manage] （your）stress? ◆苦情処理手続き complaints[grievance] procedure 《加工処理する》process ◆データを処理する process data ◆画像処理 image processing ◆データ処理 data processing ◆リアルタイム処理 real-time processing 《処分する》dispose （of） ◆汚物処理室 dirty utility room / （尿・便などの）soiled （linen）utility room / （汚染物質の）utility

room for contaminants

しょるい 書類 （用紙）form, paper （正式の）document ◆この書類に記入して下さい Please fill out[in] this form. ◆この書類を持って心電図室へ行って下さい Please take this form with you to the EKG room. ◀添付書類 accompanying[attached] document

しょろう 初老（の） presenile （年配の）elderly （中高年の）late middle-aged ▶初老期 late middle age 初老期うつ病 presenile depression 初老期認知症 presenile dementia

しらが 白髪 （白髪混じり）gray hair （白髪）white hair ◀若白髪 premature gray hair / premature （hair）graying

しらこ 白子 （白皮症）albinism

しらせ 知らせ （ニュース）news （報告）report （情報）information ☞巻末付録：悪い診断結果を伝える時 ◆良いお知らせがあります I have some good news for you. / I have a piece of good news for you. ★news は数えられないので，1つのニュースは a piece of news という． ◆残念ですが，良いお知らせではありません I'm afraid the news isn't good. / I'm sorry to have to tell you that the news isn't good. ◆残念ですが，悲しいお知らせです I'm sorry, but *I have[there's] some sad news for you.

しらせる 知らせる let a person know （話す）tell （報告する）inform ◆ご気分が悪い時にはこのコールボタンを押して知らせて下さい If you feel sick, please let us know by pushing[pressing] this call button. ◆ご用のある時は，私に知らせて下さい Please let me know if you need any help. ◆検査結果は来週お知らせします I'll let you know the test results next week. ◆彼女の病状については随時お知らせいたします I'll keep you informed about her condition.

しらべる 調べる （調査する）examine （図examination） （確認する）check （知る・突き止める）find out （原因究明する）investigate, look into ◆胃に異常な組織がないか調べましょう Let's examine[check]

your stomach for any abnormal tissues.
◆検体を顕微鏡で調べる examine the specimen under[through] a microscope ◆しこりを詳しく調べる do[carry out] a detailed[thorough] examination of a lump ◆耳鳴りの原因を調べるために，聴力検査を行いましょう Let's do[run] a hearing test to find out what's causing the ringing in your ears. ◆事故の原因を調べる *look into[investigate] the cause of the accident

シラミ lice（圈louse）◆シラミを取る remove[get rid of] lice ◆シラミがわく get lice ◀アタマジラミ head lice 毛ジラミ crab[pubic] lice コロモジラミ body lice ▶シラミ症 pediculosis

しり 尻 buttocks /bʌ́təks/ ◆通例，複数形で．bottom, gluteal region ☞尻もち

じりき 自力（で） on one's own, by oneself （助けを借りずに）without help ◆自力で呼吸する breathe on one's own / breathe by oneself ◆自力で立ち上がる stand on one's own two feet ◆自力でトイレに行く walk to the bathroom without help

シリコーン （ケイ素系樹脂）silicone ★元素のシリコン（ケイ素）は silicon．▶シリコーンインプラント silicone implant シリコーンチューブ silicone tube

じりつ 自立する （自活する）support oneself, live by oneself （図self-support）（独立する）live independently （圏independent）◆息子さんはすでに自立していますか Is your son already *supporting himself[living by himself]？ ◆退院後に自立した生活を送るためのサービスを必要としますか Do you need any services to help you *support yourself[live independently] after leaving the hospital? ▶自立生活 independent living；IL

じりつくんれん 自律訓練 autogenic training

じりつしんけい 自律神経 autonomic nerve ▶自律神経系 the autonomic nervous system；ANS 自律神経障害 autonomic disturbance 自律神経ニュー

ロパチー autonomic neuropathy

しりつびょういん 市立病院 city hospital （市営・町営の）municipal hospital

しりめつれつ 支離滅裂 ◆彼は時に支離滅裂なことを言うことがありますか Does he sometimes say things that don't make any sense? /（ろれつが回らず話し続ける）Does he sometimes ramble incoherently? ◆支離滅裂になる（考えなどが混乱する）get muddled

しりもち 尻もち ◆尻もちをつく fall on one's bottom[buttocks]

しりやく 止痢薬 （止瀉薬）antidiarrheal （medication, drug, agent）

しりょう¹ 資料 （データ）data （素材）material ◆薬の有効性と安全性についての資料を集める collect[gather] data on the effectiveness and safety of a medication ◀参考資料 reference data[material] 統計資料 statistical data

しりょう² 試料 （標本）sample （調合した薬品）preparation ☞検体, サンプル

しりょく 視力 eyesight, vision, visual acuity；VA ◆遠くの物〈近くの物〉が見えにくいなど，視力に何か問題がありますか Do you have any problems with your vision[eyesight], such as with seeing objects that are *far away〈close at hand〉? ◆最近視力が変化しましたか Have you recently noticed any changes in your eyesight[vision]? ◆視力が落ちているのですか Is your vision failing[getting weak]? ◆急に視力が低下しましたか Has your eyesight[vision] suddenly *become worse[changed for the worse]? ◆視力を測る measure[evaluate] a person's eyesight[vision] ◆視力がいい〈弱い〉have good〈poor〉eyesight[vision] ◆あなたの視力は正常です You have normal eyesight[vision]. ◆あなたの視力は右目が 1.2 で左目が 0.8 です Your eyesight is[You have a visual acuity of] 1.2 [one-point-two] in the right eye and 0.8 [(zero-)point-eight] in the left eye. ◆視力は両目とも 1.0 です Your visual acuity is 1.0[one-point-zero] in both eyes. / You have 20/20[twenty-twenty] vision in both eyes. ★視力「1.0」は，英語圏では一般に「20/20」と表現される．「20/20」は慣用的に「あなたの視力は正常です」という意味にも用いられる． ◆視力を失う lose *one's* eyesight / suffer loss of (*one's*) vision ◆視力を回復する recover[regain / restore] *one's* eyesight[vision] ◀矯正視力 corrected vision[visual acuity]　近距離視力表 near vision test chart　近見視力 near visual acuity　中心視力 central vision　裸眼視力 naked[uncorrected] vision[visual acuity]　両眼視力 binocular vision[visual acuity]　▶視力障害 vision[visual] disorder / vision[visual] impairment　視力測定 measurement of vision　視力測定器 optometer　視力調節 visual adaptation　☞視力検査

視力の分数表記
fractional visual acuity

わが国では視力は「1.5」「1.0」などの小数で表記されるが，アメリカやイギリスなど英語圏では「20/10」「30/20」「20/20」（フィート表記）や「6/3」「9/6」「6/6」（メートル表記）などの分数で表記されるのが一般的である．例えば，20/40（6/12）は 20 フィート（6 メートル）離れた物があたかも 40 フィート（12 メートル）離れたもののように見える（つまり視力が悪い）という意味で，わが国で言う 0.5 に相当する．

しりょくけんさ　視力検査　eye test, vision test, eyesight test, visual acuity test
◆視力検査をしましょう Let's do[run] *an eye[a vision] test. ◆視力検査を受ける have *an eye[a vision] test　▶視力検査表 eye chart / vision[visual acuity] (test) chart / Snellen chart

しる　知る　(一般的に)know　(情報を得る・学ぶ)learn　(気づく)notice, find　(経験する)experience ◆吸入器の使い方を知っていますか Do you know how to use the inhaler? ◆最初に心臓に問題があることを知ったのはいつですか When did you first learn[notice] that you have a heart problem? ◆あなたの国の文化についてもっと知りたいです I'd like to learn [know] more about the culture of your country.

しるし¹　印　(照合の✓印)check　(圖check)，《英》tick　(圖tick)　(記号)mark　(圖mark)
◆この問診票のあてはまる項目に印をつけて下さい Please check[mark] the items that apply (to you) in this questionnaire.

しるし²　徴　(徴候)sign　(証拠)proof, evidence ◆(手術後)ガスが出るのは腸が正常に戻ってきているしるしです Passing gas (after surgery) *is a sign[is proof] that your intestines are returning to normal.
☞おしるし

シルマーしけん　―試験　Schirmer test

じれい　事例　☞症例

しれつきょうせい　歯列矯正　teeth-straightening, straightening of the teeth
◆娘さんは歯列矯正が必要です Your daughter needs to have her teeth straightened. / (歯列矯正器の装着)Your daughter needs to have braces. ▶歯列矯正医 orthodontist　歯列矯正学 orthodontics ☞歯列矯正器

しれつきょうせいき　歯列矯正器　(dental) braces　★通例，複数形で． ◆歯列矯正器をつけている wear (dental) braces

ジレンマ　dilemma ◆彼は同僚と仲良くできないというジレンマを抱えています He has the dilemma of not being able to get along well with his colleagues. ◆彼女は手術すべきかどうかというジレンマに陥っています She is in a dilemma about whether to have the surgery. ◆彼女は帰国するか日本にとどまるかでジレンマに陥っています She is torn[caught (up) in a dilemma] between returning home and staying in Japan.

しろい　白い　white　(肌が)fair　☞白っぽい ◆白い便 white stools

しろう　脂漏(症)　seborrhea　(圏seborrheic)　▶脂漏性角化症 seborrheic keratosis　脂漏性湿疹 seborrheic eczema　脂漏性皮膚炎 seborrheic dermatitis　脂漏性疣贅 seborrheic wart

じろう¹　痔瘻　anal fistula

じろう² 耳漏 ear discharge, otorrhea ☞耳だれ

しろうと 素人 (専門家に対して)layperson (圏laypeople) (アマチュア)amateur ◆応急処置は素人にもできる緊急援助です First aid is emergency help that can be given by a layperson. ◆診断について医師は素人にもわかる言葉で説明すべきです Doctors should explain a diagnosis *in terms a layperson can understand[in layperson's terms].

シロップ syrup /sírəp/ ◆お子さんには(咳止め)シロップ剤をお出しします I'm going to[Let me] prescribe some (cough) syrup for your child. ◆シロップは1回1目盛与えて下さい Please give him〈her〉a unit[portion] of syrup each time. ◆シロップを小さじ一杯飲む take one teaspoon of syrup ◀ビタミンK₂シロップ vitamin K₂ syrup

しろっぽい 白っぽい whitish ◆白っぽい痰〈分泌物〉whitish phlegm〈discharge〉

しろめ 白目 the white(s) of one's eye(s)

しわ 皺 wrinkle (圏wrinkled), crease ◆皮膚のしわ wrinkles in the skin ◆しわの寄った皮膚 wrinkled skin ◆しわを取る remove wrinkles ◆シーツのしわを伸ばす straighten the bed sheets / smooth [straighten] out the wrinkles in the bed sheets ◆しわ取り整形する have a face-lift ◀小じわ fine wrinkles /(目尻の)crow's feet ▶しわ取り術 facelift surgery / facial rhytidoplasty

しわがれごえ しわがれ声 (がらがら声) hoarse voice (かすれた声)husky voice (擦過音の)scratchy voice ◆しわがれ声で話す speak in a hoarse[husky] voice ◆しわがれ声のようですが，いつから続いていますか Your voice sounds hoarse. How long has it been that way?

しわがれる (声ががらがらになる)get[become] hoarse ◆声がしわがれたのはいつからですか Since when has your voice been hoarse?

しん 心 heart ☞心臓 ◀滴状心 drop heart 肺性心 cor pulmonale 肥大心 hy-pertrophic heart ▶心アミロイドーシス cardiac amyloidosis ☞心陰影, 心エコー, 心音, 心外膜, 心拡大, 心悸亢進, 心機能, 心筋, 心係数, 心血管, 心原性, 心雑音, 心室, 心疾患, 心静止, 心尖, 心タンポナーデ, 心調律, 心停止, 心電計, 心電図, 心毒性, 心内膜, 心囊, 心肺, 心拍, 心破裂, 心肥大, 心不全, 心房, 心膜, 心マッサージ

じん 腎 kidney ☞腎臓 ◀アミロイド腎 amyloid kidney 萎縮腎 atrophic[con-tracted] kidney 移植腎 transplanted kidney 痛風腎 gouty kidney ドナー腎 donor kidney 馬蹄腎 horseshoe kidney 無機能腎 nonfunctioning kidney 融合腎 fused kidney 遊走腎 floating[wander-ing] kidney 矮小腎 dwarf[miniature] kidney ▶腎アミロイドーシス renal amy-loidosis ☞腎移植, 腎盂, 腎炎, 腎機能, 腎クリアランス, 腎結核, 腎血管, 腎結石, 腎硬化症, 腎後性, 腎細胞癌, 腎疾患, 腎周囲膿瘍, 腎症, 腎障害, 腎シンチグラフィ, 腎性, 腎生検, 腎切石, 腎前性, 腎疝痛, 腎損傷, 腎摘除, 腎動静脈瘻, 腎動脈, 腎毒性, 腎尿管摘除, 腎尿管膀胱部単純撮影, 腎尿細管性アシドーシス, 腎囊胞, 腎膿瘍, 腎破裂, 腎バンク, 腎不全, 腎瘻造設

じんあい 塵埃 dust ☞粉塵

しんい 真意 ◆真意がうまく伝わらなかったようです I'm afraid I haven't made myself clearly understood. / I'm afraid you haven't understood what I really [truly] meant.

じんいしょく 腎移植 kidney transplant [transplantation], renal transplant[trans-plantation]

じんいてき 人為的(な) human ◆人為的なミスによる有害事象 adverse events due to *human error[an error caused by human carelessness] ◆薬で人為的に陣痛を起こす induce labor with[by using] drugs

しんいんえい 心陰影 heart shadow, car-diac shadow

しんいんせい 心因性(の) psychogen-ic /sàikədʒénik/ ▶心因性胸痛 psycho-genic chest pain 心因性下痢 psychogenic diarrhea 心因性疾患 psychogenic disease 心因性失声症〈発声障害〉psychogenic aphonia〈dysphonia〉 心因性咳 psychogenic cough 心因性多飲 psychogenic polydipsia 心因(性)反応 psychogenic reaction

じんう 腎盂 renal pelvis, pelvis of the kidney（略語pyel(o)-） ◀逆行性腎盂造影 retrograde pyelography；RP 静脈性腎盂造影 intravenous pyelography；IVP／X-ray recording of the kidneys and urinary tract ▶腎盂がん renal pelvic cancer 腎盂結石 renal pelvic stone 腎盂腎炎 pyelonephritis 腎盂尿管形成術 pyeloureteroplasty

しんエコー 心エコー(検査) (ultrasonic) echocardiography；UCG, ultrasound recording of the heart ◀経食道心エコー検査 transesophageal echocardiography ▶心エコー図 echocardiogram

じんえん 腎炎 nephritis /nɪfráɪtɪs/（略語 nephritic） ◀間質性腎炎 interstitial nephritis ループス腎炎 lupus nephritis 腎炎症候群 nephritic syndrome ☞糸球体腎炎

しんおん 心音 heart sound[tone], cardiac sound[tone] ◀胎児心音 fetal heart tone ▶心音図 phonocardiogram

しんがいまく 心外膜 epicardium

じんかく 人格 personality ☞パーソナリティ ◆最近，彼女の人格に変化はありましたか Have you noticed any changes in her personality? ▶多重人格 multiple personality 二重人格 double[dual] personality ▶人格検査 personality test 人格変化 personality change

しんかくだい 心拡大 heart[cardiac] enlargement, enlargement of the heart, cardiomegaly （心拡張）heart[cardiac] dilatation, dilatation of the heart （心肥大）cardiac hypertrophy ◆心拡大がある have an enlarged heart

しんがた 新型 new type （新しい系統・菌の）new strain ▶新型インフルエンザ new strain[type] of influenza[flu]

しんかぶつう 心窩部痛 epigastric pain, upper abdominal pain, epigastralgia

シンガポール Singapore（略語Singaporean） ◎国籍 ▶シンガポール人(の) Singaporean

しんかん¹ 新患 new patient, first visit patient ▶新患受付 new patient registration counter[desk]

しんかん² 新館 new building （旧館に対して別館）annex ◆放射線科は病院新館地下にあります The radiology department is located in the basement of the new building.

しんきこうしん 心悸亢進 （動悸）palpitations ★通例，複数形で. （速脈）rapid pulse, accelerated heart beat

しんきしょう 心気症 hypochondriasis

しんきのう 心機能 heart[cardiac] function ◆心機能に問題はありません You have no problem with your heart function. ▶心機能評価 evaluation[assessment] of heart[cardiac] function

じんきのう 腎機能 kidney[renal] function ◆腎機能が弱りつつあるようです It appears that your kidney function is getting worse. ▶腎機能検査 kidney[renal] function test 腎機能障害 renal dysfunction

しんきもうそう 心気妄想 hypochondriac delusion

しんきゅう 鍼灸 acupuncture and moxibustion ☞灸, 鍼(はり) ▶鍼灸師 acupuncture and moxibustion practitioner

しんきょう 心境 state of mind ◆退院が決まった今のご心境はいかがですか How do you feel now that your discharge date has been set[decided]? ◆現在の心境をお聞かせ下さい What's your state of mind now? / Please tell me about your current[present] state of mind. ◆彼女は心境の変化で手術を受けないことにしました She changed her mind and decided not to have the surgery.

しんきん¹ 心筋 heart[cardiac] muscle, myocardium（略語myocardial） ◀ウイルス性心筋炎 viral myocarditis ▶心筋炎 myocarditis 心筋虚血 myocardial

ischemia　心筋血流シンチグラフィ myocardial perfusion scintigraphy　心筋血流 SPECT myocardial（perfusion）SPECT［single photon emission computed tomography］　心筋損傷 myocardial damage　心筋保護 myocardial protection
☞心筋梗塞，心筋症

しんきん²　伸筋　**extensor**

しんきん³　真菌　**fungus**（㊂**fungal**）, **mycete**　◆抗真菌薬 antifungal（medication / drug / agent）　深在性真菌症 deep mycosis　肺真菌症 pulmonary mycosis　表在性真菌症 superficial mycosis　▶真菌学 mycology　真菌感染症 fungal infection / mycosis　真菌球 fungus ball

しんきんこうそく　心筋梗塞　**myocardial infarction** /mɑ̀iəkɑ́ə·diəl ɪnfɑ́ə·kʃən/；**MI**　★一般的には heart attack という。　☞心臓発作　◆心筋に酸素を送る動脈の一部が詰まって心筋梗塞が起こっています（起こした）You've had a myocardial infarction because a part of your heart's arteries that carry oxygen to the heart muscle is blocked.　◆ご家族に狭心症や心筋梗塞の方はいますか Is there anyone in your family who has a history of angina or heart attack?　◀急性心筋梗塞 acute myocardial infarction；AMI　陳旧性心筋梗塞 old myocardial infarction；OMI / previous myocardial infarction

しんきんしょう　心筋症　**cardiomyopathy**　◆心筋症とは，心臓の異常により心機能障害を来す疾患の総称です Cardiomyopathy is the general term for any disease in which abnormality of the heart muscle causes impairment of heart function.　◀拡張型心筋症 dilated cardiomyopathy；DCM　拘束型心筋症 restrictive cardiomyopathy；RCM / constrictive cardiomyopathy　肥大型心筋症 hypertrophic cardiomyopathy；HCM

じんクリアランス　腎クリアランス　**renal clearance**

しんけい　神経　**nerve**（㊂神経の・神経質な **nervous**　神経系の **neural**　神経症的な **neurotic**　神経原性・神経因性の **neurogenic**　神経障害的な **newopathic**　神経学的な **neurologic, neurological**）
《神経系》　◆指のしびれなど，神経に問題がありましたか Have you had any nerve problems such as numbness in your fingers?　◆神経を抜く extract a nerve　◆神経を傷める damage[injure] the nerves / （傷めている）have damage[an injury] to one's nerves
《精神状態》　◆神経を鎮める calm[soothe] one's nerves　◆神経の緊張を和らげる relieve[ease] nervous tension　◆彼女は慣れない環境で神経が参っているようです It seems she's having[suffering] a nervous breakdown due to being in an unfamiliar environment.　◆神経をすり減らすようなお仕事に就いているのですか Does your work *wear on your nerves[wear you down (mentally)]? / Is your work stressful on your nerves?　◆神経の疲れ nervous fatigue[exhaustion]

◀運動神経 motor nerve　感覚神経 sensory nerve　顔面神経 facial nerve　交感神経 sympathetic nerve　坐骨神経 sciatic nerve　三叉神経 trigeminal nerve　視神経 optic nerve　自律神経 autonomic nerve　知覚神経 sensory nerve　中枢神経 central nerve　中枢神経系 the central nervous system；CNS　聴（覚）神経 auditory[acoustic] nerve　脳神経 cranial nerve；CN　副交感神経 parasympathetic nerve　末梢神経 peripheral nerve　末梢神経系 the peripheral nervous system；PNS　迷走神経 vagus nerve　迷走神経反射 vagal reflex　肋間神経 intercostal nerve

▶神経圧迫症候群 nerve compression syndrome　神経学 neurology　神経学的診察 neurologic examination　神経芽腫 neuroblastoma　神経筋疾患 neuromuscular disease　神経系 the nervous system　神経原性腫瘍 neurogenic tumor　神経原性ショック neurogenic shock　神経膠細胞 neuroglia　神経膠腫 glioma　神経細胞 nerve cell / neuron　神経支配 innervation　神経障害 neurologic disorder /

neuropathy　神経症状 neurologic symptom　神経性過食症 bulimia nervosa；BN ★一般的には bulimia のみ．　神経生検 nerve biopsy　神経線維 nerve fiber　神経線維腫症 neurofibromatosis　神経損傷 nerve injury　神経伝達 neural transmission　神経伝達物質 neurotransmitter　神経伝導速度 nerve conduction velocity　神経毒 nerve poison／neurotoxin　神経特異性エノラーゼ neuron-specific enolase　神経内分泌腫瘍 neuroendocrine tumor　神経ブロック nerve block　神経麻痺 neuroparalysis ☞神経因性疼痛，神経因性膀胱，神経炎，神経過敏，神経根，神経質，神経症，神経心理学，神経衰弱，神経性やせ症，神経節，神経痛，神経内科

しんけいいんせいとうつう　神経因性疼痛　neurogenic pain, neuropathic pain

しんけいいんせいぼうこう　神経因性膀胱　neurogenic bladder, neuropathic bladder　◀無緊張性神経因性膀胱 atonic neurogenic bladder　無抑制性神経因性膀胱 uninhibited neurogenic bladder

しんけいえん　神経炎　neuritis /njuːráɪtɪs/　◀前庭神経炎 vestibular neuritis　多発根神経炎 polyradiculoneuritis　多発神経炎 polyneuritis　単神経炎 mononeuritis　葉酸欠乏性神経炎 folic acid deficiency neuropathy[neuritis]

しんけいかびん　神経過敏（な）（過度に敏感な）oversensitive, hypersensitive （神経症的な）neurotic

しんけいこん　神経根　nerve root　◀神経根圧迫 nerve root compression　神経根障害 radiculopathy　神経根徴候 radicular[root] sign　神経根痛 radiculalgia／radicular[root] pain　神経根ブロック nerve root block

しんけいしつ　神経質（な）（傷つきやすい）sensitive （緊張した）nervous （過度に敏感な）oversensitive （興奮しやすい）high-strung　◆神経質な人 a sensitive[high-strung] person　◆神経質な気質 nervous temperament

しんけいしょう　神経症　neurotic disorder, neurosis　◀強迫神経症 obsessive-

compulsive neurosis　心臓神経症 cardiac neurosis　不安神経症 anxiety neurosis　▶神経症患者 neurotic patient

しんけいしんりがく　神経心理学　neuropsychology （㉂neuropsychological）　▶神経心理学的検査 neuropsychological test

しんけいすいじゃく　神経衰弱　nervous breakdown[exhaustion], neurasthenia　◆神経衰弱になる suffer[have] a nervous breakdown

しんけいすう　心係数　cardiac index

しんけいせいやせしょう　神経性やせ症　anorexia nervosa；AN；*an eating disorder that makes people, especially young women, suppress the urge to eat to the point of malnutrition and even starvation* ★一般的には anorexia のみ．

しんけいせつ　神経節　ganglion （㉂ganglia）　◀傍神経節 paraganglion

しんけいつう　神経痛　neuralgia　◀坐骨神経痛 sciatic neuralgia／sciatica　三叉神経痛 trigeminal neuralgia　大後頭神経痛 greater occipital neuralgia　ヘルペス後神経痛 postherpetic neuralgia；PHN　肋間神経痛 intercostal neuralgia

しんけいないか　神経内科　the department of neurology, the neurology department　▶神経内科医 neurologist　神経内科学 neurology

じんけっかく　腎結核　renal tuberculosis, tuberculosis of the kidney

しんけっかん　心血管（の）　cardiovascular /kàə-diovǽskjulə-/　▶心血管系 the cardiovascular system　心血管疾患 cardiovascular disease　心血管造影 cardiac angiography／angiocardiography

じんけっかん　腎血管（の）　renovascular, renal vascular　▶腎血管疾患 renovascular[renal vascular] disease　腎血管性高血圧 renovascular hypertension　腎血管造影 renal angiography

じんけっせき　腎結石　kidney stone[calculus（㉂calculi）], renal stone[calculus（㉂calculi）], nephrolith

しんげんせい　心原性（の）　cardiogenic

▶心原性失神 cardiogenic syncope　心原性ショック cardiogenic shock　心原性脳塞栓症 cardiogenic cerebral[brain] embolism　心原性浮腫 cardiogenic edema

しんこう¹　**信仰（心）**　**religious belief, faith**　☞宗教　◆信仰上の理由により彼女は豚肉を食べません She doesn't eat pork *because of her religious beliefs[because it's against her religious beliefs].　◆神に対する信仰心 one's faith in God

しんこう²　**進行する**
《病状が進む》**progress** /prəgrés/ （図**progression, prógress**　図**進行性の progressive**　病状が進行した **advanced**）　◆この病気は進行が速い This disease progresses [becomes worse] quickly. / The progression of this disease is quick.　◆この病気は何年にもわたり徐々に進行します This disease progresses[becomes worse] gradually over many years. / The progression of this disease takes place gradually and over many years.　◆彼女の病気は進行しています Her disease is in an advanced stage.　◆病気が進行した段階 the advanced stages of the disease
《がんなどの発育・進展》**development, growth**　◆病気の進行を抑える control the disease / stop the development of the disease　◆がんの進行を遅らせる delay the development[growth] of cancer / slow (down) the progression of cancer　◆がんの進行を早める speed up the development[growth] of cancer　◆この種のがんは進行が速い This type of cancer spreads [becomes worse] quickly.
《進行・継続中の》**underway, ongoing**　◆その薬の臨床試験は進行中です The clinical trial of that medication is now underway [ongoing].

▶進行がん advanced cancer　進行期 advanced state　進行性核上性麻痺 progressive supranuclear palsy；PSP　進行性球麻痺 progressive bulbar palsy[paralysis]；PBP　進行性筋ジストロフィー progressive muscular dystrophy；PMD　進行性多巣性白質脳症 progressive multifo-

cal leukoencephalopathy；PML　進行流産 inevitable abortion / abortion in progress

じんこう¹　**人口　population**　◆あなたの国の人口はどれくらいですか What's the population of your country? / How large is the population of your country?　◀高齢者[老年]人口 elderly population　生産年齢人口 working-age population　年少人口 young[child] population　▶人口統計 population statistics

じんこう²　**人工（の）　artificial**　（人工器官・臓器の）**prosthetic**　（合成の）**synthetic**　（機械式の）**mechanical**　◆夫の精子で人工授精を行う artificially inseminate with [using] the husband's sperm　▶人工栄養 artificial feeding[nutrition] / （乳児の）bottle-feeding / （調合乳）formula (milk)　人工換気 artificial[mechanical] ventilation　人工関節 artificial joint　人工器官[装具] prosthesis　人工血管 artificial blood vessel / prosthetic (vascular) graft / synthetic graft　人工喉頭 artificial larynx　人工骨 artificial bone　人工歯根 artificial tooth[dental] root　人工心臓 artificial[mechanical] heart；AH　人工心肺（装置）heart-lung machine　人工臓器 artificial organ　人工唾液 artificial saliva　人工多能性幹細胞 *induced pluripotent stem[iPS] cell　人工知能 artificial intelligence；AI　人工内耳 cochlear implant / artificial cochlea　人工妊娠中絶（induced）abortion　人工破水 artificial rupture of the membranes　人工皮膚 artificial skin　人工涙液 artificial tears　☞人工甘味料，ストーマ，人工呼吸，人工授精，人工弁

しんこうがいれつ　**唇口蓋裂　cleft lip and（cleft）palate**

じんこうかしょう　**腎硬化症　nephrosclerosis**　◀高血圧性腎硬化症 hypertensive nephrosclerosis

しんこうかんせんしょう　**新興感染症　emerging communicable[infectious] disease**

じんこうかんみりょう　**人工甘味料　arti-**

じんこうかんみりょう **365** **しんさつ**

ficial sweetener ◆紅茶に人工甘味料を入れる put artificial sweeteners in *one's* tea ◆人工甘味料を使う use artificial sweeteners

じんこうこうもん **人工肛門** ☞ストーマ

じんこうこきゅう **人工呼吸** **artificial respiration[ventilation, breathing]** ◆（患者に）人工呼吸を施す give[perform] artificial respiration on *a patient* ◆機械式人工呼吸 mechanical ventilation 口対口人工呼吸 mouth-to-mouth ventilation [breathing] 用手人工呼吸 manual artificial ventilation ☞人工呼吸器

じんこうこきゅうき **人工呼吸器** **artificial respirator[ventilator], mechanical respirator[ventilator], breathing machine** ◆末期の病状になった場合，人工呼吸器の装着を希望されますか If you become terminally ill[In case of terminal illness], do you wish[want] to be put on *an artificial respirator[life support]? ◆（患者に）人工呼吸器を着ける put *the patient* on an artificial respirator / connect *the patient* to an artificial respirator ◆（患者が）人工呼吸器を着けている be on an artificial respirator ◆人工呼吸器を取り外す take *the patient* off an artificial respirator / remove *the patient* from an artificial respirator / unplug an artificial respirator ▶人工呼吸器回路 ventilator circuit 人工呼吸器関連肺炎 ventilator-associated pneumonia；VAP

じんこうじゅせい **人工授精** **artificial insemination** （動inseminate artificially） ◆人工授精で子供を生む have a baby through artificial insemination ◆人工授精を行う perform artificial insemination / inseminate artificially ◀配偶者間人工授精 artificial insemination *by (the) husband[with husband's semen]；AIH 非配偶者間人工授精 artificial insemination *by (the) donor[with donor's semen]；AID

じんこうべん **人工弁** **artificial (cardiac) valve, prosthetic heart valve, valve prosthesis** ◆人工弁には機械弁と生体弁があ

ります There are two types of artificial valve: mechanical and biologic. ▶人工弁置換術 valve replacement / heart valve prosthesis implantation

しんこきゅう **深呼吸する** **breathe deeply, take a deep[big] breath** ◆深呼吸して下さい Please take a deep[big] breath. ◆お腹の力を抜いてゆっくりと深呼吸して下さい Relax the muscles of your abdomen, and breathe deeply and slowly.

しんこく **深刻（な）** （重い）**serious** （重大な）**grave** ◆深刻な病状ではありません This is not a serious condition. ◆深刻な病状です I'm afraid this is a serious condition. / I'm afraid he⟨she⟩ is seriously[gravely] ill. ◆深刻な問題を抱えている have a serious problem[worry]

じんごせい **腎後性（の）** **postrenal** ▶腎後性血尿 postrenal hematuria 腎後性腎不全 postrenal failure 腎後性乏尿 postrenal oliguria

しんこんすい **深昏睡** **deep coma**

しんさ **審査** （検討・考察）**examination** （判断・判定）**judgment** （見直し・再検討）**review** （選考）**screening** （業務などの監査）**audit** ◀介護認定審査会 committee for the certification of long-term care needs 治験審査委員会（施設内の）institutional review board；IRB 倫理審査ethics[ethical] review 倫理審査委員会 ethics[ethical] review board；ERB ▶審査委員会 judging[review / screening / audit] committee

しんざいせいしんきんしょう **深在性真菌症** **deep mycosis**

じんさいぼうがん **腎細胞癌** **renal cell carcinoma**

しんさつ **診察** （身体の診察）**examination [exam]** （動examine） （受診）**consultation** （動consult） ☞診療
《診察する》 ◆医師がまもなく診察いたします The doctor will see[examine] you soon. ◆それでは診察しましょう Now, let's do your physical exam. ◆喉を診察しましょう I'm going to examine your throat. ◆診察中にご気分が悪くなったら

言って下さい Please let me know if you feel sick during the examination. ◆診察したところ悪いところはありません After examining you, I can't find anything wrong.

《診察を受ける》 ☞受診 ◆心臓専門医の診察を受けたほうがよいと思います I think you should *go and see[consult] a heart specialist.

◀産科診察 obstetric examination 神経学的診察 neurologic examination 身体診察 physical examination；PE／physical 予備的診察 preliminary examination ▶診察時間 office[consultation] hours 診察料 doctor's[consultation] fee ☞診察券, 診察室, 診察台, 診察申込書

しんさつおん 心雑音 heart murmur
◀器質性心雑音 organic（heart）murmur 機能性心雑音 functional（heart）murmur 無害性心雑音 innocent（heart）murmur

しんさつけん 診察券 hospital ID[identification, identity] card, patient ID[identification, identity]card, consultation card
◆診察券をお出し下さい May I see your（hospital）ID card? ／ Your（hospital）ID card, please.

しんさつしつ 診察室 （doctor's）office, consulting room, consultation room ◆クロスさん, 診察室3番にお入り下さい Mrs Cross, please come into room 3. ▶診察室高血圧 office hypertension／（白衣高血圧）white-coat hypertension

しんさつだい 診察台 exam table, examination table, examining table 特にカウンセリング用の couch ◆診察台の上に仰向けに寝て下さい Please lie down on your back on the exam table.

しんさつもうしこみしょ 診察申込書
（patient）consultation form, application form for examination[consultation] ◆この診察申込書に記入して下さい Please fill out[in] this application form for the examination. ◆診察申込書は保険証と一緒に出して下さい Please hand in the consultation form along with your insurance card.

しんしつ 心室 ventricle /véntrɪkl/（形 ventrícular） ◆左心室が少し肥大しています Your left ventricle is slightly enlarged. ◀右心室 right ventricle；RV 左心室 left ventricle；LV ▶心室肥大 ventricular hypertrophy；VH 心室性不整脈 ventricular arrhythmia；VA 心室調律 ventricular rhythm ☞心室期外収縮, 心室細動, 心室粗動, 心室中隔欠損症, 心室頻拍, 心室瘤

しんしっかん 心疾患 heart disease
◀虚血性心疾患 ischemic heart disease；IHD 高血圧性心疾患 hypertensive heart disease；HHD 先天性心疾患 congenital heart disease チアノーゼ性心疾患 cyanotic heart disease リウマチ性心疾患 rheumatic heart disease

じんしっかん 腎疾患 kidney disease

しんしつきがいしゅうしゅく 心室期外収縮 premature ventricular contraction；PVC, ventricular premature contraction；VPC ★contraction は, beat, complex, systole にも置き換え可能.

しんしつさいどう 心室細動 ventricular fibrillation；VF[V-fib]

しんしつそどう 心室粗動 ventricular flutter

しんしつちゅうかくけっそんしょう 心室中隔欠損症 ventricular（heart）septal defect；VSD

しんしつひんぱく 心室頻拍 ventricular tachycardia；VT

しんしつりゅう 心室瘤 ventricular aneurysm ◀梗塞後心室瘤 postinfarction ventricular aneurysm

じんしゅ 人種 race （形racial） ▶人種差 racial difference 人種差別 racial discrimination／racism 人種的素因 racial predisposition 人種的偏見 racial prejudice

しんしゅう 侵襲 invasion （形invasive）, invasiveness ◆彼女の年齢を考えるとできるだけ侵襲性の低い手術法を選択する必要があります Considering[Given] her age, we need to choose the least invasive surgery possible. ◀最小侵襲[低侵襲]手

術 minimally invasive surgery　手術侵襲 surgery stress / stress of surgery　リンパ管侵襲［浸潤］lymphatic permeation[invasion]　▶侵襲性肺アスペルギルス症 invasive pulmonary aspergillosis

じんしゅういのうよう　腎周囲膿瘍　perirenal abscess

じんじゅうきょうつうかんせんしょう　人獣共通感染症　zoonosis

しんじゅしゅせいちゅうじえん　真珠腫性中耳炎　otitis media with cholesteatoma

しんしゅつ　滲出　exudation　(形exudative), effusion　◀漿液性滲出液 serous effusion　▶滲出液［物］exudate / effusion　滲出性胸水 exudative pleural effusion　滲出性中耳炎 middle ear effusion / otitis media with effusion；OME / secretory otitis media；SOM

しんじゅん　浸潤　(浸入)infiltration　(形infiltrate, 形infiltrating), permeation　(侵襲)invasion　(形invasive)　◆がん細胞が胃壁に浸潤しています The cancer cells have infiltrated the stomach wall.　◀局所浸潤 local infiltration　白血球浸潤 leukocytic infiltration　リンパ管浸潤 lymphatic permeation[invasion]　▶浸潤影 consolidation　浸潤麻酔 infiltration anesthesia

しんじょう　信条　(行動規範)principle　(信念)belief, faith　☞主義, 信仰, 信念

じんしょう　腎症　kidney disease, nephropathy　◀IgA 腎症 IgA nephropathy　カドミウム腎症 cadmium nephropathy　シスプラチン腎症 cisplatin nephropathy　糖尿病腎症 diabetic nephropathy　膜性腎症 membranous nephropathy

じんじょう　尋常(性の)　vulgaris　(普通の)common　(単純な)simple　▶尋常性乾癬 psoriasis vulgaris　尋常性痤瘡 acne vulgaris / common[simple] acne　尋常性天疱瘡 pemphigus vulgaris；PV　尋常性白斑 vitiligo vulgaris

じんしょうがい　腎障害　kidney disorder, nephropathy

しんじる　信じる　(本当だと思う)believe　(神などの存在を信じる)believe in　(信頼する)trust　(確信する)be sure that …　☞信

頼　◆どうぞ私を信じて下さい Believe me, please. / (私の言うことを)Please believe what I say.　◆あなたは神の存在を信じますか Do you believe in God?　◆佐々木先生は腕のいい外科医ですから信じていただいていいですよ Dr Sasaki is a skilled surgeon, so you can trust him.　◆この治療はうまくいくと信じています I'm sure that this treatment will be successful.

しんしん　心身　mind and body　(形physical and intellectual[mental])　◆心神喪失状態である be not of sound mind / be of unsound mind　◆心身障害児 child with a physical and intellectual[mental] disability / physically and intellectually [mentally] disabled child　心身負荷 physical and mental burden　☞心身症

しんしんしょう　心身症　psychosomatic disease[disorder]；PSD

じんシンチグラフィ　腎シンチグラフィ renal scintigraphy

しんすいなんこう　親水軟膏　hydrophilic ointment

シンスプリント　(過労性脛部痛)shin splints　★通例, 複数形で.

しんせい[1]　申請する　apply (for), make an application (for)　◆最寄りの保健所に行って特定疾患の医療費公費負担の申請をする go to the nearest public health center and apply for *public assistance[subsidies] for medical expense benefits for treatment of designated intractable diseases　◆保健所に申請(書)を提出する submit[(送る)send in] an application (form) to the health center　▶申請書 application form / (保険金支払いなどの請求書)(insurance) claim form

しんせい[2]　真性(の)　(本当の)true　(偽物ではない)genuine　▶真性クループ true croup　真性赤血球増加症 true erythrocytosis[polycythemia]　真性大動脈瘤 true aortic aneurysm　真性半陰陽 true hermaphroditism　真性包茎 true[genuine] phimosis

じんせい[1]　人生　life　◆人生に満足していますか Are you happy[satisfied] with your life? ◆人生に興味を失う lose interest in life ◆楽観的な人生観をもつ have an optimistic *view of life[outlook on life] ◆人格は個人の遺伝子構造と人生経験の両方から作られます Personality depends on an individual's genetic makeup and life experiences. ◆彼女は人生経験が豊富です She has had a rich and varied life. / She has seen a great deal in her life.

じんせい² 腎性(の) **renal** ▶腎性高血圧 renal hypertension 腎性貧血 renal anemia 腎性浮腫 renal edema

じんせいけん 腎生検 **renal biopsy** ◀経皮的腎生検 percutaneous renal biopsy

しんせいし¹ 新生歯 **neonatal tooth**

しんせいし² 心静止 **cardiac standstill, asystole**

しんせいじ 新生児 **newborn (baby), neonate (形neonatal)** ☞ライフステージ ◆新生児初期の異常 a problem in the early *newborn stage[neonatal period] ◀ハイリスク新生児 high-risk newborn[neonate] ▶新生児黄疸 newborn[neonatal] jaundice / jaundice of the newborn 新生児学 neonatology 新生児仮死 neonatal asphyxia 新生児期 neonatal period [stage] 新生児室 newborn[neonatal] nursery 新生児死亡 neonatal death 新生児集中治療室 neonatal[newborn] intensive care unit；NICU 新生児搬送 neonatal transport[transfer] 新生児マススクリーニング検査 newborn mass screening 新生児用コット newborn's cot [crib]

しんせいぶつ 新生物 **neoplasm** ◀悪性新生物 malignant neoplasm

しんせき 親戚 **relative** ☞血縁 ◆ご親戚のどなたかに糖尿病の人はいますか Do you have a relative with diabetes? ◆血のつながった親戚 a (close) blood relative / a relative by blood / a person related by blood ◆ごく近い親戚 an immediate relative ◆遠い親戚 a distant relative ◆父方の〈母方の〉親戚 a relative on one's father's〈mother's〉side

しんせつ 親切(な) **kind, nice** ◆ご親切ありがとうございます Thank you very much. It was very kind[nice] of you (to do so).

じんせっせき 腎切石(術) **nephrolithotomy** ◀経皮的腎切石術 percutaneous nephrolithotomy

しんせん¹ 振戦 **tremor, trembling** ◀企図振戦 intention tremor 静止時振戦 resting[static] tremor 動作時振戦 action[kinetic] tremor パーキンソン振戦 parkinsonian tremor 羽ばたき振戦 flapping tremor / asterixis 微細振戦 fine tremor 本態性振戦 essential tremor ▶振戦せん妄 delirium tremens；DT

しんせん² 心尖 **apex of the heart** ▶心尖拍動 apex beat

しんせんけつ 新鮮血 **fresh blood**

じんぜんせい 腎前性(の) **prerenal** ▶腎前性血尿 prerenal hematuria 腎前性腎不全 prerenal failure 腎前性乏尿 prerenal oliguria

じんせんつう 腎疝痛 **renal colic**

しんせんとうけつけつしょう 新鮮凍結血漿 **fresh frozen plasma；FFP**

しんぞう 心臓 **heart (形cardiac)** ☞心 ◆心臓の具合が悪いのですか Do you have any problems[Is there anything wrong] with your heart? ◆今までに心臓の病気にかかったことがありますか Have you ever had any heart disease before? /(異常を指摘されたことがあるか)Have you ever been told that you have a problem with your heart? ◆心臓の辺りが痛むことがありますか Do you ever have (a) pain around your heart? ◆心臓がドキドキしますか Does your heart beat fast? / Do you feel your heart pounding? / Do you have palpitations? ◆心臓の診察をしましょう I'm going to examine[(聴診) listen to] your heart. ◆心臓が少し肥大し負担がかかっています The heart is slightly enlarged and overworked. ◆赤ちゃんの心臓は元気に拍動しています Your baby's heart is beating strongly. ◆心臓への負担を軽減する薬を飲む take a medication

[drug] to reduce the heart's workload ◆心臓のリズムを安定させる stabilize the heart rhythm / make the heart rhythm stable ◆心臓の鼓動 a[the] heartbeat ◀人工心臓 artificial[mechanical] heart；AH 補助人工心臓 ventricular assist system；VAS ▶心臓移植 heart transplant [transplantation] 心臓カテーテル検査 cardiac catheterization 心臓外科 the department of cardiac surgery / the cardiac surgery department 心臓外科医 heart [cardiac] surgeon 心臓血管系 the cardiovascular system；CVS 心臓血管外科 the department of cardiovascular surgery / the cardiovascular surgery department 心臓血管外科医 cardiovascular surgeon 心臓手術 heart[cardiac] surgery 心臓切開手術[開心術] open-heart surgery 心臓専門医 cardiologist / heart specialist 心臓病患者 heart patient 心臓病食 cardiac[heart-healthy] diet 心臓ペーシング（artificial）cardiac pacing 心臓壁運動 heart[cardiac] wall motion 心臓弁膜症 heart valve disease / valvular heart disease 心臓リハビリテーション heart[cardiac] rehabilitation ☞心臓発作

じんぞう 腎臓 kidney（㊥renal, nephric） ☞腎 ◆腎臓か膀胱の具合が悪いのですか Do you have any problems[Is there anything wrong] with your kidneys or bladder? ◆今までに腎臓の病気にかかったことがありますか Have you ever had any kidney disease before? /（異常を指摘されたことがあるか）Have you ever been told that you have a problem with your kidney(s)? ◆腎臓は老廃物を尿として排出する働きをしています The kidneys get rid of waste products that the body does not need by making urine. / Waste products are eliminated from the body in urine, which is made in the kidneys. ◀人工腎臓 artificial kidney ▶腎臓学 nephrology 腎臓がん kidney cancer 腎臓摘出術 nephrectomy 腎臓内科 the department of nephrology / the nephrology department 腎臓内科医 nephrologist /

kidney specialist ☞腎臓病

じんぞうびょう 腎臓病 kidney disease ◀慢性腎臓病 chronic kidney disease；CKD ▶腎臓病食 renal[kidney-healthy] diet

しんぞうほっさ 心臓発作 heart attack ☞狭心症, 心筋梗塞 ◆心臓発作を起こす have[suffer] a heart attack ◆心臓発作を予防する prevent a heart attack ◆軽い心臓発作 a mild[minor] heart attack ◆重い心臓発作 a severe[major / massive] heart attack ◆致命的な心臓発作 a fatal heart attack

じんそく 迅速（な）（速い・急速な）quick, rapid, fast （すぐ・即座の）prompt ◆患者のクレームに対して迅速に対応する deal with patient complaints quickly [promptly] ◀術中迅速診断 intraoperative rapid diagnosis ▶迅速組織診 rapid histodiagnosis

じんそんしょう 腎損傷 kidney injury, renal injury

しんたい 身体 body （㊥physical, bodily） ☞体 ◆身体の発育[発達]physical development ◆病気のため身体に苦痛がある be physically suffering from an illness ◆身体の診察を行う do[perform] a physical examination ◆身体が不自由である（障害がある）be physically disabled [challenged] ◆身体に影響を及ぼす affect *one's* body ▶身体介護 physical care / care for physical needs 身体活動 physical activity 身体機能 bodily function 身体言語 body language 身体所見 physical findings 身体診察 physical examination；PE / physical 身体測定 body[（身長・体重の）height and weight] measurement 身体的苦痛 physical pain 身体的特徴 physical characteristic(s) [feature(s) / trait(s)] 身体部位 part of the body / body part[region] ☞身体障害

じんたい¹ 人体 human body ▶人体解剖図 human anatomical chart

じんたい² 靱帯 ligament （㊥ligamentous） ◆靱帯に損傷を受ける injure [hurt] *one's* ligament ◆靱帯を切る tear a ligament ◀外側側副靱帯 lateral collateral ligament；LCL / lateral ligament of the knee 後十字靱帯 posterior cruciate ligament；PCL 膝蓋靱帯 patellar ligament 前十字靱帯 anterior cruciate ligament；ACL 鼠径靱帯 inguinal ligament トライツ靱帯 Treitz ligament 内側側副靱帯 medial collateral ligament；MCL / medial ligament of the knee ▶靱帯損傷 ligamentous injury 靱帯断裂 desmorrhexis / rupture of a ligament 靱帯縫合術 syndesmorrhaphy / suturing of a ligament ☞靱帯骨化

じんたいこつか 靱帯骨化 **ligament ossification** ◀黄色靱帯骨化症 ossification of the ligamentum flavum 後縦靱帯骨化症 ossification of the posterior longitudinal ligament；OPLL

しんたいしょうがい 身体障害 **physical disability[disorder]** ▶身体障害者〈児〉 person〈child〉with a physical disability / physically disabled[challenged] person〈child〉 身体障害者手帳 physical disability handbook

しんたつど 深達度 **depth of invasion** ◆がんの深達度 depth of cancer invasion ◆胃がんの深達度 depth of invasion in stomach cancer

しんだん 診断 **diagnosis** /dàɪəgnóʊsɪs/（動diagnose 形diagnostic）（査定）**assessment** ◆喘息と診断されたのはいつですか When was your asthma diagnosed? / When were you diagnosed as having asthma? ◆正確な診断を行うために検査が必要です For us to be able to make[get] an accurate diagnosis, you need to undergo some tests. ◆診断するために生検を行います I'm going to do a biopsy for diagnostic purposes. ◆脳性麻痺と診断する have[obtain] a diagnosis of cerebral palsy / diagnose cerebral palsy ◀遺伝子診断 genetic[gene] diagnosis 確定診断 definitive[definite] diagnosis ★diagnosis のみでもよい。画像診断 diagnostic imaging 仮診断 provisional[tentative] diagnosis 鑑別診断 differen-

tial diagnosis 血清学的診断 serologic diagnosis 健康診断（health）checkup /（physical）checkup / physical 誤診断 diagnostic error / misdiagnosis / wrong diagnosis 最終診断 final diagnosis 出生前診断 prenatal[fetal] diagnosis 術中迅速診断 intraoperative rapid diagnosis 除外診断 diagnosis by exclusion 早期診断 early diagnosis 総合診断 comprehensive diagnosis 病理診断 pathologic diagnosis 放射線診断 radiodiagnosis 臨床診断 clinical diagnosis ▶診断基準 diagnostic criteria / the criteria of diagnosis 診断群分類別包括評価支払制度 *Diagnosis Procedure Combination-based[DPC] Payment System 診断未確定 not yet diagnosed / undiagnosed ☞診断書

しんだんしょ 診断書 **medical certificate**〈健康診断書〉**health certificate** ▶死亡診断書 death certificate

しんタンポナーデ 心タンポナーデ **cardiac tamponade**

じんちくきょうつうかんせんしょう 人畜共通感染症 **zoonosis**

シンチグラフィ **scintigraphy** ◀骨シンチグラフィ bone scintigraphy 心筋血流シンチグラフィ myocardial perfusion scintigraphy 動態シンチグラフィ dynamic scintigraphy 肺血流シンチグラフィ pulmonary perfusion scintigraphy

シンチグラム **scintigram**

しんちゅう 心中 ☞気持ち，察する

しんちょう¹ 身長 （高さ）**height** （背丈）**stature** ☞背 ◆身長と体重を計りましょう I'm going to[Let me] measure your height and weight. ◆赤ちゃんの身長は55 cm，体重は3,800 g です Your baby is fifty-five centimeters *tall[in length] and weighs three thousand eight hundred grams. ◆身長はどのくらいありますか How tall are you? / What's your height? ◀高身長 tall stature 低身長 short stature ▶身長計 height gauge[scale / measurer] / stand scale with a height rod

しんちょう² 慎重（な）（注意深い）**careful**

しんちょう²

（用心深い）cautious　（真剣な）serious
◆この器具は慎重に取り扱って下さい Be careful with this instrument. / You should be careful when you handle this instrument.　◆後で後悔することがないよう慎重に決断して下さい Think (over it) carefully[seriously] before you make a decision so that you won't have any regrets later.

しんちょうりつ　心調律　cardiac rhythm, heart rhythm

しんちんたいしゃ　新陳代謝　metabolism /mətǽbəlìzm/（㋳metabólic）　☞代謝　◆新陳代謝を高める improve *one's* *metabolic rate[metabolism]

じんつう　陣痛　labor pains, (labor) contractions　★通例，複数形で．◆破水し陣痛が始まったら知らせて下さい Please let me know when your waters break and *you go into labor[your contractions start].　◆陣痛の間隔はどのくらいですか How far apart are your contractions? / How close are your contractions[labor pains]?　◆彼女の陣痛は今5分間隔です Her contractions are coming every five minutes now. / Her contractions[labor pains] are five minutes apart now.　◆陣痛がある be in labor　◆陣痛を促進する accelerate labor / induce labor　◀過強陣痛 uterine hypercontraction　後陣痛 afterpains / afterbirth pains　前駆陣痛 premonitory pains　微弱陣痛 weak *labor pains[contractions]　▶陣痛間欠 interval between contractions[labor pains]　陣痛室 labor room　陣痛周期 cycle of labor pains　陣痛誘発 induction of labor　☞陣痛促進，陣痛抑制

じんつうそくしん　陣痛促進　augmentation of labor　◆陣痛を誘発するために陣痛促進薬を使用する use an oxytocic[ecbolic] (medication / drug / agent) to induce[promote] labor

じんつうよくせい　陣痛抑制　suppression of preterm labor　▶陣痛抑制薬 tocolytic (medication / drug / agent)

しんていし　心停止　cardiac arrest；CA

◆彼女はほぼ完全な心停止の状態で救急搬送されてきました She was rushed to the hospital by ambulance in almost complete cardiac arrest.　◆彼は職場で心停止を起こしました He *went into[developed] cardiac arrest while at work.　◆心停止状態の患者 a patient in cardiac arrest / a CA patient　◀来院時心停止 cardiac arrest on arrival　▶心停止液 cardioplegic solution　☞心肺停止

しんてき　心的　（精神的な）mental　（心理的な）psychological, psychologic　（情動的な）emotional　▶心的葛藤 psychological[emotional] conflict　心的過程 mental[psychological] process　心的緊張 psychological tension　心的状態 mental[psychological] state　☞心的外傷

しんてきがいしょう　心的外傷　psychological trauma　◆心的外傷となる経験 a traumatic experience　▶心的外傷後ストレス障害 posttraumatic stress disorder；PTSD

じんてきじょ　腎摘除（術）　nephrectomy

しんてん¹　伸展する　extend（㋳extension）, stretch（㋳stretching）　◎伸ばす　◆下肢を伸展させる stretch[extend] *one's* legs　◀過伸展 hyperextension　▶伸展運動 extension movement　伸展拘縮 extension contracture　伸展体操 extension exercise

しんてん²　進展する　（発症する）develop　（病状などが進む）progress /prəgrés/（㋳prógress）　◆風邪をこじらせて肺炎に進展したようです It seems that your cold got worse and developed into pneumonia.　◆状況は特に進展がみられません There hasn't been much progress in the situation. / The situation hasn't made any progress.

しんでんけい　心電計　electrocardiograph；EKG[ECG]　★米国では EKG を用いることが多い．◆心電計を着けます Let me attach the EKG[（電極）electrode pads] to your body.　◆（患者が）ホルター心電計を24時間着ける wear a Holter monitor[electrocardiograph] for twenty-four hours

しんでんず　心電図　electrocardiogram；EKG[ECG]　★米国では EKG を用いることが多い．　◆心電図検査が必要です You need to have an EKG[electrocardiogram]．◆心電図をとりましょう I'm going to do [take] your EKG. / Let's do[run] your EKG.　◆あなたの心電図は正常です Your EKG is normal[within normal limits].　◀携帯型心電図検査 portable[ambulatory] electrocardiography　トレッドミル心電図 treadmill EKG　24 時間心電図検査 twenty-four-hour EKG / Holter monitoring　負荷心電図 stress[load] EKG　▶心電図異常 abnormal electrocardiogram　心電図検査 electrocardiography　心電図室 EKG room　心電図モニター EKG monitor

しんど　深度　depth　◀熱傷深度 depth of a burn / burn depth　麻酔深度 depth of anesthesia

しんとう　振盪　concussion　▶眼球振盪 nystagmus　脳振盪（brain）concussion

しんどう　振動　vibration　◆振動を感じる feel a vibration　▶振動感覚 vibration sense / pallesthesia　振動器 vibrator　振動障害 vibration syndrome

しんとうあつ　浸透圧　osmotic pressure　◀血漿浸透圧 plasma osmotic pressure　尿浸透圧 urine osmotic pressure

じんどうじょうみゃくろう　腎動静脈瘻　renal arteriovenous fistula

じんどうみゃく　腎動脈　renal artery（囲 renal arterial）　▶腎動脈血栓症 renal arterial thrombosis　腎動脈粥状硬化症 atherosclerosis of the renal artery　腎動脈造影 renal arteriography　腎動脈瘤 kidney[renal] aneurysm

しんどくせい　心毒性　cardiotoxicity

じんどくせい　腎毒性　renal toxicity, nephrotoxicity　◆この薬剤は腎毒性があります This medication *is toxic to[damages] the kidneys.　◀リチウム腎毒性 lithium nephrotoxicity

シンナー　(paint) thinner　◆シンナーを吸う sniff[inhale] paint thinner /（接着剤を嗅ぐ）sniff glue　▶シンナー中毒 paint thinner addiction[poisoning]

しんないまく　心内膜　endocardium　◀感染性心内膜炎 infective endocarditis；IE

じんにょうかんてきじょ　腎尿管摘除（術）　nephroureterectomy

じんにょうかんぼうこうぶたんじゅんさつえい　腎尿管膀胱部単純撮影　KUB X-ray；X-ray of the kidneys, ureters, and bladder

じんにょうさいかんせいアシドーシス　腎尿細管性アシドーシス　renal tubular acidosis；RTA

しんねん　信念　(信条・信仰) belief, faith　(確信) conviction　◆彼は病気を克服するという固い信念を持っています He has a firm belief that he'll overcome the disease.

しんのう　心嚢　heart sac

じんのうほう　腎嚢胞　kidney cyst, renal cyst

じんのうよう　腎膿瘍　kidney abscess, renal abscess

しんぱい¹　心肺　heart and lungs（囲 heart-lung, cardiopulmonary）　◆残念ですが，彼女の心肺機能は低下しています I'm sorry, but her heart and lungs are failing.　◆心肺機能を高める improve (the) heart-lung[cardiopulmonary] function　◆来院時心肺機能停止 *cardiopulmonary arrest[CPA] on arrival　◀経皮的心肺補助装置 percutaneous cardiopulmonary support；PCPS　人工心肺装置 heart-lung machine　▶心肺系 the cardiopulmonary system　心肺同時移植 heart-lung transplant[transplantation]　☞心肺蘇生，心肺停止

しんぱい²　心配する　(気にかける) be concerned (about), have *a concern[concerns] (about)（囲懸念 concern）　(思い悩む) worry[be worried] (about)（囲悩み worry）　(成り行きを案ずる) be anxious (about)（囲不安 anxiety）　(危惧する) be afraid (of)　☞悩み，悩む，不安　◆心配事 a matter of[for] concern　◆何か心配なこ

とがありますか Are you worried[anxious] about anything? ◆何がご心配ですか What kind of concerns are you having? / What's worrying you? ◆お仕事で, ご家庭で, あるいは個人的に何か心配なことがありますか Are you anxious[worried / concerned] about something at work, at home, or in your personal life? ◆心配なことがあるようですが, どうなさいましたか You seem to be worried. What's the matter? ◆心配なことがあれば遠慮なくおっしゃって下さい Please don't hesitate to let us know if you have any concerns. ◆あなたは心配性のほうですか Do you tend to be an anxious or nervous person? / Do you worry a lot? ◆再発作を起こしそうで心配なのですか Are you afraid of having another attack? / Are you afraid that you'll have an attack again? ◆CT から判断すると心配なことはありません Judging from the CT scans, there's nothing to worry about. ◆心配はないでしょう I don't think there's anything to *worry about[be afraid of]. ◆検査は痛くありませんから心配しないで下さい The test is painless, so *don't worry[don't be afraid / just relax]. ◆私がそばにいますから, 心配しないで下さい. 大丈夫ですよ I'll be right here beside you, so don't worry. You'll be fine. ◆心配なことがあれば電話して下さい Please call us if you have any concerns. ◆心配な症状が出たら受診して下さい If you have any symptoms that cause you concern, come and see me again.

じんぱい 塵肺 pneumoconiosis

しんぱいそせい 心肺蘇生 cardiopulmonary resuscitation；CPR ◆心肺蘇生を行う perform CPR on *the patient* / give *the patient* CPR ◆心肺蘇生不要 Do Not Attempt Resuscitation[to Resuscitate]；DNAR

しんぱいていし 心肺停止 cardiopulmonary arrest；CPA, cardiac (and) respiratory arrest ◆心肺停止状態の患者 a patient in CPA[cardiopulmonary arrest] / a CPA patient / a patient in cardiac (and) respiratory arrest

しんぱく 心拍 heartbeat, cardiac beat ◆心拍が速い〈遅い〉The heartbeat is rapid 〈slow〉. ◆不規則な心拍 an irregular heartbeat ▶胎児心拍数 fetal heart rate 低心拍出量症候群 low (cardiac) output syndrome ▶心拍出量 cardiac output；CO 心拍数 heart[cardiac] rate；HR

しんはれつ 心破裂 heart rupture, cardiac rupture

じんはれつ 腎破裂 kidney rupture, renal rupture

じんバンク 腎バンク kidney bank

しんぴ 真皮 dermis, corium；*the layer of the skin just below the epidermis, the true skin*

しんひだい 心肥大 cardiac hypertrophy ☞心拡大

しんぶ 深部(の) (深い位置の) deep (↔superficial) (体内の) internal (↔external) ◆深部の痛み *(a) deep[(an) internal] pain ▶深部感覚 deep sense[sensation] 深部腱反射 deep tendon reflex；DTR 深部静脈血栓症 deep vein thrombosis；DVT

しんふぜん 心不全 heart[cardiac] failure ◆彼女は心不全の状態です She is suffering (from) heart failure. ◆心不全を起こす develop[have / suffer] heart failure ◆心不全で死ぬ die of heart failure ◆左心不全が進行すると肺がうっ血して呼吸困難が起こります When left-sided [left] heart failure develops, it results in congestion of the lungs, which makes breathing difficult. ◀右心不全 right-sided[right] heart failure うっ血性心不全 congestive heart failure；CHF 慢性心不全 chronic heart failure

じんふぜん 腎不全 kidney[renal] failure ◀腎後性腎不全 postrenal failure 腎前性腎不全 prerenal failure 慢性腎不全 chronic renal failure；CRF

しんぺん 身辺 ☞身の回り

しんぽ 進歩 progress /prάgrés/ (圖prógréss), advance (改善) improvement (圖

improve） ◆最近の医学の進歩は目覚ましい The recent progress in medicine is remarkable. ◆以前と比較してリハビリは着実に進歩しています Your rehabilitation is *progressing more steadily[making steadier progress] than before. / You're improving more steadily in rehabilitation than before. ◆再生医療はすでに皮膚，骨などの分野で著しい進歩を遂げています Regenerative medicine has already made [achieved] significant advances[progress] in the field of tissues such as skin and bone.

しんぼう¹ 心房 atrium /éɪtriəm/ （圏atrial） ◀右心房 right atrium；RA 左心房 left atrium；LA ▶心房血栓 atrial thrombus 心房性不整脈 atrial arrhythmia 心房調律 atrial rhythm ☞心房期外収縮, 心房細動, 心房性ナトリウム利尿ペプチド, 心房粗動, 心房中隔欠損症, 心房頻拍

しんぼう² 辛抱 patience （圏patient） ☞我慢 ◆もう少し辛抱して下さい．すぐ終わりますから Please *be patient[hold on] a little longer. It'll be finished soon. ◆しばらく辛抱してお待ち下さい Please wait patiently for a while.

しんぼうきがいしゅうしゅく 心房期外収縮 premature atrial contraction；PAC, atrial premature contraction；APC ★contraction は，beat, complex, systole にも置き換え可能．

しんぼうさいどう 心房細動 atrial fibrillation；AFL ▶弁膜症性心房細動 valvular atrial fibrillation 発作性心房細動 paroxysmal atrial fibrillation；PAF

しんぼうせいナトリウムりにょうペプチド 心房性ナトリウム利尿ペプチド atrial natriuretic peptide；ANP

しんぼうそどう 心房粗動 atrial flutter；AF

しんぼうちゅうかくけっそんしょう 心房中隔欠損症 atrial septal defect；ASD

しんぼうひんぱく 心房頻拍 atrial tachycardia；AT ◀異所性心房頻拍 ectopic atrial tachycardia 発作性心房頻拍 paroxysmal atrial tachycardia；PAT

しんまく 心膜 pericardium （圏pericardial） ▶心膜液 pericardial fluid[effusion] 心膜開窓術 pericardial fenestration 心膜切開 pericardiotomy 心膜切除 pericardiectomy 心膜穿刺 pericardiocentesis 心膜ドレナージ pericardial drainage ☞心膜炎

しんまくえん 心膜炎 pericarditis ◀癌性心膜炎 carcinomatous pericarditis 感染性心膜炎 infectious pericarditis 収縮性心膜炎 constrictive pericarditis

じんましん 蕁麻疹 hives /háɪvz/, **urticaria**, 《英》**nettle rash** ◆蕁麻疹が出ますか，出たことがありますか Do you have or have you ever had hives? ◆特定の食べ物で蕁麻疹が出たことはありますか Have you ever *gotten hives[broken out in hives] from eating any specific food? ◆エビを食べた後に蕁麻疹が出る break out in hives after eating shrimp ◆蕁麻疹が出たら直ちに薬の使用を中止して下さい Please stop the medication at once if you develop[get] hives. ◀温熱蕁麻疹 heat urticaria 寒冷蕁麻疹 cold urticaria 日光蕁麻疹 solar urticaria

しんマッサージ 心マッサージ chest compression, heart[cardiac] massage ◆心マッサージをする perform[do] chest compressions / perform[give] (a) heart [cardiac] massage

しんや 深夜（に） （真夜中に）in the middle of the night （夜遅く）late at night ◆深夜によく目が覚めますか Do you often wake up in the middle of the night? ◆深夜に物を食べるのは身体に良くありません It's not good for your health to eat late at night. ☞深夜勤務

しんやきんむ 深夜勤務 late-night shift ◆深夜勤務で働く work a late-night shift

しんやく 新薬 new medication[drug] ▶新薬臨床試験 clinical trial[test] of a new drug

しんらい 信頼 （一般的に）trust （圏信用しておける trustworthy） （信頼性）reliability （圏頼りにできる reliable） （信任・信用）

confidence ☞信じる ◆医師と患者の関係は信頼の上に築かれねばなりません The doctor-patient relationship should be based on trust. ◆患者の信頼を得る gain [win] the patient's trust[confidence] ◆彼女は担当医を信頼しきっています She has complete confidence in her doctor. ◆信頼を裏切るような結果となり大変残念です I'm very sorry that I let down the trust you'd put in me. ◆信頼を失う lose confidence in … ◆三上先生は信頼できる医師です Dr Mikami is a reliable[trustworthy] physician. ◆信頼できる情報 reliable information ☞信頼関係

しんらいかんけい　信頼関係 relationship of trust　（ラポール）rapport　（信頼のきずな）bond of trust　（法律的に）fiduciary relationship　◆患者との信頼関係を築く establish[build up] a rapport[bond of trust] with patients ◀医師-患者の信頼関係 doctor-patient relationship of trust

しんり　心理　（心の状態）state of mind, mental state　（精神的傾向）mentality （㊟ mental）　（心理学的課程・心の働き）psychology /saikάləʒɪ/ （㊟psychológical） ☞精神 ◆このような心理状態はどのくらい続いていますか How long have you been in this state of mind? ◆職場でいつもより多く心理的な圧力〈ストレス〉を受けていますか Have you been under more psychological[mental] pressure〈stress〉than usual at work? ◆音楽を聴くと心理的な効果があってリラックスできます Listening to music can *have a psychological effect[affect you psychologically] and will help you relax. ◀患者心理 the patient's mental[（情動の）emotional] state / patient psychology　臨床心理士 clinical psychologist ▶心理過程 psychological process　心理検査 psychological test　心理相談 psychological counseling　心理療法 psychotherapy

しんりがく　心理学 psychology /saikάləʒɪ/ ◀集団心理学 group psychology　発達心理学 developmental psychology　臨床心理学 clinical psychology ▶心理学

者 psychologist

しんりょう　診療　（診察・専門家の助言）consultation　（治療）medical treatment　（業務）medical practice[service]　（ケア）medical care ☞診察, 治療 ◆診療時間は9時から17時までです Our office[consultation] hours are from nine am to five pm. / Our clinic[hospital] is open from nine am to five pm. ◆本日の診療担当は石川先生です Today Dr Ishikawa will see [treat] patients. ◆診療内容についてご質問があれば遠慮なくお訊き下さい If you have any questions about your treatment, please don't hesitate to ask me. ◆佐田先生はただいま診療中ですが，お急ぎのご用向きは何でしょうか Dr Sada *is seeing [is with] patients now. What is it that you want to see him urgently for[What do you want to urgently see him for]? ◀一般診療 general practice　外来診療 outpatient treatment[care / service]　外来診療部門 outpatient department　緊急診療 emergency medical treatment　混合診療 treatments partially covered by insurance / mixed treatments　自費診療 medical services not covered by health insurance / medical services at *the patient's* own expense　初期診療 primary care　訪問診療 house call / home visit　保険診療 health care services covered by health insurance ▶診療ガイドライン clinical practice guidelines　診療義務（legal）obligation to provide medical treatment　診療記録 medical record　診療計画 treatment[care] plan　診療情報管理士 medical records clerk　診療内容明細書 attending physician's (itemized) statement of services rendered　診療部長 medical director of physicians　診療放射線技師 medical radiation[radiologic] technologist：MRT ☞診療所, 診療費, 診療報酬明細書

診療部門［診療科］Clinical Division［Department］

☞専門医(囲み：専門医)

■内科系

●内科 Internal Medicine ●総合診療内科 General (Internal) Medicine ●呼吸器内科 Respiratory Medicine ●循環器内科 Cardiology ●消化器内科 Gastroenterology ●代謝・内分泌内科 Metabolism and Endocrinology ●腎臓内科 Nephrology ●神経内科 Neurology [Neuroscience] ●血液内科 Hematology ●リウマチ科 Rheumatology ●免疫・アレルギー内科 Immunology and Allergy ●老年内科 Geriatrics ●心療内科 Psychosomatic Medicine ●腫瘍内科 Oncology ●緩和ケア科 Palliative Care ●小児科 Padiatrics ●感染症科 Infectious Diseases

■外科系

●一般外科 General Surgery ●外傷外科 Trauma Surgery ●心臓血管外科 Cardiovascular Surgery ●呼吸器外科 Thoracic Surgery ●消化器外科 Gastroenterological Surgery ●乳腺・内分泌外科 Breast and Endocrine Surgery ●脳神経外科 Neurosurgery ●整形外科 Orthopedic Surgery ●形成外科 Plastic Surgery ●小児外科 Pediatric Surgery ●産科 Obstetrics ●婦人科 Gynecology ●産婦人科 Obstetrics and Gynecology ●泌尿器科 Urology ●眼科 Ophthalmology ●耳鼻咽喉科 Otorhinolaryngology / ENT(Ear, Nose, and Throat)

■その他

●精神科 Psychiatry ●皮膚科 Dermatology ●放射線科 Radiology ●麻酔科 Anesthesiology ●リハビリテーション科 Rehabilitation ●病理診断科 Diagnostic Pathology ●遺伝子診療部 Medical Genetics ●救急部 Emergency and Critical Care ●健診センター Health Screening Center ●歯科 Dentistry ●歯科口腔外科 Oral (and Maxillofacial) Surgery

しんりょうじょ　診療所　clinic, doctor's

office ◀一般診療所 general practice clinic　急患診療所 emergency clinic　休日診療所 out-of-hours[after-hours] clinic

しんりょうないか　心療内科　psychosomatic medicine　（診療科）the department of psychosomatic medicine, the psychosomatic medicine department

しんりょうひ　診療費　medical expenses [fees], fees for medical services, hospital fees　★いずれも複数形で. ☞医療費

しんりょうほうしゅうめいさいしょ　診療報酬明細書　itemized medical bill, itemized billing statement of medical expenses　（健康保険金の請求書）health insurance claim, medical billing claim　◆これが診療報酬明細書です Here's your itemized medical bill. / Here's the itemized billing statement of your medical expenses.

しんるい　親類　relative　☞親戚

しんれつ　唇裂　cleft lip

しんろう　心労　worry　（不安）anxiety　☞心配, 不安

じんろうぞうせつ　腎瘻造設　nephrostomy　◀経皮腎瘻造設術 percutaneous nephrostomy

しんわせい　親和性　affinity　◆…に親和性をもつ have an affinity for …　◆水銀は神経組織に高い親和性をもっている Mercury has a high affinity for nerve tissues.

す

す　酢　vinegar /vínɪɡɚ/　◆食事の塩分を控えるにはお酢や柑橘類の酸味を生かすとよいでしょう To cut down on salt (intake) in your food, you should season it with tangy[tart] tastes such as vinegar or citrus fruits.　☞酢の物

ず　図　(線画)drawing (🔲draw)　(図形・図式)diagram /dáɪəɡræm/　(幾何学的図形)figure　(一覧にした図表)chart　(挿絵)illustration　(絵画)picture　◆心臓の図を描いてご説明しましょう Let me draw a diagram of the heart to explain it.　◆この図は何を表していますか What does this drawing represent? / What is this a drawing of?

すあし　素足　☞裸足(はだし)

すい　膵　pancreas /pǽŋkrɪəs/　(🔲pancreátic)　☞膵移植, 膵液, 膵壊死, 膵炎, 膵外分泌, 膵仮性嚢胞, 膵管, 膵がん, 膵機能, 膵酵素, 膵腫瘍, 膵臓同時移植, 膵石, 膵切除術, 膵全摘出術, 膵臓, 膵損傷, 膵島細胞, 膵頭十二指腸切除術, 膵内分泌腫瘍, 膵嚢胞, 膵瘻

すい　推移　☞経過

ずい　随意(の)　voluntary /vάləntèri/　(↔involuntary)　▶随意運動 voluntary movement　随意筋 voluntary muscle　随意収縮 voluntary contraction

すいいしょく　膵移植　pancreas transplant[transplantation]

すいえい　水泳　swimming　◆水泳は有効な運動療法です Swimming is an effective exercise therapy. / Swimming is an effective way to exercise.　◆水泳後に耳の感染症にかかったことがありますか Have you ever had swimmer's ear?　◀(水泳)プール結膜炎 swimming pool conjunctivitis　▶水泳肩 swimmer's shoulder

すいえき　膵液　pancreatic juice　▶膵液消化 pancreatic digestion　膵液分泌 secretion of pancreatic juice

ずいえき　髄液　cerebrospinal fluid；CSF,

spinal fluid　◆髄膜炎の検査のために髄液を採って調べます I'm going to collect a sample of your spinal fluid to test[examine] it for (the presence of) meningitis.　▶髄液圧 cerebrospinal fluid pressure　髄液検査 cerebrospinal fluid examination[analysis]　髄液シャント cerebrospinal fluid shunt　髄液瘻 cerebrospinal fluid fistula　髄液漏出 cerebrospinal fluid leakage

すいえし　膵壊死　pancreatic necrosis

すいえん　膵炎　pancreatitis　◀アルコール性膵炎 alcoholic pancreatitis　急性〈慢性〉膵炎 acute〈chronic〉pancreatitis

ずいがいぞうけつ　髄外造血　extramedullary hematopoiesis

すいがいぶんぴつ　膵外分泌　pancreatic exocrine secretion

ずいかく　髄核　nucleus pulposus, vertebral pulp　▶髄核ヘルニア nuclear[nucleus] herniation

すいかせいのうほう　膵仮性嚢胞　pancreatic pseudocyst

すいがら　吸い殻　cigarette butt　◆吸い殻を誤って飲み込む accidentally swallow a cigarette butt

すいかん　膵管　pancreatic duct　◀内視鏡的膵管ドレナージ endoscopic drainage of the pancreatic duct　▶膵管拡張 pancreatic duct dilatation　膵管癌 pancreatic ductal carcinoma　膵管狭窄 pancreatic duct stenosis　膵管内乳頭粘液性腫瘍 intraductal papillary-mucinous neoplasm；IPMN

すいがん　膵がん　pancreatic cancer, cancer of the pancreas

すいきのう　膵機能　pancreatic function　▶膵機能検査 pancreatic function test　膵機能不全 pancreatic insufficiency

すいぎん　水銀　mercury　◀メチル水銀 methylmercury / methyl mercury　有機水銀化合物 organic mercury compound　▶水銀中毒 mercury poisoning

すいくち　吸い口　☞マウスピース

すいけいかんせん　水系感染　waterborne infection

すいこうそ 膵酵素 pancreatic enzyme

すいこむ 吸い込む （気体を）breathe in （気体・液体を）inhale, suck in[up] ☞吸引, 吸う ◆口を閉じて鼻からゆっくり大きく息を吸い込んで下さい Please *breathe in[inhale] slowly and deeply through your nose, keeping your mouth closed. ◆吐物を吸い込まないように，彼の体を横に向けて下さい Please place him on his side to prevent him from inhaling[breathing in] any vomit. ◆食べ物を気管に吸い込むと誤嚥性肺炎を起こします If you inhale[take] food into your windpipe, you could develop aspiration pneumonia.

すいざい 水剤 solution （薬液）liquid medication

すいさんか 水酸化（物） hydroxide ▶水酸化アルミニウムゲル aluminum hydroxide gel 水酸化ナトリウム sodium hydroxide

すいし 水死 drowning ☞溺れる

ずいじ 随時（の） （不定期の）casual （無作為の）random ▶随時血圧 casual blood pressure 随時血糖 random blood glucose[sugar]；RBG 随時尿 random urine

ずいしつ 髄質 medulla （㊥medullary） ◀腎髄質 renal[kidney] medulla 大脳髄質 cerebral medullary substance 副腎髄質 adrenal medulla

すいしつおだく 水質汚濁 water pollution

すいじゃく 衰弱 （一般的に体力の衰え）weakness （㊥weak） （特に病気による衰え）debility （㊙衰弱した debilitated 衰弱させる debilitating） ◆脱水のため〈高熱が続いて〉衰弱する become[get] weak from dehydration〈a continuous high fever〉 ◆衰弱が激しいものの彼女の容態は安定しています Her condition is stable though she feels very weak[debilitated]. ◆彼は衰弱がひどくて手術をするのは無理です He is too weak to have surgery. ◆極端なダイエットは衰弱をきたします Excessive dieting can cause *extreme weakness[debility / extreme thinness]. ◆慢性で衰弱性の病気 a chronic debilitating disease ▶神経衰弱 nervous breakdown / neurasthenia 全身衰弱 general weakness[debility]

すいしゅ 水腫 （浮腫）edema （水瘤）hydrocele ▶肺水腫 pulmonary[lung] edema

すいしゅよう 膵腫瘍 pancreatic tumor

すいじゅん 水準 （程度）level （標準）standard ◆この分野の医療技術は日本が世界屈指の水準です Japan has one of the highest levels of medical technology in this field. ◀生活水準 the standard of living / living standards 有意水準 significance level / level of significance

ずいしょう 髄鞘 myelin sheath ▶髄鞘変性 myelin degeneration

すいしょうたい 水晶体 （crystalline） lens ◆水晶体が濁っているので像がぼんやりして見えるのです The image looks blurry to you because your lens is cloudy. ◀人工水晶体 artificial lens 超音波水晶体乳化吸引術 ultrasound phacoemulsification and aspiration；PEA ▶水晶体混濁 clouding of the lens / lens cloudiness[opacity] 水晶体嚢外摘出術 extracapsular lens extraction 水晶体偏位 lens dislocation

すいじんしょう 水腎症 hydronephrosis

すいじんどうじいしょく 膵腎同時移植 simultaneous pancreas–kidney transplant [transplantation]，SPK transplant[transplantation]

スイス Switzerland （㊥Swiss） ☞国籍 ▶スイス人（の） Swiss

すいせき 膵石 pancreatic stone[calculus]

すいせつじょじゅつ 膵切除術 pancreatectomy

すいせん 推薦する recommend ☞薦める

すいぜんてきしゅつじゅつ 膵全摘出術 total pancreatectomy

すいそ 水素 hydrogen ◀過酸化水素 hydrogen peroxide 脱水素酵素 dehydrogenase 炭酸水素ナトリウム sodium bicarbonate 硫化水素 hydrogen sulfide

すいぞう 膵臓 pancreas /pǽŋkriəs/ (形 pancreátic) ▶膵臓がん pancreatic cancer 膵臓疝痛 pancreatic colic

すいそく 推測 guess (動 guess), conjecture, speculation ☞推定, 想像 ◆伺ったお話と症状から推測するとおそらく食中毒でしょう From what you've told me and from your symptoms, *my guess is[I guess] (that) you probably have food poisoning. ◆推測の域を出ません It's mere guesswork[conjecture]. / It's a matter of guessing[speculation].

すいそんしょう 膵損傷 pancreatic injury

すいたい 錐体 pyramid (形 pyramidal) (円錐) cone ▶錐体外路徴候 extrapyramidal sign 錐体路 pyramidal tract 錐体路徴候 pyramidal sign

すいだす 吸い出す (引き出す) draw out (液体・気体を) suck out ◆このチューブで痰を気管から吸い出します Let me[I'm going to] draw the phlegm out of your windpipe using this tube.

すいちゅう 水中 ▶水中ウォーキング water walking 水中運動 underwater exercise

すいちょく 垂直(の) vertical (↔horizontal) ▶垂直眼振 vertical nystagmus 垂直感染 vertical infection / (垂直伝播) vertical transmission 垂直[上下]斜視 vertical strabismus 垂直注視麻痺 vertical gaze palsy 垂直方向 vertical direction 垂直面 vertical plane

スイッチ switch (動 スイッチを入れる turn on, switch on スイッチを切る turn off, switch off) ◆テレビのスイッチを切って下さい Please turn[switch] off the TV.

すいてい 推定する estimate (図 estimation) ☞推測 ◆最終月経の初日の日付から赤ちゃんの産まれる日を推定することができます We can estimate the date your baby will be born based on the first day of your last period. ◀死亡推定時刻 the estimated time of *a person's* death ▶推定児体重 estimated fetal body weight；

EFBW 推定値 estimate 推定量 estimator

すいている 空いている ☞空く(すく)

すいとう 水痘 chicken pox, chickenpox, varicella ☞予防接種 ▶水痘帯状疱疹ウイルス varicella-zoster[chicken pox] virus；VZV 水痘ワクチン chicken pox [varicella] vaccine

すいとうさいぼう 膵島細胞 islet cell ▶膵島細胞移植 islet cell transplant [transplantation] 膵島細胞癌 islet cell carcinoma

すいとうじゅうにしちょうせつじょじゅつ 膵頭十二指腸切除術 pancreaticoduodenectomy

すいとうしょう 水頭症 hydrocephalus ◀交通性水頭症 communicating hydrocephalus 正常圧水頭症 normal pressure hydrocephalus 非交通性水頭症 noncommunicating hydrocephalus

ずいないしゅよう 髄内腫瘍 intramedullary tumor

ずいないてい 髄内釘 intramedullary nail [rod] ▶髄内釘固定法 intramedullary nailing

すいないぶんぴしゅよう 膵内分泌腫瘍 pancreatic endocrine tumor

すいのうほう 膵嚢胞 pancreatic cyst

すいのみ 吸飲み (convalescent) feeding cup, spouted water cup

ずいはんしょうじょう 随伴症状 accompanying symptom, accessory symptom, concomitant symptom

すいぶん 水分 water (液体) liquid, fluid (水分補給) hydration ◆水分は1日にどのくらい摂りますか How much water [liquid / fluid] do you drink[take] during the day? ◆水分をこまめにとって下さい Be sure to drink water[liquids] as often as possible throughout the day. ◆あなたは水分を1日800 mL程度に控える必要があります You need to cut down on your fluids[water], to about eight hundred milliliters a day. ◆運動中は十分な水分補給が必要です Adequate *fluid intake[hydration] during exercise is necessary. /

It's important to take adequate fluids during exercise. ▶水分過剰 overhydration 水分摂取量 fluid[water] intake 水分貯留 fluid[water] retention 水分不足 dehydration / excessive loss of body water

すいへい 水平(な) **horizontal** (↔vertical) ◆両腕を左右に広げて水平に保って下さい Please extend both arms straight out to your sides[Please raise both arms to the sides to shoulder level] and hold them horizontally. ▶水平眼振 horizontal nystagmus 水平感染 horizontal infection /(水平伝播) horizontal transmission 水平注視麻痺 horizontal gaze palsy 水平面 horizontal plane

すいほう 水疱 **blister** (形**blistery**) (小さい水疱) **vesicle** (形**vesicular**) (大きめの水疱) **bulla** (形**bullous**) ◆体中に小さな水疱ができる develop small blisters all over the body ◆足に水疱ができる have[get / develop] blisters on *one's* foot ◆やけどで水疱ができています The burn has formed blisters. / Blisters have formed from the burn. ◆感染を起こすので水疱はつぶさないで下さい Don't break[pop] the blister because it can lead to infection. ◆水疱状の発疹 blistery rash ▶水疱音 coarse crackle / bubbling 水疱症 bullosis 水疱性皮膚疾患 bullous skin disease

すいま 睡魔 **sleepiness** (形**sleepy**) ☞眠い ◆日中睡魔にたびたび襲われますか Do you often feel[get] sleepy during the day? / Do you often suffer from excessive sleepiness during the day?

ずいまく 髄膜 **meninx** (複**meninges**) (形**meningeal**) ▶髄膜刺激症状 meningeal irritation[irritable] symptom 髄膜腫 meningioma ☞髄膜炎，髄膜瘤

ずいまくえん 髄膜炎 **meningitis** / mènɪndʒáɪtɪs/ ◀ウイルス性髄膜炎 viral meningitis 化膿性髄膜炎 purulent meningitis クリプトコッカス性髄膜炎 cryptococcal meningitis 細菌性髄膜炎 bacterial meningitis 無菌性髄膜炎 aseptic meningitis ▶髄膜炎菌 meningococcus /(学名) *Neisseria meningitidis*

ずいまくりゅう 髄膜瘤 **meningocele** ◀髄膜脊髄瘤 meningomyelocele

すいみん 睡眠 **sleep** (動**sleep**) ☞眠り ◆睡眠に何か問題がありますか Do you have any problems sleeping? ◆1日の睡眠時間を教えて下さい How many hours a night do you usually sleep? / How many hours of sleep do you usually get at night? ◆睡眠をよくとっていますか Are you getting[Do you get] enough sleep? ◆十分な睡眠をとった後目覚めはすっきりしますか Do you usually wake feeling refreshed after a good night's sleep? ◆睡眠中にいびきをかくと言われたことがありますか Have you ever been told that you snore in your sleep? ◆睡眠の質が悪いのかもしれません You may have poor sleep quality. / The quality of your sleep *may not be good[may be poor]. ◆お酒は睡眠の質に影響を与えます Drinking alcohol can affect the quality of your sleep. ◆適度の睡眠をとる get a proper amount of sleep / sleep properly ◆睡眠中歯軋りをする grind *one's* teeth *in *one's* sleep [during sleep] ◆睡眠中に歩き回る sleepwalk ◀終夜睡眠ポリソムノグラフィ(overnight) polysomnography；PSG 徐波睡眠 slow-wave sleep 深睡眠 deep sleep ノンレム睡眠 nonrapid eye movement sleep / non-REM[NREM] sleep 賦活睡眠 activated sleep レム睡眠 *rapid eye movement[REM] sleep ▶睡眠呼吸障害 sleep-disordered breathing；SDB 睡眠時間 hours of sleep / sleeping hours 睡眠習慣 sleep[sleeping] habit 睡眠周期 sleep cycle 睡眠障害 sleep disorder[disturbance] 睡眠段階 sleep stage 睡眠パターン sleep pattern 睡眠量 amount of sleep ☞睡眠時無呼吸，睡眠不足，睡眠薬

すいみんじむこきゅう 睡眠時無呼吸 **sleep apnea** ◆睡眠時無呼吸がある have sleep apnea / stop breathing during sleep ◆睡眠時無呼吸を指摘されたことがありますか Have you ever been told that you stop breathing *while you sleep[in your sleep]? ◀中枢性睡眠時無呼吸症候群 central sleep apnea syndrome；CSAS 閉塞性睡眠時無呼吸症候群 obstructive sleep apnea syndrome；OSAS

すいみんぶそく 睡眠不足 **lack of sleep, shortage of sleep** ◆この症状は睡眠不足が原因です This symptom *is caused by [results from] lack of sleep. ◆睡眠不足ですか Are you not getting[having] enough sleep? / Are you not sleeping enough? ◆睡眠不足の原因はご自分では何だと思われますか What do you think is causing your lack of sleep?

すいみんやく 睡眠薬 **sleeping pill, sleep medication** (睡眠導入薬)**sleep-inducing medication[drug, agent]** (催眠薬) **hypnotic (medication, drug, agent), soporific** ◆睡眠薬を飲む take[use] sleeping pills ◆睡眠薬を常用していますか Do you take sleeping pills regularly? ◆どうしても眠れないようでしたら睡眠薬をお出ししましょう If it's just that you can't sleep, let me prescribe some sleeping pills for you. ◆睡眠薬を大量に飲む take a large [heavy] dose of sleeping pills / take an overdose of sleeping pills ◆睡眠薬自殺する kill *oneself* by taking sleeping pills / commit suicide with sleeping pills ▶睡眠薬依存 sleeping pill dependence[addiction]

ずいようがん 髄様癌 **medullary carcinoma**

すいようせい¹ 水溶性(の) **water-soluble** ▶水溶性軟膏 water-soluble ointment 水溶性ビタミン water-soluble vitamin

すいようせい² 水様性(の) **watery, aqueous** ◆鼻汁は水様性ですか Is the nasal discharge watery? ▶水様性下痢 watery diarrhea 水様便 watery stool

すいようび 水曜日 **Wednesday；Wed.** ◆水曜日に on Wednesday ◆水曜日ごとに on Wednesdays

すいりゅう 水瘤 **hydrocele** ◀陰嚢水瘤 scrotal[testicular] hydrocele 精索水瘤

spermatic cord hydrocele

すいろう 膵瘻 **pancreatic fistula**

すう¹ 吸う 《呼吸する・吸入する》(息を)**breathe in** /bríːð-/ **take a breath** /bréθ/ (空気や煙を)**inhale** (喫煙する)**smoke** ☞吸入, 吸い込む ◆大きく息を吸って下さい Please *breathe in deeply[take a deep breath]. ◆息を鼻から吸って口から吐いて下さい Please breathe in through your nose and breathe out through your mouth. ◆タバコを吸いますか Do you smoke? 《液体をすすり込む》**suck (in, up)** ◆お子さんは母乳をうまく吸えないのですか Does your baby have any difficulty sucking breast milk? 《吸収する》**absorb** ☞吸収 ◆このタオルは汗をよく吸ってくれます This towel absorbs sweat well.

すう² 数 (数値)**number** (測定値)**count** (率)**rate** ☞数字 ◆入院患者数 the number of inpatients ◀呼吸数 respiratory rate；RR / breathing rate 心拍数 heart rate；HR / cardiac rate 白血球数 *white blood cell[leukocyte] count 脈拍数 pulse rate；PR ☞数値, 数量

すう³ 数— (だいたい2～3の)**a few** (だいたい4～7の)**several** (漠然と数をぼかしていくらかの)**some** ◆一度にはできませんので数日お待ち下さい We can't do this all at once, so please wait for *a few[several / some] days. ◆数人 *a few[several / some] people ◆数百人 hundreds of people ◆数千人 thousands of people ◆数分 *a few[several / some] minutes ◆数週間 *a few[several / some] weeks ◆数か月 *a few[several / some] months ◆数年 *a few[several / some] years

スウェーデン Sweden (图スウェーデンの・スウェーデン人の **Swedish**) ☞国籍 ▶スウェーデン人 Swede

すうじ 数字 **number** (特に表記された数字)**figure** (検査の値)**data** ◆時計の絵を描いて数字をすべて書き入れ, それから時計の針を9時15分にして下さい Please draw a clock and put in all the numbers, and then set the hands at nine fifteen.

◆よく頑張られたことがこの検査結果の数字に現れています That you really worked hard is evident in the actual data of this test result. / It's obvious from the test result's data that you worked very hard.

数字の読み方

■電話番号や診察券・クレジットカードの番号など長い数字が続くもの
数字を1つずつ順に読んでいく.
- 03-3451-6208 ⇒ zero-three, three-four-five-one, six-two-zero-eight ★0はアルファベットの O/óu/とも読む.

■時刻
数字をそのままの順序でいう.
- 8：00 ⇒ It's eight o'clock. / It's eight.
- 9：15 ⇒ It's nine fifteen. / It's a quarter past[after] nine.
- 9：30 ⇒ It's nine thirty. / It's half (past) nine.
- 9：45 ⇒ It's nine forty-five. / It's a quarter to[till] ten.
- 3：10 ⇒ It's three ten. / It's ten past [after] three.
- 3：55 ⇒ It's three fifty-five. / It's five to[till] four.

■日付
- 5月12日 ⇒ May (the) twelfth ★英国では the twelfth of May という. 書き言葉では May 12, 2018 のように書く.

■西暦年号
一般に, 二桁ずつ分けていう.
- 1965年 ⇒ nineteen sixty-five
- 2000年 ⇒ the year two thousand
- 2018 年 ⇒ twenty eighteen / two thousand (and) eighteen

■病室番号
百の位で分けていうか, あるいは1つずついう.
- 外科病棟 321 号室 ⇒ room *three

twenty-one[three-two-one] on the Surgical Ward.

■検査値, 計測値, 薬用量
一般に, 一の位より上は桁どりして読む. 小数点以下は数字を1つずつ順に読む.
- 224 ⇒ two hundred (and) twenty-four
- 5.6 ⇒ five point six
- 0.8 ⇒ (zero) point eight ★0を読まないことが多い.
- 1.52 ⇒ one point five two
- 130 mg/dl ⇒ one hundred (and) thirty milligrams per deciliter
- 183 cm ⇒ one hundred (and) eighty-three centimeters ★例えば 5'10" は five feet ten inches と読む.
- 78 kg ⇒ seventy-eight kilos

■救急車
数字を1字ずつ順に読んでいく.
- 119 ⇒ one-one-nine

■温度
- 38.2℃ ⇒ thirty-eight point two degrees Celsius
- 96.5°F ⇒ ninety-six point five degrees Fahrenheit

■その他の大きい数字の読み方
数の後ろに名詞が来る時には hundred や thousand を複数形にしない.
- 13,450 円 ⇒ thirteen thousand four hundred (and) fifty yen
- (病床) 674 ⇒ six hundred (and) seventy-four beds
- (症例) 10,000 人 ⇒ ten thousand cases
- (人口)100,000 人 ⇒ a[one] hundred thousand population / a population of one hundred thousand

(『そのまま使える病院英語表現 5000』第 2 版, 医学書院, 2013)

すうじつ **数日** ☞数(すう)―

すうち **数値** （測定値）**count** （計測器の表示値）**reading** （数の上の値）**numerical value** ◆血糖の数値が正常値を超えています Your blood sugar count is above normal. ◆中性脂肪の数値が高いです The triglyceride count is high. ◆血圧の数値は上が145, 下が90です Your blood pressure reading is a[one] hundred (and) forty-five over ninety. ◆尿酸の数値が下がりました Your uric acid counts have fallen. ◆数値が異常なレベルにまで上がっています The counts have risen[increased] to abnormal levels. ◆具体的な数値目標を設定する set specific numerical targets / target specific numerical values [counts] ◀痛みの数値評価尺度 *Numerical Rating Scale[NRS] for pain measurement ▶数値データ numerical data

すーっと ☞すっきりする ◆ガムを噛んだり歯を磨くと口の中がすーっとします If you chew gum or brush your teeth, your mouth will feel refreshingly cool. ◆この冷湿布には消炎鎮痛薬の他にメントールなどが含まれているのですーっとします This cold compress contains not only antiinflammatory painkiller, but menthol as well, so you'll feel a cool sensation.

すうねん **数年** ☞数(すう)―

スープ **soup** ◆スープを飲む have[eat] (some) soup / （カップから直接飲む）drink (some) soup ◆濃い〈薄い〉スープ thick 〈thin〉soup ◀チキンスープ chicken soup 野菜スープ vegetable soup

すうりょう **数量** （物の分量）**quantity** （↔quality） （総量）**amount** ☞量

スカート **skirt** ◆スカートを下げてお腹を見せて下さい Please *lower your skirt[roll your skirt down] and show me your abdomen.

ずがい **頭蓋** ☞頭蓋(とうがい)

すがた **姿** 《容姿》 （外見）**appearance** （体形）**figure** ◆姿形で判断する judge a person by his 〈her〉appearance ◆ほっそりした姿の女性 a woman with a slender figure / a slender woman 《存在》 ◆先ほど奥様のお姿を売店でお見かけしました I saw your wife at the hospital shop a little while ago. ◆お子さんのありのままの姿を受け入れて下さい Please try to accept your child as he〈she〉is.

すき **好き** **like** （…の方を好む）**prefer** （🗷お気に入りの **favorite**） ◆相撲を観るのはお好きですか Do you like watching sumo? ◆パンとご飯ではどちらが好きですか Which do you prefer[like better], bread or rice? ◆好きな食べ物は何ですか What's your favorite food? / What kind of food do you like? ◆どうぞお好きな席にお座り下さい Please sit wherever you like. ◆好きな時に来ていただいて構いません It's all right for you to come whenever *you like[it's convenient for you]. ◆好きにやっていいですよ You can do as you like[please]. ☞好き勝手, 好き嫌い

―すぎ **―過ぎ** ☞し過ぎる, 一過ぎる

すきかって **好き勝手** ◆好き勝手をされては困ります Please don't just do as you please. / Please don't do whatever you like[please].

スギかふん **―花粉** *sugi* **pollen, Japanese cedar pollen** ◆スギ花粉にアレルギーを起こす have[develop] an allergy to *sugi*[Japanese cedar] pollen ▶スギ花粉症 *sugi*[Japanese cedar] pollen allergy

すききらい **好き嫌い** **likes and dislikes** （好み）**preference** ☞偏食 ◆食べ物に好き嫌いがありますか Do you have any food likes and dislikes? / Do you have any food preferences? / （食べられないものはあるか）Is there anything you can't eat? ◆食べ物の好き嫌いは変わりましたか Have you developed a change in *food likes and dislikes[food preferences]?

ずきずき **ずきずきする** **throb** （with pain） ☞痛み ◆頭がずきずき痛む have a throbbing pain in *one's* head / have a throbbing headache ◆傷がずきずき痛む The wound is throbbing with pain.

すぎない （—に）**過ぎない** ◆医師として当然の務めを果たしたに過ぎません（医師であれば誰でも同じことをした）Any doctor would have done the same. / （義務を果たしただけ）I only did my duty as a doctor. ◆まだ治療計画全体の1/3を終了したに過ぎません We've finished only[no more than] one-third of the whole treatment schedule.

すきま **隙間** （割れ目）**gap** （ひび）**crack** （穴）**opening** ◆歯の間に隙間がある have a gap between *one's* teeth

スキムミルク **skim milk**,《英》**skimmed milk**

スキャン **scan** ◀CTスキャン CT[computed tomography] scan PETスキャン PET[positron emission tomography] scan

スキル **skill** ☞技術 ◀ソーシャルスキル social skills

すぎる **過ぎる** ◆もう寝る時間を過ぎています It's already past your bedtime.

—すぎる **—過ぎる** ☞し過ぎる ◆甘いものを食べ過ぎないで下さい Please be careful not to eat too many sweets. ◆働き過ぎる overwork / work too hard / work too much ◆食べ過ぎる eat *too much[over-eat]* ◆飲み過ぎる drink *too much[excessively]* ◆太り過ぎる become[get / be] overweight ◆やせ過ぎる become [get / be] too thin

スキン （皮膚）**skin** （コンドーム）**condom** （インフォーマル）**rubber** ☞コンドーム，皮膚 ◀ドライスキン dry skin / （乾皮症）xeroderma ▶スキンクリーム〈ローション〉skin cream〈lotion〉 スキンケア skin care スキンシップ close physical[personal] contact（with） / （親子間のきずな）bonding between parent and child through physical contact / （母子間の親密さ）closeness between mother and child ★'skinship' は和製英語。 スキンバンク skin bank

ずきんずきん ☞ずきずき

すく¹ **好く** ☞好き

すく² **空く** ◆水曜日が比較的空いています Relatively speaking, we're not so busy on Wednesdays. / The hospital is rela-tively uncrowded[quiet] on Wednes-days. ◆お手空きの時にこの質問紙に記入をお願いします Please fill out this form when *you have time[you have a moment / you're free]*. ◆お腹が空きましたか Are you hungry?

すぐ （即座に）**right away, at once, immediately**,《英》**straightaway** （速く）**quickly** （まもなく）**soon** ◆今すぐこの薬を飲んで下さい Please take this medication right away. ◆予期しない副作用が見られる時にはすぐ連絡して下さい Please call[con-tact] us *right away[at once / immediately]* if you notice any unexpected side effects. ◆この薬はすぐ効きます This medication will start working at once. / This medication will take effect immediately. ◆この傷はすぐ治りますので，焦ることはありません This type of wound heals quickly, so *don't worry about it [don't be in a rush about it]*. ◆担当医はすぐ到着します Your doctor will be coming to see you soon. ◆今すぐうかがいます I'm coming right away. ◆失礼します，すぐ戻ります Excuse me, I'll *be right back [be back soon]*.

すくう **救う** **save** （救出する）**rescue** ◆命を救う save *a person's* life ◆救いのない状況 a hopeless situation

スクール **school** ☞学校 ▶スクールカウンセラー school counselor スクールカウンセリング school counseling

すくない **少ない** （増減がわずかな）**slight** （重量が軽い）**light** （数がほとんどない）**few** （数が少しある）**a few** （量がほとんどない）**little** （量が少しある）**a little** （量が乏しい）**low, poor** ☞少々，少し ◆少ない出血 slight bleeding ◆彼女は月経の出血量が少ない Her menstrual periods are light in flow. / She has light menstrual bleeding. ◆食事を少なめにして下さい Please eat *light meals[lightly / （適量に）moderately]*. / （量を減らす）Please reduce the amount of food you eat. ◆カリウムが少ない食べ物 foods low in potassium / low-potassium foods[diet]

すくなからず　少なからず（かなりの数）quite a few, not a few　（かなりの量）quite a little, not a little　（大いに）greatly　◆残念ながら，がんが再発する患者さんは少なからず存在します Unfortunately[I'm afraid to say], there are quite a few patients whose cancer *comes back[returns].　◆幼少期の親子関係は，後の対人姿勢に少なからず影響します The parent-child relationship in early childhood greatly affects a person's attitudes toward other people later in life.

すくなくとも　少なくとも　at least　☞せめて　◆少なくとも3か月経たないと治療効果は判定できません We have to wait at least three months before we can assess the effectiveness of the treatment.　◆少なくとも5 kg減量して下さい You need to lose at least five kilograms.

すくみあしほこう　すくみ足歩行　frozen gait

スクラッチテスト　scratch test

スクリーニングけんさ　―検査　screening test

すぐれない　◆気分がすぐれない feel sick[ill] / feel poorly / don't feel well　◆顔色がすぐれない look pale

スクワット　squat　◆スクワットは注意して行って下さい Be careful when you do squats[squat exercises].　◆スクワットで下半身の筋肉を鍛える strengthen the muscles of *one's* lower body by doing squats[squat exercises]

ずけい　図形　☞図

スケジュール　（予定・計画）schedule　（予約・約束）appointment　☞予定　◆病院生活のスケジュールをお話ししましょう Let me tell you about the *typical daily hospital schedule[(日課)routine of hospital life / schedule of hospital life].　◆来週はスケジュールが詰まっています My schedule is full[tight] next week.　◆今日のスケジュールはどうなっていますか What's on the schedule today?　◆手術をスケジュールどおりに行う do[perform] the surgery *as scheduled[on schedule]　◆来月のスケジュールを立てる set up a schedule for next month / set up next month's schedule　◆予防接種のスケジュール（推奨スケジュール）(recommended) vaccination[immunization] schedule　◀服薬[投薬]スケジュール dosing schedule　▶スケジュール帳 appointment[schedule] book　スケジュール表 schedule（chart[table]）

すごい
《素晴らしい》really great, fantastic　◆1回目で禁煙できてしまうなんてすごいですね You succeeded in quitting smoking on your first try. That's really great! / You quit smoking on your first attempt. That's fantastic!
《ひどい》terrible, very bad, really awful　◆すごい物音がしましたが，大丈夫ですか I heard a terrible noise. Are you all right?　◆すごく大変な経験をなさいましたね You had a *very bad[really awful] experience, didn't you?

すこし　少し　☞少々，少ない，ちょっと
《数が少ない》a few, some　◆個室はあいにくいっぱいですが，4人部屋に少し空きがあります Unfortunately, the private rooms are all occupied, but a few four-bed rooms are available.
《量が少ない》a small amount of, a little, some　◆少しの水 *a small amount of[a little] water
《程度が少ない》a little　（わずかな）slight　◆英語は少しなら話せます I speak a little English.　◆血圧が少し高いですね Your blood pressure is *a little[slightly] high.　◆少し痛む have some slight pain　◆少しずつ回復するでしょう You'll get better *little by little[(徐々に)gradually].
《短い時間》　◆（リハビリなどで）少し休みましょう Let's take a short break. / Let's take a rest for a while.　◆少しお待ち下さい Just a moment, please. / （電話で）Please hold on for a moment.

すごす　過ごす　（時を過ごす）spend　（休息する）rest　◆休日はどのようにお過ごしですか How do you spend your *days off

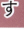

[holidays]? / What do you do on your *days off[holidays]? ◆こちらでしばらくゆっくりお過ごし下さい Please rest here a while and make yourself comfortable. ◆楽しい〈つらい〉時を過ごす have a good〈difficult〉time ◆クリスマスは楽しく過ごされましたか Did you have a good Christmas?

スコットランド **Scotland** （形スコットランドの・スコットランド人の **Scottish**） ▶スコットランド人 Scot /（男性）Scotsman /（女性）Scotswoman

すじ 筋
《筋肉》**muscle** /mʌsl/ （腱）**tendon** ☞筋肉, 腱 ◆足の筋を切る〈傷める〉tear〈injure〉a leg muscle ◆足首の筋を違える sprain *one's* ankle ◆首の筋を違える get a crick in *one's* neck
《線》**line** （色・汚れのついた筋・しま）**streak** ◆筋状の血がついた痰が出る bring up blood-streaked phlegm
《条理》（意味・道理）**sense** （形妥当な **reasonable** 理にかなった **logical**） ◆彼女の主張は筋が通っていない Her claim *doesn't make sense[isn't reasonable]. ◆彼の意見は筋が通っていますが，同意できません His opinion is logical, but I can't agree with him. ☞筋違い

ずじゅうかん 頭重感 dull headache

すすぐ **rinse** ◆（水で）口をすすぐ rinse *one's* mouth （with water）

すずしい 涼しい **cool** ◆この薬は涼しい所に保管して下さい Keep this medication in a cool place. ◆日本の夏は蒸し暑いので，エアコンなどを効果的に使って涼しくお過ごし下さい Japanese summer is hot and humid, so be sensible about using an air conditioner to stay cool.

すすむ 進む
《進展する》**progress, come along** （悪化する）**get worse** （症状が深刻になる）**advance** （形 **advanced**） ☞進行 ◆彼女のがんはかなり進んでいます Her cancer is pretty advanced. /（悪くなっている）Her cancer is getting worse. ◆あなたの肝硬変はそれほど進んでいません（まだ初期段階）Your cir-

rhosis is still in its early stage. ◆リハビリは順調に進んでいます I'm glad your rehabilitation is *coming along[progressing] well[smoothly].
《気持ちが前向きである》（快く…する）**ready** （…する気がある）**willing** ◆彼は進んでその治療を受けています He is ready[willing] to get the treatment. ◆手術をするのは気が進まないのですね You're reluctant[unwilling] to have surgery, aren't you? /（手術を受けたくない）You'd rather not have surgery, wouldn't you? ◆最近，食が進んでいますか〈進まないのですか〉Has your appetite been good〈poor〉recently? / Have you had a good〈poor〉appetite recently?

スズメバチ （攻撃的な狩りをするハチ全般）**wasp** （やや大型）**hornet** ◆スズメバチに刺される get stung by a wasp[hornet] ◆スズメバチ刺傷によるアレルギー反応 allergic reactions *caused by[due to] wasp[hornet] stings ▶スズメバチ毒 wasp[hornet] venom

すすめる 勧める・薦める **recommend** （提案する）**suggest** （奨励する）**encourage** （強く勧める・忠告する）**advise** ☞助言, 忠告 ◆もっと運動して体重を減らすこと〈規則正しい食生活をすること〉をお勧めします I recommend that you *exercise more to lose weight〈eat regularly〉. / I'd like to advise you to *lose weight by exercising more〈eat regularly〉. ◆整形外科医の診察を受けることを強くお勧めします I strongly advise you to see an orthopedic surgeon. ◆ご主人には毎日軽い運動をするよう勧めました I advised[encouraged] your husband to do some light exercise every day. ◆退院後すぐに出勤なさるのはあまりお勧めできません I'd rather not recommend that you[I can't advise you to] go back to work right after *leaving the hospital[you get out of the hospital].

スタート **start** ◆新しいスタートを切る make a new[fresh] start

スタイ （よだれ掛け）**bib**

スタッフ **the staff** （個々のスタッフ）**staff**

スタッフ　387　ずっと

member, member of (the) staff　☞職員
◆スタッフが超音波検査室までご案内します One of our staff will take you to the ultrasound room.　◆ご質問やご不安な点は医療〈病院〉スタッフにお尋ね下さい If you have any questions or concerns, don't hesitate to ask any member of the medical〈hospital〉staff.　◆英語を話す看護スタッフを呼んできますので，ここで少しお待ち下さい Please wait here for a while. I'm going to get one of our nursing staff who can speak English.　◆英語を話すスタッフのいる医院 a clinic *with English-speaking staff[that has English-speaking staff]

スタミナ　stamina　◆スタミナをつける *build up[develop] one's stamina / boost one's stamina

スタンダードプリコーション　(標準的予防策) standard precautions　★通例，複数形で.

スタンド　stand　◆電気スタンド(卓上の)a table lamp /(床置きの)a floor lamp　◆点滴スタンド an IV stand

スチールげんしょう　―現象　steal phenomenon

スチューデントアパシー　student apathy

スチルびょう　―病　Still disease

―ずつ　―ずつ　◆この薬は1回に2錠ずつお飲み下さい Please take two tablets [pills] each time. / Please take two of these tablets[pills] at a time.　◆彼女の容態は少しずつ好転しています Her condition is improving[She's improving] little by little.　◆1人ずつお入り下さい Please enter the room one at a time.

ずつう　頭痛　headache, cephalalgia
☞痛み(囲み：痛みの表現)　◆頭痛はありますか Do you have a headache?　◆頭痛はたいていいつ起こりますか When do you usually get the headaches?　◆頭痛はどのくらいの間続きますか How long do the headaches last?　◆頭痛は頻繁に起こりますか，まれにですか Do you get headaches frequently, or hardly ever?　◆頭痛の起こり方に決まったパターンがありますか Do

your headaches seem to follow a (fixed) pattern?　◆頭痛の場所は額全体〈こめかみに沿って / 目の後ろ / 後頭部 / 頭全体〉ですか Do you have the headache *across your forehead〈along your temples / behind your eyes / in the back of your head / all over your head〉?　◆ひどい頭痛 a bad[severe / intense] headache　◆軽い頭痛 a slight[mild] headache　◆頭が割れそうな頭痛 a splitting headache　◆締め付けられるような頭痛 a tightening band-like sensation around the head　◀筋収縮性頭痛 muscle contraction headache　緊張性頭痛 tension-type headache　群発頭痛 cluster headache　早朝頭痛 morning headache　拍動性頭痛 throbbing[pulsating] headache　片頭痛 migraine (headache)　▶頭痛薬 headache medication / anticephalalgic (medication / drug / agent)

すっかり　(完全に) completely　(まったく) quite　◆ごめんなさい！そのことをすっかり忘れていました I'm so sorry! I completely[quite] forgot about it.　◆すっかりお元気になられてよかったですね I'm (really) happy that *you've completely recovered.

すっきりする　(気分がさわやかになる) feel refreshed　(頭などをはっきりさせる) clear ☞すーっと　◆目覚めた時に気分がすっきりしますか Do you feel refreshed when you wake up?　◆アイスティーを飲むとすっきりします Iced tea will refresh you.　◆新鮮な空気を吸いながら散歩をすると頭がすっきりします Going for a walk in the fresh air will clear your head.

ずっと
《はるかに》much, a lot　◆顔色が昨日よりずっと良くなりましたね You look much better than yesterday, don't you?
《長い時間・距離連続して》(ある期間ずっと) all the time　(一日中) all day　(ある距離ずっと) all the way　(以前からずっと) always　◆明日はずっと病院にいますから，いつでもおいでいただいて結構です I'll be in the hospital all day tomorrow, so come and

see me anytime. ◆突き当たりまでずっとまっすぐ歩いて下さい Walk straight all the way〈till you come〉to the end. ◆あなたはずっと同じ会社で働いているのですか Have you always worked for the same company? ◆夏の間ずっと日本にいますか Are you planning to stay in Japan the whole summer?

すっぱい 酸っぱい **sour** /sáʊɚ/ （酸性の）**acidic** ☞酸味 ◆口の中は酸っぱい味がしますか Do you have a sour taste in your mouth? ◆酸っぱいにおいの便 acidic-smelling[sour-smelling] stools

すっぱり **once and for all** ◆すっぱりタバコ〈酒〉をやめる quit[give up] smoking〈drinking〉once and for all

すで 素手 **bare hands** ◆素手で他の人の血液に触るのは危険です It's dangerous for you to touch someone else's blood with your bare hands. ◆吐物は素手で触れないように十分気をつけて処理してください When you deal with vomit, *take good care[be careful] not to touch it with your bare hands.

スティーブンス・ジョンソンしょうこうぐん ―症候群 **Stevens-Johnson syndrome**

ステイプラー **stapler** ☞ホチキス

スティルびょう ―病 ☞スチル病

ステッキ **walking stick** ☞杖

ステップファミリー **step family**

すでに
《前に》《もう・とっくに》**already** （以前に）**before** ◆この書類はすでにお出しいただいていますか Have you already handed in this form[paper]? ◆息子さんはすでに手術が終わり ICU に入室しています Your son's surgery is already finished, and he's now in the intensive care unit. ◆先日すでに申し上げましたが，輸血が必要になるかもしれません As I told you before, you'll most likely need a blood transfusion.
《もはや…ない》**no longer, not … any longer[more]** ◆原先生はこの病院にはすでにいません（退職している）Dr Hara is no longer at this hospital. / Dr Hara isn't at this

hospital any longer[more].

すてる 捨てる
《不用な物を処分する》**throw away** （廃棄する）**dispose of** ◆インスリンの使用済み注射針は専用容器に入れて捨てて下さい Please *throw away[dispose of] used insulin needles in a special container.
《あきらめる》**give up** ◆どうぞ希望を捨てないで下さい Please don't give up hope.

ステレオタイプ **stereotype** （固固定観念にとらわれた **stereotyped** 紋切り型の **stereotypic, stereotypical**） ▶ステレオタイプ行動 stereotyped[stereotypic] behavior

ステロイド **steroid, steroidal drug** ◆経口ステロイドを内服していますか Are you taking oral steroids? ◆ステロイドを使っている be on steroids ◆このステロイド薬を吸入したら口をすすいでうがいして下さい Rinse your mouth and gargle after *inhaling this steroid[using this inhaled steroid]. ◀吸入ステロイド薬 inhaled steroid / inhaled corticosteroid；ICS 蛋白同化ステロイド protein anabolic steroid 非ステロイド系抗炎症薬 nonsteroidal anti inflammatory drugs；NSAIDs ▶ステロイド依存性喘息 steroid-dependent asthma ステロイド潰瘍 steroid ulcer ステロイド外用薬 topical steroid /〈軟膏〉steroid ointment /〈クリーム〉steroid cream ステロイド含有外用薬 steroid-containing external medication ステロイド筋障害 steroid myopathy ステロイド痤瘡 steroid acne ステロイド糖尿病 steroid diabetes ステロイドパルス療法 steroid pulse therapy ステロイド補充療法 steroid replacement therapy ステロイド離脱症候群 steroid withdrawal syndrome ステロイド緑内障〈白内障〉steroid-induced glaucoma〈cataract〉☞ステロイドホルモン

ステロイドホルモン **steroid hormone** ◀性ステロイドホルモン sex steroid hormone

ステント **stent** ◆ステントを動脈に挿入する insert[place] a stent in an artery ◀冠動脈ステント術 coronary stenting 尿管ステント ureteral stent ▶ステントグ

ラフト stent graft　ステント留置 stent placement / stenting

ストーマ　（人工肛門の開口部）**stoma**（圏**stomal**）　（人工肛門）**ostomy, artificial anus**　◆ストーマを作成する create[make] a stoma　▶ストーマケア stoma care　ストーマ周囲皮膚炎 peristomal dermatitis　ストーマ造設術 colostomy / construction of *a stoma[an artificial anus]　ストーマ閉鎖術 stoma closure　ストーマリハビリテーション stoma[ostomy] rehabilitation　ストーマ療法士 enterostomal therapist；ET / stoma therapist

ストッキング　**stockings**　★複数形で．（パンティストッキング）**hose**　◆ストッキングを脱いで下さい Please take your stockings off.　◆ストッキングを履く put on stockings　◆ストッキングを履いている wear stockings　◀加圧ストッキング compression stockings　サポートストッキング support stockings　塞栓防止用ストッキング antiembolism stockings　弾性ストッキング elastic stockings

ストライド　**stride**　◆大きな〈小さな〉ストライドで歩く walk with long〈short〉strides

ストレス　**stress**　《種　類》◆身体的ストレス physical stress　◆精神的ストレス mental[（心理的）psychological /（情動的）emotional] stress　◆育児ストレス child-care stress　◆仕事上のストレス job[work-related / occupational / workplace] stress　◆人間関係のストレス people-related stress / stress in human relations　◆ストレスの多い仕事 a stressful[stress-filled] job　《ストレスの有無・程度を尋ねる》◆最近ストレスがたまっていますか Have you been under much[a lot of] stress recently? / Have you had much stress recently?　◆家庭や仕事でストレスを感じていますか Do you feel stressed at home or at work?　◆あなたのストレスの程度は高いですか Is your stress level high? / Do you have a high level of stress?　《ストレスへの対応》◆ストレスを処理することができますか Can you manage[control / cope with] stress? / Do you know how to deal with stress?　◆何でストレスを発散していますか What do you do to release[get rid of / let off]（your）stress? /（ストレスを減らしているか）What do you do to relieve[reduce]（your）stress?　《有害作用の説明》◆ストレスが喘息の発作を誘発することがあります Stress may trigger an asthma attack.　◆ストレスは過食症の誘因の1つです Stress is one of the triggers for[of] bulimia nervosa.　◆ストレスが痛みを悪化させる可能性があります Stress may make the pain worse.　◆ストレスによる高血圧 stress-induced hypertension　◆ストレスに関連した症状 a stress-related symptom　◀拘束ストレス restraint stress　酸化ストレス oxidative stress　テクノストレス technostress　▶ストレス応答 stress response　ストレス潰瘍 stress[stress-related] ulcer　ストレス過剰 overstress　ストレス管理 stress management　ストレス関連障害 stress-related disorder　ストレス検査 stress test　ストレス対処行動 stress-coping behavior　ストレス反応 stress reaction

ストレッサー　**stressor**

ストレッチ　**stretching**（動**stretch**）☞伸ばす　◆肩〈脚〉の筋肉を十分にストレッチして下さい Stretch your shoulder〈leg〉muscles completely[fully].　▶ストレッチ体操 stretching exercise

ストレッチャー　**stretcher**　（車輪付きの担架）**gurney,**（英）**trolley**　◆ストレッチャーに乗せる move[put / place] *a patient* on a stretcher /（抱き上げて乗せる）lift *a patient* onto a stretcher　◆これからストレッチャーでお子さんを手術室にお連れします We're going to transport your child by stretcher to the operating room now.

スナック　**snack**　◆ケーキやクッキーなどのスナック菓子は糖分や脂肪分が多いので注意が必要です You have to be careful about eating snacks such as cakes and cookies because they are high in sugar and fat. ◆スナック食品 snack food

すね 脛 （向こう脛）shin （脚の部分）leg ▶脛当て shin guard

ずのう 頭脳 （脳）brain （知力）brains ★通例，複数形で．▶頭脳労働 brainwork / mental work 頭脳労働者 brainworker

すのもの 酢の物 vinegared dish ☞酢 ◆酢の物は体にいい Vinegared food is good for health. ◆きゅうりの酢の物 cucumbers marinated in vinegar / vinegared cucumbers

スパズム spasm ☞攣縮

すばらしい 素晴らしい great, wonderful （すぐれた）excellent ◆それはすばらしいですね That's great[wonderful]! ◆何とすばらしい考えでしょう What *a great[a wonderful / an excellent] idea! ◆すばらしい結果が出ています You've got *an excellent[a wonderful] result.

スピーチセラピー ☞言語療法

スピード speed （㊄speedy) ◆スピード感をもって問題解決にあたります We'll solve the problem *at top speed[speedily]. ◆回復のスピードが予想以上に速くて驚いています I'm surprised at your quicker-than-expected recovery. / I'm surprised at how much more quickly you recovered than I expected.

スピロヘータ spirochete （㊄spirochetal) （学名)*Spirochaeta* ▶スピロヘータ感染症 spirochetal infection

スプーン spoon ◆スプーンを使って食事をする eat with a spoon ▶スプーンネイル spoon nail

スプリント splint ☞副子

すべ 術 ☞手段，方法

スペイン Spain （㊄スペインの・スペイン人のSpanish) ☞国籍 ▶スペイン人 Spaniard

スペクト SPECT, （単光子放出コンピュータ断層撮影法) single-photon emission computed tomography ◀心筋血流 SPECT myocardial perfusion SPECT

スペクトル spectrum ◀広域スペクトル抗菌薬 broad-spectrum antibiotics 抗菌スペクトル antibacterial[antimicrobial] spectrum

すべて 全て （全部)all （全体の中の１つ１つ)everything ☞全部 ◆すべてうまくきました All[Everything] went well. / （よい結果に終わる)All[Everything] turned out well. ◆患者のニーズすべてを満足させることは難しい It's hard to satisfy *all our patients' needs[our patients' every need]. ★every の後は単数形で．私はあなたを治すために持てるすべてを尽くします I'm going to do everything in my power to cure your disease.

すべりしょう （脊椎)すべり症 spondylolisthesis

すべる 滑る 《意図せず滑る)slip, blurt ◆滑らないように注意して下さい Be careful not to slip. ◆歩道で滑って転ぶ slip and fall on the sidewalk ◆このことは誰にも口を滑らせません I'll make sure not to blurt this out to anyone. / I won't blurt this out to anyone. 《滑らかに移動させる)slide ◆文字に沿ってゆっくり指を滑らせると単語が出てきます Just slide your finger along the letters, and the words will appear.

スペル spelling ☞綴り

スポイト （点眼などに用いる)dropper, instillator

スポーツ sport （㊄運動競技の athletic) ☞運動 ◆何かスポーツをしていますか Do you play any sports? ◆どんなスポーツをしますか What (kind of) sports do you play[do]? ◆お好きなスポーツは何ですか What are your favorite sports? ◀野外スポーツ outdoor sports ▶スポーツ医 sports physician[doctor] / sports medicine specialist スポーツ医学 sports medicine スポーツ飲料 sports drink スポーツ外傷 sports[athletic] injury スポーツ心 athlete's[athletic] heart スポーツ番組 sports program スポーツ用サポーター athletic supporter / （男性用局部サポーター)

jockstrap

すぼめる ◆口〈唇〉をすぼめる purse [pucker] *one's* mouth〈lips〉 ☞口すぼめ呼吸

ズボン pants, 《英》trousers ★slacks はカジュアルなズボン. ◆ズボンを下げてお腹を見せて下さい Please lower[roll down] your pants and show me your abdomen. ◆ズボンをまくりあげて傷を見せて下さい Please roll up your pants and show me the wound. ◆ズボンを脱ぐ take *one's* pants off / take off *one's* pants ◆ズボンを履く put *one's* pants on / put on *one's* pants

すまい 住まい address ☞住宅 ◆お住まいはどちらですか Where do you live? / What's your address? ◆お住まいはアパートですか，一戸建てですか Do you live in an apartment or a house?

すます 済ます finish, complete （口語で）get done （with） ◆朝食は済ませましたか Have you finished your breakfast? ◆手術の前にいくつかの検査を済ませておく必要があります Several tests need to be completed before your surgery. / You'll need to get done with several tests before your surgery. ◆検査の1時間前までに軽い昼食を済ませておいて下さい Please eat a light lunch at least an hour before the test.

すみ 隅 corner ◆部屋〈廊下〉の隅にこの車椅子を置いておきます I'll put this wheelchair in the corner of the room 〈corridor〉.

すみごこち 住み心地 ◆この町の住み心地はいかがですか How do you like living in this town[city]?

すみません
《依頼》 ◆すみませんが，もう一度言って下さい Excuse me? / Pardon? / I beg your pardon? / Could you please say that again? ★すべて語尾を上げる口調で.
《謝罪》 ☞謝る，申し訳，詫びる ◆この間はすみませんでした I'm so sorry about the other day. ◆お待たせしてすみません I'm sorry to have kept you waiting.

すむ¹ 住む live ◆どこに住んでいますか Where do you live? / What's your address? ◆一人で住んでいますか Do you live alone? / Are you living alone? ◆誰と一緒に住んでいますか Who do you live with? ☞住み心地

すむ² 済む
《終わる》be over, be finished （活動などを終えた）be through ☞終わる ◆この検査は2，3分で済みます This test will be over in a few minutes. / This test won't take more than two or three minutes. ◆朝食〈昼食 / 夕食〉はもうお済みですか Are you finished[through] with your breakfast〈lunch / dinner〉? ◆それはもう済んだことです It's over now. / It's already done [settled].
《気がおさまる》 ◆気が済む（気分がよくなる）feel better / （気持ちが落ち着く）feel[be] settled, feel[be] calm

すむ³ 澄む become clear （醫clear） ◆尿は澄んでいます The urine is clear.

スムーズ smooth （圖smoothly） ◆すべてスムーズに運んでいます Everything is going along smoothly[well]. ◆血液が血管の中をスムーズに流れる Blood flows smoothly through the blood vessel. / The blood flow through the vessel is smooth.

スモーカー （喫煙者）smoker

スモッグ smog ◀光化学スモッグ photochemical[oxidant] smog

スモン SMON, （亜急性脊髄視神経障害）subacute myelooptic neuropathy

ずらす ◆薬の相互作用を避けるため，この薬は他の薬と少なくとも1時間ずらして服用して下さい To avoid medication interactions, take this medication at least one hour before or after taking any other medications. ◆インスリン注射は毎回少なくとも3 cmずつ場所をずらして下さい When you inject your insulin, use a different site for each injection, at least three centimeters away from the previous injection site.

すらすら （容易に）easily （流暢に）fluently ◆質問にすらすらと答える answer

the questions easily[fluently]

すりあし 摺り足 shuffle (動shuffle) ◆彼は歩く時に摺り足になりますか Does he walk with a shuffle? / Does he shuffle when he walks?

すりガラスいんえい ―陰影 ground-glass opacity

すりきず 擦り傷 (擦りむいてできた傷) scrape (動scrape), graze (動graze, skin) (引っかき傷) scratch (動scratch) (擦過傷) abrasion ☞傷, 擦り剝く

すりこむ 擦り込む rub (in, into) ◆軟膏はよく擦り込んで下さい Please rub the ointment in well.

ずりばい ずり這いする crawl on one's hands and knees

すりへる 磨り減る (骨などが) wear out [away], thin (動thin) ◆膝関節の軟骨が磨り減っています The cartilage of your knee joints has *worn out[become thinner].

すりむく 擦り剝く (こすって傷をつける) scrape, graze, skin (引っかく) scratch ◆転んで肘を擦りむく fall and scrape [graze / skin] one's elbow

スリランカ Sri Lanka (動Sri Lankan) ☞国籍 ▶スリランカ人(の) Sri Lankan

する 《行う》(一般的に実行する・遂行する) do, get, take (検査などを行う) run (手術・仕事を遂行する) perform (競技をする) play (経験する・受ける) have, undergo (契約・判断などを行う) make (相手に施す) give ◆今日はどんなトレーニングをしましたか What workout did you do today? ◆運動する exercise / do[get / take] exercise ◆深呼吸する take a deep breath ◆検査する do[run] a test / (検査を受ける) have a test ◆手術する perform[do] surgery / (手術を受ける) have[undergo] surgery ◆食事をする have a meal / eat ◆テニスをする play tennis ◆ゲームをする play a game ◆予約する make an appointment ◆診断する diagnose / make a diagnosis ◆援助する support / give support ◆訓練する(訓練を施す) train / give

training 《知覚する》◆頭痛がする have a headache ◆変なにおい〈味〉がする smell 〈taste〉 bad / have an offensive[unpleasant] odor〈taste〉 《害を被る》◆やけどする have[suffer] a burn ◆怪我をする have an injury / get [become / be] injured

するどい 鋭い (激しい) sharp (甲高くつんざくような) piercing (刺すような) stabbing (ピーンと走るような) shooting ◆頭に鋭い痛みがある have a sharp[piercing / stabbing / shooting] pain in one's head ◆鋭い音 a piercing sound

ずれ (相違) difference (動different 動differ) (隔たり) gap ◆意見のずれがあるようです I'm afraid *we have different opinions[our opinions differ]. ◆お子さんとの間に世代間のずれがありますか Is there a generation gap between you and your children?

すれる 擦れる rub against ◆傷に服が擦れないよう気をつけて下さい Please take care that your clothes don't rub against the wound.

ずれる (関節などが外れる) dislocate (位置が動く) move (軌道を外れる) get off track ◆あごの関節がずれています You've dislocated your jaw. / You've got a dislocated jaw. / Your jaw joint has moved out of its normal position. ◆話がずれたので元に戻しましょう We've gotten off track. Let's get back to what we were talking about.

すわる 座る (腰を下ろす) sit (down) (席につく) take a seat (臥位の状態から座る) sit (up) ◆どうぞお座り下さい Please sit down. / Take a seat, please. ◆(寝ている人に)ベッドに座ってもいいですよ You can sit up in bed. ◆枕に寄りかかって座ると楽になります You'll feel better if you sit propped against pillows. ◆ベッドサイドに座る sit (up) on the side of the bed ◆(乳児が)お座りする sit up without support ◆(生活様式が)座りがちなライフスタイル a sedentary lifestyle

スワン・ガンツカテーテル Swan-Ganz catheter ▶スワン・ガンツカテーテル法 Swan-Ganz catheterization

スワンネックへんけい —変形 swan-neck deformity

すんなり （大変うまく）very well （順調に）smoothly （滞りなく）without a hitch （快く）readily （自発的に）willingly ◆手術はさしたる困難もなくすんなり終わりました The surgery went *very well[smoothly / without any problems]. ◆彼女は私の頼みをすんなり受け入れてくれました She readily[willingly] consented[agreed] to my request.

せ

せ　背
《身長》height /háit/, stature　☞身長　◆背を測りましょう Let's measure[take] your height.　◆背が高い〈低い〉be tall〈short〉(in stature)　◆背が伸びる grow (taller)　◆背が縮む shrink in height
《背中》back　☞背筋(せすじ), 背中, 背骨
◆背を伸ばして下さい Please straighten your back.　◆背を丸めて歩く walk with a stoop / walk with stooped shoulders
◀猫背 stooped shoulders /〈円背〉round [rounded upper] back

せい¹　生　life　☞命, 生命　◆生への執着を失う lose *one's* attachment to life / let go of life　◆生に執着する *hold on[cling] to life　◆生と死の間をさまよう hover between life and death　▶生の本能 life instinct

せい²　性　(生物学的な性別)sex　(形sexual)
(社会的・文化的に形成される性別)gender
▶性愛 sexual love　性関係 sexual relationship[relations]　性行動 sexual behavior　性差別 sex[sexual] discrimination / sexism　☞性感, 性感染症, 性器, 性機能障害, 性教育, 性交, 性行為, 性差, 性生活, 性成熟, 性腺, 性染色体, 性体験, 性徴, 性的, 性転換, 性同一性, 性犯罪, 性別, 性ホルモン, 性本能, 性毛, 性欲

せい³　姓　family name (↔given name), **surname**　(特に欧米人の姓) **last name** (↔first name)　☞名前　◆姓はどのように綴りますか〈発音しますか〉How do you spell〈pronounce〉your family name?

せい⁴　所為　(原因で)**because of, due to**
◆病気のせいで仕事を失うのではないか不安ですか Are you concerned that you may lose your job *because of[due to] your illness?　◆物事がうまくいかないのは自分のせいだと気がとがめますか When things go wrong, do you blame yourself for everything? / Do you feel guilty when things go wrong?

せいいき　声域　voice range, vocal range

せいいく　生育・成育　growth　☞成長
◆子供の成育環境を整える provide[create] a good child-rearing[parenting] environment　▶生育歴 personal history

せいいっぱい　精一杯　◆このように腕を精一杯伸ばして下さい Extend your arms all the way out (as much as you can), like this.　◆それが精一杯ですか Is that all you can do?　◆毎日を精一杯生きる make the most of each day / live each day to the full[fullest]　☞できるだけ

せいえき　精液　semen, sperm, seminal fluid　◆精液を採取する collect sperm / collect[take] a semen sample　◀血精液症 hemospermia　▶精液検査 semen examination[analysis]　精液保存 semen storage　精液瘤 spermatocele

せいか　成果　(結果)**result, outcome, fruit**
(効果)**effect**　(形effective)　◆あなたの上司は成果を出すことを絶えず要求しますか Does your boss always demand that you achieve good results[outcomes] in your work?　◆この新薬は長年にわたる研究の成果です This new medication is the result[fruit] of years of research.　◆これまでの治療では思うような成果は出ていません So far, the treatment hasn't been as effective as we expected. / So far, we haven't got the results we'd expected from the treatment.　◆成果主義 a results-oriented approach

せいかい　正解　correct answer, right answer　◆正解はどれですか What[Which] is the correct[right] answer?　◆この問題にただ1つの正解というものは存在しません There isn't only one correct[right] answer to this problem. / There's more than one correct[right] answer to this problem.　◆救急車で来院されたのは正解でした Coming to the hospital by ambulance was the right choice[decision].

せいかがく　生化学　biochemistry　◀血液生化学検査 biochemistry blood test

せいかく¹　正確(な)　(正しい)**correct**　(事

せいかく¹ 実に基づいて確かな **accurate** （ぴったりの） **exact, precise** ◆正確にお答え下さい Please give the correct answer. / Please answer correctly ◆より正確に言うと彼女の脳卒中はくも膜下出血です To put it more accurately[To be more exact], her stroke is subarachnoid hemorrhage. ◆正確な診断をするためにいくつか検査をする必要があります To obtain an accurate diagnosis, we need to run some tests. ◆このタイプの問題を診断するには CT よりも MRI のほうがより正確です MRI is more accurate than CT scanning for diagnosing this type of problem. ◆ポリープの正確なサイズを測る measure the exact size of the polyp ◆正確な情報を得る have[obtain] correct[accurate] information

せいかく² **性格** （個性・人格）**personality** （特性）**character** （生来の性質）**nature** ◆性格が変化したことに気づきましたか Have you noticed any changes in your personality? ◆あなたは性格的に楽天家のほうですか Are you optimistic by nature? ◆性格を分析する analyze *a person's* character[personality] ◆性格上の特徴 a character[personality] trait ◆性格が几帳面である be meticulous by nature / be precise in everything *one* does ◆外向的〈内向的〉な性格 an extroverted〈introverted〉personality ◆穏やかな〈攻撃的な〉性格 *a calm〈an aggressive〉personality ◆短気な性格 a hot-tempered personality ◆せっかちな〈のんびりした〉性格 an impatient〈easy-going〉personality ◆優しい性格の人 a good-natured person ◆強迫的な性格 a compulsive personality ◀異常性格 abnormal character[personality] A 型性格 type A personality てんかん性格 epileptic personality[character] ヒステリー性格 hysterical personality 病前性格 premorbid character ▶性格検査 personality test 性格変化 personality change

せいかつ **生活** **life** （動**live**）（毎日の活動） **daily activity** （生計）**living** （生活様式）**life-**

style ◆日本での生活にはもう慣れましたか Have you got used to living[life] in Japan? ◆検査後は普段通りの生活をして結構です After the test, you can go about your normal daily activities. ◆日常生活で一番困っておられることは何ですか What bothers you most in your everyday life? / What gives you the most trouble day to day? ◆生活費のことがご心配ですか Are you concerned about the cost of living? ◆彼女は日常生活を送るうえで全介助が必要です She needs full assistance with the activities of daily living. ◆ソーシャルワーカーが退院後の生活を立て直す手助けをしてくれます Your social worker will help you rebuild your life after you're discharged from the hospital. ◆生活習慣を改善すれば治療目標を達成することができます Change[Improve] your way of life[living], and you'll be able to reach your treatment goal. ◆彼の生活リズムは乱れています His daily rhythm[routine] is disturbed. ◆健康的な〈不健康な〉生活を送る live *a healthy〈an unhealthy〉life[lifestyle] ◆生活が苦しい（生計が立たない）find it difficult to make a living / （金に困っている）be badly off（for money）◀家庭生活 family[home] life 結婚生活 married life 食生活 eating habits 自立生活 independent living；IL 内的生活 inner life 入院生活 life in the hospital / hospital life ▶生活活動指数 index of living activity 生活サイクル life cycle 生活史 life history 生活支援施設 assisted living facility 生活状態 living conditions 生活水準 the standard of living / living standards 生活相談 life consultation[counseling] 生活費 living expenses[costs] / the cost of living 生活歴 life history ☞生活環境, 生活習慣, 生活の質, 生活保護, 性生活, 日常生活

せいかつかんきょう **生活環境** **living environment, the environment** *one* **lives in** （暮らしの状況）**living conditions** ★通例，複数形で．◆生活環境を改善する improve *one's* living conditions[environment]

◆生活環境を整える put *one's* living conditions in order　◆大気汚染が進み生活環境が悪化している The living environment is deteriorating[getting worse] due to air pollution.　◆体によくない都会の生活環境 an unhealthy urban environment

せいかつしゅうかん　生活習慣 （日課）daily routine （日常活動）daily activities ★通例，複数形で．（毎日の習慣）daily habit ☞習慣　◆生活習慣についておうかがいします Let me ask you some questions about your daily routine[activities].　◆どうすれば生活習慣を変えられるか考えて下さい Please think about how you can change[improve] your daily habits.　▶生活習慣病 lifestyle[lifestyle-related] disease[illness]

せいかつのしつ　生活の質　quality of life：**QOL**　◆生活の質を保つ〈向上させる〉 maintain〈improve〉*one's* quality of life　◆生活の質が低下する the quality of life decreases

せいかつほご　生活保護　public assistance, welfare （手当）public assistance[welfare] payment　◆生活保護を受ける receive public assistance payments　◆生活保護を受けている be on public assistance[welfare]　◆生活保護の申請をする *apply for[claim] public assistance[welfare] （payments）　▶生活保護受給者 welfare recipient　生活保護世帯 family on welfare

せいかん¹　性感　sexual feeling[sensation]　▶性感極期 orgasm　性感帯 erogenous zone

せいかん²　精管　ductus deferens, vas deferens, deferent duct, spermatic duct　▶精管炎 vasitis / deferentitis　精管結紮術 vasoligation　精管切除術 vasectomy / deferentectomy

せいかんせんしょう　性感染症　sexually transmitted disease：**STD, sexually transmitted infection**：**STI**　☞巻末付録：訊きにくい質問のコツ　◆性感染症の診断を受けたことがありますか Have you ever been diagnosed as having *an STD[a sexually

transmitted disease]?　◆性感染症に対してどんな予防措置を講じていますか What precautions do you take against contracting STDs?

せいき　性器　genitals, genitalia, genital [sex] organs （生殖器）reproductive organs　★いずれも通例，複数形で．◆女性〈男性〉性器 female〈male〉 genitals[genitalia / genital organs]　◆性器がただれている have genital sores　◆性器いじりをする play with *one's* genitals　◀外〈内〉性器 external〈internal〉 genitals[genitalia / genital organs]　▶性器奇形 genital anomaly　性器クラミジア感染症 genital chlamydiosis　性器出血 genital bleeding　性器ヘルペス genital herpes

せいきさん　正期産　term birth, labor at term　▶正期産児 full-term newborn / term baby[infant]

せいきのうしょうがい　性機能障害　sexual dysfunction

せいきぶんぷ　正規分布　normal distribution

せいきゅう　請求する （要求する）request （図request）（頼む・求める）ask for （補償などを請求する）claim （図claim）　◆請求額はトータルで2万円になります Your bill comes to twenty thousand yen in total. / The total amount of your bill is twenty thousand yen.　◆申請書は市役所〈区役所〉でご請求下さい Please request[ask for / （手に入れる）obtain] the application form at the city〈ward〉 office.　◆カルテの開示請求には個人情報保護のため患者さんご本人による申請が必要です To release a patient's chart[medical records], we need to obtain the request from the patient himself〈herself〉 to protect his 〈her〉 right to privacy. / We'll release a patient's chart[medical records] only if requested by the patient in person.　◆彼女の請求に応じる meet[comply with] her request　▶請求書 bill / （保険金などの請求書）（insurance）claim form

せいきょ　逝去する　die （婉曲的に）pass away　☞死，死ぬ，死亡，亡くなる

せいぎょ 制御する （管理・コントロールする）control （調節する）regulate ☞コントロール ◆感情を制御するのが難しい have difficulty controlling *one's* feelings ◆負の制御 a negative control ▶制御装置 control device[equipment]

せいきょういく 性教育 sex education

せいきん 静菌（の）bacteriostatic ◆静菌作用がある have a bacteriostatic action / be capable of inhibiting the growth and reproduction of bacteria ▶静菌性抗菌薬 bacteriostatic antibiotics

せいけい¹ 生計 living ◆どのようにして生計を立てているのですか How do you make[earn] a living? / How do you support yourself?

せいけい² 整形 （整形手術）orthopedic surgery （形成手術）plastic surgery （美容手術）cosmetic surgery ◆顔を整形する have plastic[cosmetic] surgery on *one's* face ▶整形靴 orthopedic shoe(s) / （矯正靴）corrective shoe(s) ☞整形外科

せいけいげか 整形外科 orthopedics /ɔ̀ə-θəpíːdɪks/ （🔊orthopedic） （診療科）the department of orthopedics[orthopedic surgery], the orthopedics department ▶整形外科医 orthopedic surgeon / orthopedist 整形外科手術 orthopedic surgery 整形外科病棟 orthopedic ward[floor / unit]

せいけつ 清潔（な） clean （衛生的な）sanitary ◆清潔なタオル a clean towel ◆部位を清潔に乾かしておいて下さい Please keep the area clean and dry. ▶清潔間欠導尿 clean intermittent catheterization 清潔区域 clean area

せいけん 生検 biopsy /báɪɑpsi/：Bx ◆結腸の生検をします I'm going to do a biopsy of your colon. / （生検のために結腸から組織を採る）I'm going to remove some tissue from your colon for biopsy. ◆生検の結果は1週間後に出ます The results of the biopsy should be available in a week. ◆乳房の生検をする do[take] a breast biopsy ◆生検サンプルを採取する collect samples for biopsy ◆皮膚の病変

を生検する biopsy the skin lesion ◀鉗子生検 forceps biopsy 肝生検 liver biopsy 筋生検 muscle biopsy 経皮的生検 percutaneous biopsy 骨髄生検 bone marrow biopsy 子宮内膜生検 endometrial biopsy 神経生検 nerve biopsy 腎生検 kidney biopsy 切開生検 incision[incisional] biopsy 穿刺吸引生検 fine needle aspiration biopsy；FNAB 超音波ガイド下生検 ultrasonography[ultrasonically] guided biopsy 直視下生検 open[directvision] biopsy 摘出生検 excision[excisional] biopsy 内視鏡下生検 endoscopic biopsy 肺生検 lung biopsy 針生検 needle biopsy 皮膚生検 skin biopsy リンパ節生検 lymph node biopsy ▶生検鉗子 biopsy forceps

せいげん 制限する （限定する）limit （🔊limit, limitation） （規制する）restrict （🔊restriction） （制御する）control （🔊control） ◆集中治療室のご面会はご家族に制限させていただきます Visiting in the ICU is limited [restricted] to family members. ◆宗教上の食事制限がありますか Do you have any religious dietary (food) restrictions? ◆活動を院内に制限する limit[restrict] *one's* activities to inside the hospital ◆塩分を制限する limit[restrict] salt (intake) ◆カロリーを1日約1,500 kcal に制限する restrict[keep / limit] *one's* calorie intake to about one thousand five hundred (kilocalories) per day ◆食事制限をしている be on a restricted diet ◀運動制限 movement limitation 塩分制限 salt restriction 塩分制限食 low-salt[low-sodium / sodium-restricted] diet 活動制限 activity restriction 可動域制限 limited range of motion カリウム制限食 low-potassium[potassium-restricted] diet カロリー制限 caloric restriction / calorie control 気流制限 airflow limitation 産児制限 birth control 脂肪制限食 low-fat[fat-restricted] diet 食事制限 dietary restriction 蛋白制限食 low-protein[protein-restricted] diet 年齢制限 age limit 水制限 water restriction

せいご 生後 after birth ◆今，お子さんは生後何か月ですか How many months old is your baby? ◆生後9か月の乳児 a nine-month-old baby ◆生後4か月健診 a four-month (health) checkup after birth

せいこう¹ 成功 success (↔failure) (動 succeed, work out well 形 successful) ◆彼女の手術は成功しました Her surgery *was successful[was a success]. ◆この手術の成功率は高いです This surgery has a high success rate. / The success rate of this surgery is high. / (成功する見込みが高い) This treatment has a good chance of success.

せいこう² 性交 (sexual) intercourse, sex, coitus ☞巻末付録：訊きにくい質問のコツ ◆性交時に痛みや不快感がありますか Do you have (any) pain or discomfort during intercourse? ◆性交後に腟から出血することがありますか Do you ever have vaginal bleeding after intercourse? ◆無防備な性交 unprotected sex ▶性交痛 painful intercourse / pain during intercourse 性交不能 (sexual) impotence

せいこうい 性行為 sexual activity, intercourse, sex (act) ☞巻末付録：訊きにくい質問のコツ ◆性行為はして構いません You can continue having sex[sexual activity]. ◆しばらくの間性行為は控えて下さい Please refrain from sexual activity for a while. ◆性行為をする have (sexual) intercourse (with) ◆性行為の相手 one's sex partner

せいこつ 整骨 ☞整復 ▶整骨医学 osteopathic medicine 整骨院 osteopathic clinic 整骨療法 osteopathy / osteopathic therapy

せいさ¹ 精査 ☞精密検査

せいさ² 性差 difference between the sexes, sex difference (社会・文化における男女差) gender difference

せいざい 製剤 (製品) product (化合物) compound (薬剤) agent, drug (調合した薬品) preparation (分離・精製物) derivative ◀加熱血液製剤 heat-treated blood product 血漿分画製剤 plasma derivative [product] 生物学的製剤 biologic product[drug / agent] 白金製剤 platinum drug マグネシウム製剤 magnesium preparation

せいさく 精索 spermatic cord ▶精索静脈瘤 varicocele 精索水瘤 spermatic cord hydrocele 精索捻転 spermatic cord torsion

せいさん¹ 青酸 (シアン化物) cyanide / sáiənàid/ ▶青酸カリ potassium cyanide 青酸ソーダ sodium cyanide 青酸中毒 cyanide poisoning

せいさん² 精算する (支払う) settle ◆退院する前に会計窓口で入院費をご精算下さい Before leaving the hospital, please settle your (hospital) bill at the cashier counter.

せいさんねんれいじんこう 生産年齢人口 working-age population

せいさんやく 制酸薬 antacid

せいし 精子 sperm, spermatozoon ◆精子数が少ない have a low sperm count ◀殺精子薬 spermatocide / spermatocidal agent / spermicide 乏精子症 oligospermia / oligozoospermia 無精子症 azoospermia ▶精子運動能 sperm motility 精子奇形 abnormal spermatozoa / malformed sperm 精子頸管粘液適合試験 sperm-cervical mucus compatibility test 精子検査 sperm analysis 精子無力症 asthenozoospermia / asthenospermia

せいしき 清拭する (清潔にする) clean (ベッドの上で体を拭く) give a bed bath (患者を寝かせたまま体を拭く) give a blanket bath (スポンジで体を拭く) give a sponge bath ◆清拭いたしましょう I'm going to [Let me] give you a bed bath. ◆陰部の清拭はご自分でなさいますか Would you like to clean your private areas by yourself?

せいしじしんせん 静止時振戦 resting tremor, static tremor

せいししょう 青視症 cyanopsia, blue vision

せいしつ 性質 （性格）character （生来の性質）nature （特性・属性）property （資質）quality ☞性格, 性状

せいじゅく 成熟する mature （図maturity, maturation 図mature） ▶成熟期 (the period of) maturity / maturation period 成熟細胞 mature cell 成熟児 mature infant 成熟乳 mature milk

せいしゅんき 青春期 adolescence （図adolescent） ☞ライフステージ ◆青春期には in *one's* *young days[youth] ▶青春期危機 adolescent crisis

せいじょう¹ 正常（な） normal （図正常化する normalize） ◆尿は正常です Your urine is normal. ◆血液検査はすべて正常です Your blood test shows that everything is normal. ◆血糖値は正常です Your blood sugar levels are normal. / You have normal blood sugar levels. ◆コレステロール値は正常の範囲内です Your cholesterol levels are normal[within the normal range / within normal limits]. ◆高血圧を正常にする normalize high blood pressure ▶正常圧水頭症 normal pressure hydrocephalus 正常眼圧緑内障 normal-tension glaucoma；NTG 正常組織 normal tissue 正常妊娠 normal pregnancy 正常分娩 normal childbirth[delivery] / eutocia ☞正常値

せいじょう² 性状 （物の属性）property （物の硬度・粘度）consistency （質感・触感）texture （特性）characteristic, character ◆有毒ガスの性状を分析する analyze the properties of toxic gases ◆おりものの性状が変化する The consistency of vaginal discharge changes. ◆どのような痛みですか What's the pain like? / Can you describe the pain? / How would you describe the pain?

せいじょう³ 清浄（な） （清潔な）clean （不純物を含まない）pure ◀空気清浄器 air purifier ▶清浄作用 cleaning action 清浄綿 antiseptic wipe 清浄薬 sanitizer / antiseptic wash

せいじょうち 正常値 （測定値）normal （count） （測定レベル）normal level （基準値）normal value ◆血圧は正常値よりやや高い〈低い〉です Your blood pressure is slightly above〈below〉normal. ◆尿酸は正常値の範囲内です Your uric acid is within normal range[limits]. ◆血圧が正常値まで下がっています Your blood pressure has dropped[fallen] to normal. ◆彼女の白血球数は正常値を超えて〈下回って〉います Her white blood cell counts are above〈below〉normal. ◆正常値の上限〈下限〉the upper〈lower〉limit of normal [the normal value]

せいしょうどう 性衝動 ☞性欲

せいじょうひしゅ 精上皮腫 seminoma

せいしょく¹ 生殖 reproduction （図reproductive） ◆生殖能力は一般に加齢によって低下します Generally, the[a person's] reproductive potential gradually decreases[weakens] with age. ▶生殖機能 reproductive function 生殖細胞 germ [reproductive] cell 生殖周期 reproductive cycle 生殖腺 gonad / reproductive [sex] gland 生殖補助技術[生殖医療] assisted reproductive technology；ART ☞生殖器

せいしょく² 青色（の） blue ▶青色強膜 blue sclera 青色鼓膜 blue eardrum[tympanic membrane] 青色母斑 blue nevus

せいしょくき 生殖器 ☞性器, 性腺 ◀女性生殖器系〈男性生殖器系〉the female 〈male〉reproductive system

せいしん 精神 mind （図mental 情動的な emotional 心理的な psychological 精神医学の・精神障害の psychiatric / sàɪkɪætrɪk/ 精神病性の psychotic） ☞心理 ◆精神疾患 psychiatric[mental] disease[illness] / （精神病）*psychotic disorder[psychosis] ◆精神疾患の患者 a psychiatric[mentally ill] patient ◆精神衛生 mental health ◆精神状態 mental[psychological] condition[state] ◆彼女の精神状態は悪化しています Her psychological condition is *getting worse[deteriorating]. ◆彼は精神的に不安定です He is *emotionally unstable[mentally unbalanced]. ◆これまでに感情面や精神面で

問題がありましたか Have you ever had any emotional or psychiatric problems in the past?　◆精神的疲労 mental fatigue ◆精神的に疲れている be mentally tired[exhausted]　◆精神的なケアをする give mental[psychological / psychiatric] care　◆彼女は精神的な援助を必要としています She needs emotional support. /（励ましを必要とする）She needs moral support.　◁向精神薬 psychotropic（medication / drug / agent）　集団精神療法 group psychotherapy　▶精神安定薬 tranquilizer　精神運動発達遅滞 psychomotor retardation　精神運動発作 psychomotor seizure　精神活動 mental activity　精神看護 psychiatric and mental health nursing　精神鑑定 psychiatric examination[test]　精神腫瘍学 psychooncology　精神身体症[心身症] psychosomatic disease[disorder]；PSD　精神遅滞 mental retardation；MR　精神年齢 mental age；MA　精神発達 mental development　精神賦活薬 psychostimulant / psychic energizer　精神分析 psychoanalysis　精神変調 mental aberration　精神療法 psychotherapy　☞精神医学, 精神科, 精神障害, 精神病, 精神保健

せいじん　成人　**adult**　（子供から見た大人）**grown-up**　☞ライフステージ　▶成人看護 adult（health care）nursing　成人Ｔ細胞白血病 adult T-cell leukemia；ATL　成人保健 adult health

せいしんいがく　精神医学　**psychiatry**　◁思春期精神医学 adolescent psychiatry　児童精神医学 child psychiatry　犯罪精神医学 criminal psychiatry　リエゾン精神医学 liaison psychiatry

せいしんか　精神科　**psychiatry** /saɪkáɪə-tri/（形**psychiátric**）（診療科）**the department of psychiatry, the psychiatry department**　▶精神科医 psychiatrist　精神科病院 psychiatric[mental] hospital

せいしんしょうがい　精神障害　**mental disability[disorder]**　（精神病性の）**psychotic disorder**　◆精神障害者 a person with a mental disability / a mentally

disabled[challenged] person　▶精神障害者保健福祉手帳 mental disability handbook

せいしんびょう　精神病　**psychotic disorder, psychosis**　◁アルコール精神病 alcoholic psychosis　抗精神病薬 antipsychotic（medication / drug / agent）/ major tranquilizer　産褥精神病 puerperal psychosis　心因性精神病 psychogenic psychosis　内因性精神病 endogenous psychosis　薬剤誘発性精神病 drug-induced psychosis　▶精神病質 psychopathy /（精神病質者）psychopath　精神病質パーソナリティ psychopathic personality

せいしんほけん　精神保健　**mental health**　▶精神保健福祉士 psychiatric social worker；PSW　精神保健福祉センター mental health and welfare center　精神（障害者）保健福祉手帳 mental disability handbook　精神保健福祉法 the Mental Health and Welfare Law

せいせい¹　生成する　（生産する）**produce**（図**production**）（生体物質などを合成する）**synthesize**（図**synthesis**）　◆ホルモンの生成 production of hormones　◁尿酸生成抑制薬 uric acid synthesis inhibitor　▶生成物 product

せいせい²　精製する　（純化する）**purify**（図**purification**）（純度を高める）**refine**（図**refinement**）　▶精製水 purified water　精製ツベルクリン purified protein derivative of tuberculin；PPD

せいぜい　**at**（**the**）**most**　◆熱は長引いてもせいぜい3日ぐらいです The fever will continue[drag on] for three days at（the）most.

ゼイゼイ　（ゼイゼイいう音）**wheeze**（動**wheeze**　形**wheezy**）（息がゼイゼイすること）**wheeziness**　◆ゼイゼイしたり, 息苦しかったり, 胸が締め付けられるようなことがありますか Do you experience any wheezing, difficulty breathing, or chest tightness?　◆ゼイゼイし始めたのはいつですか When did this wheeziness start? / Since when have you been feeling wheezy?　◆ゼイゼイする咳 a wheezy cough

せいせいかつ　性生活　sex life ☞巻末付録：訊きにくい質問のコツ　◆性生活についてお聞かせ下さい I'm going to ask you some questions[Please tell me] about your *sex life[〈性的志向〉sexual preferences].　◆性生活に満足していますか Are you satisfied with your sex life?　◆最近，性生活をしていますか Are you currently sexually active? / Are you having sexual relations?

せいせいじゅく　性成熟　sexual maturation　▶性成熟期 reproductive age

せいせき　成績　(結果)outcome, result (予後)prognosis　(記録)record　(学業の評価)grade　(点数)score, mark　◆患者のおよそ 95％は術後の成績が良好です About ninety-five percent of all patients have a good outcome[result] after surgery.　◆肺がんⅣ期の治療成績は不良です Stage four lung cancer has a poor[bad] prognosis[treatment outcome].　◆リハビリで期待通りの成績をあげて満足でしょう You must be happy to have achieved *what you wanted to achieve[the outcome you expected] with your rehabilitation.　◀検査成績 test result　手術成績 surgical outcome[result] / outcome[result] of surgery　治療成績 treatment outcome[result]

せいせん　性腺　gonad, sex gland　▶女性〈男性〉性腺 female〈male〉gonad　▶性腺機能低下症 hypogonadism　性腺刺激ホルモン gonadotropin；Gn　性腺刺激ホルモン放出ホルモン gonadotropin-releasing hormone；GnRH / luteinizing hormone-releasing hormone；LH-RH

せいせんしょくたい　性染色体　sex chromosome　▶性染色体異常 sex chromosome disorder[aberration / abnormality]

せいせんしょくひん　生鮮食品　fresh food

せいそう[1]　精巣　testicle（形testicular），**testis**（複testes），**orchis**　◆精巣に痛みがある have (a) pain in *one's* testicle(s) / have testicular pain　◆精巣が痛んで腫れていますか Are your testicles painful and

swollen?　◀停留精巣 retained testicle[testis] / undescended testicle[testis] / cryptorchidism　ムンプス精巣炎 mumps orchitis　遊走精巣 migratory[retractile] testis　▶精巣炎 testitis / orchitis　精巣機能不全 testicular insufficiency　精巣固定術 orchiopexy　精巣腫瘍 testicular tumor　精巣上体 epididymis　精巣上体炎 epididymitis　精巣女性化症候群 testicular feminization syndrome　精巣摘除術 orchiectomy / orchidectomy　精巣ホルモン testicular hormone

せいそう[2]　清掃する　clean ☞掃除　◆ポータブルトイレを清掃する clean a portable toilet　◆毎日午前中に清掃員が病室の清掃に伺います Our cleaning staff will come and clean your room every morning.　◆口腔清掃で誤嚥性肺炎のリスクを減らせます Good oral care[Mouth cleaning] can reduce the risk of developing aspiration pneumonia.

せいぞう　製造　(生産)production　(大量生産)manufacture　◆インフルエンザワクチンの製造 the manufacture of influenza vaccine　◆その薬は製造中止になっていて手に入りません The drug[pharmaceutical] company stopped producing[making] that medication, so it's no longer available.

せいぞん　生存する　(生き残る)survive（名survival）　(存在する)exist（名existence）(生きる)live ☞生きる　◆手術をしないと彼女が生存できる見込みは 10％しかありません I'm afraid that without the surgery she has only a ten percent chance of survival.　◆赤ちゃんは子宮外でも生存可能です The baby can survive outside the womb.　◆この病気の 5 年生存率は 90％です The five-year survival rate for this disease is ninety percent.　◀累積生存率 cumulative survival rate　▶生存可能性[能力] viability　生存期間 survival period

せいたい[1]　声帯　vocal cords　★複数形で．　◆声を使い過ぎると声帯を傷めます Overuse[Misuse] of the voice can damage your vocal cords.　◆声帯に小さな結

せいたい¹ 節ができていますが，特に切除は必要ありません You have a small nodule on your vocal cords, but there's no need for it to be removed. ◀ポリープ様声帯 polypoid vocal cords ▶声帯炎 (vocal) chorditis 声帯結節 vocal (cord) nodule 声帯ポリープ vocal cord polyp 声帯麻痺 vocal cord paralysis[(不全麻痺)paresis]

せいたい² 生体(の) (生存している)living (生物学上の)biologic, biological (生命維持の)vital ◆生体肝移植 living[living-donor] liver transplant[transplantation] ▶生体応答 biologic response 生体応答修飾物質 biologic response modifier；BRM 生体工学 bioengineering 生体臓器提供者 living donor 生体時計 biological clock 生体弁 biologic[tissue / bioprosthetic] valve

せいたいけん 性体験 sexual experience

せいたいじゅつ 整体術 *seitai* (massage) therapy, chiropractic；*traditional therapy using the fingers, hands, and elbows to adjust the spine and manipulate the joints*

せいちゅう 正中(の) median, midline ▶正中頸囊胞 median cervical cyst 正中神経麻痺 median nerve paralysis 正中切開 midline[median] incision 正中線 median line 正中面 median plane

せいちょう¹ 成長 growth (圖grow) ☞発育, 発達 ◆成長を促すホルモン a hormone that promotes[contributes to] growth ◆お子さんは順調に成長しています Your child is growing well[properly]. ◆子供の成長の早さには個人差があります Children grow at different rates. / Each child has his or her own growth rate. ◆子供の成長が遅れていると心配しているのですか Are you concerned about your child's *delayed growth[growth delay]*? ◀上皮成長因子 epidermal growth factor；EGF ▶成長因子 growth factor 成長過程 growth process 成長曲線 growth curve 成長線 growth line 成長速度 growth rate 成長痛 growing pains ☞成長ホルモン

せいちょう² 性徴 sexual characteristics ★通例，複数形で. ◆二次性徴が現れ始める年齢には個人差があります The age at which a child's secondary sexual characteristics begin to develop differs from child to child. / There are individual differences in the age at which children begin to develop secondary sexual characteristics. ◀一次性徴 primary sexual characteristics

せいちょうホルモン 成長ホルモン growth hormone；GH ▶成長ホルモン産生腺腫 growth hormone-producing adenoma 成長ホルモン分泌不全症 growth hormone deficiency；GHD 成長ホルモン放出ホルモン growth hormone-releasing hormone；GHRH[GRH] 成長ホルモン補充療法 growth hormone replacement therapy

せいちょうやく 整腸薬 intestinal regulator

せいてき¹ 性的(な) sexual ☞巻末付録：訊きにくい質問のコツ ◆ここ数か月で何人と性的関係を持ちましたか How many partners have you had in the past several months? ◆パートナーには性的に何か不満はありますか Are you sexually unhappy [dissatisfied] with your partner? ◆性的衝動に問題がありますか Do you have any problems with your sex drive? ▶性的虐待 sexual abuse 性的興奮 sexual excitement 性的刺激 sexual stimulation 性的志向 sexual orientation[preference] 性的倒錯 sexual inversion[perversion] 性的不感症 sexual frigidity 性的暴行 sexual violence / (強姦)sexual assault

せいてき² 静的(な) static (↔dynamic) ▶静的作業 static work[action] 静的姿勢 static posture

せいてんかん 性転換 ☞性別適合手術

せいど¹ 制度 system ◆日本の医療制度では正常な妊娠や健康診断には保険が使えません In the Japanese medical insurance system, normal pregnancy and health checkups are not covered by insurance. ◀教育制度 educational sys-

せいど¹ tem　公的介護制度 public care system　措置制度 welfare referral system

せいど²　精度　◆この測定方法は非常に精度が高いです This measurement method is very accurate[precise].

せいとう　正当（な）　（十分な）good　（当然の）due, justifiable　◆化学療法を中止する正当な理由があります We have good reason for discontinuing[stopping] the chemotherapy. / There's due[justifiable] cause to discontinue[stop] the chemotherapy.

せいどういつせい　性同一性　gender identity　▶性同一性障害［性同一不合］gender identity disorder；GID / gender incongruence

せいとやく　制吐薬　antiemetic（medication, drug, agent）

せいねん¹　成年　adult（age）　（法定年齢）legal age　▶成年後見制度 adult guardianship[conservatorship]（system）　成年後見人 guardian[conservator] of an adult

せいねん²　青年　（男性）young man　（女性）young woman　▶青年期 youth / adolescence

せいねんがっぴ　生年月日　date of birth；DOB　◆生年月日はいつですか What's your date of birth? / When were you born?

せいのう　精嚢　seminal vesicle　▶精嚢炎 seminal vesiculitis

せいはんざい　性犯罪　sex crime, sex offense

せいびょう　性病　☞性感染症

せいひん　製品　（産物・生成物）product　（物）object　（品物・商品）goods　★複数形で．◆大豆製品 soy products　◆乳製品 dairy[milk] products　◆金属製品 metal[metallic] object　◆綿製品 cotton goods

せいふく　整復する　set　（位置を復元する）reposition（図reposition）　（還元・縮小する）reduce（図reduction）　◆折れた骨を整復する set a broken bone　◆脱臼した肩を整復する reposition a dislocated shoulder　◀観血的〈非観血的〉整復 open〈closed〉reduction　徒手整復 manual reposition

[correction]

せいぶつ　生物　（生き物）living thing　（有機体）organism　（生命体）life　（接頭bio-）　▶生物活性 biological activity / bioactivity　生物時計 biological clock　生物物理学 biophysics　☞生物学

せいぶつがく　生物学　biology（形biologic, biological）　◆生物学上の父親〈母親〉biological father〈mother〉/ birth father〈mother〉　◀分子生物学 molecular biology　▶生物学的製剤 biologic product[drug / agent]

せいぶん　成分　《構成部分》component, constituent, element　◆血液成分 blood components[constituents]　◆血球成分 cellular components of blood　◆分泌成分 secretory components

《混合物の材料》ingredient　◆睡眠薬の成分 sleeping pill ingredients　◆有効成分 an active ingredient

《物質》substance　◆この薬には眠くなる成分が入っています This medication contains a substance that will make you sleepy.

▶成分栄養剤 elemental diet　成分献血 blood component donation　成分分析 constituent analysis　成分輸血（blood）component transfusion　成分輸血製剤 blood component derivative　成分ワクチン component vaccine

せいべつ　性別　（生物学的な男女の別）sex　（社会的・文化的に形成される男女の別）gender　（性による区別）sex distinction　◆（妊婦に）お子さんの性別をお知りになりたいですか Would you like to know your baby's sex?　▶性別不合［性同一性障害］gender incongruence / gender identity disorder；GID　性別判定 sex determination　☞性別適合手術

せいべつてきごうしゅじゅつ　性別適合手術　sex change surgery, sex reassignment surgery；SRS　◆性別適合手術を受ける undergo *sex change surgery[sex reassignment surgery]

せいホルモン　性ホルモン　（性ステロイドホ

せいホルモン ルモン) sex steroid hormone

せいほんのう 性本能 sexual instinct

せいみつけんさ 精密検査 （徹底的な）thorough test[examination] （詳細な）detailed test[examination] （網羅的な）complete test[examination] ◆精密検査をする *carry out[do / run] a thorough[detailed] examination ◆精密検査を受ける have[undergo] a thorough[complete] examination ◆この件に関して他の病院で精密検査を受けたことがありますか Have you ever had a thorough[detailed] test for this problem at another hospital? ◆診断するためにさらに精密検査をしましょう We need to do some more detailed tests before we can make a diagnosis. ◆前立腺の精密検査を受けることをお勧めします I recommend that you have a thorough examination of your prostate.

せいみつど 精密度 ☞精度

せいめい¹ 生命 life ☞命, 生 (せい) ▶生命科学 life science / (生物科学)bioscience 生命徴候 vital signs 生命力(活力)vitality 生命倫理 bioethics ☞生命維持, 生命保険

せいめい² 姓名 (full) name ☞名前 ◆姓名をお聞かせ下さい Could you tell me your name, please? ◆ここに姓名を活字体で記入し署名して下さい Please print your name here and add your signature.

せいめい³ 清明(な) ◆彼女の意識は清明です She is fully conscious[alert].

せいめいいじ 生命維持 life support ☞延命 ◆生命維持処置を行う〈行わない〉provide〈withhold〉*life support[life-sustaining procedures] ◆生命維持処置を中止する withdraw a person's *life support [life-sustaining procedures] ☞生命維持装置

せいめいいじそうち 生命維持装置 life support system[machine], life sustaining equipment ◆彼女は生命維持装置をつけています She is (being kept) on life support. ◆生命維持装置をつける place [put] the patient on *a life support machine[a life support system / life sup-

port] ◆生命維持装置を取り外す remove the patient from life support / take the patient off life support ◆生命維持装置を止める turn[switch] off the life support machine[system]

せいめいほけん 生命保険 life insurance ◆生命保険の支払請求のために診断書が必要であれば，用紙を窓口にご提出下さい If you need a copy of a medical certificate to claim life insurance, hand in the necessary form[paper] at the counter.

せいもう 性毛 pubic hair

せいもん 声門 glottis

せいやく 制約 restriction, limitation （条件)condition ☞制限

せいやくがいしゃ 製薬会社 drug company, pharmaceutical company

せいやくしょ 誓約書 （承諾書）(written) consent form ◆この誓約書を読んで，同意していただけた場合はサインして下さい Please read this consent form and if you agree with its contents, sign below. ◀入院誓約書 consent form for hospital admission

せいよう 静養 rest ◆静養する take a rest / rest quietly ◆自宅で十分に静養する take a good rest at home

せいようどうさ 整容動作 grooming activity

せいよく 性欲 （欲望)sexual desire （衝動)sex drive, sexual impulse[urge] （リビドー)libido ☞巻末付録：訊きにくい質問のコツ ◆性欲はありますか Are you interested in sexual activity? / Do you have a normal sex drive? ◆性欲をなくしたのですか Have you noticed any loss of libido [interest in sex]?

せいり¹ 生理 （月経)(menstrual) period, menstruation （略menstrual) ☞月経 ◆直近で生理があったのはいつですか When was your last period? ◆いま生理中ですか Are you having your period now? ◆生理は重いほうですか Do you tend to have heavy periods? / Do your periods tend to be heavy? ▶生理休暇

menstrual leave 生理痛 period pains / menstrual pains[cramps] 生理不順 menstrual disorder / irregular period 生理用タンポン tampon 生理用ナプキン sanitary pad[napkin] / pad 生理用品 sanitary goods

せいり[2] **生理** (生物体の現象)physiology (㊒physiologic, physiological) ▶生理機能検査 physiologic function test 生理機能検査室 physiology laboratory 生理現象 physiologic phenomenon 生理食塩水 physiologic saline[salt] solution 生理的黄疸 physiologic[neonatal] jaundice 生理的体重減少 physiologic[neonatal] weight loss ☞生理学

せいり[3] **整理する** (片付ける)tidy (up), straighten (up) (整理整頓する)put … in order ◆部屋の整理をお手伝いしましょうか Shall I help you tidy up the room? ◆身の回りをきちんと整理する keep oneself neat and tidy ◀身辺整理 putting one's affairs in order ▶整理運動 cooldown 整理券(先着順の)numbered slip [ticket](given to patients in order of their arrival) 整理番号(参照番号)reference number / (先着順番号)number given to patients in order of their arrival

せいりがく **生理学** physiology (㊒physiologic, physiological) ◀運動生理学 exercise[sport(s)] physiology 電気生理学的検査 electrophysiologic test 病態生理学 pathophysiology ▶生理学者 physiologist

せいりょういんりょうすい **清涼飲料水** soft drink(s) ☞ジュース

せいりょく **精力** (元気・活気)energy, vigor (体力)strength (生命力)vitality ☞活力, 元気, 体力

ゼーゼー ☞ゼイゼイ

セーフティネット safety net ◆在日外国人のためのセーフティネット a safety net for *foreign residents of Japan[Japan's foreign population]

せかいほけんきかん **世界保健機関** the World Health Organization；(the) WHO

セカンドオピニオン second opinion

◆治療のことでセカンドオピニオンを希望しますか. すべての診療録, 画像, 検査データをお渡しします Would you like to have [get] a second opinion about your treatment? I'll provide you with all your medical records, films and lab test data. ◆セカンドオピニオン外来は予約制になっております Second opinion consultations [visits] are by appointment only. ◆セカンドオピニオンを求める ask for a second opinion ▶セカンドオピニオン外来 second opinion clinic

せき **咳** cough (㊒cough) ☞咳嗽 ◆咳を止める suppress[stop] a cough ◆咳を鎮める relieve a cough

《診察の基本表現》 ◆咳が出ますか Do you have a cough? / Do you cough? ◆咳はかなり出ますか Do you cough a lot? / Do you have a bad cough? ◆どの程度の咳ですか How severe is your cough? ◆どのくらいの頻度で咳が出ますか How often do you cough? ◆どんな時に咳が出ますか. 昼間, 夜間, それとも運動中ですか When do you cough—during the day, during the night, or while exercising? ◆咳がひどくなるのはどんな時ですか What situations make your cough worse? / In what situations does your cough become worse? ◆どんな咳が出ますか What's your cough like? ◆咳をする時痰が出ますか Do you bring up phlegm[sputum] when you cough? / Do you cough up phlegm[sputum]? ◆(手術後など)できるだけ咳をして下さい Please try to cough as much as you can.

《程度・頻度などの表現》 ◆ひどい〈少し〉咳が出る have a bad〈slight〉cough ◆激しく咳をする cough *very hard[violently] ◆急に咳込む have a fit of coughing ◆発作的に咳が出る have coughing spasms ◆持続的に咳が出る cough constantly [continuously] ◆頻繁に咳が出る cough often[frequently] ◆時折咳が出る cough occasionally

◀心因性咳 psychogenic cough 遷延性咳 persistent cough 百日咳 whooping

cough / pertussis ▶咳失神 cough[tussive] syncope / cough fainting 咳喘息 cough variant asthma；CVA 咳止め cough medication /（ドロップ）cough drop /（シロップ）cough syrup 咳反射 cough reflex 咳発作 coughing spasm / spasm of coughing

咳の表現

★以下 cough にはすべて a か an をつける.

■咳の性状
●乾性咳 dry[nonproductive] cough ●湿性咳 wet[productive] cough ●犬吠様咳 barking cough ●ゼイゼイする咳 wheezy[wheezing] cough ●喘息様の咳 asthmatic cough ●短く頻発する空咳 hacking cough ●むせるような咳 choking cough ●発作的な咳 spasmodic cough ●慢性の咳 chronic cough

■咳の程度
●少々の咳 slight[little] cough ●軽い咳 mild cough ●中程度の咳 moderate cough ●ひどい咳 bad cough ●激しい咳 severe[intense] cough ●ものすごく激しい咳 violent cough

■咳の頻度・時間帯
●時折出る咳 occasional cough ●断続的な咳 intermittent cough ●持続的な咳 constant[persistent] cough / continuous[nonstop] cough ●繰り返す咳 recurrent cough ●夜間の咳 nighttime[nocturnal] cough ●就寝中の咳 cough during sleep / cough while sleeping ●早朝の咳 early morning cough

せきがいせん 赤外線 infrared ray ▶赤外線照射 infrared radiation 赤外線療法 infrared therapy

せきがきゅう 赤芽球 erythroblast ◀巨赤芽球性貧血 megaloblastic anemia ▶赤芽球癆 pure red cell aplasia；PRCA

せきかっしょく 赤褐色（の）reddish brown （さび色の）rusty ◆赤褐色の痰 *reddish brown[rusty] phlegm

せきじゅうじ 赤十字 the Red Cross ◀国際赤十字社 the International Committee of the Red Cross；ICRC 日本赤十字社 the Japanese Red Cross Society

せきずい 脊髄 spinal cord （腰髄myel(o)-）◀脳脊髄液漏 cerebrospinal fluid leakage 脳脊髄損傷 cerebrospinal injury 脳脊髄膜炎 cerebrospinal meningitis 皮質脊髄路 corticospinal tract ▶脊髄圧迫（spinal）cord compression 脊髄運動ニューロン spinal motor neuron / spinal motoneuron 脊髄液 spinal fluid 脊髄空洞症 syringomyelia 脊髄くも膜下麻酔 spinal anesthesia 脊髄疾患 spinal cord disease 脊髄腫瘍 spinal cord tumor 脊髄小脳失調症 spinocerebellar ataxia；SCA 脊髄小脳変性症 spinocerebellar degeneration；SCD 脊髄神経 spinal nerve 脊髄性進行性筋萎縮症 spinal progressive muscular atrophy；SPMA 脊髄造影 myelography 脊髄損傷 spinal（cord）injury 脊髄中心症候群 central cord syndrome 脊髄反射 spinal reflex 脊髄麻痺 spinal paralysis / myeloparalysis 脊髄レベル診断 spinal cord level diagnosis / diagnosis of the level of spinal cord injury ☞脊髄炎, 脊髄症

せきずいえん 脊髄炎 myelitis ◀横断性脊髄炎 transverse myelitis 脳脊髄炎 encephalomyelitis

せきずいしょう 脊髄症 myelopathy ◀頸椎症性脊髄症 cervical spondylotic myelopathy 脊椎症性脊髄症 spondylotic myelopathy

せきちゅう 脊柱 spinal column, vertebral column （口語）spine, backbone ☞脊椎 ▶脊柱管 spinal[vertebral] canal 脊柱管狭窄症 spinal canal stenosis 脊柱後彎 kyphosis /（円背）round back 脊柱前彎 lordosis 脊柱装具 back brace 脊柱側彎 scoliosis 脊柱長 spinal length；SL 脊柱変形 spinal curvature

せきちん 赤沈 （赤血球沈降速度）erythrocyte[blood] sedimentation rate；ESR, sedimentation rate ◆赤沈を測る check[test] *a person's* sedimentation rate / do

[run] *a blood[an erythrocyte] sedimentation rate test

せきつい 脊椎 spine /spáin/ (㊤spinal) ☞脊柱 ◀二分脊椎 spina bifida 肋骨脊椎角 costovertebral angle ▶脊椎カリエス spinal caries 脊椎後方固定術 posterior spinal fusion 脊椎骨折 spinal fracture 脊椎すべり症 spondylolisthesis 脊椎穿刺 spinal tap[puncture] 脊椎装具 spinal[spine] brace 脊椎分離症 spondylolysis 脊椎麻酔 spinal anesthesia ☞脊椎炎, 脊椎症

せきついえん 脊椎炎 spondylitis /spàndiláɪtɪs/ ◀化膿性脊椎炎 pyogenic spondylitis 乾癬性脊椎炎 psoriatic spondylitis 強直性脊椎炎 ankylosing spondylitis 結核性脊椎炎 tuberculous spondylitis

せきついしょう 脊椎症 spondylosis (㊤spondylotic) ◀腰部脊椎症 lumbar spondylosis ▶脊椎症性脊髄症 spondylotic myelopathy

せきにん 責任 responsibility (㊤responsible) (説明・報告する責任)accountability (㊤accountable) (賠償などに対する法的責任) liability (㊤liable) ◆責任感が強い have a strong sense of responsibility ◆当院は病室内の私物には責任を負いません We can't be responsible for personal belongings in your room. ◆医師は病状を説明する責任があります Your doctor is responsible[accountable] for explaining your condition to you. ◆すべての病院職員は患者の安全に責任があります All the hospital staff *have a responsibility[are responsible] for patient safety. ◆自己責任でやって下さい You should do this on your own responsibility. / You should take the responsibility for doing this. ◆責任を果たす fulfill a responsibility ◆過失責任を負う *accept liability[take responsibility] for one's error[misconduct] ▶病棟責任者 person in charge of the ward[floor / unit] ▶責任者 person in charge (of) / responsible person 責任能力 the mental capacity to distinguish

right from wrong / sufficient mind and understanding to be held responsible for one's actions / (刑事・民事上の責任能力) criminal responsibility

せきめんきょうふ 赤面恐怖 erythrophobia, fear of blushing

せきめんはい 石綿肺 asbestos lung, asbestosis, pulmonary asbestosis

せきり 赤痢 dysentery ◀赤痢に罹る have[get / come down with] dysentery ◀アメーバ赤痢 amebic dysentery 細菌性赤痢 bacillary dysentery ▶赤痢アメーバ Entamoeba histolytica 赤痢菌 Shigella

せきりょくしきかくいじょう 赤緑色覚異常 red-green (color) blindness, red-green color vision defect

セクシャルハラスメント sexual harassment ◆セクシャルハラスメントの被害者 a victim of sexual harassment ◆おやめ下さい, それはセクシャルハラスメントに当たります Don't do that. It's considered[It's a form of] sexual harassment.

セクレチン secretin

―せざるをえない ―せざるを得ない ◆残念かとは思いますが, ご旅行計画は断念していただかざるを得ません You may feel disappointed to hear this, but you *have to[have no choice but to] give up your travel plans. ◆申し訳ありませんが見舞客の人数を制限せざるを得ません We're sorry, but we have to restrict the number of visitors.

せすじ 背筋 (背中)back (背柱)spine (背骨)backbone ☞背, 背中, 背骨 ◆背筋を伸ばして下さい Straighten your back, please. ◆背筋を伸ばして座って下さい〈立って下さい〉Sit〈Stand〉upright, please. ◆曲がった背筋を伸ばす運動をする do exercises to straighten a rounded back

ぜせい 是正する correct ◆この点滴は電解質のバランス異常を是正するために行っています I'm giving you this IV drip to correct your electrolyte imbalance.

せたい 世帯 (家族)family (一家)household ◆お宅は何人世帯ですか How many people are there in your family? ◆世帯主はどなたですか Who is the head of your family[household]? ◀生活保護世帯 family on welfare

せだい 世代 generation (瞬generational) ◆親子の間に世代のギャップがある There is a generation gap between parents and children. ◆何世代にも渡って受け継がれてきた特質 traits passed down *from generation to generation [through the generations] ▶世代交代 generational[generation] change / alternation of generations

せたけ 背丈 height ☞身長

せつ¹ 説 （意見）opinion, view （学説）theory ☞意見 ◆あなたの説には賛成しかねます I can't agree with you[your opinion]. ◆その問題に関してはさまざまな説があります There are a variety of views on that issue. ◆笑いは免疫を高めてくれるという説があります One theory says that laughter boosts the immune system.

せつ² 癤 boil, furuncle

ぜつ 舌 tongue /tʌŋ/, lingua (瞬lingual 暖頭gloss(o)-) ☞舌（した） ◀いちご舌 strawberry tongue 巨大舌 macroglossia 亀裂舌 fissured[furrowed] tongue 苔舌 coated[furred] tongue 毛舌 hairy tongue ▶舌潰瘍 tongue[lingual] ulcer 舌咬傷 bite on the tongue 舌尖 the tip of the tongue 舌損傷 lingual injury / injury to the tongue 舌痛 glossalgia / glossodynia / pain in the tongue 舌乳頭 lingual [tongue] papilla 舌白板症 lingual [tongue] leukoplakia 舌扁桃 lingual tonsil ☞舌圧子, 舌咽神経, 舌炎, 舌下, 舌がん, 舌骨, 舌根, 舌小帯, 舌神経, 舌苔

ぜつあつし 舌圧子 tongue depressor, tongue blade

ぜついんしんけい 舌咽神経 glossopharyngeal nerve ▶舌咽神経痛 glossopharyngeal neuralgia

ぜつえん 舌炎 glossitis

ぜっか 舌下（の）sublingual, hypoglos-

sal ▶舌下温 sublingual temperature 舌下錠 sublingual tablet 舌下腺 sublingual gland 舌下投与 sublingual administration ☞舌下神経, 舌下腺

せっかい 切開する make an incision, cut … open, lance （暖風-tomy) ◆膿を出すために切開する make an incision to release[drain] the pus ◆鼓膜を切開して中耳内の液を出す make an incision in the eardrum to drain fluid from the middle ear ◆おできを切開する open[cut open / lance] a boil ◆気管切開を行う perform a tracheotomy / open up the windpipe surgically ◆皮膚に小切開を加えて組織を採取する make a small incision in the skin and collect a tissue sample ◀会陰切開 episiotomy / perineotomy 横切開 transverse incision 鼓膜切開 myringotomy 正中切開 midline[median] incision 帝王切開 cesarean section[delivery]； CS / C-section 膿瘍切開 abscess incision 皮膚切開 skin incision ▶切開生検 incision[incisional] biopsy 切開排膿 incision and drainage

せっかいか 石灰化 calcification (瞬石灰化した calcified) ▶石灰化組織 calcified tissue

ぜっかしんけい 舌下神経 hypoglossal nerve

ぜっかせん 舌下腺 sublingual gland

ぜつがん 舌がん tongue cancer, cancer of the tongue, lingual cancer

せつがんえん 雪眼炎 snow ophthalmia

せつがんレンズ 接眼レンズ eye lens

せっきょくてき 積極的（な）（前向きの）positive （↔negative）（能動的な）active （↔passive）（意欲的な）aggressive, active （↔inactive）（自己主張する）assertive ◆積極的な態度をとる have a positive attitude / be positive ◆積極的な治療 aggressive[active / (疾病を治すための)curative] treatment ◆この治療はあなた自身がどれだけ積極的に病気と向きあうかが鍵になります Your own positive attitude toward the disease is the key to this treatment. / The key to this treatment's success is whether you can face your disease positively. ◆彼女のお年を考えると積極的には手術をお勧めしません Considering her age, *I'd rather not[I'm not willing to] recommend surgery.

セックス sex, sexual activity, sexual intercourse ☞性交, 性行為, 性生活 ▶セックスカウンセリング sex counseling

せっけっきゅう 赤血球 red blood cell ; RBC, erythrocyte, red corpuscle ◆赤血球数は正常範囲内です The number of the red blood cells is within normal range. ◆赤血球数を測定する measure[check] *a person's* red blood cell counts ▶遺伝性球状赤血球症 hereditary spherocytosis 鎌状赤血球症 sickle cell disease ; SCD 真性赤血球増加症 true erythrocytosis [polycythemia] 洗浄赤血球 washed red cell ; WRC 濃厚赤血球 concentrated [packed] red (blood) cell ; CRC 白血球除去赤血球 leukocyte-poor red cell ; LPRC ▶赤血球円柱 *red (blood) cell [erythrocytic] cast 赤血球凝集反応 hemagglutination[HA] reaction 赤血球凝集抑制試験 *hemagglutination inhibition / [HI] test 赤血球沈降速度[赤沈] erythrocyte[blood] sedimentation rate ; ESR 赤血球輸血 *red blood cell[erythrocyte] transfusion

せっけん 石鹸 soap ◆最近, お使いの石鹸や洗剤を変えましたか Have you recently changed the soaps or detergents that you use? ◆刺激の少ない〈低刺激性の〉石鹸を使って下さい Please use a mild 〈hypoirritant〉 soap. ◀逆性石鹸 invert [cationic] soap 洗顔石鹸 face[facial] soap 薬用石鹸 medicated[medicinal] soap

せっこう 石膏 plaster (ギプス)gypsum ▶石膏副木 plaster[gypsum] splint 石膏模型 plaster cast[model]

ぜっこう 絶好(の) (申し分のない)perfect (最も良い)the best ◆心身を休める絶好の機会と考えてみてはいかがですか How about thinking that this is *a perfect[the best] opportunity to get some rest mentally and physically?

せっこつ 接骨 ☞整骨
ぜっこつ 舌骨 lingual bone, hyoid bone
ぜっこん 舌根 root of the tongue ▶舌根沈下 airway obstruction by the tongue

せっし¹ 切歯 incisor, incisor tooth, incisive tooth (圏teeth)

せっし² 摂氏 Celsius /sélsiəs/, centigrade ; C ★華氏は Fahrenheit ; F. 摂氏の換算式は℃=(°F−32)×5/9. ◆熱は摂氏38度7分です Your temperature is thirty-eight point seven degrees Celsius. ▶摂氏温度計 Celsius thermometer

せっし³ 鑷子 thumb forceps
せっしゅ¹ 接種 ☞予防接種
せっしゅ² 摂取 (食べ物の)ingestion (薬物の)dose ◆砂糖の摂取を減らすようにして下さい Please try to reduce your sugar intake. ◆塩分の摂取は控えめにして下さい Please be moderate in your salt intake. ◆アルコールの大量摂取 heavy alcohol intake ◀栄養摂取 nutrient[nutritional] intake / nutrition 過剰摂取 excessive intake / (薬物の)overdose カルシウム摂取量 calcium intake カロリー摂取量 caloric[calorie] intake 酸素摂取量 oxygen intake 脂肪摂取量 fat intake 食事摂取量 dietary intake 水分摂取量 fluid[water] intake ▶摂取不足 deficient intake

せっしゅ³ 節酒する (適度に飲む)moderate *one's* drinking, drink in moderation (酒量を減らす)cut down on *one's* drinking ◆節酒の必要性についてはご理解されていますか Do you understand why you need to *cut down on[moderate] your drinking? ◆今日からでも節酒を始めて下さい Starting from today, try cutting down on your drinking. ◆節酒すれば必ず検査結果は良くなってきます Once you start cutting down on your drinking, your test results will definitely improve.

せつじょ 切除する (除去する)(surgically) remove, cut out[off] (臓器などの摘出する) excise (臓器などを一部摘出する)resect (圏 removal, surgical removal, excision,

せつじょ

resection 略尾-ectomy) ☞摘出 ◆胃のポリープを切除する remove a polyp from the stomach ◆腫瘍が拡がっているかをみるためリンパ節を切除する必要があります The lymph nodes need to be removed [excised] to see if the tumor has spread to them. ◆肝臓を部分的に切除する remove part of the liver ◆胃の3分の2を切除する remove two-thirds of the stomach ◆胃切除 gastrectomy　合併切除 combined resection　肝切除 hepatectomy　広範切除 wide resection　根治切除 radical excision[resection]　腫瘍切除 tumor excision[resection]　創縁切除 debridement　虫垂切除 appendectomy　内視鏡的切除 endoscopic resection　乳房切除 mastectomy　肺葉切除(pulmonary) lobectomy　部分切除 partial removal[resection] ▶切除断端 surgical margin / resection stump[margin]　切除標本 resected specimen

ぜつしょうたい　舌小帯　frenulum of the tongue, lingual frenulum ▶舌小帯切除術 frenotomy　舌小帯短縮症 ankyloglossia / tongue-tie

せっしょく¹　摂食　eating　(乳・食べ物をとること)feeding ▶摂食行動 eating[feeding] behavior　摂食障害 eating disorder　摂食中枢 the feeding center

せっしょく²　接触する　make contact (with)　(曝される)be exposed (to) ◆結核にかかっている人に接触したことがありますか Have you ever *come in contact[had contact] with anyone who had tuberculosis? / Have you ever been exposed to anyone with tuberculosis? ◆有害な物に接触してから発疹が出ましたか Did the rash come on after you were exposed to something harmful? ◆インフルエンザ患者との接触を避ける avoid contact with flu patients ▶接触によって感染する病気 a contagious disease ▶接触アレルギー contact allergy　接触感染 contact infection　接触皮膚炎 contact dermatitis

せっしょく³　節食する　(ダイエットする)go on a diet　(適度に食べる)eat in moderation

ぜったい²

(食べる量を減らす)cut down on *one's* food (intake)　☞節制 ◆節食を心がけて下さい You should *go on a diet[eat in moderation]. ◆節食の具体的な方法についてご一緒に考えてみましょう Let's work together and plan a specific way to cut down on your food (intake).

ぜっしょく　絶食　fasting, fast ★医療者への指示は NBM[nothing by mouth], NPO [nothing per os / non per os / nil per os] などを用いる. ◆今日から2日間の絶食となります Starting from today for two days, *you won't be able to eat any food[you'll have to go on a fast]. ▶絶食療法 fasting therapy

ぜつしんけい　舌神経　lingual nerve

せっせい¹　摂生する　(健康に注意する)be careful about *one's* health, take good care of *oneself* ◆療養中なので摂生に努めて下さい You're still under medical treatment, so *be careful about your health [take good care of yourself].

せっせい²　節制する　(食べる量を減らす)cut down on *one's* food (intake)　(適度にする)be moderate (in)　☞節食 ◆暴飲暴食は体によくありませんので節制して下さい Overeating and overdrinking aren't good for your health. Try to *cut down on[be moderate in] the amount you eat and drink.

せっそう　切創　incised wound

ぜったい¹　舌苔　fur on the tongue, coat on the tongue ◆舌苔が付着している The tongue is furred[furry / coated].

ぜったい²　絶対(の)　complete, absolute ◆1週間絶対安静が必要です You need to take[go on] complete bed rest for one week. ◆彼女は絶対安静です She is on complete bed rest. ◆絶対に禁煙して下さい You absolutely must stop smoking. / Be sure to quit smoking. ◆私たちが患者さんの個人情報を漏らすことは絶対にありません We never leak patients' personal information. ▶絶対安静 complete bed rest；CBR / absolute bed rest；ABR

せつだん 切断する **amputate** (図**amputation**), **cut** ◆足の指は壊死しているので切断せざるを得ません As gangrene has set in because of necrosis, we *have to[have no choice but to] amputate the toes. ◀外傷性切断 traumatic amputation 下肢切断 lower limb amputation 下腿切断 below-the-knee[BK] amputation 上腕切断 above-the-elbow[AE] amputation 大腿切断 above-the-knee[AK] amputation 指切断 digital amputation / (手の指) *finger amputation[amputation of the finger] / (足の指) *toe amputation[amputation of the toe] ▶切断端 amputation stump

せっち 設置する (装置・設備などを)**install**, **set up** (組織などを)**establish**, **organize** (備える)**provide** ◆監視装置を設置する install[set up] a monitoring device ◆医療安全推進委員会〈医療事故対策本部〉を設置しました We established[set up / organized] *a medical safety promotion committee〈headquarters to cope with medical accidents〉.

せっちゃく 接着 (粘着)**adhesion** (歯の接合)(dental) **bonding** ◆接着剤で傷口を閉じる close the wound with an adhesive ◆歯の接着 teeth[dental] bonding

せってい 設定 **setting** (動目標などを定める **set** 準備する・設置する **set up**) ◆空調の温度は25℃に設定されていますが、寝苦しければおっしゃって下さい The (temperature of the) air conditioner is set at[to] twenty-five degrees (Celsius). Let us know if you can't sleep well. ◆長期的な目標を設定する set a long-term goal[target] ◆医師との面談日を設定する set up an appointment *to see the doctor[to have an interview with the doctor] ◀目標設定 goal setting

セット **set** ◀輸液セット infusion set

せっとく 説得する (説得して仕向ける)**persuade** (図説得力のある **persuasive**, **convincing**), **talk into** (強く促す)**urge** (説得して断念させる)**talk out of** ◆手術を受けるよう患者を説得する persuade the patient

to have the surgery / talk the patient into having the surgery ◆禁煙するよう患者を説得する urge the patient to give up smoking / talk the patient out of smoking ◆説得力のある説明 a convincing[persuasive] explanation ◆説得力に欠ける証拠 unconvincing evidence

せっぱく 切迫(した) (緊急の)**urgent** (図**urge**, **urgency**) (危険が差し迫った)**threatened** (間近に迫った)**imminent**, **impending** ◆事態は切迫していて一刻の猶予も許されませんでした Matters were so urgent that there was no time *to lose[for delay]. ◀尿意切迫 urinary urgency / urge to urinate 切迫心筋梗塞 impending myocardial infarction 切迫性尿失禁 urge[urgency] incontinence 切迫早産 threatened premature delivery 切迫流産 threatened[imminent] abortion[miscarriage]

せつび 設備 (装置・機器など)**equipment** (建物など)**facilities** ★複数形で. ◀貯蔵設備 storage facilities

せっぺん 切片 (部分)**section** (薄切り)**slice** ◀凍結切片 frozen section

ぜつぼう 絶望する **despair** (of) (図**despair** 膨絶望して自暴自棄の **desperate**) (望みを失う)**lose hope** (望みを捨てる)**give up hope** (図**hopelessness** 膨**hopeless**) ◆ずっと絶望的な気持ちになっていますか Do you feel desperate[hopeless] most of the time? ◆彼女は治療に絶望しています She is in despair over the treatment. ◆何が起ころうとも決して絶望しないで下さい Whatever may happen, you should never *give up hope[despair]. ◆将来が絶望的だと感じることがありますか Do you ever feel hopeless about your future? ◆絶望の淵に落ちる fall into the depths of despair ▶絶望感 feeling of despair

せつめい 説明する **explain** (図**explanation**) (言葉で描写する)**describe** (図**description**) (話す)**tell** (示す)**show** (実例・図を示して説明する)**illustrate** 《基本的な表現》 ◆詳しく説明する explain in detail ◆繰り返し説明する explain repeatedly ◆十分に説明する(納得がいくように)explain satisfactorily ◆納得のいく説明 a satisfactory[convincing] explanation ◆曖昧な説明 an unclear[ambiguous] explanation ◆適切な〈不適切な〉説明 an adequate〈inadequate〉 explanation ◆説明のつかない体重減少 unexplained weight loss

《よく使う会話表現》 ◆この器具の使い方をご説明します Let me show you how to use this device[instrument]. ◆検査結果をご説明しましょう Let me explain[tell you] the test results. ◆病状についてこれまでどんな説明を受けましたか What have you been told about your condition so far? ◆手順について詳しい説明を受けましたか Did you get[receive] a detailed explanation about the procedure? / Did somebody describe the details of the procedure for you? ◆簡潔に説明するのは難しいので，図で骨折部位をご説明しましょう It's difficult (for me) to describe[explain] it briefly, so let me illustrate the fracture site. ◆麻酔については麻酔医が後で詳しく説明いたします Your anesthesiologist will explain the anesthesia to you in detail later. ◆今の説明でおわかりになりましたか Was my explanation clear? / Did I explain clearly? / Did you understand my explanation? ◆今の説明で納得していただけましたか Have I explained things well enough? / Are you satisfied with my explanation? ◆追加の説明が必要でしたらいつでもおっしゃって下さい Let me know if *there's anything else I should explain[you need any additional explanation]. ◆受傷された状況について説明していただけますか Could you describe[tell me] how the injury occurred? ◆そのことを他の言葉で説明して下さい Could you explain it in another way?

▶説明義務 (legal) obligation to explain 説明責任 accountability ☞説明書

せつめいしょ　説明書 （小冊子）**brochure** （取扱い手引書）**(instruction) manual[handbook]** （薬の）**medication leaflet** （添付文書）**drug package insert[insertion]** ◀入院説明書 (hospital) admissions brochure [booklet / leaflet] / brochure[booklet / leaflet] on admission

せつもう　雪盲 ☞雪眼炎

せなか　背中　back ☞背，背筋(せすじ)，背骨 ◆背中が痛む have (a) backache [back pain / pain in the back] ◆背中が丸い have a rounded upper back / be stoop-shouldered ◆背中に赤い発疹がある have a red rash on *one's* back ◆背中や膝に問題がありますか Do you have any back or knee problems? ◆背中に痛みはありますか Do you have (a) backache? ◆背中を押します Let me[I'm going to] press your back. ◆背中を叩きます Let me[I'm going to] tap your back. ◆背中を伸ばして下さい Straighten your back, please. ◆背中に手を回せますか Can you slide[stretch] your arms behind[around] your back? ◆背中をさすりましょうか Shall I rub[massage] your back? / Shall I give you a back rub[massage]?

せばまる　狭まる （狭くなる）**narrow** （限定する）**limit** ☞狭い ◆動脈の内腔がプラークで狭まって血流が悪くなっています The inner walls of your arteries have become narrow because of a buildup of plaque, so the blood does not flow smoothly. ◆彼は全身状態が不良なため治療の選択肢が狭められています Due to his poor general condition, the treatment options are limited.

ぜひ　是非 ◆今日からでも是非禁煙なさって下さい Be sure to[You must / I really want you to] quit smoking, starting today.

せぼね　背骨　spine /spáɪn/, **backbone** ☞背，背筋(せすじ)，背中 ◆背骨を叩きます Let me[I'm going to] tap your spine[(脊柱) spinal column]. ◆背骨を傷める injure *one's* spine

せまい　狭い （幅が狭い）**narrow** (↔wide, broad) （面積が小さい）**small** (↔large) （寸法が短い）**short** (↔long) ☞狭まる ◆視野が狭くなっているように感じますか Do you feel that your visual field *is narrow[has become narrow]? ◆軟骨がすり減って関節の間が狭くなり痛みが誘発されています The cartilage has become thinner, making the joint space narrow, and that's what's causing the pain. ◆骨盤が狭い have a small pelvis / one's pelvis is small ◆彼は歩く時歩幅が狭く足を引きずる When he walks, his steps are short and shuffling.

せめて
《少なくとも》at least ☞少なくとも ◆せめてあと 2 日は自宅で安静にしていて下さい Stay home in bed for at least two more days.
《せめても》 ◆入院中，見舞客とのおしゃべりが彼女にとってせめてもの慰めになっています（唯一の楽しみ）Having a chat with visitors is the only pleasure she can find in the hospital.

セメント cement ▶セメント固定 cement fixation

せもたれ 背もたれ backrest, support for the back

セラチア serratia （学名）*Serratia* ▶セラチア感染症 serratia infection

ゼラチン gelatin

セラピー therapy ☞治療，療法

セラピスト therapist ☞療法士

セラミックス ceramics ★通例複数形で.

ゼリー （商標名）Jell-O，《英》jelly ★米での jelly はジャムをさす. （ゲル・ゼリー状態）gel /dʒél/ ★超音波検査などで使用するゼリーは，英語では gel という. ◆お腹にゼリーを塗ります I'm going to[Let me] *spread gel on[apply gel to] your abdomen. ◆ゼリーを拭きとりましょう Let's wipe off the gel. ◆いちごゼリー状の便 strawberry jelly-like stool ▶膣用ゼリー vaginal gel ▶ゼリー状物質 jelly-like substance[matter]

セルフケア self-care

セルフコントロール self-control

セルフヘルプグループ self-help group

セルフモニタリング self-monitoring

セルロース cellulose

セレウスきん ―菌 *Bacillus cereus* ▶セレウス菌食中毒 *Bacillus cereus* food poisoning

ゼロ zero /zíːrou/ ◆明日 357-5004 番にお電話を下さい Please call[ring] me tomorrow at three-five-seven, five-zero-zero-four[five-oh-oh-four]. ◆糖類ゼロの甘味料〈飲み物〉sugar-free sweetener〈drinks〉 ◆完治の可能性はゼロではありませんから希望を持ちましょう It's not that you have a zero chance of making a full recovery[It's still medically possible for you to make a full recovery], so you must *keep up hope[not give up hope]. ▶ゼロ歳児 baby aged less than *one year [twelve months]

ゼロコンバージョン seroconversion

セロトニン serotonin ◀選択的セロトニン再取込み阻害薬 selective serotonin reuptake inhibitor；SSRI ▶セロトニン(受容体)拮抗薬 serotonin (receptor) antagonist セロトニン・ノルアドレナリン再取り込み阻害薬 serotonin-norepinephrine reuptake inhibitor；SNRI

せわ 世話 care （㊂take care of, look after） 援助 help （㊂help） ▶介護, ケア ◆自宅で世話をしてくれる人がいますか Do you have anyone who can *look after [take care of] you at home? ◆何かお世話できることがあればおっしゃって下さい Please let me know if you need any help. ◆患者の排泄の世話をする help the patient use the toilet[(ベッド上便器) bed-pan] ◆患者の入浴の世話をする help the patient *take a bath[bathe]

せん¹ 栓 （穴の詰め物）plug （瓶のふた）cap, stopper （コルク栓）cork ◀粘液栓 mucous plug 膿栓 pus plug 耳栓 ear-plug(s)

せん² 腺 gland ◀外分泌〈内分泌〉腺 exocrine〈endocrine〉gland 汗腺 sweat gland 消化腺 digestive gland 生殖腺 reproductive[sex] gland 粘液腺 mucous gland 皮脂腺 sebaceous gland

せん³ 線 line （流れ）stream ◆真っ直ぐな線を引いて下さい Please draw a straight line. ◆この真っ直ぐな線の上を歩く walk along[on] this straight line

◆尿線 a urinary stream　☞曲線，線状

ぜん — 前 — former （接頭ex-, pre-↔post-）☞前（まえ）

せんい[1] 船医　ship's doctor

せんい[2] 線維・繊維　fiber /fáɪbə/ （形fibrous）◆食事で繊維を十分摂っていますか Are you getting enough fiber in your diet?　◆繊維の多い食べ物 food high [rich] in fiber / a high-fiber diet　◀筋線維 muscle fiber　膠原線維 collagenous fiber　合成繊維 synthetic fiber　植物繊維 vegetable fiber　食物繊維 dietary fiber　神経線維 nerve fiber　弾性線維 elastic fiber　▶線維芽細胞 fibroblast　線維筋痛症 fibromyalgia　線維細胞 fibrocyte　線維腫 fibroma　線維性骨異形成症 fibrous (bone) dysplasia　線維性収縮 fibrillation　線維性癒着 fibrous adhesion　線維腺腫 fibroadenoma；FA　線維束性収縮 fasciculation　線維組織 fibrous tissue　線維肉腫 fibrosarcoma　☞線維症，線維素

せんいしょう 線維症　fibrosis　◀骨髄線維症 myelofibrosis　囊胞性線維症 cystic fibrosis　肺線維症 pulmonary[lung] fibrosis

せんいそ 線維素　fibrin　▶線維素原 fibrinogen　線維素沈着 fibrin deposit　線維素溶解現象 fibrinolysis　線維素溶解薬 fibrinolytic medication[drug / agent]

ぜんいん 全員　◆スタッフ全員 the entire staff / all staff members / all the members of the staff

せんえん 遷延性（の）（長期に及ぶ）prolonged（持続性の）persistent　◀分娩遷延 prolonged labor[delivery]　▶遷延性昏睡 prolonged coma　遷延性植物状態 persistent vegetative state；PVS　遷延性咳 persistent cough

ぜんかい[1] 全快　complete recovery　☞全治，治る　◆2，3か月もすれば全快するでしょう You'll make a complete recovery [You'll be completely well again] in a few months.　◆この病気が全快するにはもう少し時間がかかるでしょう It will take a little more time to recover completely from this disease.

ぜんかい[2] 前回　(the) last time　◆前回の検診はいつでしたか When was your last checkup?

ぜんかい[3] 全開する（子宮口・血管などが完全に拡がる）dilate ... fully（大きく開く）open wide　◆子宮口は全開しています The cervix is fully dilated.　◆傷口は全開しています The wound is wide open.

ぜんかいじょ 全介助　full assistance

ぜんがく[1] 全額　all one's expenses, the total cost of one's expenses　◆医療費を全額支払う pay all one's medical expenses / pay one's medical expenses in full

ぜんがく[2] 前額　forehead （形frontal）▶前額断 frontal section

せんがん[1] 洗眼　eye irrigation, eye-bathing　▶洗眼薬 eyewash / collyrium

せんがん[2] 洗顔　face[facial] washing, face[facial] cleansing　▶洗顔クリーム facial cleansing cream　洗顔石鹼 face [facial] soap

せんがん[3] 腺癌　adenocarcinoma　◀管状腺癌 tubular adenocarcinoma　高分化型〈低分化型〉腺癌 well-differentiated〈poorly differentiated〉adenocarcinoma　漿液性腺癌 serous adenocarcinoma　囊胞腺癌 cystadenocarcinoma

ぜんがん 前がん（性の）　precancerous　▶前がん期 precancerous stage　前がん状態 precancerous condition　前がん病変 precancerous lesion

せんかんびょう 潜函病　☞潜水病

ぜんき 前期　the early stage[period]（1年の前半）the first half, the earlier half　▶前期高齢者 (65～74 歳) (elderly) person aged 65[sixty-five] to 74[seventy-four] years, junior senior /（総称的に）young-old　前期破水 premature rupture of membranes；PROM

せんきあんてん 閃輝暗点　scintillating scotoma；a blind spot in the visual field containing flashing lights

せんきょせいびょうへん 占拠性病変　space-occupying lesion；SOL　◀頭蓋内占拠性病変 intracranial space-occupying lesion

せんきんしゅしょう 腺筋腫症 adeno-myomatosis

せんきんしょう 腺筋症 adenomyosis ◀子宮腺筋症 uterine adenomyosis

ぜんくしょうじょう 前駆症状 （予兆の）premonitory symptom （事前の）advance symptom ☞先行，前兆

ぜんくじんつう 前駆陣痛 premonitory pain

ぜんくたい 前駆体 （前駆物質）precursor ◀ドパミン前駆体 dopamine precursor

ぜんくつ 前屈する bend forward ◀子宮前屈 anteflexion of the uterus ▶前屈姿勢 stooped[forward-bent] posture

せんけいコンジローマ 尖圭コンジローマ condyloma acuminatum, genital[venereal] wart

ぜんけいしせい 前傾姿勢 stooped posture, forward-bent posture

ぜんけいぶ 前頸部 the front of the neck ◀前頸部のこのしこりは悪性のものではありません This lump on the front of your neck is not malignant. ◆前頸部が痛みますか Do you have any pain in the front of your neck?

ぜんけいほこう 前傾歩行 frontal gait

せんけつ¹ 先決 the first thing to do （圏first） ◆原因を突き止めることが先決です The first thing we need to do is find out what is causing the problem. / First, we have to try to find the cause of the problem.

せんけつ² 潜血 occult blood, occult bleeding ◆便〈尿〉に潜血反応が出ています Blood was detected in your stool 〈urine〉. / We've detected what's known as occult blood in your stool〈urine〉. ◀尿潜血 occult blood in urine / occult hematuria　便潜血 occult blood in stool / fecal occult blood；FOB ▶潜血検査 occult blood test　潜血反応 occult blood reaction

せんけつ³ 鮮血 （bright red）blood ◆トイレットペーパーに鮮血が付いている

There is bright red blood on the toilet paper. ◆鮮血便に気づく notice bright red blood in *one's* stool

せんげつ 先月 last month

ぜんけつ 全血 whole blood ▶全血輸血 whole blood transfusion

ぜんげん 漸減 waning （↔waxing） ▶漸減現象 waning phenomenon

ぜんけんぼう 全健忘 total *memory loss [amnesia]

せんこう¹ 穿孔 perforation （圏穿孔性の perforative, perforating　穿孔した perforated） （能動的に穴を開けること）piercing ◆穿孔した虫垂 a perforated appendix ◀鼓膜穿孔 perforation of the eardrum / tympanic membrane perforation　消化管穿孔 perforation of the digestive tract　腸〈胃〉穿孔 intestinal〈stomach / gastric〉perforation ▶穿孔性潰瘍 perforated [perforating] ulcer　穿孔性腹膜炎 perforative peritonitis

せんこう² 閃光 flashing light, flash of light ◆脳波検査の途中，閃光で脳に刺激を与えます．目を閉じてリラックスしていて下さい During the EEG[electroencephalography] we're going to use flashing lights to stimulate the activity in your brain, so please relax and keep your eyes closed. ◆頭痛がする前に視野に閃光が見えることがありますか Just before your headache starts, do you ever see flashing lights in your field of vision?

せんこう³ 先行する precede （圏preceding, previous） ◆発疹に先行して風邪症状はありましたか（発疹が出る前に）Did you have any cold symptoms before the rash developed? ◆先行する感染 a preceding infection

ぜんこうけんぼう 前向健忘 anterograde amnesia

せんこうしょく 鮮紅色（の） scarlet, bright red

せんこきゅう 浅呼吸 shallow breathing [respiration] ◆患者は浅呼吸になっています The patient is breathing shallowly. / The patient's breathing is shallow.

ぜんごけい 前後径 anteroposterior diameter, AP diameter

せんこく 宣告 (話す)tell (通知する)inform (宣言する)pronounce ☞告知 ◆がんを宣告する tell[inform] *the patient that he*⟨she⟩ *has cancer* ◆(医師が)死亡を宣告する pronounce *the patient dead*

せんこつ 仙骨 sacral bone, sacrum ▶仙骨(硬膜外)麻酔 sacral[caudal](epidural) anesthesia

せんこつしんけい 仙骨神経 sacral nerve ◆仙骨神経叢 sacral plexus

センサー sensor ◆バイオセンサー biosensor

せんざい¹ 洗剤 detergent ☞石鹸

せんざい² 潜在(的な) (可能性のある)potential (意識下の)subconscious (潜伏している)latent, occult (無症状の)silent, asymptomatic, subclinical ☞潜伏 ◆それぞれの治療の潜在的なリスクと利点について話し合いましょう Let's discuss the potential risks and benefits of each treatment. ◆誰しも長生きしたいという潜在的な欲望を持っています Everybody has a subconscious[隠れた)hidden] desire to live long. ▶潜在意識 the subconscious (mind / awareness) 潜在出血 occult bleeding 潜在性結核感染症 latent tuberculosis infection 潜在性甲状腺機能低下症 subclinical hypothyroidism 潜在性胆石 silent[asymptomatic] gallstone(s) 潜在能力 potential (capacity)

せんざいせいしんきんしょう 浅在性真菌症 superficial mycosis

せんし 穿刺 (穴開け)puncture (体液の吸い取り)paracentesis ◀関節穿刺 arthrocentesis 胸腔穿刺 thoracentesis / thoracic paracentesis 経皮的穿刺 percutaneous puncture 骨髄穿刺 bone marrow puncture 試験穿刺 exploratory puncture 超音波ガイド下穿刺術 ultrasonically guided puncture 動脈穿刺 arterial puncture 腹腔穿刺 abdominocentesis / abdominal paracentesis[puncture] 羊水穿刺 amniocentesis 腰椎穿刺 lumbar puncture ▶穿刺液 puncture fluid 穿刺

吸引組織診 fine needle aspiration biopsy；FNAB

せんじ 潜時 latency

ぜんしきもう 全色盲 (1色覚)achromatopsia, total color blindness

せんじぐすり 煎じ薬 (生薬を煮出した薬液)decoction (熱湯に浸した薬液)infusion

せんじつ 先日 the other day (2, 3日前) a few days ago (少し前) some days ago, some time ago ◆先日お願いした書類はお持ちいただいていますか Did you bring the forms[documents] I requested the other day? ◆先日も申し上げましたように As I said *the other day[a few days ago / some days ago]*, …

ぜんじつ 前日 the day before, the previous day ◆手術の前日に入院して下さい I'd like you to be admitted to the hospital the day before the surgery.

ぜんしつご 全失語(症) total aphasia, global aphasia

ぜんしゃかくきん 前斜角筋 anterior scalene muscle

せんしゅ 腺腫 adenoma (形adenomatous) ◆生検の結果，胃のポリープは腺腫でした The biopsy results show that the polyp in your stomach was an adenoma. ◀アルドステロン産生腺腫 aldosteronoma / aldosterone-producing⟨-secreting⟩ adenoma 胃腺腫 gastric adenoma 下垂体腺腫 pituitary adenoma 成長ホルモン産生腺腫 growth hormone-producing adenoma 線維腺腫 fibroadenoma；FA 大腸腺腫症 adenomatosis polyposis 微小腺腫 microadenoma 副腎腺腫 adrenal adenoma プロラクチン産生腺腫 prolactin-producing adenoma / prolactinoma ▶腺腫症 adenomatosis 腺腫内癌 carcinoma in adenoma 腺腫様過形成 adenomatous hyperplasia；AH 腺腫様甲状腺腫 adenomatous goiter

せんしゅう 先週 last week ◆事故は先週の木曜日のことでしたね The accident happened last Thursday, didn't it?

ぜんじゅうじじんたい 前十字靱帯 anterior cruciate ligament；ACL ▶前十字

靭帯断裂 rupture of the anterior cruciate ligament

せんじょう¹　洗浄する　(洗う)**wash (out)** (きれいにする)**clean**　(傷口などを洗浄する) **cleanse, irrigate**　(汲み出して洗う)**pump** (すすぎ洗いをする)**rinse**　(腟などを洗浄する) **douche**　(器官やある部位を洗浄する)**lavage** (図**cleansing, irrigation, douche, lavage**) ◆傷を洗浄する *wash out[clean / cleanse] the wound　◆胃を洗浄する pump the stomach　◆腸を洗浄する cleanse[irrigate] the bowels　◀胃洗浄 gastric lavage[irrigation] / stomach pumping　口内洗浄剤 mouthwash　創傷 洗浄 wound cleansing　超音波洗浄 ultrasonic cleaning　腸洗浄 bowel irrigation / intestinal lavage　鼻洗浄 nasal douche [irrigation]　▶洗浄液 liquid cleaner / cleaning solution /（レンズの）lens cleaner [cleaning solution]　洗浄赤血球 washed red cell；WRC

せんじょう²　線状・線条(の)　(すじ・溝状 の)**streaky, striated, striate**　(直線状の)**linear**　(皮膚などが伸長した)**stretch**　◆線状 の血液が痰に混じっている Streaky blood is mixed in with the phlegm.　◀皮膚線条 stretch mark　▶線状骨折 linear fracture 線条体 striatum / striate body　線状瘢痕 linear scar　線状萎縮症 linear atrophy

せんしょく　染色　**staining**　(圖**stain**) (布・髪の毛などの染色)**dyeing**　(圖**dye**)　(染 料・着色剤)**stain, dye**　◆組織標本を染色す る stain tissue samples　◀グラム染色 Gram stain　チール・ニールセン染色 Ziehl–Neelsen stain　パス染色 *periodic acid–Schiff[PAS] stain　パパニコロー染 色 Papanicolaou[Pap] stain　ヘマトキシ リンエオジン染色 hematoxylin–eosin [HE] stain　ペルオキシダーゼ染色 peroxidase stain　ルゴール染色 Lugol iodine staining

せんしょくたい　染色体　**chromosome** /króuməsòum/　◀X染色体 X chromosome　常染色体 autosome　常染色体優 性〈劣性〉遺伝 autosomal dominant〈recessive〉inheritance　脆弱X染色体 fragile X

chromosome　性染色体 sex chromosome　フィラデルフィア染色体 Philadelphia chromosome　Y染色体 Y chromosome　▶染色体異常 chromosome abnormality[aberration]　染色体検査 chromosome test[testing]　染色体疾患 chromosome disorder　染色体分析 chromosome analysis

せんしん　専心する　☞専念

ぜんしん　全身(の)　(体中の)**overall**　(圖圖 **all over**)　(総合的な)**general**　(全身性の) **systemic**　(広範囲にわたる)**widespread** (症状などが全身にわたる)**generalized**　(圖**the whole body, the entire body, every part of the body**)　☞全体　◆だるいのは全身です か、体の一部ですか Do you feel tired all over or in just one part of your body? ◆彼女の全身状態は安定しています Her overall[general] condition is stable. ◆患者は全身の痛みを訴えています The patient is complaining of（widespread） pains.　◆全身を冒す病気 a disease affecting the whole[entire] body　◆全身 に拡がる spread all over the body　◆全身 運動 whole body exercise　全身管理 general care　全身倦怠感 general malaise 全身衰弱 general weakness[debility]　全 身性アミロイドーシス systemic amyloidosis　全身性エリテマトーデス systemic lupus erythematosus；SLE　全身性炎症反 応症候群 systemic inflammatory response syndrome；SIRS　全身性強皮症 systemic sclerosis；SSc　全身性疾患 systemic disease　全身麻酔 general anesthesia　☞全身不随

せんしんいりょう　先進医療　**advanced medicine**　(先端技術を駆使した)**high–tech medicine**　◆(高度)先進医療技術（highly） advanced medical technology　◆先進医 療技術を駆使して治療を行う make full use of advanced medical technology to treat patients　◆この治療法は先進医療に指定 されていますので医療費が全額個人負担と なります This type of treatment is designated（by the government）as advanced medicine, so you have to pay all of the medical expenses yourself.

ぜんじんてきいりょう 全人的医療 holistic medicine[medical care]

ぜんしんふずい 全身不随 full body paralysis, paralysis of the whole body ◆全身不随になる the whole body is paralyzed / be paralyzed from the neck down

せんずい 仙髄 sacral cord

せんすいびょう 潜水病 divers' disease, caisson disease （減圧症）decompression sickness；DCS

ぜんせいぞんきかん 全生存期間 overall survival period

ぜんせきずいどうみゃくしょうこうぐん 前脊髄動脈症候群 anterior spinal artery syndrome

ぜんぜん 全然 （まったく…ない）not[no] … at all （本当に）really ◆食欲が全然ないのですか Do you have no appetite at all? ◆彼女はその言葉の意味が全然わかっていないようです She doesn't seem to understand the meaning of the word at all. / It seems she doesn't really understand the meaning of the word.

ぜんぞう 漸増（の） （徐々に増大する）waxing （↔waning） （段階的に進む）progressive ▶漸増現象 waxing phenomenon 漸増抵抗運動 progressive resistance exercise；PRE

せんそく 尖足 equinus foot ▶尖足歩行 equinus gait

ぜんそく 喘息 asthma /ǽzmə/ （形asthmátic） ◆喘息患者 a patient with asthma / an asthma patient ◆アレルギーによる喘息 asthma brought on by allergy / allergic asthma ◆喘息様の咳 an asthmatic cough ◆喘息にかかったことがありますか Have you ever had asthma? ◆小児喘息がぶり返したようですね I'm afraid your childhood asthma has returned. ◆喘息発作を起こす have *an asthma attack[asthma attacks] / （発作を引き起こす）trigger asthma attacks ◆喘息発作はどのくらいの頻度で起こりますか．毎日ですか How often do you have (the) asthma attacks? Every day? ◆喘息は，発作を抑

える薬と気道の炎症を軽減するステロイド薬との組み合わせで対処していきます I'm going to give you a combination of medications: a medication to get the attack under control and a steroid to reduce the inflammation in the airway.

◀アスピリン喘息 aspirin asthma / aspirin-induced asthma；AIA / aspirin-sensitive asthma アトピー〈非アトピー性〉性喘息 atopic〈nonatopic〉 asthma 運動誘発喘息 exercise-induced asthma；EIA 抗喘息薬 antiasthmatic （medication / drug / agent） 小児喘息 childhood asthma 職業性喘息 occupational asthma ステロイド依存性喘息 steroid-dependent asthma 成人発症喘息 adult-onset asthma 咳喘息 cough variant asthma；CVA 通年性喘息 perennial asthma 難治性喘息 intractable asthma ▶喘息死 asthma[asthma-related] death 喘息発作重積状態 status asthmaticus 喘息発作薬 medication for asthma attacks

センター center ◀医療センター medical[health] center がんセンター cancer center 健診センター health screening center / comprehensive physical examination center デイケアセンター day care center リハビリテーションセンター rehabilitation center

ぜんたい 全体（の） whole, entire （すべての）all （圏all over, throughout） ☞全身，全般 ◆病気は体全体に拡がっています The disease has spread throughout the body. ◆お腹全体が痛む have (a) pain all over *one's* abdomen ◆体全体がかゆい feel itchy all over *one's* body ◆胃全体を切除する必要があります The entire [whole] stomach needs to be removed. ◆検査成績は全体的に良好ですが，いくつか気になる数値が見られます（概して）On the whole[Generally], your test results are good[favorable], but there are a few counts I'm concerned about. ◆全体的に見るとこの治療がベストだと思います All things considered, I think this treatment is best for you.

ぜんだいのうどうみゃく　前大脳動脈
anterior cerebral artery；ACA

せんたく¹　選択　choice（圏choose）（より慎重な選択）**selection**（圏select **selective**）（自由裁量の選択）**option**（圏opt 圏**elective**）☞選ぶ　◆治療の選択はよくお考え下さい Please think carefully before you choose which treatment to take. ◆重大な選択ですので迷うのは当然です This is going to be a very important choice for you, so it's natural that you can't make up your mind. ◆選択はあなたにお任せします The choice is yours. / I'm leaving the choice up to you. ◆どちらを選択しますか Which have you decided on? / What's your choice? / Which option will you take? ◆帝王切開を選択するなら直ちに手術日の予定を入れる必要があります If you opt to have a cesarean section, we'll need to schedule the date for the surgery right away. ◆負の選択 a negative selection ▶選択基準 selection criteria　選択性緘黙 selective[elective] mutism　選択的[待機的]手術 elective surgery　選択的セロトニン再取込み阻害薬 selective serotonin reuptake inhibitor；SSRI ☞選択肢

せんたく²　洗濯する　do the laundry, do the washing, do the wash　◆入院中の洗濯はコインランドリーをご利用になれます If you have washing to do during your hospital stay[If you need to do any laundry while you're in the hospital], you can use the (hospital) Laundromat[coin-operated laundry]. ◆コイン式洗濯機と乾燥機は地下にあります Coin-operated *washing machines[washers] and dryers are located in the basement. ◆有料の洗濯サービスがあります Laundry services are available at an additional charge. ◆何か洗濯物はありますか Do you have any laundry[washing]? ◆花粉の量が多い日は洗濯物を室外に干さないようにして下さい Don't hang washing outside to dry on days of high pollen counts.

せんたくし　選択肢　choice（自由裁量の）

option（代案の）**alternative**　◆この病気には治療の選択肢が３つあります You have [There are] three treatment choices[options] for this illness. ◆手術ではなく放射線治療も選択肢の１つです Radiation treatment is one of the alternatives to surgery. ◆最善の選択肢 the best option

ぜんだまコレステロール　善玉コレステロール　good cholesterol, *high-density lipoprotein[HDL] cholesterol

せんたん　先端（先の部分）**tip**（端の部分）**end**（尖った部分）**point**　◆点眼容器の先端が目の表面に触れるのを避ける avoid touching the surface of the eye with the tip of the eyedropper ▶先端恐怖 aichmophobia　先端巨大症 acromegaly

せんたんいりょう　先端医療 ☞先進医療

ぜんち　全治する　heal completely, recover completely (from) ☞全快, 治る　◆傷は全治２週間です Your injury will take two weeks to heal completely. / You will completely recover from the injury in two weeks. ◆全治３か月の怪我 an injury requiring three months *to heal completely [for complete recovery]

ぜんちたいばん　前置胎盤　placenta previa

センチネルリンパせつ　―節　sentinel lymph node

センチメートル　centimeter /séntəmíːtə/；cm ☞巻末付録：単位の換算

せんちゃくじゅん　先着順　◆先着順にお名前をお呼びします Patients will be called [seen] in order of arrival. / Patients will be called[seen] on a first-come, first-served basis. / We'll call your name in order of arrival.

せんちゅう　線虫　nematode ▶線虫感染症 nematode infection

ぜんちゅう　蠕虫（一般的に）**worm**（寄生虫）**helminth**（圏**helminthic**）▶蠕虫症 helminthiasis / helminthic infection

せんちょう　洗腸　intestinal lavage, colonic irrigation

ぜんちょう　前兆（警告徴候）**warning sign**（前駆症状）**premonitory symptom, aura**

◆心臓発作の前兆 warning signs of a heart attack　◆片頭痛の前兆 early〈warning〉signs of migraine　◆前兆のある〈ない〉片頭痛 migraine with〈without〉aura　◆頭痛が起こる前に何か前兆を感じましたか Did you have[feel] any warning signs before the headache began?　▶前兆感覚 warning sensation

せんちょうかんせつ　仙腸関節　sacroiliac joint

せんつい　仙椎　sacral vertebra

せんつう¹　疝痛　colic, colicky pain　◀胃疝痛 gastric colic／colic in the stomach　胆石疝痛 biliary[gallstone] colic　腸疝痛 intestinal colic　尿管疝痛 ureteral colic　反復性疝痛 recurrent colic　▶疝痛性腹痛 colicky abdominal pain

せんつう²　穿通(性の)　penetrating　▶穿通性潰瘍 penetrating ulcer　穿通性損傷 penetrating injury　穿通創 penetrating wound

ぜんてい　前庭　(耳の)vestibule (形vestibular)　▶鼻前庭 nasal vestibule　▶前庭炎 vestibulitis　前庭機能 vestibular function　前庭神経炎 vestibular neuritis[neuronitis]　前庭性めまい vestibular vertigo

ぜんてき　全摘(術)　total removal[excision, extraction], complete removal[excision, extraction]　(接尾-ectomy)　☞切除, 摘出　▶胃全摘術 total gastrectomy　結腸全摘術 total colectomy

せんてんせい　先天性(の)　congenital　(性質などが生まれながらに備わっている, 先天的な)natural, innate　◆心臓に先天性の障害がある have a congenital heart problem [disorder]　◆先天性の心臓疾患 congenital heart disease　▶先天性異常 congenital abnormality　先天性奇形 congenital anomaly　先天性筋ジストロフィー congenital muscular dystrophy；CMD　先天性股関節脱臼 congenital dislocation of the hip joint；CDH　先天性風疹症候群 congenital rubella syndrome；CRS

ぜんとう　前頭(部)　forehead, frontal region　▶前頭骨 frontal bone　前頭前野 prefrontal area　前頭洞 frontal sinus　前頭洞炎 frontal sinusitis　前頭面 frontal plane　前頭連合野 frontal association area　☞前頭葉

ぜんどう　蠕動(運動)　peristaltic movement, peristalsis　◆腸の蠕動運動が亢進しているようです It seems your peristaltic movements have increased[become too fast].／It seems that food is moving through your digestive tract too fast.　▶蠕動亢進 hyperperistalsis　蠕動低下 hypoperistalsis

せんとうじゅつ　穿頭術　burr hole opening, trepanation, trepanning

ぜんとうやく　前投薬　premedication

ぜんとうよう　前頭葉　frontal lobe　▶前頭葉症候群 frontal lobe syndrome

ぜんにゅう　全乳　whole milk

せんねん　専念する　concentrate　◆しばらくリハビリに専念して下さい I'd like you to concentrate on your rehabilitation for a while.

ぜんのう　全納する　pay in full　◆お支払いは全納でお願いします You are requested to pay in full.

せんぱつ　洗髪する　wash one's hair, shampoo one's hair　◆今日洗髪をして差し上げましょうか Shall I wash[shampoo] your hair?

ぜんぱん　全般(の)　(すべての)all　(全体の)whole, overall, general　(症状などが全身にわたる)generalized　☞全体　◆全般的にご主人の状態は上向いています All in all [All things considered／On the whole], your husband's condition is *getting better[improving].　◆入院全般に関してご質問がありますか Do you have any questions about your admission in general?　▶全般性不安障害 generalized anxiety disorder；GAD　全般てんかん generalized epilepsy　全般発作 generalized seizure

ぜんぶ¹　全部(の)　(すべての)all　(1つ1つの)every　(全体の)whole, entire, overall　(完全な)complete　(十分な)full　☞すべて　◆服は全部脱いで下さい Please take all your clothes off.／Please remove all your clothes. ◆腫瘍は全部きれいに取り除きました The entire tumor was removed. / The tumor was completely removed. ◆思っていることを全部お話し下さい Please tell me everything that's going through your mind. ◆医療費は全部で 20,000 円になります Your medical charges will be twenty thousand yen *in all[altogether]. ◆それで全部ですか Is that all?

ぜんぶ² 前部 the front (↔the back) (㊎anterior (↔posterior))

ぜんふか 前負荷 preload ◆前負荷を減少させる decrease the preload

せんぷく 潜伏(している) (隠れている)latent /léitənt/, occult (㊎incubation) ☞潜在 ◆潜伏性の病気 a latent disease ◆この病気の潜伏期は通常 2, 3 週間です The incubation[latent] period for this disease is usually two to three weeks. ▶潜伏感染 latent infection 潜伏時間 latent time

ぜんぼうぐうかく 前房隅角 anterior chamber angle

ぜんぽうじょうきたい 全胞状奇胎 complete hydatidiform[hydatid] mole

ぜんめい 喘鳴 wheeze ☞ゼイゼイ

せんめん 洗面 washing one's face (and hands) ▶洗面器 washbowl / washbasin 洗面道具 toiletries

せんめんじょ 洗面所 ☞トイレ

ぜんめんてき 全面的(な) (完全な)complete, entire (全体の)overall, whole (十分な)full ◆治療計画の全面的な見直しが必要です The treatment plan needs to be reviewed[reexamined] completely[entirely]. ◆この問題はまだ全面的には解決していません We still haven't entirely solved this problem. / We haven't worked out the overall solution to this problem. ◆彼女は脳の機能が全面的に停止して脳死状態にあります Her brain has completely stopped functioning, so she's now brain-dead. ◆全面的なご協力をお願いいたします We ask for your full cooperation.

せんもう¹ 線毛 cilia (㊎cilium) ★通例,

複数形で. (㊎ciliary, ciliated) ▶線毛運動 ciliary movement 線毛運動障害 ciliary motility disorder 線毛細胞 ciliated cell 線毛不動症候群 immotile cilia syndrome

せんもう² 譫妄 delirium /dəlíriəm/ (㊎delirious) ☞意識混濁 ◆ご主人はせん妄に陥っていますので, ベッドからの転倒を予防するために拘束具を使ってもよろしいでしょうか Your husband is delirious, so is it all right if we use a physical restraint to prevent him from falling out of bed? ◀術後せん妄 postoperative delirium 夜間せん妄 nocturnal[night] delirium

ぜんもう 全盲 total blindness ◆全盲である be totally blind

せんもん¹ 泉門 fontanelle ◆泉門はたいてい 2 歳くらいまでに閉じます The fontanelle usually closes about two years after birth.

せんもん² 専門 specialty (㊎specialize ㊎special, specialized 専門職の professional) ▶専門分野 specialty / specialized field ◆私は腎臓の病気が専門です I specialize in kidney diseases. / Kidney disease is my specialty. ◆この病気は私の専門外なので, 専門医をご紹介しましょう This disease is *not my field[(範囲外)outside my field / (よく知らない領域)an area I don't know much about]. Let me refer you to a specialist. ◆当院はがん治療を専門としている病院です This hospital specializes in the treatment of cancer. / This is a cancer hospital. ◆なるべく専門用語を使わないようにしますが, もし分かりにくければおっしゃって下さい I try not to use technical words[terms] if I can help it, but let me know *when it is hard to understand. ◆高度に専門化した分野 a highly specialized field ◀医療専門職 the medical professions 介護支援専門員 care manager ▶専門外来 special outpatient clinic 専門学校 vocational school[college] 専門看護師 certified nurse specialist：CNS 専門職協働医療チーム interprofessional health care team ☞専門医

せんもんい 専門医 **specialist** ◆心臓〈肺〉の専門医をご紹介します I'm going to *refer you[give you a referral] to a heart 〈lung〉 specialist for consultation. ◆専門医の診察を受けたことがありますか Have you ever been examined by a specialist? ◆専門医の意見を聞いてみましょう Let's hear what the specialists have to say. / Let's get some professional advice from the specialists. ◆このしこりが気になりますので, 専門医に診てもらう必要があります I'm concerned about this lump, and I think you need to have it seen by a specialist. ◆言語療法の専門医にかかる see a specialist in speech therapy

---

専門医

専門医は, 通常[専門＋-ist / -an]あるいは[専門＋specialist / surgeon]で表す. ☞診療(囲み：診療部門)

■内科系
●内科医 internist ●小児科医 pediatrician ●呼吸器科医 pulmonologist / lung specialist ●循環器科医 cardiologist / heart specialist ●消化器科医 gastroenterologist ●腎臓内科医 nephrologist / kidney specialist ●内分泌科医 endocrinologist ●リウマチ科専門医 rheumatologist ●神経科医 neurologist ●血液内科医 hematologist ●アレルギー専門医 allergist ●睡眠科専門医 sleep (disorders) specialist ●感染症専門医 infectious disease specialist ●感染症対策専門医 infection control doctor ●緩和ケア専門医 palliative medicine specialist ●老年病専門医 geriatrician

■外科系
●外科医 surgeon ●一般外科医 general surgeon ●小児外科医 pediatric surgeon ●心臓血管外科医 cardiovascular surgeon ●胸部外科医 thoracic surgeon ●乳腺外科医 breast surgeon ●形成外科医 plastic surgeon ●脳神経外科医 neurosurgeon ●泌尿器科医 ur-

ologist ●産科医 obstetrician ●婦人科医 gynecologist ●産科婦人科医 obstetrician-gynecologist；OB/GYN ●耳鼻咽喉科医 otorhinolaryngologist / ENT doctor ●眼科医 ophthalmologist ●整形外科医 orthopedist / orthopedic surgeon

■その他
●精神科医 psychiatrist ●皮膚科医 dermatologist ●放射線診断医 diagnostic radiologist ●放射線治療医 interventional radiologist ●病理医 pathologist ●麻酔科医 anesthesiologist ●救急専門医 emergency medicine specialist ●腫瘍専門医 oncologist / cancer[tumor] specialist ●スポーツ医 sports physician [doctor] / sports medicine specialist ●リハビリテーション科専門医 rehabilitation physician / physiatrist ●歯科医 dentist ●歯科矯正医 orthodontist ●口腔外科医 oral surgeon

---

せんよう¹ 専用 （唯一…だけ）**only** （独占的に）**exclusively** （🔲私用の **private** 特殊化した **specialized**） ◆こちらは救急専用の入り口ですので, あちらの正面玄関をご利用下さい This entrance is for emergency use only, so please use the main entrance over there. ◆一階に車椅子専用のトイレがあります There is a toilet for wheelchair users on the first floor. ◆女性専用外来 a women's-only clinic / a clinic exclusively for women ◆このタイプの病室には専用トイレとシャワーがついています This type of room has a private toilet and shower. ◆この方法のメリットは高価な専用器具が不要であるということです The advantage of this method is that it doesn't require expensive specialized instruments.

せんよう² 線溶 （線維素溶解）**fibrinolysis** （🔲**fibrinolytic**） ▶抗線溶療法 antifibrinolytic therapy ▶線溶系 the fibrinolytic system 線溶亢進 excessive fibrinolysis 線溶療法 fibrinolytic therapy

せんようぞうしょくしょう 腺様増殖症

adenoidism ☞アデノイド

せんようのうほうがん　腺様嚢胞癌　adenoid cystic carcinoma

せんりつ　戦慄　shiver　◀悪寒戦慄 chills and shivering

ぜんりつせん　前立腺　prostate〔gland〕〔㊜prostatic〕　◆前立腺疾患 prostatic disease　◆前立腺が少し肥大しています Your prostate gland is slightly enlarged.　◆前立腺の手術をする operate on *a person's* prostate　◆肥大した前立腺 an enlarged prostate　◀経尿道的前立腺切除術 transurethral resection of the prostate；TURP　▶前立腺炎 prostatitis　前立腺酸性ホスファターゼ prostatic acid phosphatase；PAP　前立腺摘除術 prostatectomy　前立腺特異抗原 prostate-specific antigen；PSA　前立腺肥大 benign prostatic hyperplasia[hypertrophy]；BPH　前立腺マッサージ prostatic massage　☞前立腺がん

ぜんりつせんがん　前立腺がん　prostate cancer　▶前立腺がん検診 prostate cancer screening[checkup]　前立腺がんマーカー prostate cancer marker

せんりょう　線量　dose　◀最大許容線量 the maximum permissible dose；MPD　最大耐容線量 the maximum tolerated [tolerance] dose；MTD　照射線量 exposure dose　組織線量 tissue dose　致死線量 lethal dose　治癒線量 curative dose；CD　被曝線量 exposed dose　累積吸収線量 cumulative[accumulated] dose　▶線量計 dosimeter　線量限度 dose limit　線量当量 dose equivalent　線量分布 dose distribution

ぜんりょく　全力　◆全力を尽くす do *one's* best / do all *one* can do

せんれい　先例　〔先行事例〕precedent　〔前の例〕previous example　◆この問題には規則や先例がありません There is no rule or precedent for this problem.　◆先例にならってその問題を処理しました We dealt with the problem by following previous examples.

ぜんろう　全聾　total deafness[hearing

loss]　◆全聾である be totally deaf

ぜんわん　前腕　forearm, antebrachium　▶前腕義手 below-elbow[BE] prosthesis　前腕骨 forearm bone

そ

そいん 素因 predisposition, predisposing factor, diathesis ☞体質 ◆乳がんの遺伝的素因がある have a genetic predisposition to breast cancer ◀アトピー素因 atopic predisposition[diathesis] 出血性素因 hemorrhagic diathesis 人種的素因 racial predisposition

そう¹ 《軽い受け答え：相槌，軽い驚き・念押し，会話の間（ま）など》 ◆そうですか I see. / Well. / Oh. / Really? / Is that so? / Let me see. / Let's see. ★一般的に，語尾を上がり調子で言うと驚きや関心を表す．ただ単に相手の話に調子を合わせる場合には，下がり調子で言う．I see. など頻繁に使いすぎると関心が薄いと思われるので注意．
《同意》 ◆そうです（その通り）(That's) right. / Exactly. / You're right. ◆そう思います（願う）I hope so. / (賛成する)I agree. / (考える)I think so, too. / (残念ながら)I'm afraid so. ◆そうは思いません I don't think so. ◆そうして下さい Please do so. / Please do that.
《それほど》 ◆そう大変でもありません It won't be so hard. ◆今回はそう長くはかからないでしょう It won't take so[very] long this time.

そう² 相 （時期・局面）phase （物の側面）aspect ◀吸息相 inspiratory phase 高温相 hyperthermic phase 呼息相 expiratory phase 低温相 hypothermic phase

そう³ 巣 （焦点・中心）focus （病変）lesion ◀感染巣 infection[infectious] focus 原発巣 primary focus 散布巣 satellite lesion 転移巣 metastatic lesion ☞巣状，病巣

そう⁴ 層 （重なり）layer （集団）group （範囲）range ◀角質層 horny layer 低エコー層 hypoechoic layer 二層 double layer 年齢層 age group[range]

そう⁵ 添う （要求を満たす）meet （満足させる）satisfy （要求をかなえる）answer ◆残念ですが，ご要望に添うことができません I'm sorry to tell you that we can't meet [satisfy] your request. ◆ご意向に添うように努力いたします We'll try to meet your wishes.

ぞう 像 （姿・印象）image （画像）picture （視界）view ◆X線検査では疾患の特徴的な像が見られます Characteristic images of the disease can be seen on X-ray. ◀鏡面像 mirror image 血液像 blood picture / hemogram 硬化像 consolidation 残像 afterimage / postimage 敷石像 cobblestone appearance 自己像 self-image 正面像 anterior view 身体像 body image 側面像 lateral view 透亮像 translucency / translucent area ニボー像 niveau / air-fluid level

ぞうあく 増悪させる （より悪くさせる）make *things* worse （病気・状況を悪化させる）aggravate, exacerbate （病気・状況が悪化する）get worse ☞悪化 ◆痛みを増悪させるものがありますか Does anything make the pain worse? ▶増悪因子 aggravating[exacerbating] factor

そうい¹ 相違 （差異）difference （区別）distinction ☞差，違い ◀質的相違 qualitative difference 量的相違 quantitative difference

そうい² 総意 consensus ◆この決断はご家族全員の総意ですか Did all the members of your family agree with this decision? / Was this decision made by family consensus? ◆日本では脳死や尊厳死などに関して国民の総意形成が進んでいません In Japan, there is still no consensus of opinion on issues involving brain death or death with dignity.

そういえん 爪囲炎 paronychia

そういれば 総入れ歯 complete dentures ★複数形で．☞入れ歯

そううつびょう 躁うつ病 ☞双極性

ぞうえい 造影 （造影検査）contrast study ◆このMRI造影検査の同意書をよく読んでサインして下さい Please read this *consent form for an MRI contrast study

[MRI contrast consent form] carefully before signing it. ◆それでは，造影検査の結果について詳しくお話ししましょう Now, I'd like to discuss the details of this contrast study with you. ◀下部消化管造影 lower gastrointestinal[GI] series[radiography] / barium enema；BE / contrast enema　関節造影 arthrography　冠動脈造影 coronary angiography[arteriography]；CAG　逆行性腎盂造影 retrograde pyelography；RP　逆行性尿道造影 retrograde urethrography；RUG　血管造影 angiography　上部消化管造影 upper gastrointestinal[GI] series[radiography] / barium swallow　脊髄造影 myelography　胆管造影 cholangiography　デジタルサブトラクション血管造影 digital subtraction angiography；DSA　内視鏡的逆行性胆道膵管造影 endoscopic retrograde cholangiopancreatography；ERCP　尿路造影 urography　肺動脈造影 pulmonary arteriography　▶造影 MRI〈CT〉contrast enhanced MRI〈CT〉　造影効果 contrast enhancement　☞造影剤

ぞうえいざい　造影剤　contrast material[dye, medium]　◆血管の中に造影剤を入れます I'm going to inject a contrast material[dye] into the blood vessel. ◆これまでに造影剤でアレルギー反応を起こしたことはありますか Have you ever had any allergic reactions to a contrast material[dye]? ◆造影剤を入れると少し体が熱くなるような感覚がありますが心配ありません Your body may become[feel] slightly hot when the contrast material[dye] is injected, but there's no need to worry. ◀バリウム造影剤 barium contrast material[dye]

そうえん¹　爪炎　onychia, onychitis
そうえん²　創縁　wound margin　▶創縁クリップ wound clip　創縁切除 debridement　創縁接着剤 wound adhesive / adhesive for wound closure　創縁縫合 wound suture[suturing]
そうおん　騒音　noise　◆騒音に曝される be exposed to（loud）noise　▶騒音外傷

noise trauma　騒音性難聴 noise-induced *hearing loss[deafness]　騒音損傷 noise damage　騒音程度 noise level

ぞうか　増加する　（数・量が増す）increase /ɪnkríːs/（↔decrease）（図increase）（重量を増す・増幅する）gain（↔lose）（図gain）（上昇する）rise（↔fall）（図rise），elevate（図elevation）☞増える　◆白血球の数が増加しています The number of white blood cells is increasing[rising]. ◆検診で PSA が軽度増加している所見が見られました The screening test shows that the PSA levels are slightly elevated. ◆体重の増加を抑える control weight gain[increase]　◆白血球数の急激な増加 a sharp increase in the number of white blood cells

そうがく　総額　the total amount[expenses]　◆今月の医療費は総額 28 万円になります Your total medical expenses [The total amount of your medical expenses] for this month are[is] two hundred and eighty thousand yen.

そうかこうか　相加効果　additive effect
そうかん¹　相関する　be correlated（with），correlate（with）（図correlation）　◆肺がんと喫煙の間にはかなりの相関関係があります Lung cancer is highly[closely] correlated with smoking. / There is a close correlation between lung cancer and smoking. ◀逆相関 inverse correlation / negative correlation

そうかん²　挿管する　insert a tube, intubate（図intubation）　◆気管内に挿管する insert[place] a tube into the trachea [windpipe]　◀気管挿管 tracheal[endotracheal / intratracheal] intubation　経鼻挿管 nasal intubation　▶挿管不要 Do Not Intubate；DNI

そうかんかん　総肝管　common hepatic duct

ぞうかんざい　増感剤　sensitizer　◀放射線増感剤 radiosensitizer / radiosensitizing agent

そうカンジダしょう　爪カンジダ症　nail candidiasis

そうき　早期(の)　early (stage) （通常より早い）**premature** （予定日前の）**preterm** ☞初期　◆がんは早期に発見することが重要です It is important to find[detect] cancer *in its early stages[at an early stage]. / Early detection of cancer is important.　◆この病気は早期に治療すれば治ります If treated early, this disease is curable.　◆早期に治療を受ける have [get] early treatment　▶早期がん early [early-stage] cancer　早期産児 preterm baby[infant]　早期射精 premature ejaculation　早期手術 early surgery　早期診断 early diagnosis　早期破水 premature rupture of membranes；PROM　早期離床 early ambulation

そうぎ　葬儀　funeral (service, ceremony)　◆彼の葬儀は土曜日に西葬儀場で行われます His funeral will be held at Nishi Funeral Home on Saturday.　◆葬儀に参列する attend a funeral　▶葬儀場 funeral home[parlor]　葬儀屋 funeral director / undertaker

ぞうき　臓器　organ （内臓）**internal organ**　◆生命維持に不可欠の臓器 vital organs　◀実質臓器 parenchymal organ　人工臓器 artificial organ　生体臓器提供者 living donor　多臓器不全 multiple organ failure；MOF　摘出臓器（切除した臓器）removed organ / （分離した臓器）isolated organ　標的臓器 target organ　▶臓器提供 organ donation　臓器提供意思表示カード (organ) donor card　臓器提供者 organ donor　臓器バンク organ bank　☞臓器移植

ぞうきいしょく　臓器移植　organ transplant[transplantation]　◆臓器移植を行う perform an organ transplant　▶生体臓器移植 living-donor organ transplant[transplantation]　日本臓器移植ネットワーク the Japan Organ Transplant Network　脳死臓器移植 organ transplant[transplantation] from a brain-dead donor

そうぎし　総義歯　complete dentures　★複数形で.　☞入れ歯

ぞうきょう　増強する （鍛える・強固にする）**strengthen** （増大・増加させる）**build up, increase**　◆グレープフルーツはこの薬の作用を増強することがあるので召し上がるのを控えて下さい Grapefruit strengthens [increases] the effect of this medication, so please refrain from eating it.　◀筋力増強訓練 muscle-strengthening exercise　筋肉増強剤 muscle-building drug / （同化ステロイド）anabolic steroid

そうきょくせい　双極性(の)　bipolar　◆双極性障害はかつて躁うつ病として知られていました Bipolar disorder was formerly known as manic-depressive illness.

そうぐ　装具 （固定具）**brace** （矯正器具）**orthosis** （圏orthoses） （人工装具）**prosthesis**　◆頸椎の装具をつけている wear a *neck brace[cervical collar / cervical orthosis]　◀下肢装具 lower limb orthosis　義肢装具士 prosthetist and orthotist；PO　機能装具 functional brace　靴型装具 corrective shoe(s)　膝装具 knee brace　脊柱装具 back brace　補助装具（日常生活用具）assistive[supportive] device / （備品）auxiliary equipment　免荷装具 non-weight-bearing orthosis　立位支持装具 standing brace

そうげい　送迎　☞送り迎え

そうけいどうみゃく　総頸動脈　common carotid artery；CCA

ぞうげしつ　象牙質　dentin

ぞうけつ　造血　blood formation, hematopoiesis （圏hematopoietic）**, hemopoiesis**　▶造血幹細胞 hematopoietic[blood-forming] stem cell　造血幹細胞移植 hematopoietic stem cell transplant[transplantation]　造血器 hematopoietic [blood-forming] organ　造血器腫瘍 hematologic neoplasm　造血機能 hematopoietic[blood-forming] function / hematopoietic capacity　造血薬 blood-forming medication / hematinic

ぞうげん　増減する （上下する）**go up and down** （増加・減少する）**increase and〈or〉decrease** （変動する）**fluctuate, vary**　◆最近, 体重は増減しましたか Has your weight *gone up and down[fluctuated] recently? / Has your weight increased and⟨or⟩ decreased recently? ◆検査値に多少の増減はありますが正常の範囲内ですので，心配ありません Your test counts may fluctuate[go up and down / vary] slightly, but they're within the normal range, so there's no need to worry.

そうご　相互（の）　reciprocal, mutual
▶相互関係 reciprocal[mutual] relationship　相互転座 reciprocal translocation　相互理解 mutual understanding　☞相互作用

そうこう　爪甲　nail plate　▶爪甲剥離症 onycholysis

そうごう　総合（的な）（一般的な・多面的な）**general**（包括的な）**comprehensive**　◆総合的な医療 comprehensive medical care　▶総合案内 general information counter[desk]　総合受付 general reception counter[desk]　総合感冒薬 common cold medication　総合診断 comprehensive diagnosis　総合ビタミン剤 multivitamin tablet[pill / supplement]　総合病院 general hospital　☞総合診療

そうごうしんりょう　総合診療　general medicine　◆原因不明の体調不良でお悩みでしたら，まず総合診療科にかかって下さい If you feel sick and aren't sure what the problem is, the first thing you should do is visit[go to] the department of general medicine.　▶総合診療医 general practitioner；GP　総合診療科 the department of general medicine

そうごさよう　相互作用　interaction（**interact**）　◆この薬は他の薬と相互作用を起こすことがあります This medication may interact with other medications. /（有害な相互作用）This medication may cause adverse interactions with other medications.　◆薬によっては相互作用により副作用を起こすかもしれませんので，新しい薬を飲む前に必ずご相談下さい Certain medications, if taken together, may interact and cause harmful side effects, so be sure to check with me before taking a

new medication.　◀薬物食品相互作用 drug-food interaction / interaction between foods and medications　薬物相互作用 drug interaction

ぞうこつ　造骨（性の）　▶造骨[骨芽]細胞 osteoblast　造骨性病変 osteoblastic lesion　造骨性変化 osteoblastic change

そうコレステロール　総コレステロール　total cholesterol：TC　☞コレステロール

そうさ¹　走査する　scan　▶走査型電子顕微鏡 scanning electron microscope；SEM　走査型レーザー検眼鏡 scanning laser ophthalmoscope

そうさ²　操作する　operate（図operation）（巧みに手を使って操る）**manipulate**（図manipulation）**, control**（図control）　◀遺伝子操作 genetic[gene] manipulation　遠隔操作 remote control

そうざん　早産　premature birth, preterm birth（分娩）**premature delivery, preterm delivery**　◆その子は6週間の早産でした The baby was born six weeks premature.　◀切迫早産 threatened premature delivery　▶早産児 preterm baby[infant] /（未熟児）premature baby[infant]

そうじ　掃除する　clean（掃く）**sweep**（掃除機をかける）**vacuum** /ˈvækjuːm/（水拭きする）**wipe**（埃を払う）**dust**（モップをかける）**mop**　☞清掃　◆お部屋を掃除させて下さい Let me clean[（掃除機で）vacuum] your room.　◆耳掃除をする clean one's ears

そうしき　葬式　☞葬儀

そうしつ　喪失する　lose（図loss）　◆記憶を喪失する lose one's memory　◆自信を喪失する lose one's self-confidence / lose confidence in oneself　◆喪失感を味わう feel a sense of loss　◀意識喪失 loss of consciousness：LOC / unconsciousness　感覚喪失 sensory loss / loss of sensation　記憶喪失 memory loss / loss of memory /（健忘）amnesia　自信喪失 loss of confidence

そうじゅく　早熟　precocity（図precocious）　◆早熟な子供 a precocious child　◀性的早熟 sexual precocity

そうしゅしょくしん 双手触診 bimanual palpation

そうしょう¹ 爪床 nail bed

そうしょう² 創傷 wound （切り傷）cut
▶創傷感染 wound infection　創傷洗浄 wound cleansing[toilet]　創傷治癒 wound healing　創傷治療 wound treatment[care / management / therapy]　創傷被覆材 wound dressing　創傷離開 wound dehiscence

そうじょう¹ 相乗（作用） synergism
◀薬物相乗作用 drug synergism[potentiation]　☞相乗効果

そうじょう² 巣状（の） focal ▶巣状糸球体硬化症 focal glomerulosclerosis；FGS　巣状糸球体腎炎 focal glomerulonephritis

そうじょうこうか 相乗効果 synergistic effect, synergy ◆この２つの薬の相乗効果 the synergistic effect of[between] these two medications

そうじょうたい 躁状態 manic state
☞躁病　◆躁状態である be in a manic state

ぞうしょく 増殖 （増大・成長）growth （🔲grow）（増加）increase /ínkri:s/（🔲incréase）（大幅な増加）multiplication （🔲multiply）（急増・繁殖する）proliferation （🔲proliferate, 🔲proliferative）（過形成）hyperplasia ◆細胞の異常増殖 an abnormal growth[multiplication] of cells / an abnormal increase in the number of cells ◆網膜で毛細血管が増殖しており，放置すると失明する危険があります The number of capillaries in your retina has increased. *If we leave them untreated[If we don't do anything], there's a risk you'll *go blind[lose your sight]. ◀細胞増殖 cell growth　子宮内膜増殖症 endometrial hyperplasia　歯肉増殖症 gingival hyperplasia ▶増殖因子 growth factor　増殖曲線 growth curve　増殖性糸球体腎炎 proliferative glomerulonephritis；PGN　増殖性硝子体網膜症 proliferative vitreoretinopathy；PVR　増殖速度 growth rate

そうしょくひん 装飾品 ornament ☞装身具

ぞうしん 増進する （増す）increase （促進する）promote （改善する）improve ◆食欲を増進する increase[improve] one's appetite ◆健康を増進する promote[improve] one's health

そうしんぐ 装身具 （宝飾品）jewelry （アクセサリー）accessories ★通例，複数形で. ◆装身具はすべて取って下さい Please remove all of your jewelry and accessories.

そうしんやく 痩身薬 weight loss drug, antiobesity medication[drug, agent]

ぞうせいきのう 造精機能 spermatogenic function ▶造精機能障害 spermatogenic dysfunction

そうせいじ¹ 双生児 twins （双子の１人）twin ☞双胎，双子（ふたご）◀一卵性双生児 identical[monozygotic / uniovular] twins　二卵性双生児 fraternal[dizygotic / biovular] twins

そうせいじ² 早生児 preterm baby[infant]　（未熟児）premature baby[infant]　☞早産

ぞうせつじゅつ 造設術 –ostomy ◀胃瘻造設術 gastrostomy　経皮的内視鏡下胃瘻造設術 percutaneous endoscopic gastrostomy；PEG　結腸瘻造設術 colostomy　腎瘻造設術 nephrostomy

そうぞう 想像する imagine （🔲想像上の imaginary）☞推測 ◆検査は想像していたよりずっと楽だったでしょう The test must have been much easier than you had imagined. ▶想像妊娠 imaginary pregnancy

そうぞうしい 騒々しい noisy ☞うるさい ◆少し騒々しいようです．他の患者さんの迷惑になりますので静かにしていただけませんか It's a little noisy in here. For the sake of the other patients, could I ask you to keep the noise down?

そうたい¹ 相対（的な） relative ◆様々な要因を相対的に見る consider various factors relative to one another / look at various factors relatively ▶相対概念 relative concept　相対危険度 relative risk；RR　相対湿度 relative humidity

そうたい²　双胎　twins　★通例，複数形で．☞双生児，双子(ふたご)　◀一絨毛膜双胎 monochorial twins　一絨毛膜二羊膜双胎 monochorionic diamniotic twins　▶双胎間輸血症候群 twin-to-twin[twin-twin] transfusion syndrome；TTTS　双胎妊娠 twin pregnancy

ぞうだい　増大する　(徐々に上昇・増加する)**build up**　(☞**buildup**)　(数量・程度が増加する)**increase** /ɪnkríːs/　(☞**íncrease**)　(成長する)**grow**　(☞**growth**)　(増大・拡大する)**enlarge**　(☞**enlargement**)，**expand**　(☞**expansion**)　◆プラークの増大 buildup of plaque　◆糖尿病の血糖コントロールが悪いと心血管疾患発症のリスクが増大します Poor glycemic control in diabetes can increase the risk of developing cardiovascular disease.　◆この画像は腫瘍の増大を示しています This film shows that the tumor has grown (larger).

そうだん　相談する　(意見を訊く)**consult**　(助言を求める)**ask[go to] for advice**　(話し合う)**talk (with, to)**　(チェックする)**check (with)**　(☞**consultation**　カウンセリング **counseling**)　◆どなたか相談にのってくれる人がいますか Do you have anyone to consult with? / Do you have anyone you can go to for advice?　◆悩みをカウンセラーに相談する consult a counselor about *one's* problems / ask[go to / see] a counselor for advice about *one's* problems　◆困ったことがあれば相談に来て下さい If you're ever in trouble[If you have any problem], come and talk to me.　◆その件についてはかかりつけ医に相談するほうがいいでしょう You should go and see your family doctor about it.　◆ご相談したいことがありますので，ナースステーションにおいで下さい I have something I need to talk about with you, so please come to the nurses' station.　◆お食事については栄養士と相談しましょう Let's talk[check] with the dietitian about your diet.　◆新しい薬を飲み始める前には私に相談して下さい Please check with me before you begin taking any new medication.　◀医療相談 medical counseling[consultation]　医療福祉相談室 medical social work[services] office[unit]　健康相談 health consultation[counseling]　子育相談 counseling for parent(s)　児童相談所 child guidance center / counseling clinic for children　生活相談 life consultation[counseling]　不妊相談 infertility consultation　▶相談員 counselor　相談室 counseling room

そうたんかん　総胆管　common bile duct　▶総胆管結石 common bile duct stone(s) / choledocholithiasis　総胆管切開術 choledochotomy

そうたんぱく　総蛋白　total protein

そうち　装置　(特別な使用目的のある機器)**device**　(機器・備品)**equipment**, **apparatus**　(大がかりな機械装置)**system**　(監視装置)**monitor**　(道具・手段)**tool, instrument**　◆これは心拍を調整してくれる装置です This is a device used to regulate the heartbeat.　◀安全装置 safety device　換気装置 ventilator　監視装置 monitoring device / (設備)monitoring equipment / (機器)monitoring instrument　警報装置 alarm system　酸素供給装置 oxygen supply equipment　歯科矯正装置 orthodontic appliance　生命維持装置 life support system[machine]　/life-sustaining equipment　分析装置 analyzer　防火装置 fire prevention equipment　冷却装置 cooling apparatus / cooler

そうちゃく　装着する　(取り付ける)**attach … (to)**　(身につける)**put (on)**　◆心電計などのモニターを装着します I'm going to attach an EKG and other monitors to your body.　◆(患者に)人工呼吸器を装着する put *the patient* on an artificial respirator / attach *the patient* to an artificial respirator　▶(義肢の)装着訓練 prosthetic training

そうちょう　早朝　early morning　(☞**early in the morning**)　◆早朝の咳 an early morning cough / a cough in the early morning　▶早朝嘔吐 morning vomiting[sickness]　早朝覚醒 early morning awakening[arousal]　早朝血圧 morning blood pressure 早朝高血圧 morning hypertension 早朝頭痛 morning headache 早朝尿 first[early] morning urine

そうとう 相当（な・に）
《大変な・に》（かなり）**pretty, considerably**（圏**considerable**）（とても）**very** ☞かなり ◆これまで相当つらい思いをなさったでしょう I guess you've been having a pretty hard time. ◆医療費はご家族にとって相当な負担になるでしょう Medical expenses can be a considerable burden on the family.
《十分な》**good, sufficient** ◆手術を勧める相当な理由があります There is good[sufficient] reason to recommend surgery.
《ほぼ等しい》（対応する）**correspond**（to）（ほぼ同価値である）**be equal**（to）**, be equivalent**（to）◆0 から 10 のスケールで，痛みの程度はどのくらいですか。0 は「無痛」，10 は「耐えられない痛み」に相当します Can you describe your pain rate on a scale of zero to ten? Zero corresponds to 'no pain' and ten corresponds to 'unbearable pain.' ◆グラニュー糖の小匙一杯はおよそ 4 g に相当します One teaspoon of granulated sugar is roughly equal to four grams of sugar.

そうどう 相同 **homology**

そうにゅう 挿入する **insert, put …**（into）（埋め込む）**implant** ◆この坐薬は肛門に挿入して下さい Please insert this suppository into your *back passage[bottom]. ★anus（肛門）という語は患者に不快な思いを抱かせるので避けたい．◆…にカテーテルを挿入する insert[put] a catheter into … ◆鼻から胃管を挿入する insert[put] a stomach tube through the nose ▶挿入物 insert /（埋入物）implant

そうねん 壮年 （人生の最盛期）**prime** （中年）**middle age** ◆壮年期 the prime of life

そうは 掻爬する **curet, curette** ▶掻爬術 curettage / curettement

そうはく 蒼白（な）**pale**（圏**pallor**）◆患者は顔面が蒼白です The patient looks pale. ◆蒼白になる turn pale ◀口囲蒼白 perioral[circumoral] pallor ▶蒼白乳

頭 optic disc pallor

そうはつせい 早発性（の） （早熟の）**premature, precocious** （早期の・初期の）**early** ▶早発月経 premature menstruation 早発思春期 premature[precocious] puberty 早発性脱毛症 premature alopecia[balding] 早発性認知症 premature dementia / dementia praecox 早発閉経 premature menopause

そうはんげつ 爪半月 **half-moon of the nail, lunule of the nail, nail lunula**

ぞうびじゅつ 造鼻術 **rhinoplasty**

ぞうひびょう 象皮病 **elephantiasis**

そうびょう 躁病 **mania, manic disorder** ☞躁状態 ◆躁病患者 a manic（patient）

そうぼうきん 僧帽筋 **trapezius muscle**

そうぼうしつにん 相貌失認 **prosopagnosia, face blindness**

そうぼうべん 僧帽弁 **mitral valve** ▶僧帽弁逸脱症 mitral valve prolapse；MVP 僧帽弁逆流症 mitral（valve）regurgitation；MR 僧帽弁狭窄症 mitral（valve）stenosis；MS 僧帽弁修復術 mitral valve repair 僧帽弁断裂 mitral valve rupture[tear] 僧帽弁置換術 mitral valve replacement；MVR 僧帽弁閉鎖不全症 mitral（valve）insufficiency；MI 僧帽弁輪形成術 mitral annuloplasty 僧帽弁膜症 mitral valve disease

そうよう 掻痒 **itch**（圏**itchy**）**, itching, pruritus** ☞痒み ◀外陰掻痒症 vulvar pruritus[itching] 肛門掻痒症 anal pruritus[itching] /（口語）itchy bottom 皮膚掻痒症 pruritus cutaneous / itching[itchy] skin ▶掻痒感 itch[itchy] sensation 掻痒性丘疹 itching papule

そうろう¹ 早老 **premature aging, premature senility, presenility**（圏**presenile**）

そうろう² 早漏 **premature ejaculation**

そえぎ 添え木・副え木 **splint**（動添え木を当てる splint）◆骨折した腕に添え木を当てる splint[apply a splint to / place a splint on] a fractured arm ◆添え木が当てられている be in a splint

ソーシャルスキル **social skills** ★通例,

複数形で.

ソーシャルワーカー social worker ◀医療ソーシャルワーカー medical social worker；MSW

ソーダ （炭酸飲料）soda （ナトリウム）sodium ◀青酸ソーダ sodium cyanide

そがい 阻害する （妨げる）inhibit （図inhibition 図inhibitory）（低下させる）impair （図impairment）☞抑制 ◆この薬は胃酸分泌を阻害する働きをします This medication works by *inhibiting the production of stomach acid[preventing the stomach from making acid]. ◆干渉のし過ぎはお子さんの健全な発達を阻害する恐れがあります Parental overinterference may inhibit[impair] a child's healthy development. ▶阻害作用 inhibitory action 阻害物質 inhibitor / inhibitory substance [agent] ☞阻害薬

そがいかん 疎外感 sense of alienation ◆疎外感に苦しむ suffer from a sense of alienation ◆疎外感をもつ feel alienated / have a sense of alienation /（無視されたと感じる）have a feeling of being neglected ◀社会的疎外 social alienation

そがいやく 阻害薬 inhibitor ◀アンギオテンシン変換酵素阻害薬 *angiotensin-converting enzyme[ACE] inhibitor 核酸合成阻害薬 nucleic acid synthesis inhibitor 競合的阻害薬 competitive inhibitor セロトニン・ノルアドレナリン再取込み阻害薬 serotonin-norepinephrine reuptake inhibitor；SNRI 選択的セロトニン再取込み阻害薬 selective serotonin reuptake inhibitor；SSRI ドパミン取り込み阻害薬 dopamine uptake inhibitor プロテアーゼ阻害薬 protease inhibitor プロトンポンプ阻害薬 proton pump inhibitor；PPI ベータラクタマーゼ阻害薬 β-lactamase inhibitor

そくおう 即応 ◆緊急時に即応できる体制を整えています We have a system in place to deal with emergency cases. /（即座にケアを行う用意がある）In cases of emergency, we're well prepared to take care of patients immediately[instantly]. ◆患者

の容態の変化に即応した治療を行う adjust the treatment *according to[in response to] changes in a patient's condition

そくがい 側臥位 side position, side-lying position, lateral position ☞左向き，右向き ▶側臥位像 lateral decubitus view

そくかんせつ 足関節 ankle joint ▶足関節骨折 ankle fracture 足関節捻挫 ankle sprain

そくけい 側頸(部) the side of the neck, the lateral cervical region （図lateral cervical）▶側頸囊胞 lateral cervical cyst

そくこん 足根 ☞足根(そっこん)

そくざ 即座(に) ☞すぐ

そくし 即死 （瞬間の死）instant death, instantaneous death （その場での死）death on the spot ◆お子さんは軽傷ですが，ご主人は即死でした Your child suffered a mild injury, but I'm afraid your husband was killed instantly.

そくじ 即時(の) immediate, instant ▶即時型反応 immediate[immediate-type] reaction 即時記憶 immediate memory

そくじつ 即日 (the) same day ▶即日手術 same day surgery 即日入院 same day admission

そくしん 促進する promote （急がせる）precipitate （加速する）accelerate ◆発毛を促進する promote hair growth ◆分泌を促進する promote[help / increase] secretion ◆分娩を促進する accelerate labor /（陣痛促進薬で誘発する）induce labor ◀分娩促進薬 ecbolic （medication / drug / agent）▶促進因子 promoting [precipitating] factor

そくせん 塞栓 embolus （図embolic）▶塞栓摘出術 embolectomy ☞塞栓術，塞栓症

そくせんじゅつ 塞栓術 embolization ◀経カテーテル肝動脈塞栓術 transcatheter hepatic arterial embolization 経カテーテル動脈塞栓術 transcatheter arterial embolization；TAE 脳動脈瘤コイル塞栓術 coil embolization of a cerebral aneurysm

そくせんしょう 塞栓症 embolism ◀アテローム血栓性塞栓症 atherothrombotic embolism 冠動脈塞栓症 coronary embolism 奇異性塞栓症 paradoxical embolism 空気塞栓症 air embolism 血栓塞栓症 thromboembolism 脂肪塞栓症 fat embolism 心原性脳塞栓症 cardiogenic cerebral[brain] embolism 肺血栓塞栓症 pulmonary thromboembolism；PTE 羊水塞栓症 amniotic (fluid) embolism

ぞくぞく ◆体中がぞくぞくする（寒気がする）feel chilly all over *one's* body / feel cold and shivery all over *one's* body

そくてい¹ 足底（の） plantar（图足の裏・靴底 sole (of the foot)）▶足底板 insole / footplate 足底反射 plantar[sole] reflex 足底部 plantar region 足底疣贅 plantar wart

そくてい² 測定する measure（图measurement 腰尾-metry）, take, check ☞測る ◆血糖値を測定する measure[take / check] *a person's* blood sugar level ◆筋力を測定する measure *a person's* muscle strength ◆毎朝起床後すぐに体温を測定して下さい Please take your temperature as soon as you get up every morning. ◀眼圧測定 tonometry 血圧測定 measurement of blood pressure / sphygmomanometry 血糖自己測定 self-monitoring of blood glucose；SMBG 視野測定 perimetry 視力測定 vision measurement / measurement of visual acuity 身体測定 body[（身長・体重）height and weight] measurement 体温測定 measurement of body temperature 体力測定 physical strength[fitness] test / test of physical strength and fitness ▶測定感度 sensitivity of measurement 測定誤差 measurement error 測定値 measured value[（計数値）count] 測定特異度 specificity of measurement ☞測定器

そくていき 測定器 measuring instrument, measuring device （量を示す計器）meter ◀血糖値測定器 glucose meter / glucometer 自動血圧測定器 automatic blood pressure measuring device / automated sphygmomanometer

そくど 速度（速さ）speed, velocity （ある時間内に起こる回数・割合）rate （歩調）pace ◆脈の速度が速い〈遅い〉have a fast〈slow〉pulse rate ◆このタイプのがんの進行速度は比較的遅い〈速い〉This type of cancer develops at a relatively slow〈fast〉speed. ◆ゆっくりとした速度で歩いて下さい Please walk at a slow pace. ◀赤血球沈降速度 erythrocyte sedimentation rate；ESR 増殖速度 growth rate 反応速度 reaction rate[velocity] 輸液速度 infusion speed

そくとう 側頭（の） temporal ▶側頭筋 temporal muscle 側頭筋膜 temporal fascia 側頭骨 temporal bone 側頭部 temples (of the head) / temporal region[part] (of the head) 側頭葉 temporal lobe

そくのうしつ 側脳室 lateral ventricle

そくはいどうみゃく 足背動脈 dorsalis pedis artery, dorsal artery of the foot ▶足背動脈拍動 dorsalis pedis pulse

ぞくはつせい 続発性（の） secondary ▶続発症 secondary disease / sequela 続発性貧血 secondary anemia 続発緑内障 secondary glaucoma

そくばん 足板 footplate

そくふく 側副（の） collateral ▶側副血行 collateral circulation 側副靱帯 collateral ligament 側副靱帯断裂 collateral ligament rupture 側副路 collateral pathway / bypass

そくふくぶ 側腹部 flank, the lateral abdominal region ▶側腹部痛 flank pain

そくぶはくせん 足部白癬 athlete's foot, tinea pedis

そくぶへんけい 足部変形 foot deformity

そくみゃく 速脈 quick pulse, rapid pulse, pulsus celer

そくめん 側面 side（图lateral）◆この治療にはプラスとマイナスの側面があります There are both positive and negative sides to this treatment. ◀外側面 lateral surface ▶側面像 lateral view

そくよく 足浴 foot bath

ぞくりゅうけっかく　粟粒結核　miliary tuberculosis

そくわんしょう　側彎症　scoliosis　◀学童期側彎症 juvenile scoliosis　胸椎側彎症 thoracic scoliosis

そけい　鼠径（部）　groin, inguinal region　◆鼠径部を触診しましょう I'm going to palpate your groin.　◆鼠径部に痛みやしこりがありますか Do you have any pain or lump in your groin?　◆鼠径部が腫れている have a swelling in the groin　▶鼠径管 inguinal canal　鼠径靭帯 inguinal ligament　鼠径ヘルニア inguinal hernia　鼠径リンパ節 inguinal lymph node

そけつ　阻血　☞虚血

そこ　there　（ちょうどそこに）right there　（向こうに）over there　◆そこに仰向けになって下さい Please lie （down） there on your back.　◆（脱いだ）衣類はそこのかごに入れて下さい Please put your clothes in the basket right there.　◆自動販売機はそこのロビーにあります There's a vending machine in the lobby over there.　◆そのままそこにいて下さい Please stay where you are.　◆治療についてそこまではご理解いただけましたか Have you understood so far about your treatment?　◆そこまで主張されるのでしたら何か別の治療を考えましょう If you insist that much, let's consider another treatment option.

そこうしょう　鼠咬症　rat-bite fever[disease], sokosho

そこねる　損ねる　（害する）damage　（傷つける）injure　（台なしにする）ruin　◆過度のダイエットはかえって健康を損ねます Excessive[Too much] dieting can damage [injure / ruin] your health.

そしき　組織　（体組織）tissue　（構造）structure　（圏structural）　（組織学）histology　（圏histologic, histological）　◆肝臓から組織検体を採る take[obtain / remove] tissue samples from the liver　◆異常な組織 abnormal tissue　◀遺残組織 remnant tissue　筋組織 muscle[muscular] tissue　結合組織 connective tissue　骨組織 bone tissue　脂肪組織 fatty[adipose] tissue

上皮組織 epithelial tissue　正常組織 normal tissue　石灰化組織 calcified tissue　線維組織 fibrous tissue　軟部組織 soft tissue　粘膜下組織 submucosal tissue　皮下組織 subcutaneous tissue　リンパ組織 lymphatic[lymphoid] tissue　▶組織型分類 histologic typing　組織適合試験 histocompatibility test[testing]　組織培養 tissue culture　組織バンク tissue bank　組織プラスミノゲン活性化因子 tissue plasminogen activator；tPA　◆組織化学，組織学, 組織球症, 組織診

そしきかがく　組織化学　histochemistry　◀免疫組織化学 immunohistochemistry

そしきがく　組織学　histology　（圏histologic, histological）　◀病理組織学 pathologic histology　▶組織学検査 histologic examination

そしききゅうしょう　組織球症　histiocytosis

そしきしん　組織診　histologic diagnosis　◀迅速組織診 rapid histodiagnosis

そしつ　素質　（力量）making　（適性・才能）aptitude, capability　（疾病素因）predisposition　◆彼女はまだ未熟ですが，よい看護師になる素質があります She's still immature, but has the makings of a good nurse.　◆日本語がお上手ですね。あなたは語学の素質があります You speak Japanese fluently, don't you? You have a natural aptitude for languages.

そしゃく　咀嚼する　chew, masticate　（图mastication　圏masticatory）　☞噛む　◆食べたものをよく咀嚼すれば胃への負担を減らせます If you chew your foods well, it will reduce the burden on your stomach.　◆咀嚼できる軟らかさに茹でる boil foods until they are soft and easy to chew　▶咀嚼運動 chewing[masticatory] motion　咀嚼困難 difficulty[trouble]（in）chewing / chewing difficulty　咀嚼障害 disorder[dysfunction] of mastication　咀嚼力 chewing force / force of mastication /（噛み切る力）biting force

そしょう　訴訟　（law）suit　（圏sue）　◆医

療過誤で病院に対し訴訟を起こす sue a hospital for medical malpractice / file a suit against a hospital for medical malpractice ▸医療訴訟 medical (malpractice) lawsuit

そせい¹　組成　composition

そせい²　蘇生　resuscitation（翻蘇生させる resuscitate, revive　蘇生する come back to life, revive　◆彼を蘇生させる努力を続ける continue *one's* attempts to resuscitate him　◆心肺蘇生 cardiopulmonary resuscitation；CPR　心肺蘇生不要 Do Not Attempt Resuscitation；DNAR　▸蘇生薬 analeptic（medication / drug / agent）蘇生用カート resuscitation cart

そだいうんどう　粗大運動　gross motor（↔fine motor）

そだち　育ち　growth（翻grow）☞成長

そだてる　育てる　bring up, raise　◆どこで生まれ育ったのですか Where were you born and brought up?　◆お子さんは母乳で育てましたか Did you breastfeed your baby?

そち　措置　measure　◆インフルエンザに対して緊急措置を講じる take emergency measures against the flu　◆これはあくまでも暫定的な措置です This is only a temporary[（仮の）provisional] measure.　◀延命措置 life support measure(s)　予防措置 preventive[（念のための）precautionary] measure(s)　▸措置入院 involuntary admission

ソックス　socks　★通例，複数形で．　◆ソックスを脱ぐ take *one's* socks off / take off *one's* socks　◆ソックスをはく put *one's* socks on / put on *one's* socks

そつご　卒後（の）　postgraduate　▸卒後教育 postgraduate education　卒後研修 postgraduate training

そっこう　即効・速効　immediate effect, instant effect　（即座の緩和）immediate relief　◆この薬は胸痛に即効性があります This medication will have an immediate[instant] effect on your chest pain. / This medication will provide immediate relief for your chest pain.　▸速効型インスリン

short-acting insulin　☞即効薬

そっこうやく　即効薬　fast-acting[rapid-acting] medication　（治療薬）quick cure, instant remedy　◆この症状には即効薬はありません There is no *fast-acting medication[quick cure / instant remedy] for this symptom.

そっこつ　足骨　foot bone(s), bone(s) of the foot

そっこん　足根　tarsus　（足根骨）tarsal bone　▸足根管 tarsal tunnel　足根管症候群 tarsal tunnel syndrome

そっちょく　率直（に）　（ざっくばらんに）frankly　（隠し立てをしないで）openly　◆率直に言えば喫煙がこの病気の主たる原因です Frankly speaking[To be frank with you], smoking is one of the leading causes of this disease.　◆もしご心配なことがあれば率直なお気持ちをお話し下さい If you are concerned or worried about something, please talk about your feelings openly[frankly].

そっと　（優しく）softly, gently　（軽く）lightly　（静かに）quietly　◆皮膚にそっと触るだけでも痛いですか Does it hurt even to touch the skin softly[gently / lightly]?　◆他の患者さんが眠っておられますので，病室のドアはそっと閉めて下さい Please close the door of your room quietly[softly / gently] because the other patients are sleeping.　◆しばらくそっとしておいてあげましょう Let's leave him〈her〉alone[to himself〈herself〉] for a while.

そっとう　卒倒する　☞失神

そで　袖　sleeve　◆袖をまくって腕を出して下さい Please roll up your sleeve and stretch out your arm.

そどう　粗動　flutter　◀心室粗動 ventricular flutter　心房粗動 atrial flutter；AF

そとがわ　外側　the outside, the outer side [part]　（外側面）lateral side[part]　☞外側（がいそく）　◆右膝の外側が痛みますか Do you have any pain on the outer side of your right knee?

そなえつける　備え付ける　（設備する）be equipped（with）　（用意・提供する）provide ◆各病室にはケーブルテレビが備え付けてあります Each hospital room is equipped with cable television. ◆衣類は備え付けのロッカーに入れて下さい Please put your clothes in the locker provided.

そなえる 備える （準備する）**prepare** (**for**), **get ready** (**for**) ◆手術に備えてこの小冊子を読んで下さい Please read this brochure to prepare[get ready] for your surgery. ◆最悪の事態に備える prepare for the worst

そのうち （すぐに）**soon** （近いうちに）**before long** ◆傷痕はそのうち目立たなくなります The scar will fade soon[before long]. / It won't take long for the scar to fade.

そのご その後 （その時以来）**since then** （その後で）**after that** ◆体調はその後いかがでしたか How have you been feeling since then?

そのつど その都度 **each time** （…な時はいつでも）**whenever** ◆頭痛がつらかったらその都度この薬を服用して下さい Please take this medication each time your headache becomes unbearable. ◆薬の投与量は血糖値に合わせてその都度決定します Whenever[Each time] your blood sugar levels go up or down, I'm going to change the dose of your medication.

そのつもり （準備する）**be ready** (**for**), **prepare** *oneself* ◆手は尽くしていますが，今日が峠かと思いますので，どうぞそのつもりでいて下さい We're doing all[everything / as much as] we can, but today will be a critical stage, so please *be ready for that[prepare yourself]*.

そのとおり その通り （正しい）**right** ◆その通りです You're absolutely right. / That's exactly right.

そのぶん その分 （それだけ）**that many**, **that much** ◆この薬は劇的な効果を示しますが，その分副作用も出やすいことをご承知下さい This medication has dramatic effects, but may have that many more side effects. ◆前もって予約をしていただ

ければ，その分待ち時間が少なくてすみます If you make an appointment beforehand, you'll save yourself that much waiting time. ◆リハビリを頑張らないと，その分退院が遅れます If you don't work harder on your rehabilitation, it'll take you that much longer to get discharged.

そのまま ◆（検査などで）服はそのままで大丈夫です You can keep your clothes on. ◆検査が終わったらそのままお帰りいただいて結構です As soon as the test is over [After the test], you can go home without waiting. ◆症状は落ち着いていますので少しそのまま様子を見ましょう Your condition is stable, so let's wait a while and see how it goes. ◆スタッフが部屋を片づけますのでどうぞそのままにしておいて下さい Please leave your room as it is. Our staff will tidy it up. ◆（電話で）そのままお待ち下さい Hold the line[Hang on], please.

そば 傍 **beside** ◆心配しないで下さい，おそばについていますよ Don't worry! I'll be here beside[for] you. / Don't worry! I'll just sit with you.

そばかす **freckles** ◆通例，複数形で.

そびれる （忘れる）**forget** （…し損なう）**miss** ◆重要なことを訊きそびれた〈言いそびれた〉のですが I'm afraid that I forgot [missed] to *ask you*〈mention / let you know〉something important. ◆この薬を飲みそびれたら，気がついた時すぐに飲んで下さい If you miss a dose of this medication, take it as soon as you remember.

そふ 祖父 **grandfather** ◆母方〈父方〉の祖父 *one's* grandfather on *one's* mother's〈father's〉side / *one's* maternal〈paternal〉grandfather

ソフトコンタクトレンズ **soft** (**contact**) **lens**

ソフトドリンク **soft drink**(**s**) ☞ジュース

そぼ 祖母 **grandmother** ◆父方〈母方〉の祖母 *one's* grandmother on *one's* father's〈mother's〉side / *one's* paternal〈maternal〉grandmother

ソマトスタチン **somatostatin**

そめる 染める **dye** ◆髪を染めています

か Is your hair dyed? / Did you dye your hair?

そらす 反らす （傾ける）lean （曲げる）bend ◆上体を後ろに反らす lean[bend] backward

ゾリンジャー・エリソンしょうこうぐん ―症候群 Zollinger–Ellison syndrome；ZES

そる 剃る shave （図shave） （むだ毛などを取り除く）remove ◆手術準備のためにお腹の部分の毛を剃りましょう To prepare for your surgery, I'm going to shave your abdomen. ◆ご自分で手術の部位を剃って下さい Please shave *the surgical area [the area where you're going to have the surgery] by yourself. ◆剃るのをお手伝いしましょうか Would you like assistance with shaving? ◆私が剃って差し上げましょうか Would you like me to give you a shave? ◆胸毛を剃る shave[remove] *a person's* chest hair ◆頭の毛を剃る shave *a person's* head ◆ひげを剃る shave / get a shave

それぞれ each ◆その件についてはご家族それぞれにご意見があるでしょう Each member of your family will have a different opinion on that matter. ◆痛みや不安の感じ方は人それぞれです How we feel pain or anxiety differs[is different] from person to person. ◆朝晩それぞれ2錠ずつお飲み下さい Please take two tablets in the morning and in the evening.

それで ◆それで？（相手の発言を促して）Go on. / And then? / Yes? / And? / Uh huh? / Mmm, hmm?

それでは then, well ◆それでは，また明朝〈あとで〉お目にかかります I'll be off then. I'll come to see you again *tomorrow morning〈later〉. ◆それでは今日の訓練はこれまでにしましょう Well, that's all [enough] for today's training.

そろえる 揃える （配置する）arrange, put （用意する）get[make]... ready ◆カードを順番に揃えて下さい Please arrange[put] the cards in order. ◆足を揃えて立って下さい Please stand with your feet togeth-

er. ◆次回の診察までに必要書類一式を揃えておいて下さい Please get[have] all the necessary forms[documents] ready before your next visit.

そろそろ 《適度の頃合い》any time, about time ◆そろそろ彼女の麻酔が切れてくる頃です She should be coming out of the anesthesia any time now. / It's about time for the anesthesia to be wearing off. ◆退院後どんなケアが必要になるか，そろそろ話し合いましょう Let's discuss what kind of care you'll need after your discharge from the hospital, shall we? 《ゆっくり》slowly ◆そろそろ歩く walk slowly

そんがい 損害 （物理的な損害）damage （経済的な損失）loss

そんきょ 蹲踞 squatting ☞しゃがむ

そんげんし 尊厳死 death with dignity / dígnəti/ ☞安楽死 ◆尊厳死は患者さんご本人の明確な意思が示されている必要があります To carry out death with dignity, the patients' wishes and intentions must be (made) very clear. / To allow death with dignity, patients must make their own intentions[wills] clear. ◆わが国では尊厳死はまだ法制化されておらず，臨床現場ではかなり慎重な扱いです Since Japan has no "death with dignity" law, it has to be dealt with very carefully in clinical practice[settings].

そんざい 存在する exist, be present (in) ◆ウイルスや細菌はあらゆる所に存在しています Viruses and bacteria exist [are present] everywhere. ◆回復のしかたは合併症の存在に左右されます How you recover depends on whether there are any complications. ◆糖尿病が進むと末梢神経が障害され足に怪我をしてもその存在に気づきにくくなります Advanced-stage diabetes causes peripheral nerve damage, so you'll lose your sense of feeling and may not even be aware of a foot injury. ◆愛犬の存在が大きな支えですね Your dear doggy gives you a lot of emotional support, doesn't he⟨she⟩?

そんしつ　損失　loss　◀聴力損失 hearing loss

そんしょう　損傷　(怪我) **injury** (動 **injure**), **wound**　(物理的な損害) **damage**　(筋肉などの断裂) **tear** /téɚ/　☞傷, 怪我　◆肋骨を損傷したことがありますか Have you ever had a rib injury?[injured your ribs?]　◆頭部に損傷を受ける injure *one's* head / have some head injury[damage] / have some injury[damage] to the head　◆回復不能な損傷 irreversible[permanent] damage[injury]　◀圧挫損傷 crush injury　開放性⟨非開放性⟩損傷 open⟨closed⟩ injury　肝損傷 liver injury　顔面損傷 facial injury　胸部損傷 chest[thoracic] injury[wound]　筋損傷 muscle injury　頸椎損傷 cervical spine injury　血管損傷 vascular injury　産道損傷 birth canal injury[tear]　神経損傷 nerve injury　穿通性損傷 penetrating injury　内臓損傷 visceral injury　脳損傷 brain injury[damage]　肺損傷 lung injury　腹部損傷 abdominal injury　物理的損傷 physical injury　鞭打ち損傷 whiplash injury

そんちょう　尊重する　respect　(図 **respect**)　◆もちろん患者さんのご意見を尊重しています We certainly respect our patients' opinions.　◆人命尊重の観点から患者さんの治療にあたっています Respect for human life is at the heart of our medical treatment[care].

そんな　so, such　(そのような) **like that**　◆そんなに無理しなくていいのですよ You don't have to work so hard.　◆そんな時にはボタンを押して看護師を呼んで下さい At such times[At times like that], push[press] the button to call the nurse.　◆そんなつもりで申し上げたわけではありません I didn't mean it[what I said].

た

ターナーしょうこうぐん ―症候群 Turner syndrome

ターミナルケア terminal care ☞終末期

タールべん ―便 tarry stool

タイ Thailand（㏄Thai） ☞国籍 ▶タイ人（の）Thai

だい[1] 大（の）（形・数量が大きい）large, big（↔small）（事柄が重大な・容易でない）major（↔minor） ◆バストバンドには大中小があります Chest binders are available in three sizes：small, medium, and large. ★この場合は，通例，small を先にする． ◆湿布は大小どちらがよいですか What size compress would you like to have, large or small? ▶大手術 major surgery

だい[2] 台 table （支えるもの）support ◆この台の上に左を下にして寝て下さい Please lie on this table, on your back on your left side. ◆（眼科などで）あごと額をこの台の上に載せて下さい Please put your chin and forehead on this support. ◀起立台 standing table 傾斜台 tilt[tilting] table 手術台 operating table 床頭台 bedside cupboard[table] 診察台 exam[examination / examining] table /（特にカウンセリング用の）couch 内診台 gynecological exam table

たいい[1] 体位 （体の位置）(body) position （姿勢）posture（㏄postural） ☞姿勢 ◆痛みは体位を変えると悪化しますか〈和らぎますか〉Does the pain get worse〈better〉when you change your (body) position? ◆褥瘡ができないよう2時間ごとに体位交換をいたします We'll[We're going to] turn you every two hours to prevent *pressure sores[bedsores]. ◆頻繁に体位を変える change *one's* position frequently ◀手術体位 surgical[operative] position ショック体位 shock position トレンデレンブルグ体位 Trendelenburg position ファウラー体位 Fowler position

分娩体位 posture in labor ▶体位性血圧調節反射 postural blood pressure reflex 体位性失神 postural syncope 体位ドレナージ postural drainage 体位交換 postural change

体位・動作の指示

■体位交換
●体の向きを変えるのをお手伝いしましょう Let me help you change (your) position. / Let me help you move onto the other side.
●右に向きを変えます You're going to *move onto your right side[move so that you're facing right].
●まず，左腕を右上の方に持ち上げて下さい First, move your left arm over to your right.
●次に，左膝を曲げて右足に交差させて下さい Now, bend your left knee and cross it over to the right.

■寝る lie
●台の上に仰向け〈うつ伏せ〉に寝て下さい Please lie on your back〈stomach〉on the table.
●右〈左〉向きに寝て下さい Please lie on your right〈left〉side.

■向く look, turn
●こちらを向いて下さい（視線を向ける）Please look this way. /（体を向ける）Please turn over this way.
●前を向いて立って下さい Please stand with your head facing the front.
●横を向いて立って〈寝て〉下さい Please stand〈lie〉turning sideways.
●後ろを向いて下さい Please turn around.
●反対側を向いて下さい Please turn over.
●右〈左〉を向いて下さい Please turn to the right〈left〉. / Please look to your right〈left〉.
●上を向いて下さい Please look up[upward].
●下を向いて下さい Please look down[downward].

■**向ける　turn**
●両方の手のひらを上に向けて下さい Please turn both palms up. /（腕を伸ばしたまま）Please hold your arms out,（with）both palms up.
●こっちに顔を向けて下さい Please turn your face toward me.

■**回す・回る　turn, rotate**
●首を左に回して下さい Please turn your head to the left.
●首をぐるっと回せますか Can you *turn your neck all the way around[rotate your neck]?
●腕〈肩〉は後ろに回りますか Can you rotate your arms〈shoulders〉back?

■**上げる　raise, lift**
●両手を上に高く上げて下さい Please raise[lift] both hands high above your head.
●手を上げて頭の上に載せて下さい Please *lift up[raise] your hands and put them on your head.
●つま先〈かかと〉を上げて下さい Please lift up your toetips〈heels〉.
●あごを少し上げて下さい Lift your jaw forward slightly.
●ベッドの頭のほうを少し上げましょうか Shall I raise the head of your bed a little?

■**下ろす・下げる　put down**
●手を下ろしてもいいですよ You can put your hands down. / Hands down, please.

■**かがむ**　（上体を曲げる）**bend over**　（しゃがむ）**squat down, crouch down**
●かがめますか Can you *bend over[squat down / crouch down]?

■**曲げる　bend, flex**
●膝〈肘〉を曲げて下さい Please bend[flex] your knees〈elbows〉.
●体を前に曲げて下さい Please bend over[forward at the waist].
●体を左右に曲げて下さい Please bend

from side to side.
●首を曲げると痛みますか Does it hurt when you bend your head[neck]?

■**伸ばす　stretch, extend**　（まっすぐにする）**straighten**
●膝を伸ばしてもいいですよ You can stretch[extend] your knees.
●足〈手〉を伸ばす stretch[extend] *one's* legs〈arms / hands〉
●背筋を伸ばす straighten *one's* back / make *one's* back straight
●背筋を伸ばして座る sit upright

たいい²　胎位　(fetal) presentation ◀分娩 胎位 labor[delivery] presentation ▶胎位異常 malpresentation　胎位矯正 correction of malpresentation

たいいく　体育　physical education；PE
◆体育の授業はしばらく見学して下さい You have to sit out physical education class[You should not do PE] for a while.

だいいち　第一・第1(の)　(the) first（圖first），**primary** ☞一次，1度 ◆まず第一に空床があるか確かめてみましょう First (of all), let's make sure we have some vacant[unoccupied] beds available.
◆COPD の治療としてまず第一に禁煙することが大切です With COPD, *first and foremost, you should quit smoking[first it's important that you quit smoking].
▶第1期 first stage　第1子 *one's* first [first-born] child　第Ⅰ度熱傷 a first-degree burn

たいいん　退院する　leave the hospital（退院させる）**discharge** /dɪstʃάɚdʒ/（圖discharge）；**DC[dc]** ◆傷が治り次第退院できます Once the wound has healed satisfactorily, you can leave the hospital.
◆もうすぐ退院できます You'll be able to leave the hospital soon. / You can go home soon.　◆退院するには早すぎます You're not well[You haven't recovered] enough to *leave the hospital[go home] yet. ◆退院は術後の回復次第です Your discharge will be decided depending on

*how quickly you recover[how you're doing] after the surgery. ◆退院後1週間経ってから外来へおいで下さい Please come to the outpatient department for a follow-up visit one week after being discharged (from the hospital). ◆今日ご退院ですね。おめでとうございます You're leaving today. Congratulations! ◆退院の手続きは病棟の事務職員に確認して下さい Please check with a ward clerk about the discharge procedures. ▶退院計画 discharge plan 退院指示 discharge instructions 退院指導 discharge guidance 退院時要約 discharge summary

だいいんしん 大陰唇 labium majus（圏 labia majora）

だいうつびょうせいしょうがい 大うつ病性障害 major depressive disorder

たいえき 体液 body fluid （精液）semen ◆体液量 body fluid volume ◆体液貯留 fluid retention

ダイエット diet（圏diet 圏dietary 規定食用の dietetic）☞食事制限, 食事療法 ◆ダイエット食品 diet[dietetic] food ◆ダイエット療法 diet[dietary] therapy ◆ダイエットをしていますか Are you on a diet? ◆ダイエットを始めたのはいつですか When did you first try to diet[go on a diet]? ◆過度のダイエットは体によくありません Excessive[Too much] dieting is bad for your health.

たいおう 対応する （手助けする）help, assist （奉仕する）serve （世話をする）attend (to) （応じる）respond (to) （対処する）treat, deal (with), cope (with) ☞応じる, 応対, 処理, 対処 ◆その件については受付の事務が対応します A clerk at the reception desk will help[assist] you in that matter. ◆英語を話せる者が対応しますのでしばらくお待ち下さい An English-speaking member of staff will be here to help[assist] you, so could you wait for a little while? ◆対応が悪かった点はお詫びします We apologize for any *poor service you may have received[inconvenience we have caused]. ◆不適切な対応 inad-

equate response ◆その件に関してはできるだけ速やかに対応します We are trying to deal with the matter as promptly [quickly] as we can. ◆一人ひとりの患者に対して誠実に対応する treat each patient with sincere care

だいおうけい 大横径 biparietal diameter；BPD

ダイオキシン dioxin

たいおん 体温 (body) temperature；T [temp.] ☞熱 ◆体温を測りましたか Did you take your temperature? ◆体温を測りましょう Let me[I'm going to] take your temperature. ◆今朝の体温は何度でしたか What was your temperature this morning? ◆体温は平熱〈37.6℃〉です Your temperature is normal〈thirty-seven point six degrees Celsius〉. ◆体温が平熱より高い〈低い〉one's temperature is above〈below〉normal ◆体温を下げる *bring down[lower / reduce] one's temperature ◆毎日の体温を記録する record one's daily temperature ◀基礎体温 basal body temperature；BBT 基礎体温表 BBT chart[record] 高体温 hyperthermia 低体温 hypothermia ▶体温調節 thermoregulation / body temperature regulation 体温表 temperature chart ☞体温計

たいおんけい 体温計 thermometer /θəˈmɑmətə/ ◆この体温計が鳴るまで腋の下にはさんで下さい Please keep this thermometer under your arm until it beeps. ◀水銀体温計 mercury thermometer デジタル体温計 digital thermometer

たいがい¹ 大概 ☞たいてい

たいがい² 体外（の）extracorporeal （外部の）external ▶体外式除細動器 external defibrillator 体外式膜型人工肺 extracorporeal membrane oxygenation；ECMO 体外式ペースメーカ external pacemaker 体外受精 in vitro fertilization；IVF 体外循環 extracorporeal circulation 体外衝撃波砕石術 extracorporeal shock wave lithotripsy；ESWL 体外心マッサージ

external cardiac massage；ECM

たいかく 体格 **build** ☞体型 ◆標準的な体格 an average build ◆その患者さんは平均的な体格でした(中肉中背だった)The patient was of average height and build. ◆お子さんは年齢の割に体格がいいですね Your child *has a good build[is well built] for his〈her〉age. ◆筋肉質の体格 a muscular[sturdy] build

だいがく 大学 (総合大学)**university** (単科大学)**college** ◀医科大学 medical university[school/college] ★medical school[college] は医学部のこともいう。 看護大学 college of nursing／nursing university[college] ▶大学院 graduate school 大学生 university student ☞大学病院

だいがくびょういん 大学病院 **university hospital**

たいかん 体幹 **trunk** (医truncal), **torso** ▶体幹運動失調 truncal ataxia 体幹ギプス body cast 体幹装具 spinal orthosis

たいき 待機する (近辺にいる)**be on hand** (場所にとどまる)**remain, stay** (事に備えて待つ)**stand by, be on standby** ◆彼は容態が非常に不安定ですので，急変に備えて病院内で待機していて下さい His condition is very unstable, so we'd like you to *be on hand[remain] somewhere in the hospital in case there's a turn for the worse. ◆少なくとも2，3日は自宅に待機して症状が出ないことを確認して下さい You should stay [remain] at home for at least a few days to make sure that you don't come down with any symptoms. ◆スタッフが24時間待機しています The staff is available *twenty-four hours a day[around-the-clock]. ◆ご退院に備えて介護タクシーを待機させております We have a care taxi [cab] standing by for when you're ready to leave the hospital. ▶待機患者 patient on the waiting list 待機手術 elective [planned／nonemergency] surgery

たいきあつ 大気圧 **atmospheric pressure, barometric pressure**

たいきおせん 大気汚染 **air pollution** ▶大気汚染物質 air pollutant

だいきぼ 大規模(な) **large-scale, mass** (接頭mega-) ▶大規模災害 large-scale [mass] disaster 大規模試験 megatrial

たいきゅう 耐久 **endurance** ◆耐久性 durability ▶耐久力訓練 endurance training[exercise]

だいきゅういんし 第IX因子 **factor IX** ▶第IX因子欠乏症 factor nine deficiency／(血友病B)hemophilia B

だいきゅうし 大臼歯 **molar** (**tooth**)

だいきょうきん 大胸筋 **pectoralis major** (**muscle**), **greater**[**larger**] **pectoral muscle** ▶大胸筋皮弁 pectoralis major myocutaneous[musculocutaneous] flap

たいくう 体腔 **body cavity**

たいくつ 退屈 **boredom** (医bored) ◆床上安静でさぞ退屈なことでしょう You must feel[be] really bored lying in bed all the time. ◆退屈をまぎらすために何をしたいですか What would you like to do to *kill the time[relieve the boredom]?

たいげ 帯下 (vaginal) **discharge** ☞おりもの ◀黄色帯下 yellow[yellowish] discharge 血性帯下 bloody discharge 膿性帯下 purulent discharge

たいけい 体型 (骨格) **build** (体つき) **body shape** ☞体格 ◆痩せ型の体型 a thin[slender] build ◆太めの体型 a heavy build ◆若い時からだいぶ体型が変わりましたか Has your body shape changed a lot since you were young?

だいけっかん 大血管 **great artery[vessel]** ◀完全大血管転位 complete *transposition of the great arteries[TGA]

たいけん 体験 **experience** ☞経験 ◆子供の頃の体験についてお話し下さい Please tell me about your childhood (experiences). ◆日本で何か不快な体験をしたことがありますか Have you ever had any unpleasant experience in Japan? ◆貴重な体験をする have a valuable experience ◀性体験 sexual experience 臨死体験 near-death experience

たいこう 退行 **involution** (医involutional) ▶退行期うつ病 involutional depression 退行期精神病 involutional psychosis

だいこう 代行する substitute〔for〕 ☞代理 ◆今日は私が星先生を代行いたします I'm going to substitute for Dr Hoshi today.

だいこうとうこう 大後頭孔 foramen magnum, great foramen ▶大後頭孔ヘルニア foraminal herniation

だいこうとうしんけい 大後頭神経 greater occipital nerve ▶(大)後頭神経痛 (greater) occipital neuralgia

たいこうはんしゃ 対光反射 light reflex

たいこばち 太鼓ばち(の) clubbed ▶太鼓ばち指 clubbed finger／(親指の) clubbed thumb 太鼓ばち爪 clubbed nail

たいざい 滞在する stay〔図stay〕 ◆どのくらい日本に滞在しますか How long〔(何日くらい)How many days〕are you going to stay in Japan? ◆東京のどちらにご滞在ですか Where are you staying in Tokyo? ◀短期〈長期〉滞在 short-term〈long-term〉stay〔residence〕 短期〈長期〉滞在者 short-term〈long-term〉resident 不法滞在 illegal stay ▶滞在期間 the length of one's stay〔visit〕

たいさいぼう 体細胞 somatic cell, body cell ▶体細胞突然変異 somatic (cell) mutation 体細胞分裂 somatic (cell) division

たいさく 対策 measure ◆院内感染に適切な対策を講じる take appropriate〔adequate〕measures against hospital-acquired infections ◆万全の対策 all possible measures ◀安全対策 safety〔security〕measure(s) 感染症対策 measure(s) to control infectious diseases 感染対策専門医 infection control doctor〔physician〕

だいさん 第三・第3(の) (the) third〔図third〕, tertiary ☞三次, 3度 ▶第3期 third〔tertiary〕stage 第三世代抗菌薬 third-generation antibiotics 第Ⅲ相試験 phase three trial 第3度 third degree

たいし 胎脂 vernix caseosa

たいじ 胎児 fetus /fíːtəs/〔図fetal〕 睡頭胎児・胎芽の embry(o)- ◀アルファ胎児

性蛋白質 alpha-fetoprotein；AFP 癌胎児性抗原 carcinoembryonic antigen；CEA 死胎児 dead fetus 母体・胎児集中治療室 maternal-fetal intensive care unit；MFICU ▶胎児アルコール症候群 fetal alcohol syndrome 胎児機能不全 non-reassuring fetal status；NRFS 胎児月齢 gestational period 胎児姿勢 fetal posture 胎児児頭大横径 biparietal diameter；BPD 胎児死亡 fetal death 胎児心音 fetal heart tones；FHT／fetal heart sound 胎児診断 fetal〔(出生前の)prenatal〕diagnosis 胎児心拍数 fetal heart rate；FHR 胎児性癌 embryonal carcinoma 胎児聴診器 fetal〔Traube〕stethoscope 胎児治療 fetal therapy 胎児頭殿長 crown-rump length；CRL 胎児発育不全 fetal growth restriction 胎児-母体間輸血症候群 *fetomaternal transfusion〔FMT〕syndrome 胎児モニター fetal monitor

だいじ 大事 《重要である》important （影響力のある・大切な）significant ☞重要 ◆ここは大事な点ですから、よく聞いて下さい Please listen carefully, because this is very important. ◆喘息の治療で大事なのは、発作のない時にも定期的にステロイド薬を吸入することです The important thing about asthma treatment is *to keep using the inhaler〔to take inhaled steroids〕regularly even if you're not having attacks. ◆ご自分にとって最も大事なことはなんですか For you, what's the most important thing in life? ／ What do you value most of all? ◆あなたにとっていちばん大事な人は誰ですか Who is the most important person for you? ◆集中治療室の面会は近親者と(患者さんにとって)大事な方に限らせていただきます Visiting in the ICU is restricted to immediate family and significant others. ★significant other は配偶者、同棲するパートナー、恋人などを指す。 《重大な結果》 ◆事故現場での適切な救急処置のおかげでお子さんは大事に至らずにすみました(命が救われた)Your child's life was saved thanks to the appropriate emergency treatment at the scene of the accident.

《用心・安全》（予防対策）**precaution** （安全）**safety** （㊙**safe**）　◆怪我は大したことはありませんが，大事をとって今晩は入院して下さい Your injury is not so serious, but I want you to remain in the hospital for tonight *just as a precaution[just to be on the safe side].

《体調を整える》　◆どうぞお大事に(Please) take (good) care of yourself. / Take care! / Get well soon!

たいしかん　大使館　embassy　◆母国の大使館に出生届を出す必要があります You need to submit a report of birth to the embassy of your home country.　◆手続きの詳細については大使館に問い合わせて下さい For further information on procedures, please contact[inquire at] your embassy.

たいした　大した（深刻な・重い）**serious**　◆貧血は大したことはありません Your anemia is nothing serious.

たいしつ　体質（疾病素因）**predisposition**（傾向）**tendency**（素質・身体の健康度）**constitution**（㊙**constitutional**）☞素因　◆アレルギー体質ですか Do you have allergies? / Do you tend[have a tendency] to get allergies? / Do you have a predisposition toward allergies?　◆肥満体質を遺伝的に受け継ぐ inherit a tendency toward [to] obesity　◆体質を改善する improve *one's* physical constitution　◆生まれつきの体質 *a natural[an innate] predisposition*　◀虚弱体質 weak[delicate] constitution　特異体質 idiosyncrasy　▶体質性黄疸 constitutional jaundice　体質性要因 constitutional factor

たいしぼう　体脂肪　body fat　◆体脂肪を減らす reduce[take off / lose] *one's* body fat　▶体脂肪率 body fat percentage

たいしゃ　代謝　metabolism /mətǽbə-lìzm/（㊙**metabólic**）　◆定期的に運動することで代謝が良くなります You can improve your body's metabolism by exercis-ing regularly. / Your body's metabolism will be improved by regular exercise.

◀アミノ酸代謝異常 disorder of amino-acid metabolism　エネルギー代謝 energy metabolism　基礎代謝 basal metabo-lism；BM　基礎代謝率 basal metabolic rate；BMR　プリン代謝拮抗薬 purine antagonist　薬物代謝酵素 drug-metabo-lizing enzyme　▶代謝異常 metabolic disorder　代謝産物 metabolic product　代謝性アシドーシス metabolic acidosis　代謝性アルカローシス metabolic alkalosis　代謝性疾患 metabolic disease　代謝当量 metabolic equivalents；METS　代謝内分泌内科 the department of metabolism and endocrinology / the metabolism and endocrinology department　代謝率 met-abolic rate；MR

たいしゅう　体臭　body odor；**BO**　◆体臭がきついと言われたことがありますか Have you ever been told that you have a strong body odor?

たいじゅう　体重　weight（㊙**weigh**）

≪体重の測定≫　◆今体重はどのくらいありますか How much do you weigh? / What's your weight?　◆身長と体重を計りましょう Let me measure your height and weight.　◆あなたの体重は 65 kg です You weigh sixty-five kilos[kilo-grams]. / You're sixty-five kilos[kilo-grams] in weight.

≪体重の評価≫　◆身長の割に体重がありますね〈ありませんね〉You are overweight〈underweight〉for your height.　◆あなたの体重は標準です You are of standard weight.　◆これくらいの体重増加〈減少〉は普通ですから心配しないで下さい This much weight gain〈loss〉is quite normal, so don't worry.　◆お子さんは年の割に体重が重い〈軽い〉です Your child is heavy〈light〉for his〈her〉age. / Your child *weighs a lot〈doesn't weigh much〉for his〈her〉age.

≪体重の変動について尋ねる≫　◆最近，体重は変化しましたか Has your weight changed recently?　◆体重が 3 kg 増える

〈減る〉gain〈lose〉three kilos[kilograms] ◆最近，体重は増えたり減ったりしましたか Have you gained or lost weight recently? ◆最近，体重の減少〈増加〉に気づきましたか Have you noticed any weight loss〈gain / increase〉recently? ◆どのくらい体重が増加〈減少〉しましたか How much[How many kilos] have you gained〈lost〉? ◆これまでの最高〈最低〉の体重はいくらですか What is the most〈least〉you've (ever) weighed? ◆体重の変動が激しいですか Does your weight fluctuate dramatically?

≪体重への認識を促す≫ ◆ベストな体重はいくらですか What's your optimal weight? / What weight do you feel healthiest at? ◆ご自分の体重をどうお考えですか How do you feel about your weight? ◆体重を減らす lose[take off] weight ◆体重を増やす gain[put on] weight ◆現在の体重を維持する maintain *one's* present weight / maintain the weight *one* has at present ◆（太らないように）体重に注意する watch *one's* weight /（管理する）control *one's* weight

◀過体重 overweight　推定児体重 estimated fetal body weight；EFBW　生理的体重減少 physiologic weight loss　低体重 underweight / low body weight　標準体重 standard (body) weight　理想体重 ideal (body) weight　▶体重曲線 weight curve　体重測定 weight measurement　体重負荷運動 weight-bearing exercise　体重変化 weight change　☞体重計

たいじゅうけい　体重計　scale〈英〉scales ◆靴を脱いで体重計に乗って下さい Please take your shoes off and step[stand] on the scale. / Please step[stand] on this scale with your shoes off. ◆体重計で体重を計る（患者本人が）weigh *oneself* on the scale /（医療者などが）weigh *a person* on a scale

たいしゅうやく　大衆薬　over-the-counter drug, OTC drug

たいしゅく　退縮　involution　◀胸腺退縮 thymic involution

だいしゅっけつ　大出血　☞大量出血

たいしょ　対処する　（うまく切り抜ける）cope（with）, manage　（取り扱う）deal（with）, handle　☞処理, 対応 ◆問題に柔軟に対処する cope with the problem flexibly ◆ストレスにどう対処していますか How do you *cope with[manage]* stress? ◆その件に関してはできるだけ早く対処いたします We'll try to deal with the matter as soon as we can.　▶対処行動 coping behavior

たいしょう¹　対称　symmetry（↔asymmetry）（㊕symmetric, symmetrical）

たいしょう²　対象　object　（的・働きかける相手）target　（影響・支配を受けるもの）subject ◆関心の対象 an object of interest ◆対象となるグループ a target group ◆術後患者を対象にしたリハビリプログラム a rehabilitation program for patients who have had[undergone] surgery ◆残念ですがあなたは介護保険の対象とはなりません I'm sorry, but you're not *covered by*[（資格がない）eligible for] long-term care insurance.　◀研究対象者 research participant[patient]　★被験者が人間の時には subject は用いないほうがよい。▶対象喪失 object loss

たいしょう³　対照　（対比する相手）control ◆対照群 controls[a control group]/（患者）control patients（動物）control animals ◆この臨床試験では，1つのグループは新規治療を受け，対照となるグループは標準治療を受けます In this clinical trial, one group will receive the new treatment while the control group will receive the standard treatment.　◀症例対照研究 case-control study

だいしょう　代償　compensation（㊕compensatory, compensated）　◀機能代償 functional compensation　▶代償運動[動作] compensatory movement　代償機能 compensatory function[mechanism]　代償性アシドーシス〈アルカローシス〉compensatory[compensated] acidosis〈alkalosis〉　代償性過膨張 compensatory hyperinflation　代償性〈非代償性〉肝硬変

compensated〈decompensated〉(liver) cirrhosis 代償性肥大 compensatory[vicarious] hypertrophy

だいじょうぶ　大丈夫　all right, okay, OK
◆大丈夫ですか Are you *all right[okay / OK]?／(苦痛などがないか) Are you comfortable enough?　◆大丈夫ですよ You'll [It'll] be all right. / You're going to be just fine. /(すべてうまくいっている) Everything is all right. /(万事うまく運ぶだろう) Everything is going to be all right.　◆(注射の前などで)アルコール消毒は大丈夫ですか Is it *all right[safe] to use alcohol wipes on your skin?　◆心配ありません。大丈夫ですよ There's nothing to worry about. You'll be fine.　◆彼女はもう大丈夫です(危機を脱している)She's out of danger now.

たいじょうほうしん　帯状疱疹　shingles, herpes zoster　◆帯状疱疹になったことがありますか Have you ever had shingles?　◀水痘帯状疱疹ウイルス chickenpox virus / varicella-zoster virus；VZV　▶帯状疱疹後神経痛 postherpetic neuralgia；PHN

だいじょうみゃく　大静脈　vena cava
◀下大静脈 inferior vena cava；IVC　下大静脈フィルター IVC filter　上大静脈 superior vena cava；SVC

たいしょうりょうほう　対症療法　symptomatic treatment[therapy]　◆対症療法は症状を和らげますが，治すものではありません Symptomatic treatment relieves the symptoms of a disease, but does not cure the disease itself.　◆この処置は対症療法にすぎません This procedure is only to treat the symptoms of your disease.　◆感冒に有効な抗ウイルス薬はないので，対症療法しかできないのです There are no effective antiviral drugs against the common cold, so the only thing we can do is provide treatment that will relieve the symptoms.

たいしょく¹　大食　◆普段から大食なほうですか Are you usually a big[heavy] eater? / Do you usually eat a lot?　◆大食は体によくありません Eating a lot of food can't be good for your health.

たいしょく²　退職する　retire (from) (图 retirement)　◆退職していますか Are you retired?　◆退職者 a retired person / a retiree / a person who has retired

だいしん　代診　◆今日は私が林先生の代診を務めます I'm substituting for Dr Hayashi today. / I'm going to examine you instead of Dr Hayashi today.

たいじんかんけい　対人関係　(human) relationships[relations], interpersonal relationships[relations]　★いずれも通例，複数形で。　◆対人関係はどうですか How are your relationships with other people?　◆対人関係がうまくいかないのですか Do you have difficulty *getting along[maintaining good relationships] with other people?

たいじんきょうふ　対人恐怖　anthropophobia；*fear of meeting people*

だいず　大豆　soybean　◆大豆にアレルギーがありますか Are you allergic to soybeans?　▶大豆製品 soy products

たいすいせい　耐水性(の)　water-resistant, waterproof

たいせい¹　耐性　(許容度)tolerance (↔intolerance) (图tolerant)　(抵抗性)resistance (图resistant)　◆がん細胞は時に抗がん剤に耐性を獲得することがあります Cancer cells sometimes acquire[develop] resistance to anticancer drugs.　◆ストレスへの耐性が弱い〈強い〉have a low〈high〉tolerance to[for] stress　◆この細菌は多くの抗菌薬に耐性を持っています These bacteria are resistant to multiple antibiotics.　◀多剤耐性 multidrug resistance；MDR　乳糖耐性検査 lactose tolerance test　薬剤耐性 drug resistance[tolerance]　薬剤耐性菌 drug-resistant bacteria　▶耐性遺伝子 resistance gene　耐性因子 resistance factor

たいせい²　胎勢　fetal attitude[posture]
たいせい³　体性(の)　somatic　▶体性感覚 somatic sensation　体性感覚野 somatosensory area　体性神経 somatic nerve

体性痛 somatic pain

たいせつ **大切** ☞重要，大事

たいぜつ **苔舌** coated tongue, furred tongue

たいせん **苔癬** lichen ◀扁平苔癬 lichen planus

だいせんもん **大泉門** anterior fontanelle ☞泉門

たいそう **体操** exercise ◀産褥体操 puerperal exercise 柔軟体操 calisthenics（exercise） ストレッチ体操 stretching exercise 妊娠体操 pregnancy [maternity] exercise 腰痛体操 exercise for lower back pain

たいそく **対側（の）** contralateral 図反 対側部位に及ぶ衝撃の）contrecoup ▶対側損傷 contrecoup injury 対側片麻痺 contralateral hemiplegia

だいたい¹ **大体** （ほとんど）almost, just about （おおよそ）roughly, approximately （そのくらい）… or so （たいてい）usually ☞おおよそ，大抵，約 ◆大体終わりました You're almost[just about] finished. ◆入院は大体5日間になります Your hospital stay will be roughly[approximately] five days. / Your hospital stay will be five days or so. ◆大体安静により数日でよくなるでしょう If you stay in bed, you *will usually[should] *be well again[recover / feel better again] within several days.

だいたい² **大腿** thigh /θáɪ/ （図大腿・大腿骨の femoral） ▶大腿義足 above-knee [AK] prosthesis 大腿四頭筋 quadriceps muscle of the thigh / quadriceps femoris （muscle） 大腿静脈 femoral vein 大腿切断 above-knee[AK] amputation 大腿動脈 femoral artery 大腿二頭筋 biceps muscle of the thigh / biceps femoris （muscle） 大腿ヘルニア femoral hernia

だいたい³ **代替（の）** （別の選択肢の）alternative （補足的な）complementary ◀補完代替医療 complementary and alternative medicine；CAM ▶代替薬 alternative medication[drug] 代替療法 alternative therapy[treatment]

だいたいこつ **大腿骨** femur （図femoral），

thigh bone ▶大腿骨頸部骨折 femoral neck fracture 大腿骨骨折 femoral fracture 大腿骨頭壊死 femur head necrosis 大腿骨頭すべり症 slipped capital femoral epiphysis

たいちょう **体調** （physical）condition ☞具合，調子 ◆今日，体調はいかがですか How are you feeling today? / How's your condition today? ◆どことなく体調がおかしいと感じることはありますか Do you feel that something in your body is wrong? ◆治療後体調に変化がありましたか Did you have anything wrong with you after the treatment? ◆体調がよくない時には早めに休息をとって下さい Please *take an early rest[get some rest as early as you can] if you don't feel well. ◆寒暖差が激しい時には体調を崩しやすいので注意が必要です Extreme fluctuations in temperature can be bad for the body, so please be careful about that. ◆体調がよい be in good condition[shape] / feel well ◆体調が悪い be in bad[poor] condition[shape] / don't feel well ◆体調を整える get *oneself* in good shape[condition] ◆体調を維持する keep[stay] physically fit

だいちょう **大腸** large intestine[bowel] （結腸）colon （図colonic） ◆大腸の検診を受ける have a colon *screening test [checkup] ◀胃大腸反射 gastrocolic reflex 肛門温存大腸切除術 restorative proctocolectomy ▶大腸腺腫症 adenomatous polyposis 大腸ポリープ polyp of the large intestine / （結腸の）colonic polyp / （結腸直腸の）colorectal polyp ☞大腸炎，大腸がん，大腸菌，大腸憩室，大腸内視鏡

だいちょうえん **大腸炎** colitis /koʊˈláɪtɪs/ ◀潰瘍性大腸炎 ulcerative colitis 出血性大腸炎 hemorrhagic colitis

だいちょうがん **大腸がん** （結腸の）colon cancer （結腸・直腸の）colorectal cancer ▶大腸がん検診 colorectal cancer screening

だいちょうきん **大腸菌** *Escherichia coli*,

E. coli /íːkóʊlaɪ/ ◀腸管出血性大腸菌 enterohemorrhagic *Escherichia coli*；EHEC 毒素原性大腸菌 enterotoxigenic *Escherichia coli*；ETEC 病原性大腸菌 pathogenic *Escherichia coli*

だいちょうけいしつ　大腸憩室 diverticulum of the *large intestine[colon] ▶大腸憩室炎 colonic diverticulitis　大腸憩室症 colonic diverticulosis

だいちょうないしきょう　大腸内視鏡 colonoscope （検査）colonoscopy /kòʊlənáskəpi/ ◆結腸と直腸の異常の有無を視覚的に調べるために大腸内視鏡検査を行います I'm going to perform a colonoscopy to visually examine your colon and rectum for any abnormalities.

たいてい　大抵 usually, generally, mostly, in most cases ☞大体 ◆ステロイド薬を毎日吸入すれば喘息症状は大抵良くなります Asthmatic symptoms will usually improve[In most cases, asthmatic symptoms will improve] with daily use of inhaled corticosteroids.

だいでんきん　大殿筋 gluteus maximus （muscle）

だいでんし　大転子 greater trochanter

たいど　態度 （心構え・姿勢）attitude （行動・ふるまい）behavior （圏behave） ◆治療に積極的な〈消極的な〉態度をとる take[have] a positive〈negative / passive〉attitude toward *one's* treatment ◆態度を変える change *one's* attitude ◆生活態度を改める change *one's* attitude toward life / change *one's* way of living ◆態度が悪い be badly behaved / have bad behavior

たいどう　胎動 baby's movement, fetal movement, the quickening ◆赤ちゃんの胎動を感じましたか Have you felt your baby moving? ◆胎動がなくなった時にはお電話を下さい Please call us if the baby's movements stop.

たいとうのう　耐糖能 glucose tolerance ◆耐糖能障害 impaired glucose tolerance；IGT

だいどうみゃく　大動脈 aorta /eɪɔ́ɚtə/, the main artery （圏aortic） ◀胸部大動脈 thoracic aorta　上行〈下行〉大動脈 ascending〈descending〉aorta　腹部大動脈 abdominal aorta ▶大動脈炎症候群 aortitis syndrome　大動脈解離 aortic dissection　大動脈弓 arch of the aorta / aortic arch　大動脈粥状硬化症 aortic atherosclerosis　大動脈洞 aortic sinus　大動脈内バルーンパンピング intraaortic balloon pumping；IABP ▶大動脈弁, 大動脈瘤

だいどうみゃくべん　大動脈弁 aortic valve ◆大動脈弁がうまく閉じないため血液が逆流しています Your aortic valve doesn't close properly, *so the blood in your heart is flowing backward[so there's a backflow of blood into your heart]. ▶大動脈弁逆流症 aortic（valve）regurgitation；AR / （大動脈弁閉鎖不全症）aortic（valve）insufficiency；AI　大動脈弁狭窄症 aortic（valve）stenosis；AS　大動脈弁形成術 aortic valvuloplasty　大動脈弁置換術 aortic valve replacement　大動脈弁膜症 aortic valve[valvular] disease

だいどうみゃくりゅう　大動脈瘤 aortic aneurysm /eɪɔ́ɚtɪk ǽnjʊrìzm/ ◆お腹に大動脈瘤が見つかりました We've found *an aortic aneurysm in your abdomen[an aneurysm in your abdominal aorta]. ◆大動脈瘤が破裂すると大出血を起こします If an aortic aneurysm ruptures, it will lead to massive bleeding. ◆腹部大動脈瘤破裂の危険性はサイズと膨らむ速度によります The risk of an abdominal aortic aneurysm rupturing depends on its size and the rate at which it expands. ◀解離性大動脈瘤 dissecting aortic aneurysm 胸腹部大動脈瘤 thoracoabdominal aortic aneurysm　胸部大動脈瘤 thoracic aortic aneurysm；TAA　真性大動脈瘤 true aortic aneurysm　腹部大動脈瘤 abdominal aortic aneurysm；AAA ▶大動脈瘤破裂 aortic aneurysm rupture

たいない¹　体内（に） in the body, inside the body ◆ペースメーカを体内に埋め込む place[insert] a pacemaker inside *a person's* body ◆チタンは体内に入れても

安全な金属です Titanium is a metal that can be safely implanted in the body. ◆体内に金属が入っている方は MRI 検査を受けることができません If you have any metal implants in your body, you can't have an MRI. ▶体内式[植込み型]除細動器 implantable (cardioverter) defibrillator；ICD　体内式[植込み型]ペースメーカ implantable pacemaker　体内時計 biological[body] clock　体内被曝 internal exposure

たいない[2]　胎内(に・で)　(子宮内で)in the uterus, in the womb　◆胎内で死ぬ die in the uterus[womb]

だいに　第二・第2(の)　(the) second (圏 second), secondary　☞二次，2度　◆この薬を処方するのは，第1に効果があること，第2に副作用がほとんどないからです I prescribe this medication because first (of all) *it's effective[it works well], and second it has very few side effects. ▶第2期 second stage　第二次性徴 secondary sex characteristic　第二世代 second generation　第II相試験 phase II trial　第II度熱傷 second-degree burn

たいねつ　耐熱(性の)　heat-resistant, heat-stable, thermostable　▶耐熱ガラス heat-resistant glass　耐熱性毒素 heat-stable[thermostable] toxin

たいねんれい　体年齢　physical age

たいのう　胎嚢　gestational sac；GS

だいのう　大脳　cerebrum /sərí:brəm, sérə-/ (圏cerebral)　▶大脳萎縮 cerebral atrophy　大脳鎌 cerebral falx　大脳基底核 basal ganglia　大脳脚 cerebral peduncle　大脳溝 cerebral sulci　大脳髄質 cerebral medullary substance　大脳白質 cerebral white matter　大脳半球 cerebral hemisphere　大脳皮質 cerebral cortex　大脳辺縁系 the (cerebral) limbic system

だいのうどうみゃく　大脳動脈　cerebral artery　☞脳動脈

だいはちいんし　第VIII因子　factor VIII　▶第VIII因子欠乏症 factor eight deficiency／(血友病A)hemophilia A

たいばん　胎盤　placenta (圏placental)　◆胎盤を出すためにもう一度いきんで下さい Please give one more push to expel the placenta. ◀常位胎盤早期剝離 abruptio placentae　前置胎盤 placenta previa　低位胎盤 low-lying placenta　癒着胎盤 adhesive placenta　▶胎盤機能検査 placental function test　胎盤機能不全 placental dysfunction[insufficiency]　胎盤残留 retained placenta　胎盤剝離 placental separation　胎盤娩出 placental delivery

たいひょう　体表　body surface　▶体表面積 body surface area；BSA

たいびょう　大病　serious illness, major illness　◆これまでに大病を患ったことはありますか Have you ever had a serious [major] illness?

たいぶ　体部　body, corpus　▶胃体部 the gastric body　子宮体部 the uterine body　▶体部白癬 ringworm of the body／tinea corporis

タイプ　type　☞型

だいぶ　☞かなり

たいへき　体壁　body wall

たいへん　大変
《辛い・難儀な》hard　◆大変でしたね You had a hard time, didn't you?　◆お仕事で大変とは思いますが体のケアも怠らないで下さい I know your work must be hard, but please don't neglect to take good care of yourself.
《重大な》(深刻な)serious　(ひどい・恐ろしい)terrible, awful　◆今の食生活を続けると大変なことになりかねません If you continue these eating habits, the consequences could be serious.　◆大変な事故に遭われましたね You really had *a terrible[an awful] accident.
《とても》very, really　◆大変よくできました Very good.／Excellent.／You did really well.　◆大変残念です I'm very sorry.　◆あなたの回復が早いので大変嬉しく思います I'm very[really] happy that you're getting better quickly.

たいべん　胎便　meconium；*a baby's first stool*　▶胎便吸引症候群 meconium aspiration syndrome；MAS　胎便性肺炎

meconium pneumonia

だいべん 大便 stool, feces ★feces は専門用語なので患者には用いないほうがよい. ☞便 ◆大便をする have a bowel movement / move[empty] *one's* bowels

だいほっさ 大発作 （激しい発作）major attack （全般性強直間代発作）grand mal （seizure）, *generalized tonic-clonic[GTC] seizure ▶大発作てんかん major[grand mal] epilepsy

たいま 大麻 marijuana /mǽrəwά:nə/, marihuana, cannabis, hashish （インフォーマルに）joint, weed, pot, grass, dope ◆大麻を吸う smoke marijuana[a joint] ◆日本では大麻の使用は法律で禁じられています The use of marijuana in Japan is prohibited by law. / It's illegal to use marijuana in Japan. ▶大麻依存 marijuana[cannabis] dependence 大麻中毒 marijuana[hashish] intoxication / marijuana addiction[abuse] / cannabism

タイミング timing ☞時期 ◆手術は患者さんの状態を見ながら最適なタイミングを図って行います By monitoring the patient's condition carefully, we'll find *just the right timing[the most suitable time] to perform surgery.

たいめんしやけんさ 対面視野検査 confrontation （visual field）test, confrontation （visual field）method

たいもう[1] 体毛 （body）hair ☞毛
たいもう[2] 大網 greater omentum

だいよう 代用する substitute （図substitute） ◆詰まってしまった心臓の血管を足の血管で代用します A blood vessel taken from your leg will substitute for the blocked vessel in your heart. / The blocked vessel in the heart will be replaced with a blood vessel taken from the leg. ◆砂糖の代用品 a sugar substitute ▶代用音声 alternative voice 代用血液 blood substitute 代用血漿 plasma substitute 代用硬膜 dural substitute 代用膀胱 substitute bladder

だいようきん 大腰筋 psoas major （muscle）, greater psoas muscle

たいようせきしすう 体容積指数 body mass index；BMI ☞ビーエムアイ

たいようせんりょう 耐容線量 tolerated dose；TD ◆最大耐容線量 maximum tolerated dose；MTD

たいようねんすう 耐用年数 ◆この装置の耐用年数はおよそ 10 年です This device has a life of[will last] about ten years.

たいら 平ら（な） （薄くて平たい）flat （図flat） （均等で平らな）even （でこぼこがない）smooth ◆ベッドに平らに寝るのは辛いですか Do you have difficulty lying flat in bed? ◆平らな面 *a flat[an even / a smooth] surface

だいり 代理（人） surrogate （略surrogate）, proxy ☞代行 ◆患者さんに意思決定能力がない場合、患者さんの代理としてご家族に同意書にサインしていただきます When patients do not have （the）capacity to make their own decisions, we ask one of their family members to sign the consent form *on their behalf[as their proxy]. ▶代理決定人 surrogate decision-maker / health care proxy 代理出産 surrogate birth 代理母 surrogate mother

たいりょう 大量（の） a large amount of （↔a small amount of）, a large quantity of （大規模な・膨大な）massive （豊富な）copious （喫煙・飲酒などが多量の）heavy ☞多い, 多く, 沢山, 多量 ◆大量に出血する lose a large amount of blood / bleed massively [copiously] ◆大量に食べる eat[binge on] large amounts of food ◆アルコールを大量に摂取する drink alcohol heavily ▶大量[高用量]化学療法 high-dose chemotherapy ☞大量出血

たいりょうしゅっけつ 大量出血 （膨大な出血）massive bleeding[hemorrhage] （激しい出血）severe bleeding[hemorrhage] （多量の出血）heavy bleeding[hemorrhage] ◆消化管に大量出血が起こっています Massive bleeding has occurred in the digestive tract.

たいりょく 体力 （physical）strength （エネルギー）energy （level） （運動能力などの体

力)physical performance （持久力）stamina ◆体力がある have *good physical strength[a lot of energy / a lot of stamina] ◆体力がない do not have enough physical strength / lack stamina / have poor stamina ◆体力をつける *build up[develop] one's strength ◆体力を回復する recover one's strength ◆体力が衰える one's strength declines / one's energy levels decrease ◆体力が消耗する one's strength ebbs away ◆体力を維持する maintain one's strength ◆彼女には手術に耐えるだけの体力がありません She is not strong enough for the surgery. / She doesn't have enough physical strength to withstand the surgery. ◆最近，体力が落ちたと感じますか Do you feel you have less energy than you used to? / Do you feel your energy levels have *gone down[declined]? ◆歩くことで徐々に体力をつける *build up[develop] one's strength little by little by walking ▶体力回復訓練 convalescence[convalescent] exercise 体力測定 physical strength test / test of physical strength and fitness 体力評価 evaluation of physical fitness

たいわ　対話　☞会話，話す

たいわん¹　大彎　greater curvature of the stomach

たいわん²　台湾　Taiwan　（㊞Taiwanese）
▶台湾人（の） Taiwanese

たいん　多飲　excessive thirst, polydipsia　◀心因性多飲 psychogenic polydipsia

たいんし　多因子（の）　multifactorial
▶多因子遺伝病 multifactorial inheritance disease

ダウンしょうこうぐん　─症候群　Down syndrome, trisomy 21 syndrome　◆ダウン症児 a Down syndrome child / a child with Down syndrome

だえき　唾液　saliva /səláɪvə/　（㊞sálivary）　◆唾液の分泌 salivary secretion / salivation　◆唾液を飲み込む時喉がつかえますか Do you choke when you swallow your saliva?　◆唾液が出にくいと感じ

ますか Do you feel that your saliva doesn't flow easily?　◆以前と比べて唾液の量が減りましたか Do you have less saliva than you used to?　◆唾液の減少 a decrease in saliva　◀人工唾液 artificial saliva　▶唾液分泌検査 test for salivary secretion　唾液分泌障害 disturbance of salivary secretion　唾液分泌不全 hyposalivation / hypoptyalism　☞唾液腺

だえきせん　唾液腺　salivary gland　▶唾液腺疾患 salivary gland disease　唾液腺シンチグラフィ salivary gland scintigraphy　唾液腺造影 sialography　唾液腺ホルモン salivary gland hormone

たえまない　絶え間ない　（一定の）constant　（連続した）continuous　◆その痛みは絶え間なく続いていますか Is the pain constant? / Do you have the pain constantly[continuously]? / （常に）Are you always in pain? / Do you always have the pain?

たえる　耐える　bear, tolerate, stand, withstand, put up with　（長期にわたって）endure　☞我慢，持ちこたえる　◆苦痛に耐える bear[stand / put up with] the pain　◆化学療法に耐える endure[put up with] chemotherapy　◆お母様は年齢，体力的に手術には耐えられないと思います Considering her age and physical strength, I'm afraid your mother isn't well enough to withstand the surgery.　◆耐えられる痛み（a) bearable[tolerable] pain　◆耐えがたい痛み (an) unbearable[intolerable / excruciating] pain

タオル　towel /táʊəl/　（顔や手を拭く小型のタオル）washcloth, facecloth　◆このタオルで顔を拭いて下さい Dry[Wipe] your face with this washcloth.　◆タオルで体を拭く dry oneself with a towel　◆清潔なタオルで with a clean towel　◆濡れたタオルで with a wet[moist] towel

たおれる　倒れる　（転ぶ）fall over, fall down　（卒倒する）collapse, faint　（病気になる）get[fall] sick, break down　◆失神して倒れる *fall down[collapse] in a faint　◆うつ伏せに倒れる fall flat on one's face　◆仰向けに倒れる fall on one's back　◆過労で倒

たおれる れる *become sick[break down] from overwork

たかい 高い high (↔low) （程度・水準が）elevated （身長が）tall (↔short) （値段が）expensive, costly ◆血圧が高いと言われたことがありますか Have you ever been told *you have high blood pressure[your blood pressure is high]? ◆血圧が高いですね You have high blood pressure. / Your blood pressure is high. ◆LDL コレステロール値が正常値より高めです Your LDL cholesterol is *higher than[high above] normal. ◆高い音や声が聞き取りにくいですか Do you have difficulty hearing high[high-pitched] sounds and voices? ◆残念ながらⅢa 期の肺がんは高い割合で再発します Unfortunately, stage-three-a lung cancer has a high rate of recurrence. ◆緑内障を放置すると高い確率で視力を失い失明に至ります If not treated in time, there's a high probability that glaucoma will lead to loss of vision and, ultimately, to blindness. ◆平均より背が高い be taller than average / have taller than average height ◆この薬剤はかなり値段が高いのが難点です The trouble[drawback] with this medication is that it's *fairly expensive[quite costly].

たかく 他覚(的な) objective (↔subjective) ▶他覚症状 objective symptom 他覚的所見 objective findings[signs]

たかまる 高まる ◆この軟膏は風呂上がりに塗ると効果が一層高まります This ointment is more effective if applied right after taking a bath. / If you apply[use] this ointment right after your bath, it'll be all the more effective. ◆この新薬は臨床試験で有効性が示され，期待が高まっている薬剤です This new drug has been shown to be effective in clinical trials, so we have high hopes[expectations] for it. ◆…に対する不満が高まっている There are increasing complaints[There is growing frustration] about …

たかめる 高める （上げる）raise （増やす）increase （改善する）improve ◆脂肪分の摂りすぎは心臓病の危険性を高めます Too much fat raises[increases] the risk of heart disease. ◆心肺機能を高める improve (the) heart-lung[cardiopulmonary] function ◆検査の精度を高める improve the test's accuracy / make the test more accurate

たかやすどうみゃくえん 高安動脈炎 Takayasu arteritis, Takayasu disease （大動脈炎症候群）aortitis syndrome

たかん 多汗 excessive sweating ▶多汗症 hyperhidrosis

だきおこす 抱き起こす ◆抱き起こして座らせる help *the person* sit up by putting *one's* arms around him〈her〉

だきぐせ 抱き癖 ◆抱き癖は一時的なものですから、できるだけ抱っこしてあげて下さい Your baby's wanting to be held all the time[Your baby's clinging tendency] isn't going to last forever, so please hold [carry] him〈her〉 in your arms whenever you can.

だく 抱く （抱きかかえる）hold … (in *one's* arms) （抱きしめる）hug ◆お子さんをしっかり抱いて下さい Please hold your child firmly[tightly]. ◆赤ちゃんをたくさん抱いてあげて下さい．甘やかすことにはなりませんから Hold your baby a lot. It won't spoil him〈her〉.

たくさん 沢山(の) （数が多い）a lot of, lots of, many （量が多い）a lot of, lots of, much （十分な）plenty of ☞多い，多く，大量，多量 ◆水分をたくさん摂って下さい Please drink *a lot[lots] of water. / Please take plenty of fluids. ◆緑黄色野菜をたくさん食べる eat plenty of dark green or yellow vegetables

たくしあげる たくし上げる roll up ◆ズボン〈シャツの袖〉をたくし上げて下さい Please roll up your *pant leg(s)〈shirt sleeve(s)〉.

タクシー taxi, cab ◆タクシーを呼びましょうか Shall I call a taxi for you? ◆タクシーに乗る take a taxi ◆タクシーで帰る get[catch] a taxi home / go home by taxi ◀介護タクシー care taxi[cab]

▶タクシー乗り場 taxi stand

たくじじょ 託児所 （child）day care facility[center]，《英》day nursery （託児室）（child）day care room ☞保育園

ダグラスか 一窩 Douglas pouch （直腸子宮窩）rectouterine pouch ▶ダグラス窩穿刺術 paracentesis[puncture] of the Douglas pouch ダグラス窩膿瘍 Douglas pouch abscess

たけい 多形・多型 polymorph （形multiform, pleomorphic） ◀一塩基多型 single nucleotide polymorphism；SNP ▶多形紅斑 erythema multiforme 多形細胞癌 pleomorphic cell carcinoma 多形滲出性紅斑 erythema multiforme exudativum

たけいとう 多系統 multiple system ▶多系統萎縮症 multiple system atrophy；MSA 多系統変性症 multiple system degeneration

たけつしょう 多血症 （赤血球増加症）polycythemia

たこ （胼胝）callus ◆それは指しゃぶりのしすぎでできたたこです It's a callus that has formed because of excessive sucking of his〈her〉finger[（親指）thumb].

たこいぼびらん varioliform erosion

たこう 多幸 euphoria

だこう 蛇行 tortuosity （形tortuous） ▶蛇行動脈 tortuous artery

たこきゅう 多呼吸 polypnea

たざいたいせい 多剤耐性 multidrug resistance；MDR ▶多剤耐性菌 multidrug-resistant bacteria 多剤耐性結核 multidrug-resistant tuberculosis；MDR-TB 多剤耐性緑膿菌 multidrug-resistant *Pseudomonas aeruginosa*；MDRP

たざいへいようかがくりょうほう 多剤併用化学療法 combination chemotherapy

たしか 確か（な） sure, certain （正確な）accurate （明確・確実な）definite （正しい）correct, right ◆（残念ですが）確かなことは言えません（I'm sorry, but）I can't say for sure. ◆それは確かです I'm sure[certain] of it. / That's for sure[certain]. ◆確かですか Are you sure? ◆確かな診断を出す make an accurate diagnosis

◆井出先生の腕は確かです Dr Ide is definitely a very skilled doctor. ◆飲酒が悪影響を及ぼすことは確かです Drinking alcohol is definitely *bad for health[harmful]. ◆確かに理論上はおっしゃる通りなのですが，実際にはそううまく運ばないのです In theory, what you say is right, but in practice, things don't work out that way. ◆確か水曜日は都合が悪いとおっしゃっていましたね If I remember correctly[rightly], you said *Wednesday is inconvenient for you[you aren't available on Wednesdays], right?

たしかめる 確かめる （確信する）make sure, be certain （チェックする）check （確認する）confirm ◆確かめるための検査が必要です We need to run some tests to *make sure[be certain]. ◆お名前を確かめて下さい Please confirm that this is your name. ◆渡辺先生に訊いて確かめてみましょう I'll check with Dr Watanabe. ◆新薬の安全性を確かめる check the safety of a new drug

たししょう 多指症 polydactyly

たじゅう 多重（の） multiple ▶多重がん multiple cancer 多重感染 multiple infection 多重人格[解離性同一症] multiple personality / dissociative identity disorder

たしょう 多少 ☞少し

たしょくしゅ 多職種 ☞多専門職

たしょくしょう 多食症 polyphagia （過食症）hyperphagia

だしん 打診する （指先で軽く叩く）tap （叩いて診察する）sound, examine by percussion （考えを探る）sound out ◆胸部の打診をさせて下さい Let me sound your chest. / Let me tap on your chest. ◆治療についてはまず患者さんの考えを打診する必要があります We have to sound out the patient's feelings about the treatment first.

だす 出す ☞出る 《外に移す・送る》（排泄する）pass （液体などを排出する・抜く）drain （流す・垂らす）run, dribble （外に出す）put out, take out （汲み

出す）pump （動かす）move （押し出す）push ◆ガスを出す pass gas ◆尿を出す *pass water[urinate] ◆傷口から膿を出す drain pus from a wound ◆鼓膜を切開して中耳内の液を出す make an incision in the eardrum to drain fluid from the middle ear ◆(上部消化管内視鏡検査で)唾は口から流れるままに出して下さい Please let the saliva run[dribble] from your mouth. ◆ごみは廊下に出さず，スタッフにお申し付け下さい Please don't put the trash out in the hallway. Let the staff[Ask one of the staff to] take care of it. ◆病院の備品を持ち出すことはできません You can't take hospital equipment out. ◆食べ物を腸に送り出す胃の動きが鈍っているのです Your stomach's ability to pump [move] food into the bowel *is poor[has weakened].

《見せる・露出させる》let a person see, show （差し出す・伸ばす）put out, hold out ◆診察券をお出し下さい May I see your ID card? / Your ID card, please. ◆手〈舌〉を出して見せて下さい Let me see your hand (s)〈tongue〉. ◆肺〈お腹〉を診察しますので胸〈お腹〉を出していただけますか I'm going to examine your lungs〈abdomen〉, so could you show me your chest〈abdomen〉? ◆袖をまくって腕を出して下さい Please roll up your sleeve and put out your arm. ◆唇をすぼめて前にぐっと出して下さい Please purse your lips and hold them out as far as you can.

《提示する》 （提出する）hand in, submit （公表する）disclose ◆承諾書〈入院申込書〉をお出しいただけますか Could you *hand in [submit] your written *consent form〈application for admission〉? ◆断りなく患者さんの個人情報を出すことは決してありません We never disclose a patient's personal[private] information without his〈her〉consent. ◆結論を出すのはもう少し先でも大丈夫です It's all right if you need[take] a little more time to come to a decision. / It's all right if you put off coming to a decision. ◆助言はいたしま

すが，答えを出すのはご自分です I can give you (some) advice, but *only you can find the answer to this problem[the answer lies within yourself]. / I'm going to give you a piece of advice, but you have to *solve the problem[find the answer to the problem] yourself. ◆ご意見やご要望があれば遠慮なく出して下さい If you have any questions or requests, please feel free to tell us. / Please feel free to ask questions or make any requests.

《発揮する・発生させる》 ◆思い切り力を出して下さい Please give it all *your strength [the strength you've got]. ◆元気を出しましょう，私たちがサポートしますよ Cheer up! We're here to support[help] you. ◆大声を出すのはやめて下さい Please stop shouting[yelling]. ◆手術後熱を出すのは珍しいことではありません It's not unusual to develop[run] a fever after surgery.

《働きかけを行う》 ◆胃炎の薬をお出しします I'm going to *give you a medication[(処方箋を書く)write a prescription] for your gastritis. ◆指示を出す give instructions [directions]

たすかる 助かる live （図life）, survive （図survival） （回復する）recover （図recovery） （救助される）be saved[rescued] （助けになる）be helpful （図help） ◆彼女は意識が戻ったのできっと助かるでしょう She's regained consciousness, so I'm sure she'll live. ◆彼は助からないかもしれません I'm afraid he may not survive. ◆彼は助かる可能性があると思います I think there's some hope of his recovery. ◆この手術をしないと彼女が助かる見込みはありません Without this surgery, she has no chance of survival. ◆彼が助かる見込みは五分五分です He has a fifty-fifty chance of survival. / His chances of recovering are fifty-fifty. ◆そうしていただけると助かります If you could do that (for me), *it would be a great help[I'd really appreciate it].

たすける 助ける （援助する）help （図help）, aid （補助する）assist （図assistance） （支

援する）give support（図support）（救助する）save, rescue ☞援助, 支える, サポート, 支援 ◆困った時近くに助けてくれる人がいますか If you have any trouble[In times of difficulty], do you have anyone nearby who can help you? ◆助けを求める ask for help ◆助けがいる時はおっしゃって下さい Please let me know when you need any help. ◆患者の歩行を助ける help[assist] the patient to walk ◆これは消化を助けてくれる薬です This medication aids digestion. / This medication is good[effective] for digestion. ◆救急患者を助ける save an emergency patient

たずねる　尋ねる　ask（問い合わせる）inquire ☞訊く ◆お尋ねしたいことがあるのですが May I ask you some questions? ◆病気や治療について質問があれば担当医に遠慮なくお尋ね下さい If you have any questions about your illness or treatment, please feel free to ask your doctor. ◆手続きについては看護師にお尋ね下さい Please ask the nurse about the procedure.

だせき　唾石　salivary stone[calculus]
▶唾石症 sialolithiasis / salivolithiasis

たせんもんしょく　多専門職（の）　interprofessional　▶多専門職（連携）協働 interprofessional work；IPW　多専門職協働医療チーム interprofessional health care team

たぞうきふぜん　多臓器不全　multiple organ failure；MOF ◆彼は多臓器不全という，体中の臓器機能が障害される危険な状態にあります He's in critical condition due to multiple organ failure, meaning that *various organs of his body are not functioning[the function of various organs of his body has failed].

ただ　just, only ☞単なる ◆恐らくただの風邪ですね It's probably just a (common) cold. / You probably just have a cold. ◆ただ食事の摂取量を減らすのではなく, 軽い運動も組み合わせてみて下さい Rather than just cutting down on the amount of food you eat, you should also do light

exercise.

たたい　多胎（の）　multiple　▶多胎児 multiplets / multiple birth offspring　多胎出産 multiple birth　多胎妊娠 multiple pregnancy　多胎分娩 delivery of multiple fetuses / multiple births

だたい　堕胎　illegal abortion, criminal abortion

たたかう　闘う（果敢に挑む）fight（against), battle（with）（困難に対して奮闘する）struggle（with） ◆彼女は勇敢にがんと闘っています She is fighting bravely against cancer. / She is struggling[battling] bravely with cancer. ◆心筋梗塞や脳梗塞の治療は時間との闘いです The treatment of myocardial or cerebral infarction is a race against *the clock [time].

たたく　叩く（指先で軽く打つ）tap（こぶしなどで）knock（平手で）slap（強く打ちつける）hit, strike ◆背骨を軽く叩きます Let me[I'm going to] tap your spine[spinal column]. ◆膝を軽く叩いて反射を調べます Let me[I'm going to] check the reflexes by tapping your knee.

ただしい　正しい（誤りのない）right, correct（良い）good（正確な）accurate（適切な）proper ◆あなたの言うことはまったく正しいです What you say is quite right [correct]. ◆正しい姿勢をとる assume a good posture ◆吸入器の正しい使い方を説明する explain how to use the inhaler properly / explain the proper way to use the inhaler ◆もっと正しい情報が必要である need more accurate[correct] information

ただちに　直ちに　right away, at once, immediately,《英》**straightaway** ☞すぐ

ただれる　爛れる（傷・かぶれを起こして痛む）become sore（図sore）（化膿する）fester（図festering）（炎症を起こす）become inflamed（図inflammation）（粘膜を侵食する）become erosive（図びらん erosion） ◆皮膚が火傷でただれている The skin has become sore from the burn. ◆性器にただれがある have genital sores ◆右足に

ただれができている have a sore on *one's* right leg ◆床ずれがただれてきています（化膿しはじめている）The bedsore has begun to fester. ◆瞼がただれている（炎症をおこしている）The eyelids have become inflamed.

たちあいしゅっさん　立会い出産 ◆立会い出産をご希望ですか（妊婦に対して）Would you like to have your husband〈partner〉in the delivery room? / （夫やパートナーに対して）Would you like to be with your wife〈partner〉in the delivery room *when the baby is being born[for the birth]?

たちあう　立ち会う　be with, be present (at) ◆彼の手術に立ち会う be with him during the surgery ◆彼女の最期に立ち会いました I was with her *in her last moments[when she passed away]. / I was present at her deathbed.

たちあがる　立ち上がる　stand up, get up, rise ☞立つ ◆急に立ち上がるとめまいがしますか Do you feel dizzy when you stand up quickly[suddenly]? ◆椅子から立ち上がる get[stand] up from a chair ◆座った状態から立ち上がるのは難しいですか Do you have difficulty rising *from a chair[from a sitting position]?

たちいる　立ち入る ◆立ち入ったことを伺うようですが，私からの質問は診断や治療を行う上で重要です I'm sorry if I'm being too personal, but my questions are important for diagnosing and treating your illness.

たちくらみ　立ちくらみする　get dizzy, feel dizzy ☞めまい ◆立ちくらみを起こしやすいですか Do you often get[feel] dizzy when you stand up suddenly?

たちば　立場 （観点）**standpoint, point of view** （置かれた状況・位置）**position, place** ◆専門医の立場から助言する give advice *from the standpoint of a specialist[from a specialist's point of view] ◆私の立場では明確にお答えできませんので，そのことについては主治医に訊いて下さい I'm not in a position to say anything definite, so please ask your doctor about that. ◆延

命治療については，彼女の立場になってお考え下さい When deciding about life support measures, ask yourself what she would want[choose]. / Regarding life support measures, please put yourself in her place.

たちむかう　立ち向かう　face … with determination, fight against … with determination ★determination は「決意」「やる気」を意味する. ◆敢然と病気に立ち向かう勇気を持てば必ず克服できます If you courageously face[fight against] your illness with determination, you'll certainly conquer[overcome] it.

たつ[1]　立つ　stand (up) ☞立ち上がる ◆支えなしにお独りで立てますか Can you stand alone without support? ◆立ち続けるのが難しいですか Do you find it difficult to keep standing? ◆前を向いて真っ直ぐ立って下さい Please stand straight with your head facing forward. ◆目を閉じて片足で立って下さい Please stand on one leg with your eyes closed. ◆横を向いて立って下さい Please stand turning sideways.

たつ[2]　経つ　go by, pass by ◆時が経つにつれて痛みは和らぐでしょう As time goes[passes] by, it will be less painful. ◆その手術をしてからどのくらい経ちましたか How long has it been since you had the surgery? ◆1週間経ったらまた来て下さい Please come and see me again in a week.

たつ[3]　絶つ （断ち切る）**break (off)** （やめる）**give up, stop, quit** ◆悪い習慣を断つ break bad habits ◆酒を断つ quit[stop / give up] drinking ◆命を断つ take *one's* own life / commit suicide

だついかご　脱衣かご　clothes basket
だつかんさ　脱感作 ☞減感作
だっき　脱気する （ガスを抜いてしぼませる）**deflate** ◆バルーンカテーテルを脱気する deflate the balloon catheter ◆気胸腔を脱気する remove the air from the pleural cavity

だっきゅう　脱臼する　dislocate （図dislocation, luxation), become dislocated (関節が外れる) slip out of joint[place] ◆脱臼したことがありますか Have you ever dislocated a bone? ◆右肩を脱臼しています You've dislocated your right shoulder. / Your right shoulder has slipped out of joint[place]. ◆脱臼した肘を整復する reposition the dislocated elbow / manipulate the dislocated elbow back into position ◀亜脱臼 subluxation / incomplete[partial] dislocation 顎関節脱臼 jaw dislocation 肩関節脱臼 shoulder dislocation 環軸椎脱臼 atlantoaxial dislocation 頸椎脱臼 cervical dislocation 股関節脱臼 hip dislocation 習慣性脱臼 habitual dislocation 肘関節脱臼 elbow dislocation 反復性脱臼 recurrent dislocation ▶脱臼骨折 dislocation fracture

だっこ 抱っこ ☞抱く

だっこう 脱肛 anal prolapse

だっしにゅう 脱脂乳 skim milk, 《英》skimmed milk ▶脱脂粉乳 powdered skim milk / dried skim milk

だっしめん 脱脂綿 absorbent cotton, 《英》cotton wool （綿球）cotton ball

だっしゅうざい 脱臭剤 deodorant, deodorizer, odor remover

だっしゅつ 脱出 prolapse （⇒prolapsed） ◀臍帯脱出 umbilical cord prolapse ▶脱出痔核 prolapsed hemorrhoids

ダッシュボードそんしょう ―損傷 dashboard injury

だっすい 脱水(症) dehydration （⇒dehydrated） ◆軽度〈中程度 / 重度〉の脱水症です You have mild〈moderate / severe〉dehydration. / You're mildly〈moderately / severely〉dehydrated. ◆体がだるいのや心拍が速くなるのは脱水症の徴候です Physical fatigue[weakness] and a rapid heart beat are signs of dehydration. ◆下痢が続いて脱水症状を起こす *become dehydrated[lose a lot of water] due to continuous diarrhea ◆脱水で弱っている be weak from dehydration[(喉の渇き)thirst] ◆脱水症にならないよう水

分と塩分を適度に摂って下さい To avoid becoming dehydrated, please drink lots of fluids and take enough salt. / Please take the right[proper] amount of fluids and salt so that you won't get dehydrated. ◀低張性脱水 hypotonic dehydration

だつずい 脱髄 demyelination （⇒demyelinate） ▶脱髄疾患 demyelinating disease 脱髄性多発ニューロパチー demyelinating polyneuropathy 脱髄性脳脊髄炎 demyelinating encephalomyelitis

だっする 脱する come out of ◆危篤状態を脱する come out of critical condition / be no longer in critical condition

たった just, only 《わずか》 ◆たった 2, 3 分の我慢ですよ. すぐ終わりますから Please *hold on[be patient] for just a few minutes more. You'll be finished soon. 《ちょうど》 ◆上田先生はたった今戻られました Dr Ueda has just *come back[returned] (to his office).

だっちょう 脱腸 ☞ヘルニア

たっぷり plenty of, lots of, a lot of （気前良い）generous （いっぱい・最大の）full ☞十分 ◆野菜をたっぷり食べて下さい Please eat *plenty of[lots of] vegetables. ◆皮膚の乾燥を防ぐために保湿剤をたっぷり塗って下さい Please apply a generous amount of moisturizer to your skin to prevent it from drying. ◆傷は治るまでたっぷり 3 日はかかります It'll take three full days for the wound to heal.

だつもう 脱毛 （脱毛症）hair loss, baldness, balding, alopecia （脱毛術）hair removal ☞禿げ ◆脱毛がみられますか Have you noticed any hair loss? ◆治療中にたぶん脱毛するでしょう You'll probably lose your hair during the treatment. ◆脱毛は化学療法の一時的な副作用で, 髪の毛は治療が終われば生えてきます The hair loss is a temporary side effect of the chemotherapy; it will grow back after the treatment. ◆脱毛の原因はまだ十分にわかっていません The cause of hair loss is not fully understood yet. ◆脱毛剤

を使った跡がかぶれているようですね I'm afraid you've got[developed] a skin rash from using a hair removal product. ◆むらのある脱毛 patchy hair loss ◀円形脱毛症 alopecia areata /（口語的に）spot baldness / patchy hair loss　早発性脱毛症 premature alopecia[baldness]　男性型脱毛症 male pattern alopecia[baldness]　レーザー脱毛 laser hair removal ▶脱毛薬 depilatory

だつりょく　脱力 ▶情動脱力発作 cataplexy ▶脱力発作 drop attack / atonic [drop] seizure ☞脱力感

だつりょくかん　脱力感 （極度の疲労）excessive fatigue[tiredness]　（疲労感）feeling of exhaustion　（力が入らないこと）weakness　（筋無力）adynamia ◆脱力感がありますか Do you feel excessively tired? ◆筋肉に脱力感がありますか Do your muscles feel weak? / Do you feel weakness in your muscles? ◆筋肉の脱力感 muscle weakness

たて　縦（の） （垂直の）vertical　（縦方向の）longitudinal　（幅・距離が長い）long ★英語では長いほうを縦，短いほうを横とする. ◆縦方向 a vertical[longitudinal] direction ◆縦軸 a longitudinal axis ◆この機器は縦15 cm，横10 cm，奥行き3 cmで，重さは500 gです This apparatus is fifteen centimeters long, ten centimeters wide, three centimeters deep, and weighs five hundred grams. ▶縦アーチ（足の）longitudinal arch (of the foot)　縦ひだ（十二指腸の）longitudinal fold (of the duodenum)

たてこむ　立て込む ◆順番を待つ多くの患者さんで立て込んでいますので，もう少しお待ちいただけませんか A lot of patients are still waiting their turn, so could you wait just a bit more? ◆来週は立て込んでいて予約をお受けできません We're busy[（予約がいっぱいで）fully booked] all next week, so I'm afraid we can't give you an appointment.

たてもの　建物　building

たてる　立てる
《起こす》put up, set up ◆仰向けに寝て膝

を立ててお腹の力を抜いて下さい Please lie on your back, put your knees up, and relax your abdomen.
《構築する》set up, build, establish ◆手術の予定を立てる set up a schedule for the surgery ◆まずは実現の難しくない短期目標を立てましょう First, let's set up a short-term goal that won't be so difficult to achieve. ◆仮説を立てる *set up[build / establish] a hypothesis ◆筋道を立てて考えてみましょうか Let's think about this logically. / Shall we think logically?
《怒る》☞怒る ▶腹を立てる get angry [upset] / lose *one's* temper ◆何に腹を立てているのですか What are you angry at [about]?

たどう¹　他動（性の）　passive ▶他動運動 passive movement　他動運動訓練 passive exercise　他動関節可動域 passive range-of-motion；PROM

たどう²　多動（性の） （活動亢進の）hyperactive （图hyperactivity）　（運動亢進の）hyperkinetic ◀注意欠如・多動症 attention deficit hyperactivity disorder；ADHD　注意欠如・多動症児 child with ADHD ▶多動症候群 hyperkinetic syndrome　多動性障害 hyperkinetic disorder

だとう　妥当（な） （事実に基づいて正当な）valid（图validity）　（状況や目的に適った）appropriate（图appropriateness）　（筋の通った）reasonable ◆その判断は妥当でした The judgment was valid. ◆大川先生のとった緊急処置は妥当だったと思います I think the emergency treatment[care] Dr Okawa gave was appropriate[reasonable]. ◆検査の妥当性 the validity of the test / the test's validity

たとえば　例えば　for example, for instance （…のような）such as ◆最近服用した薬がありますか，例えば鎮痛薬など Have you recently taken any medications? Any painkillers, for example? ◆胃に何か問題はありませんでしたか，例えば吐き気や嘔吐など Have you had any stomach trouble, such as nausea or vomiting? ◆他に気になることがあればお

話し下さい，例えば家庭生活や仕事など Please let me know if you have any other concerns—for example, about your family life or work.

たどたどしい **unsteady, faltering** ◆たどたどしい足取りで歩く walk with unsteady [faltering] steps / walk with *an unsteady [a faltering] gait

ダニ **mite** （マダニ）**tick** ◆ダニに刺されたのかもしれません You may have been bitten by a tick. ◆お宅に住むダニの糞や死骸などがアレルギーの原因になっている可能性があります The droppings and carcasses of dust mites in your house may be causing your allergy. ◀室内塵ダニ house dust mite ▶ダニアレルギー mite allergy　ダニ媒介疾患 tick-borne disease

たにょう **多尿（症）** **polyuria**; *passage of excessive amounts of urine* ◆夜間多尿 nocturia / nycturia

たにんきょうふ **他人恐怖** **xenophobia**; *fear of strangers*

たのうほう **多嚢胞（性の）** **polycystic, multicystic** ▶多嚢胞腎 polycystic kidney disease；PCKD［PKD］　多嚢胞性異形成腎 multicystic dysplastic kidney　多嚢胞性卵巣症候群 polycystic ovary［ovarian］syndrome；PCOS

たのしい **楽しい** **happy** ◆一番楽しいと感じるのはどんな時ですか When are you at your happiest? / When do you feel most happy? ◆何をしても楽しくないと感じることはありますか Do you ever feel unhappy *no matter what you do［whatever you do］? / Do you ever feel that whatever you do, you can't *cheer up［feel happy］? ◆コンピュータゲームをするのは楽しいですか Do you enjoy playing computer games? ◆楽しい休暇を！ Have a good vacation!

たのしみ **楽しみ** 《楽しいこと》（喜び）**joy, pleasure** （気晴らし）**pastime** （趣味）**hobby** ◆患者さんの笑顔を見るのが私たちの楽しみです Seeing our patients smile is our joy. / It's our pleasure to see patients smile. ◆今楽し

みにしていることは何ですか What do you most enjoy doing? / What's your favorite pastime［hobby］?

《心待ち》**look forward to …** ◆またお会いするのを楽しみにしています I'm looking forward to seeing you again. ◆久しぶりにお家に帰るのが楽しみでしょう You must be really happy to go home［You must be looking forward to going home］after such a long time.

たのみ **頼み** （願い事）**favor** （要望）**request** ☞依頼 ◆頼みがあるのですが Could［Can］you do me a favor? / I have a favor to ask of you.

たばこ **煙草・タバコ** （紙巻き煙草）**cigarette** （刻み煙草）**tobacco** ◆煙草の煙 cigarette smoke ◆煙草の灰 cigarette ash ◆煙草の吸い殻 cigarette butt ◆院内でのお煙草はご遠慮下さい Smoking is prohibited［not allowed］anywhere inside the hospital.

《喫煙状況を訊く》 ◆煙草を吸いますか Do you smoke? ◆煙草を吸ったことがありますか Have you ever smoked? ◆煙草を吸い始めたのは何歳の時ですか How old were you when you started smoking? ◆煙草は 1 日に何本〈何箱〉吸いますか How many cigarettes〈packs of cigarettes〉a day do you smoke? ◆煙草を大量に吸う be a heavy smoker / smoke heavily

《禁煙を勧める》 ◆煙草は吸わないで下さい You should not smoke. ◆煙草はやめるべきです You should quit［give up］smoking. ◆煙草はあらゆる面で体に害があります Smoking is bad for your health in every respect. ◆煙草は心臓病やがんのリスクを高めます Smoking increases the risk of heart disease and cancer. ◆煙草は周囲の人にも害になるということを認識して下さい You should realize that smoking is also harmful［dangerous］to those around you. ◆煙草をやめるのを助けてくれる薬があります There are medications that can help you quit smoking. ◆煙草の量を減らす cut down on smoking

▶タバコ依存 tobacco dependence　タバコ嗜癖 tobacco addiction　タバコ中毒 tobacco poisoning

たはつ　多発(性の)　multiple（多病巣性の）**multifocal**（多中心性の）**multicentric**（接頭poly-）　▶多発外傷 multiple trauma　多発がん multifocal[multicentric] cancer　多発関節痛 polyarthralgia　多発奇形 multiple anomalies[malformations]　多発血管炎 polyangiitis　多発骨折 multiple fractures　多発根神経炎 polyradiculoneuritis　多発神経炎 polyneuritis　多発性関節炎 polyarthritis　多発性筋炎 polymyositis；PM　多発性硬化症 multiple sclerosis；MS　多発性骨髄腫 multiple myeloma　多発性内分泌腫瘍 multiple endocrine neoplasia；MEN　多発単ニューロパチー multiple mononeuropathy　多発ニューロパチー polyneuropathy

ダブる　☞重複(ちょうふく)　◆物がダブって見えますか Do you see double?　◆申し訳ありません，同じ検査がダブって予約されていますので片方をキャンセルします I'm sorry, but the same tests have been booked for the same time slot, so I'm going to cancel one of them.　◆他の先生からのお薬とダブるようでしたら，調整して処方します If you've already been given this medication by another doctor, I'm going to adjust the prescription.

たぶん　☞恐らく

たべあわせ　食べ合わせ　◆この薬はグレープフルーツとの食べ合わせが悪いので注意して下さい（食べないで下さい）Do not take grapefruit with this medication as harmful problems[side effects] might occur.

たべさせる　食べさせる　let[help] *a person* eat（食べ物を与える）**feed**　◆子供にファーストフードをあまり食べさせるのはよくありません It's not wise[a good idea] to let children eat a lot of fast food.　◆息子さんが固形物を飲み込みづらいようでしたらゼリーやプリンなど軟らかいものを食べさせて下さい If your son has difficulty swallowing solid foods, please feed[give]

him soft foods such as jello or pudding.　◆食べさせる時にはゆっくり彼女のペースに合わせるよう心掛けて下さい When you help her eat, you should always try to *take your time and adjust to her eating pace[feed her at a rate that is comfortable for her].

たべすぎる　食べ過ぎる　overeat, eat too much　◆食べ過ぎで腹痛を起こす get [have] (a) stomachache from overeating

たべもの　食べ物　food　★特定の食べ物の種類について言う場合は数えられる名詞として foods とするが，食べ物全般をさす場合には，'s' を付けずに food のみにする。☞食，食事，食品，食物(しょくもつ)　◆食べ物にアレルギーがありますか Are you allergic to any foods? / Do you have any food allergies?　◆宗教上，制限のある食べ物はありますか Are there any foods you shouldn't eat for religious reasons? / Do you have any religious food restrictions?　◆食べ物はどんなものがお好きですか What kind of food do you like? / What's your favorite kind of food?　◆食べ物に好き嫌いはありますか Do you have likes and dislikes in food? / Are there any foods you won't eat?　◆体に合わない食べ物がありますか Do you have foods that don't agree with you[your stomach]?　◆食べ物をよく噛む chew food well　◆固形の食べ物(a) solid food　◆栄養価の高い食べ物(a) highly nutritious[nourishing] food　◆鉄分の多い食べ物(an) iron-rich food　◆消化に良い食べ物(an) easily digestible food / (a) food that is easy to digest　◆塩辛い食べ物(a) salty food　◆辛い食べ物(a) spicy food　◆脂っこい食べ物(a) fatty[greasy / oily] food /(しつこい) heavy food

たべる　食べる　eat, have　☞食事，食べさせる，食べ過ぎる，食べ物　◆ふだん何を食べていますか What do you usually eat?　◆朝食には何を食べましたか What did you eat[have] for breakfast?　◆食べられないものがありますか Is there anything you can't eat?　◆検査前の2時間は食べたり

飲んだりしないで下さい Please don't eat or drink anything for two hours before the test. ◆一度に少しずつ食べる eat a little at a time ◆大量に食べる eat[(暴食する)binge on] large amounts of food ◆食べることに気がとがめる feel guilty about eating ◆食べ始めるとやめられなくなる find it difficult to stop eating ◆食べた後無理に吐く induce vomiting after eating

たぼう¹ 多忙(な) busy ☞忙しい

たぼう² 多房(性の) multilocular ▶多房性膿瘍 multilocular abscess

だぼくしょう 打撲傷 bruise /brúːz/ (圏打撲傷を負う be[get, become] bruised), contusion ☞あざ ◆打撲傷ですね, 骨には特に異常はありません You're bruised, but there's nothing wrong with the bone. ◆右足に打撲傷を受ける get a bruise on one's right leg / be[get] bruised on one's right leg ◆全身にひどい打撲傷を負う be[get] badly bruised all over

たまご 卵 egg ◆卵にアレルギーがありますか Are you allergic to eggs? ◆卵の白身 the white of an egg ◆卵の黄身 the yolk of an egg ▶卵過敏症 egg sensitivity[hypersensitivity]

たまたま ☞偶発

たまる 溜まる build up (図buildup), accumulate (図accumulation) (積み重なる) pile up ◆膝にかなり水がたまっているので抜いて痛みをとりましょう A large amount of water has *built up[accumulated] in your knee, so let's remove[drain] it to help relieve the pain. ◆傷口に膿がたまっているようです Pus seems to have *built up[accumulated] in the wound. ◆疲労がたまっていて朝起きられないのですか Do you have difficulty getting out of bed in the morning *because you're too tired[because of severe fatigue]? ◆ストレスがたまっているようですね It seems you've had[built up] a lot of stress. / I'm afraid you've been under a lot of stress. ◆入院中に仕事がたまらないか気掛かりなのですね You're concerned

that your work may pile up while you're in the hospital, aren't you? ◆趣味を持つことでたまったストレスを解消する release[get rid of] built-up stress by having a hobby ◆歯垢がたまっている have a buildup of plaque on one's teeth ◆お腹にガスがたまる have gas in one's bowels / have intestinal gas

だまる 黙る 《言葉を発しない》not say anything ◆彼の訴えを黙って聴いてあげるだけで十分慰めになります Just listening to his complaints quietly[without saying anything] *gives him a lot of comfort[is a great comfort to him]. ◆息子さんは部屋に閉じこもって黙り込んでいることがよくありますか Does your son often stay in his room *without saying anything to anyone[refusing to talk]? 《口外しない》not mention (秘密にする) keep … a secret ◆ご家族にはこのことは黙っていたほうがよいですか Would you rather I didn't mention this to your family? / Do you want me to keep this a secret from your family? 《圏許可を得ないで》without permission ◆黙って外出されては困ります Please don't leave the hospital without permission.

ため 為 for ◆エレベーターではなく階段を使うと健康のためになります It'll be good for your health if you take the stairs instead of the elevator. ◆激しい運動はあなたのためになりません(よくない)Strenuous exercise will do you no good.

だめ 駄目 (役に立たない)no good, no use (するべきではない)shouldn't ◆いろいろ試してみましたが駄目でした I tried various approaches, but they were no good. ◆今晩はお酒を飲んでは駄目です You shouldn't drink alcohol tonight.

ためいき 溜め息 sigh

ダメージ damage /dǽmɪʤ/ ☞損傷 ◆喫煙は心臓に深刻なダメージを与えます Smoking can cause[do] serious damage to your heart. ◆大きな精神的ダメージを

ためす 試す　try（図try 試用 trial）（試してみる）give *something* a try, try out　◆試しにこの薬で様子を見て下さい Please *try out this medication[give this medication a try] and see how it works.　◆試しにやってみましょう Let's give it a try.

ためらいきず ためらい傷　hesitation mark[cut], tentative wound　◆手首のためらい傷 hesitation mark on *one's* wrist

ためらう hesitate　◆手術をためらわれる一番の理由は何ですか What's the biggest [most important] reason *that makes you hesitate[for you to hesitate] to have the surgery?

ためる 溜める　store　◆尿はすべてこの蓄尿器にためて下さい Please use this bag [storage container] to store all your urine. / Please store all your urine in this bag[container].

たもう 多毛　excessive growth of hair （男性型多毛）hirsutism　▶多毛症 hypertrichosis

たもつ 保つ　（ある状態を維持する）keep, hold, maintain　（同じ場所にとどまる）stay, remain　◆健康を保つ keep healthy / *stay in[maintain] good health　◆バランスを保つ keep *one's* balance　◆血圧を一定に保つ keep *one's* blood pressure stable [steady]　◆冷静さを保つ keep[stay / remain] calm / stay[keep] cool　◆腕を横に伸ばして肩の位置に保って下さい Please stretch your arms out to the sides and hold them at shoulder level.　◆院内は1年中快適な温度を保つよう設定されています This hospital is kept at a comfortable temperature *year-round[throughout the year]. / The temperature of this hospital is kept at a comfortable level year-round.

たようせい 多様性　diversity　◆文化的多様性 cultural diversity / multiculturalism　◆民族的多様性 ethnic diversity

たよる 頼る　（助けを求める）turn to *a person*（for help）（依存する）depend（on）（当てにする）rely（on）　◆頼れる人がいます

か Do you have someone⟨anyone⟩ you can *turn to for help[rely on]?

たらす 垂らす　drip（絞って入れる）squeeze（into）（よだれを）drool, dribble （鼻水を）have a runny nose　◆この点眼液を1日4回，1滴ずつ両眼に垂らして下さい Please squeeze one drop of this eye lotion into each eye four times a day.　◆この時期の赤ちゃんがよだれを多く垂らすのはごく普通のことです It is quite normal for a baby to drool a lot at this age.

タリウム thallium　▶タリウム中毒 thallium poisoning

たりない 足りない　lack, be deficient （in）　☞足りる，不足　◆鉄分が足りないようです It seems you have an iron deficiency. / It seems you lack[are deficient in] iron.　◆足りないものは病院内の売店で買うことができます（必要なもの）You can buy any items you may need at the hospital shop.　◆母乳の出が足りない do not produce enough breast milk / have a low breast milk supply

たりょう 多量（の）　a lot of, lots of, a large amount of, a large quantity of, much （豊富な）abundant　（過度の）excessive　☞多い，多く，大量，沢山　◆痰は多量に出ますか Do you cough up a lot of phlegm?　◆多量に吐く vomit a large amount　◆この果物はビタミンCを多量に含んでいます This fruit is rich in vitamin C.　◆出血多量で死ぬ die from *loss of blood[heavy bleeding] / bleed to death　◆多量の睡眠薬を飲む take a large[heavy] dose of sleeping pills / take an overdose of sleeping pills

たりる 足りる　be enough（for）, be sufficient（for）　☞足りない　◆入院中パジャマは2，3枚で足りるでしょう Two or three pairs of pajamas will be enough[sufficient] during your stay in the hospital.　◆次回の外来まで足りるようにお薬を処方します I'm going to prescribe you（with） enough medications to last until your next visit to the outpatient clinic.　◆母乳は足りていますか Is the baby getting enough breast milk? / Are you producing

[Do you have] enough breast milk to feed the baby?

だるい （疲れている）feel tired[exhausted] （動作などが鈍い）feel sluggish （無気力な）feel lethargic （弱っている）feel weak （重い）feel heavy ◆体がだるいのですか Do you feel tired and sluggish? ◆足がだるいのですか Do your legs feel heavy[tired / weak]？ ◆だるいと感じ始めたのはいつからですか Since when have you been feeling sluggish[lethargic]?

タルク talc

たるじょうきょうかく 樽状胸郭 **barrel chest, barrel-shaped chest**

だれ 誰 ☞どなた

《誰が》who （誰でも）whoever ◆今日面会にいらっしゃったのは誰ですか Who came to see you today? ◆付き添うのは誰ですか Who's going to accompany[be with] you? / （面倒を見る）Who's taking care of you? ◆それは誰が聞いても驚くでしょう Whoever hears that will be surprised.

《誰か》（肯定文で）somebody, someone （疑問文・否定文で）anybody, anyone ★疑問文でも yes の答えを想定している場合には someone, somebody を用いる。 ◆あなたはそのことを誰かと相談しましたか Did you talk that over with anybody? ◆誰か病院への送り迎えをしてくれる人がいますか Is there someone[anyone] who can come with you to the hospital and take you home again? ◆誰か頼れる人はいますか Do you have someone[anyone] to *rely on[turn to]? / Do you have someone[anyone] you can depend on? ◆誰か一緒にお話を聞いて欲しい方はいますか Is there anyone[someone] who you'd like to *be with you[have with you] during this talk? ◆私が誰かわかりますか Do you know who I am? / Can you tell me who I am?

《誰にも・誰でも》anybody, anyone ◆この件は誰にも話しませんのでご安心下さい I won't tell this to anybody, so please don't worry. ◆ご家族の方でしたら誰でも結構です Any family member will be fine. / As long as it's a family member, anyone will be fine. ◆普通は誰でもそうするでしょう Anybody would do the same thing.

《誰と》who ◆誰と一緒に住んでいますか Who do you live with? ◆昨日誰と話したか覚えていますか Do you remember who you talked with yesterday? ★会話では whom ではなく、通例 who を用いる。

《誰の》whose ◆誰の許可〈承諾〉が必要ですか Whose permission〈consent〉do you need?

《誰を》who ◆誰を探しているのですか Who are you looking for? ★会話では whom ではなく、通例 who を用いる。

たれあし 垂れ足 **foot drop, drop foot**

たれて 垂れ手 **drop hand**[（手首）**wrist**], **hand**[（手首）**wrist**] **drop**

たれゆび 垂れ指 **drop finger**

たれる 垂れる （滴る）**drip** （流れ出る）**drain** （垂れ下がる）**hang** ◆鼻汁が喉のほうに垂れる *the mucus from the nose[the nasal discharge] drains into the throat

たん 痰 **phlegm** /flém/, **sputum** /spjúː-təm/ ★sputum は主に専門用語として用いる。 ◆悪臭のある痰 foul-smelling phlegm ◆痰がからむ咳 a productive cough / a cough that brings up phlegm ◆少量の痰 *a small amount[a little bit] of phlegm ◆痰を吐く cough up[out] phlegm ◆痰を切る *get rid of[remove / clear] phlegm ◆咳をすると痰が出ますか Do you cough up phlegm? / Do you bring up phlegm when you cough? ◆1日にどのくらい痰が出ますか How much phlegm do you cough up each day? ◆痰に血が混じっていますか Have you coughed up bloody phlegm? / Does the phlegm contain blood? / Is the phlegm mixed with blood? ◆痰が彼女の喉にからんでいます There's phlegm caught in her throat. / Her throat is clogged with phlegm. ◆痰のサンプルは朝早く食事前に採って下さい Please collect the phlegm sample in the early morning before breakfast. ◆このコップに痰を入れて下さい Please cough up some phlegm into this cup. ◆喉にた

まった痰を吸引しましょう I'm going to draw the clogged-up phlegm out of your throat. /（取り除く）Let me clear the congested phlegm from your throat. ◀去痰薬 expectorant　血痰 bloody phlegm [sputum]　粘液痰 mucous phlegm[sputum]　▶痰吸引器 sputum aspirator　痰検査 sputum examination[test]　痰細胞診 sputum cytology　痰培養 sputum culture

痰に関する基本的な表現

■色

どんな色をしていますか What color is the phlegm?

●透明な clear / transparent　●白い white　●白っぽい whitish　●緑色の green　●黄緑色の greenish yellow　●黄色味を帯びた yellowish　●ピンクがかった pinkish　●鮮血の bright red　●暗赤色の dark red / dark-colored　●赤褐色の reddish brown　●赤さび色の rusty　●赤い red　●灰色の gray

■性状

どんな感じの痰ですか What is the[your] phlegm like? / Can you describe the [your] phlegm?

●さらさらした（水様性の）thin /（漿液性の）serous　●どろどろした thick　●ねばねばした sticky / viscous　●粘液性の mucous, mucoid　●膿性の purulent /（膿のような）pus-like　●泡状の frothy / foamy　●点状の血液が混じった blood-stained　●筋状の血が混じった blood-streaked

■におい

痰はどんなにおいがしますか How does the [your] phlegm smell?

●無臭の odorless　●不快な unpleasant　●悪臭がする foul-smelling / bad-smelling

■頻度

どのくらいの頻度で痰が出ますか How often do you bring up phlegm?

●いつも most of the time　●頻繁に often / frequently　●時折 occasionally

たんい　単位　（度量衡の単位）unit　（測定の尺度）measure　☞巻末付録：単位の換算　◀国際単位系 International System of Units / SI units

たんいつ　単一の　single （腰頭mon(o)-）　▶単一遺伝病 monogenic disease　単一刺激 single stimulus

たんおうしょく　淡黄色（の）　light yellow　▶淡黄色野菜 light yellow vegetables

たんか　担架　stretcher　（特に車輪付きの）gurney,《英》trolley　◆（患者を）担架で運ぶ carry *a patient**on a stretcher[by stretcher]

だんかい　段階　（ある過程の時期）stage, period　（歩み・ステップ）step　（局面）phase　◆がんはまだ初期の段階です The Cancer is still in its early stages.　◆段階を踏んで治療を進めていきましょう Let's take the treatment one step at a time. /（ゆっくり慎重に）Let's take it slow and proceed down the treatment path step by step.　◆治療の次の段階に進む go to the next stage of *a person's* treatment / take the next step toward *a person's* treatment　◆最終段階 the end[final] stage[period]　初期段階 the first[initial] stage[period]　睡眠段階 sleep stage　発達段階 stage of development / developmental stage

たんかくきゅう　単核球　mononuclear cell　◀伝染性単核球症 infectious mononucleosis；IM

たんかしそうぐ　短下肢装具　short leg brace；SLB, ankle-foot orthosis；AFO

たんかん　胆管　bile duct （腰頭cholangi(o)-）　☞胆道　◀肝外〈肝内〉胆管 extrahepatic〈intrahepatic〉bile duct　内視鏡的逆行性胆管膵管造影 endoscopic retrograde cholangiopancreatography；ERCP　内視鏡的逆行性胆管ドレナージ endoscopic retrograde biliary drainage；ERBD　▶胆管拡張 bile duct dilatation　胆管狭窄 bile

duct stricture　胆管結石 bile duct stone
☞胆管炎, 胆管がん

たんがん[1]　担がん(の)　**tumor-bearing**
▶担がん患者 tumor-bearing patient　担
がん状態 tumor-bearing condition

たんがん[2]　単眼(の)　**monocular**　▶単眼
視 monocular vision　単眼斜視 monocular strabismus　単眼複視 monocular diplopia

たんかんえん　胆管炎　**cholangitis**　◀原
発性硬化性胆管炎 primary sclerosing
cholangitis；PSC

たんかんがん　胆管がん　**bile duct cancer,
cholangiocarcinoma**　◀肝内胆管癌 intrahepatic bile duct carcinoma　肝門部胆
管癌 hepatic hilar carcinoma

たんき[1]　短期　**short time, short period of
time**（㊣短期間の **short-term**　短期滞在の
short-stay）　◆短期間で体重を減らす
lose weight in a short time　◆短期的な目
標を設定する set a short-term goal　◆日
本での滞在は短期間ですか Are you plan-
ning to stay in Japan for a short period of
time?　◆適切に治療すれば短期間で治り
ます If treated properly, you'll recover
from your illness in a short period of
time.　▶短期記憶 short-term memory；
STM　短期ケア short-term[(急性期の)
acute] care　短期滞在 short-term stay
[residence]　短期滞在者 short-term resident　短期滞在ビザ short-stay visa　短期
入院 short-term[short-stay] hospitalization　短期入院患者 short-stay patient
短期入所施設 short-stay[short-term] facility / (一時的な介護の代行施設)respite
care facility　短期療法 short-term therapy[remedy]

たんき[2]　短気(な)　(すぐかっとなる)**short-
tempered, quick-tempered**　(いらいらし
た)**impatient**　◆ご自分で短気なほうだと
思いますか Do you *see yourself as[con-
sider yourself] a short[quick] -tempered
person?　◆短気を起こさず根気よく治療
を続けていきましょう(そんなに急がないで)
Please don't be in such a rush. Let's
continue[persevere] patiently with the

treatment.

たんきゅう　単球　**monocyte**（㊣**monocytic**）　▶単球性白血病 monocytic leukemia

たんきょく　単極(性の)　**unipolar, mo-
nopolar**　▶単極性うつ病 unipolar[mo-
nopolar] depression　単極性躁病 unipolar[monopolar] mania

たんご　単語　**word**　(語彙)**vocabulary**
☞語, 言葉

たんこうしょく　淡紅色(の)　**pink**　(淡い
ピンク色の)**light pink**

たんこうふはい　炭鉱夫肺　**coal miner's
lung**

たんこぶ　たん瘤　☞瘤(こぶ)

たんさ　胆砂　(胆泥)**biliary sludge**

だんさ　段差　◆段差がありますからご注意
下さい(床が平らでないので)The floor is uneven, so please watch your step. / (掲示)
Uneven Floor (Surfaces). Watch Your
Step.

たんさん　炭酸　**carbonic acid**（㊣飲み物が
炭酸入りの **carbonated**）　▶炭酸飲料 carbonated beverage / soda　炭酸カルシウ
ム石 calcium carbonate stone　炭酸水
soda / carbonated[carbonic] water　炭
酸水素ナトリウム sodium bicarbonate　炭
酸脱水酵素阻害薬 carbonic anhydrase inhibitor / carbonate dehydratase inhibitor
炭酸リチウム lithium carbonate　☞炭酸ガ
ス

たんさんガス　炭酸ガス　**carbon dioxide**
◀動脈血炭酸ガス分圧 partial pressure of
carbon dioxide in arterial blood；$PaCO_2$ /
arterial partial pressure of carbon dioxide　▶炭酸ガスナルコーシス carbon di-
oxide narcosis　炭酸ガスレーザー carbon
dioxide laser

だんし　男子　(男性)**boy**　(男性)**man**（㊣**men**　㊣
male）　☞男性　◆男子学生 a male stu-
dent

たんじかん　短時間(で)　**in a short time**
(短い間)**for a short time**　◆手術は短時間
で終わります The surgery will be over in a
short time. / The surgery won't take so
long.　◆短時間しか眠れないのですか Do

you feel like you sleep for only a short time? ◆時間がなければ短時間でできる運動を行うとよいでしょう If you are short on time, *you can do a short workout[you can try an exercise that you can do in a short time].

だんじき　断食　☞絶食

だんしゅ　断酒　☞禁酒

たんじゅう　胆汁　bile /báɪl/ （㊒biliary, bilious　喉頭chol(e)-）▶胆汁うっ滞 cholestasis　胆汁うっ滞性黄疸 cholestatic jaundice　胆汁うっ滞性肝炎 cholestatic hepatitis　胆汁うっ滞性肝硬変 cholestatic cirrhosis　胆汁酸 bile acid　胆汁色素 bile pigment　胆汁性嘔吐 bilious vomiting　胆汁性腹膜炎 biliary peritonitis　胆汁分泌 bile secretion　胆汁漏出 biliary leak / bile leakage

たんしゅく　短縮　shortening （㊒shorten）◆入院期間を短縮する shorten *one's* hospital stay　◀骨短縮 bone shortening / shortening of a bone　舌小帯短縮症 ankyloglossia / tongue-tie

たんじゅん　単純（な）（簡単な・平易な）simple　（造影剤を用いない）plain　（通常の）ordinary　（未熟練の）unskilled ◆単純な計算問題をしていただきます I'm going to ask you some simple arithmetic questions. / Please answer these simple arithmetic questions.　▶単純X線撮影 plain radiography　単純型 simple type　単純骨折 simple fracture　単純酩酊 ordinary drunkenness　単純労働 unskilled labor ☞単純ヘルペス

たんじゅんヘルペス　単純ヘルペス　herpes simplex ▶単純ヘルペスウイルス herpes simplex virus；HSV　単純ヘルペスウイルス感染症 herpes simplex infection　単純ヘルペス角膜炎 herpes simplex keratitis　単純ヘルペス脳炎 herpes simplex encephalitis；HSE

たんじょう　誕生　birth ◆お子さんのお誕生おめでとうございます Congratulations on (the birth of) your new baby! ◆お誕生日おめでとう Happy birthday (to you)! / Many happy returns of the day!

◆お誕生日はいつですか When is your birthday?

たんしょういんけい　短小陰茎　small penis, micropenis

たんしょくし　探触子　probe

だんじょさ　男女差　（性差）gender differences, differences between the sexes

たんしん　単身で　（独力で）by *oneself* （独りで）alone ◆彼は日本に単身赴任しています He has taken a new post and lives in Japan *by himself*[leaving his family behind].　▶単身世帯 one-person household

たんしんかてい　単親家庭　single-parent family

たんしんけいえん　単神経炎　mononeuritis

たんすいかぶつ　炭水化物　carbohydrate ☞糖質

だんせい¹　男性　man （㊒men ㊒male, virile, masculine　喉頭andr(o)-）◆高齢男性 an elderly man ◆男性看護師 a male nurse　◀副腎性男性化 adrenal virilism ▶男性化 virilism / masculinization　男性型脱毛症 male pattern alopecia　男性更年期 andropause / male menopause[climacteric]　男性不妊症 male infertility　男性ホルモン male sex hormone / androgen

だんせい²　弾性　elasticity （㊒elastic）▶弾性固定 elastic fixation　弾性線維 elastic fiber　弾性ストッキング elastic stockings　弾性組織 elastic tissue　弾性包帯 elastic bandage

たんせき　胆石　gallstone, biliary stone ［calculus （㊒calculi）], cholelith ◆胆石があるようです I'm afraid you have gallstones.　◀コレステロール胆石 cholesterol gallstone　潜在性胆石 silent[asymptomatic] gallstone　浮遊胆石 floating gallstone　▶胆石症 cholelithiasis / gallstone disease　胆石疝痛 gallstone[biliary] colic　胆石破砕術 cholelithotripsy　胆石溶解薬 gallstone-dissolving medication[drug / agent]　胆石溶解療法 gallstone dissolution (therapy)

たんそ¹ 炭素　carbon

たんそ² 炭疽　anthrax　◀皮膚炭疽 skin [cutaneous] anthrax　▶炭疽菌 anthrax bacillus /（学名）*Bacillus anthracis*

だんそう¹ 断層　▶断層画像 scan (image)　断層撮影 tomography

だんそう² 弾創　bullet wound

たんそうきゅう 淡蒼球　globus pallidus, pallidum

だんぞく 断続（的 な）　intermittent, discontinuous（副長い期間にわたって時々 on and off）　◆咳が断続的に出る have an intermittent cough / cough on and off ◆断続的に頭が痛む The headache comes and goes.　▶断続性発語 scanning speech 断続性ラ音 discontinuous (adventitious) sounds / crackles　断続痛 intermittent pain

だんたん 断端　stump　▶断端再発 stump recurrence　断端痛 stump pain

たんたんふんごう 端々吻合　end-to-end anastomosis

たんちょう 単調（な）（変化のない）monotonous（退屈な）dull　◆単調な話し方 monotonous speech　◆単調な生活を送る have[lead] a monotonous[dull] life

たんでい 胆泥　biliary sludge

たんでんい 単殿位　frank breech presentation, single breech presentation

たんとう 担当する　take charge (of)（担当している）be in charge (of)　◆あなたの看護を担当する加藤陽子です I'm your nurse, Yoko Kato.　◆担当の医師は上田俊男です Your doctor will be Dr Toshio Ueda.　◀保健担当者 health officer　☞担当医

たんどう 胆道　biliary tract　☞胆管 ◀経皮経肝胆道ドレナージ percutaneous transhepatic cholangiodrainage；PTCD 先天性胆道閉鎖症 congenital biliary atresia　点滴静注胆道造影 drip infusion cholangiography；DIC　▶胆道がん biliary tract cancer　胆道感染 biliary (tract) infection　胆道ジスキネジア biliary dyskinesia　胆道閉塞症 biliary obstruction

たんとうい 担当医　doctor in charge, one's doctor, attending doctor[physician]　◆担当医の鈴木です My name is Dr Suzuki,（and I'm going to be）the doctor in charge of your care.　◆直ちに担当医を呼んでまいります I'll call your doctor right away.　◆詳しいことは担当医に訊いて下さい Please ask your doctor for further details.　◆担当医の指示に従って下さい Please follow your doctor's[attending physician's] instructions.　◆来週の月曜日から担当医が変わります You'll have a new doctor from next Monday.

たんどく¹ 丹毒　erysipelas

たんどく² 単独（の）　single（副独力で by oneself）　◆単独行動はお控え下さい You shouldn't do things by yourself.　◆抗がん剤を単独で使うより異なる種類を組み合わせたほうがよりよい効果が期待できます You can expect a much better outcome if you use a combination of a few different anticancer medications rather than a single medication.

たんなる 単なる　just, only　☞ただ　◆片頭痛を単なる頭痛と侮ってはいけません Don't dismiss a migraine as just a headache. / Don't *make light of[underestimate] a migraine as just a headache.　◆それは単なる噂にすぎません It's just[only] a rumor.

だんにゅう 断乳する　stop breastfeeding, discontinue breastfeeding　☞離乳 ◆無理に断乳する必要はありません You don't have to stop breastfeeding if you don't want to.

タンニン tannin（形tannic）　▶タンニン酸 tannic acid

だんねん 断念する　give up, abandon ☞あきらめる　◆残念ながら手術〈これ以上の積極的な治療〉は断念せざるを得ません I'm sorry, but we must give up surgery〈more aggressive treatment〉. / I'm afraid surgery〈more aggressive treatment〉is no longer an option.

たんのう 胆囊　gallbladder, cholecystis（接頭cholecyst(o)-）　◀無石胆囊炎 acalculous cholecystitis　▶胆囊炎 cholecystitis 胆嚢管 cystic duct 胆嚢がん cancer of the gallbladder / gallbladder cancer 胆嚢管遺残残症候群 cystic duct remnant syndrome 胆嚢結石 gallbladder stone / cholecystolithiasis 胆嚢摘出術 cholecystectomy 胆嚢ポリープ gallbladder polyp

たんぱく 蛋白 protein /próuti:n/ ◆尿に蛋白が出ています There is some protein in your urine. ◆高蛋白低カロリーの食事を摂るよう心がけて下さい Please try to eat *meals that are high in protein and low in calories[high-protein, low-calorie foods]. ◀血漿蛋白分画 plasma protein fraction；PPF 高〈低〉蛋白 high〈low〉 level of protein / high〈low〉 protein 高〈低〉蛋白血症 hyperproteinemia〈hypoproteinemia〉 高〈低〉蛋白食 high-protein〈low-protein / protein-restricted〉 diet 植物性〈動物性〉蛋白 vegetable〈animal〉 protein 総蛋白 total protein 糖蛋白 glycoprotein 尿蛋白 urinary protein ヘム蛋白 heme protein ベンス・ジョーンズ蛋白 Bence Jones protein リポ蛋白 lipoprotein ▶蛋白合成 protein biosynthesis 蛋白必要量〈daily〉 protein allowance 蛋白代謝 protein metabolism 蛋白同化ステロイド〈ホルモン〉 protein anabolic steroid〈hormone〉 蛋白分解 protein degradation / proteolysis 蛋白分解酵素 protease / proteolytic enzyme 蛋白変性 protein denaturation 蛋白漏出性胃腸症 protein-losing gastroenteropathy ☞蛋白尿

たんぱくにょう 蛋白尿 proteinuria, protein in urine ◀起立性蛋白尿 orthostatic [postural] proteinuria 偶発性蛋白尿 accidental[chance] proteinuria 無症候性蛋白尿 asymptomatic proteinuria

ダンピングしょうこうぐん ―症候群 dumping syndrome

たんぷんちんちゃく 炭粉沈着 anthracosis

だんぼう 暖房 heating ◆暖房を入れる〈切る〉turn the heater on〈off〉 ▶暖房器具 heater

タンポナーデ tamponade ◀心タンポナーデ cardiac tamponade

タンポン tampon

だんめん 断面 cross section, cross-section (㊕cross-sectional) ◆脳の断面図 a cross-sectional image[diagram] of the brain

だんりょくせい 弾力性 ☞弾性

だんれつ 断裂 rupture, tear /téɚ/ ◀アキレス腱断裂 Achilles tendon rupture 筋断裂 muscle rupture 腱断裂 tendon rupture 靱帯断裂 rupture of a ligament / ligament rupture 側副靱帯断裂 collateral ligament tear[rupture] 乳頭筋断裂 papillary muscle rupture 半月板断裂 meniscus tear[rupture]

だんわしつ 談話室 lounge, day room

た

ち

ち 血 **blood** /blʌ́d/ （血**bleed**） ☞血液
≪出血≫ ☞出血 ◆血が出る bleed ◆血が吹き出る blood spurts (from) ◆血を吐く(咳とともに)cough up blood /(消化管から)vomit blood /(口から唾とともに)spit up blood ◆血が滲む(血が筋になって)be streaked with blood /(血の色を帯びて)be tinged with blood ◆血が滲み出る blood oozes (from / out of) ◆血が筋状に滲んだ痰 blood-streaked phlegm ◆血が滲んだ分泌物 blood-tinged discharge ◆血が混じった尿 blood-stained urine ◆尿に血が混じっています There is some blood mixed in the urine. ◆歯茎から血が出ています Your gums are bleeding. / You have bleeding gums. ◆包帯に血が付いています The bandage is stained with blood. / There is some blood[There are some blood stains] on the bandage.
≪凝血・止血≫ ◆血が固まる blood clots / blood coagulates ◆傷口の血は止まっています The wound has stopped bleeding. ◆血が止まりません The bleeding doesn't stop. ◆血の固まり a blood clot / (血栓)a thrombus
≪処置≫ ☞採血 ◆血を止める stop [staunch / stem] the bleeding ◆血を採る take a blood sample / do a blood draw
≪血縁≫ ◆血のつながった家族 a blood-related family member ◆血のつながった親戚 a (close) blood relative / a relative related by blood

チアノーゼ **cyanosis** /sàɪənóʊsɪs/ （形**cy-anotic**） ▶チアノーゼ性心疾患 cyanotic heart disease チアノーゼ発作 cyanotic attack

ちいき 地域 (市町村)**community** （形**re-gional** 地元の **local**） ▶地域医療 com-munity medical[health] care 地域社会 local community 地域住民 local[com-munity] resident 地域病院 community

hospital 地域包括支援センター regional comprehensive support center 地域保健 community health 地域リハビリテーション community-based rehabilitation

ちいさい 小さい **small, little** (音・声が) **low, soft** ◆腎臓に小さな石があります There is a small stone in your kidney. ◆テレビの音を小さくして下さい Please turn down the TV. ◆他の患者さんの迷惑にならないように小さい声でお話しいただけますか Could you speak in a lower voice so as not to disturb the other patients? ◆このあざは小さい時からあったものですか Have you had this mark ever since you were little[a child]?

チーズ **cheese** （形**cheesy**） ★cheesy には「どろどろした」と「臭い」という両方の意味がある. ◆チーズのような(乾酪性の)分泌物がある have (a) cheesy discharge

チーフ ☞主任

チーム **team** ◆医療チームの一員 a member of the medical team ◀医療チーム health[medical] care team 災害派遣医療チーム disaster medical assis-tance team；DMAT 専門職間協働医療チーム interprofessional health care team ▶チーム医療 team[team-based] medical care / team (health) care チームワーク teamwork

チェコ **the Czech Republic** （形**Czech**） ☞国籍 ▶チェコ人(の) Czech

チェック
≪検査・照合・確認≫**check** （動**check**） ◆検査の際は,お名前と生年月日をチェックさせていただきます Before you have the test, let me just check[confirm] your name and date of birth. ◆記載もれがないかチェックして下さい Please check that *there are no omissions[you haven't missed anything].
≪マーク≫**check** (mark),《英》**tick** ◆当てはまる症状があればチェックを入れて下さい Please check any of the following symp-toms you are experiencing. /(横のボックスに)Please put a check[check mark] in the box next to any symptoms you have.

◀メディカルチェック medical checkup

ちえねつ 知恵熱 （生歯熱）teething fever

ちえん 遅延(性の) （遅発の）delayed （長引いている・先延ばしになっている）prolonged （図発育などの不良・遅れ restriction, retardation 排尿などの躊躇 hesitancy） ◀覚醒遅延 prolonged awakening 発育遅延 delayed growth ▶遅延型アレルギー delayed-type allergy 遅延型過敏反応 delayed-type hypersensitivity reaction 遅延射精 delayed ejaculation 遅延性[遷延性] 排尿 urinary hesitancy / difficulty starting the urinary stream 遅延反応 delayed reaction[response]

ちか 地下 （地下室）basement ◆売店は地下にあります The hospital shop is located in the basement. ◆地下2階の検査室へはエレベーターをお使い下さい Please use the elevator to get to the laboratory on basement level two.

ちかい 近い

《距離》close, near, nearby ◆近くの物が見えにくいですか Do you have difficulty seeing things close up? ◆もっと近くに寄って下さい Please come closer. ◆テレビ画面のすぐ近くに座る sit *very close to [near] the TV screen ◆目が近い（近視である）be nearsighted[myopic] ◆近くの病院に通院する go to one's nearby hospital as an outpatient

《時間・程度・間隔》 （ほとんど）almost, nearly （約・おおよそ）about, approximately （間もなく）soon （頻繁に）often, frequently ◆出産が近い It's almost time for the baby to be born. / The baby is due soon. ◆この病状で飛行機に乗るのは不可能に近いです It's almost[nearly] impossible for you to fly[take an airplane] in[with] this medical condition. ◆治療費は10万円近くかかるでしょう Your medical expenses will cost about[approximately] one hundred thousand yen. / It will cost you about[approximately] one hundred thousand yen for your treatment. ◆トイレが近い have to go to the bathroom often [frequently] / *pass urine[urinate] often

[frequently] ◆訓練というよりもレクリエーションに近いですよ This is more like a recreational activity than a training activity.

ちがい 違い difference ☞差 ◆この2つの方法には大した違いはありません There isn't a big difference between these two methods. ◆この2つの治療には明らかな違いがあります There is a distinct difference between these two treatments. ◆意見の違い a difference of opinion ◆正常な細胞と異常な細胞の違い the difference between normal cells and abnormal ones ◆大きな違い a big [major] difference ◆著しい違い a marked difference

ちがう 違う differ, be different （from）, vary ◆症状は似ていますが，気管支喘息は COPD とは違います Although they share many of the same symptoms, *asthma and COPD are different[asthma differs from COPD]. ◆症状は人によって違います The symptoms differ[vary] from person to person. ◆その点はあなたと違う考えをもっています I don't *agree with you[think the same as you] on that point. / I have a different opinion on that point.

ちがえる （筋を）違える （ひねる）twist （筋肉などを無理に伸ばして痛める）pull （捻挫する）sprain ◆首の筋を違える twist one's neck / （筋肉が痙攣する）crick one's neck / get a crick in one's neck ◆足首の筋を違える sprain one's ankle

ちかく¹ 近く ☞近い

ちかく² 知覚 （感覚）sensation, sense, esthesia （認知）（sensory） perception ☞感覚 ◆知覚に異常はありますか Have you noticed any abnormal sensations (anywhere in your body)? ◀空間知覚 space perception[sense] 妄想知覚 delusional perception ▶知覚異常 abnormal sensation[perception] / paresthesia 知覚過敏症 hyperesthesia 知覚神経 sensory nerve 知覚低下 decreased sensation / hypoesthesia

ちかちか ◆目がちかちかして痛みますか Are your eyes irritated and painful? ◆ひどい頭痛がする前にちかちかするような目の症状がありますか Do you have any visual symptoms such as flashing lights followed by severe headache?

ちかづく 近づく (時間的に近づく)**come soon, get close** (接近する)**approach** (そばへ来る) **come near** (そばに行く) **go near** ◆出産予定日が近づいてきましたが何か不安なことがありますか Your due date is *coming soon[getting close / approaching]. *Are you worried about anything[Is there anything you're worried about]?

ちから 力
《体力・筋力》**strength** ◆栄養を沢山とって力をつけて下さい Please eat a lot of nutritious food to build up your strength. ◆足に力が入らない感じがしますか Do your legs feel weak? / Do you have weakness[no strength] in your legs? ◆筋肉の力をつける build up *one's* muscle strength ◆(筋肉に)力が入らない feel weak in *one's* muscles ◆腕にぐっと力を入れて下さい Please tighten your arm muscles. ◆私の手を力いっぱい押して下さい Please push my hands with all your strength. ◆体の力を抜いて下さい Please relax (your muscles). ◆手足の力を抜く relax *one's* arms and legs ◆お腹の力を抜く relax the muscles of *one's* abdomen ◆体の力を抜いて深呼吸して下さい Please let your body go limp and take a deep breath.
《能力》**ability, power** ◆力の限り努力いたします I'll do *to the best of my ability[as hard as I can]. / I'll do everything[all] in my power. ◆できるだけのことをしたのですが, 力が及ばず蘇生できませんでした We did everything we could, but I'm sorry we weren't able to revive him〈her〉. ◆この病気を治すのに一番大切なのは, あなた自身の治そうとする意思の力です The most important thing to cure this illness is your own determination[will-power] to

*overcome it[get well]. ★determination は「決意」を意味する. ◆自分の力でやってごらんなさい Please do it *by yourself[on your own].
《支え, 助け》**support** (動**support**), **help** (動**help**) ◆彼女のそばにいて力になってあげて下さい Please stay *beside her[by her side] to support her. ◆何かお力になれることがございましたらおっしゃって下さい Please let us know if there's anything we can do for you. ◆お力になれず申し訳ありません I'm sorry (that) I can't help you.

ちかん 置換する (整復する)**replace** (図**replacement**) (代用する)**substitute** (図**substitution**) ☞置き換える ◀関節置換術 joint replacement 股関節置換術 hip replacement 人工弁置換術 valve replacement / implantation of a heart valve prosthesis

ちくせき 蓄積する **accumulate** (図**accumulation** 形**accumulated, cumulative**), **build up** ▶蓄積効果 accumulated[cumulative] effect 蓄積線量 accumulated[cumulative] dose 蓄積疲労 accumulated fatigue

チクチクする **tingle** (形**tingling**), **sting, prickle** (形**prickly, prickling**), **prick, smart** ◆チクチクするような痛み(a) tingling[prickly] pain ◆目がチクチクしている *one's* eyes are stinging[smarting]

チクッ **prick** (動**prick, sting**) ◆(注射で)ちょっとチクッとしますよ There'll be a little prick. / You'll feel a slight prick. / It will sting a little.

ちくにょう 蓄尿する **collect and store urine** (図**urine collection**) ◆検査のためにこれから3日間蓄尿して下さい For the *urine test[urinalysis], please collect and store all your urine for the next three days. ◆尿はこのコップに採って蓄尿瓶に貯めて下さい Please collect your urine in this cup and store it in the container [bottle] provided. ◀24時間蓄尿 twenty-four-hour urine collection ▶蓄尿器 urinal

ちくのうしょう 蓄膿症 (慢性副鼻腔炎)

ちくのうしょう 471 **ちち²**

chronic sinusitis

ちくび 乳首 nipple ☞乳頭 ◆サイズ，形，色など乳首に何か変化がありましたか Have you noticed any changes in your nipples, such as changes in the size, shape, or color? ◆乳首から分泌物が出ますか Have you noticed any discharge from your nipples? ◆乳首からの分泌物は何色ですか．What's the color of the nipple discharge? / What color is the nipple discharge? ◆乳首をつまんで分泌物を調べます Let me just pinch[squeeze] your nipples to check for any discharge. ◆乳首が陥没している have *an inverted nipple[a nipple that turns inward]

ちけん 治験 clinical trial ◆治験に参加する participate[take part] in a clinical trial ◆治験へのご協力をお願いできないでしょうか Would you mind participating [taking part] in a clinical trial? ▶治験コーディネーター clinical trial coordinator 治験審査委員会 institutional review board；IRB 治験薬 investigational new drug；IND

ちこう¹ 恥垢 smegma ▶恥垢菌 smegma bacillus

ちこう² 遅効 delayed effect（圏遅効性の delayed, slow-acting） ▶遅効性作用 delayed action 遅効性製剤 delayed-action preparation

ちこつ 恥骨 pubic bone, pubis ▶恥骨結合 pubic symphysis

ちし¹ 致死（性の）（致命的な）fatal（圏fatality）（薬などで致死の）lethal（圏lethality） ◆致死的な傷を負う be fatally wounded ◀過失致死 manslaughter / accidental [involuntary] killing ▶致死率（case）fatality[lethality] rate 致死量 lethal dose；LD

ちし² 智歯 wisdom tooth, third molar（tooth） ☞親知らず ◆智歯が生えてきている one's wisdom tooth is erupting[coming out] ◀埋伏智歯 impacted wisdom tooth ▶智歯周囲炎 pericoronitis (of a wisdom tooth)

ちしき 知識（一般的に）knowledge ☞情報 ◆その病気について正確な知識を得る get accurate knowledge about[of] the disease ◀最新知識 the latest[newest / most up-to-date] knowledge 背景知識 background knowledge 予備知識 preliminary knowledge

ちず 地図 map ◆地図が当院のウェブサイトに掲載されていますのでご覧ください For directions to the hospital, visit the map and directions page on the hospital's website. / Please access the hospital's website to view the map carried on it.

ちずじょうぜつ 地図状舌 geographic tongue

ちたい 遅滞（遅延・遅発）delay（成長などの不良・遅れ）restriction, retardation ◆学業遅滞児 slow learner 子宮内胎児発育遅滞 intrauterine growth restriction[retardation]；IUGR 精神遅滞 mental retardation；MR

ちだらけ 血だらけ（の） bloody, (be) covered with blood

チタン titanium ◆体内にチタンが埋め込んであっても MRI 検査を受けることができます It's OK to have an MRI even though you have titanium implants in your body.

ちち¹ 父 father, male parent（圏fatherly, paternal） ◆父方の祖母 one's grandmother on one's father's side / one's paternal grandmother

ちち² 乳 milk（母乳）breast milk（調合乳）formula（乳房）breast ☞乳（にゅう），乳房，母乳，ミルク ◆赤ちゃんにお乳をあげる breastfeed one's baby / nurse one's baby ◆赤ちゃんはどのくらいお乳を飲んでいますか How much formula[breast milk] does your baby drink? ◆お子さんがお乳をうまく吸ってないとご心配なのですか Are you concerned that your baby is not breastfeeding[sucking] well? ◆お乳の出が十分でない時には哺乳瓶での授乳になります You'll have to bottlefeed your baby if your breasts don't produce enough milk. ◆離乳するとお乳は出なくなります As you wean your baby off breast milk, your breasts will stop producing milk. ◆お乳が張るようなら絞って下さい Please express your (breast) milk if your breasts become (too) full. ◆お乳が張りすぎると腫れたり痛んだりするかもしれません If your breasts become *too full[engorged], they may become swollen and painful. ◆左側のお乳のところに小さなしこりがあります You have a small lump in your left breast.

ちちおや 父親 **father** ☞父

ちぢむ 縮む （小さくなる）**shrink** （虚脱する）**collapse** （短くする）**shorten** ◆気胸のために肺が縮んでいます Your lung has collapsed due to pneumothorax. ◆加齢で背が縮む shrink in height with age ◆寿命を縮める shorten *one's* life

ちちゅうかいねつ 地中海熱 **Mediterranean fever**

ちつ 膣 **vagina** /vədʒáinə/ （膣**váginal**）◆膣からおりものが出ますか Do you have any *vaginal discharge[discharge from the vagina]? ◆膣からの出血がありますか Do you have any vaginal bleeding [hemorrhage]? ◆膣の乾燥 vaginal dryness ◆膣のかゆみ vaginal itching ◆性交後に膣から出血する have vaginal bleeding after intercourse ▶膣鏡 vaginal speculum / vaginoscope 膣トリコモナス症 vaginal trichomoniasis 膣内診 vaginal exam[examination] 膣用ゼリー vaginal jelly ☞膣炎

ちつえん 膣炎 **vaginitis** ◀カンジダ膣炎 *Candida* vaginitis / vaginal candidiasis 淋菌性膣炎 gonococcal vaginitis

チック tic ◆お子さんに顔のチックがありますか Does your child have any (facial) tics? ◆チックの回数を減らす reduce the frequency of the tics ◀顔面チック facial tic 痙攣性チック convulsive tic 習慣性チック habit[habitual] tic ▶チック症 tic disorder

ちっそ 窒素 **nitrogen** （窒**nitric, nitrous**）◀亜酸化窒素 nitrous oxide / （笑気）laughing gas 一酸化窒素 nitric oxide / nitrogen monoxide 液体窒素 liquid nitrogen 過酸化窒素 nitrogen peroxide 血液尿素窒素 blood urea nitrogen；BUN 高窒素血症 hyperazotemia / azotemia 二酸化窒素 nitrogen dioxide ▶窒素酸化物 nitrogen oxide

ちっそく 窒息する （気道が塞がれて息が止まる）**choke** （酸素不足で死ぬ）**suffocate** （窒**suffocation**）◆もちが喉に詰まって窒息する choke on a piece of rice cake ◆窒息死する choke to death / suffocate ◆火事で窒息死する die of[from] suffocation in a fire ▶窒息死 death from suffocation

ちてき 知的（な）**intellectual** ▶知的障害 intellectual disability[disorder / impairment] / mental retardation 知的障害者〈障害児〉child〈person〉with an intellectual disability / intellectually challenged child〈person〉 知的能力 intellectual ability

ちのう 知能 **intelligence, intellectual ability** ◆知能を測る measure intelligence ◆高い〈低い〉知能 high〈low〉intelligence ◆知能の発達には個人差がありますから心配する必要はありません Intelligence develops at different rates in different people[Intelligence development varies from person to person], so don't worry. ◆人工知能 artificial intelligence ▶知能検査 intelligence test / *intelligence quotient[IQ] test 知能障害 impairment of intelligence / mental disturbance 知能年齢 intelligence age 知能発達 intellectual development ☞知能指数

ちのうしすう 知能指数 **intelligence quotient；IQ** ◆知能指数を測る measure *a person's* IQ ◆知能指数の数値が高い〈低い〉have a high〈low〉IQ score

ちばしる 血走る （充血した）**bloodshot** ◆彼女の目は血走っている Her eyes are bloodshot. / She has bloodshot eyes.

ちはつ 遅発（性の）**late, delayed** ◀思春期遅発 delayed puberty ▶遅発型アレルギー反応 late-phase allergic reaction 遅発月経 delayed menstruation 遅発効果 delayed[late] effect

チフス （腸チフス）typhoid fever （パラチフス）paratyphoid fever （発疹チフス）epidemic typhus

チベット Tibet （形Tibetan）▶チベット人（の）Tibetan

ちほう¹ 地方 ☞地域

ちほう² 痴呆 ☞認知症

ちまめ 血豆 blood blister （斑状出血）blot hemorrhage ◆指に血豆ができる get a blood blister on *one's* finger

ちみゃく 遅脈 slow pulse, pulsus tardus

ちめいしょう 致命傷 fatal injury［wound］ ◆頭に致命傷を受ける suffer a fatal *injury to the head［head injury］ ★最終的に助かる場合には a very serious injury という.

ちめいてき 致命的（な） fatal ☞致死 ◆肺がんが脳に転移したのが致命的でした It was fatal that the cancer had spread［metastasized］to the brain.

ちもう 恥毛 pubic hair

ちゃ 茶 tea （日本茶）green tea, Japanese tea （紅茶）black tea ◆お茶をいかがですか How about a cup of tea? ★この場合, ふつうは紅茶を指す. ◆薬はコーヒー, お茶, ジュースと一緒に飲まないで下さい Please don't take the medication with coffee, tea, or juice.

チャイルドシート child （safety） seat

ちゃいろ 茶色（の） brown ◆コーヒーかす様の濃い茶色の吐物 dark brown vomit that looks like coffee grounds ◀薄茶色 light brown 焦げ茶色 dark brown

ちゃくじつ 着実（に） steadily ◆肝機能は着実に改善しています Your liver function is improving steadily.

ちゃくしょう 着床 （embryo） implantation ▶着床前診断 preimplantation assessment［diagnosis］ 着床部位 implantation site

ちゃくしょくりょう 着色料 coloring （matter） ◀人工着色料 artificial coloring

ちゃくよう 着用する （体に着ける）put on （↔take off） （着ている）wear ◆集中治療室の中ではマスク, 帽子, ガウンを着用して下さい Please *put on［wear］a mask, cap,

and gown in the intensive care unit.

チャペル chapel ◀院内チャペル hospital chapel

ちゃんと （確かに・間違いなく）definitely （正しく・正確に）exactly （適切に）properly （規則的に）regularly ☞きちんと ◆頑張れば結果にちゃんと表れます If you work［try］hard, *good results will definitely follow［your efforts will be well rewarded］. ◆口を利くことはできませんが, 彼にはこちらの声はちゃんと聞こえているはずです Even though he's unable to speak, he should be able to hear exactly what we're saying. ◆院内規則をちゃんと守って下さい Please follow the hospital （rules and） regulations properly. ◆3度の食事は毎日ちゃんと食べていますか Do you eat regularly three times a day? / Do you eat［have］three regular meals a day? ◆この薬はちゃんと服用して下さい Please be sure to take this medication exactly as directed. ◆ちゃんと座れますか（姿勢正しく）Can you sit up properly［straight］?

ちゆ 治癒 （病気が治ること）cure （形治癒力がある curative 治癒可能な curable） （傷が癒えること）healing ◀回復, 治る ◀完全治癒 complete cure 自然治癒 spontaneous cure／natural healing ▶治癒手術 curative surgery 治癒率 curative ratio

チュアブルじょう ―錠 chewable tablet ◆チュアブル錠は飲み込む前に完全に口の中で溶かして下さい Please allow these chewable tablets to completely melt in your mouth before swallowing.

ちゅう 中（の） （平均）average （図average） （中くらい・Mサイズ）medium （真ん中）middle ◆中の上〈下〉である be above〈below〉average ◆ガウンは大中小のどのサイズにしますか What size gown do you want? Small, medium, or large? ★この場合は, 通例 small を先にする.

―ちゅう ―中 in （…の間）during, while ◆午前中に in the morning ◆食事中に during a meal／while *one* is having a meal ◆睡眠中に during sleep ◆運動中に during exercise ◆鈴木先生

は今外来患者さんの診察中です Dr Suzuki is now *seeing outpatients[on duty in the outpatient clinic].

ちゅうい 注意する (気を配る)be careful (of, to do), take care (of, to do) (用心・警戒する)pay attention (to), watch (注意をひく)get attention, attract attention ◆体重が増えすぎないように注意して下さい Please be careful not to gain too much weight. ◆風邪をひかないように十分注意して下さい Please *take good care[be careful] not to catch a cold. ◆健康に十分注意して下さい Please take good care of yourself. ◆注意して Be careful! ◆大変申し訳ありません。私の注意不足でした I'm awfully sorry. *I wasn't careful enough (with that)[I should have been more careful]. ◆足元にご注意下さい Please watch your step. ◆転ばないように注意して歩く walk carefully so as not to fall down ◆あなたの血圧は要注意です Your blood pressure requires careful medical attention. / You should watch your blood pressure. ◆彼女の血圧を注意深くモニターする必要があります Her blood pressure needs to be carefully monitored. ◆最近注意力が低下していると感じますか Do you feel that *you have a shorter attention span[your attention span has decreased] recently? ◆お子さんが騒いだのは注意を引くためだったかもしれません Your child must have made a fuss just *to attract attention[because he ⟨she⟩ wanted some attention]. ☞注意欠如多動症，注意事項

ちゅういけつじょたどうしょう 注意欠如多動症 attention deficit hyperactivity disorder；**ADHD** ▶注意欠如多動症児 child with ADHD

ちゅういじこう 注意事項 (指示)instructions (心に留め置くべきこと)things to note ★いずれも通例，複数形で．◆注意事項をよくお読み下さい Please read the instructions carefully. ◆注意事項は必ず守って下さい Please make sure to follow the instructions.

ちゅういんとう 中咽頭 oropharynx (圏oropharyngeal) ▶中咽頭がん oropharyngeal cancer / mesopharyngeal cancer；MPC

ちゅうおう 中央 (中心点)the center (圏central) (中心部)the middle (圏middle 中央値の median) ◆ナースステーションは病棟の中央にあります The nurses' station is located in the center of the ward. ◆胸部の中央に限局した痛み pain localized to the center[middle] of the chest ◆生存期間の中央値 median survival

ちゅうかん 中間(の) (真ん中の)middle (中くらいの)medium (程度・段階が中の)intermediate (場所・地点が途中の)halfway, midway ▶中間位 intermediate position 中間型インスリン intermediate-acting insulin 中間管理職 middle management 中間施設 halfway house / rehabilitation facility ☞中間尿

ちゅうかんにょう 中間尿 midstream urine

ちゅうき 中期 the middle stage[period] ▶妊娠中期 the middle stage of pregnancy / the second trimester of pregnancy

ちゅうこく 忠告 advice /ədváıs/ (動advise /ədváız/) ★advice は数えられない名詞なので，1つの情報は a piece of advice という．☞助言，勧める ◆一言忠告しておきますが，決して無理はしないで下さい Let me give you a piece of advice; *don't overdo things[don't push yourself too hard]. ◆禁煙するように忠告します My advice (to you) is to stop[quit] smoking. / I'd like to advise you not to smoke. ◆市販薬を飲まないように忠告する advise *a person *not to take[against taking] over-the-counter drugs ◆忠告に従う follow [take] someone's advice ◆担当医の忠告に従って1週間学校を休む stay home from school for a week on the advice of one's doctor

ちゅうごく 中国 China (圏Chinese) ☞国籍 ▶中国医学 Chinese medicine 中国人(の) Chinese

ちゅうさつもうそう 注察妄想 delusion of observation

ちゅうし[1] 注視 gaze ◀上方注視麻痺 upward gaze palsy 垂直注視麻痺 vertical gaze palsy 水平注視麻痺 horizontal gaze palsy ▶注視眼振 gaze nystagmus

ちゅうし[2] 中止する stop （中断する）discontinue （一時的に中断する）suspend （断念する）give up （破棄・解消する）cancel ☞止める(やめる) ◆吐き気や嘔吐がある時は直ちに薬の使用を中止して下さい Please stop the medication at once if you experience any nausea or vomiting. ◆症状が改善しないので化学療法は一時中止しましょう Let's discontinue[stop] the chemotherapy[We have to cancel your chemotherapy] because your condition hasn't improved.

ちゅうじ 中耳 middle ear ☞中耳炎

ちゅうじえん 中耳炎 otitis media /oʊˈtaɪtɪs míːdiə/, middle-ear infection ◀化膿性中耳炎 suppurative otitis media 航空中耳炎 aerotitis media 滲出性中耳炎 otitis media with effusion；OME / secretory otitis media；SOM

ちゅうししょう 虫刺症 insect bite

ちゅうしゃ[1] 注射 injection, shot ◆左腕に注射をしましょう I'm going to[Let me] give you *an injection[a shot] in your left arm. ◆インフルエンザの予防注射は受けましたか Did you have a flu shot[injection]? ◆これは痛み止めの注射です This shot is for your pain. / This is a shot of pain medication. / This shot is to ease your pain. ◆注射は痛くありません The injection isn't going to hurt you at all. ◆注射した部位をこすらないで下さい Please *avoid rubbing[don't rub] the injection site[area]. ◆インスリンを自分で注射する self-inject insulin ◀インスリン自己注射 self-injection of insulin 関節内注射 intraarticular injection 筋肉内注射 intramuscular[IM] injection 持続性剤注射 depot injection 静脈内注射 intravenous[IV] injection 髄腔内注射 spinal injection 点滴静脈内注射 intravenous

[IV] drip 皮下注射 subcutaneous[hypodermic] injection 皮内注射 intracutaneous[intradermal] injection 腹腔内注射 intraperitoneal injection 予防注射 vaccination / immunization / inoculation ▶注射液[薬] injection 注射器 syringe / injector ☞注射針

ちゅうしゃ[2] 駐車する park ◆ここは駐車禁止ですのであちらの有料駐車場を利用して下さい This is a no-parking area, so please use the pay[paid] parking lot over there. ◀無料駐車区域 Free-Parking Area 有料駐車場 Pay Parking Lot ▶駐車施設 parking facilities 駐車場 parking lot /《英》car park

ちゅうしゃばり 注射針 injection needle, syringe needle ◆誰かと同じ注射針を使ったことはありますか Have you ever shared needles with another person? ◆使用済み注射針は病院へ持ってきて下さい Please bring used needles to the hospital. ◀滅菌注射針 sterile needle ▶注射針刺傷 needlestick injury

ちゅうしゅこつ 中手骨 metacarpal bones, the metacarpals

ちゅうしゅつ 抽出する draw, extract, sample ◆無作為にサンプルを抽出する draw samples at random ◆ペニシリンは青カビから抽出されました Penicillin was extracted from blue mold. ◀無作為抽出 random sampling 無作為抽出標本 random sample ▶抽出調査 sampling survey 抽出物 extract

ちゅうしょく 昼食 lunch ◆昼食をとる have[eat] lunch ◆昼食を抜く skip lunch ◆昼食後30分に薬を飲む take the medication thirty minutes after lunch

ちゅうしん 中心
《中央の位置》（中心点）the center （類central）（中心部）the middle （類middle）
◆ご紹介する病院は市の中心部にあります The hospital I recommend is in the center of the city. ◆心臓は胸の中心部にあります The heart is located in the middle of the chest.
《最も重点を置く部分》 ◆当病院は患者中心

の医療を心がけております We strive to provide patient-centered medical care in this hospital. ◆魚と野菜中心の食事(主成分とする)a fish and vegetable[vegetable-based] diet / a diet based on fish and vegetables ◆食事はお肉が中心ですか Is your diet primarily meat-based? / Do you have a primarily meat-oriented diet? ▶中心暗点 central scotoma 中心暗点計 scotometer 中心視 central vision 中心視野 central visual field / field of central vision 中心視野計 campimeter 中心性肥満 central obesity

ちゅうしんじょうみゃく 中心静脈 central vein ▶中心静脈圧 central venous pressure；CVP 中心静脈栄養[完全静脈栄養] total parenteral nutrition；TPN 中心静脈カテーテル *central venous[CV] catheter 中心静脈穿刺 central venous puncture

ちゅうすい 虫垂 appendix ◆虫垂の切除手術を受けたことがありますか Have you had your appendix (taken) out? / Have you had an appendectomy? ▶虫垂切除術 appendectomy 虫垂糞石 stercolith of the appendix ☞虫垂炎

ちゅうすいえん 虫垂炎 appendicitis /əpèndəsáɪtɪs/

ちゅうすう 中枢 center (圏central) ◆この部位に言語に関わる中枢があります In this region there is *a language-related center[a center involved in language processing]. ◀嚥下中枢 the swallowing [deglutition] center 言語中枢 the speech[language] center 呼吸中枢 the respiratory center 視覚中枢 the visual center 摂食中枢 the feeding center 聴覚中枢 the auditory[acoustic] center 満腹中枢 the satiety center ▶中枢作用 central action 中枢性睡眠時無呼吸 central sleep apnea；CSA 中枢性鎮痛薬 centrally acting analgesic (medication / drug / agent) ☞中枢神経

ちゅうすうしんけい 中枢神経 central nerve (圏central nervous) ◆中枢神経を冒す damage[affect] the central nerves

▶中枢神経系 the central nervous system；CNS 中枢神経興奮薬 central nervous system stimulant / (蘇生薬)analeptic (medication / drug / agent) 中枢神経抑制薬 central nervous system depressant

ちゅうせい 中性(の) neutral ▶中性洗剤 neutral detergent ☞中性子，中性脂肪

ちゅうせいし 中性子 neutron

ちゅうせいしぼう 中性脂肪 neutral fat, triglyceride；TG ◆中性脂肪の値は動脈硬化などいろいろな疾患のリスクの目安になります Neutral fat levels indicate risk factors for various diseases, including arteriosclerosis. ◆中性脂肪を減らす reduce *neutral fats[triglycerides]

ちゅうぜつ 中絶 ☞妊娠中絶

ちゅうそくこつ 中足骨 metatarsal bones, metatarsals

ちゅうだいのうどうみゃく 中大脳動脈 middle cerebral artery；MCA

ちゅうだん 中断する (作業・過程を中途停止する)interrupt (圏interruption) (中止する)discontinue (圏discontinuation) (一時停止する)suspend (圏suspension) (断ち切る)break ☞中止 ◆眠りが中断するので夜のお酒はやめたほうがよいでしょう You should avoid drinking alcohol at night because it can interrupt sleep. ◆重い副作用が出るようなら治療を一時中断しましょう If any severe side effects appear, we're going to temporarily discontinue the treatment. ◆連続性を中断する break[interrupt] the continuity ◀排尿中断 interruption of micturition

ちゅうちょう 注腸 enema /énəmə/ ▶注腸造影検査 contrast enema / barium enema；BE / (下部消化管造影)lower gastrointestinal[GI] series[radiography]

ちゅうていど 中程度(の) (程度が中くらいの)moderate (平均の)average ◆中程度の痛みがある have (a) moderate pain

ちゅうでんきん 中殿筋 gluteus medius (muscle)

ちゅうと 中途(の) ☞途中 ▶中途覚醒 waking up several times during[in] the night / (frequent) nighttime awakening

ちゅうとう 肘頭 elbow point, olecranon

ちゅうとうど 中等度 ☞中程度

ちゅうどく 中毒
《化学物質による有害反応》（毒物・ガスなどによる中毒）poisoning（圏poisonous, toxic）（酒などによる酩酊）intoxication（圏intoxicating）（薬物の過剰摂取）overdose ◆急性アルコール中毒 alcohol poisoning[intoxication] ◆毒キノコの中毒症状 symptom of mushroom poisoning ◆野生のキノコを食べて中毒を起こす be poisoned by eating wild mushrooms / have wild mushroom poisoning
《依存の形成》（麻薬などの嗜癖）abuse, addiction（圏addicted）（中毒者）abuser, addict（腰尾-holic）◆アルコール中毒である be an alcoholic ◆仕事中毒である be a workaholic[work addict] ◆覚醒剤中毒である be addicted to stimulant drugs / be a stimulant addict ◆シンナー中毒になる become addicted to paint thinner
◀一酸化炭素中毒 carbon monoxide poisoning　覚醒剤中毒 stimulant addiction　ガス中毒 gas poisoning　仕事中毒 workaholism / work addiction　食中毒 food poisoning / foodborne disease / (飲料水による中毒)waterborne disease　シンナー中毒 paint thinner addiction[poisoning]　タバコ中毒 tobacco poisoning / (急性ニコチン中毒)nicotine poisoning　ニコチン中毒 nicotine addiction / (依存症者)nicotine addict　農薬中毒 agricultural chemical poisoning / (殺虫剤中毒)pesticide poisoning　ベンゾジアゼピン中毒 benzodiazepine poisoning[intoxication / (過量服薬)overdose]　麻薬中毒 narcotic (drug) addiction / (依存症者)narcotic drug addict[user], (インフォーマルに)junkie[junky]　モルヒネ中毒 morphine poisoning[intoxication / addiction] / (依存症者)morphine addict　薬物中毒 drug poisoning / poisoning by a drug ▶中毒学 toxicology　中毒学者 toxicologist　中毒死 death by poisoning[poisonous substances]　中毒症 toxicosis　中毒症状 poisoning[toxic] symptom　中毒疹 toxicoderma / toxic eczema　中毒性[毒素性]ショック toxic shock　中毒反応 toxic reaction　中毒量 toxic[intoxicating] dose

ちゅうないしょう 肘内障 pulled elbow

ちゅうにゅう 注入 （注射）injection（圏inject）（輸液）infusion ◆血管に造影剤を注入する inject the contrast medium into the blood vessels （肝動脈注入療法(hepatic) transcatheter arterial infusion；TAI ▶注入器 injector / infuser　注入部位 injection site

ちゅうねん 中年 （年齢層）middle age（圏middle-aged), midlife （中年者）middle-aged person （総称的に）people of middle age ◆中年の女性 a middle-aged woman ◆中年の初期 early middle age ◆中年の危機 a midlife crisis ◆中年になると筋力がだんだん衰えてきます Muscle strength gradually deteriorates *with middle age[as we reach middle age]. ◆これは中年に多い病気です This medical condition is common[prevalent] among middle-aged people. ▶中年期 middle age / the middle years of *one's* life　中年太り middle-age spread

ちゅうのう 中脳 mesencephalon, midbrain

ちゅうびこうかい 中鼻甲介 middle nasal concha

ちゅうひしゅ 中皮腫 mesothelioma
◀胸膜中皮腫 pleural mesothelioma / (悪性中皮腫)malignant mesothelioma

チューブ tube ☞管（くだ）◆呼吸用のチューブを口に挿入する put[place / insert] a breathing tube into the mouth ◆栄養チューブを取り外す remove[take out] a feeding tube ◀栄養チューブ feeding tube / nutritional tube　気管チューブ tracheal tube　吸引チューブ suction tube　胸腔チューブ chest tube　シリコーンチューブ silicone tube　ドレナージチューブ drainage tube ▶チューブ[経管]栄養 tube feeding

ちゅうや day and night ◆昼夜逆転している have *one's* days and nights reversed / have day-night sleep reversal

ちゅうよう　中葉　middle lobe　▶中葉症候群 middle lobe syndrome

ちゅうらん　虫卵　parasite egg　▶虫卵検査〈寄生虫検査〉parasite examination

ちゅうわ　中和する　neutralize（図neutralization）　▶中和試験 neutralization test；NT　中和薬 neutralizer

ちょう　腸　（内臓）bowel /báʊəl/（医頭enter(o)-）（大腸・小腸）intestine /ɪntéstɪn/（医intestinal）（結腸）colon /kóʊlən/（医colonic）　◆腸の具合が悪いのですか Do you have any bowel trouble? / Is there anything wrong with your intestines?　◆腸の中を空にするための下剤を差し上げます I'm going to give you a laxative drug to empty[clear] your bowels[intestines].　◆腸を洗浄する cleanse[irrigate] the bowels　◆腸の働きを活発にする stimulate bowel activities / promote regular bowel function　◀十二指腸 duodenum　小腸 small intestine[bowel]　大腸 large intestine[bowel]　直腸 rectum　盲腸 cecum　▶腸運動 intestinal movement /（腸蠕動）intestinal peristalsis, peristaltic movement　腸液 intestinal juice　腸音 bowel sound /（腸雑音）intestinal murmur　腸狭窄 intestinal stenosis　腸憩室 intestinal diverticulum　腸結核 intestinal tuberculosis　腸出血 intestinal bleeding[hemorrhage]　腸上皮化生 intestinal metaplasia　腸生検 intestine[intestinal] biopsy　腸切除術 intestinal resection　腸穿孔 intestinal perforation　腸洗浄 bowel[colonic] irrigation / intestinal lavage / colon cleansing　腸疝痛 intestinal colic　腸通過時間 bowel transit time　腸内ガス bowel gas　腸捻転 intestinal volvulus / twisting of the intestines[bowels] /（捻転した腸）twisted bowels　腸粘膜 intestinal mucosa　腸壁 intestinal wall　腸溶錠 enteric-coated tablet　腸瘻 intestinal fistula　☞腸炎, 腸管, 腸間膜, 腸球菌, 腸重積, 腸癌候群, 腸チフス, 腸内細菌, 腸閉塞, 腸ヘルニア

ちょうい　弔意　☞お悔やみ

ちょうえん　腸炎　（小腸結腸炎）enterocoli-tis /èntəroʊkoʊláɪtɪs/　（特に小腸の炎症）enteritis　▶感染性腸炎 infectious enterocolitis　カンピロバクター腸炎 Campylobacter enterocolitis　偽膜性腸炎 pseudomembranous enterocolitis　虚血性腸炎 ischemic enteritis　▶腸炎ビブリオ Vibrio parahaemolyticus

ちょうおんぱ　超音波　ultrasound /ʌ́ltrəsàʊnd/；US, ultrasónics, ultrasonic waves　★通例, 複数形で.　▶超音波ガイド下生検〈穿刺術〉ultrasonically guided biopsy〈puncture〉　超音波写真 ultrasound film　超音波診断 ultrasound[ultrasonic] diagnosis / echography　超音波洗浄 ultrasonic cleaning　超音波内視鏡検査 endoscopic ultrasound[ultrasonography]；EUS　超音波ネブライザー ultrasonic nebulizer　超音波白内障手術 ultrasonic phacoemulsification　☞超音波検査

ちょうおんぱけんさ　超音波検査　ultrasound（test, exam, examination）, ultrasonography, echography　◆超音波検査をしましょう Let me[I'm going to] do an ultrasound.　◆超音波検査はお腹の赤ちゃんに安全です An ultrasound test is safe for your unborn baby.　◆超音波検査で小さな胆石が2つ見つかりました We found two small gallstones during the ultrasound. / Two small gallstones were found[detected] during the ultrasound.　◀カラードプラ超音波検査 color Doppler ultrasound　経腟超音波検査 transvaginal ultrasound；TVUS　経直腸超音波検査 transrectal ultrasound　経尿道的超音波検査 transurethral ultrasound　心臓超音波検査 cardiac ultrasound　乳房超音波検査 breast ultrasound　腹部超音波検査 abdominal ultrasound　▶超音波検査技師 ultrasound technician[technologist] / sonographer　超音波検査室 ultrasound（scanning）room　超音波内視鏡下吸引針生検 endoscopic ultrasound-guided fine-needle aspiration；EUS-FNA

ちょうか　超過する　exceed, go over　☞オーバー, 超過勤務

ちょうかきんむ　超過勤務　overtime

(**work**) ◆あなたは週に何時間超過勤務をしていますか How many hours' overtime do you work a week?

ちょうかく 聴覚 (the sense of) hearing, auditory sense, auditory perception (形 auditory, acoustic) ☞聴力 ◀言語聴覚士 speech-language-hearing therapist；ST ▶聴覚過敏症 hyperacusis／hyperacusia 聴覚検査 hearing test 聴覚検査技師 audiometrist 聴覚刺激 acoustic stimulation 聴覚失認 auditory agnosia 聴覚障害 hearing disorder[impairment] 聴覚障害者 person with a hearing impairment[disorder]／deaf[hard-of-hearing] person ★the deaf には差別的なニュアンスがあるので，総称的には deaf people を用いる. 聴覚消失 anacusis 聴覚中枢 the auditory [acoustic] center 聴覚反射 acoustic reflex 聴覚野 auditory area 聴覚路 auditory pathway

ちょうかしギプスほうたい 長下肢ギプス包帯 long leg cast；LLC

ちょうかしそうぐ 長下肢装具 long leg brace；LLB, knee-ankle-foot orthosis；KAFO

ちょうかん 腸管 intestinal tract ▶腸管過敏症 irritable bowel 腸管出血性大腸菌 enterohemorrhagic *Escherichia coli[*E. coli*]；EHEC 腸管破裂 intestinal rupture 腸管病原性大腸菌 enteropathogenic *Escherichia coli[*E. coli*]；EPEC 腸管ベーチェット病 intestinal Behçet disease 腸管麻痺 intestinal paresis 腸管癒着 intestinal adhesion

ちょうかんまく 腸間膜 mesentery (形 mesenteric) ▶腸間膜虚血 mesenteric ischemia 腸間膜血栓症 mesenteric thrombosis 腸間膜塞栓症 mesenteric embolism 腸間膜動脈閉塞症 mesenteric artery occlusion

ちょうき 長期 long time, long period of time (長期間の long-term, long-range 長引く protracted, prolonged 長期滞在の long-stay) ◆経口避妊薬を長期間飲んでいますか Have you been taking the pill for a long time?／Have you been on the pill

for a prolonged period of time? ◆関節リウマチは良好にコントロールされるまでに長期間かかります It takes a long time for rheumatoid arthritis to be well controlled.／Bringing rheumatoid arthritis under control takes a long time. ◆この薬は長期間飲み続ける必要があります You need to continue taking this medication for a long time. ◆長期的な目標を設定する set a long-term goal ▶長期記憶 long-term memory；LTM 長期ケア long-term care 長期計画 long-term[long-range] plan 長期滞在 long-term stay [residence] 長期滞在者 long-term resident 長期滞在ビザ long-term visa 長期毒性 long-term toxicity 長期入院 long-term[long-stay] hospitalization 長期入院患者 long-stay patient 長期療法 long-term therapy[remedy] 長期療養 long-term medical care

ちょうきどくせい 聴器毒性 ototoxicity

ちょうきゅうきん 腸球菌 enterococcus (複enterococci) (学名)*Enterococcus*

ちょうけいいんえい 蝶形陰影 butterfly shadow

ちょうけいこうはん 蝶形紅斑 butterfly erythema (蝶形発疹)butterfly rash

ちょうけいこつ 蝶形骨 sphenoid (bone) (形sphenoidal) ▶蝶形骨洞 sphenoid[sphenoidal] sinus

ちょうこう 徴候 sign, indication ☞症状 ◆血液検査で炎症の徴候が見られます The blood test shows signs of inflammation. ◆皮膚が黄色になるのは黄疸の徴候です Yellowing of the skin[Yellow-colored skin] is *a sign[an indication] of jaundice. ◆お産の徴候がある have a sign of the onset of labor／(おしるしがある) have *a bloody show[one's show] ◆死の徴候 signs of death ◀アップルコア徴候 apple core sign 局在徴候 focal signs 自覚的〈他覚的〉徴候 subjective〈objective〉signs 錐体外路徴候 extrapyramidal signs 錐体路徴候 pyramid[pyramidal] signs 生命徴候 vital signs；VS 妊娠徴候 signs of pregnancy

ちょうごう 調合する **prepare**（特に薬局で）**dispense**（処方箋の薬を）**fill a prescription** ☞調剤 ▶調合乳 formula (milk)

ちょうこうおんさっきん 超高温殺菌 **ultrahigh temperature sterilization**

ちょうこうれいしゃかい 超高齢社会 **super-aged society**

ちょうこつ¹ 腸骨 **ilium, iliac bone**

ちょうこつ² 長骨 **long bone**

ちょうさ 調査（実態調査）**survey** /sɚ́:veɪ/（原因・事実関係などの評価）**investigation**（問い合わせ）**inquiry**（研究調査）**research, study** ◆肺がん患者の実態調査を行う *carry out[conduct] a survey of patients with lung cancer ◆喫煙が寿命短縮に与えるリスクについての医学的な調査を行う do[carry out / conduct] medical research on the risks of smoking in decreasing life expectancy ◆原因は現在調査中です The cause is now under investigation. / We're in the process of investigating what's causing this. ▶患者調査 patient survey 製造販売後［市販後］調査 post-marketing surveillance；PMS 抽出調査 sampling survey 追跡調査 follow-up survey 予備調査 pilot study[survey] ▶調査委員会 fact-finding committee

ちょうざい¹ 長座位 **long sitting (position)**

ちょうざい² 調剤する **fill a prescription, dispense**（a prescription）◆この処方箋の薬はどこの薬局でも調剤してもらえます You can have this prescription filled at any pharmacy. ◆薬を調剤する prepare[dispense] a medication ▶（病院内の）調剤室 (hospital) pharmacy / dispensary 調剤薬局 outside pharmacy 調剤料金 dispensing fee

ちょうし 調子 《具合》**condition, state**（of health）☞具合, 体調 ◆調子はいかがですか How are you feeling[doing]? / How's your condition now? ◆眼の調子はどうですか How are your eyes? ◆胃の調子が悪いのですか Do you have stomach trouble? / Is there something wrong with your stomach?

◆彼は調子が良くなっています There has been some improvement in his condition. ◆体の調子がいい be in good condition[shape] / feel well ◆体の調子が悪い be in bad[poor] condition[shape] / not feel well / feel[be] poorly 《やり方》**way** ◆こういう調子でやってみて下さい Please try it this way. ◆そう, その調子です That's it. / That's the way. ◆調子はいいですよ（順調にやっている）You're doing fine[well].

ちょうじが 超自我 **the superego**

ちょうじかん 長時間 **long hours** ◆パソコンの画面を長時間見つめるようなことは控えて下さい Please avoid staring at the computer screen for long hours. ◆この薬はより長時間効果が持続します The effect of this medication will last *more hours[longer].

ちょうしゅ 聴取する ☞聞く ◀病歴聴取 (medical) history-taking

ちょうじゅ 長寿 ☞長生き

ちょうじゅうせき 腸重積 **intussusception**（of the intestine）

ちょうしょうこうぐん 腸症候群 **bowel syndrome** ◀過敏性腸症候群 irritable bowel syndrome；IBS

ちょうしょく 朝食 **breakfast** ◆朝食は7時になります Breakfast is served at seven. ◆朝食に何を食べましたか What did you eat for breakfast? ◆次回は朝食抜きでご来院下さい Next time, please come to the hospital without having breakfast. ◆軽い朝食をとる have a light breakfast ◆朝食を抜く skip breakfast ◆朝食の30分後に薬を飲む take a medication thirty minutes after eating breakfast

ちょうしん 聴診 **auscultation**（動**auscultate** 形**auscultatory**）◆それでは胸の聴診をします Well, let me listen to your chest. ◆聴診音 auscultatory sound ☞聴診器

ちょうしんき 聴診器 **stethoscope** /stéθəskòup/ ◆聴診器を胸に当てる put[apply] a stethoscope to *a person's chest ◆聴診器で胸の音を聴く listen to a *person's* chest and heart with a stethoscope ◀胎児聴診器 fetal[Traube] stethoscope

ちょうしんけい　聴神経　**auditory nerve, acoustic nerve**　▶聴神経腫瘍 acoustic tumor[neuroma]　聴神経障害 auditory neuropathy　聴神経鞘腫 acoustic neurinoma[schwannoma]

ちょうせい¹　調整する・調製する
《合わせる》**adjust**（図**adjustment**）☞調節　◆なるべく早く手術ができるよう日程を調整します We'll be happy to adjust the schedule so that you can have the surgery as soon as possible.　◆義足のアライメントを調整する必要があります We need to adjust the alignment of your prosthetic leg. / The alignment of your artificial leg needs to be adjusted.
◀咬合調整 occlusal adjustment
《調合する》**formulate**（図**formula**）▶調整食（既定食・処方食）formula diet, formulated food /（均衡食）balanced diet　調製粉乳 formula（milk）/ infant formula

ちょうせい²　聴性（の）　**auditory**　▶聴性脳幹反応 auditory brainstem response；ABR　聴性誘発電位 auditory evoked potential；AEP / auditory evoked response

ちょうせつ　調節する　（制御する）**control**（調整する）**regulate, modulate**　（修正する・適合させる）**adjust**（図**control, regulation**　順応 **adaptation**）☞調整　◆体温を調節する control[regulate] *one's* body temperature　◆ご自分で点滴の速度を調節しないで下さい Please don't adjust the drip rate yourself.　◆ベッドはこの調節つまみで下げることができます You can use this control（button）to lower your bed.　◆調節機能つきのベッド an adjustable bed
◆目の遠近調節 accommodation of the eye ◀換気調節 ventilatory regulation[control] 起立性調節障害 orthostatic dysregulation；OD　受胎調節 birth control　視力調節 visual adaptation　体温調節 thermoregulation / regulation of body temperature　ネガティブフィードバック調節機構 negative feedback regulation

排便調節 bowel control　免疫調節薬 immunomodulator　▶調節換気 controlled mechanical ventilation；CMV　調節器 regulator　調節幅 range of accommodation　調節弁 control valve

ちょうせん　挑戦する　**try, challenge**　◆これを機に禁煙に挑戦されてみてはいかがですか How about taking this opportunity to try to quit smoking?

ちょうそっこうがたインスリン　超速効型インスリン　**ultra rapid-acting[short-acting] insulin**

ちょうチフス　腸チフス　**typhoid fever**

ちょうつがいかんせつ　蝶番関節　**hinge joint**

ちょうていしゅっせいたいじゅうじ　超低出生体重児　**extremely low birth-weight infant；ELBWI**　（出生体重 1,000 g 未満）infant weighing less than one thousand grams at birth

ちょうていひじゅう　超低比重　**very low density**　▶超低比重リポ蛋白 very low-density lipoprotein；VLDL

ちょうど　**exactly, just**
《ぴったり合致する》◆体重は 60 kg ちょうどです Your weight is[You weigh] exactly sixty kilos[kilograms].　◆子宮筋腫はちょうどこぶしぐらいの大きさです The（uterine）fibroid[myoma] is just the size of a fist.　◆ちょうどいいサイズがなくてご不便をおかけします I'm sorry for the inconvenience, but we don't have just the right size for you.
《まさによいタイミングで》◆ちょうど今日ベッドが空いたところでした Just today, *an empty bed[one of the beds] became available.

ちょうどうけん　聴導犬　**hearing dog（for deaf people）**

ちょうないさいきん　腸内細菌　**intestinal bacteria**　▶腸内細菌叢 intestinal（bacterial）flora / gut flora

ちょうにゅう　調乳　（調合乳）**formula（milk）**

ちょうのうくんれん　聴能訓練　**auditory training**　▶聴能訓練士 audiologist

ちょうふ 貼付する （薬などを貼る）apply … to （くっつける）put[place]… on, attach … to ☞貼る ▶貼付試験 patch test

ちょうふく 重複（の） （2つの・二重の）double （多重・多発の）multiple （上に重なった）overlapping （図overlap） （複製の・ダブっている）duplicate, duplicated ☞ダブる ◆同じ薬効の薬を2種類以上重複して服用するのは危険です It's dangerous to take two or more different medications that have the same effect[efficacy]. ◆2つの感染症が同時に重複して起こっています You have developed two infections [infectious conditions] at the same time. ▶重複がん double cancer 重複感染 multiple infection 重複子宮 double uterus 重複障害 multiple disabilities 重複症候群 overlap syndrome

ちょうふやく 貼付薬 ☞湿布

ちょうへいそく 腸閉塞 ileus, bowel obstruction, intestinal obstruction ◀痙攣性腸閉塞 spastic ileus[bowel obstruction] 術後腸閉塞 postoperative ileus 糞便性腸閉塞 fecal ileus

ちょうヘルニア 腸ヘルニア intestinal hernia

ちょうみりょう 調味料 seasoning （香辛料）spice ◀化学調味料 artificial seasoning[（香味料）flavoring]

ちょうめい 長命 ☞長生き

ちょうやく 調薬 ☞調剤

ちょうようきん 腸腰筋 iliopsoas （muscle）

ちょうりつ 調律 （心拍の）rhythm ◀異所性調律 ectopic rhythm 心室調律 ventricular rhythm 心房調律 atrial rhythm 正常洞調律 normal sinus rhythm；NSR 房室接合部調律 atrioventricular[AV] junctional rhythm 補充調律 escape[escaped] rhythm 奔馬調律 gallop rhythm

ちょうりょく¹ 張力 tension, tensile strength ◀表面張力 surface tension

ちょうりょく² 聴力 （the sense of）hearing, hearing acuity ☞聴覚 ◆最近，聴力に変化がありましたか Have you noticed any changes in your hearing? ◆聴力の衰えで日常生活に不便を感じていますか Do you feel inconvenience in your daily life because your hearing is *getting worse[getting weaker / declining]? ◆聴力が低下する get[become] hard of hearing ◆聴力を失う lose *one's* hearing ◆聴力を改善させる improve *one's* hearing ▶聴力閾値レベル hearing threshold level 聴力計 audiometer 聴力障害 hearing disorder[impairment] 聴力損失 hearing loss / deafness 聴力低下 decreased hearing / （部分的な低下）partial hearing 聴力レベル hearing level；HL ☞聴力検査

ちょうりょくけんさ 聴力検査 hearing test, audiometry ◆聴力検査をしましょう Let's do[run] a hearing test. / Let's test [check] your hearing. ◆聴力検査を受ける have a hearing test ◀純音聴力検査 pure-tone audiometry

ちょくげきそんしょう 直撃損傷 coup injury

ちょくご 直後（に） immediately after, right after, just after ◆立ち上がった直後にめまいが起こったのですか Did you feel dizzy immediately[right] after you stood up? ◆食直後に immediately[right] after meals[eating]

ちょくしかせいけん 直視下生検 direct-vision biopsy, open biopsy

ちょくしゃにっこう 直射日光 direct sunlight ◆強い直射日光か高温に曝されていましたか Have you been exposed to strong (direct) sunlight or high temperatures? ◆この薬は直射日光を避けて保管して下さい Please keep this medication away from direct sunlight. ◆直射日光に当たらないようにして下さい Please avoid[keep away from / don't expose your skin to] direct sunlight.

ちょくしん 直進する go straight, walk straight ◆エレベーターを降りたらそのまま廊下を直進して下さい When you get out of the elevator, go[walk] straight down the hallway.

ちょくせつ 直接（の） direct, immediate

◆直接の原因 *a direct[an immediate] cause ◆直接の死因 the immediate[direct] cause of death ◆傷口に直接軟膏を塗って下さい Please apply the ointment directly to the cut. ◆次回は直接検査室においで下さい Please come directly to the laboratory next time. ◆ご主人に直接お目にかかりたいのですが(他人を介さずに)I'd like to see your husband *in person[personally]. ▶直接圧迫止血 direct hemostatic pressure / arrest of bleeding [hemorrhage] by *application of direct pressure[direct compression] 直接X線撮影 direct radiography 直接感染 direct (contact) infection 直接クームス試験 direct Coombs test 直接対光反射 direct light reflex 直接的関係 direct connection[relation] 直接ビリルビン direct bilirubin

ちょくせん 直線 straight line (形linear) ▶直線加速器 linear accelerator；LINAC

ちょくぜん 直前(に) immediately before, right before, just before (形immediate) ◆この薬は食事の直前に飲んで下さい Please take this medication immediately[right] before meals[eating]. ◆直前の記憶を失う lose one's immediate memory / experience immediate memory loss

ちょくたつけんいん 直達牽引 direct (skeletal) traction

ちょくたつこっせつ 直達骨折 direct fracture

ちょくちょう 直腸 rectum (形rectal 接頭proct(o)-) ▶直腸炎 proctitis 直腸潰瘍 rectal ulcer 直腸がん rectal cancer 直腸鏡検査 rectoscopy / proctoscopy 直腸指診 digital rectal examination；DRE / digital examination of the rectum 直腸出血 rectal bleeding 直腸脱 rectal prolapse 直腸ポリープ rectal polyp / polyp of the rectum

ちょくめん 直面する face ◆多くの難しい問題に直面している be faced with various difficult problems

ちょくりつ 直立する stand upright, stand up straight

ちょくりゅうじょさいどうき 直流除細動器 direct current defibrillator, DC defibrillator

ちょくりゅうつうでんショック 直流通電ショック direct current shock, DC shock

ちょけつ 貯血 ◆手術前にご自分の貯血が必要です We will need to store[bank] some of your own blood before the surgery. ◀自己貯血 autologous blood donation / donation of one's own blood (for one's own later use)

チョコレートのうほう ─嚢胞 chocolate cyst

ちょぞう 貯蔵 storage (動store) ☞保管, 保存 ▶貯蔵血 stored blood 貯蔵設備 storage facility 貯蔵鉄 storage iron

ちょっけい 直径 diameter /daɪǽmətə/ ◆ポリープは直径7 mm です The polyp is seven millimeters across[in diameter]. / The polyp has a diameter of seven millimeters.

ちょっと
《少し》(少し)a little (ほんの少しの時間)just a moment[minute] (もう少しで)almost ☞少し ◆ちょっと気になる検査所見があります There are some lab findings I'm a little concerned about. ◆ちょっとお待ち下さい Just a moment[minute], please. ◆ちょっといいですか Do you have a moment[minute]? ◆もうちょっとで終わりです You're almost finished [done]. / It's almost over. ◆もうちょっとゆっくり話してくれませんか Could you speak a little more slowly? ◆(注射で)ちょっとチクッとしますよ There'll be a little prick.
《気軽に・簡単に》just ◆ちょっと試飲してみませんか Could you just try and drink this? / How about tasting this? ◆それにはちょっとお応えできません I'm sorry, but we just can't do that.

ちょりゅう 貯留 retention ◀水分貯留 fluid[water] retention ▶貯留嚢胞 retention cyst

ちらちら ◆目の前にちらちらする光が見え

ますか Do you see flickering lights in front of your eyes?

ちり 塵 **dust** ☞埃 ▶塵ダニ dust mite

チリ Chile（形Chilean） ☞国籍 ▶チリ人（の）Chilean

ちりがみ 一紙 **tissue**

ちりょう 治療 **treatment**, **cure**（動cure）, **therapy**（形therapeutic）, **care**, **remedy** （介入）**intervention** ☞処置

《基本表現》 ◆…の治療を受ける have[receive / undergo / get] treatment for … ◆治療を受け入れる accept treatment ◆治療を拒否する reject treatment ◆彼の怪我を治療する treat him for his injuries ◆あなたの症状はこの薬で治療できます Your symptom can be treated with this medication.

《治療歴を尋ねる》 ◆どんな治療を受けましたか What kind of treatment did you receive? / How was it[the symptom] treated? ◆治療を受けたのはいつですか When was it[the symptom] treated? ◆現在治療中ですか Are you currently under[receiving / undergoing] any treatment? ◆現在他院で狭心症の治療を受けていますか Are you currently under treatment for angina at another hospital?

《治療の必要性を説明する》 ◆特別な治療は必要ありません You don't need any special treatment. ◆膀胱炎の治療を受ける必要があります You need to have[undergo] treatment for cystitis. ◆抗菌薬を用いてすぐに治療する必要があります Early treatment with antibiotics is vital. / You must be treated immediately with antibiotics. ◆一連のがん治療が必要です You need to have[undergo] a course of treatment for your cancer. ◆この治療にはあなた自身の前向きな取り組みが必要です You need to be positively *involved in [committed to] this treatment. / Your own positive involvement is essential for this treatment.

《治療内容・予定・予後を説明する》 ◆治療の計画を立てましょう Let's make[draw up / decide on] your treatment plan. ◆乳が

んの最適な治療を選ぶ choose the most appropriate treatment for breast cancer ◆この方法は現在選択できる最も効果的な治療法です This is the most effective treatment available now. ◆私はそれが最善の治療法だと思います In my opinion, it's the best (treatment) option. ◆この病気はおよそ半年の治療が必要です This disease requires about six months' treatment. ◆残念ですが, この症状には有効な治療法がありません I'm sorry[Unfortunately], there's no effective treatment [cure] for this symptom.

◀維持治療 maintenance treatment[therapy] 遺伝子治療 gene therapy インスリン治療 insulin treatment 遠隔治療 teletherapy / teletreatment 延命治療（生命を維持するための）life-support[life-supporting / life-sustaining] treatment / （手段）life-support measures / （生命を引き延ばすための）life-prolonging treatment 外来[通院]治療 outpatient[ambulatory] treatment[care] 隔離治療 isolation treatment 緩和治療 palliative treatment [care] 救急治療 emergency treatment [care] 外科的治療 surgical treatment 研究的治療 experimental[investigational] treatment 根治治療 radical[curative] treatment 歯科治療 dental treatment 集学的治療 multidisciplinary treatment 集中治療 intensive care 初期治療 early[initial] treatment 積極的治療 aggressive[active] treatment 創傷治療 wound treatment[management] 胎児治療 fetal therapy 対症的治療 symptomatic treatment[care] 内科的治療 medical[nonsurgical] treatment 内視鏡的治療 endoscopic treatment 入院治療 hospital treatment 標準治療 standard treatment / （従来の治療）conventional treatment 不妊治療 infertility treatment 放射線治療 radiation therapy[treatment] / radiotherapy 保存的治療 conservative treatment[therapy] 予防的治療 preventive treatment レーザー治療 laser treatment[therapy] ▶治療計画

treatment plan[program] /（あらかじめ定められた治療計画）protocol　治療効果 therapeutic effect　治療室 treatment room　治療食 therapeutic diet[food]　治療成績 treatment outcome　治療費 medical expenses / doctor's fee　治療方針 treatment policy　治療目標 therapeutic goal[objective]　治療薬 therapeutic medication[drug / agent]　治療用装具 therapeutic orthosis

ちんがいやく　鎮咳薬　cough medicine, cough suppressant, antitussive (medication, drug, agent)　（ドロップ）cough drop　（シロップ）cough syrup

ちんきゅうせい　陳旧性（の）　（古い）old　（以前の）previous　▶陳旧性心筋梗塞 old[previous] myocardial infarction；OMI　陳旧創 old wound

ちんけいやく　鎮痙薬　antispasmodic (medication, drug, agent)　（抗痙攣薬）anticonvulsant

ちんこう　沈降　sedimentation, precipitation (🈑precipitate)　◀赤血球沈降速度 erythrocyte sedimentation rate；ESR / blood sedimentation rate　▶沈降抗体 precipitating antibody

チンしょうたい　―小帯　Zinn zonule　（毛様小帯）ciliary zonule

ちんせい　鎮静　sedation (🈑sedate 🈑sedative)　◆胃内視鏡検査を受ける際，鎮静をご希望なさいますか Would you like to receive sedation when you have the endoscopy?　◆大量の鎮静薬を飲んで自殺を図る attempt (to commit) suicide by taking an overdose of sedatives　▶鎮静効果 sedative effect[（作用）action]　鎮静薬 sedative (medication / drug / agent) /（精神安定薬）tranquilizer　鎮静薬依存 sedative dependence / addiction to sedatives

ちんちゃく　沈着　（堆積）deposition　（蓄積）accumulation, storage　◆コレステロールの沈着を防ぐ prevent cholesterol accumulation[deposits]　◀色素沈着 pigmentation / accumulation[deposits] of pigments　歯石沈着 tartar deposition　炭粉沈着症 anthracosis　ヘモジデリン沈着症

hemosiderosis　▶沈着物 deposit

ちんつう　鎮痛　analgesia (🈑analgesic), pain relief　◀自己調節鎮痛法 patient-controlled analgesia；PCA　▶鎮痛解熱薬 analgesic-antipyretic (medication / drug / agent) / pain-fever medication　鎮痛効果 analgesic effect　☞鎮痛薬

ちんつうやく　鎮痛薬　painkiller, pain reliever, medication for pain, analgesic (medication, drug, agent)　☞痛み止め　◆この鎮痛薬はよく効きます This painkiller works very well. / This painkiller is very effective.　◀麻薬性鎮痛薬 narcotic analgesic (medication / drug / agent)　▶鎮痛薬依存 analgesic dependence / painkiller dependence[addiction]

ちんでん　沈殿する　（沈降する）precipitate　（堆積する）deposit　▶沈殿物 precipitate / deposit

ちんとやく　鎮吐薬　antiemetic (medication, drug, agent)

ちんもくりょうほう　沈黙療法　vocal rest, voice rest

つ

ついか 追加する add（to）（圏addition 圏additional）（効果を強化する）boost（圏booster）☞加える ◆何か追加したいことはありますか Is there anything you want to add? ◆痛みがとれない時はもう1錠追加して下さい Please take one more tablet if you still have the pain. ◆追加の情報が必要です I need additional[more / further] information. ▶追加処置 additional procedure 追加接種 booster shot[injection] / booster[additional] vaccination 追加免疫 booster immunization ☞追加料金

ついかりょうきん 追加料金 additional charge, additional expenses （別料金）extra charge ◆特別室は追加料金をいただきます You would have to pay an additional charge for a special[deluxe] room.

ついかんかんせつ 椎間関節 apophyseal joint （小関節）facet（joint）▶椎間関節固定術 facet fusion

ついかんこう 椎間孔 intervertebral foramen （圏foraminal）▶椎間孔拡大術 foraminotomy 椎間孔狭窄 foraminal encroachment

ついかんばん 椎間板 intervertebral disc[disk] ◆頸椎〈胸椎 / 腰椎〉椎間板ヘルニア cervical〈thoracic / lumbar〉disc hernia[herniation] ▶椎間板症 discopathy / disc lesion 椎間板切除術 discectomy[diskectomy] 椎間板造影 discography[diskography] 椎間板ヘルニア（intervertebral）disc hernia[herniation] /（滑脱した椎間板）slipped[herniated] disc

ついきゅう¹ 追究する （解明する）find out （調査する）investigate ◆アレルギーの治療ではその原因を追究することがとても大切です To treat allergies, it's important that we *find out[investigate] what's causing them.

ついきゅう² 椎弓 vertebral arch ▶椎弓形成術 laminoplasty 椎弓切除術 laminectomy

ついこつ 椎骨 vertebra（圏vertebrae）（圏vertebral）▶椎骨動脈 vertebral artery 椎骨脳底動脈循環不全 vertebrobasilar insufficiency

ついし 追視 tracking eye movement, pursuit eye movement

ついせき 追跡 chase, pursuit （検証のために行う作業）follow-up （かすかな痕跡などの探知）tracing ▶追跡研究 follow-up study 追跡検査 follow-up test[examination] 追跡子 tracer 追跡調査 follow-up survey

ついたい 椎体 vertebral body ▶椎体圧迫骨折 compression fracture of the vertebral body 椎体間固定術 interbody fusion

ついたて 衝立 screen （間仕切り）partition（圏仕切る partition）◆衝立でベッドを仕切る partition off the beds with a screen

ついていく 付いて行く （一緒に行く）go with （同行する）accompany ◆私がリハビリ室まで付いて行きます I'll *go with[accompany] you to the rehab room.

ついてくる 付いて来る （あとをつける）follow （一緒に来る）come with ◆私に付いて来て下さい Please follow[come with] me.

ついに 遂に finally （努力のかいあって）at last ◆ついに禁煙に成功しましたね I'm glad that you finally[at last] succeeded in quitting smoking.

ついまひ 対麻痺 paraplegia ◀痙性対麻痺 spastic paraplegia

つういん 通院する visit[go to, come to] the hospital as an outpatient （医院・診察室に行く）go to a doctor's office （医師に診てもらう）see[visit] a doctor ★go to the hospital は「入院する」という意味にもなるので注意．◆しばらく定期的に〈毎月〉通院して下さい Please come here[to the hospital] regularly〈every month〉for a while. / Please see[visit] me regularly〈every month〉for a while. ▶通院患者 outpatient / ambulatory patient / day patient

つういん 487 **つうやく**

通院手術 outpatient[day / ambulatory] surgery　通院治療 outpatient[ambulatory] treatment[care]

つうか　**通過する**　pass（図passage）, transit（図transit）　◆食べ物や飲み物が通過しづらいことはありますか（胸から胃にかけて）Do you ever feel that it's difficult for foods and liquid to pass through your *chest to the stomach[（食道を）esophagus]?　◀卵管通過障害 blockage of the fallopian tube　▶通過時間 transit time

つうかく　**痛覚**　pain sensation, pain sense　◀ピン刺激痛覚検査 pinprick test　▶痛覚過敏 hyperalgesia　痛覚受容器 pain receptor　痛覚消失 analgesia　痛覚鈍麻 hypoalgesia / hypalgesia

つうがく　**通学**　go to school　☞通勤

つうき　**通気**　（換気）ventilation　（膨らませること）inflation　（吹き入れること）insufflation　◀耳管通気法 tympanic inflation[insufflation]　卵管通気法 tubal insufflation

つうきん　**通勤する**　go to work, commute　◆ふだん通勤にはどんな交通手段を利用しますか How do you commute[go] to work? / What kind of transportation do you usually take to go to work?　◆通勤は徒歩ですか，電車ですか Do you walk to your office or go to work by train?　◆通勤にどのくらい時間がかかりますか How long does it take to commute[get] to your office?　▶通勤拒否 refusal to go to work　通勤時間 commuting time

つうじ　**通じ**　☞排便，便通

つうしょ　**通所**　▶通所介護施設 day care facility　通所リハビリテーション outpatient[ambulatory] rehab[rehabilitation]

つうじょう　**通常**　（いつもの）usual　（定期的な）regular, routine　（普通の）ordinary　☞いつも，普段，普通　◆それは通常のやり方です It's the usual method.　◆月経は通常何日続きますか How long do your periods usually last?　◆通常ならば鎮痛解熱薬の作用は6時間くらい持続します Pain-fever medications[Analgesic-antipyretics] usually work for about six hours.

▶通常勤務 regular duty

つうじる　**通じる**　（言いたいことをわからせる）make *oneself* understood　（意味が通じる）make sense　◆言葉が通じないのはストレスになるでしょう You must feel stressed when you can't make yourself understood.　◆私の英語で通じていますか Do you understand my English? / Does my English make sense?

つうてん　**痛点**　pain spot[point]

つうねん　**通年（性の）**　perennial　▶通年性アレルギー性鼻炎 perennial allergic rhinitis　通年性喘息 perennial asthma

つうふう　**痛風**　gout /ɡáʊt/（図gouty）　◆痛風になったことがありますか Have you ever had gout?　◀偽痛風 pseudogout　▶痛風結節 *gouty node[tophus]　痛風食 gout diet　痛風腎 gouty kidney　痛風性関節炎 gouty arthritis　痛風治療薬 gout suppressant　痛風発作 attack of gout / gouty attack

つうやく　**通訳する**　interpret /ɪntɚ́ːprɪt/（図通訳者 interpreter　通訳・解釈 interpretation）　◆通訳が必要ですか Do you need an interpreter?　◆通訳をしてくれる人がいますか Do you have anyone who can interpret for you?　◆通訳をしてくれる人がいたらお名前と電話番号を書いて下さい If you have someone who could interpret for you, please write his⟨her⟩ name and telephone number here.　◆通訳が必要ならば医療ソーシャルワーカーに手配してもらって下さい If you need an interpreter, ask the medical social worker to make the arrangements for you.　◆通訳サービスは無料です Interpreting services are offered free of charge.　◆通訳サービスは有料となっております Patients *must pay[are charged] for interpreting services. / We offer paid interpreting services.　◆通訳サービスを受けるには最低3,000円の料金をお支払いいただきます You'll be asked to pay a three thousand yen minimum charge for interpreting services.　◆彼女があなたの通訳をしてくれる田中さんです This is Ms Tanaka. She will interpret for you. ◀医療通訳 medical interpretation /（通訳者）medical interpreter　ボランティア通訳者 volunteer interpreter

つうれい　通例 ☞通常

つうろ　通路　passage, passageway
◆通路に物を置かないで下さい Please don't put things in the passage[passageway].

つえ　杖　cane, walking stick ◆いつも杖か歩行器を使っていますか Do you usually use a cane or a walker? ◆杖をついて歩く walk with a cane ◆杖をつかずに歩く walk without the help of a cane ◆杖で体を支える support oneself with a cane ◀三脚杖 tripod cane　T字杖 T-handle [T-shaped] cane　（視覚障害者用の）白杖 white cane　四脚杖 quad[quad-point] cane ☞松葉杖

つかいすぎ　使いすぎ　overuse, excessive use ◆この炎症は手指の使いすぎが原因です This inflammation is caused by overuse[excessive use] of the fingers and thumbs. ◆目の使いすぎで頭痛がする have a headache from overuse[excessive use] of the eyes ▶使いすぎ症候群 overuse syndrome

つかいすて　使い捨て（の）　disposable
◆使い捨ての注射針 a disposable injection needle

つかう　使う　use ☞使用, 利用 ◆吸入器の使い方を説明する explain[show] how to use an inhaler ◆病室ではコンピュータが使えます You can use your computer in your room. 〔◆当医院ではクレジットカードは使えません（受け付けない） We don't accept credit cards at this clinic. ◆どうぞ気を使わないで下さい Please don't bother yourself.

つかえる　（物が引っかかる）**get[be] stuck, get[be] caught**　（物が中に食い込む）**get[be] lodged**　（窒息する）**choke**　（言葉に詰まる）**stumble** ◆何かが喉につかえている感じがしますか Do you feel as if something is stuck in your throat? / Does your throat feel as if there's something stuck [lodged] in it? ◆食べ物が喉につかえる

food gets stuck in one's throat / choke on food ◆胸がつかえる（窒息しそうな感じがする）have a choking feeling /（胸に圧迫感がある）feel pressure in one's chest ◆言葉がつかえる stumble over one's words

つかさどる　司る　control ☞支配

つかまりだち　つかまり立ちする　stand with support, stand holding onto something

つかまる　掴まる　hold on (to) ◆この手すりにつかまって下さい Please hold on to this handrail. ◆腕につかまって歩く walk along holding on to a person's arm ◆しっかりつかまる hold on tight[tightly]

つかむ　掴む　hold　（強く握る）**grasp**
◆右手でバーをしっかりつかんで下さい Please hold[grasp] the bar firmly with your right hand.

つかれ　疲れ　tiredness, fatigue /fətíːg/　（極度の疲れ）**exhaustion** /ɪgzɔ́ːstʃən/ ☞疲れる, 疲労 ◆休息すると疲れがとれますか Does rest relieve your tiredness[fatigue]? ◆疲れを覚える feel tired ◆疲れがたまる get too tired[exhausted] ◆疲れがとれない can't shake off one's tiredness[fatigue] / can't get over one's tiredness[fatigue] ☞疲れ目

つかれめ　疲れ目　tired eyes ★複数形で.（眼精疲労）**eyestrain**

つかれる　疲れる　get tired, tire　（くたくたになる）**be exhausted, worn out**　（仕事などが疲れさせる **tiring**） ☞疲れ, 疲労 ◆疲れていますか Are you tired? / Do you feel tired[exhausted / worn out]? ◆以前より疲れやすいですか Do you *get tired [tire] more easily than you used to? ◆疲れていると感じるのはいつですか When do you feel tired? ◆どんな活動が原因で疲れると感じましたか What type of activity *made you[caused you to] feel tired? ◆目がすぐ疲れますか Do your eyes get tired easily? ◆お仕事はすごく疲れますか Is your work very tiring? ◆お疲れでしょう. リハビリ頑張りましたね You must be tired. You've worked hard with the rehab[rehabilitation]. ◆疲れて

だるい feel tired and sluggish
つき 月 (暦の) month (略monthly) ◆月1回の検査 a monthly test ◆月に1回 once a month ◆毎月 every month / each month ★同義として用いられることもあるが，every month は「あらゆる月」を意味し，each は「個別の・各々の月」を意味する. ◆月の初め〈終わり〉に at the beginning〈end〉 of the month
つぎ 次 (the) next (以下の) the following ◆次の方，どうぞ Next person, please. ◆次は三浦さんで，その次があなたの番です It's Mrs Miura's turn next, and your turn after that. ◆次の来院時に検査結果をお話しします I'll tell you the test results when you come in for your next visit. ◆次の文を読んで質問にお答え下さい Please read the following passage and answer the questions.
つきあう 付き合う (友人と交わる) make friends with (仲良くする) get on[along] with (友好関係を維持する) maintain good relationships (ストレスなどに対処する) manage, cope with ◆職場での付き合いは大変ですか Is it difficult to make friends with people at work? / Do you have difficulty *getting on with people[maintaining good relationships] at work? ◆ストレスとうまく付き合うようにして下さい You need to learn to manage[cope with] stress. ◆付き合いやすい〈付き合いにくい〉easy〈difficult〉 to get along with
つぎあしほこう 継ぎ足歩行 tandem gait [walking] ◆このように継ぎ足歩行をしてみましょう (踵をつま先につけながら歩く) Please walk heel to toe, *like this[in this way].
つききず 突き傷 stab (wound)
つきささる 突き刺さる ☞刺さる
つきそい 付き添い (手伝い) (private) helper (介護者) caregiver ◆当院では付き添いは必要ありません You don't have to have a helper to take care of you in this hospital. ◆お子さんの付き添いをご希望でしたら看護師にご相談下さい Please check with a nurse if you'd like to stay with your child.
つきそう 付き添う (面倒をみる) take care (of) (医療者が患者の世話をする) attend (ついて行く) accompany ◆看護師が付き添いますので心配しないで下さい A nurse will *be with[take care of / attend to] you, so don't worry. ◆通院の際に付き添ってくれる人がいますか Do you have anyone who can accompany you when you come to the hospital?
つぎて 継手 joint
つきとめる 突き止める determine, find out (場所を) locate (原因・痕跡を) trace ◆熱の原因を突き止める determine[find out] the cause of the fever
つぎば 継ぎ歯 post crown ◆継ぎ歯をする (治療を行う) put in a post crown / (治療を受ける) have a post crown put on *one's* tooth
つきものもうそう 憑きもの妄想 delusion of possession, possession delusion
つきゆび 突き指 sprained finger (親指の) sprained thumb ◆右の人差し指を突き指する sprain *one's* right index finger
つく¹ 付く (付属する) have, be equipped (with) ◆各病室にはロッカーが付いています Each room has a locker. / Each room is equipped with a locker. ◆骨折した肋骨はうまく付きました Your fractured rib has healed well. ◆心配しないで下さい. 私がそばに付いていますから Don't worry. I'll be right with you.
つく² 着く arrive (at), get to, reach ◆病院に着いたらすぐ受付に行って下さい Please go to the reception desk as soon as you arrive at the hospital. ◆処方箋を事前に FAX しておけば，調剤薬局に着いたら待つことなく薬を受け取れます If you fax this prescription *in advance[beforehand], you can receive your medication at the outside pharmacy without waiting. ◆さあ(病室に)着きましたよ Here we are (at your room).
つくす 尽くす ◆最善を尽くします I'll do my best. ◆全力を尽くす do all *one* can ◆あらゆる手を尽くす try *everything

possible[every possible means]

つくる　作る　make　(調理する)**cook, prepare**　(確立する)**build (up)**　(発展させる)**develop**　◆食事はご自分で作りますか Do you cook for yourself?　◆誰が食事を作っていますか Who prepares your meals?　◆時間を作って相談しましょう Let's make time to discuss[talk over] things.　◆彼女との信頼関係を作る *build (up)[develop] a rapport[bond] with her

つけぐすり　付け薬　☞塗り薬

つけくわえる　付け加える　☞加える, 追加

つける¹　付ける　(付着させる)**put**　(薬品などを塗る)**apply**　(筋肉などを増やす・鍛える)**increase, build up**　(印をつける)**put on, mark**　◆傷口に軟膏を付ける apply (an) ointment to a cut / put (an) ointment on a cut　◆筋力を付ける increase[build up] *one's* muscle strength　◆持ち物すべてに名前を付ける put *one's* name on all *one's* belongings / mark all *one's* things with *one's* name

つける²　点ける　turn on (↔turn off)　◆明かり〈テレビ〉を点けるにはこのスイッチを使います You can use this switch to turn on the lamp〈TV〉.

つける³　着ける　put on　(着用している)**wear**　☞装着　◆かつらを着ける *put on a wig / (着けている)wear a wig　◆生命維持装置を着ける place[put] *the patient* on *life support[a life-support machine]

つける⁴　漬ける　soak　◆哺乳瓶の殺菌には, 煮沸するか専用の薬液に漬けるか電子レンジ消毒器を利用するとよいでしょう You can sterilize baby bottles by boiling them, soaking them in a baby-bottle [specialized / formulated] liquid cleanser, or using a microwave sterilizer.

つごう　都合
《具合・好都合》**convenience**　(形都合がいい)**convenient** (↔inconvenient)　◆ご都合がつき次第私のオフィスにおいで下さい Please come to my office at your earliest convenience.　◆ご都合のよろしい時においで下さい Please come and see me whenever it's convenient for you.　◆明日は都合がいいですか Is tomorrow convenient for you?　◆ご都合はいつがいいですか When is (it) convenient for you?　◆ご都合は何時がいいですか What time is good for you?　◆ご都合は何曜日がいいですか What day of the week would be convenient for you?　◆私は今度の土曜日でしたら都合がいいですよ I'm free this Saturday.　◆明日は都合がつきません I'm afraid that I can't make time tomorrow.　《事情》**circumstances**　★通例, 複数形で.　◆鈴木先生は来週の月曜日は都合により休診となります Owing to personal circumstances, Dr Suzuki will not (be available to) see patients next Monday.

つたいあるき　伝い歩きする　◆お子さんは伝い歩きしますか(家具につかまって歩くか) Does your child walk holding on to furniture?

ツタウルシ　poison ivy　▶ツタウルシ過敏症 poison ivy hypersensitivity

つたえる　伝える　(知らせる)**tell, inform**　(情報などを伝達する)**communicate, convey**　(話などを理解させる)**make *oneself* understood[clear]**　(刺激などを伝達する)**pass, transmit**　☞巻末付録: 悪い診断結果を伝える時　◆残念ですが, 悲しい知らせをお伝えしなければなりません I'm sorry, but *I have to tell you some sad news[I have some sad news for you].　◆ご家族の方には私からお伝えしましょうか Shall I tell[inform] your family about that?　◆日本語で自分の気持ちを伝えるのは難しいですか Do you have difficulty making yourself understood in Japanese? / Is it hard for you to communicate in Japanese?　◆私の話を正確にお伝えできなかったのではないかと思います I'm afraid I couldn't *make myself clear to you[communicate clearly].　◆この病気の遺伝子がお子さんに伝わる確率は 50%です The probability of the gene for this disease being passed [transmitted] to your children is fifty percent.

つちけいろ　土気色(の)　(蒼白の)**deadly pale**　(灰白色の)**ashen**　(血色の悪い)

sallow　◆顔が土気色になる turn deadly pale / become ashen-faced

ツチこつ　ツチ骨　malleus（bone）, hammer（bone）

つちふまず　土踏まず　the arch of the foot, foot[plantar] arch

つちゆび　槌指　mallet[hammer] finger（親指の）mallet[hammer] thumb

ツツガムシびょう　―病　tsutsugamushi disease[fever], scrub typhus

つづく　続く　continue　（特定の期間続く）last　（しつこく続く）persist　☞持続，連続　◆熱は1日中続いていましたか Did the fever continue all day long?　◆熱は何日続いていますか How many days have you had the fever? / How many days has the fever continued[lasted]?　◆毎回どのくらい続きますか How long does it last each time?　◆痛みはずっと続いていますか Is the pain constant?　◆副作用はしばらく続くかもしれません The side effects may continue for a while.　◆痛みが続くようであれば救急外来を受診して下さい If the pain persists, please go to the emergency room.　◆この薬は効き目が長く続きます This is a long-acting medication.

つづける　続ける　（継続する）continue, keep　（…し続ける）go[keep] on …　☞継続　◆お仕事は続けてもいいでしょう You can keep working.　◆この治療を続けていきましょう Let's continue[go on with] this treatment.　◆調子が良くなってもこの薬を飲み続けて下さい Please *continue to take[continue taking] this medication even if you feel better.　◆この治療は3回続けてやる必要があります You need to have this treatment *three times in a row [three consecutive times].　◆（リハビリなどで）その調子！続けて下さい That's it! Keep going[Keep it up].

つつしむ　慎む　refrain（from）　☞控える　◆お酒はしばらく慎んで下さい Please refrain from drinking alcohol for a while.　◆他の患者さんの迷惑となるような行為は慎んで下さい Please refrain from any behavior that may disturb the other patients.

つっぱる　突っ張る　（硬直する）stiffen（up）（國stiff 图stiffness）　◆どこか突っ張っているところがありますか Do you have any stiffness anywhere?

つづり　綴り　spelling（國spell）　◆お名前の綴りを言って下さい How do you spell your name? / Please spell out your name for me.

つとめる¹　努める　try　◆無理をせず体調管理に努めて下さい Please don't *overdo things[push yourself too hard], but try to stay in good condition.　◆努めて水分を摂るようにして下さい Be sure to *take lots of fluids[drink water as often as possible].

つとめる²　勤める　work　（雇われている）be employed　☞仕事，職業　◆お勤めですか Do you work? / Are you employed?　◆どちらにお勤めですか What company [Who] do you work for? / Where do you work?　◆勤め先の電話番号をここに書いて下さい Please write your office phone number here.

つながる　繋がる　（結ばれる）be connected to　（達する）get　◆このコンピュータはインターネットにつながっています This computer *is connected to the internet[has internet connection].　◆このボタンを押すとナースステーションにつながります Push[Press] this button, and you'll get [be connected to] the nurses' station.　◆血のつながったご家族で，同じ病気の方はいますか Do you know of any blood relative who has or has had this same problem[illness]?

つば　唾　saliva /səláivə/（國唾を吐く spit）　◆唾をゆっくり飲み込んで下さい Please swallow some saliva slowly.　◆唾をごくんと飲み込む swallow *one's* saliva *in one gulp[（一度に）in one go].

つぶす　潰す　（押しつぶす）crush　（割る）break　（水疱などをポンと割る）pop　◆この薬は潰したり噛んだりしないで下さい Please don't crush[break] or chew this medication.　◆火傷の水疱は潰さないで下さい Please avoid popping[breaking] the burn blisters.

つぶる **close** ◆両眼をぎゅっとつぶって下さい Please close both your eyes very tightly.

つぶれる 潰れる （押しつぶされる）**be crushed** ◆腰椎が圧迫されて潰れています One of *your lumbar vertebrae[the bones in your lower back] is crushed.

ツベルクリン **tuberculin** /tʊbɝːkjʊlɪn/ ◆ツベルクリン検査を受けたことがありますか Have you ever had a tuberculin test? ◆ツベルクリン検査をして48時間から72時間後に反応を調べます I'm going to do a tuberculin test and then check the response forty-eight to seventy-two hours later. ◆ツベルクリン反応は陰性〈陽性〉です The tuberculin reaction is negative〈positive〉. ◀精製ツベルクリン purified protein derivative of tuberculin；PPD ▶ツベルクリン反応陽転 tuberculin conversion

つぼ （鍼の）**acupuncture point** （指圧の）**acupressure[finger-pressure] point** （灸の）**moxibustion point**

つぼめる **purse, pucker** ◆口〈唇〉をつぼめてゆっくり息を吐き出して下さい Please purse[pucker] your mouth〈lips〉 and breathe out slowly. ☞口すぼめ呼吸

つま 妻 **wife**

つまさき 爪先 **tiptoe** ▶爪先立ち standing on tiptoe 爪先歩行 toe gait / walking on tiptoe

つまずく （足をとられる）**trip**（over, on） （つまずいてよろめく）**stumble**（over, on） ◆頻繁につまずいたり転んだりしますか Do you often trip or fall? ◆段差がありますのでつまずかないよう注意して下さい The floor isn't even, so please watch your step so that you don't trip[stumble]. / （掲示）Uneven Floor. Watch Your Step. ◆階段でつまずく stumble over the steps

つまむ （指先ではさむ）**pinch** （ぎゅっと握る）**squeeze** （つまんで持ち上げる）**pick** ◆乳頭をつまんで分泌物が出ないかをチェックして下さい Please pinch[squeeze] your nipples to make sure that there's no

discharge coming out of them. ◆この豆粒を1つずつつまんでこちらの皿に移して下さい Please pick these beans up one by one and put them onto this plate.

つまり 詰まり **clotting** ◆血管の詰まり clotting in the blood vessels ◆鼻詰まり a stuffy[congested] nose

つまる 詰まる
《つかえる・通じなくなる》（物が引っかかる）**get[be] stuck, get[be] caught** （詰まる）**get[be] blocked, get[be] plugged, get[be] clogged, get[be] congested, get[be] stopped up, get[be] stuffy** （物が中に食い込む）**get[be] lodged** （窒息する）**suffocate, choke** （言葉に詰まる）**stumble** ◆喉に何か詰まっていますか Is there something stuck[caught] in your throat? ◆耳が詰まった感じがしますか Do you feel as if your ears are blocked[clogged / plugged] up? ◆異物が外耳道に詰まっています A foreign object is lodged in the outer ear canal. ◆よく鼻が詰まりますか Do you often have a stuffy[blocked (up) / congested] nose? / Does your nose often get stuffy? ◆血管がプラークで詰まっています The blood vessels are blocked[clogged] by plaque. ◆息が詰まりそうですか Do you feel as if you are suffocating? ◆胸が詰まったような感じがしますか Do you have a sense of fullness or heaviness in your chest? ◆言葉に詰まる stumble over *one's* words / be stuck[at a loss] for words
《いっぱいで余裕がない》（いっぱいの）**full** （きつい）**tight** （多忙な）**busy** ◆来週は予定が詰まっています I have a full[tight / busy] schedule next week. / My schedule is full next week.

つみ 罪 （法律上の罪）**crime** （違反行為）**offense** （宗教上・道徳上の罪）**sin** ◆罪を犯す commit *a crime[an offense]* ◆それをしたら罪に問われます（責められる）You'll be blamed if you do that. ◆あなたが罪の意識を感じる必要は全くありません You don't have to feel guilty at all.

つめ 爪 **nail** （手の爪）**fingernail** （足の

つめ 爪)**toenail** (親指の爪)**thumbnail** ◆爪がどうかしましたか Do you have any problems with your nails? ◆爪に何か変化がありましたか Have you noticed any changes in your nails? ◆爪が剥がれたのですか Has the nail (plate) separated from the nail bed? ◆爪を見せて下さい Let me look at your nails. ◆お子さんは爪を嚙みますか Does your child bite his ⟨her⟩ nails? ◆きつい靴のせいで足の爪が陥入してしまうことがよくあります Tight shoes often cause ingrown toenails. ◆爪を切る cut one's nails ◆深爪する cut one's nails[(手の爪)fingernails / (足の爪)toenails] too short / (嚙んで) bite one's nails down to the quick ◆爪を割る break[split] a nail ◆指の爪が変色して黒い the fingernails become discolored and turn black ◆肥厚した爪 a thickened nail ◆肉に食い込んだ爪 an ingrown[ingrowing] nail ◀匙状爪 spoon nail 太鼓ばち爪 clubbed nail ▶爪痕 nail mark / (ひっかき傷)scratch 爪床 nail bed 爪板[爪甲] nail plate 爪かみ(癖) nail biting / onychophagia 爪切り nail clippers[scissors] 爪白癬 tinea unguium / ringworm of the nails 爪やすり nail file

爪の性状
●弯曲した curved / (内側に曲がった)inward ●太鼓ばち状の clubbed ●スプーン状の spoon-shaped ●隆起した ridged ●肥厚した thickened ●溝のある(くぼんだ)pitted ●陥入した ingrown ●剥がれた separated from the nail bed ●亀裂の入った split ●もろい brittle ●変色した discolored

つめしょ 詰所 (拠点)**station** (場所)**room** ◀看護師詰所 nurses'[nurses] station 警備員詰所(hospital) guard office [room]

つめたい 冷たい **cold** (冷たくて快い)**cool** (ひんやりした)**chilly** (態度が無愛想な)**cold, unfriendly** ◆手足が冷たくなることがありますか Do your hands or feet ever feel cold? ◆この器具は少し冷たいかもし

れません This instrument may feel a little cold. ◆冷たい飲み物 cool[cold] drink ◆…に対して冷たい態度をとる be cold [unfriendly] toward …

つめもの 詰め物 (歯の)**(dental) filling** ◆歯の詰め物がとれています Your filling has come out. ◆虫歯に詰め物をする fill a decayed tooth

つめる 詰める 《充塡する》 (詰め込む)**pack, stuff** (管・穴を塞ぐ)**plug** (歯の穴を塞ぐ)**fill** ◆持ち物を詰めるのをお手伝いしましょうか Shall I help you pack your things? ◆虫歯の穴を詰める fill a cavity[decayed tooth] 《待機する》**be on standby** ◆看護師が24時間ナースステーションに詰めています Nurses are on standby at the nurses' station twenty-four hours a day.

つもり ◆そういうつもりで言ったのではありません I didn't mean that. ☞意図

つや 通夜 **wake** ◆通夜に参列する attend a wake

つよい 強い 《強力な》 (一般的に強い)**strong** (度合・程度が激しい)**intense** (作用が強い)**powerful** (痛みなどが激しい)**severe** (圖強く **strongly** 力を込めてぎゅっと **firmly, tightly** 圖 **strengthen**) ◆効果の強い薬 a powerful [strong] medication ◆強い不安 strong [intense] anxiety ◆強い痛み *(a) severe[(an) intense] pain ◆黄疸が強い have a severe form of jaundice ◆日差しが強い時にはサングラスをしたほうがよいでしょう You should wear sunglasses when the sunlight is intense[very strong]. ◆このレバーを強く握って下さい Please grasp this lever firmly. ◆飲食物の食べ合わせによってはこの薬の効果が強くなることがありますので注意して下さい You need to be careful with this medication, because when taken together, some foods and drinks strengthen its effect. ◆痛みが徐々に強くなるかもしれません The pain may gradually become worse[more severe]. ◆事情を考えるとあまり強くも言えません (主張できない) As things stand

[Under the circumstances], I can't insist on my opinion. 《丈夫で抵抗力がある》 ◆ストレスには強いほうですか(抵抗力があるか)Do you tend to have a high tolerance for stress?

つよみ 強み advantage ☞有利

つらい 辛い (不快な)uncomfortable, (ひどい)terrible, awful, tough (痛い)painful (困難な)difficult, hard (耐えられない)unbearable (気に障る)annoying 《身体が苦しい》 ◆この検査は少しつらいかもしれません I'm sorry if this test makes you a little uncomfortable. ◆頭痛はつらかったでしょう This headache must have been terrible[very tough / painful] for you. ◆目を開けるのがつらいのですか Is it difficult (for you) to open your eyes? / Do you have difficulty opening your eyes? ◆薬の副作用がつらい時にはご相談下さい If the side effects of the medication become unbearable, please tell us. ◆(出産・手術後などで)つらかったでしょうが，よく頑張りましたね You really had a hard time[You've had a really hard time], but you've made it through. 《耐えがたい心地である》 ◆おつらいでしょう This must be terrible[awful] for you. ◆今一番つらいことは何ですか What's giving you the most difficulty right now? / What's the hardest thing for you (to deal with) right now? / What's the most painful or annoying thing for you right now? ◆申し上げるのはつらいのですが，腫瘍は悪性です I'm sorry to (have to) tell you this, but the tumor is malignant.

つりほうたい 吊り包帯 (手・腕用の吊り包帯)sling (陰嚢などに用いる懸垂包帯)suspensory bandage ◆吊り包帯で腕を吊る have *one's* arm in a sling ◀腕吊り包帯 arm sling

つる¹ 吊る (掛ける)hang (包帯などで)put[have]... in a sling ◆骨折した腕を包帯で吊りましょう I'm going to[Let me] put your broken arm in a sling.

つる² 攣る get a cramp, have a cramp ◆足がつることがありますか Do you ever get[have] cramps in your legs?

つれる 連れる (連れて行く)take (連れて来る)bring (同行する)accompany ◆私がリハビリ室にお連れいたします I'm going to take[accompany] you to the rehabilitation room. ◆次回の診察にご主人を連れてきていただけますか Could you bring your husband with you at your next visit?

つわり (早朝嘔吐)morning sickness (重症妊娠悪阻)hyperemesis gravidarum；HG ◆つわりはまだありますか Do you still have morning sickness? ◆つわりはあと2, 3週間で治まるでしょう Your morning sickness will go away in a few weeks.

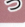

て

て 手 （手首から先）hand （腕）arm
《診察の基本表現》 ◆手が荒れた原因は何か思い当たりますか What do you think is causing your rough and chapped hands? ◆手にしびれがありますか Do you have any numbness in your hands? ◆手がこわばりますか Do your hands get stiff? ◆手が震える have shaky hands / one's hands shake[tremble] ◆手の上げ下げが困難ですか Do you have difficulty raising and lowering your arms? ◆両手を上げて頭の上に載せて下さい Please raise both hands and put them on your head. ◆ゆっくり手を下ろして下さい Please lower your hand(s)[arm(s)] slowly. ◆左手を差し出して下さい Please hold out your left hand. ◆あなたはどちらの手をよく使いますか Which hand do you use more often than the other? / （利き手はどちらか）Which is your dominant hand? ◆（血液検査などで）手を握って下さい Please make a tight fist. ★fist は握りこぶし. ◆私の手をしっかり握って下さい Please grip[hold / grasp] my hand firmly. ◆手を伸ばす stretch (out) one's hand[arm] ◆手すりから手を離さないで下さい Don't let go of the handrail. ◆手を離して下さい Please let go (of your hand). ◆握った手を緩める〈離す〉loosen〈release〉one's grip
《慣用表現》 ◆お子さんぐらいの年齢がちょうど手のかかる頃です A child of about your child's age still needs a lot of looking after. ◆すみませんが，どうしても今が手が離せません I'm sorry, but *my hands are full[I'm tied up / I'm too busy] right now. ◆あらゆる手を尽くしたのですが，大変残念です We've tried *everything possible[every possible means]. I'm very sorry. ◆彼は当院到着時点ですでに脳の損傷がひどく手のつけようがない状態でし

た When he arrived at the hospital, the injuries to his brain were so serious that nothing could be done to save him.
◀利き手 dominant hand ☞手関節（しゅかんせつ），手指（しゅし），手足，手洗い，手首，手先，手湿疹，手の甲，手のひら，手袋

てあし 手足 （腕と脚）arms and legs （手首の先と足首の先）hands and feet （四肢）the limbs ◆彼女は手足が不自由です She has difficulty using her arms[hands] and legs. ◆手足が勝手に動く one's hands, arms, or legs move involuntarily[uncontrollably] ◆手足が震える have shaky hands and feet / one's hands and feet shake[tremble] ◆手足を伸ばす stretch one's limbs[arms and legs] ☞手口病

てあしくちびょう 手足口病 hand, foot and mouth disease, hand-foot-and-mouth disease；HFMD

てあつい 手厚い tender ◆できる限り手厚い介護を提供します We'll provide *the most tender care possible[the very best of care]. ◆手厚く介護する care for a person tenderly

てあて 手当
《治療》treatment （動treat）（世話）care ☞治療 ◆すぐに傷の手当をしましょう I'll treat[take care of] your injury *right away[immediately]. ◆別室で手当を受けて下さい Please go to another room to receive the treatment.
《給付》benefit /bénəfit/, allowance /əláʊəns/ ◆外国籍の方でも支援手当の対象になる場合があるので，市役所〈区役所〉の担当に問い合わせてはいかがですか Foreign residents may be eligible for (medical) benefits, so why don't you make inquiries at the city〈ward〉office?
◀応急手当 first aid / emergency care[treatment] 児童手当 child benefit[allowance] 児童扶養手当 child care benefit / child-rearing allowance 出産手当 maternity allowance 障害手当 disability allowance 傷病手当 injury and disease allowance

てあらい 手洗い hand washing （手術前

の手洗い）**scrubbing** （個人の家のトイレ）**bathroom** （公共の場所のトイレ）**restroom, rest room** ☞トイレ ◆手洗いはインフルエンザ予防にとても大切です Hand washing is very important to prevent flu. / Hand washing can help you avoid catching flu. ◆こまめな手洗いを心がけて下さい You should wash your hands frequently. ◆お手洗いに頻繁に行きますか Do you have to go to the bathroom often?

ていあくせいど 低悪性度（の）**low-grade** ▶低悪性度リンパ腫 low-grade lymphoma

ていあつ 低圧 **low pressure**

ていアルブミンけっしょう 低アルブミン血症 **hypoalbuminemia**

ていあん 提案する （勧める・示唆する）**suggest** （図suggestion）（積極的に提案する）**propose** （図proposal）◆別の治療法を提案いたします I'd like to suggest another treatment. ◆1つご提案があるのですが May I make a suggestion? / Let me make a suggestion. ◆この前の提案についてご検討いただけましたか Did you think over what I proposed[suggested] the other day?

ていい 定位（の）**stereotactic** ▶定位脳手術 stereotactic brain surgery 定位放射線治療 stereotactic radiotherapy；SRT

ディーエヌエー DNA （デオキシリボ核酸）**deoxyribonucleic acid** ▶DNA ウイルス DNA virus DNA 鑑定 DNA test[testing / analysis] / DNA-based test / DNA profiling / genetic[DNA] fingerprinting DNA 合成阻害薬 DNA synthesis inhibitor DNA 修復 DNA repair DNA 診断 DNA diagnosis DNA 損傷 DNA damage

ティーさいぼう T 細胞 **T cell**

ていいたいばん 低位胎盤 **low-lying placenta**

ティーリンパきゅう T リンパ球 **T lymphocyte**

ていインスリンけっしょう 低インスリン血症 **hypoinsulinemia**

ていえいよう 低栄養 （栄養失調・栄養障害）**malnutrition** （栄養不足）**undernutrition**

（授乳不足）**underfeeding** ▶低栄養患者 undernourished patient

ていエコー 低エコー（の）**hypoechoic** ▶低エコー域 hypoechoic area

ていエネルギー 低エネルギー ☞低カロリー

ていえんしょく 低塩食 **low-salt[low-sodium] diet, sodium-restricted diet**

ていおうせっかい 帝王切開 **cesarean** （**delivery**）/sɪzériən-/, **cesarean** (**section**)；**CS, C-section** ◆（患者が）帝王切開を受ける have[undergo] a cesarean section[delivery] / （口語的に）have a cesarean ◆（医師が）帝王切開する perform a cesarean section[delivery] / deliver (a baby) by cesarean section ◆お産は自然分娩でしたか，それとも帝王切開でしたか Did you have a natural delivery or a cesarean? ◆赤ちゃんは帝王切開で産まれましたか Was the baby born[delivered] by cesarean section? ◆母子の安全のため帝王切開による出産をお勧めします For the safety of the mother and baby, I'd like to recommend a cesarean (delivery / section).

ていおん¹ 低音 **low[low-pitched] sound** (↔high[high-pitched] sound) （音色の）**low[low-pitched] tone** （声の）**low[low-pitched] voice** （低周波の）**low frequency** ☞音 ◆低音が聞こえにくいですか Do you have difficulty hearing low [low-pitched] sounds? ▶低音域障害型難聴 low-frequency[low-tone] hearing loss

ていおん² 低温 **low temperature** （低体温）**hypothermia** （図hypothermic）◆低体温にして脳のダメージを防ぐ prevent the risk of brain damage by cooling *a person's* body down to a low temperature ◀脳低温療法 brain hypothermia therapy ▶低温相(基礎体温の)hypothermic phase[period] 低温やけど low-temperature burn ☞低体温

ていか 低下する

《減少する》（下がる）**drop** （図drop）, **lower** 《衰える》**fall off, decline** ◆血圧の急激な

〈わずかな〉低下がある have a sudden〈slight〉drop in *one's* blood pressure / the blood pressure has dropped suddenly〈slightly〉 ◆脂質を低下させる薬(a) lipid-lowering medication[drug / agent] ◆食欲が低下する *one's* appetite *falls off [declines] 《悪化する》（衰える）**fail** （悪化する）**get worse, deteriorate, worsen** （弱まる）**weaken, lower** ◆彼女の心肺機能は徐々に低下しています Her heart and lungs are slowly failing. / Her heart and lung functions are gradually *getting worse[deteriorating]. ◆感染に対する抵抗力を低下させる weaken[lower] *one's* resistance to infection ◆視力が低下する *one's* eyesight worsens ◆聴力が低下する（難聴になる）get[become] hard of hearing

◀意識低下(傾眠)drowsiness /（低下した意識）impaired consciousness　運動低下 hypokinesia / hypokinesis　活動低下 hypoactivity　機能低下 hypofunction　筋力低下 muscle weakness　血圧低下 *fall in [drop in / lowering of] blood pressure　食欲低下 poor appetite / loss of appetite　知覚低下 decreased sensation　注意力低下 decreased attentiveness　聴力低下 decreased hearing　反射低下 hyporeflexia

ていがくばらい　定額払い　flat sum payment, fixed sum payment

ていカリウム　低カリウム　low potassium ▶低カリウム血症 hypokalemia / hypopotassemia　低カリウム血性周期性四肢麻痺 hypokalemic periodic paralysis　低カリウム食 low-potassium diet

ていカルシウムけつしょう　低カルシウム血症　hypocalcemia

ていカロリー　低カロリー　low calorie （脂肪分の少ない）**light calorie** ◀高蛋白低カロリー食品 high-protein, low-calorie food　▶低カロリー食 low-calorie diet [food]；LCD / calorie-restricted[calorie-restriction] diet

ていかんき　低換気　hypoventilation ◀肺胞低換気症候群 alveolar hypoventilation syndrome

ていき　定期(的な)　**（規則的な）regular** （いつも通りの）**routine** （周期的な）**periodical, periodic** ◆定期的に通院する visit[go to / come to] the hospital regularly ★come to the hospital は視点が医療者側にある. ◆定期的に運動していますか Do you exercise regularly[routinely]? / Do you do[get / take] regular exercise? ◆歯科医へは定期的に通っていますか Do you visit the dentist regularly? ◆乳房自己触診を定期的にしていますか Do you do regular breast self-exams? ◆どんなサプリメントを定期的に飲んでいますか What supplements do you take routinely[regularly]? ▶定期検査 regular[routine / periodical] test　定期検診 regular[routine / periodical] (medical) checkup[screening]　定期健康診断 regular (health) checkup / regular physical (examination)　定期予防接種 routine vaccination [immunization]

ていぎ　定義　definition （動define）

ていきょう　提供する　provide （与える）**give** （差し出す）**offer** （臓器などを）**donate** （図donation） ◆当院ではリハビリテーションを提供しています We provide rehabilitation in this hospital. ◆乳がんの情報を提供する provide[give / offer] information about[on] breast cancer ◆幅広い範囲の患者サービスを提供する offer [provide] a wide range of patient services ◀血液を提供する donate[give] blood　◀臓器提供 organ donation　☞提供者

ていきょうしゃ　提供者　donor ◀血液[輸血]提供者 blood[transfusion] donor　骨髄提供者 bone marrow donor　臓器提供者 organ donor

デイケア　day care, daycare ▶デイケアサービス day care service　デイケアセンター day care center

ていけいせい　低形成　hypoplasia （形hypoplastic）

ていけつあつ　低血圧　low blood pressure, hypotension （形hypotensive） ☞血圧　◀起立性低血圧 orthostatic[postural]

hypotension

ていけっとう 低血糖 low blood sugar, hypoglycemia （形hypoglycemic） ☞血糖 ◀空腹時低血糖 fasting hypoglycemia ケトン性低血糖 ketotic hypoglycemia ▶低血糖昏睡 hypoglycemic coma

ていこう 抵抗 resistance （形resistant, resistive） ◆感染症に対する身体の抵抗力が低下していますので，風邪を引かないように十分注意して下さい Your body's resistance to infection has decreased[weakened], so *take good care[be careful] not to catch a cold. ◆ストレスに対する身体の抵抗力を高める improve the body's resistance to stress ◀インスリン抵抗性 insulin resistance 抗菌薬抵抗性 antibiotic resistance 呼吸抵抗 respiratory resistance 漸増抵抗運動 progressive resistance[resistive] exercise；PRE 放射線抵抗性 radioresistance 薬物抵抗性 drug resistance ▶抵抗運動(訓練) resistance[resistive] exercise / (動き・動作) resistive movement

ていこきゅう 低呼吸 hypopnea；*abnormally shallow breathing* ◀無呼吸低呼吸指数 apnea-hypopnea index；AHI

ていゴナドトロピンせいせいせんきのうていかしょう 低ゴナドトロピン性性腺機能低下症 hypogonadotropic hypogonadism

ていコレステロール 低コレステロール low cholesterol, hypocholesterol ▶低コレステロール血症 hypocholesterolemia 低コレステロール食 low-cholesterol diet

デイサージェリー （same） day surgery, outpatient surgery, ambulatory surgery

デイサービス ☞デイケア

ていざんさしょく 低残渣食 low-residue diet；LRD, low-fiber diet；LFD

ていさんそ 低酸素 hypoxia ▶低酸素血症 hypoxemia

ていし 停止する stop （形stop） （一時的に） suspend （形suspension） 图 (停止状態) arrest ◆分娩の取り扱いを停止します（サービスを提供できない）The hospital will no longer be able to provide maternity

services. / The hospital will stop[suspend] maternity services. ◆入院患者の受け入れを一時停止している The hospital is suspending[temporarily stopping] new patient admissions. ◆インフルエンザに罹った子は，解熱した後 2 日を経過するまで通学できません Any children with flu will not be allowed to attend school until they have been fever-free for two days. ◀呼吸停止 respiratory arrest / (無呼吸) apnea 思考停止 thought stopping 心停止 cardiac arrest；CA / heart arrest 心肺停止 cardiopulmonary arrest；CPA / cardiac (and) respiratory arrest

ていしきそせいひんけつ 低色素性貧血 hypochromic anemia

ていしげき 低刺激 (の) （皮膚に優しい） mild （刺激の少ない）hypoirritant ◆低刺激性の石鹸 mild soap

ていしぼう 低脂肪 (の) low-fat （低カロリーの）light ▶低脂肪牛乳 low-fat[light] milk / (乳脂肪 2% の) two-percent milk 低脂肪高蛋白食品 low-fat, high-protein food 低脂肪食 low-fat diet

ていじゅう 定住(の) permanent ▶定住外国人 permanent foreign resident 定住地 permanent abode[place of residence]

ていしゅうは 低周波 low frequency ▶低周波療法 low-frequency therapy

ていしゅつ 提出する submit, turn in （手渡す）hand in （報告書などを）present ◆この同意書をよく読んでサインしてからご提出下さい Please read this (informed) consent form carefully and sign it before *handing it in[submitting it]. ◆出生届を大使館に提出して下さい Please submit the forms[necessary documents] for registration of your baby's birth to the embassy. / (大使館に登録して下さい)Please register the birth of your baby at the embassy.

ていしゅっせいたいじゅうじ 低出生体重児 low birth weight infant；LBWI （出生体重 2,500 g 未満）infant weighing less than twenty-five hundred grams at birth ☞未

熟児 ◀極低出生体重児 very low birth weight infant；VLBWI／(出生体重 1,500 g 未満) infant weighing less than fifteen hundred grams at birth 超低出生体重児 extremely low birth weight infant；ELBWI／(出生体重 1,000 g 未満) infant weighing less than one thousand grams at birth

でいじょう 泥状(の) muddy ◆泥状の便 muddy stools

ていしょとく 低所得 low income ◆低所得の家族 a low-income family

ていしりょく 低視力 low vision

ていしんしゅうしゅじゅつ 低侵襲手術 minimally invasive surgery

ていしんちょう 低身長 short stature ▶低身長症 dwarfism

ていしんはくしゅつりょうしょうこうぐん 低心拍出量症候群 low (cardiac) output syndrome

ていせい 定性(の) qualitative (↔quantitative) ▶定性分析 qualitative analysis

ていせつ 定説 (広く認められている説・意見) widely accepted theory[opinion], widely held theory[opinion] (立証された説) established theory ◆この病気の原因について定説はありません There is no widely accepted[established] theory about the causes of this disease.

ていたいおん 低体温 low temperature, hypothermia (形 hypothermic) ▶低体温症 hypothermia 低体温麻酔 hypothermic anesthesia 低体温療法 hypothermia therapy／therapeutic hypothermia

ていたいじゅう 低体重 low body weight (形 underweight) ◆お子さんはやや低体重です You child is slightly underweight. ☞低出生体重児

ていたんぱく 低蛋白 low protein, hypoprotein ▶低蛋白血症 hypoproteinemia 低蛋白食 low-protein[protein-restricted] diet

ていちょうせいだっすい 低張性脱水 hypotonic dehydration

ティッシュペーパー tissue (商標名) Kleenex (ウェットティッシュ) wet wipe, towelette ◆ティッシュペーパーを使う

use a tissue[Kleenex] ◆このティッシュペーパーでお口を拭いて下さい Here's a tissue[Kleenex] to wipe your mouth. ◆ティッシュペーパー 1 箱 a box of tissues [Kleenex]

ていど 程度 (レベル・水準・高さ) level (標準) standard (数量・度合いの単位) degree (範囲) extent ☞レベル ◆あなたのストレスの程度は高いですか Is your stress level high?／Do you have a high level of stress? ◆痛みの程度はどのくらいですか How severe[bad] is the pain? ◆めまいの程度はどのくらいですか How bad is your dizziness? ◆生活程度が高い have a high standard of living ◆彼女の脱水の程度は軽度〈中程度／重度〉です The degree of her dehydration is mild〈moderate／severe〉. ◆あなたはご自分の病気をどの程度理解していますか What[How much] do you know about your illness? ◆ライフスタイルを変えることで心臓病をある程度予防することができます Heart disease can be prevented to some extent by changing *one's* lifestyle.

ていナトリウムけっしょう 低ナトリウム血症 hyponatremia

ていねい 丁寧(な) (詳細な) detailed (注意深い・綿密な) careful (徹底的な) thorough /θ́ːrə/ (礼儀正しい) polite ☞詳しい ◆担当医は丁寧に説明してくれましたか Did your doctor give you a detailed [careful] explanation about this?／Did your doctor explain this *in detail[carefully]* to you? ◆傷口は丁寧に水洗いして下さい Please wash the wound thoroughly with water. ◆丁寧な対応 a polite response

ていねんたいしょくしゃ 定年退職者 retired person, retiree

ていのうど 低濃度 low concentration

ていひじゅう 低比重(の) low-density ▶超低比重リポ蛋白 very low-density lipoprotein；VLDL 低比重リポ蛋白 low-density lipoprotein；LDL／bad cholesterol

ていぶんか 低分化(の) poorly differenti-

ated ▶低分化癌 poorly differentiated carcinoma　低分化腺癌 poorly differentiated adenocarcinoma

ていぶんしヘパリン　低分子(量)ヘパリン low molecular weight heparin；LMWH

ていマグネシウムけっしょう　低マグネシウム血症　hypomagnesemia

ていみつど　低密度　☞低比重

ていもう　剃毛　shaving（動shave）　◆手術前の剃毛 preoperative shaving　◆手術前の剃毛はご自分でしますか，それとも私がしましょうか Before the surgery, will you shave yourself or shall I do it for you? ◆下腹部の剃毛をしますので，動かないで下さい I'm going to shave your lower abdomen, so please stay still.　◀陰部剃毛 shaving of the pubic hair[region]

ていようりょう　低用量(の)　low dose, low dosage　★dose は1回の摂取量，dosage は一定期間に渡る摂取量をいう．　▶低用量アスピリン low-dose[low-dosage] aspirin　低用量ピル low-dose[low-dosage] pill

ていヨードしょく　低ヨード食　low-iodine diet

でいり　出入りする　go into (and out), enter　◆こちらは病院関係者以外出入りできません We're sorry, but only the hospital staff[personnel] *can go into[are permitted to enter] this area.　◆小さいお子さんの出入りはご遠慮願っております Small children are not allowed to enter this area.　◀緊急出入り口 emergency entrance

ていりゅうせいそう　停留精巣　undescended testicle[testis], retained testicle [testis], cryptorchidism, cryptorchism

ていりょう　定量(の)　quantitative （↔qualitative）　▶定量分析 quantitative analysis

ていリンさんけっしょう　低リン酸血症 hypophosphatemia（形hypophosphatemic）　▶低リン酸血症性ビタミンD抵抗性くる病 hypophosphatemic vitamin D–resistant rickets

ていリンしょく　低リン食　low-phospho-

rus diet

データ　data /déitə/　◆データはここにお示しします Your data are shown here. ★data は複数形だが単数扱いにもなる．　◆治療成績や副作用に関するデータを集める collect[gather] data on treatment outcomes and adverse effects　◆データを保存する save[store] the data　◆データを処理する process the data　▶検査データ test data　数値データ numerical data　電子データ electronic data　統計データ statistical data　生データ raw data　臨床データ clinical data　▶データ解析 data analysis　データ収集 data collection データ処理 data processing　データベース database

テーピング　taping　◆右足首をテーピングする tape a person's right ankle

テープ　tape（動テープを貼る tape）　◆傷口にガーゼを当ててテープで留める place a gauze pad over[on top of] the wound and tape it down　◆テープをそっと剥がす *take off[remove] the tape gently　◀粘着テープ adhesive tape

テーブル　table　◆(ベッドの)テーブルを出しましょう Let me pull up the (overbed) table.　◆(ベッドの)テーブルをしまう *push back[put away] the (overbed) table　◆テーブルの上に朝食のお膳を置きます I'm going to put your breakfast tray on the table.　◀ベッドサイドテーブル bedside table

テーラーメイド　tailor-made　▶テーラーメイド医療〈治療〉 tailor-made medicine 〈treatment / therapy〉

デオキシリボかくさん　―核酸　☞DNA

ておくれ　手遅れ　too late　◆手遅れにならないうちに心臓の専門医に診てもらって下さい Please see a heart specialist before it's too late.

でかける　出掛ける　go out (of)　☞外出

てがみ　手紙　letter,《英》post（郵便物） mail　◆シムさん，お手紙ですよ Mrs Sim, here's a letter for you.　◆問い合わせの手紙を書く write a letter of inquiry (to) ◆紹介の手紙を書く write a *referral letter

[letter of referral]（to）

てき　滴　drop　◆目薬を1日に2回2, 3滴ずつ差して下さい Please put[apply] a few drops into[to] your eyes twice a day.

できあがる　出来上がる　（用意が出来る）be ready　（完成する）be finished　◆入れ歯ができあがるのに約2, 3週間かかります It will take a few weeks (or so) before your dentures are ready[finished].

てきおう　適応　（順応）adaptation　（國 adapt　國adaptive, adaptable）, adaptability　（調整）adjustment（↔maladjustment）（國adjust）　（治療上の必要性・妥当性）indication　（適格性）eligibility（國eligible）☞順応　◆日本の生活に適応する adapt [adjust] *oneself* to life in Japan　◆この症状は薬で改善しない時には手術の適応になります If this symptom does not improve with medication, *it will be an indication that surgery is necessary[surgery is indicated].　◆あなたは肝移植の適応です You are eligible for a liver transplant.
◀過剰適応 excessive adaptation / overadaptation　社会適応 social adaptation [adjustment]　社会不適応 social maladjustment　宿主適応 host adaptation　手術適応 surgical indication / indication for surgery　心理的適応 psychological adaptation　▶適応行動 adaptive behavior　適応障害 adjustment disorder；AD　☞適応外

てきおうがい　適応外　off-label　▶適応外使用 off-label use[indication]　適応外薬 off-label medication[drug]

てきおん¹　適温　（中等度の温度）moderate temperature　（適切な温度）suitable temperature　（至適温度）optimal temperature, optimum temperature

てきおん²　笛音　（ゼイゼイする音）wheeze　（ヒュー・ピーという音）whistle

てきごう　適合(性)　（互換性）compatibility （國compatible）　（一致）match, congruity　◆提供された血液と患者の血液との適合性を輸血前に調べる test the compatibility *between the donor and recipient blood[of a donor's and a recipient's

blood] before transfusion　◆HLA型が適合したドナーが見つかりました An HLA-matched donor was found.　◀血液交差適合試験 blood cross-matching (procedure)　☞不適合

できごと　出来事　event　（思いがけない出来事）happening, incident, occurrence　◆最近の出来事の記憶を失う lose *one's* memory of recent events　◆最近の出来事より遠い過去の出来事のほうをはっきり覚えている remember distant past events more clearly than recent past events

できし　溺死　drowning, death by drowning　☞溺れる

てきしゅつ　摘出する　（除去する）remove （國removal）　（臓器・組織を切除する）excise （國excision 國excisional）　（抜き取る）extract （國extraction）　（接尾-ectomy）☞切除　◆胆嚢〈扁桃腺〉を無事に摘出しました The gallbladder was 〈The tonsils were〉 successfully removed.　◆腫瘍を摘出する手術 surgery to remove a tumor
◀胸腺摘出術 thymectomy　筋腫摘出術 myomectomy　結石摘出術 lithectomy / stone extraction / extraction[removal] of *a stone[stones]　子宮摘出術 hysterectomy　腎摘出術 nephrectomy　水晶体嚢外摘出術 extracapsular lens extraction　胆嚢摘出術 cholecystectomy　脾摘出術 splenectomy　副甲状腺摘出術 parathyroidectomy　扁桃摘出術 tonsillectomy / tonsil removal surgery　卵巣摘出術 ovariectomy / oophorectomy　▶摘出生検 excision[excisional] biopsy　摘出臓器(切除した臓器)removed organ / (分離した臓器) isolated organ

できすい　溺水　near drowning, submersion　☞溺れる

てきする　適する　（良い）be good（for, to *do*）　（ふさわしい）be suitable（for, to *do*）, be fit（for, to *do*）　（適当である）be adequate（for, to *do*）　（適格である）be eligible（for, to *do*）　（合う）suit, fit　◆日本の水は飲用に適しています Water in Japan is good[fit] to drink.　◆最小侵襲手術はすべての患者さんに適しているわけではありませ

ん Minimally invasive surgery *does not suit[is not suitable for] all patients. / Not all patients are eligible candidates for minimally invasive surgery.

てきせい¹　**適正（な）**　proper　（最適の）optimal　☞適切　▶適正体重 optimal [healthy] weight

てきせい²　**適性**　（素質）aptitude　（健康状態の良好さ）fitness　◀体力適性テスト physical fitness test　▶適性検査 aptitude test

てきせつ　**適切（な）**　（よい）good　（目的にかなった）appropriate　（ふさわしい）suitable, adequate　（妥当な）proper, reasonable　◆適切な助言を与える give a person good [appropriate] advice　◆救急患者に適切な処置を施す give the emergency patient appropriate treatment　◆適切なカロリー量を摂取することが大切です It is important to get a proper amount of calories.

できだかばらい　**出来高払い**　fee for services

てきど　**適度（な）**　（ほどよく中くらいの）moderate　（圀moderation）　（適性な）proper　（ふさわしい）suitable　☞適切, 適量　◆適度な運動と食事は病気のリスクを下げます Proper exercise and diet will lower[reduce] the risk of illness.　◆適度に運動する get[do] moderate[（軽い）light] exercises / exercise in moderation　◆お酒を適度に飲む drink moderately / drink alcohol in moderation　◆適度の睡眠をとる have[get] a proper amount of sleep

てきとう　**適当（な）**　☞適切

できない　cannot, can't, be unable to …　☞できる　◆ご要望に応じることができない場合もありますのでご了承下さい Please understand that we are sometimes unable to meet[satisfy / fulfill] patients' requests.　◆入院できない理由〈事情〉は何ですか What are the reasons〈circumstan­ces〉preventing you from *being hospitalized[going into the hospital]?

てきひ　**摘脾**　splenectomy

できもの　（おでき）boil　（突発的な発疹）eruption　◆首にできものがある have a boil on one's neck / a boil has formed on one's neck

てきよう　**適用する**　（当てはめる）apply（to）　（圀application　圀applicable）　（保険対象とする）cover（圀coverage）　◆この指針は主に冠動脈性心疾患の患者に適用されます These guidelines apply primarily to patients with coronary heart disease.　◆この薬は保険適用ではありません This medication is not covered by health insurance. / Health insurance does not cover the cost of this medication.　◆国民健康保険に加入していれば，外国の方にも様々な医療給付サービスが適用されます Various medical（care）benefits are also applicable to foreign residents who have National Health Insurance. / （権利が与えられる）Non-Japanese patients who have National Health Insurance are also entitled to receive various medical（care）benefits.

てきりょう　**適量**　moderate amount　（投薬量）optimal dose, optimum dose　☞適度　◆適量のお酒を飲む drink a moderate amount of alcohol　◆お酒は適量であればかまいません You can drink alcohol in moderation.　◆この薬の適量は血液検査によって決定されます The optimal[optimum] dose of this medication is determined by a blood test.

できる

《可能である》can, be able to …, be possible　☞可能, できるだけ, できれば　◆何か私にできることはありますか What can I do for you? / Is there anything I can do for you?　◆お子さんはお座りができますか Is your child able to[Can your child] sit up without support?　◆来週の金曜日に受診できますか Is it possible for you to come and see me next Friday?

《上手に行える》（首尾よく完了する）do a good job　（上手である）be good at　◆（軽い口調で）よくできましたね（You did a）good job.　◆彼女は日本語がよくできます She is very good at Japanese.

《物・状況が生じる》（病変が生じる）have, get

できる 503 **てすり**

（発症する）develop （ある事態が生じる）**come up** ◆水疱ができる have[get / develop] blisters ◆首に湿疹ができる get eczema on the neck ◆急用ができたので，少しここでお待ちいただけませんか An emergency[Something] just came up, so could you please wait here for a while?

できるだけ ☞精一杯 ◆できるだけ早くご来院下さい Please get[come] to the hospital[clinic /（こちらへ）here] as soon as possible. ◆できるだけのことは行いましたが，大変残念です We did everything *we could[possible]. I'm very sorry. ◆スタッフができるだけお手伝いします Our staff will help you in every way possible.

できれば **if possible** ◆できれば明日にでもお会いしたいのですが I would like to see you tomorrow, if possible. ◆できれば予約を木曜日に変更していただけるとありがたいのですが I'd really appreciate it if you could change your appointment to Thursday. ★could を用いて「可能なら」という依頼の気持ちを表す.

でぐち **出口** （建物の）**exit, way out** （開口部）**opening, orifice** （流出口）**outlet** ◆出口はあちらです The exit[way out] is over there. ◆自動販売機はカフェテリアの出口近くにあります The vending machines are located near (the entrance of) the cafeteria. ★英語では exit を使うと不自然になる. entrance は入口. ◆尿道の出口付近が痛む have (a) pain around the urethral opening[orifice]

てくび **手首** **wrist** /ríst/ ◆ID バンドを手首に付けます Let me attach your ID band to your wrist. ◆手首を骨折〈捻挫〉する break〈sprain〉*one's* wrist ◆かみそりで手首を切る cut[slit / slash] *one's* wrist(s) with a razor ◆手首の損傷 wrist injury ▶手首自傷症候群 wrist-cutting syndrome

てさき **手先** （手）**hand** （指）**finger** ◆彼は手先が器用〈不器用〉です He is good 〈clumsy〉with his hands[fingers].

デジタル（の） **digital** ▶デジタルX線撮影 digital radiography；DR　デジタル画像 digital imaging　デジタル・サブトラクション血管造影法 digital subtraction angiography；DSA

てしっしん **手湿疹** **hand eczema, eczema on the hand(s)**

デシベル **decibel；dB[db]**

デシリットル **deciliter；dL**

てじゅん **手順** （進行の順序）**procedure** （段階）**step** ◆手術の手順をご説明しましょう Let me explain *the procedure for your surgery[the surgical procedure]. ◆きちんと手順を踏む必要があります We need to follow the proper steps[procedures]. ◀看護手順 nursing procedure

てすう **手数** ◆手数をかける trouble / give you (much) trouble ◆お手数をおかけしますが，診断書の受け取りは後日ご来院下さい I'm sorry to have to ask you this [I hate to trouble you with this], but could you come to the hospital[clinic] some other day to pick up your medical certificate? ☞手数料

てすうりょう **手数料** （報酬）**(processing) fee** （料金）**(processing) charge** ◆手数料を請求する charge a (processing) fee ◆手数料を支払う pay a (processing) fee ◆診断書1通につき 2,000 円の手数料をいただきます A processing fee of two thousand yen will be charged for each medical certificate.

テスト **test, examination** ☞検査, 試験 ◀診断テスト diagnostic test　体力テスト physical strength test　知能テスト intelligence test / *intelligence quotient[IQ] test　パッチテスト patch test　メンタルテスト mental test

テストステロン **testosterone**

てすり **手摺** （移動・歩行用の）**handrail,** （support）**rail** （立ち座り用の）**(grab) bar** ◆安全用の手すり a safety rail ◆手すりにおつかまり下さい Please hold onto the handrail. ◆手すりをしっかり握って下さい Please grab (onto) the bar firmly. ◆手すりから手を離さないで下さい Don't let go of the handrail. ◆手を離して下さ

い Please let go〈of your hand〉. ◆手すりにつかまって歩く walk holding onto the handrail / walk with the support of the handrail ◆階段〈トイレ〉に手すりを付ける install handrails *on the staircase〈in the bathroom〉

テタニー tetany

てちょう **手帳** （記録）record （手引き書）handbook （メモ帳）notebook （日誌）diary, log ◆お薬手帳 personal medication record[history handbook] 血圧手帳 blood pressure diary[log] 健康手帳 personal health record 身体障害者手帳 physical disability handbook / handbook for the physically disabled 精神障害者保健福祉手帳 mental disability handbook / handbook for the mentally disabled 年金手帳 pension handbook 母子（健康）手帳 mother and child health handbook / Boshi-techo 療育手帳 intellectual disability handbook / handbook for children with an intellectual disability

てつ **鉄** iron /áiən/ ▶貯蔵鉄 storage iron ▶鉄吸収 iron absorption 鉄欠乏 iron deficiency 鉄欠乏性貧血 iron-deficiency anemia 鉄剤 iron （preparation） ☞鉄結合能, 鉄分

てつけつごうのう **鉄結合能** iron-binding capacity ◀総鉄結合能 total iron-binding capacity；TIBC 不飽和鉄結合能 unsaturated iron-binding capacity；UIBC

てつだう **手伝う** help （図help）, assist （図assistance） ◆お手伝いしましょう Let me *help you[give you a hand]. ◆何かお手伝いすることはありますか Do you need any help? / Is there anything I can do for you? ◆体の向きを変えるのをお手伝いします I'm going to[Let me] help you change your position. ◆着替えを手伝いましょうか Shall I help you change your clothes? / Shall I help you with your clothes? ◆手伝いが必要でしたら遠慮なくお申し出下さい If you need any help, please don't hesitate to ask us. ◆喜んでお手伝いいたします I'll be glad to help you.

てつづき **手続き** procedure （段取り）arrangements ★通例，複数形で. ☞手配 ◆入院の手続きについては病院事務で訊いて下さい Please ask about admission[admitting] procedures at the hospital business office. ◆窓口のクラークが手続きをしてくれます The clerk at the reception desk will take care of you. ◆入院手続きは済ませましたか Have you already finished the admission procedure? / Have you already completed the admission forms[paperwork]? ◆退院の手続きをする必要があります You need to complete some discharge procedures. ◆必要な手続きはこちらで行います We'll make the necessary arrangements.

てつぶん **鉄分** iron （content） /áiən-/ ☞鉄 ◆この食品は鉄分に富んでいます This food is high in iron. / This food has a high iron content. ◆鉄分の不足は貧血の原因になります Lack of iron causes anemia. ◆もっと鉄分の多い食事を心がけて下さい Please try to eat more iron-rich foods. ◆十分な鉄分を補給する supply [provide] sufficient iron ▶鉄分不足 iron deficiency / lack of iron 鉄分補給剤 iron supplement

テトロドトキシン tetrodotoxin

テニスひじ **―肘** tennis elbow （上腕骨外側上顆炎）lateral （humeral） epicondylitis

てのこう **手の甲** the back of the hand

てのひら **手のひら** palm /páːm/, the palm of the hand ◆右手を出して手のひらを上に向けて下さい Please hold out your right hand with the palm facing upward. ◆手のひらを上に向ける turn *one's palm up ◆手のひらを差し出す hold out *one's palm

では then, OK[Okay] then, now then, well, well then, so ◆では，始めましょう OK then[Now then], let's start. ◆ではまた月曜日の朝にお会いしましょう See you 〈on〉 Monday morning. / Well then, I'll see you 〈on〉 Monday morning. ◆では今日はこのへんでおしまいにしましょう That's all for today.

てはい　**手配する**　(前もって準備する)**arrange**（for）, **make arrangements**（for）(用意する)**prepare**（for）, **make preparations**（for）(予約する)**reserve, book** ☞準備, 用意　◆すぐに入院の手配をしましょう I'm going to arrange[make arrangements] for you to be admitted to the hospital right away.　◆できるだけ早く彼の手術の手配をいたします We'll arrange for him to have the surgery as soon as possible.　◆臨床心理士との面会の手配をする arrange an interview with a clinical psychologist　◆ご希望なら個室を手配いたします If you want[like], I'll reserve a private room for you.　◆介護タクシーの手配をする arrange[book] a care taxi[cab]

てはじめ　**手始め(に)**　(まず最初に)**first**（of all）(慣)**first**, **at the beginning**　(始めるに当たって)**to begin with**　☞最初　◆手始めに間食を控えることからなさってはいかがですか As a first step[To begin with], how about cutting back on eating between meals? / How about cutting back on eating between meals first[at the beginning]?

てはじめる　**出始める**　(発症する)**start, begin, come on**　(現れ始める)**start to appear, begin to appear**　◆熱はいつ出始めましたか When did the fever start[come on]?　◆認知症の症状が出始めています Symptoms of dementia have started to appear.

てぶくろ　**手袋**　**gloves**　(二股の手袋)**mittens**　★いずれも通例, 複数形で.　◆手袋をはめる put *one's* gloves on / put on *one's* gloves　◆手袋を脱ぐ take *one's* gloves off / take off *one's* gloves　◆手袋をしている wear gloves　◀ゴム手袋 rubber gloves 防護手袋 protective gloves　ラテックス手袋 latex gloves　▶手袋靴下型感覚消失 glove-and-stocking anesthesia

でべそ　**出臍**　**protruding navel**

てまわりひん　**手回り品**　☞持ち物

てみじか　**手短(に)**　(簡潔に)**briefly**　(要するに)**in brief, in short**　◆手短にお話しいたします Let me *explain this matter briefly

[speak briefly about this].

デュシェンヌがたきんジストロフィー　**―型筋ジストロフィー**　**Duchenne muscular dystrophy ; DMD**

てゆび　**手指**　☞手指(しゅし)

デリケート　(繊細で壊れやすい)**delicate** /délikət/ (過敏な)**sensitive**　◆デリケートな肌 delicate[sensitive] skin　◆デリケートな問題 a delicate problem　◆神経がデリケートな人 a sensitive person / (興奮しやすい人)a high-strung person

でる　**出る**　☞出す
《症状などが出る》**have, get**　(始まる)**start**　(生じる)**come on**　(現れる)**appear**　(発疹・汗などが突然出る)**break out**　(膿・血液などがしみ出る)**ooze**（out）　◆その症状が出たのはいつからですか When did the symptom start[first come on / appear]?　◆鼻血がよく出ますか Do you often have nosebleeds? / Does your nose bleed often?
◆熱が出るのはいつも夕方ですか Does the fever usually come on in the evening? / Do you usually have the fever in the evening?　◆彼は体中に赤い斑点が出ています He's got red spots all over his body. / Red spots have appeared all over his body.　◆傷口から膿が出ています The wound is oozing pus. / Pus is oozing [draining] *out of[from] the wound.
◆わけもなく涙が出ますか Do your eyes water[tear] for no particular reason?
◆血尿が出ています There is blood in your urine. / Blood was detected in your urine.　◆発疹が出る break out in a rash　◆蕁麻疹が出る break out in hives / get[have] hives　◆咳が出る cough / have a cough　◆アレルギー症状が出る have an allergic reaction　◆鼻水が出る have a runny nose / *one's* nose is running　◆歯茎から血が出る the gums bleed / have bleeding gums　◆食欲は出てきましたか Did your appetite *come back[return]? / Did you get your appetite back?
《その他》◆田中先生は診察中ですので電話口には出られません Dr Tanaka can't

come to the phone right now because he ⟨she⟩ is seeing a patient. ◆検査結果が出ました Your test results have come back [through]. / I've got your test results.

テレビ television；TV （テレビ番組）TV program ◆テレビは有料でレンタルすることができます Televisions are available for rent. / A rental television is available. ◆テレビの貸出をご希望の場合は病棟の事務員にお申し出下さい If you want to arrange a rental TV, please contact a floor clerk. ◆各ベッドに有料テレビがついていますので，プリペイドカードを前もってお求め下さい Each bed has *a pay TV[a rental TV service], so please buy a TV card beforehand. ◆テレビの音が大きすぎます I'm afraid that your TV is too loud. ◆テレビをつける⟨消す⟩ turn on ⟨off⟩ the TV ◆テレビの音を小さく⟨大きく⟩する turn down⟨up⟩ the (volume on the) TV ◆お子さんはテレビ画面のすぐ近くに座りますか Does your child sit very close to the TV screen? ◆お子さんは1日にどれくらいテレビを見ますか How many hours a day does your child watch TV? ◆テレビを見る時はイヤホンを使用して下さい When watching TV, please use the earphones provided. ◆お好きなテレビ番組は何ですか What's your favorite TV program? ◀ポータブルテレビ portable TV[television] set ▶テレビカード prepaid TV card　テレビてんかん television epilepsy

てん 点 《小さな円（で示されたところ）》（斑点）spot （小さいしみ）speck （ピリオドなどの点）dot （特定の点）point, punctum （部位）site ◆目を大きく開けたままピカピカ光る点を追いかけて下さい Keep your eye open wide, and follow the flashing spot. ◆目の前に黒い点や光が見えたことがありますか Have you ever seen black spots or lights in front of your eyes? ◆視野の中に黒い点が浮かんでいますか Do black specks float about in your field of vision? 《着目・話題の箇所》point ◆その点ではあな

たと同じ意見です I agree with you on that point. ◆この薬の良い点は副作用がほとんどないことです The good point of this medication is that it has few side effects. ◆わからない点は遠慮なく訊いて下さい If there's anything you don't understand, please don't hesitate to ask.

◀圧迫点 pressure point　作用点 point of action／working point／（薬物の作用部位）site of action　痛点 pain spot[point]／punctum dolorosum　転換点 turning point　臨界点 critical point　類似点 point of similarity[resemblance]／point in common／similarity　涙点 lacrimal point[punctum]

てんい[1] 転位 transposition （転座）translocation ◀完全大血管転位 complete *transposition of the great arteries [TGA] ▶転位歯 displaced[malposed] tooth

てんい[2] 転移 （がんなどの）metastasis／mətǽstəsɪs／（複 metastases 転 metastatic 転 metastasize 広がる spread） ★metastasize は専門用語なので，患者によっては spread を用いるほうがよい．◆がんが肺に転移しています The cancer has spread [metastasized] to the lung(s). ◆骨への転移 metastasis to *a bone[bones] ◆転移の恐れがあるのでリンパ節の切除を行う必要があります We need to remove the lymph nodes because *there's a risk the cancer may spread[we think the cancer may spread]. ◆転移の徴候はありません There is no sign that the cancer has spread[metastasized] to any other parts of your body. ◀遠隔転移 distant[remote] metastasis　血行性転移 hematogenous metastasis　骨転移 bone metastasis　リンパ行性転移 lymphogenous metastasis　リンパ節転移 lymph node metastasis ▶転移性骨⟨脳／肺／肝⟩腫瘍 metastatic bone⟨brain／lung／liver⟩ tumor　転移巣 metastatic lesion

でんい[1] 電位 （electric）potential ◀活動電位 action potential；AP　誘発電位 evoked potential

でんい² 殿位 breech presentation ◀単
殿位 frank[single] breech presentation

てんいん 転院する transfer（to） ◆ご自
宅の近くの病院への転院を希望なさいます
か Would you like to transfer[be trans-
ferred] to a hospital nearer your home?

でんおんなんちょう 伝音(性)難聴（聴力
消失）**conductive hearing loss**（聴力障害）
conductive hearing impairment

てんか 転化 ☞転換

でんかいしつ 電解質 electrolyte ◆電
解質バランスが崩れているようです Your
electrolytes seem to be out of balance. /
Your electrolyte levels seem to be unbalanced. ▶電解質平衡 electrolyte balance
電解質平衡障害 electrolyte imbalance

てんかぶつ 添加物 additive ◀食品添
加物 food additives 人工添加物 artificial
additives

てんかん¹ 癲癇 epilepsy /épələpsi/（形
てんかん性の epiléptic てんかん様の epilép-
toid） ◆てんかん患者 a patient with epilepsy / an epileptic patient ◆てんかん発
作 an epileptic seizure ◆てんかんの発作
を起こす have an epileptic seizure ◆て
んかん発作は薬で抑えられます Epileptic
seizures can be controlled with medication. ◀外傷後てんかん posttraumatic
epilepsy 局在関連性てんかん localization-related epilepsy 欠神てんかん absence epilepsy 抗てんかん薬 antiepilep-
tic（medication / drug / agent） 症候性
てんかん symptomatic epilepsy 小発作
てんかん minor[petit mal] epilepsy 全般
てんかん generalized epilepsy 大発作て
んかん major[grand mal] epilepsy テレ
ビてんかん television epilepsy 点頭てん
かん(乳児痙攣)infantile spasm 特発性て
んかん idiopathic epilepsy 光過敏性てん
かん photosensitive epilepsy；PSE ヒス
テリーてんかん hysteroepilepsy 部分て
んかん partial epilepsy ミオクローヌスて
んかん myoclonus[myoclonic] epilepsy ▶てんかん重積状態 status epilepticus てんかん焦点 epileptic focus てん
かん性格 epileptoid personality[charac-

ter] てんかん性人格変化 epileptic personality change てんかん性脱力発作
atonic[drop] seizure てんかん発作後麻
痺 postepileptic paralysis

てんかん² 転換（変化）**change**（変換）
conversion（接頭**trans-**） ◆気分転換に散
歩する take a walk *to have a change[for
a change of mind] / take a walk to
refresh *oneself* ◆積極的治療から緩和治
療へと方針を転換する move[shift] *a pa-
tient* from curative treatment to palliative
treatment[care] ◆転換点 a turning
point ◀性転換[性別適合]手術 sex
change[reassignment] surgery ▶転換
障害 conversion disorder 転換神経症
conversion neurosis 転換ヒステリー
conversion hysteria

てんがん 点眼する apply *eye drops[eye-
drops], **put** *eye drops[eyedrops] ★目薬
は複数形で. ☞目薬 ◆目薬を1日2回,
両目に1, 2滴点眼して下さい Please apply
one or two eye drops into[to / in] both
eyes twice a day. ◆瞳孔を広げるために目
薬を点眼します I'm going to put eye drops
in your eye(s) to dilate the pupil(s).
▶点眼薬 eye drops / eyedrops /（点眼液）
ophthalmic solution

てんき¹ 転帰 outcome

てんき² 天気 weather ◆今日はいいお
天気ですよ It's fine today. / The weather
is good[fine] today. / It's a beautiful day
today. ◆症状は天気の影響を受けますか
Do certain weather conditions affect your
symptoms? ◆あなたのお国の天気はどう
ですか What's the weather like[How's
the weather] in your country?

でんき 電気（電灯）**light**（電気エネルギー）
electricity（形**electric**） ◆電気を点ける
〈消す〉turn on〈off〉the light ◆電気は点
けたままにしておきましょうか Shall I leave
the light on? ◆電気が明るい〈暗い〉The
light is bright〈dim〉. ◀静電気 static
electricity ▶電気泳動 electrophoresis
電気刺激 electric stimulation 電気焼灼
術 electric cauterization / electrocautery
電気ショック療法 *electric shock[electro-

shock] therapy；EST／(電気痙攣療法) electroconvulsive therapy；ECT　電気生理学的検査 electrophysiologic test　電気的除細動 electric defibrillation／cardioversion　電気メス electric[cautery] knife／electrotome

でんきょく　電極　electrode　◆胸, 腕, 足にこの電極パッチを付けます I'm going to apply[attach] these electrode pads to the skin of your chest, arms, and legs.　◀表面電極 surface electrode

てんきん　転勤　transfer（國transfer to）　◆彼は今度シンガポール支店に転勤します He is being transferred to the Singapore branch (office).　◆お勤め先には転勤がありますか Are there job transfers in your company?

デングねつ　―熱　dengue（fever）　▶デング出血熱 dengue hemorrhagic fever；DHF　デングショック症候群 dengue shock syndrome；DSS

てんけい　典型(的な)　typical（↔atypical）　◆典型的な症状 a typical symptom　◆典型的な特徴 a typical feature [characteristic]

でんげき　電撃　electric shock　◆電撃性の痛み(an) electric shock-like pain　▶電撃損傷 electric injury　電撃熱傷 electric burn

てんけん　点検する　☞確認, 調べる

でんげん　電源　power（source）　(コンセント)（electrical）outlet, socket　◆携帯電話の電源を切って下さい Please turn [switch] off (the power on) your mobile phone.　◆電源を入れる turn[switch] on the power　◆コンピュータの電源を入れる plug in the computer　◆電源のプラグを抜く pull the plug from[out of] the socket

てんこう　天候　weather　☞天気

でんごん　伝言　message　◆奥様からのご伝言です You have a message from your wife.　◆あなたに至急の伝言があります I have an urgent message for you.　◆ご伝言がございましたら承ります Can I take a message? / Would you like to leave a message?　◆伝言を受け取る get[re-

ceive] a message　◆伝言を残す leave *someone* a message / leave a message for *someone*

てんざ　転座　translocation　◆相互転座 reciprocal translocation　▶転座型トリソミー translocation trisomy

てんじ　点字　braille, Braille /bréil/　◆点字を読む read braille　◆点字の本 a braille book / a book in braille

でんしカルテ　電子カルテ　(電子診療記録) computer-based patient record, electronic medical record；EMR, electronic health record；EHR

でんしけんびきょう　電子顕微鏡　electron microscope　◆走査型電子顕微鏡 scanning electron microscope；SEM　透過型電子顕微鏡 transmission electron microscope；TEM

でんじは　電磁波　electromagnetic wave

てんしゃ　転写　transcription

てんじやく　点耳薬　ear drops, eardrops　★通例, 複数形で. ◆点耳薬を1日2回, 右耳に1, 2滴さして下さい Please put one or two ear drops in your right ear twice a day.

てんじょう　点状(の)　stained　(ぽつぽつの) spotted　◆血液が点状についた痰 blood-stained phlegm　▶点状出血 petechiae／petechial hemorrhage

てんしょく　転職する　change *one's* job [occupation]　◆転職を考えてみてはいかがですか How[What] about changing jobs?

テンション　tension　◆テンションが非常に高い be in a state of extreme tension／(興奮しやすい)be high-strung

でんしレンジ　電子レンジ　microwave （oven）　◆電子レンジでスープを温める warm up the soup in the microwave

でんせん　伝染　infection　(接触による) contagion（國infectious, contagious　國病気が移る be transmitted to）　☞感染　◆この病気は伝染します This disease is infectious[contagious].　◆食品〈水／便／空気〉で伝染する be transmitted through food〈water／feces／the air〉　◆直接接触

により伝染する be transmitted by direct contact ◆伝染力が強い be highly infectious[contagious] ▶伝染性紅斑 erythema infectiosum /〔第 5 病〕fifth disease 伝染性単核球症 infectious mononucleosis；IM 伝染性軟属腫 molluscum contagiosum；MC 伝染性膿痂疹 contagious impetigo

でんたつ 伝達 transmission, conduction ◀神経伝達 neural transmission ▶伝達麻酔 conduction anesthesia

デンタルクリニック dental clinic

デンタルケア dental care

デンタルフロス dental floss（覆floss） ◆歯にデンタルフロスを使う floss *one's* teeth / use dental floss ◆健康的な歯と歯肉のためには毎日デンタルフロスで掃除することが大切です It's important to floss daily for healthy teeth and gums.

てんちりょうよう 転地療養 health resort therapy, therapeutic change of residence ◆転地療養をお勧めします I recommend that you take a holiday somewhere for the sake of your health. / I recommend that you visit a health resort.

てんてき 点滴 （点滴静注）intravenous drip, IV drip, drip, drip infusion ◆点滴を施す give *the patient* *an IV drip[a drip] / put *the patient* on *an IV drip[a drip] ◆点滴を受ける have an IV（drip） ◆これから点滴します．2 時間くらいかかります Now, I'm going to *put you on[give you] *an IV drip[a drip]. It'll take about two hours. ◆点滴部位は痛みますか Does the IV site hurt? ◆ご自分で点滴の速度を調整しないで下さい Please don't adjust[control] the drip rate yourself. ◆点滴が終わりましたら，ナースコールでお知らせ下さい When the drip *is finished[is empty / has emptied]，please push[press] the button to call a nurse. ◆抗菌薬の点滴を 1 日 2 回，1 週間続ける give an intravenous drip [infusion] of antibiotics twice a day for a week ◆点滴の滴下速度が速い〈遅い〉 The flow rate of the（IV）drip is fast 〈slow〉. ◆経口摂取ができるようになるま

で点滴で栄養を摂ることになります You'll *be fed[receive nourishment] through *an IV drip[a drip] till you can consume nutrients *by mouth[orally]. ◆点滴で栄養を与える feed[provide nourishment] through *an IV drip[a drip] ◀持続的点滴 continuous drip infusion ▶点滴静注腎盂造影 drip infusion pyelography；DIP 点滴静注胆道造影 drip infusion cholangiography；DIC 点滴スタンド IV stand [pole] 点滴バッグ IV bag 点滴ボトル IV bottle

てんとう 転倒する fall（down）（つまずいて転ぶ）stumble（over, on），trip（over, on）（転げ落ちる）tumble（down）☞転ぶ ◆よく転倒しますか Do you often fall down? / Do you have a tendency to fall? ◆転倒しないように気をつけて下さい Please be careful not to fall[have a fall]. ◆転倒して左足を骨折する fall and break *one's* left leg ◆すべって転倒する slip and fall ◆自転車で転倒する fall off *one's* bike ◆転倒して死ぬ fall to *one's* death ◆不慮の転倒 an accidental fall ▶転倒傾向 tendency to fall 転倒事故 fall[falling] accident / accident from a fall 転倒発作 drop attack

でんどう¹ 伝導 conduction ◀神経伝導速度 nerve conduction velocity；NCV 直流伝導除細動器 *direct current[DC] defibrillator 副伝導路 accessory（conduction）pathway / bypass tract 房室伝導 atrioventricular[AV] conduction ▶伝導時間 conduction time 伝導障害 conduction defect 伝導性失語 conduction aphasia

でんどう² 電動（の）（電気の）electric （電子の）electronical ◆このベッドは電動式です This bed is electronically operated. ▶電動義手 electric arm 電動車椅子 electric[electric-powered] wheelchair 電動歯ブラシ electric toothbrush 電動ベッド electric[electronically operated] bed

てんねんとう 天然痘 smallpox, variola

てんびやく 点鼻薬 nose drops, nose-

drops ★通例，複数形で．（噴霧液）**nasal spray** ◆1日2回両方の鼻孔に点鼻薬を1，2滴さして下さい Please put one or two nose drops in both nostrils twice a day.

てんぷ　添付する　attach ◆ご請求のあった資料を添付いたします I'm attaching the information you requested. ◆詳細については添付ファイルをご覧下さい For detailed information, please see the attached file. ▶添付書類 accompanying [attached] document　添付ファイル attached file / attachment　（医薬品の）添付文書（medication）information leaflet

でんぶ　殿部　buttocks /bʌ́təks/ ★通例，複数形で．**gluteal region**

でんぷう　癜風　tinea versicolor

てんぽうそう　天疱瘡　pemphigus ◀尋常性天疱瘡 pemphigus vulgaris；PV

デンマーク　Denmark（㊫デンマークの・デンマーク人の **Danish**）☞国籍　▶デンマーク人 Dane

てんめつ　点滅する（ピカピカ光る）**flash**（on and off）（ライトなどが点滅する）**blink** ◆赤く点滅する光を目で追いかけて下さい Please follow the red flashing lights with your eye.

てんらく　転落する　fall ▶転落死 fall [falling] death　転落事故 fall[falling] accident / accident from a fall

でんりほうしゃせん　電離放射線　ionizing radiation ◀非電離放射線 nonionizing radiation　非電離放射線障害 nonionizing radiation injury[disorder]

でんわ　電話（電話機）**telephone, phone**（通話）（phone）**call**（電話番号）**phone number**（㊙call, phone）☞巻末付録：電話応対の表現 ◆ご自宅〈勤務先〉の電話は何番ですか What's your *phone number〈business[office] phone number〉? ◆熱や痛みがある時にはお電話を下さい Please call[phone] us if you have any fever or pain. ◆明日もう一度お電話をいただけますか Could you call[phone] us back tomorrow? / Could you give us a call back tomorrow? ◆後でこちらからお電話します I'll call you back later. ◆電話の

声が聞こえにくいですか Do you have difficulty hearing on the phone? ◆病室には電話が付いていて直接かけられます Your room is equipped with a direct-dial telephone. ◆国際電話をかける時には0の番号を押してオペレーターにご連絡下さい To make an international（phone）call, please contact the hospital operator by dialing zero. ◆この場所では携帯電話を使用できません You can't use your mobile phone in this area. / Mobile phones may not be used in this area of the hospital. ◆申し訳ありませんが，電話での予約は受け付けておりません I'm sorry, but we can't [don't] accept appointments by phone. ◆電話で予約を変更できます You can change your appointment by phone. ◀緊急電話 emergency call　緊急電話番号 emergency（phone）number /（緊急連絡先の）emergency contact number　公衆電話 public telephone / pay phone　▶電話ボックス（public）phone booth ☞携帯電話，国際電話

と

と 戸 door ☞ドア

ど 度

《温度など数量の単位》**degree** ☞巻末付録：単位の換算 ◆熱は何度ありましたか What was your temperature? / How high was your temperature? ◆熱は摂氏38度3分です Your temperature is 38.3[thirty-eight point three] degrees Celsius.

《程度》**degree** （強度・矯正度）**strength** （節度）**moderation** （㊥**moderate**） （レベル・水準）**level** ◆Ⅰ〈Ⅱ／Ⅲ〉度の熱傷を受ける have a first〈second／third〉-degree burn ◆あなたの眼鏡は度が合っていません The lenses of your glasses are not the right strength for your eyes. ◆眼鏡の度を上げる increase the strength of *one's* glasses ◆度の強い眼鏡をかける wear high-strength[strong／thick] glasses ◆近視の度が進む become more near-sighted. ◆飲酒の度を越してはいけません You must be moderate in drinking (alcohol). / If you drink alcohol, you must do so *in moderation[moderately]. ◆運動は結構ですが，度を越つと体に良くありません Exercise is OK, but too much is bad for you. / Exercise is good, but it's not good for your body if you overdo it.

《回数》**time** ◆1度 once ◆2度 twice／two times ◆3度 three times ◆一晩に何度もトイレに起きますか Do you wake up several times at night to go to the bathroom?

◀安静度 level[degree] of bed rest　重症度（disease) severity　手術危険度 surgical risk　ストレス度 stress level　熱傷度 degree of the burn (injury)／burn degree　肥満度 degree of obesity／(指標) obesity index　要介護度 care level／the level of care needs

ドア door ◆医師が名前をお呼びするまでドアは開けないで下さい Please don't open the door until the doctor calls your name. ◆病室のドアは開けたままにしていただけますか Could you please leave [Would you mind leaving] your room door open?

といあわせる 問い合わせる （連絡を取る）**contact** （尋ねる）**ask, inquire, make an inquiry** （確認する）**check** （**with**） ☞照会 ◆前の手術の詳細について問い合わせる手紙を書いてもいいですか Do you mind if I contact[write to] your surgeon for details about your previous surgery? ◆詳細については最寄りの保健所に問い合わせて下さい For further information, please contact[inquire at／check with] the local health center. ◆問い合わせの手紙 a letter of inquiry

ドイツ Germany （㊥**German**） ☞国籍
▶ドイツ人（の）**German**

トイレ （公共の場所の）**restroom, rest room,** 《英》**toilet** （個人の家の）**bathroom** （便器）**toilet** （**bowl**） ☞尿, 排泄, 排尿, 排便 ◆トイレに行きたいのですか Do you want to go to the restroom? ◆トイレを我慢する control *one's* need to go to the bathroom [restroom] ◆トイレが近いですか（頻繁に行くか）Do you need to go to the bathroom [restroom] *very often[frequently]? / Do you have to *pass urine[urinate] *very often[frequently]? ◆夜間, トイレに何回起きますか How many times do you wake up to go to the bathroom during the night? ◆トイレは廊下の突き当たり〈ナースステーションの隣〉にあります The restroom is *at the end of the corridor〈next to the nurses' station〉. ◆トイレに歩いて行くことは許可されていません You are not allowed to walk to the restroom. ◆トイレ以外はベッドで安静にしていて下さい Please stay in bed at all times except when you need to *use the toilet[go to the restroom]. ◆検査前にトイレを済ませてきて下さい Please go to the restroom before we start the test. ◆自力でトイレに座ることができますか Can you sit on the toilet without any help? ◆トイレの水を

流す flush the toilet ◀携帯用トイレ portable toilet / (室内便器)commode　洋式トイレ Western-style toilet　和式トイレ Japanese-style toilet　☞トイレトレーニング

トイレットペーパー　toilet paper[tissue]
トイレトレーニング　toilet-training (動toi-let-train), potty-training　◆お子さんはトイレトレーニングが済んでいますか Is your child toilet-trained?　◆トイレトレーニングを急ぐ必要はありません。お子さんのペースでやればいいのです There's no hurry[rush] to toilet-train your child. Just take it at his〈her〉pace.

とう　糖　sugar　(ブドウ糖)glucose　(総称として)carbohydrate　☞砂糖, 糖質, 糖分　◆尿に糖が出ています There is sugar in your urine.　■血糖 blood sugar[glucose]　尿糖 urinary[urine]　sugar[glucose]　☞糖衣錠, 糖原病, 糖脂質, 糖代謝, 糖尿病, 糖負荷試験

どう¹　☞どういたしまして, どんな
《いかが(質問)》(何・どんなこと)what　(どのように)how　◆今日はどうなさいましたか How can I help you today? / What can I do for you today? / What problems have brought you here today?　◆どうされましたか What seems to be the problem[trouble]? / (怪我などの患者に)What happened to you?　◆ご気分はどうですか How are you feeling now? / How do you feel now?　◆この前診察してから具合はどうですか How have you been since I last saw you?　◆首をどうかしたのですか What's wrong with your neck?　◆どういう時に痛みますか In what situations do you get the pain?　◆どういう症状がありますか What kind of symptoms do you have?　◆この治療方針をどう思いますか What do you think of this treatment plan?
《いかが(提案)》how about, what about
◆ご家族の考えも伺ってみてはどうですか How[What] about asking your family what they think (about this)?　◆もう一度挑戦してみてはどうですか How about giving it one more try? / I recommend

that you try one more time.
《いかに…しても》no matter how, even if
◆どう姿勢を変えても痛みは変わりませんか No matter how you change your position[posture], do you still have the pain? / Does it make no difference to the pain even if you change position?　◆どうしてもご承諾いただけませんか(絶対だめか) Is there no way (at all) that you'll give your consent?

どう²　洞　sinus　◀篩骨洞 ethmoid[ethmoidal] sinus　上顎洞 maxillary sinus　前頭洞 frontal sinus　大動脈洞 aortic sinus　蝶形骨洞 sphenoid[sphenoidal] sinus　▶洞徐脈, 洞調律, 洞停止, 洞頻脈, 洞不整脈, 洞不全症候群, 洞房

どう³　胴　(身体)body　(体幹)trunk, torso
とうい¹　頭囲　head circumference
とうい²　頭位　(胎位の)cephalic presentation (of the fetus)　☞頭位眼振
どうい　同意　(承諾)consent　(意見の一致)agreement　(動agree)　◆この手術をするにはあなたの同意が必要です I need your consent to do this surgery.　◆早期の退院には同意しかねます I'm afraid I don't agree with you about your being discharged early.　◆患者の同意を得る obtain[get] the patient's (informed) consent　☞同意書
どういう　☞どんな
とういがんしん　頭位(性)眼振　positional nystagmus　◀方向交代性頭位眼振 direction-changing positional nystagmus　方向固定性頭位眼振 direction-fixed positional nystagmus　▶頭位変換性眼振 positioning nystagmus

どういげんそ　同位元素　isotope　☞放射性同位元素
どういしょ　同意書　(十分な説明を受けた上での承諾書)(informed) consent form　(契約書)agreement　◆この同意書をよく読んで署名し日付を入れて下さい Please read this consent form carefully before signing and dating it.　◆どなたか同意書にサインしてくれる人はいますか Do you have anyone who can sign the consent form for

you？◆血液製剤を使用するためにはこの同意書にサインが必要です I need your signature on this consent form to use blood products. ◆これは差額ベッド利用に関する同意書です This is a written agreement regarding the *extra-charge bed[special charge room]. ◀HIV 検査同意書 consent form for HIV blood testing / HIV test consent form　手術同意書 consent form for surgery / surgery consent form　輸血同意書 consent form for blood transfusion / blood transfusion consent form

とういじょう　糖衣錠　sugar-coated tablet[pill]

どういたしまして　◆(患者から「ありがとう」と御礼を言われて)どういたしまして(軽い口調で) That's okay. / No problem. / Not at all. / Don't mention it. / Any time. / (改まって) You're (quite) welcome. / (It's) my pleasure.

どういつせい　同一性　identity　◀性同一性障害[性別違和] gender identity disorder　▶同一性危機 identity crisis

とういん　当院　(病院)this hospital　(クリニック)this clinic　◆当院では敷地内はすべて禁煙です Smoking is not allowed anywhere inside this hospital. ◆当院では職員への謝礼はお断りしております We are not allowed to accept (thank-you) gifts from patients to the staff in this hospital. / In this hospital, gifts from patients to staff are not allowed.

とうえい　投影　projection　☞投射

とうか¹　透過　(浸透・浸潤)permeation　(伝達)transmission　▶透過型電子顕微鏡 transmission electron microscope；TEM　透過性 permeability

とうか²　等価　equivalent　☞同等

どうか¹　☞どうぞ

どうか²　同化　(物質代謝の)anabolism (㊅anabolic), assimilation　◀蛋白同化ステロイド[ホルモン] protein anabolic steroid [hormone]　▶同化作用 anabolism

どうが　動画　dynamic image　(画像化)dynamic imaging　(㊅cine-)　◀冠動脈造影撮影 cinecoronary angiography　▶動

画 CT　cine CT（scan）

とうがい　頭蓋　skull, cranium（㊅cranial）　▶頭蓋咽頭腫 craniopharyngioma　頭蓋顔面外傷 craniofacial trauma　頭蓋牽引 skull traction　頭蓋底 cranial base　☞頭蓋骨, 頭蓋内

とうがいこつ　頭蓋骨　skull, cranial bones, bones of the cranium　★通例，複数形で．▶頭蓋骨骨折 skull fracture / fracture of the skull

とうがいない　頭蓋内(の)　intracranial　▶頭蓋内圧 intracranial pressure；ICP　頭蓋内圧亢進 intracranial hypertension / increased intracranial pressure　頭蓋内出血 intracranial bleeding[hemorrhage]　頭蓋内占拠性病変 intracranial space-occupying lesion

とうがらし　唐辛子　red pepper

とうかん　盗汗　night sweats　★通例，複数形で．☞寝汗

どうかん　導管　conduit　(体液・涙などの排泄管)(excretory) duct　◀回腸導管 ileal conduit；IC

どうがんしんけい　動眼神経　oculomotor nerve　▶動眼神経麻痺 oculomotor nerve paralysis

どうき¹　動悸　palpitations　★通例，複数形で．◆動悸を感じたことがありますか Have you noticed *any palpitations? [your heart pounding hard and fast]? ◆階段を上る時動悸がしますか Do you feel your heart *beats fast[pounds] when you go up stairs? ◆動悸が激しいのですか Do you feel your heart pounding[throbbing]? ◆異常な動悸がする have abnormal palpitations　◆動悸が鎮まる the palpitations subside

どうき²　動機　motive　(意欲・動機づけ)motivation　◆生きる動機を失う lose one's motivation for living

とうきゅう　等級　(程度)degree　(段階)grade　(階級・部類)class　◀障害等級 degree of disability[invalidity]

どうきょにん　同居人　roommate, housemate,《英》flatmate

どうぐ　道具　(機器)instrument　(手仕事の

どうぐ 道具）tool （道具一式）kit ◀遊び道具 plaything / （子供用の玩具）toy 洗面道具 toiletries 髭そり道具 shaving things [items] / （道具一式）shaving kit

とうげ 峠 crisis, critical stage ☞危機 ◆彼にとってこの一両日が峠でしょう The next one or two days will be critical for him. ◆彼女の容態は峠を越えました She's past the critical stage.

とうけい 統計 statistic （㊂statistical） ◆統計によれば According to the statistics, … ◆統計上の事実 a statistical fact ◀死亡統計 mortality statistics 人口統計 population statistics ▶統計資料 statistical data 統計的有意性 statistical significance 統計分析 statistical analysis

とうけいぶがん 頭頸部がん head and neck cancer

とうけつ 凍結させる freeze （㊂凍結した frozen ㊟㊙cry(o)-） ☞冷凍 凍結乾燥した食品 freeze-dried food ◀新鮮凍結血漿 fresh frozen plasma；FFP ▶凍結肩 frozen shoulder 凍結剤 freezing mixture / cryogen 凍結手術 cryosurgery / cryogenic surgery 凍結切片 frozen section 凍結保存 cryopreservation 凍結療法 cryotherapy

とうけっしゅ 頭血腫 cephalohematoma

とうけつしょうこうぐん 盗血症候群 steal syndrome ◀鎖骨下動脈盗血症候群 subclavian steal syndrome

とうげんびょう 糖原病 glycogenosis, glycogen-storage disease；GSD

どうこう 瞳孔 pupil （㊂pupillary） ◆瞳孔を広げるために目薬をさします I'm going to put eye drops in your eye(s) to dilate your pupil(s). 彼女は瞳孔が開いています Her pupils are dilated. ◆散大した瞳孔 dilated pupils ◆縮小した瞳孔 constricted pupils ◀針穴瞳孔 pinhole[pinpoint] pupil ▶瞳孔散大 pupil[pupillary] dilatation / mydriasis 瞳孔縮小 pupil[pupillary] constriction / miosis 瞳孔反応[反射] pupil[pupillary] reaction [reflex] 瞳孔不同 anisocoria

とうこうきょひ 登校拒否 refusal to go to school, school[classroom] refusal ☞不登校 ◆息子さんは登校拒否を起こしているのですか Does your son refuse to go to school? ◆お子さんの登校拒否でお困りですか Are you concerned about your child's *school refusal[refusal to go to school]?

とうごうしっちょうしょう 統合失調症 schizophrenia /skìtsəfrí:niə\ （㊂schizophrenic） ◆統合失調症患者 a patient with schizophrenia / a schizophrenic patient ◀解体型[破瓜型]統合失調症 disorganized[hebephrenic] schizophrenia / hebephrenia 緊張型統合失調症 catatonic schizophrenia 妄想型統合失調症 paranoid schizophrenia ▶統合失調質パーソナリティ障害 schizoid personality disorder

とうこつ¹ 橈骨 radius （㊂radial） ▶橈骨骨折 radial fracture 橈骨神経 radial nerve 橈骨神経麻痺 radial nerve paralysis 橈骨反射 radial reflex

とうこつ² ☞頭蓋骨（とうがいこつ）

どうさ 動作 （動き）movement, motion （具体的な行為・活動）action, activity ☞動き, 体位（囲み：体位・動作の指示） ◆動作に何か問題がありますか Do you have any problems with movement? ◆どんな動作がしにくいですか What kind of movement *gives you difficulty[is difficult for you]? ◆日常の動作はスムーズにできますか Can you perform everyday movements smoothly? ◆どんな動作をすると痛みますか What kind of movement causes you to feel pain? ◆動作がぎこちない be awkward[clumsy] in one's movements ◆動作がゆっくりで最初の一歩が踏み出せない be slow in one's movements and have difficulty taking the first step ◆異常な動作をする exhibit[make] unusual movements[actions] ◆落ち着きのない動作をする have restless movements / move restlessly ◆無意識の動作 an involuntary movement[action] ◆手を洗うなどある一定の動作を繰り返さないと気がすまないことがありますか Do you feel a need to repeat certain actions, such as washing your hands? ◀移乗動作 transfer activity[movement] 床上動作 bed activity 整容動作(personal) grooming / grooming activity 日常生活動作 activities of daily living；ADL(s) 反響動作 echopraxia ▶動作訓練 movement exercise 動作時振戦 action[kinetic] tremor 動作時ミオクローヌス action myoclonus

とうさく 倒錯 perversion ◀性的倒錯 sexual perversion

とうし¹ 凍死 death due to freezing, death by freezing (類freeze to death) (致命的低体温症)fatal hypothermia

とうし² 透視 (X線透視検査)fluoroscopy /flɔːráskəpi/ (形fluoroscópic) ◆X線透視下で腫瘍生検を行う perform a fluoroscopy-guided tumor biopsy / perform a tumor biopsy using[under] fluoroscopy

どうじ 同時(に) at the same time, simultaneously, concurrently (…するとすぐに) as soon as …, the moment (that) ◆下痢と嘔吐が同時に起こる時は脱水に特に注意して下さい Please be especially careful about dehydration when diarrhea and vomiting occur *at the same time[simultaneously]. ◆寒気がすると同時に熱が出る chills and fever *come on[appear] at the same time / have a fever as soon as chills come on ◀膵腎同時移植 *simultaneous pancreas-kidney[SPK] transplant[transplantation] ▶同時併用化学放射線療法 concurrent chemoradiotherapy 同時視 simultaneous perception；SP 同時性がん simultaneous cancer

とうししつ 糖脂質 glycolipid

とうしつ¹ 糖質 sugar (ブドウ糖)glucose (総称として)carbohydrate ☞砂糖, 糖, 糖分 ▶糖質吸収 carbohydrate absorption 糖質コルチコイド glucocorticoid 糖質消化不良 sugar[carbohydrate] indigestion / disorder of sugar[carbohydrate] digestion

とうしつ² 等質(の) homogeneous (↔heterogeneous)

とうじつ 当日 the day of ◆検査当日は予約時刻の15分前においで下さい Please come to the hospital fifteen minutes before the appointment on the day of your examination[test]. ◀手術当日 the day of the surgery

どうしつ 同室 ◆同室の方をご紹介しましょう．こちらは渡辺さんです Let me introduce you to your roommate. This is Mrs Watanabe. ◀母子同室 rooming-in

どうして ☞なぜ

どうしても ☞どう

とうしゃ 投射 projection (形projective) ▶投射法 projective method[technique / test]

とうしゃく 等尺(性の) isometric ▶等尺性訓練 isometric exercise 等尺性収縮 isometric contraction

どうしゅ 同種(の) (相同性の)homologous (同種異系の)allogenic, allogeneic (等質・均質の)homogeneous (↔heterogeneous) ◀不規則同種抗体 irregular[unexpected] alloantibody ▶同種移植 homologous transplant[transplantation] / allotransplantation 同種移植片 allograft 同種骨髄移植 allogenic bone marrow transplant[transplantation] 同種植皮 allogenic skin grafting

とうしょう 凍傷 frostbite (軽度の霜焼け)chilblains ★通例, 複数形で. (寒冷損傷)cold injury

どうじょうみゃく 動静脈(の) arteriovenous；AV ▶動静脈奇形 arteriovenous malformation；AVM 動静脈シャント arteriovenous shunt 動静脈瘤 arteriovenous aneurysm 動静脈瘻 arteriovenous fistula

どうじょみゃく 洞徐脈 sinus bradycardia

どうせいあい 同性愛 homosexuality, homosexual love (男性の)male homosexuality (女性の)female homosexuality ▶同性愛カップル same-sex couple 同性愛者(男性)homosexual[gay] man / (女性)*homosexual woman[lesbian] ★総称としての homosexual は差別的な表現.

LGBT は lesbian（女性同性愛者），gay（男性同性愛者），bisexual（両性愛者），transgender（心と体の性が一致しない人）の頭文字をとった総称．

とうせき 透析 **dialysis** /daɪǽləsɪs/（圏 **dialýtic**） ◆透析を行う perform dialysis ◆透析を受ける have[receive / undergo] dialysis / go on dialysis ◆透析を受けている be on dialysis ◆腎臓の働きが悪いので透析が必要でしょう Your kidneys aren't working properly[correctly], so you'll have to start[go on] dialysis. ◀維持透析 maintenance dialysis 間欠的腹膜透析 intermittent peritoneal dialysis；IPD 血液透析 hemodialysis；HD 在宅透析 home dialysis 腹膜透析 peritoneal dialysis；PD 連続携行式腹膜透析 continuous ambulatory peritoneal dialysis；CAPD ▶透析アミロイドーシス dialysis-related amyloidosis；DRA 透析患者 dialysis patient / patient on dialysis 透析器 dialysis machine / dialyzer

どうせき 同席する **sit with** ◆医師の細川と看護師の加藤が同席してもよろしいですか Is it all right if Dr Hosokawa and Nurse Kato sit with me? ◆どなたかこの話し合いに同席してもらいたい人がいますか Is there anyone you would like to have with you for this discussion?

とうぜん 当然（な）（もっともな）**natural**（妥当な）**reasonable** ◆今後の生活のことで不安をお持ちなのは当然です It's（quite）natural for you to have concerns about how this is going to affect your life. ◆あなたの要求は当然です I think your request is reasonable.

どうぞ **please**
《相手を促す》 ◆どうぞおかけ下さい Please sit down. / Sit down, please. ◆どうぞこちらへ Come[Walk] this way, please. ◆（人を先に行かせる時）どうぞお先に（Please）go ahead. / After you.
《どうか》 ◆どうぞがっかりしないで下さい Please don't be disappointed. ◆（旅行に出かける人に）どうぞ気を付けて行ってらっしゃい Have a safe trip[journey]. ★相手

の利益になるようなことを勧める場合には please をつけなくても失礼にならない．
《物を勧める・提供する》 ◆さあどうぞ There you go. / There you are.
《承諾・承知の返答する》 ◆（相手の求めに応じて物を渡す時）ええ，どうぞ Sure. Here you are. / Here you go. / Here it is. / Here's your … . ◆（相手から「…をしてもいいですか」と訊かれて）ええ，どうぞ Sure. / Certainly. / Of course. / Go ahead.

とうそう¹ 凍瘡 **frostbite** ☞凍傷
とうそう² 痘瘡 **smallpox, variola**
とうそくせい 等速性（の）**isokinetic**
▶等速性運動 isokinetic exercise
どうたい¹ 胴体 ☞胴
どうたい² 動態 **dynamic state, dynamics, kinetics** ★いずれも単数扱いで．◀血行動態 hemodynamics 尿流動態検査 urodynamic study；UDS 薬物動態 pharmacokinetics ▶動態機能検査 dynamic function study[test] 動態シンチグラフィ dynamic scintigraphy

とうたいしゃ 糖代謝 **carbohydrate metabolism**

とうたつ 到達する（達成する）**reach, attain**（接近する）**approach** ◆目標に到達する reach[attain] the target ◀経腹的腹膜到達法 *transabdominal preperitoneal [TAPP] approach

とうちゃく 到着する ☞着く
どうちゅうかがくりょうほう 動注化学療法 **intraarterial infusion chemotherapy**
とうちょう¹ 頭頂 **the top of the head, crown of the head**（圏**parietal**）▶頭頂骨 parietal bone 頭頂部 the parietal region ☞頭頂葉
とうちょう² 等張（性の）**isotonic** ▶等張液 isotonic solution 等張性訓練 isotonic exercise 等張性収縮 isotonic contraction 等張尿 isotonic urine
とうちょうよう 頭頂葉 **parietal lobe**
▶頭頂葉症候群 parietal lobe syndrome 頭頂葉てんかん parietal lobe epilepsy
どうちょうりつ 洞調律 **sinus rhythm**
◀正常洞調律 normal sinus rhythm；NSR
とうちょく 当直（で）**on duty** ☞当番

医 ◆今晩は佐藤先生が当直です Dr Sato is on duty tonight. ▶当直医 doctor on (night) duty 当直看護師 charge nurse on (night) duty 当直室 on-call room / (医師の)room for doctors on night duty

とうつう 疼痛 pain ☞痛み ◀がん性疼痛 cancer pain がん性疼痛治療ラダー ladder for cancer pain relief 自己疼痛管理 patient-controlled analgesia；PCA 神経因性疼痛 neuropathic pain 慢性疼痛 chronic pain ▶疼痛外来 pain clinic 疼痛管理 pain management[control] 疼痛緩和 pain relief 疼痛許容レベル pain tolerance level 疼痛ケア pain care 疼痛性障害 pain disorder

どうていし 洞停止 sinus arrest

どうてき 動的(な) dynamic (↔static) ▶動的運動 dynamic exercise

どうてん 動転する get upset, become upset ☞動揺

どうとう 同等(の) (同価値の)equivalent (比較可能な)comparable ☞同じ, 等しい ◆このタイプの経口抗菌薬は注射薬と同等の生物活性を示します This type of oral antibiotic produces bioactivity equivalent [comparable] to that of the parenteral form.

とうにゅう 豆乳 soybean milk, soya milk

どうにゅう 導入する (実施する)implement (図implementation) (誘発する)induce (図induction) (制度・技術などを取り入れる)introduce (図introduction) ◆先進医療技術を導入する implement advanced medical technology ◆当院では電子カルテを導入しています We have implemented use of computer-based patient records in this hospital. ◀寛解導入 remission induction 睡眠導入薬 sleep-inducing medication[drug / agent] ▶導入化学療法 induction chemotherapy 導入麻酔 induction of anesthesia

どうにょう 導尿 (尿管の)urinary catheterization (尿道の)urethral catheterization ◆自分で導尿する self-catheterize ◆トイレに行くのがおつらいようでしたら, 導尿しましょうか If it's difficult for you to

go to the restroom, *do you want to have a urinary catheter put in place[should I place a tube into your bladder to drain the urine]? ◀自己導尿 self (urinary) catheterization ▶導尿用カテーテル urinary [urethral] catheter

とうにょうびょう 糖尿病 diabetes (mellitus) /dàɪəbíːtiːz-/ (形diabetic) ◆糖尿病の疑いがあります We suspect (that you have) diabetes. / There's a suspicion of diabetes. ◆ご家族に糖尿病の方がいますか Does anyone in your family have diabetes? ◆これは糖尿病でよくみられる合併症です This is a common complication of diabetes. ◆糖尿病患者のための教育プログラムへの参加をお勧めします I'd like to recommend that you take part in the education program for people with diabetes. ◆彼女は糖尿病です She is diabetic. / She has diabetes. ◆糖尿病の合併症を防ぐ prevent[avoid] *diabetes complications[the complications of diabetes] ◀1型〈2型〉糖尿病 type 1〈type 2〉diabetes 境界型糖尿病 borderline diabetes 若年型糖尿病 juvenile diabetes ステロイド糖尿病 steroid diabetes 妊娠糖尿病 diabetes in[during] pregnancy / gestational diabetes mellitus；GDM ▶糖尿病IDカード diabetic ID card / (腕輪)diabetic ID bracelet 糖尿病患者 patient with diabetes / diabetic patient 糖尿病教室 diabetes class / class for people with diabetes 糖尿病食 diabetic diet 糖尿病性壊疽 diabetic gangrene 糖尿病性ケトアシドーシス diabetic ketoacidosis；DKA 糖尿病性昏睡 diabetic coma 糖尿病性神経障害 diabetic neuropathy 糖尿病性腎症 diabetic nephropathy 糖尿病性網膜症 diabetic retinopathy

とうはつ 頭髪 ☞髪, 毛

とうばんい 当番医 doctor on duty ☞当直 ◀救急当番医 doctor on duty in the emergency room 休日当番医 doctor on holiday duty 夜間当番医 night-duty doctor / doctor on night duty

とうひ¹ 頭皮 scalp ◆頭皮を掻く scratch the scalp

とうひ² 逃避する（回避する）escape（図 escape）（引き籠る）withdraw（図withdrawal）◆現実から逃避する escape from reality ◆社会から逃避する withdraw from society ▶逃避行動 escape behavior　逃避反射 withdrawal reflex

とうびょう 闘病する fight against *one's* illness, struggle[battle] with *one's* illness ◆外国で闘病生活を送るのはさぞ不安でしょう It must make you feel very anxious[uneasy] to be living in a foreign country while *fighting against[struggling with] your illness.

どうひんみゃく 洞頻脈 sinus tachycardia

とうぶ 頭部 head ☞頭 ◆頭部の CT 検査をする do a CT scan of *a person's* head ◆頭部の CT 検査を受ける have a CT scan of *one's* head ◆頭部に重傷を負う have a serious head injury / have a serious injury to the head ▶頭部圧迫試験 head compression test　頭部外傷 head injury[trauma]　頭部外傷後遺症 sequelae of traumatic head injury / posttraumatic sequelae　頭部後屈法 head-tilt method　頭部白癬 scalp ringworm / ringworm of the scalp / tinea capitis ★scalp は頭皮.

どうぶ 胴部 ☞胴

とうふかしけん 糖負荷試験 glucose tolerance test；GTT

どうふせいみゃく 洞不整脈 sinus arrhythmia

どうふぜんしょうこうぐん 洞不全症候群 sick sinus syndrome；SSS

どうぶつ 動物 animal ◆動物の毛アレルギーがある *have an allergy[be allergic] to *animal fur[dander] / have an allergy brought on by *animal fur[dander] ◀媒介動物 vector　有毒動物 poisonous [toxic] animal ▶動物恐怖 zoophobia / fear of animals　動物咬傷 animal bite　動物実験 animal experiment / experiment using animals　動物性脂肪 animal

fat　動物性蛋白 animal protein　動物媒介疾患 animal-borne disease

とうぶん 糖分 sugar （ブドウ糖）glucose （総称として）carbohydrate ☞砂糖, 糖, 糖質 ◆この食品には糖分が多い This food has a high sugar content. / This food contains a lot of sugar. ◆糖分をとり過ぎています You're getting too much sugar. ◆糖分を控えて下さい Please cut down (on) your sugar intake. ◆尿に糖分が出る have sugar in *one's* urine ◆糖分の多い〈少ない〉ソフトドリンク a soft drink high〈low〉in sugar ◆低糖分〈糖分ゼロ〉のジュース low-sugar〈sugar-free〉juice

どうぼう 洞房（の）sinoatrial ▶洞房結節 sinoatrial[SA] node　洞房ブロック sinoatrial[SA] block

どうまわり 胴回り ☞腰, 腹囲

どうみゃく 動脈 artery /άɚtəri/（↔vein）（図arterial）◀冠動脈 coronary artery　総頸動脈 common carotid artery；CCA　大動脈 aorta / the main artery　肺動脈 pulmonary artery ▶動脈圧 arterial pressure　動脈系 the arterial system　動脈血 arterial blood　動脈血ガス分析 *arterial blood gas[ABG] analysis　動脈血酸素分圧 *arterial partial pressure of oxygen[partial pressure of oxygen in arterial blood]；PaO₂　動脈血酸素飽和度 arterial (blood) oxygen saturation；SaO₂　動脈血栓症 arterial thrombosis　動脈血炭酸ガス分圧 *arterial partial pressure of carbon dioxide[partial pressure of carbon dioxide in arterial blood]；PaCO₂　動脈性出血 arterial bleeding[hemorrhage]　動脈穿刺 arterial puncture　動脈造影 arteriography　動脈塞栓症 arterial embolism　（経カテーテル的）動脈注入療法 transcatheter arterial infusion；TAI　動脈拍動 arterial pulse　動脈閉塞 arterial occlusion　動脈閉塞性疾患 arterial occlusive[obstructive] disease；AOD ☞動脈炎, 動脈管, 動脈硬化, 動脈瘤

どうみゃくえん 動脈炎 arteritis ◀巨細胞性動脈炎 giant cell arteritis　結節性多発動脈炎 polyarteritis nodosa；PN　側頭

どうみゃくえん 動脈炎 temporal arteritis；TA　大動脈炎症候群 aortitis syndrome

どうみゃくかん　動脈管　arterial duct
▶動脈管開存症 patent ductus arteriosus；PDA

どうみゃくこうか　動脈硬化　arteriosclerosis　(アテローム性の)atherosclerosis　(形arteriosclerotic, atherosclerotic)　◆動脈硬化が進んでいますので注意が必要です You need to be more careful because *your arteriosclerosis is getting worse[the hardening in your arteries is progressing].　◆動脈硬化があるので塩分や脂質の摂取は控えめにして下さい You've got hardening of the arteries, so please be moderate in your salt and fat intake.
◆アテローム性動脈硬化による心血管〈脳血管〉疾患 atherosclerotic cardiovascular〈cerebrovascular〉disease　◀高血圧性動脈硬化症 hypertensive arteriosclerosis　閉塞性動脈硬化症 arteriosclerosis obliterans；ASO

どうみゃくりゅう　動脈瘤　aneurysm /ǽnjərìzm/　◆検査で脳に小さな動脈瘤があるのがわかりました The test results show that you have a small aneurysm in the brain.　◆動脈瘤が破裂して脳内出血を起こしています The aneurysm has ruptured[burst] and caused *bleeding in the brain[an intracerebral hemorrhage].
◆破裂した動脈瘤 a ruptured aneurysm　◆動脈瘤の破裂を予防する prevent an aneurysm from rupturing　◀大動脈瘤 aortic aneurysm　脳動脈瘤 cerebral[brain] aneurysm　脳動脈瘤クリッピング cerebral aneurysm clipping　▶動脈瘤破裂 aneurysm rupture / rupture of an aneurysm

とうめい　透明(な)　(液体が澄んだ)clear　(無色の)colorless　(透けて見える)transparent　(↔opaque)　(形transparency)　◆透明な分泌物が出る have a clear[colorless] discharge　◆透明な尿 clear urine　◆透明度が高い have a high degree of transparency　◆透明性のある情報開示 transparent disclosure

どうめいはんもう　同名半盲　homonymous hemianopia

とうやく　投薬　give (a) medication, administer (a) medication　(図administration)　☞処方, 投与　◀前投薬 premedication

とうゆ　灯油　kerosene

とうよ　投与する　give (a) medication, administer (a) medication　(図administration)　(処方する)prescribe　(図prescription)　◆この薬は発症から4時間半以内に投与する必要があります This medication must be given[administered] within four hours and thirty minutes of the onset of symptoms.　◆抗凝固薬を投与していますので, 怪我に気をつけて下さい Since you are on an anticoagulant, please be careful not to *get injured[injure yourself].　◆1日1回〈2回〉服用する降圧薬を投与しましょう I'm going to[I'll] give you a once-daily〈twice-daily〉 antihypertensive.
◀過剰投与 overdose / overmedication / overdosage　吸入投与 inhalation administration　経験的投与 empirical administration　経口投与 oral administration　自己投与 self-medication / self-administration　舌下投与 sublingual administration　鼻腔内投与 intranasal administration　▶投与間隔 dosing interval　投与期間 dosing period　投与計画 dosage schedule　投与経路 route of administration　投与量 a dose / a dosage　★dose は1回分の投与量, dosage は一定期間の総投与量をいう.

どうよう¹　同様　☞同じ, 同等
どうよう²　動揺(した)
《気が動転した》upset　(ショックで震えた)shaken　(興奮した)agitated, worked up　◆彼女は検査結果を聞いてひどく動揺しています She is very upset at the test results. / She is badly shaken by the test results.　◆彼を動揺させないように気をつけて下さい Please be careful not to give him a shock.
《身体がぐらつく》(体の部位が激しく揺れた)flail　(関節などが緩んだ)loose　(歩行がよた

よたの）**waddling**

◀胸壁動揺 flail chest ▶動揺肩 loose [flail] shoulder 動揺関節 flail[loose] joint 動揺性歩行 waddling gait 動揺病 [乗物酔い] motion[travel] sickness

とうよういがく 東洋医学 **Oriental medicine, East Asian medicine** ◆当院では東洋医学を取り入れた治療も行っています Oriental medicine is also practiced[offered] in this hospital.

とうりょう 等量 **equal amount[quantity], the same amount[quantity]**

とうるい 糖類 ☞砂糖, 糖, 糖質, 糖分

どうろ 道路 （車道）**road** （街の通り）**street** （歩道）**pavement, sidewalk** ◆正面玄関を出て道路を渡ったところに薬局があります There's a drugstore across the street[road] from the main entrance. ◆道路の段差でつまずかないよう注意して下さい Please be careful not to trip on uneven pavements[sidewalks].

とうろく 登録 **registration** （動**register**） ◆当院は初めてですか. それではまず登録をお願いします Is this your first visit to this hospital? Then, you'll need to register first. ◆この登録用紙に記入をお願いします Would you fill out this registration form? ◆お待たせしました. これがあなたの登録カードです Thank you for waiting. Here's your registration card. ◀外国人登録 alien[foreign resident / non-Japanese] registration 患者登録 patient registration がん登録 cancer registration ▶登録看護師 （米）registered nurse；RN

とうろん 討論する （話し合う）**discuss** （口論・議論する）**argue** ◆検査結果と治療方針についてカンファレンスで討論する discuss the test results and treatment plan at a[the] conference

とおい 遠い

《距離が離れている》**far, distant** （図**distance**） ◆勤務先はご自宅から遠いですか Is your office far from your house? ◆当病院はご自宅から遠いですね This hospital is *a long way[far] from your house, isn't

it? ◆遠くの物が見えにくいですか Do you have difficulty seeing things at a distance?

《時間的に隔たっている》**distant** （図ずっと前に **a long time ago**） ◆遠い過去の記憶はありますか Do you *have memories of[remember] things that happened a long time ago? ◆このぶんだと退院できるのもそう遠くなさそうですね As things stand now, you ought to be able to leave[be discharged from] the hospital soon.

《機能が弱っている》 ◆耳が遠くなりましたか Are you hard of hearing?

とおす 通す **pass**

《話を》 ◆担当医にはこちらから話を通しておきます I'll pass this information along to your doctor.

《目を》 ◆注意書きにざっと目を通しておいて下さい Please have a quick look over [through] the instructions.

《火を》 ◆食べ物はよく火を通して早く召し上がって下さい（入念に調理して）Please cook food thoroughly and eat it *promptly [while it is still hot].

とおのく 遠のく （気を失う）**faint** （頭がくらくらする・気を失いそうになる）**feel faint** ◆動悸がする時, 意識が遠のきますか Do you feel faint when *your heart is pounding[you have palpitations]?

ドーパミン ☞ドパミン

ドーピング **doping** ◆ドーピングの検査をする give a *doping test[test for doping] ◆ドーピング検査を受ける take a doping test ◆ドーピング検査に合格する〈不合格になる〉pass〈fail〉a doping test ▶ドーピング疑惑 suspicion of doping

とおる 通る **pass, move, go through** ☞通過 ◆食べ物が喉を通りづらい感じがしますか Do you feel as if food doesn't pass[move] through your throat smoothly? ◆ここは通り抜けできません I'm sorry, but you can't go through here.

とかす¹ 溶かす

《液状にする》 （熱で液状にする）**melt** （溶解する）**dissolve** ◆錠剤は舌の下に入れたままゆっくり溶かして下さい Please place the tablet under your tongue and allow it to melt[dissolve] slowly. ◆この薬は水かジュースで溶かして飲めます This medication may be taken dissolved in water or juice. ◆血の塊を溶かす dissolve the blood clot ◆薬をぬるま湯で溶かす dissolve the medication in lukewarm water 《解凍する》thaw, defrost ◆冷凍した母乳をぬるま湯で溶かす thaw[defrost] frozen breast milk in lukewarm water

とかす² 梳かす （櫛で）comb /kóum/ （ブラシで）brush ◆髪をとかす comb [brush] *one's* hair

とがめる 咎める （心に痛みを感じる）feel guilty （about） （責める）blame, reproach ◆気がとがめることがありますか Do you ever feel guilty about things? ◆病気になったことで自分をとがめないで下さい Please don't blame[reproach] yourself for getting ill.

とがん 兎眼 lagophthalmos （㊫lagophthalmic） ▶兎眼性角膜炎 lagophthalmic keratitis / exposure keratitis

トキソイド toxoid ◆破傷風トキソイド tetanus toxoid

トキソプラズマ toxoplasma （㊫toxoplasmic） （学名）*Toxoplasma gondii* ◀眼トキソプラズマ症 ocular toxoplasmosis ▶トキソプラズマ脳炎 toxoplasmic encephalitis トキソプラズマ肺炎 toxoplasmic pneumonia

ときどき 時々 sometimes （たまに）occasionally （やや定期的に）once in a while （不定期に）from time to time （間隔を置いて）at intervals ◆時々喘息の発作を起こしますか Do you sometimes have asthma attacks? ◆時々痛むのですか，それともずっと痛いですか Does the pain come on occasionally[once in a while / at intervals] or is it constant?

ドキドキする （心臓が速く鼓動する）beat fast （心臓が激しく鼓動する）pound, throb （動悸する）have palpitations ☞動悸 ◆心臓がドキドキしますか Does your heart beat fast? / Do you feel your heart pounding[throbbing]? / Do you have palpitations?

とぎれる 途切れる （途中で止まり，また出始める）stop and start （中断する）become [get, be] interrupted （断続的になる）become[get, be] intermittent ◆尿線が途中で途切れることがありますか Do you ever experience stopping and starting during urination? / Does your urinary stream sometimes become interrupted? ◆脈が途切れる the heart skips beats / have an intermittent pulse / the pulse is intermittent

とく 溶く （溶解する）dissolve ☞溶かす

どく 毒 《毒物》 （一般的に毒物）poison （㊫poisonous） （細菌由来の毒素）toxin （㊫toxic） （ヘビ・昆虫などの毒液）venom （㊫venomous） ◆毒を飲む take poison ◆この植物には強い毒があります This plant is very poisonous. ◆毒キノコで中毒症状を起こす have symptoms of mushroom poisoning 《有害なこと》 ◆ほぼ毎晩のように深酒をするのは体に毒です Drinking a lot almost every evening *is bad[isn't good] for your health.

◀貝毒 shellfish poison[toxin] 神経毒 neurotoxin / nerve poison ハチ毒 hornet[wasp / bee] venom フグ毒 fugu poison[toxin] ヘビ毒 snake venom ▶毒蛾 poisonous[venomous] moth 毒ガス poison[toxic / poisonous] gas / （毒煙）toxic smoke 毒キノコ poisonous [toxic] mushroom 毒グモ poisonous [venomous] spider 毒ヘビ poisonous [venomous] snake ☞毒性，毒素，毒針，毒物，毒薬，猛毒，有毒

とくい¹ 特異（的な） （特定の・固有の）specific （↔nonspecific） （独特な）peculiar （他に類のない）unique ◀前立腺特異抗原 prostate-specific antigen；PSA ▶特異体質 idiosyncrasy 特異的免疫療法 specific immunotherapy 特異度 specificity

とくい² 得意（な） （上手な）good （大好きな）favorite （図強み strength） ◆料理が得意なのですね You're good at cooking, aren't you? / You're a good cook, aren't you? ◆〈学校での〉得意科目は何ですか What's your favorite subject (at school)? ◆仕事上の得意分野は何ですか What are your strengths at work?

どくご 独語 monologue ☞独り言

どくじ 独自(の) 〈自分自身の〉own 〈他に類のない〉unique 〈独創的な〉original ☞独特 ◆患者は誰でも独自の悩みを抱えています Every patient has his〈her〉own problems to worry about. ▶独自性〈個性〉identity / 〈独創性〉originality / 〈ユニークさ〉uniqueness

どくじしょうがい 読字障害 reading difficulty[disorder, disturbance] 〈難読症〉dyslexia (形dyslexic) ◆読字障害がある have dyslexia[reading difficulty] / be dyslexic

とくしゅ 特殊(な) 〈特別な〉special 〈類のない〉unique 〈独特な〉particular ☞独特, 特別 ◆特殊なニーズを持つ子供 a special-needs child / a child with special needs ▶特殊外来 special outpatient clinic 特殊教育 special education 特殊健康診断 special health checkup (for workers)

どくしょ 読書する read (a book) ◆読書はふだんよくなさるのですか Do you usually read a lot (of books)? ▶読書用眼鏡 reading glasses[spectacles]

とくしょく 特色 〈特徴〉characteristic 〈特異さ〉peculiarity ☞特徴

どくしん 独身(の) single 〈未婚の〉unmarried ◆独身ですか, 結婚していますか Are you single or married? / 〈パートナーがいるか〉Do you have a partner? ▶独身者 single person / 〈独身男性〉single man, bachelor / 〈独身女性〉single woman

とくせい 特性 〈特徴〉characteristic 〈性状〉property ☞特徴

どくせい 毒性 〈細菌由来の〉toxicity (↔nontoxicity)(形toxic) 〈一般的に毒物の〉poison (形poisonous) ☞毒 ◆毒性が高い物質 a highly toxic[poisonous] substance ◀肝毒性 hepatotoxicity 残留毒性 residual toxicity 心毒性 cardiotoxic-

ity 腎毒性 renal toxicity / nephrotoxicity 長期毒性 long-term toxicity 聴器毒性 ototoxicity 薬物毒性 drug toxicity ▶毒性試験 toxicity test[testing] 毒性物質 toxic substance

どくそ 毒素 〈細菌由来の〉toxin 〈有毒な物質〉poisonous substance 〈ヘビ・昆虫などの毒液〉venom ☞毒 ◀外毒素 exotoxin 抗毒素 antitoxin / antivenom 耐熱性毒素 thermostable[heat-stable] toxin 内毒素 endotoxin ベロ毒素 verotoxin ボツリヌス毒素 botulinum toxin；BTX ▶毒素型細菌性食中毒 *endotoxigenic bacterial[bacterial toxin] food poisoning 毒素血症 toxemia 毒素原性大腸菌 enterotoxigenic *Escherichia coli*；ETEC 毒素性ショック症候群 toxic shock syndrome；TSS

ドクター doctor ☞医師 ▶ドクターカー doctor's car / medic car / physician (rapid response) car ドクターショッピング doctor shopping ドクターヘリ air ambulance / doctor helicopter / *emergency medical service[EMS] helicopter

とくちょう 特徴 〈特質・特性〉characteristic (動特徴づける characterize) 〈特に目立つ点〉feature 〈人の性格・身体の特性〉trait ◆関節リウマチの特徴は朝のこわばりです A characteristic of rheumatoid arthritis is joint *stiffness in the morning[morning stiffness]. ◆メニエール病の特徴は繰り返すめまいの発作, 耳鳴り, そして難聴です Ménière disease is characterized by recurrent attacks of dizziness, ringing in the ears, and hearing loss. ◆著しい特徴 a marked[dominant] characteristic ◆遺伝的特徴 a genetic[hereditary] characteristic ◆身体的特徴 a physical characteristic[trait] ◆顔の特徴 facial features ◆性格上の特徴 character[personality] trait ◆文化的特徴 cultural characteristics ◆典型的な特徴 a typical feature[characteristic]

とくてい 特定(の) 〈ある一定の〉certain 〈明確な・具体的な〉specific, particular 〈明記された〉specified (動確定する determine

物事の本質などを明確にする **identify** （具体的にはっきり指定する **specify**） ◆症状はある特定の時期だけに出ますか Does the symptom occur just at certain[specific] times of the year? ◆痛みの真の原因を特定するために検査をしましょう I'm going to perform some tests to determine[identify] *the exact cause of your pain[what exactly is causing your pain]. ▶特定機能病院 advanced treatment hospital[facility] 特定保健用食品 food for specified health use(s) ☞特定疾患

とくていしっかん 特定疾患 （指定難病） **designated intractable disease** ◆外国籍の方でも特定疾患の医療費助成制度の対象になる場合があるので，市〈区〉の窓口に問い合わせて下さい Foreign residents may be eligible for financial support[assistance] for patients with intractable diseases, so please contact[inquire at / check with] the *city hall〈ward office〉.

とくとう 禿頭 **baldness** ☞脱毛，禿げ

どくとく 独特（の）（他に類のない）**unique** （固有の）**peculiar** （特徴的な）**characteristic** ☞独自 ◆それはあなたの国に独特の風習ですか Is that a custom that's unique to your country?

とくに 特に **particularly, in particular, especially** ◆特にご心配なことがありますか Are you afraid of anything in particular? ◆今日の午後は特に予定はありません I have no particular plans for this afternoon. ◆特に悪いところはなさそうです I don't see anything particularly wrong. ◆特に段差のある（平らでない）歩道では歩く時には気をつけて下さい Please take care when you walk, especially on uneven sidewalks.

とくはつせい 特発性（の）（原因不明の）**idiopathic** （自然発生的な）**spontaneous** ◆「特発性」とは平たく言えば「疾患の原因が特定できない」ということです Put simply, the word 'idiopathic' means that the cause of a disease is unknown. ▶特発性間質性肺炎 idiopathic interstitial pneumonia；IIP 特発性血小板減少性紫斑病

idiopathic thrombocytopenic purpura；ITP 特発性心筋症 idiopathic cardiomyopathy；ICM 特発性肺線維症 idiopathic pulmonary fibrosis；IPF

どくばり 毒針 （動物・昆虫の）（**poison**）**stinger**

どくぶつ 毒物 **poison, poisonous substance** （細菌由来の有毒物質）**toxic substance** ☞毒 ▶毒物学 toxicology

とくべつ 特別（の）**special, especial** （特定の）**particular** （追加の）**extra** （圖…以外は **except …**）◆特別料金（追加料金）an extra charge[fee] /（割引料金）a specially reduced fee ◆お子さんの食事には特別な配慮が必要です You need to pay special attention to your child's diet. ◆特別な事情がない限り，面会は午後3時から7時までです Visiting hours are from three to seven in the afternoon except in special circumstances. ◆特別な理由もないのに絶えずいらいらしたり不安になりますか Do you feel constantly on edge or worried for no particular reason? ◆申し訳ありませんが，あなたを特別扱いはできません I'm sorry, but we can't make an exception for you. ★exception は「例外」を意味する．▶特別支援学校〈学級〉 special needs[education] school〈class〉 特別室 special [deluxe] room 特別食 special diet 特別養護老人ホーム special nursing home for seniors[elderly people]

とくゆう 特有（の）（特徴的な）**characteristic** （固有の）**peculiar** ☞特徴 ◆これは蕁麻疹特有の症状です This symptom is characteristic of hives. ◆そういった行動は若者特有なものです That behavior is peculiar to young people.

とくよう 特養 （特別養護老人ホーム）**special nursing home for seniors[elderly people]**

どくりつ 独立した **independent** ◆あなたはご両親から独立して別に住んでいるのですか Are you living[Do you live] independently of[from] your parents?

とくれい 特例 **exception** ☞例外 ◆今回のみ特例として認めますが，次回は時間

内でのご面会をお願いします I'll make an exception just this once, but please come during visiting hours next time.

とげ　棘　(骨などの)**splinter**　(バラなどの)**thorn**　(植物の)**prickle**　◆指にとげが刺さる get a splinter[thorn] in *one's* finger　◆親指のとげを抜く remove a splinter[thorn] from *one's* thumb / get[take] a splinter[thorn] out of *one's* thumb

とけい　時計　(掛け時計・置時計)**clock**　(腕時計)**watch**　◆あなたの時計では何時ですか What time do you have? / What time is it by your watch?　◆時計の絵を描いて数字をすべて書き入れて下さい Please draw a clock and put in all the numbers.　◀生物[体内]時計 biological[body] clock　目覚まし時計 alarm clock　▶時計描画テスト clock drawing test；CDT

とけつ　吐血　hematemesis；*vomiting blood*

とける　溶ける　(個体が熱で液状化する)**melt**　(個体が液体の中で溶解する)**dissolve**　◆この錠剤は完全に溶けるまでそのまま舌の下に入れておいて下さい Please keep this tablet under your tongue until it melts[dissolves] completely.　◆この薬は溶けやすいので水なしでも服用できます This medication dissolves easily[quickly], so you can take it even without water.

どこ　where　(場所を限定して訊く)**which**　(漠然と場所を訊く)**what**　☞どこか
《どの場所》　◆痛むのはどこですか Where is the pain? / Where do you feel the pain? / Where does it hurt?　◆お腹のどこが痛みますか Where in the abdomen does it hurt? / Which part of the abdomen hurts?　◆どこも悪くありません There is nothing wrong with you. / I can't find anything wrong with you.　◆(認知症が疑われる相手に)ここはどこですか Where are you[we] now?　★"Where is *here*?"や"Where is *this*?"とは訊かないことに注意.
◆どこの国からおいでですか Where are you from? / Which country are you from?　◆アメリカのどこのご出身ですか What[Which] part of the United States

are you from? / Where in the United States are you from?
《何という(施設・組織)》　◆どこの病院で手術を受けましたか Which hospital did you have the surgery at?　◆どこの会社にお勤めですか What company do you work for?
《どこでも》　◆この処方箋の薬はどこの薬局でも調合してもらえます You can have the prescription filled at any pharmacy.　◆この貼り薬はどこでもお好きな場所に貼って下さい Please *put this patch on [apply this patch to] any part of your body that you like.
《どこまで》　◆リハビリはどこまで進みましたか How far have you progressed with your rehabilitation?

とこう　渡航　overseas travel, international travel　◆最近，海外渡航なさいましたか Have you recently *traveled out of Japan [gone overseas / been overseas]?

どこか
《どの場所か》**somewhere, someplace**　(疑問文・否定文で)**anywhere, anyplace**　◆彼女はどこか家の近くの病院への転院を希望しています She wishes[hopes] to be transferred to a hospital somewhere near her house.　◆ここがどこかわかりますか Do you know where you are?　◆どこか痛みますか Do you have any pain anywhere?　◆どこかご不明な点がありましたら遠慮なくご質問下さい If you have any questions or concerns, please don't hesitate to ask me.
《どことなく》　◆どこか体調がおかしいと感じることがありますか Do you feel that something in your body is wrong?　◆彼女の行動はどこか変ですか Is her behavior strange in any way? / Is her behavior somehow strange?

ドコサヘキサエンさん　―酸　docosahexaenoic acid；**DHA**

とこジラミ　床ジラミ　bed bug

とこずれ　床擦れ　bedsore, pressure sore, decubitus ulcer　☞褥瘡　◆腰に床ずれができ始めています You've started to develop

bedsores on your lower back. ◆床ずれ
ができないように体の向きを頻繁に変えて
下さい Please change your position frequently *so that you won't get bedsores [to prevent bedsores / for bedsore prevention].

ところ　所
《位置・場所》place　（部屋）room　（部位）site
（空間的な余地）room, space　◆ここは化学
療法を行う所です This is the chemotherapy room. / This is (the room) where chemotherapy treatments are given.
◆ここが胆石のある所です This is (the site) where you have a gallstone.　◆くるぶしの所が少し腫れていますね You have some slight swelling in your ankles.　◆薬は子供の手の届かない所に保管して下さい Please keep these medications out of the reach of children.　◆病室にはかばんを2つも置く所はありません There is no room [space] in your room for two pieces of baggage.
《箇所・部分》　◆わかりづらい所があれば遠慮なくお尋ね下さい If there is anything you don't understand, please don't hesitate to ask me.
《現在の状況》　◆今は内科と外科とで治療方針を検討しているところです The physicians and surgeons are now examining [reviewing] your treatment plan.　◆このところご気分はどうですか How has your mood been *these days[recently]?
《推測される程度》　◆入院期間は1週間といったところでしょう You'll be in the hospital for about a week. / Your hospital stay will be about a week or so.　◆見たところ深刻なものではなさそうです It doesn't seem to be anything serious. / Apparently[It seems that] it's nothing serious.

ところで　well, now, well then, now then, so then　（話題を変えて）by the way, incidentally　◆ところで，食欲はどうですか Well [Now] then, how is your appetite?　◆ところで，ペットを飼っていますか So[Well], do you have any pets?　★so は「それで」と相手の言葉を受けていう.

とざす　閉ざす　（人目を避ける）shut *oneself* off　（引きこもる）withdraw （into, from）
◆彼は突然心を閉ざしたのですか Did he suddenly *shut himself off[withdraw into himself / (自分の殻に)crawl into his own shell]?　◆彼女は心を閉ざして口をききません She withdrew into silence.　◆医療スタッフに心を閉ざす withdraw from the medical staff

とし　年・歳　age　（歳(さい)，年齢　◆お子さんの年はおいくつですか How old is your child? / What's your child's age?
◆年をとるにつれて代謝が落ちます As you get older, your metabolism slows down.
◆彼女は年の割には記憶力が良い Considering her age[years], she has a good memory. / She has a good memory for her age.

とじこめしょうこうぐん　閉じ込め症候群　locked-in syndrome

とじこもる　閉じこもる　（外出を拒否する）refuse to leave home　（部屋などにこもる）shut *oneself* up （in）　（終日家にいる）stay at home all day　（病気などで外出できない）be housebound, be confined to home[*one's* house]　☞引きこもる　◆彼女は何もしないでほとんど部屋に閉じこもっていた She *shut herself up[stayed] in her room most of the time without doing anything.　◆長期にわたる病気で家に閉じこもっている be housebound because of a long-term illness

としゃ　吐瀉　vomiting and diarrhea
▶吐瀉物 vomit and stools[excreta]

としゅ　徒手(の)　manual　▶徒手筋力検査法 manual muscle test[testing]；MMT 徒手整復 manual reposition[correction]

としょ　図書　book　◀医学図書 medical book　参考図書 reference book　▶図書カート book cart　図書コーナー book corner　☞図書室

としょしつ　図書室　library　（読書室）reading room　◆病院内図書室 the hospital library　◆患者用図書室 the patients' library / the patient library　◆図書室のスタッフ(司書)a librarian / (職員)the

としょしつ　library staff　◀(病院内)移動図書室(in-hospital) bookmobile

とじる　閉じる　**close, shut**　◆目を閉じて下さい Please close[shut] your eyes.　◆唇をしっかり閉じる close[shut] *one's* lips tightly

どせき　努責　☞息む, 力む

とちゅう　途中　(中間で)**halfway through**　(道のりの一部まで)**part of the way**　◆排尿の途中で尿サンプルを採って下さい Please collect a sample of urine halfway through urinating.　◆尿線が途中で途切れる the urinary stream becomes interrupted / have an interrupted urinary stream　◆途中までお供します I'll go with you part of the way.　◆お話の途中ですが, もう行かなければなりません(中断してすみませんが) Excuse me for interrupting, but I'll have to be going now.

どちょう　怒張　**engorgement**　◀頸静脈怒張 engorgement of the jugular vein

どちら　(限定して訊く)**which**　(やや漠然と訊く)**what**　(場所を訊く)**where**　(どちらか片方)**either**　(どちらも両方)**both**
《場所》☞どこ　◆ご出身はどちらですか Where are you from? / Which country are you from?　◆お勤めはどちらの会社ですか What company do you work for?
《人》☞どなた　◆どちら様ですか(受付で) May I have your name, please? / (電話口で)*May I ask who's calling[Who's calling, please]?
《択一》◆右耳と左耳のどちらが聞こえにくいですか In which ear do you have difficulty hearing, the right or the left?　◆首をどちらの方向に曲げるとめまいが起きやすいですか Which direction[way] do you bend your neck when you become dizzy?　◆朝食はパンとライス, どちらがよいですか Which would you like for breakfast, bread or rice?　◆加藤先生か私のどちらかが後で診察にまいります Either Dr Kato or I will come to see you later.　◆どちらの曜日でも検査の予約をお取りできます You can make an appointment for either day of the week.　◆どちらの薬もす

ぐに効果があるでしょう Both medications will take effect soon.

ドック　◀人間ドック comprehensive physical[health] checkup[screening] / complete physical[health] checkup [screening]　脳ドック brain screening [checkup]

とっこうやく　特効薬　**specific medication[cure]**　(驚異的な効果を示す薬)**miracle drug[cure]**　◆残念ですが, この病気には特効薬はありません Unfortunately, there's no specific medication[cure] for this disease.

とっしゅつ　突出する　**bulge, protrude**　(図**bulging, protrusion**　形突き出た**prominent**)　◆眼球が突出する have bulging eyes[eyeballs] / have abnormal bulging [protrusion] of the eyeballs　◆彼女の眼球は異常に突出しています Her eyeballs are protruding abnormally.　◀眼球突出 exophthalmos / (ocular) proptosis　前額突出 prominent forehead

とっしんげんしょう　突進現象　**pulsion**

とつぜん　突然(の)　**sudden**　(切迫した)**urgent**　(予期しない)**unexpected**　(不意の)**abrupt**　☞突発　◆痛みの起こり方は突然ですか Does the pain come on suddenly?　◆その症状が始まるのは突然ですか, 徐々にですか Does the symptom come on suddenly or gradually?　◆彼の死は突然で予期しないものでした His death was sudden and unexpected.　◆突然の心臓発作で死亡する die of a sudden heart attack　◆突然尿意を催す have *a sudden[an urgent] need to urinate　▶突然発症 sudden onset　☞突然死, 突然変異

とつぜんし　突然死　**sudden death**　(予期せぬ死)**unexpected death**　◆突然死の危険性を減らす reduce[lower] the risk of sudden death　◀乳幼児突然死症候群 sudden infant death syndrome；SIDS / crib death

とつぜんへんい　突然変異　**mutation**　(図**mutant**)　◆お子さんの障害は遺伝子の突然変異によるものです Your child's disorder is caused by a gene mutation.　▶突然

変異遺伝子 mutant gene

どっち ☞どちら

とって 取っ手 handle （車椅子などの）handlebar （ドアの）knob （レバー）lever
◆この取っ手をしっかり握ってください Please grasp this handlebar[handle] firmly.

とっぱつ 突発(性の・的な) （突然の）sudden （予期しない）unexpected ☞突然
◆突発的な出来事 *a sudden[an unexpected] incident ◆蕁麻疹の突発的発症 an outbreak of hives ▶突発性難聴 sudden hearing loss；SHL / sudden deafness 突発性発疹 roseola infantum / exanthema subitum；ES

ドップラー ☞ドプラ

とつレンズ 凸レンズ convex lens

とても
《非常に》☞実に ◆とてもよくできました Very good. / Excellent. / You did really well. ◆とても残念です I'm very sorry.
《とても…ない》 ◆これだけ全身状態が悪いと化学療法はとてもできません We can't possibly give[administer] chemotherapy when *the patient* is in such a bad general condition[state].

とどく 届く
《受け取る》receive, get ◆あなたのかかりつけ医から紹介状が届きました I received a referral letter from your regular doctor.
《手が届く》reach （図手が届く距離 reach）
◆呼び出しボタンに手が届きますか Can you reach the call button? ◆この薬は子供の手の届かないところに保管して下さい Please keep this medication out of the reach of children.

とどけ 届け(出) （登録・登記）registration （動register） （報告）report （通知）note, notification, notice ◆出生届を出す register the birth of *one's* baby ◆病気欠席の届けを学校に出す submit[send in] a sick note[excuse] to *one's* school ◆無届けで会社を休む be absent from the company without notice ◆欠席届 notice of absence 婚姻届 notification of marriage / marriage registration / （用紙）marriage registration form 死産届 notification[registration] of stillbirth 死亡届 notification[registration] of death / death registration 出生届 notice[notification / registration] of birth ▶届出伝染病 notifiable infectious disease

とどける 届ける
《持って来る》bring （手渡す）hand in （配達する）deliver （提出する）submit ◆痛み止めはできるだけ早くお届けします I'll bring the pain medication to you as soon as possible. ◆車椅子を患者の病室に届ける deliver a wheelchair to the patient's room ◆署名した同意書を担当看護師に届けて下さい Please *hand in[submit] the signed consent form to your nurse.
《通知する》report ◆結核の症例を保健所に届ける report a case of tuberculosis to the health center

ととのえる 整える・調える
《用意する》get … ready, prepare ◆必要な書類を調える get the necessary papers ready
《乱れを直す》（整備する）put … in order （良好にする）get *oneself* into good … ◆身辺を整える put *one's* affairs in order ◆住宅環境を整える put *one's* house in order ◆手術前には体調を調えておいて下さい Please get yourself into good condition[physical shape] before your surgery. / Please prepare for the surgery by getting into good condition[physical shape]. ◆髪を整える do *one's* hair ◆ベッドを整える make the beds

ドナー donor （↔recipient） ◀生体ドナー living donor ▶ドナーカード donor card ドナーコーディネーター donor coordinator ドナー腎 donor kidney

どなた who （不特定の誰か〈肯定文で〉）someone, somebody （不特定のだれか〈疑問文・否定文で〉）anyone, anybody ☞誰
◆今日の診察にはどなたが付き添ってきましたか Who accompanied[was with] you for today's examination? ◆どなた様ですか May I have[ask] your name, please? / What's your name? ★上昇口調で．"Who

are you?"は相手に失礼な言い方になるので注意. ／（電話口で）Who is calling, please?
◆ご家族のどなたかに健康上の問題や障害がありますか Does anyone in your family have any health problems or disability?

となり 隣(の) **next** ☞シャワー室は浴室のすぐ隣にあります The shower room is right next (door) to the bathroom. ◆隣の病室〈ベッド〉の患者 the patient in the next room〔bed〕

とにゅう 吐乳する **vomit milk, bring up milk, spit up milk**

どのあたり ☞どこ

どのくらい （時間・期間）**how long** （頻度）**how often** （量・重さ）**how much** （程度）**how** ◆痛みは毎回どのくらい続きますか How long does the pain last each time?
◆来日してからどのくらいになりますか How long have you been in Japan? ◆どのくらいの頻度で痛みますか How often do you have the pain? ◆お酒は1日にどのくらい飲みますか How much alcohol do you drink a day? ◆体重はどのくらいですか How much do you weigh? ◆痛みの程度はどのくらいですか How severe is the pain?

どのへん どの辺 ☞どこ

どのような ☞どんな

ドパミン **dopamine** ▶ドパミン拮抗薬 dopamine antagonist　ドパミン作動薬 dopamine agonist　ドパミン受容体刺激薬 dopamine receptor stimulant　ドパミン前駆物質 dopamine precursor　ドパミン取り込み阻害薬 dopamine uptake inhibitor

とびいしじょうびょうへん 飛び石状病変 **skip lesion**

とびおりる 飛び降りる **jump (off, from)** ◆マンションの屋上から〈橋から〉飛び降りて自殺する kill *oneself* by jumping off〔from〕*the roof of an apartment building〈a bridge〉 ▶飛び降り自殺 suicide〔killing *oneself*〕by jumping

とびなおりはんのう 跳び直り反応 **hopping reaction**

とびひ （伝染性膿痂疹）**contagious impetigo**

とふ 塗布する **apply** ☞塗る　かゆみ止め塗布薬 topical antipruritic (medication / drug / agent)　▶塗布薬(軟膏)ointment

とぶ 飛ぶ **skip** ◆脈はよくとびますか Does your heart skip beats frequently?

ドブタミン **dobutamine**

とぶつ 吐物 **vomit** ☞嘔吐物

ドプラ **Doppler** ◀超音波ドプラ法 Doppler ultrasound〔ultrasonography〕

とふんしょう 吐糞症 **fecal vomiting**

とふんじょうべん 兎糞状便 （**rabbit**） **pellet-like stools / scybalum**

とまつ 塗抹 **smear** ◆痰の塗抹検査では結核菌は検出されませんでした Your sputum smear for tuberculosis was negative.

とまる[1] 止まる
《停止する》**stop** ◆出血が止まらないことがありましたか Have you ever experienced bleeding that wouldn't stop? ◆咳が止まらないのですね You can't stop coughing, can you? ◆睡眠中に呼吸が止まることがあると指摘されたことがありますか Have you ever been told that you sometimes stop breathing in your sleep?
《症状が治まる》（消える）**go （away）** （鎮まる）**subside** ◆胃の痛みは止まりましたか Has your stomachache *gone away*〔subsided〕? ◆この薬を飲めば痛みが止まるでしょう Your pain will go away after you take this medication.

とまる[2] 泊まる **stay （with）, spend the night （with）** ◆お子さんの付き添いで泊まることをご希望でしたら看護師にご相談下さい If you want to *stay overnight*〔spend the night〕with your child, please talk〔check〕with the nurse about it.

とむ 富む **be rich （in）** ☞豊富 ◆大豆〈大豆食品〉は蛋白質に富んでいます Soybeans〈Soy foods〉are rich in protein.

とめがね 留め金 **clasp**

ドメスティックバイオレンス **domestic violence ; DV**

とめる[1] 止める
《終わらせる》**stop** ◆出血を止める stop the bleeding ◆痛みを止める薬を処方します

I'm going to prescribe some medication to stop the pain.

《こらえる》hold, suppress　◆息を大きく吸って止めて下さい Take a deep breath and hold it.　★「息を止める」には stop を用いないことに注意.　◆排尿を止める stop [hold] the flow of urine　★「尿を止める」では stop も使える.

《スイッチを切る》turn off, switch off　◆エアコンを止める turn off the air conditioner

とめる²　留める　《テープで》tape　《ホチキスで》use a stapler　◆傷口のガーゼをテープで留める tape gauze over[on] the wound　◆傷口を医療用ホチキスで留める use a surgical[medical] stapler to close a wound / close a wound with staples　★staple はホチキスの針.

ともだち　友達　friend　《仲間》companion　◆親しい友達がいますか Do you have close friends?　◆友達とはどのくらいの頻度で会って(あなたの問題について)話をする機会がありますか How often do you get a chance to meet and talk (about your problems) with a friend?　◆お子さんは友達と遊びますか Does your child play with friends?　◆日本人の友達がなかなかできない have difficulty making Japanese friends　◆頼りになる友達 a reliable[dependable] friend　◆飼っているペットがあなたの一番の友達ですか Is your pet your closest companion?　◀遊び友達 playmate

ともなう　伴う　《付随する》come with, accompany　《影響を与える》involve　《関連する》associate with　◆頭痛に発熱が伴いましたか Did a fever come with the headache?　◆脳腫瘍には痙攣を伴うことがよくあります Brain tumors are often accompanied by seizures.　◆この手術には多少危険が伴います This surgery involves[carries] some risks.　◆糖尿病に伴う合併症 diabetes-associated complications / complications associated with diabetes

ともばたらき　共働き　◆お宅は共働きですか Do both you and your wife〈husband〉work? / Do both of you work?

▶共働き家庭 dual-income[dual-worker] family / double-income family　★income は「収入」を意味する.

どもる　吃る　《言葉が詰まる》stammer　《発声・構音障害がある》stutter　☞吃音　◆どもりながら話す speak with a stammer[stutter]

どようび　土曜日　Saturday；Sat.　◆土曜日に on Saturday　◆土曜日ごとに on Saturdays

ドライアイ　dry eye　▶ドライアイ症候群 dry eye syndrome

ドライアイス　dry ice　◆ドライアイスでいぼを凍結除去する apply dry ice to freeze and remove warts

トライツじんたい　─靱帯　Treitz ligament

トラウベちょうしんき　─聴診器　Traube stethoscope

トラウマ　trauma（形traumatic）　☞外傷, 心的外傷

トラコーマ　trachoma（形trachomatous）　▶トラコーマ角膜炎 trachomatous keratitis

ドラッグストア　drugstore

トラブル　trouble　☞問題　◆仕事中にトラブルを起こす get into trouble at work

トランスジェンダー　transgender　★LGBT は lesbian（女性同性愛者）, gay（男性同性愛者）, bisexual（両性愛者）, transgender の頭文字をとった総称.

トリアージ　triage　▶トリアージシート triage sheet　トリアージタッグ triage tag

とりあつかう　取り扱う　《手で扱う》handle　《対処する》deal（with）, treat　《受け付ける》accept　☞扱う

とりいれる　取り入れる　《運動・趣味などを始める》take up　《加える》add　《採用する》adopt, incorporate　◆軽い運動を取り入れるとよいでしょう You should take up some light exercise. / It'll be good for your health if you add a light workout plan (to your daily routine).　◆東洋医学を取り入れて治療する adopt[incorporate] Oriental medicine in one's practice

トリインフルエンザ　鳥インフルエンザ

bird flu, avian flu[influenza] ◀高病原性鳥インフルエンザ highly pathogenic avian influenza

とりかえる　取り替える・取り換える　(替える)change　(交換する)exchange　☞替える・換える　◆包帯を取り替えましょう I'm going to[Let me] change the bandage [dressing].　◆生理用ナプキンを1日に何回取り替えますか How many times a day do you change your *sanitary pads[napkins]?　◆このガウンは小さすぎますので大きいのに取り換えましょう This gown is too small for you. Let me exchange it for a larger one.

トリグリセリド　triglyceride　◀中性脂肪

とりけす　取り消す　cancel　(発言などを撤回する)take back　◆受診の予約を取り消す cancel one's doctor's appointment　◆誤解があったようです．先ほどの発言は取り消します There must have been some misunderstanding. I take back what I said before.

トリコスポロン　*Trichosporon*　▶トリコスポロン症 trichosporonosis

トリコモナス　*Trichomonas*　◀腟トリコモナス症 vaginal trichomoniasis

とりしいくしゃはい　鳥飼育者肺　bird breeder's lung

とりすぎ　摂り過ぎる　eat too much, take too much　◆塩分の摂り過ぎに注意して下さい Please be careful not to eat[take] too much salt.

トリソミー　trisomy　◀転座型トリソミー translocation trisomy　21トリソミー trisomy twenty-one syndrome

とりたてて　取り立てて　☞特に

とりのぞく　取り除く　☞除去

とりはからう　取り計らう　(手配する)arrange, make the arrangements　(きちんと対処する)see to　◆通訳が必要ならこちらで取り計らいましょう If you need an interpreter, we'll *arrange that for you[make the arrangements for you].　◆必要な書類を準備しておくよう取り計らいましょう I'll see to it that you get the papers you need.

とりはずす　取り外す　remove (形removable), take off　☞外す　◆取り外しのきく入れ歯 removable dentures

とりはだ　鳥肌　goose bumps, goose pimples, gooseflesh　★bumps, pimples はいずれも複数形で．◆鳥肌が立つ get *goose bumps[gooseflesh]

トリパノソーマ　*Trypanosoma*　▶トリパノソーマ症 trypanosomiasis

トリプシン　trypsin

とりみだす　取り乱す　get[become, be] upset　◆どうか取り乱さないで落ち着いて話を聞いて下さい Please don't get upset, but listen to me calmly.

とりめ　鳥目　(夜盲症)night blindness (形night-blind), nyctalopia

とりもどす　取り戻す　(回復する)recover (元の状態になる)regain　◆冷静さを取り戻す recover one's *peace of mind[composure]　◆健康を取り戻す recover[regain] one's health　◆意識を取り戻す regain consciousness / become conscious again / come around

どりょうこう　度量衡　weights and measures　★複数形で．☞巻末付録：単位の換算

トリヨードサイロニン　triiodothyronine；T₃　◀遊離トリヨードサイロニン free triiodothyronine；free T₃

どりょく　努力する　try, make an effort (図effort 形呼吸が苦しそうな labored　強制的な forced)　◆頑張る　◆禁煙するよう努力して下さい Please try to stop smoking.　◆努力の成果が出ましたね Your efforts have finally paid off, haven't they?　◆できるだけ努力します(最善を尽くす)We'll do our best[utmost]. / We'll make our utmost efforts.　◆今それをする努力を惜しむべきではありません Now, you should work as hard as possible to achieve that. / You should do everything you can to make that happen.　▶努力呼吸 labored breathing　努力呼出 forced expiration 努力肺活量 forced vital capacity；FVC

ドリル　drill　◀歯科用ドリル dental drill

とる¹　取る・採る・摂る

《取り去る》 (除去する)remove　(脱ぐ)take

off （振り払う・治す）shake off　◆装身具を全部取って下さい Please *take off[remove] all of your jewelry.　◆包帯を取らないで下さい Please don't remove the bandage.　◆悪い癖を取る shake off a bad habit　◆ポリープを内視鏡で取る remove a polyp using an endoscope　◆痛みを取る（和らげる）relieve the pain

《採取・摂取する》（集める）collect　（手に入れる）get, take, obtain　◆このコップに尿を採って下さい Please use this cup to collect your urine. / Please collect a sample of your urine in this cup.　◆親指から血を採ります I'm going to prick your thumb and get[obtain] a blood sample.　◆この管を入れて膀胱から尿を採ります（尿を排出させる）I'm going to drain the urine from your bladder with this tube.　◆組織を採って確かめる get[obtain] tissue samples to make sure　◆パンフレットはご自由にお取り下さい Please feel free to take a brochure. / Please help yourself to a brochure.　◆栄養を摂る take (in) nourishment　◆塩分を摂りすぎる get[take in] too much salt

とる²　撮る　take　◆胸の X 線写真〈CT〉を撮りましょう Let's take *an X-ray〈a CT (scan)〉of your chest.　◆乳房 X 線写真を撮ったことがありますか Have you ever had *a mammogram[an X-ray of your breast] taken?　◆胸の写真を最後に撮ったのはいつですか When was your last chest X-ray?

トルエン　toluene

トルコ　Turkey（形トルコの・トルコ人のTurkish）☞国籍　▶トルコ人 Turk

トルコあん　─鞍　Turkish saddle, sella turcica

トルソーちょうこう　─徴候　Trousseau sign

どれ　which（どちらでも）**whichever**　☞どちら　◆この治療法の中でどれを選んでよいか決めかねているのですね You can't decide which (option) to choose among these treatment options, can you?　◆どれでもお好きなものをお取り下さい Please take whichever you like[prefer].

トレイ　tray　◆トレイを下げてもいいですか May I take your tray away?

トレーニング（運動）**exercise, workout**（訓練）**training**　☞運動, 訓練　◆散歩は格好のトレーニングとしてお勧めです I recommend walking because it's *good exercise [a good workout].　◆当院で心臓リハビリのトレーニングを受けることができます Cardiac rehabilitation is provided at this hospital. / You can receive[undergo] cardiac rehabilitation at this hospital.　◀筋力トレーニング muscle (strength) training　不安管理トレーニング anxiety management training　☞トイレトレーニング

ドレーン（排液管）**drain, drainage tube**　☞ドレナージ　◆胸腔内にたまった液体を出すためにドレーンを右胸腔内に挿入する place[insert] a (drainage) tube inside the right chest cavity to drain fluids out of the pleural space　◀留置ドレーン indwelling drain

どれくらい　☞どのくらい

トレッドミル　treadmill　◆トレッドミルは運動しながら記録する心電図検査です A treadmill test is an EKG that is recorded during exercise.　◆トレッドミル検査の 1 時間前までに軽く食事をすませて, 動きやすい服装とウォーキングシューズでおいで下さい Please eat a light meal at least an hour before the treadmill test, and wear comfortable clothes and walking shoes.　◆このトレッドミルの上を歩いて下さい Please walk on this treadmill.　▶トレッドミル運動負荷試験 treadmill exercise (stress / tolerance) test

ドレナージ　drainage　☞ドレーン　◆ドレナージチューブを胸部に挿入する place[insert] a drainage tube into the chest　◀胸腔ドレナージ thoracic[intrathoracic] drainage　経皮経肝胆汁ドレナージ percutaneous transhepatic biliary drainage；PTBD　経皮経肝胆道ドレナージ percutaneous transhepatic cholangiodrainage；PTCD　心嚢ドレナージ pericardial drainage　脳室ドレナージ ventricular drainage

脳槽ドレナージ cisternal drainage　閉鎖式ドレナージ closed drainage system

どれほど ☞どんな

とれる　取れる　（なくなる）go away, disappear　（落ちる）come out　（はがれる）come off, fall off　◆痛み〈熱〉はまもなく取れるでしょう The pain〈fever〉will go away soon.　◆このしみは完全には取れないかもしれません This stain may not come out completely.　◆かさぶたは自然に取れるまでほっておいて下さい Just leave the scab alone until it comes[falls] off by itself.

トレンデレンブルグたいい　―体位　Trendelenburg position

トレンデレンブルグほこう　―歩行　Trendelenburg gait

どろ　泥　mud　（㊥muddy）◆泥状の便 muddy stools

トローチ　troche　（薬用ドロップ）（throat）lozenge

ドロップ　drop　（薬用ドロップ）lozenge　◀咳止めドロップ cough drop

どろどろ（の）　（濃い）thick　（泥状の）muddy　◆どろどろした痰 thick phlegm　◆膿のようにどろどろした分泌物 thick pus-like discharge　◆どろどろした便 muddy stools

トロポニン　troponin

トロンビン　thrombin　▶トロンビン・アンチトロンビン複合体 thrombin–antithrombin complex；TAT　トロンビン時間 thrombin time；TT

トロンボプラスチン　thromboplastin　◀活性化部分トロンボプラスチン時間 activated partial thromboplastin time；APTT　部分トロンボプラスチン時間 partial thromboplastin time；PTT

どんきしょう　呑気症　aerophagy, aerophagia

どんきそんしょう　鈍器損傷　blunt weapon injury

どんつう　鈍痛　dull pain, ache

どんてきがいしょう　鈍的外傷　blunt trauma[injury]

どんな　（健康状態はどうか）how　（どんな種類の）what kind of　（何の）what　（方法などが

どのように）how　（たとえどんなに…でも）no matter how, however
《どのような》◆どんな具合ですか How have you been feeling?　◆どんな症状がありますか What kind of symptoms do you have?　◆どんな痛みですか What's the pain like? / Can you describe the pain (for me)?　◆どんな治療を受けましたか How were you treated?　◆どんな運動をしていますか What kind of physical exercise do you do?
《どれ程に》◆これまでどんなにかおつらかったこととお察しいたします I can understand how rough[hard] it's been for you. / I can guess what a rough[hard] time you've been having.　◆どんなに運動を頑張っても食習慣を変えなければ体重は減りません No matter how[However] hard you exercise, you won't lose (any) weight without changing your eating habits.

トンネル　tunnel　◀疥癬トンネル cuniculus

とんぷくやく　頓服薬　medication to be taken only when necessary

どんま　鈍麻　decreased sensitivity to stimuli　◀感覚鈍麻 hypesthesia / hypoesthesia　感情鈍麻 apathy / lack of interest

な

な 名 ☞名前

ナーシングホーム nursing home, home for seniors[elderly people]

ナースコール (nurse call) bell, (nurse call) button ◆ナースコールはここ枕元にあります The nurse call bell is here by the pillow. ◆ご用のある時にはナースコールで呼んで下さい Please push[press] the button to call a nurse when you need any help.

ナースステーション nurses' station, nurses station

ない 無い ◆今週は時間がないので，来週来て下さい I don't have any time this week, so please come and see me next week. ◆もう再発の恐れはないでしょう I don't think there's any fear of the illness returning[recurring]. ◆入れ歯がないのですか Have you lost your dentures? / Are your dentures missing?

―ない ―内 (中)in (内部)inside (範囲内)within ◆診察室内での携帯電話の使用はご遠慮下さい Please refrain from using mobile phones in the consulting[consultation] room. ◆病院内はすべて禁煙です Smoking is not allowed anywhere inside the hospital. ◆期限内に出生届を出す register the birth of one's baby within a specified period of time ◆病院の敷地内で散歩して下さい Please take a walk on the hospital premises.

ナイアシン niacin ▶ナイアシン欠乏症 niacin deficiency

ないいん 内因 internal cause (顆internal 生体内の endogenous, endogenic 内部から生じた原因の intrinsic) ▶内因子 intrinsic factor；IF 内因性感染 endogenous infection 内因性精神病 endogenous psychosis 内因性喘息 intrinsic asthma

ないか 内科 (内科学)internal medicine (診療部門)the department of internal medi-

cine, the internal medicine department ☞診療(囲み：診療部門) ◀一般内科 general internal medicine ▶内科医 internist / physician 内科的治療 medical [nonsurgical] treatment 内科病棟 medical[internal medicine] ward[floor / unit]

ないけい 内径 inside diameter, internal diameter

ないけいじょうみゃく 内頸静脈 internal jugular vein；IJV

ないけいどうみゃく 内頸動脈 internal carotid artery；ICA

ないこう 内向(的な) introverted (↔extroverted) ◆内向的である be introverted / be an introvert ◆内向的な性格 an introverted personality

ないこてい 内固定 internal fixation

ないじ 内耳 inner ear, internal ear ◀人工内耳(蝸牛の)cochlear implant / artificial cochlea ▶内耳炎 internal otitis / inflammation of the inner[internal] ear / (迷路炎)labyrinthitis 内耳神経 vestibulocochlear nerve 内耳性難聴 inner ear *hearing loss[deafness] / (蝸牛性難聴)cochlear *hearing loss[deafness]

ナイジェリア Nigeria (顆Nigerian) ☞国籍 ▶ナイジェリア人(の) Nigerian

ないじかく 内痔核 internal hemorrhoids [piles] ★通例，複数形で。

ないしきょう 内視鏡 (内視鏡)endoscope /éndəskòup/ (顆endoscópic) (内視鏡検査) endoscopy /endάskəpi/, endoscópic examination ◆胃の内視鏡検査をします I'm going to do[run] an endoscopy of your stomach. ◆内視鏡検査当日は朝食を摂らず，水分の摂取も控えて下さい On the day of your endoscopy, please don't eat breakfast and refrain from drinking anything. ◆この病変は内視鏡で治療できます We can treat this lesion using an endoscope. ◀拡大内視鏡 magnifying endoscope カプセル内視鏡 capsule endoscope 蛍光内視鏡検査 fluorescence endoscopy 経鼻内視鏡検査 transnasal [pernasal] endoscopy 上部消化管内視

鏡検査 upper gastrointestinal[GI] endoscopy 大腸[結腸]内視鏡検査 colonoscopy 超音波内視鏡検査 endoscopic ultrasound[ultrasonography]；EUS 立体内視鏡 stereoscopic[three-dimensional] endoscope ▶内視鏡下胃瘻造設術 endoscopic gastrostomy 内視鏡下生検 endoscopic biopsy 内視鏡検査室 endoscopy room[unit] / endoscopic examination room 内視鏡手術 endoscopic surgery [surgical procedure] 内視鏡治療 endoscopic treatment 内視鏡的逆行性胆管ドレナージ endoscopic retrograde biliary drainage；ERBD 内視鏡的逆行性胆道膵管造影 endoscopic retrograde cholangiopancreatography；ERCP 内視鏡的硬化療法 endoscopic sclerotherapy 内視鏡的止血 endoscopic hemostasis 内視鏡的膵管ドレナージ endoscopic drainage of the pancreatic duct

ないしゃし 内斜視 internal strabismus [squint], convergent strabismus[squint], esotropia；ET （寄り目）crossed eyes ★通例，複数形で．

ないしゅっけつ 内出血 internal bleeding[hemorrhage] （青あざ）internal bruising （打撲傷）bruise /brúːz/ (複bruise) ☞出血 ◆胸腔で内出血を起こしている可能性があります You may have some bleeding[There may be internal bleeding] in your chest. ◆気がつかないうちに内出血していることがよくありますか Do you often get bruises that happen before you realize it? /（内出血しやすいか）Do you bruise easily?

ないしん 内診 （骨盤診察）pelvic exam [examination], internal exam[examination] （婦人科診察）gynecologic exam[examination] （腟内診）vaginal exam[examination] ◆内診をしましょう．この診察台に上がって横になって下さい I'm going to[Let me] do a pelvic exam. Please lie down on this exam table. ▶内診台 gynecologic exam table

ないせいしょくき 内生殖器 internal genitals[genitalia, genital organs] ★いずれも複数形で．

ないせん 内旋 internal rotation, medial rotation

ないぞう 内臓 internal organ(s), viscera (複viscus 形visceral) ▶内臓感覚 visceral sense[sensation] 内臓逆位 visceral inversion / heterotaxia 内臓損傷 visceral injury ☞内臓脂肪

ないぞうしぼう 内臓脂肪 visceral fat /vísərəl-/ （日常会話で）organ fat, abdominal fat, belly fat, hidden fat ◆内臓脂肪が増えています〈減っています〉Your visceral [organ] fat has increased〈decreased〉. / You have more〈less〉 organ[abdominal] fat than before. ◆内臓脂肪を減らしたほうがよいでしょう You should lose some visceral[belly] fat. ◆内臓脂肪がつく visceral fat builds up ▶内臓脂肪型肥満 visceral fat obesity

ないそく 内側(の) medial ☞内側（うちがわ）▶内側側副靱帯 medial collateral ligament；MCL / medial ligament of the knee 内側半月 medial meniscus 内側部 medial region[part] 内側面 medial surface

ないそけいヘルニア 内鼠径ヘルニア internal inguinal hernia

ないてき 内的(な) （内側の）inner （内部の）internal （本質的な）intrinsic ◆内的な葛藤がありますか Do you have any inner [（精神的な）mental] conflict? ▶内的要因 internal factor / （内因子）intrinsic factor 内的生活 one's inner life

ないてん 内転 adduction（↔abduction）▶内転筋 adductor muscle

ないどくそ 内毒素 endotoxin（↔exotoxin）

ないにょうどうこう 内尿道口 internal urethral orifice[opening]

ないはん 内反 （四肢の）varus （瞼・唇などの）entropion ◀眼瞼内反 lid entropion ▶内反位 varus position 内反膝 bowlegs / genu varum 内反足 clubfoot / talipes varus 内反肘 cubitus varus 内反母趾 hallux varus

ないひ 内皮 endothelium（形endothelial）

▶内皮細胞 endothelial cell

ナイフ **knife** ◆ナイフで刺すような痛み knife-like, stabbing pain / sharp, knife-like pain ◆ナイフで手首を切る cut[slit / slash] *one's* wrist with a knife ◀ガンマナイフ gamma knife

ないぶ **内部(の)** **internal** ▶内部照射 internal radiation

ないふく **内服** (経口投与)**oral administration** ◆ステロイドを内服する take an oral steroid (medication) ▶内服薬 oral medication

ないぶんぴつ **内分泌** **internal secretion** (内分泌腺・内分泌物)**endocrine** ◀神経内分泌腫瘍 neuroendocrine tumor 多発性内分泌腫瘍 multiple endocrine neoplasia；MEN ▶内分泌科 the department of endocrinology / the endocrinology department 内分泌科医 endocrinologist 内分泌学 endocrinology 内分泌攪乱(化学)物質 endocrine disruptor / endocrine disrupting chemical(s)；EDC 内分泌機能検査 endocrine function test 内分泌系 the endocrine system 内分泌腺 endocrine gland 内分泌臓器 endocrine organ 内分泌療法 endocrine[hormone / hormonal] therapy

ないヘルニア **内ヘルニア** **internal hernia**

ないまく **内膜** **inner membrane** (图内部の end(o)-) ◀頸動脈内膜切除術 carotid endarterectomy；CEA 子宮内膜 endometrium 心内膜 endocardium

ないめん **内面(の)** **inner** ☞内的

ないよう **内容** (中身)**contents** (詳細)**details** ★通例，複数形で. ◆入院準備に関する内容はこの冊子に書いてあります This booklet[brochure] gives details about how to prepare for your hospital stay. ◆お仕事の内容についてお話し下さい Please tell me about (what you do in) your job. / (仕事の責務) Please tell me about the duties and responsibilities of your work. ◆胃の内容物 stomach[gastric] contents

なおす¹ **治す** (病気・病人を)**cure** (图cure) (傷・怪我を)**heal** (修復する)**fix, repair, set**

☞治療 ◆この病気は治すことができます This disease *can be cured[is curable]. ◆残念ですが，この病気は完全に治すことはできません I'm sorry, but *there's no complete cure for this disease[this disease cannot be cured completely]. ◆この薬はすぐに胸痛を治してくれます This medication will cure your chest pain right away. ◆足の怪我を治す heal[cure] a leg injury ◆骨折を治す fix[repair / set] a broken[fractured] bone ◆虫歯を治す repair tooth decay

なおす² **直す** 《悪い習慣をやめる》(断ち切る)**break** (捨てる)**get rid of** (克服する)**get over, overcome** ◆爪を嚙む癖を直す break[get rid of] the habit of biting *one's* nails ◆偏食を直す *get over[overcome] *one's* food likes and dislikes
《整える》**straighten** ◆歯並びを直す straighten *a person's* teeth ◆患者のシーツを直す straighten the patient's sheets
《元の状態に戻す》**recover** ◆機嫌を直す recover *one's* good humor[mood] / be in a good mood again

―なおす **―直す** ◆治療計画を一部見直しましょう We need to modify[alter] part of the treatment plan. ◆この問題を考え直して下さい Please reconsider this question. / Please give this question further thought. ◆5分ほど安静にしてから血圧を測定し直しましょう Please rest for about five minutes, and after that let's take your blood pressure again.

なおり **治り** **recovery** (图recover) ◆怪我の治りが早かったですね You've made a quick[speedy] recovery from your injury. / You've quickly recovered from your injury. ◆治りが遅い make a slow recovery / recover slowly

なおる **治る** (病気・病人が)**be cured** (元の状態に回復する)**recover** (from) (病気などを克服する)**get over, overcome** (よくなる)**get well, get better** (傷・怪我が治る)**heal** ☞回復，全快 ◆肺炎はすっかり治っています Your pneumonia is completely cured. / You've completely *recovered from[gotten over] your pneumonia. ◆貧血は完全には治ってはいません You haven't recovered from your anemia completely. / Your anemia is not completely cured. ◆この風邪はすぐに治るでしょう You'll *get over[get rid of] this cold soon. ◆病気が治るには少なくとも3か月はかかるでしょう It will take at least three months before your illness is cured. ◆脚の怪我はうまく治ってきています Your leg is healing nicely. ◆この傷は自然に治るのを待つしかありません There's nothing for you to do but[There's nothing that can be done except to] let this wound heal by itself. ◆彼女は治る可能性があります(望み) There's some hope of her recovery. ◆残念ですが,(彼女が)治る可能性はほとんどありません I'm afraid there's not much hope that she'll recover. / I'm afraid the chance[possibility] of her recovering is rather small.

なか 中(に・で) in (中へ)into (内側・内部に[で])inside (範囲内に)within (図内部 the inside) ◆持ち物はこのかごの中に入れて下さい Please put your things in [into] this basket. ◆どうぞ中へお入り下さい Please come in. ◆耳の中を診察しましょう I'm going to examine the inside of your ear(s).

ながい 長い long ◆痛みは毎回どのくらい長く続きますか How long does the pain last each time? ◆長くはかかりません It won't take long. ◆残念ですが,彼はもう長くはないかもしれません I'm afraid that he won't last much longer. / I'm sorry, but he may not have long to live. ◆この薬は効き目が長く続きます This medication is long-acting.

ながいき 長生き long life, longevity ◆長生きの秘訣は毎日十分な睡眠とバランスのとれた食事をとることです The secret to living a *long life[longevity] is to get *plenty of[enough] sleep and to eat a balanced diet every day. ◆長生きする live a long life / live long ◆百歳まで長生きする live to be one hundred years (old)

ながく 長く ☞長い

ながつづき 長続きする keep up for long, last long ◆完璧にやろうとすると長続きしないものです If you want to do things perfectly, you won't be able to keep things up for long. / If you *aim for perfection[try to be perfect], your efforts won't last long.

なかなか ◆なかなか熱が引かないですね I'm afraid your fever just won't come down. ◆なかなか難しい問題です That problem cannot be answered easily. / That problem is harder than I expected.

ながびく 長引く (長期に及ぶ)prolong (いつまでも治癒しない)linger ◆ひどい風邪が長引いているのですか Does it take you a long time to get over a bad cold? ◆苦しみが長引く one's suffering is prolonged ◆長引く咳 a lingering[prolonged] cough

なかまちあいしつ 中待合室 inner waiting room ☞待合室

なかみ 中身 contents ★通例,複数形で. ☞内容

なかゆび 中指 (手)middle finger (足)middle toe ☞指

ながれ 流れ flow (動flow), stream ◆これは血の流れを良くする薬です This medication improves blood flow. / This is a medication for improving[facilitating smooth] blood flow. ◆右足の血液の流れが悪くなっています The blood in your right leg is not flowing smoothly[properly].

ながれる 流れる flow, run (こぼれ出る)spill (into, out) ◆血液が血管の中をスムーズに流れないと,凝固し始めます When blood does not flow smoothly through a blood vessel, it can begin to clot. ◆血管が破れて血液がくも膜下腔に流れ出ています The brain's blood vessel has ruptured[burst] and the blood is spilling into the subarachnoid space.

なく 泣く (声を出して泣く)cry (涙を流して泣く)weep (むせび泣く)sob ◆お子さんはいつもと違って激しく泣きますか Is your child crying more excessively than usual? / Is your baby's crying shriller or more urgent than usual? ◆ひっきりなしに泣く cry incessantly ◆かん高い声で泣く cry shrilly ◆慰めようもないほど泣く cry inconsolably

なぐさめる 慰める **comfort**（図**comfort**）, **console**（図**consolation**） ◆家族と話すことが彼女にとって大きな慰めになります Talking with her family gives her great comfort[consolation]. ◆彼女を慰めようがありません There is nothing I can do or say to console her. /（慰めの言葉がみつからない）I don't know what to say to comfort her.

なくす 無くす （失う）**lose** ☞失う

なくなる[1] 亡くなる **die**（図**death**） （婉曲的に）**pass away, go** （息を引き取る）**expire** ☞死, 死ぬ, 死亡 ◆お父さんが亡くなられた原因は何でしたか What did your father die of? / What was the cause of your father's death? ◆いつ亡くなられましたか When did he die? ◆大変残念ですがお母様は今朝早く亡くなられました I'm very sorry, but your mother passed away early this morning. ◆彼は午前4時45分に亡くなりました He *passed away at four forty-five am[in the morning]. ◆彼女は眠りながら安らかに亡くなりました She died[went] peacefully in her sleep.

なくなる[2] 無くなる （使い尽くす）**run out** （**of**） （消える）**go away, disappear** ◆薬がなくなる前においで下さい Please come and see me again before your medication runs out. ◆痛みはもうすぐなくなります The pain will disappear[go (away)] soon.

なぐる 殴る **beat** （こぶしで）**punch** ◆目をどうしましたか, 誰かに殴られたのですか What happened to your eye? Did someone beat[punch] you?

なげく 嘆く （悲しむ）**feel[be] sad** （**about**） （悲嘆に暮れる）**grieve** （**for, over**） （死を悼む）**mourn** ◆自分の境遇を嘆く feel sad about *one's* circumstances ◆夫の死を嘆く grieve for her husband / mourn

her husband's death ◆病気を嘆いてばかりいないで, 今後の治療について話し合いましょう It's time to stop grieving over your illness; instead, let's discuss your treatment plan from now on.

なげる 投げる **throw** ◆ボールを投げると肩〈ひじ〉が痛みますか Do you throw your shoulders〈elbows〉hurt when you throw a ball?

なぜ 何故 **why** （どんなことが）**what** ◆今日はなぜ受診されたのですか What's brought you here today? / Why did you come to see me today? ◆なぜそう思われるのですか Why do you think so[that way]? / What makes you think so? ◆なぜそんなに腹を立てているのですか Why are you so upset? / What's making you so upset?

なつかしむ 懐かしむ **miss** ◆郷里の友人やご家族のことが懐かしいですか Do you miss your friends and family back home?

なつかぜ 夏風邪 **summer cold, summer minor illness** ☞風邪

ナッツ **nut** ◆ナッツにアレルギーがある be allergic to nuts ▶ナッツ過敏症 nut hypersensitivity

なっとく 納得する （満足する）**be satisfied** （**with**）（図**satisfaction** 圐**satisfying**） （確信する）**be convinced** （**of**）（圐**convincing**） （了解する）**understand** （図**understanding**） ◆私の説明で納得していただけましたか Are you satisfied with my explanation? / Have I explained this to your satisfaction? ◆納得のいく説明をする give a convincing[satisfying] explanation

なつばて 夏ばて **summer heat exhaustion** ◆夏ばて気味ですか Are you exhausted from the summer heat? / Is the summer heat telling on you?

なでがた 撫で肩 **sloping shoulders, round shoulders**

ナトリウム **sodium** ◀次亜塩素酸ナトリウム sodium hypochlorite 炭酸水素ナトリウム sodium bicarbonate 低ナトリウム血症 hyponatremia ☞ナトリウム利尿ペプチド

ナトリウムりにょうペプチド ―利尿ペプ

チド natriuretic peptide ◀心房性ナトリウム利尿ペプチド atrial natriuretic peptide；ANP　脳ナトリウム利尿ペプチド brain natriuretic peptide；BNP

ななめ　斜め(の)　（対角面・対角線）diagonal（圓diagonally）（斜角・斜線）oblique　◆右斜め上 diagonally to the upper right　◆身体が斜めに傾きますか Does any part of your body lean to one side?

なに　何　what　◆何が心配なのですか What's worrying[bothering] you? / What kind of concerns do you have?　◆私に何ができるか考えますね Let me see what I can do.　☞何か，何も，何(なん)

なにか　何か　（肯定文で）some, something　★相手からの Yes という返事を期待する時には疑問文にも用いる．（疑問文・否定文で）any, anything　◆何かご質問はありますか Do you have any questions?　◆体の調子が何かおかしいと感じることはありますか Do you ever feel *that something's not quite right in your body?[something is wrong with you]?　◆何かご不明な点がありましたらいつでもスタッフにお尋ね下さい If you have anything you're unsure about, please ask the staff anytime.　◆何か困ったことがありますか Is anything wrong? / Do you have trouble of any kind?　◆何かあったらすぐ連絡して下さい If anything happens, please contact us immediately.　◆何かご用でしょうか What can I do for you?

なにも　何も　not anything, nothing　◆検査当日は何も口にしないで下さい Please don't eat or drink anything on the day of your examination.　◆検査で何も異常は見つかりませんでした The tests didn't show[find] anything wrong. / The tests showed (that there is) nothing wrong with you.

なにようび　☞何曜日(なんようび)

ナノグラム　nanogram；ng

ナノテクノロジー　nanotechnology

ナプキン　（生理用品）sanitary pad[napkin]

なふだ　名札　☞ネームバンド

なま　生(の)　（加熱していない）raw　（未調理

の）uncooked　（新鮮な）fresh　（菌などが生きている）live /láɪv/　◆食べた魚は生か半生でしたか Did you eat raw or half-cooked fish?　◆生ものを食べるのを控えて下さい Avoid eating uncooked food.　▶生傷 fresh wound　生野菜 raw[fresh] vegetables　☞生ワクチン

なまえ　名前　name　◆お名前をいただけますか What's your name, please? / May I have your name?　★いずれも上昇口調で．　◆お名前を確認させて下さい Let me just confirm your name.　◆お名前はどう綴るのですか How do you spell your name?　◆名前と住所は活字体でお書き下さい Please write your name and address in block letters. / Please print your name and address.　◆お名前をお呼びするまでここでお待ち下さい Please wait here until *we call your name[your name is called].　◆持ち物にはすべて名前を付けて下さい Please put your name on all your belongings.

名前の確認と敬称

■名前の確認

●外国人の名前は発音が難しいので，最初にきちんと確認する必要がある．

発音を確認したい時には，"How do you pronounce your name?" "Could you tell me how to pronounce your name?"（お名前はどう発音するのですか）などと訊く．

●日本語では名前を「姓・名」の順序で並べるが，他の言語では国や文化によって異なる．一般的に，英語圏では日本とは逆に「名・姓」の順に並べる．中国・韓国・ハンガリー人の姓名は，日本人と同じく「姓・名」の順で記載するが，国外に出た場合には「名・姓」にすることが多い（韓国系アメリカ人など）．

姓名の区別を確認したい時には，"Please give your full name and write your *family name[surname] in capital letters."（お名前はフルネームで，姓をすべて大文字で書いて下さい）と頼むとよい．

■**名前につける敬称**
●大人の患者の場合は，相手がファーストネームで呼んでほしいと言わない限り，Mr, Mrs, Ms, Miss, Dr, Prof を付けて姓で話しかける．★最近，Mr や Dr のように敬称にピリオドを付けない人が増えている．
●再診の時，ファーストネームで呼びかけたほうが親しみがわくと判断した時には，"May I call you Peter?"などと訊いてからにする．

なまきず 生傷 （一般的に）fresh wound （切り傷）fresh cut （打撲傷）fresh bruise ☞傷

なまもの 生もの ☞生

なまり 鉛 lead /léd/ ◆この鉛入りのエプロンは放射線の被曝を防いでくれます This lead apron will shield you from exposure to the radiation. ▶鉛中毒 lead poisoning / plumbism

なまワクチン 生ワクチン live vaccine / láiv væksíːn/ ◀弱毒性生ワクチン attenuated live vaccine

なみだ 涙 tears ★通例，複数形で．(圖 tear) ◆涙が出る tears flow / the eyes water[tear] ◆涙がたくさん出ますか Do your eyes tear easily? / Do your eyes water a lot? ◆涙が出にくいと感じますか Do you feel that your tears don't flow easily[smoothly]? / Do you feel that your eyes don't produce tears easily? ◆涙が少ないですか Do your eyes produce only a small amount of tears? / Do your eyes not make many tears? ◆涙が止まらなかったことがありますか Have you ever had excess tearing? ◆涙が湧き出る(たまる)the eyes well up with tears / tear up ◆涙もろい feel tearful ◆涙でうるんだ目 watery eyes / eyes filled with tears / teary eyes

なめらかな （すべすべした）smooth （柔らかい）soft （きめの細かい）fine （油を塗ったような）lubricating ◆ゆでた野菜をミキサーにかけてなめらかにすると食べやすくなります Boiled vegetables are easier to eat if you mix them in a blender until smooth [soft]. ◆なめらかな肌 smooth[fine] skin

なめる （しゃぶる）suck on （ぺろぺろなめる）lick ◆この薬用ドロップは嚙まないでなめて下さい Just suck on this lozenge; don't chew it. ◆唇をなめる lick one's lips

なやみ 悩み （心配）worry （圖 be worried about） （困ること）trouble （問題）problem ☞心配, 悩み, 不安 ◆悩み事がある時には相談に来て下さい If you're ever worried about anything, please come to talk to me. ◆悩み事を医療ソーシャルワーカーに相談する consult a medical social worker about one's troubles ◆深刻な悩みを持つ have a serious worry[problem] / be deeply worried

なやむ 悩む （心配する）worry, be worried about, have worries （困る）trouble ☞心配, 悩み, 不安 ◆何を悩んでいるのですか What are you worried about? / What's worrying[troubling] you? ◆もし何か悩むようなことがあれば，遠慮なく相談して下さい If you have *any worries[anything you're worried about], don't hesitate to *talk it over[consult] with me. ◆手術を受けるか受けないかで悩んでいらっしゃるのですね You're worried about whether to have the surgery or not, aren't you?

ならす 鳴らす （ベルを）ring ◆呼び出しベルを鳴らして呼んで下さい Please ring (the call bell) for us.

ならぶ 並ぶ stand in line （列を作って待つ）wait in line ◆そちらに並んでお待ち下さい Please wait there in line.

ナルコレプシー narcolepsy

なるべく ☞できるだけ

なれる 慣れる （当たり前になる）get used [accustomed] (to), become used[accustomed] (to) （順応する）adjust (to) ◆じきに減塩食に慣れるでしょう You'll soon get[become] used to a low-salt diet. ◆体が薬に慣れるにつれて副作用は取れるでしょう The side effects will go away as your body adjusts to the medication. ◆日本の生活に慣れる get used to living in

Japan / adjust to life in Japan

なん 何 **what** ◆今，何とおっしゃいましたか(I beg your) pardon? / Sorry? / What did you say just now? ◆わからないことは何なりとお訊き下さい ★いずれも上昇口調で. If there's anything you don't understand, please feel free to ask. ◆彼女が完治するかどうかは何とも言えません I can't say *anything definite about[for sure] whether she'll make a complete recovery. ◆前に何という病気で治療を受けたのですか What were you treated for before? ☞何(なに)，何か，何も，何回，何階，何歳，何時，何でも，何度，何日，何人，何年，何番，何曜日

なんエックスせん 軟X線 **soft X-ray** ▶軟X線撮影 soft X-ray radiography

なんか 軟化 **softening, malacia** ◀骨軟化症 osteomalacia 膝蓋軟骨軟化症 chondromalacia patellae 便軟化剤 stool softener

なんかい¹ 何回
《どのくらいの回数》**how many times, how often** ◆夜何回トイレに起きますか How many times do you wake up to urinate at night? ◆日本へ来たのはこれで何回目ですか How many times have you come to Japan so far?
《何回も》(たびたび) **many times** (数回) **several times** ☞再三 ◆何回も吐く vomit many times ◆何回も彼女にお電話したのですがつながりませんでした I called[phoned] her several[many] times, but I couldn't get through to her.

なんかい² 何階 **what floor** ◆何階に住んでいますか What floor do you live on?

なんぎ 難儀 **difficulty** ☞困る，困難，難しい

なんご 喃語 **babble, baby's babbling** ◆喃語を話す babble

なんこう 軟膏 **ointment** ◆傷口にこの軟膏を直接塗って下さい Please apply this ointment directly to the cut. / Please put this ointment directly on the cut. ◆この軟膏は薄く伸ばして傷によくすり込んで下さい Please apply a thin layer of this

ointment to the wound and rub it in well. ◆抗菌薬の軟膏 an antibiotic ointment ◆眼軟膏 eye[ophthalmic] ointment 吸水軟膏 water-absorbing ointment 親水軟膏 hydrophilic ointment 水溶性軟膏 water-soluble ointment ステロイド軟膏 steroid ointment 油脂性軟膏 grease / oleaginous ointment

なんこうがい 軟口蓋 **soft palate** (略式soft palatal) ▶軟口蓋裂 cleft of the soft palate / soft palatal cleft

なんこつ 軟骨 **cartilage** (連結形chondr (o)-) ◆膝の軟骨が加齢で擦り減ってきています The knee cartilage is thinning [wearing thin / (劣化している) deteriorating] with age. ◀耳介軟骨 auricular cartilage 鼻翼軟骨 alar cartilage 輪状軟骨 cricoid cartilage 肋軟骨 costal cartilage ▶軟骨炎 chondritis 軟骨腫 chondroma 軟骨腫症 chondromatosis 軟骨肉腫 chondrosarcoma

なんさい 何歳 **how old** ★大人に "How old are you?" と年齢を訊くのは失礼なことがあるので注意. ◆あなたは今何歳ですか May I ask your age? / (子供の患者に) How old are you? ◆お子さんは今何歳ですか How old is your child? ◆最初の月経があったのは何歳の時でしたか How old were you when you had your first period? ◆お父さんは亡くなられた時何歳でしたか How old was your father when he died?

なんざん 難産 **difficult labor, hard labor** ◆赤ちゃんが大きくて骨盤が狭いことによる難産 a difficult labor due to a large baby and a narrow[small] pelvis

なんじ 何時 **what time** ◆すみません，今何時ですか Excuse me. Do you have the time? / Excuse me. Could you tell me what time it is? ◆いつも朝は何時に起きますか What time do you usually get up in the morning? ◆何時がご都合がいいですか What time is good for you?

なんしょく 軟食 **soft diet**

なんせいげかん 軟性下疳 **soft sore[ulcer, chancre], chancroid**

なんちせい 難治性(の) (治癒の難しい) intractable (不応性の)refractory (根深く執拗な)obstinate (薬物抵抗性の)pharmacoresistant ▶難治性潰瘍 intractable ulcer 難治性下痢intractable diarrhea 難治性喘息 intractable asthma 難治性てんかん intractable[refractory / pharmacoresistant] epilepsy 難治性疼痛 intractable pain

なんちょう 難聴 (聴力消失)hearing loss, deafness (聴力障害) hearing impairment ◆難聴がある have difficulty hearing / be hard of hearing ◆加齢による難聴と思われます I suspect you have *age-related hearing loss[hearing loss that comes with age]. ◀遺伝性難聴 hereditary *hearing loss[deafness] 感音(性)難聴 sensorineural hearing loss 高音(域)障害型難聴 high-frequency[high-tone] hearing loss 職業性難聴 occupational hearing loss 心因性難聴 psychogenic hearing loss ストレプトマイシン難聴 streptomycin(-induced) hearing loss 先天性難聴 congenital hearing loss 騒音性難聴 noise-induced hearing loss 低音(域)障害型難聴 low-frequency[low-tone] hearing loss 伝音(性)難聴 conductive hearing loss 突発難聴 sudden hearing loss；SHL / sudden deafness 内耳性難聴 inner ear hearing loss / (蝸牛性難聴) cochlear hearing loss 片側性難聴 single-sided[unilateral] hearing loss 両側性難聴 bilateral hearing loss

なんでも 何でも (どれでも)any, anything (すべて)whatever ◆お酒以外なら何でも好きな物を召し上がってもいいですよ You can eat or drink anything[whatever] you like other than alcohol.

なんど 何度 《温度》◆今朝，熱は何度ありましたか What[How high] was your temperature this morning? 《回数》how many times, how often ☞何回

なんにち 何日 《日付》what day ◆きょうは何日ですか What's today's date? / What's the date

today? 《どのくらいの日数》how many days ◆熱は何日続いたのですか How many days did the fever last[go on for]?

なんにん 何人 how many *people* ◆ご家族は何人ですか How many people are there in your family? ◆ごきょうだいは何人ですか How many brothers and sisters do you have?

なんねん 何年 《西暦》what year ◆今年は何年ですか What year is this? ◆あなたは何年生まれですか In what year were you born? 《どのくらいの年数》how long, how many years ◆日本には何年住んでいますか How long[How many years] have you lived in Japan?

なんばん 何番 what number ◆携帯電話は何番ですか What's your mobile phone number?

なんびょう 難病 (治癒が難しい病)intractable disease (重病)serious disease (不治の病)incurable disease ◆この病気は難病に指定されていますので，医療費の助成が受けられます This disease is designated as an intractable disease, so its treatment is subsidized. ◀指定難病 designated intratable disease

なんぶそしき 軟部組織 soft tissue ▶軟部組織感染(症) soft tissue infection 軟部組織腫瘍 soft tissue tumor

なんべん 軟便 (軟らかい便)soft stool (ゆるい便)loose stool (ゆるい便通)loose bowel movement ☞便

なんまく 軟膜 pia mater

なんようび 何曜日 what day of the week ◆今日は何曜日ですか What day of the week is it today? ◆何曜日がご都合がいいですか What day of the week would be convenient for you?

に

ニーズ **needs** ★通例，複数形で．　◆日常生活のニーズの世話をする take care of *a person's* daily needs　◆患者のニーズに応える meet[satisfy / address] a patient's needs

におい 匂い・臭い **smell**　（嫌なにおい）**odor** /óʊdər/　◆においがわからないのですか Have you lost your sense of smell?　◆妊娠中においを強く感じることはよくあることです It's not unusual to *have a heightened sense of smell[（においに敏感になる）become sensitive to smells] during pregnancy.　◆傷口から嫌なにおいの分泌物が出ていますか Is the wound producing a foul-smelling[bad-smelling] discharge?　◆不快なにおいがする have an offensive[unpleasant] smell / smell bad　◆腐ったにおいがする be foul-smelling / have a foul odor[smell]　◆酸っぱいにおいがする be sour-smelling / smell acidic / have an acidic smell　◆においの感覚が鋭い have *a keen[an acute] sense of smell　◆かびくさいにおい a musty smell[odor]　◆便のにおい a fecal odor

におう 臭う・匂う **smell**　◆口がにおうのですか Does your breath smell? / Do you have bad breath?　◆おりものはにおいますか Does the discharge have any odor?

にがい 苦い **bitter**　◆この薬は少し苦いかもしれません This medication may have a slightly bitter taste. / This medication may taste slightly bitter.

にがす 逃がす **miss**　☞逃す（のがす）

にがた 2型・Ⅱ型 **type 2, type Ⅱ**　▶2型糖尿病 type 2 diabetes (mellitus)

にがつ 2月 **February**；**Feb.**　☞1月

にがみ 苦味 **bitter taste, bitterness**

にき 2期 （第2の段階）**second stage** （2つの期間・時期）**two periods[terms]**　☞期

にきび **pimple** （痤瘡）**acne** /ǽkni/　★acne は数えられない名詞．　◆額ににきびができる develop pimples[acne] on *one's* forehead　◆にきびをつぶさないで下さい Please don't pop or squeeze your pimples.　◆にきびが消える the acne clears up　▶にきび痕 acne spot[pit]

にぎる 握る （こぶしを握る）**make a fist** （つかむ）**grasp, grip** （ぎゅっと握る）**squeeze**　◆（採血時など）こぶしを握って下さい Please make a fist.　◆私の手をしっかり握って下さい Please grasp[grip] my hand firmly.　◆私の指をぎゅっと強く握って下さい Please squeeze my finger(s) hard.

にく 肉 **meat**　◆（宗教的な理由で）豚や牛の肉を召し上がらない時には病院スタッフにお知らせ下さい If you don't eat pork or beef (for religious reasons), please inform the hospital staff.　◆脂の多い肉は避けて下さい You should avoid fatty meats.　◆肉を減らす *eat less[cut down on] meat　◀牛肉 beef　魚肉 fish　子牛肉 veal　鶏肉 chicken　鳥肉 poultry　豚肉 pork　羊肉 mutton　▶肉料理 meat dish

—にくい　◆治りにくい疾患 a hard-to-treat disease / （しつこい病）a stubborn disease / （不治の病）an incurable disease　◆答えにくいこともお訊きするかと思いますが治療に必要なことなので，ご理解下さい I know these questions may be difficult to answer, but I need to ask them to decide on your treatment plan. I hope you understand.

にくがん 肉眼 （略gross, macroscopic）　◆細菌は小さすぎて肉眼で見ることはできません Bacteria are too small to be seen with the naked eye.　▶肉眼的観察 gross[macroscopic] observation / macroscopy　肉眼的血尿 gross[macroscopic] hematuria / macrohematuria

にくげ 肉芽（形成） **granulation**　◆病的肉芽 abnormal granulation　☞肉芽腫

にくげしゅ 肉芽腫 **granuloma**　◀環状肉芽腫 granuloma annulare　菌状肉芽腫 granuloma fungoides

にくしゅ 肉腫 **sarcoma**　◀横紋筋肉腫

rhabdomyosarcoma　滑膜肉腫 synovial sarcoma　カポジ肉腫 Kaposi sarcoma；KS　癌肉腫 carcinosarcoma　骨肉腫 osteosarcoma　線維肉腫 fibrosarcoma　軟骨肉腫 chondrosarcoma　平滑筋肉腫 leiomyosarcoma　ユーイング肉腫 Ewing sarcoma

にくしん　肉親　(血縁の)blood relative[relation]　(直近の)immediate family　◆肉親の方ですか Are you related by blood?

にくたい　肉体(的な)　(身体の)bodily, physical　(肉体労働の)manual　☞体, 身体(しんたい)　▶肉体関係 sexual relationship[relations]　肉体労働 physical[manual] labor / physical[manual] work

にくばなれ　肉離れ　muscle strain, torn muscle, pulled muscle　◆大腿部に肉離れを起こす have *a torn muscle[muscle strain] in one's thigh

ニコチン　nicotine /níkətìːn/ (㊋nicotínic)　◆ニコチン中毒になっている be addicted to nicotine / be a nicotine addict　▶ニコチン依存 nicotine dependence　ニコチンガム〈パッチ〉nicotine gum〈patch〉　ニコチン拮抗薬 nicotinic antagonist　ニコチン作動薬 nicotinic agonist　ニコチン中毒(依存症者)nicotine addict / (状態)nicotine poisoning[addiction]　ニコチン離脱症状 nicotine withdrawal symptom(s)

ニコチンさん　―酸　nicotinic acid　☞ナイアシン

にごる　濁る　get[become, be] cloudy, get[become, be] turbid　◆水晶体が濁っています The lens has become cloudy.　◆尿が濁る have cloudy[turbid] urine

にさんか　二酸化(物)　dioxide　▶二酸化炭素 carbon dioxide　二酸化窒素 nitrogen dioxide　二酸化硫黄 sulfur dioxide

にじ¹　二次(の)　(二次性の・続発性の)secondary　(順番が二番目の)(the) second　(一次より先進的な)advanced　▶二次医療 secondary medical[health] care　二次感染 secondary infection　二次救急 secondary emergency care　二次救命処置 advanced cardiac[cardiovascular] life support；ACLS　二次性徴 secondary sex

characteristic(s)　二次予防 secondary prevention

にじ²　虹　rainbow　◆電灯の周囲に虹のような輪が見えますか Do you see rainbow-like[rainbow-colored] halos around lights?

にしきかく　2色覚　dichromatism, color blindness　☞色覚

にしブロック　二枝ブロック　bifascicular block

にじみでる　滲み出る　ooze /úːz/　◆傷口から血が滲み出ている Blood is oozing from[out of] the cut.

にじむ　滲む　(染みになって)be stained (with)　(少し色がついて)be tinged (with)　(筋になって)be streaked (with)　◆包帯に血がにじんでいます The bandage is stained with blood.　◆血がにじんでいる分泌物 blood-tinged discharge　◆血がにじんでいる痰 blood-streaked[blood-stained] phlegm

にじゅう　二重(の)　(2倍の量・数の)double (㊋圖double)　(2つの部分の)dual　(遠近両用の)bifocal　◆物が二重に見えますか Are you having any double vision? / Are you seeing double?　▶二重焦点眼鏡 bifocal glasses　二重焦点レンズ bifocal lens　二重人格 dual[double] personality　二重盲検法 double-blind test

21 トリソミー　trisomy 21[twenty-one]　☞ダウン症候群

24 じかん　24時間　24[twenty-four] hours　★インフォーマルに, 24時間, 週7日, 年がら年じゅうという意味で 24 / 7[twenty-four seven]ともいう.　◆24時間は運転をしないで下さい Please don't drive for twenty-four hours.　◆彼女には24時間体制のケアが必要です She needs *twenty-four-hour[around-the-clock / 〈英〉round-the-clock] care.　◆24時間の看護を必要とする require twenty-four-hour nursing care　▶24時間心電図検査 24-hour EKG　24時間尿 24-hour urine

にしゅこんごうワクチン　二種混合ワクチン[ジフテリア・破傷風ワクチン]　diphtheria and tetanus vaccine, DT vaccine

にせんべん 二尖弁 bicuspid valve（僧帽弁）mitral valve ☞僧帽弁

にそう 二相（性の）biphasic

にそくブロック 二束ブロック bifascicular block

にだんみゃく 二段脈 coupled pulse, bigeminal pulse, bigeminy

にち 日 day ☞何日

にちじ 日時 the time and date ◆手術の日時は後でお知らせします I'll let you know[You'll be notified of] the time and date of your surgery later. ◆予約の日時を変更していただくことは可能ですか Would it be possible to change the date of your appointment?

にちじょう 日常（の）（日々の）daily（毎日の）everyday（決まった手順で行う）routine ◆日本語は日常会話なら話しますか Do you speak everyday Japanese? / Do you speak conversational-level Japanese? ◆日常的な作業を行う perform everyday tasks ◆日常的な手術 routine surgery ☞日常生活

にちじょうせいかつ 日常生活 daily life, everyday life ☞生活 ◆不眠で日常生活に支障をきたしていますか Does your insomnia affect your daily[everyday] life? ◆日常生活ができますか Can you cope with everyday matters? ◆日常生活のニーズを満たす meet[satisfy / address] one's daily needs ☞日常生活動作

にちじょうせいかつどうさ 日常生活動作 activities of daily living；ADL（s）◆日常生活動作を維持する maintain one's ADL ◀手段的日常生活動作 instrumental ADL ▶日常生活関連動作 activities parallel to daily living；APDL 日常生活動作訓練 ADL training 日常生活動作テスト ADL test 日常生活動作能力 ability to perform ADL

にちないへんどう 日内変動（24時間変動）daily[diurnal] variation（検査値における精度）within-day[daily, intraday] precision（病状の変動）daily[intraday] fluctuation

にちようび 日曜日 Sunday；Sun. ◆日曜日に on Sunday ◆日曜日ごとに on Sundays

にっか 日課 daily routine[tasks]（日常の雑事）（daily）chores ★taskとchoreは通例, 複数形で. ☞生活 ◆何か日課にしていることはありますか Are there any tasks you do daily[routinely]?

にっきん 日勤（昼間の勤務）day duty（交替制勤務）day shift（一般的に昼間の仕事）day work, daytime work

にっけい 日系 ◆日系アメリカ人 a Japanese American ◆カナダの日系3世 a third-generation Japanese Canadian

にっこう 日光 sunlight, sunshine（太陽の solar）◆強い直射日光に当たる be exposed to strong direct sunlight ◆ぎらぎらする日光は目に良くありません Glaring sunlight is *not good[harmful] for the eyes. ◀直射日光 direct sunlight ▶日光過敏症 photosensitivity 日光蕁麻疹 solar urticaria 日光皮膚炎 solar dermatitis /（日焼け）sunburn ☞日光浴

にっこうよく 日光浴 sunbath（sunbathe /sʌ́nbèɪð/）, sunbathing（外気浴）air-bathing, air bath ◆日光浴は, 日焼け止めクリームをたっぷり塗って時間を限ってして下さい When you sunbathe[sit in the sun], use lots of sunscreen and don't spend[stay] too long in the sun.

にっさへんどう 日差変動（検査値における精度）between-day[day-to-day, inter-day] precision（病状の変動）day-to-day[interday] fluctuation

にっしゃびょう 日射病 sunstroke ☞熱中症 ◆日射病になる get[have] sunstroke

にっすう 日数 days（長さ・期間）length ◆日本にはどのくらいの日数滞在しますか How long[How many days] are you going to stay in Japan? ◀在院日数 the length of one's hospital stay

にっちゅう 日中 during the day, in the daytime（日中の間ずっと）throughout the day ◆日中に眠気を感じますか Do you feel sleepy or drowsy during the day? ▶日中傾眠 daytime drowsiness

にっちょく　日直　day duty ◆今日は山田先生が日直です Dr Yamada is on day duty today.

にってい　日程　☞スケジュール

にっぽん　日本　☞日本(にほん)

にている　似ている　☞似る

にてんほこう　二点歩行　two-point gait

にど¹　2度・Ⅱ度　(the) second degree ▶2度房室ブロック second-degree atrioventricular[AV] block

にど²　二度　(2回)twice, two times (再び)again

ニトログリセリン　nitroglycerin /nàɪtrəglísrɪn/　(インフォーマルに)nitro ◆胸の痛みを感じたらこのニトログリセリンを服用して下さい Please take this nitroglycerin[nitro] whenever you have chest pain.

にばい　2倍　(倍増する)double (▥twice, two times)　◆薬の量を2倍に増やしましょう I'm going to double your dose. ◆特別室は通常個室の2倍の広さです Special rooms are *twice the size of [twice as large as] regular private rooms. ◆この手術は通常の2倍の時間がかかるでしょう This surgery will take twice as long as usual.

にぶい　鈍い 《はっきりしない》dull ◆胸に鈍い痛みがある have[feel] a dull pain in *one's* chest 《動きがのろい》slow ◆動作が鈍い be slow in *one's* movement / *one's* movement is slow / move slowly

にぶる　鈍る　(感覚がはっきりしなくなる)get [become, be] dull　(能力が低下する)decline ◆嗅覚〈触覚〉が鈍っていますか Has your sense of smell〈touch〉become dull [less sharp]? / Has your sense of smell 〈touch〉lost some of its sharpness? ◆彼は記憶力が鈍っています His memory has declined.

にぶんせきつい　二分脊椎　spina bifida

ニボーぞう　―像　niveau (気液界面)air-fluid level

にほん　日本　Japan ◆日本にはいつ来ましたか When did you come to Japan? ◆日本に住んでどのくらいになりますか How long have you lived in Japan? ◆日本に来る前はどこに住んでいましたか Where were you living before you came to Japan? ◆これから日本にどのくらい滞在しますか How long are you going to stay in Japan? ◆日本の生活に慣れましたか Have you become[got] used to living [life] in Japan? / Have you adjusted to life in Japan? ◆日本の印象はいかがですか How do you like Japan? / What are your impressions of Japan? ☞日本語, 日本食, 日本脳炎

にほんご　日本語　Japanese (単語)Japanese word　◆日本語を話せますか Do you speak some Japanese? ◆日本語の読み書きはできますか Do you read and write Japanese? / Are you able to read and write Japanese? ◆お知り合いに誰か日本語を話せる人がいますか Do you know anyone who can speak Japanese?

にほんしょく　日本食　Japanese dish [food]

にほんのうえん　日本脳炎　Japanese encephalitis ▶日本脳炎ワクチン Japanese encephalitis vaccine

にゅう　乳　milk　☞乳(ちち), ミルク ◀移行乳 transitional milk　溢乳 regurgitation of milk　初乳 colostrum / foremilk　成熟乳 mature milk　全乳 whole milk /《英》full-fat milk　脱脂乳 skim[one-percent] milk /《英》skimmed milk　断乳 breast-feeding cessation　調合乳 formula (milk)　低脂肪乳 low-fat milk / two-percent milk /《英》semi-skimmed milk　濃縮乳 concentrated milk

にゅういん　入院　hospitalization, hospital admission (滞在)hospital stay　◆虫垂炎で入院する be hospitalized[admitted to the hospital] for[with] appendicitis ◆検査入院する*be hospitalized[go into the hospital] for a checkup[medical examination]　★入退院を表す場合,《米》では hospital に the を付けるが,《英》では通例 go into hospital のように the は省かれる. ◆入院の申し込みをする apply for admission to the hospital ◆入院時に *at the time of [upon] admission ◆入院中に during *one's* stay in the hospital / while *one* is in the hospital ◆入院中ずっと throughout [at all times during] *one's* hospital stay ◆入院中に死亡する die in the hospital

《入院歴》◆入院したことがありますか Have you ever been hospitalized[admitted to the hospital] before? ◆入院の理由は何でしたか Why were you hospitalized? / What were you hospitalized for? ◆いつどこで入院したのですか When and where were you hospitalized? ◆日本で入院したのは初めてですか Is this the first time you've been hospitalized in Japan?

《入院の指示》◆2, 3日入院していただきます I'd like you to stay in the hospital for a few days. ◆この検査をするにはひと晩の入院が必要です This test requires *an overnight hospital stay[overnight hospitalization]. ◆2週間ほどの入院が必要です You need to be hospitalized[admitted to the hospital] for about two weeks. / You have to stay in the hospital for about two weeks. ◆今すぐ入院する必要があります You need to be *admitted to the hospital[hospitalized] immediately[right away]. ◆受付で入院手続きをして下さい Please go through the admission[admitting] procedures at the admissions counter[office]. ◆入院の必要はありません You don't need to be hospitalized. / Your illness doesn't require hospitalization.

《入院時の説明》◆入院のことで何かご質問がありましたら, 入院受付でお尋ね下さい If you have any questions about your admission, please ask at the admissions counter[office]. ◆入院の際にはアクセサリー, お金(小銭を除いて), その他の貴重品は自宅に置いてきて下さい Please leave jewelry, money (other than small change), and other valuables at home before admission to the hospital. ◆入院中は常時このリストバンドをはめていて下さい You must wear this wristband[identi-

fication bracelet] throughout[at all times during] your hospital stay.

◀一泊入院 overnight hospitalization [stay in the hospital] 教育入院 educational hospitalization 緊急入院 emergency admission[hospitalization] / urgent admission[hospitalization] 検査入院 hospitalization for a checkup[medical examination] 再入院 readmission (to the hospital) / rehospitalization 措置〈任意〉入院 involuntary〈voluntary〉hospitalization 短期〈長期〉入院 short-term〈long-term〉hospitalization 短期〈長期〉入院患者 short-stay〈long-stay〉patient 保護入院 hospitalization for (medical) care and protection ▶入院案内 admission information 入院受付 admissions counter[desk] / (事務室) admissions office 入院患者 inpatient 入院関連機能障害 hospitalization-associated disability 入院時オリエンテーション preadmission (patient) orientation 入院生活 life in the hospital / hospital life 入院誓約書 consent form for (hospital) admission / hospital admission consent form 入院説明書 (hospital) admissions brochure[booklet / leaflet] / brochure[booklet / leaflet] on admission 入院費(料金) hospital expenses[charges / fees] / (請求書)hospital bill 入院保証金 deposit upon admission 入院申込書 (hospital / patient) admission form / application form for admission to the hospital ☞入院期間

にゅういんきかん **入院期間** length of hospital stay ◆以前の入院期間はどのくらいでしたか How long *were you[did you stay] in the hospital before? ◆入院期間はほぼ3日になるでしょう You'll have to be in the hospital for about three days. ◆入院期間を延長〈短縮〉する extend〈shorten〉*one's* hospital stay

にゅうか **乳化** emulsification (動emulsify) ▶乳化剤 emulsifying agent

にゅうかん **乳管** lactiferous duct, mammary duct, milk duct

にゅうがん **乳がん** breast cancer ◆ご

家族に乳がんの人がいますか Has anyone in your immediate family had breast cancer? ◆市では40歳以上の女性に乳がんの無料健診を行っています The city offers free breast cancer screening for women aged forty years and over. ◀非触知乳がん nonpalpable[impalpable] breast cancer ▶乳がん検診 breast cancer screening[checkup] / breast check-up 乳がん専門医 breast cancer specialist

にゅうきょしゃ　入居者　resident

にゅうこく　入国する　enter (a country) (図entrance[entrance] into a country) ◀再入国 reentry　再入国許可証 reentry permit　不法入国 illegal entry　密入国者 illegal entrant /（不法移民）illegal immigrant ▶入国管理局 The Immigration Bureau　入国許可証 entry permit　入国ビザ entry visa

にゅうざい　乳剤 （乳濁液）**emulsion** （クリーム）**cream**

にゅうさん　乳酸　lactic acid ▶乳酸アシドーシス lactic acidosis　乳酸カルシウム calcium lactate　乳酸菌 lactic acid bacteria　乳酸脱水素酵素 lactate dehydrogenase；LDH

にゅうし　乳歯　milk tooth, baby tooth （脱落歯）**deciduous tooth, temporary tooth**

にゅうじ　乳児　infant (図infantile) （赤ん坊）**baby** ☞子供, 小児, 乳幼児, ライフステージ ◆生後3か月の乳児 a three-month-old baby ▶乳児院 infants' home / home for infants　乳児期 infancy / babyhood　乳児下痢症 infantile diarrhea　乳児湿疹 infantile eczema　乳児死亡 infant death　乳児食 baby[infant] food　乳児保育 infant care

ニュージーランド　New Zealand (図ニュージーランドの・ニュージーランド人の New Zealand) ☞国籍 ▶ニュージーランド人 New Zealander

にゅうしゅ　入手する　get, obtain (図入手できる available) ◆予防接種の日程は市の広報から入手できます You can get[obtain] the vaccination schedule in [through] your local city bulletin. ◆その

薬は処方箋がなければ入手できません That medication is available by prescription only. / You can't get[obtain] that medication without a prescription. ◆その薬は日本では入手できません That medication is not available in Japan.

にゅうじゅう　乳汁　milk (図milky) （母乳）**breast milk** (接頭lact(o)-, galact(o)-) ◆乳房マッサージは乳汁の分泌を良くします Breast massage is effective for stimulating milk ejection. / Breast massage is effective for increasing[boosting] *the milk supply[the flow of milk]. ▶乳汁のような分泌物 milky discharge ▶乳汁分泌 lactation / milk secretion　乳汁分泌不全 lactation failure　乳汁分泌抑制 lactation suppression　乳汁漏出症 galactorrhea

にゅうしょ　入所する　enter, be admitted to ◆介護施設に入所する enter[be admitted to] a care home ◀短期入所施設 （ショートステイ）short-stay facility /（一時的な介護代行施設）respite care center

にゅうじょう　乳状(の)　milky, emulsified ☞乳糜 ◆乳状の尿 milky[（乳びの）chylous] urine

にゅうせいひん　乳製品　dairy products / milk products ★通例, 複数形で.

にゅうせん　乳腺　mammary gland ▶乳腺炎 mastitis　乳腺外科医 breast surgeon　乳腺症 mastopathy　乳腺・内分泌外科 the department of breast and endocrine surgery / the breast and endocrine surgery department

にゅうとう¹　乳頭　nipple ☞乳首 ◆乳頭をつまんで分泌物が出ないかをチェックします I'm going to pinch[squeeze] your nipple to make sure *that it's not producing any discharge[there's no discharge coming out of it]. ◆乳頭がへこんでいる（逆さになっている）have an inverted nipple ◀陥没乳頭 inverted[retracted] nipple　扁平乳頭 flat nipple ▶乳頭陥凹 nipple retraction　乳頭亀裂 cracked nipple / fissure of the nipple　乳頭出血 nipple bleeding　乳頭分泌物 nipple discharge

にゅうとう[2] （視神経）乳頭　optic disc [disk]，optic papilla （瞳頭papill(o)-）　◀うっ血乳頭 choked disc　蒼白乳頭 optic disc pallor　▶乳頭陥凹 optic disc cupping　乳頭腫脹 optic disc swelling / swelling of the optic disc　乳頭浮腫 optic disc edema / papilledema

にゅうとう[3]　乳糖　lactose, milk sugar　▶乳糖耐性検査 lactose tolerance test　乳糖不耐症 lactose intolerance

にゅうとうしゅ　乳頭腫　papilloma　◀ヒト乳頭腫ウイルス human papillomavirus；HPV

にゅうはくしょく　乳白色(の)　milky white, milky　◀乳白色の分泌物が出る have a milky white discharge

にゅうび　乳糜　chyle （瞳chylous）　▶乳び胸 chylothorax　乳び尿 chylous [milky] urine

にゅうぼう　乳房　☞乳(ちち)　breast　◆乳房は痛みますか Are your breasts painful?　◆乳房を押すと痛みますか Do your breasts feel sore[tender]?　◆サイズ，形，色，乳首など乳房に何か変化がありましたか Have you noticed any changes in your breasts, such as changes in the size, the shape, the skin color, or the nipples?　◆乳房X線検査を受けたことがありますか Have you ever had a mammogram?　◆乳房を触診します(指先の腹で) I'm going to examine your breasts *with the pads of my fingers[by palpating them with my fingers].　◆乳房に硬いしこりがある have a hard[firm] lump in *one's* breast　◆乳房の表面にくぼみがある have a dimple *on the breast[of the breast skin / of the surface of the breast]　◆乳房が張っている *one's* breasts are full and swollen　◆乳房の生検をする do[take] a breast biopsy　◆残念ですが，乳房にがんが見つかりました I'm sorry, but we found cancer in your breast.　◀女性化乳房 gynecomastia　▶乳房インプラント[プロステーシス] breast implant[prosthesis]　乳房X線検査 mammography　乳房X線写

真 mammogram　乳房温存手術 breast-conserving surgery　乳房温存療法 breast-conserving therapy；BCT　乳房再建術 breast reconstruction (surgery)　乳房切除術 mastectomy　乳房超音波検査 breast ultrasound[ultrasonography]　乳房マッサージ breast massage　☞乳房自己触診

にゅうぼうじこしょくしん　乳房自己触診　breast self-exam[self-examination]；BSE　◆これまで定期的に乳房自己触診をしていますか〈していましたか〉Do you do 〈Have you been doing〉 regular breast self-exams?　◆毎月乳房自己触診を行って下さい I recommend monthly breast self-exams.

にゅうみん　入眠　▶入眠困難 difficulty (in) falling asleep　入眠時幻覚 hypnagogic hallucination　入眠薬 soporific / sleep-inducing medication[drug / agent]

ニューモシスチスはいえん — 肺炎　*Pneumocystis* pneumonia；PCP

にゅうようじ　乳幼児　infant　★infant は狭義では乳児をさすが，広義には幼児も含める．☞乳児，ライフステージ　▶乳幼児健診 infant health checkup　乳幼児突然死症候群 sudden infant death syndrome；SIDS　乳幼児揺さぶられっ子症候群 shaken baby syndrome；SBS

にゅうようとっき　乳様突起　mastoid (process)　▶乳様突起炎 mastoiditis

にゅうよく　入浴する　take a bath, have a bath, use the bath　☞風呂　◆入浴は担当医の許可が必要です Before you take a bath, you need to get your doctor's permission.　◆今晩は入浴を控えて下さい You should not take a bath tonight.　◆入浴は差し支えありません You can take a bath. / It's OK to have a bath.　◆入浴時間は，月・水・金曜日の午後1時から8時です You can take a bath between the hours of one pm and eight pm on Mondays, Wednesdays, and Fridays.　◆クロスさん，入浴のお時間です Mr Cross, it's time for you to take a bath.　◆入浴のお世話をしましょう Let me help you take a bath.　▶入浴ケア bathing care　入浴剤 bath salts[additives]／〈泡入浴剤〉bubble bath　入浴治療 bath treatment[therapy]

にゅうりん　乳輪　**nipple areola, areola of the breast**

ニューロパチー　**neuropathy**　◀アミロイドニューロパチー amyloid neuropathy　遺伝性ニューロパチー hereditary neuropathy　脚気ニューロパチー beriberi neuropathy　腫瘍随伴性多発ニューロパチー paraneoplastic polyneuropathy　多発ニューロパチー polyneuropathy　単ニューロパチー mononeuropathy　糖尿病性ニューロパチー diabetic neuropathy　尿毒症性ニューロパチー uremic neuropathy　慢性炎症性脱髄性多発ニューロパチー[多発根ニューロパチー] chronic inflammatory demyelinating polyneuropathy[polyradiculoneuropathy]；CIDP

ニューロン　**neuron**　◀運動ニューロン疾患 motor neuron disease；MND　下位運動ニューロン lower motor neuron；LMN　上位運動ニューロン upper motor neuron；UMN

にょう　尿　**urine** /jórm/　㊥**urinary**　㊥排尿する　**urinate** /jórənèit/, **pass urine [water])**　◆尿に異常がありましたか Have you had any problems[trouble] *with your urine[with passing urine]?

《尿の性状》　☞囲み：尿の性状の表現　◆どんな尿が出ますか What is your urine like?

◆尿はどんな色をしていますか What color is your urine?　◆尿の色に何か変化がありましたか Have you noticed any changes in the color of your urine?　◆尿に血〈膿／小さい石〉が混じりますか Have you noticed any blood〈pus／small stones〉in your urine?　◆尿に蛋白が出ています There is protein in your urine. ／You have protein in your urine.

《尿量》　◆尿の量に何か変化がありましたか Have you noticed any changes in the amount of your urine?　◆尿の量はどのくらいですか About how much urine do you pass each time?　◆いつもより尿が多く出ますか Are you passing more urine than

usual?　◆尿の量が多い〈少ない〉urinate *a lot〈small amounts〉／pass excessive 〈small〉amounts of urine／have increased〈decreased〉urine output　◆尿の量を正確に把握するために，すべての尿をこの容器にためて下さい Please collect and store all urine in this container so that we can accurately measure the amount of urine your body produces.

《排尿回数》　◆尿の回数はいつもより多いですか，少ないですか Do you have to urinate more often[frequently] than usual or less often[frequently]?　◆1日に何回尿が出ますか How many times a day do you urinate?　◆尿が近い〈頻尿である〉urinate often[frequently]　◆排尿のため夜中に何回目を覚ましますか How many times do you wake[get] up in the night to urinate[pass urine]?　◆尿が近くてよく眠れないのですか Do you not sleep well because of frequent calls?

《排尿障害》　◆尿はどんなふうに出ますか How does the urine come out?　◆尿が出にくいですか Do you have difficulty passing urine?／（特に最初に）Do you have difficulty starting the urine flow?　◆尿の出が悪いのですか Is your urine flow weak and slow?／Is the force of your urine flow decreased?／Do you feel that your urine doesn't flow smoothly[naturally]?　◆尿はしたたるように出る The urine continues to dribble little by little.　◆尿がまったく出ない pass no urine　◆排尿後も尿が残っている感じがしますか Even after you've urinated, do you feel that *your bladder hasn't emptied completely[you haven't completely emptied your bladder]?　◆絶えず尿を出したくなる have a constant urge to urinate

《尿失禁》　◆尿のコントロールが難しいですか Do you have difficulty controlling your bladder[urine flow]?　◆尿漏れでお困りですか Do you have any problem with urine dribbling[leakage]?　◆くしゃみや咳をした時に尿が漏れることがありますか Do you ever leak or dribble urine when you sneeze or cough? ◆尿失禁すること がありますか Do you ever become incontinent? / Do you have any bladder incontinence? ◆尿を我慢することが難しいで すか Do you have difficulty holding your urine? ◆夜お子さんは尿を漏らすことが ありますか Does your child ever wet the bed (at night)?

《排尿痛》 ◆尿をする時痛みますか Do you have any pain when you urinate? ◆尿を する時焼けるような感じがしますか Do you have a burning sensation when you urinate?

《検尿》urine test[examination], urinalysis；UA ◆尿検査をします We need a sample of your urine. / We need to check[examine] your urine. / Let me[I'm going to] do [run] a urine test. ◆このコップに尿を 採って下さい Please use this cup to collect your urine. ◆まず, トイレに尿を少し出し てから, コップ3分の1くらいまで入れて下 さい First, urinate a small amount into the toilet and then fill the cup to about one-third with urine. ◆膀胱にこの管を入れて 尿を採りましょう Let me drain[collect] the urine from your bladder with this tube.

◀アルカリ尿 alkaluria / alkaline urine カテーテル尿 catheterized urine 血尿 hematuria / bloody urine / blood in the urine ケトン尿 ketonuria 高張尿 hypersthenuria 混濁尿 cloudy[turbid / nebulous] urine 細菌尿 bacteriuria 採 尿 urine collection / collection of a urine sample[specimen] / urine sampling 酸 性尿 acidic urine / aciduria 残尿 residual urine 残尿感 constant urge to urinate 随時尿 random urine 早朝尿 first morning urine 多尿 polyuria 蓄尿 urine collection and storage / collecting and storing one's urine 中間尿 midstream urine 等張尿 isotonic urine / isosthenuria 24時間尿 24-hour[twenty-four-hour] urine 濃縮尿 concentrated urine 膿尿 pyuria 頻尿 frequent urination / frequency of micturition 乏尿 oliguria 無尿 anuria / no urine production 夜尿 bedwetting / nocturnal enuresis

▶尿カップ urine collection cup / urine specimen[test] cup 尿検査室 urine testing[test / exam] room 尿細胞診 urine [urinary] cytology 尿サンプル urine sample[specimen] 尿しぶり urinary tenesmus 尿臭 urine odor 尿浸透圧 urine osmolarity / urine[urinary] osmotic pressure 尿潜血 occult hematuria / occult blood in urine 尿蛋白 urinary protein / proteinuria 尿沈渣 urinary sediment 尿停滞 urinary stasis 尿 培養 urine culture 尿比重 urine specific gravity 尿閉 urinary retention ☞尿意, 尿管, 尿器, 尿細管, 尿失禁, 尿線, 尿糖, 尿 道, 尿とりパッド, 尿流, 尿量, 尿路, 排尿

尿の性状の表現

■色
●澄んだ麦わら色の clear, straw-colored ●淡い黄色の light[pale] yellow ●濃い黄色の dark yellow / deep amber ●赤い red ●赤味がかった reddish ●赤褐色の reddish brown ●鮮紅色の bright red ●黒い black ●黒褐色の dark brown

■性状
●濃い concentrated ●薄い dilute ●乳状の milky ●濁った cloudy / turbid / nebulous ●血液が混じった blood-stained ●血性の bloody ●泡立った frothy / foamy

■におい
●甘い果実のような sweet and fruity ●アセトン臭の acetone-smelling ●甘 酸っぱい sweet and sour ●アンモニア臭 の ammonia-smelling ●かび臭い musty ●腐ったような bad-[decayed- / rotten-] smelling ●むかつくような foul-smelling ●糞便臭の fecal-smelling

---

にょうい 尿意 urge to urinate, need to urinate, urinary sensation ◆尿意を感じ る have[feel] the urge to urinate ◆突然

尿意を催すことがありますか Do you ever have a sudden (and urgent) need to urinate? ◆尿意を我慢できますか Can you hold your bladder[urine]? ◆尿意を我慢するのが難しいですか Do you have any trouble holding your bladder? ◆尿意が残る still feel the need to urinate ▶尿意切迫 urge to urinate / urinary urgency

にょうかん 尿管 ureter /jύrətə/（🇺🇸uréteral）◀膀胱尿管逆流 vesicoureteral reflux；VUR ▶尿管カテーテル ureteral catheter 尿管狭窄 ureteral stenosis 尿管結石 ureter stone[calculus] 尿管損傷 ureteral injury

にょうき 尿器 （しびん）urine bottle, bed bottle, urinal ◆この尿器を使って下さい Please use this urine bottle.

にょうけんさ 尿検査 urine test[examination], urinalysis；UA ☞尿《検尿》

にょうさいかん 尿細管 kidney[renal] tubule ◀遠位尿細管 distal (kidney) tubule；DT 近位尿細管 proximal (kidney) tubule；PT 腎尿細管性アシドーシス renal tubular acidosis；RTA ▶尿細管再吸収 tubular reabsorption

にょうさん 尿酸 uric acid；UA ◆尿酸値を調べましょう Let me[I'm going to] measure your uric acid level. ◆尿酸値が高い have a high uric acid level ◀高尿酸血症 hyperuricemia ▶尿酸結石 uric acid stone[calculus] 尿酸生成抑制薬 uric acid synthesis inhibitor 尿酸排泄促進薬 uricosuric medication[drug / agent]

にょうしっきん 尿失禁 urinary incontinence；UI ☞尿《尿失禁》 ◀溢流性尿失禁 overflow (urinary) incontinence 切迫性尿失禁 urge (urinary) incontinence 腹圧性尿失禁 stress (urinary) incontinence；SUI

にょうせん 尿線 urine stream, urinary stream, the stream of *one's* urine ☞尿《排尿障害》 ◆尿線は正常ですか Is the stream of your urine normal? ◆尿線のサイズや勢いに変化がありますか Have you noticed any changes in the size or force of your urine stream? ◆尿線が途中で途切れることがありますか Do you ever have an interrupted urine stream? / Does the urine stream ever become interrupted? ◆尿線が細くなる have a thin urine stream ◆尿線に勢いがなくなる have a weak urine stream / the force of the urine stream weakens[becomes weak]

にょうそ 尿素 urea ◀血中尿素窒素 blood urea nitrogen；BUN ▶尿素呼気試験 urea breath test

にょうとう 尿糖 sugar in urine, glucose in urine, urine sugar[glucose]

にょうどう 尿道 urethra /jʊríːθrə/（🇺🇸urethral）☞尿路 ◆尿道の出口付近〈尿道の中〉に痛みがある have (a) pain *around the urethral opening〈inside the urethra〉 ▶尿道括約筋 urethral sphincter 尿道(留置)カテーテル urethral (indwelling) catheter 尿道下裂 hypospadias 尿道狭窄 urethral stenosis[stricture] 尿道結石 urethral stone[calculus] 尿道口 urethral orifice[opening / meatus] 尿道損傷 urethral injury 尿道脱 urethral prolapse 尿道ブジー urethral bougie 尿道分泌物 urethral discharge 尿道膀胱鏡検査 urethrocystoscopy ☞尿炎造影，尿道造影

にょうどうえん 尿道炎 urethritis ◀クラミジア尿道炎 chlamydial urethritis 非淋菌性尿道炎 nongonococcal urethritis；NGU 淋菌性尿道炎 gonococcal urethritis；GU

にょうどうぞうえい 尿道造影 urethrography ◀逆行性尿道造影 retrograde urethrography；RUG

にょうどくしょう 尿毒症 uremia（🇺🇸uremic）◀溶血性尿毒症症候群 hemolytic uremic syndrome；HUS ▶尿毒症性ニューロパチー uremic neuropathy 尿毒症性肺症 uremic lung

にょうとりパッド 尿とりパッド (urine) incontinence pad （ベッド用の）(urine) incontinence bed pad, underpad

にょうほうしょう 尿崩症 diabetes insipidus；DI

にょうまくかん 尿膜管 urachus（形ura-chal）▶尿膜管遺残 urachal remnant

にょうもれ 尿漏れ urinary incontinence ☞尿《尿失禁》

にょうりゅう 尿流 urine flow, urinary flow ◆尿流量の検査をする do a urine flow test ▶尿流時間 urinary flow time 尿流測定法 uroflowmetry；UFM 尿流動態検査 urodynamic study；UDS 尿流パターン urinary flow pattern 尿流率 urine [urinary] flow rate

にょうりょう 尿量 the amount of urine, volume of urine, urinary output[volume], the amount[volume] of urine ☞尿《尿量》▶尿量減少（乏尿）oliguria / decreased [scanty] urinary output

にょうろ 尿路 urinary tract ☞尿道 ◀下部尿路 lower urinary tract 排泄性尿路造影 excretory urography ▶尿路感染症 urinary tract infection；UTI 尿路系 the urinary system 尿路結石 urinary stone[calculus]

にらんせいそうせいじ 二卵性双生児 dizygotic twins, biovular twins （その1人）dizygotic[biovular] twin

にる 似る look similar, resemble, be [look] like （親などに似る）take after（形類似の similar）◆似た症状 a similar symptom ◆この2つの薬は外見が似ているので飲み間違えないように注意して下さい These two medications look similar, so be very careful not to *take the wrong one [get them confused]. ◆結核の初期症状は風邪と似ています The initial symptoms of tuberculosis can *be similar to[resemble] the symptoms of the common cold. ◆お子さんはお父さんにとてもよく似ていますね Your child really takes after his father, doesn't he?

にんい 任意(の) （自分で選べる）optional （↔compulsory）（随意の）voluntary ◆この予防接種は任意です This vaccination is optional. ▶任意手術 optional surgery 任意入院 voluntary hospitalization 任意保険 voluntary insurance 任意予防接種 voluntary vaccination

にんか 認可 ☞承認，認定

にんげんかんけい 人間関係 （個人的な相互関係）(human) relationship （一般的な相互関係）(human) relation ◆職場や家族の人間関係に何か悩みがありますか Do you have any problems with relationships at work or with your family? ◆職場で人間関係によるストレスを受けている be under stress due to *unhappy relationships at work[problems with people at work] ◆人間関係がうまくいかない have difficulty keeping up good (human) relationships

にんげんドック 人間ドック comprehensive physical[health] checkup[screening], complete physical[health] checkup [screening] ◆人間ドックを受ける have [undergo] a comprehensive physical checkup ◆1泊2日の人間ドック a comprehensive physical checkup with an overnight stay in the hospital ◆日帰り人間ドック a one-day comprehensive physical[health] checkup

にんしき 認識 （理解）understanding（動understand）（意識・自覚）awareness（動be aware of）（認知）recognition（動recognize), cognition ◆自分の病気について正しい認識を持っていますか Do you fully understand about your (own) illness? / Do you have an accurate understanding of your (own) illness? ◀自己認識 self-understanding / self-awareness / self-recognition パターン認識 pattern recognition

にんしん 妊娠 pregnancy, gestation（形pregnant, gestational）◆あなたは妊娠10週です You are ten weeks pregnant. ◆妊娠していますか Are you pregnant? ◆妊娠している可能性はありますか Is there any possibility that you're pregnant? / Could you be pregnant? ◆妊娠何週目ですか How many weeks pregnant are you? ◆妊娠を考えていますか Are you planning to become pregnant? ◆妊娠を望んでどのくらいの期間になりますか How long have you been trying to get pregnant? ◆妊娠したことがありますか Have you ever been pregnant? ◆これまでに何回妊娠しましたか How many times have you been pregnant before? ◆妊娠中に何か問題がありましたか Did you have any problem during your pregnancy? ◆その時妊娠は何週でしたか How many weeks were you pregnant then? ◆望まない妊娠 an unwanted pregnancy ◆無計画妊娠 an unplanned pregnancy ◀過期妊娠 postterm pregnancy 子宮外妊娠 ectopic[extrauterine] pregnancy 正常〈異常〉妊娠 normal〈abnormal〉pregnancy 遷延妊娠 prolonged pregnancy 双胎妊娠 twin pregnancy 多胎妊娠 multiple pregnancy ハイリスク妊娠 high-risk pregnancy 母児血液型不適合妊娠 incompatibility of maternal and fetal blood types / maternal and fetal blood type incompatibility ▶妊娠悪阻 hyperemesis gravidarum；HG 妊娠嘔吐 vomiting[emesis] of pregnancy 妊娠合併症 pregnancy complication(s) / complication(s) of pregnancy 妊娠期間 the length of pregnancy / (在胎期間)gestational period[age] 妊娠(反応)検査 pregnancy (reaction) test 妊娠高血圧症候群 pregnancy-induced hypertension；PIH / gestational hypertension 妊娠時期 dating of pregnancy 妊娠週数 week(s) of pregnancy / pregnancy[gestational] week(s) 妊娠証明書 pregnancy certificate / certificate of pregnancy 妊娠線 (pregnancy) stretch marks / striae gravidarum 妊娠糖尿病 gestational diabetes mellitus；GDM / pregnancy diabetes / diabetes in pregnancy 妊娠貧血 pregnancy anemia / anemia in pregnancy 妊娠歴 obstetrical history ☞妊娠期，妊娠中絶

妊娠月数の数え方

妊娠月数，あるいは妊娠前期・中期・後期などの数え方は，日本と欧米で異なることに注意する．一方，妊娠週数については，日本を含めた多くの国で WHO 方式を採用しており，外国籍の患者を診察するときには

妊娠週数で説明したほうがよい．

にんしんき 妊娠期 stage of pregnancy, gestation period （3 か月を単位として）pregnancy trimester ▶妊娠初期 the early stage of pregnancy / the first trimester 妊娠中期 the middle stage of pregnancy / the second trimester 妊娠後期 the late stage of pregnancy / the third trimester

にんしんちゅうぜつ 妊娠中絶 （人工流産）(induced) abortion ☞流産 ◆妊娠中絶を受ける have[undergo] an abortion ◆母体の安全のために妊娠中絶する perform[carry out] an abortion to save the life of the mother

にんたいづよい 忍耐強い ☞粘り強い

にんち 認知 recognition, cognition (形 cognitive) ◆認知機能が低下している have a low degree of recognition / have low cognitive function ▶認知行動療法 cognitive-behavioral therapy；CBT 認知リハビリテーション cognitive rehabilitation ☞認知症，認知障害

にんちしょう 認知症 dementia /dɪménʃə/ ◆彼女は軽い認知症と思われます I suspect she has mild dementia. ◆認知症の徴候がある show signs of dementia ◆認知症が始まる begin to show signs of dementia ◀アルツハイマー型認知症 Alzheimer(-type) dementia / dementia of the Alzheimer type；DAT 若年性認知症 early-onset dementia 脳血管性認知症 cerebrovascular dementia / (血管性) vascular dementia；VD[VaD] まだら認知症 lacunar dementia レビー小体型認知症 dementia with Lewy bodies；DLB / Lewy body dementia

にんちしょうがい 認知障害 cognitive disorder[impairment] ◀軽度認知障害 mild cognitive impairment；MCI

にんてい 認定する （証明する）certify (名 certification) （承認する）recognize (名 recognition) （認可する）license (名 license) ☞承認 ◆アスベスト患者と認定される be (officially) certified[recognized]

as an asbestosis patient ◆過労死と認定
される be certified[recognized] as a victim of death from overwork ◆要介護 5
の認定を受ける be certified as requiring
care level five / be certified as a person
with level-five care needs ◀介護度認定
certification of long-term care needs /
certification of eligibility for long-term
care needs 介護認定審査会 certification
committee of needed long-term care
▶認定医(日本内科学会の)Board-certified
member[doctor / physician](of the Japanese Society of Internal Medicine) 認
定看護師 certified[licensed] nurse

にんぷ 妊婦 **pregnant woman** (出産予
定の母親) **expectant mother, mother-to-
be** ▶妊婦健診 pregnancy[prenatal]
checkup 妊婦体操 pregnancy[mater-
nity] exercise 妊婦服 maternity clothes
[wear]

ぬ

ぬう 縫う ☞縫合

ぬく 抜く
《不要な物を取り出す》take (out) （引き抜く) pull (out) （取り除く) remove （排出させる) drain ◆最近歯を抜きましたか Have you had any of your teeth taken[pulled] out recently? ◆髪の毛を抜く癖がある have a habit of pulling one's hair ◆電源のプラグを抜く pull the plug from the socket ◆親指のとげを抜く remove a splinter from one's thumb / pull a splinter out of one's thumb ◆右胸にたまった水を抜く drain (off) fluid from the right chest / remove[drain] the fluid that has *built up[accumulated] in the right chest ◆傷口から糸を抜きましょう I'm going to *remove your stitches[take your stitches out].
《力を抜く》 ◆体の力を抜く(リラックスさせる)relax / relax one's muscles / (だらりとさせる)let one's body go limp ◆肩の力を抜く relax one's shoulders
《省く》skip ◆朝食は抜かないで下さい Please don't skip breakfast.

ぬぐ 脱ぐ take off (↔put on) remove （さっと脱ぐ)slip off ◆服は上半身を脱いで下さい Please *take off[remove] your clothes from the waist up. / Please take[slip] off your top things. ◆ズボン以外すべて脱いで下さい Please *take all your clothes off[remove all your clothes] except your pants. ◆靴を脱いで体重計に乗って下さい Please *take your shoes off[take off your shoes] and step[stand] on the scale.

ぬけげ 抜け毛 hair loss （抜け落ちた毛)fallen hair ◆最近抜け毛が増えましたか Have you noticed unusual amounts of hair loss recently?

ぬける 抜ける （失う)lose （落ちる)fall out[off] （外れて取れる)come out ◆毛がよく抜けますか Are you losing a lot of hair? / Is your hair falling out badly? ◆化学療法で髪の毛が抜けるかもしれませんが、それは一時的なものです You may lose some of your hair during the chemotherapy, but it will only be a temporary thing. ◆歯が抜ける a tooth comes[falls] out / lose a tooth

ぬの 布 cloth ▶布おむつ cloth diaper

ぬらす 濡らす wet, get ... wet （湿らす)moisten ◆お子さんはおむつを毎日何枚濡らしますか How many diapers does your baby wet a day? ◆ギプス包帯を濡らさないで下さい Please don't get the cast wet.

ぬりぐすり 塗り薬 （軟膏)ointment （クリーム)cream （ローション)lotion ◆傷口に塗り薬をつける(軟膏を)apply some ointment to the cut / put some ointment on the cut

ぬる 塗る （薬・化粧品をつける)apply, put, spread （擦りこむ)rub （滑らかにする)lubricate ◆1日に1回、入浴後にこの軟膏を塗って下さい Please apply[use] this ointment once a day after your bath. ◆かゆいところにこの軟膏を薄く塗って下さい Please apply a thin layer of this ointment to the itchy area. ◆患部にクリームをたっぷり塗って下さい Please lubricate the affected area with a generous amount of cream. / Please apply the cream generously to the affected area. ◆お腹にゼリーを塗ります I'm going to [Let me] *spread gel on[apply gel to] your abdomen. ◆指の傷口に消毒薬を塗る put some disinfectant on one's cut finger / apply some disinfectant to one's cut finger ◆日焼け止めクリームを塗る *put on[apply] sunscreen

ぬるまゆ 一湯 lukewarm water, tepid water ◆お風呂やシャワーはぬるま湯にして下さい Please take a bath or shower in lukewarm water. ◆冷凍母乳をぬるま湯で解凍する thaw[defrost] frozen breast milk in lukewarm water ◆ぬるま湯の風呂(微温浴)a lukewarm[tepid] bath

ぬれた 濡れた **wet** (湿った)**moist** ◆おむつが濡れています The diaper is wet. ◆冷たい濡れタオルでやけどした部分を冷やす use a cold, wet towel to cool down the burned area ◆濡れタオルで顔を拭く wipe the face with a moist washcloth

ね

ねあせ 寝汗 **night sweats** /swéts/ ★通例，複数形で．☞汗 ◆寝汗をよくかきますか Do you often have night sweats? ◆寝汗をひどくかく have drenching night sweats / sweat[perspire] a lot while sleeping ◆寝汗をかいて夜中に何度も起きる wake up several times in the night dripping with sweat

ネイティブ （地元民）**native** （その言語を母語とする人）**native speaker** ◆英語のネイティブスピーカー a native speaker of English ◆ネイティブにチェックを依頼する consult a native speaker ◆ネイティブに単語の発音を訊く ask a native speaker how to pronounce a word

ネームバンド （hospital）**ID band** （識別用腕輪）**wristband, ID bracelet** ◆これはあなたのネームバンドです．お名前を確かめて下さい Here's your ID band. Please make sure that your name is correct. ◆このネームバンドは入院中ははずさないで下さい Please do not remove this ID band during your stay in the hospital.

ネームプレート （胸に付ける名札）**name tag** （ドアに付ける表札）**nameplate**

ねがい 願い 《希望》**hope** （願望）**desire** （実現の可能性が低い願い）**wish** ◆退院したいという強い願いを表明する express a strong desire to leave the hospital ◆彼の最期の願い his dying wish / his last wishes ◆早くお元気になられるよう願っております I hope you get better soon.
《依頼》 ◆お願いがあるのですが Could you do me a favor? / I need to ask you a favor. ◆お静かに願います Please be quiet. / Be quiet, please.

ねがえり 寝返りする （向きを変える）**turn over** （in bed） （転がる）**roll over** （on *one's* own） ◆寝返りのお手伝いをしましょう Let me help you turn[roll] over. ◆うつ伏せに寝がえりをして下さい Please turn over on your stomach. / Please roll onto your stomach. ◆お子さんは何か月頃に寝返りができるようになりましたか How many months〈old〉was your baby when he〈she〉started rolling over on his〈her〉own?

ネグレクト （無視・放置）**neglect** （育児放棄）**child neglect**

ねこぜ 猫背 **stooped shoulders** ★複数形で．（㊩**stoop-shouldered, round-shouldered**）◆彼は猫背です He is stoop-shouldered[round-shouldered]. / His shoulders are rounded[stooped]. ◆猫背で歩く walk with a stoop

ねごと 寝言 ◆寝言を言う talk in *one's* sleep

ねこむ 寝込む （病床に就く）**be sick in bed**

ねざけ 寝酒 **nightcap** ◆寝酒は睡眠の質を下げます Drinking a nightcap will [would] lower the quality of your sleep.

ねしょうべん 寝小便 ☞夜尿

ねじる **twist** ☞捻挫，捻る

ネズミ （はつかネズミ）**mouse** （㊤**mice**） （野ネズミ）**rat** （齧歯類）**rodent**

ねたきり 寝たきり（の） **bedridden** ◆彼女はどのくらい寝たきりになっていますか How long has she been bedridden? / （安静状態を強いられている）How long has she been confined to bed? ◆寝たきり患者〈高齢者〉a bedridden patient〈older person〉

ねちがえる 寝違える ◆首を寝違えたのですか Did you crick[（ひねったか）twist] your neck while sleeping?

ねつ 熱 （発熱）**fever** /fíːvə/, **pyrexia** （体温・温度）**temperature** ☞体温 ◆熱は摂氏 37 度 8 分です Your temperature is 37.8[thirty-seven point eight] degrees Celsius. ◆熱で体が震える shiver with [from] fever ◆熱で食欲がない have no appetite due to the fever
《熱が出る》 ◆熱はありますか Do you have a fever? / Are you running a fever? ◆微熱がある have a slight[mild / low-grade] fever ◆高い熱がある have a high fever

◆熱があるような感じがしますか Do you feel feverish? ◆最近熱が出ましたか Have you recently had a fever? ◆熱はいつ出始めましたか When did the fever start? ◆熱は決まった時間帯に出ますか Do you have the fever at a certain [specific] time of day? ◆今朝, 熱は何度でしたか What was your temperature this morning? / How high was your temperature this morning? ◆この薬は38度以上の熱がある時に飲んで下さい Please take this medication whenever you have a fever of thirty-eight degrees or more.

《熱が上がる／下がる》 ◆熱が上がっています Your fever has gone up. ◆熱が下がりました Your fever has come[gone] down. ◆熱は1日の中で変動[上下]しますか Does your temperature fluctuate [rise and fall] during the day? / Have you noticed any fluctuations in your temperature during the day? ◆熱を下げる薬を出しましょう I'm going to give you a medication to *bring down[lower / reduce] your fever.

《熱が続く》 ◆熱は何日続いていますか How many days have you had the fever? ◆3日以上熱が続くようでしたら, 医師の診察を再度受けて下さい Please see the doctor again if the fever continues [lasts] for more than three days. / Please see the doctor again if you run a fever for more than three days.

《熱を測る》 ◆熱を測りましたか Have you taken your temperature? ◆この体温計で熱を測って下さい Please take[check] your temperature with this thermometer. ◀回帰熱 relapsing[recurrent] fever 間欠熱 intermittent fever 稽留熱 continued[sustained] fever 詐(病)熱 factitious fever 産褥熱 puerperal[childbed] fever 弛張熱 remittent fever 周期熱 periodic fever 猩紅熱 scarlet fever 知恵熱[生歯熱] teething fever プール熱 pharyngoconjunctival fever 不明熱 fever of unknown[undetermined] origin；FUO 平熱 normal (body) temperature

薬剤熱 drug fever リウマチ熱 rheumatic fever ▶熱感 heat sensation / (温熱感覚) warm sensation 熱型 fever type 熱量 calorie 熱量計 calorimeter ☞加熱, 解熱薬, 熱射病, 熱傷, 熱性痙攣, 熱帯, 熱中症, 熱湯

ねつき **寝付き** ◆寝付きはいいですか Do you fall asleep easily[quickly]? ◆寝付きが悪くてお困りなのですか Do you have any difficulty falling asleep[trouble getting to sleep]? ◆これは寝付きをよくする薬です This is a medication to *help you fall asleep[induce sleep].

ネックカラー neck brace, neck collar, cervical collar

ねつさまし **熱冷まし** ☞解熱薬

ねっしゃびょう **熱射病** heatstroke, heat stroke ☞熱中症 ◆熱射病に罹る have [develop] heatstroke

ねっしょう **熱傷** (火・熱・薬品による)burn (injury), burn wound (熱湯・蒸気による) scald ☞火傷(やけど) ◆表層の熱傷を受ける have a superficial burn ◆I〈II / III〉度の熱傷を受ける have a first〈second / third〉-degree burn ◀化学熱傷 chemical burn 気道熱傷 inhalation burn 広範囲熱傷 extensive burn 重症熱傷 severe burn 電撃熱傷 electric burn 熱湯熱傷 scald burn 放射線熱傷 radiation burn ▶熱傷死 death due to burns[burn injuries] 熱傷指数 burn index；BI 熱傷ショック burn shock 熱傷深度 depth of a burn / burn depth 熱傷創感染 burn wound infection 熱傷度 degree of a burn (injury) / burn degree 熱傷面積 extent of the burn 熱傷瘢痕 burn scar

ねっする **熱する** heat (up) ☞加熱

ねっせいけいれん **熱性痙攣** febrile seizure[convulsion], fever seizure[convulsion]

ねったい **熱帯(の)** tropical ▶熱帯医学 tropical medicine 熱帯熱マラリア falciparum malaria 熱帯病 tropical disease

ねっちゅうしょう **熱中症** heat illness, heat-related illness ◆熱中症に罹る have [develop] a heat illness ◆熱中症患者の

体温を下げるには腿の付け根，首，脇の下に氷嚢を当てる *place ice packs on[apply ice packs to] the groin, neck, and armpits to lower the temperature of a patient with a heat illness

ネット （インターネット）Internet, internet, web ☞インターネット ◆ネットをよく利用しますか Do you often use the internet? ◆ネット上には不正確な医療情報があふれていますから，担当医に確かめて下さい A lot of the medical information on the internet is inaccurate, so be sure to check with your doctor. ◆医療情報をネットから入手する access[get / obtain] medical information through[over] the internet

ねっとう **熱湯** boiling water （やけどするほどの熱湯）scalding water ▶熱湯［煮沸］消毒 boiling (water) sterilization / sterilization[disinfection] *by boiling[in boiling water] 熱湯熱傷 scald burn

ネットワーク network ◆患者ネットワーク patient (support / access) network

ネパール Nepal （图Nepalese) ☞国籍 ▶ネパール人（の）Nepalese

ねばねばした sticky, viscous （图viscosity) （粘液性の）mucus-like ◆ねばねばした痰〈分泌物〉は出ていますか Do you have sticky phlegm〈discharge〉? ◆腟からねばねばした分泌物が出る have a mucus-like vaginal discharge

ねばりづよい **粘り強い** （辛抱強い）patient （图patience) （着実な）steady ◆粘り強く今の治療を続けていきましょう Let's be patient and *keep going[stick] with this treatment. ◆あなたの粘り強さに感心しています I really admire you for your patience.

ねぶそく **寝不足** lack of sleep ◆寝不足ですか Are you not getting[Didn't you get] enough sleep? / Are you short of sleep? ◆寝不足で頭が重い one's head feels heavy[dull] due to lack of sleep

ネブライザー nebulizer ◆ネブライザーを使う use a nebulizer ◀超音波ネブライザー ultrasonic nebulizer ▶ネブライザー療法 nebulization

ネフローゼ nephrosis （图nephrotic) ◀微小変化型ネフローゼ症候群 minimal-change nephrotic syndrome；MCNS

ねぼう **寝坊** ☞朝寝坊

ねぼける **寝ぼける** be half-asleep ◆寝ぼけて廊下を歩きまわる walk around the hall half-asleep[in one's sleep]

ねまき **寝間着** ☞パジャマ

ねむい **眠い** sleepy （傾眠性の・だるそうな）drowsy /dráʊzi/ （嗜眠性の）lethargic ◆眠くなる feel[get / become] sleepy[drowsy] ◆日中に眠くなることはよくありますか Do you often feel sleepy[drowsy] during the day? ◆この薬を飲むと眠くなるかもしれません This medication may make you sleepy[drowsy].

ねむけ **眠気** sleepiness, drowsiness

ねむり **眠り** sleep ☞睡眠 ◆眠りにつく fall asleep ◆眠りが浅い sleep poorly[lightly] ◆眠りが深い sleep deeply[soundly] ◆眠りが深い〈浅い〉ほうですか Are you a heavy〈light〉sleeper? ◀居眠り dozing[nodding] off (to sleep) ▶眠り薬 sleeping pill[tablet]

ねむる **眠る** sleep （寝入る）fall asleep （うたた寝する）doze （仮眠する）take a nap ☞就寝，熟眠，寝る ◆うつ伏せ〈仰向け／横向き〉に眠る sleep on one's stomach〈back / side〉 ◆眠るように息を引き取る pass away peacefully[as if one is only falling asleep]
《睡眠の質》 ◆毎日何時間眠りますか How many hours do you usually sleep every night? ◆夜はよく眠れますか Do you sleep well at night? ◆眠った後での目覚めはすっきりしますか Do you usually wake feeling refreshed? ◆ふだん昼間に眠りますか Do you usually *take a nap[sleep during the day]? ◆昨晩はよく眠れましたか Did you sleep well last night? ◆今夜はもっとよく眠れるといいですね I hope you can sleep better tonight. ◆彼はぐっすり眠っています He is sound[fast] asleep. / He's sleeping well[soundly]. ◆眠りながらいびきをかく snore in one's sleep ◆死んだように眠る

sleep like a log ★log は「丸太」を意味する.

《睡眠障害》 ◆眠れなくて困っていることがありますか Do you have any sleeping problems? ◆夜眠れないことがありますか Do you have difficulty sleeping at night? ◆眠るのに時間がかかりますか Does it take a long time for you to fall asleep? / Do you have difficulty *falling asleep[getting to sleep]? ◆ふだん一晩通して眠れますか Do you usually sleep through the night? ◆よく眠れない sleep badly / (眠りが浅い) sleep poorly[lightly] ◆断続的に眠る(眠りが切れ切れになる)sleep *on and off[fitfully] ◆夜中に目が覚めて再度眠ることができないのですか Do you wake up during the night and then have difficulty falling[getting] back to sleep? ◆眠れない時にはどのように対処していますか How do you cope with sleeplessness? ◆この薬は眠れない時に飲んで下さい Please take this medication when you can't sleep.

ねる 寝る

《床に就く》go to bed ☞就寝, 眠る ◆いつも何時に寝ますか What time do you usually go to bed? ◆寝る時間ですよ It's time to go to bed. / It's bedtime. ◆この薬は寝る前に飲んで下さい Please take this medication *before you go[before going] to bed.

《横になる》lie (**down**) ◆診察台に仰向け〈うつ伏せ〉に寝て下さい Please lie (flat) on your back〈stomach〉on the exam table. ◆右〈左〉を下にして寝る lie on *one's* right〈left〉side ◆トイレ以外はベッドに寝ていて下さい Please stay in bed at all times except when you need to use the toilet. / Please don't get out of bed except to use the bathroom.

ねん 年 **year** ◆あなたは何年生まれですか When were you born? ◆彼女は1985年生まれです She was born in 1985[nineteen eighty-five]. ◆日本に来られて何年になりますか How long have you been in Japan? ◆インドには年に何回くらい帰りますか How many times a year do you go

back to India? ◆少なくとも年に1回は健診を受けて下さい Please have[go for] a checkup[physical] at least once a year.
☞年月日, 年収, 年齢

ねんえき 粘液 **mucus** (🈩**mucous, mucus-like, mucinous**) ◆粘液が混じった下痢をする have diarrhea with mucus in it ◆粘液性の鼻汁が出る have a mucus-like nasal discharge ◀頸管粘液 cervical mucus ▶粘液癌 mucinous carcinoma 粘液栓 mucous plug 粘液腺 mucous gland 粘液痰 mucous sputum 粘液分泌 mucous secretion 粘液便 mucous stool 粘液溶解薬 mucolytic (medication / drug / agent)

ねんがっぴ 年月日 **date** ◆同意書に年月日を書き入れて下さい Please fill in the date on the consent form.

ねんきん 年金 **pension** ◆日本の公的年金をもらっていますか Are you receiving a Japanese public pension? ◆年金で暮らす live on a pension ◀遺族年金 Survivors' Pension 共済年金 Mutual Aid Pension 厚生年金 Employees' Pension 国民年金 National Pension (system) / government pension 障害年金 disability pension 傷病年金 injury and disease compensation pension 福祉年金 welfare pension 老齢年金 old-age pension ▶年金証書 pension certificate 年金生活者 pensioner 年金手帳 pension handbook

ねんけつべん 粘血便 **bloody mucous stool, bloody mucoid stool**

ねんざ 捻挫 **sprain** (🈩**sprain** 捻る **twist**) ☞捻る ◆足首を捻挫する sprain[twist] *one's* ankle ◀頸椎捻挫 neck[cervical] sprain 足関節[足首]捻挫 ankle sprain

ねんしゅう 年収 **annual income, yearly income** ◆年収はおいくらですか What's your annual income?

ねんせい 粘性 ☞ねばねばした

ねんちゃく 粘着(性の) **adhesive** ▶粘着テープ adhesive tape 粘着包帯 adhesive bandage

ねんてん　捻転　twisting（動twist），torsion　◆腸が捻転している *one's* bowels are twisted / have twisted bowels　◀茎捻転 torsion of the pedicle　精巣捻転 torsion of the testis / testicular torsion　腸捻転 intestinal volvulus / twisting of the intestines[bowels]

ねんど　粘度　☞ねばねばした

ねんどいろ　粘土色(の)　clay-colored　◆粘土色の便 clay-colored stools

ねんのため　念のため　(確かめるため)just to be certain, just to make sure　(万一に備えて)just in case　(安全のため)just to be on the safe side　◆念のために腸の生検をします I'm going to do[perform] a biopsy of your colon *just to be certain[just in case].　◆念のため脳の MRI を撮ることをお勧めします I recommend that you have a brain MRI just to *make sure[be on the safe side].

ねんまく　粘膜　mucous membrane, mucosa（形mucosal）　◆副鼻腔は粘膜に覆われています The sinus cavities are lined with mucous membranes.　◀胃粘膜 gastric mucosa / the mucosa of the stomach　口腔粘膜 oral[mouth] mucosa　腸粘膜 intestinal mucosa　▶粘膜下出血 submucosal bleeding　粘膜下組織 submucosa　粘膜疹 enanthema　粘膜内癌 intramucosal carcinoma

ねんれい　年齢　age　☞年(とし)　◆この病気はどの年齢でも発症します This disease can occur at any age.　◆がんのリスクは年齢とともに上昇します The risk of cancer increases with age.　◆この手術に年齢制限はありません There's no age limit for this type of surgery.　◆初経年齢は何歳の時ですか How old were you when you had your first (menstrual) period?　◆年齢に応じて発達する develop appropriately for *one's* age　◆年齢の割には体重が重い be heavy for *one's* age　◆年齢による難聴 age-related hearing loss / hearing loss associated with age　◀好発年齢 peak age /（発生率のピーク）peak incidence　骨年齢 bone age　実年齢 *one's* real age

精神年齢 mental age；MA　知能年齢 intelligence age　発症年齢 age of onset　閉経年齢 age of menopause　▶年齢差 age difference　年齢差別 age discrimination / ageism[agism]　年齢制限 age limit　年齢層 age group[(範囲)range]

の

ノイズ noise ☞雑音

ノイローゼ neurotic disorder, neurosis （神経衰弱）nervous breakdown ☞神経症

のう¹ 脳 brain, encephalon（图大脳の cerebral） ◆脳に異常がある have a brain disorder ◆脳に問題がある have something wrong with *one's* brain ◆脳に損傷を受ける have some brain injury[damage] / have some injury[damage] to the brain ◆脳に損傷がある be brain-damaged ◆右〈左〉脳 the right〈left〉brain [hemisphere] 血液脳関門 blood-brain barrier；BBB 小脳 cerebellum 除脳 decerebration 大脳 cerebrum 中脳 mesencephalon / midbrain ▶脳圧 intracranial pressure；ICP 脳圧迫 cerebral compression / compression of the brain 脳萎縮 cerebral atrophy 脳組織 brain tissue 脳膿瘍 brain abscess ☞脳炎，脳幹，脳機能障害，脳虚血，脳血管，脳血栓，脳血流，脳梗塞，脳挫傷，脳死，脳室，脳手術，脳出血，脳腫瘍，脳循環，脳症，脳神経，脳震盪，脳性麻痺，脳脊髄液，脳脊髄炎，脳槽，脳塞栓，脳卒中，脳損傷，脳代謝，脳低温療法，脳動脈，脳ドック，脳内，脳ナトリウム利尿ペプチド，脳膿瘍，脳波，脳浮腫，脳ヘルニア，脳瘤

のう² 膿 ☞膿（うみ），化膿

のう³ 嚢 sac, pouch （被膜）capsule ◀心嚢 heart sac 胎嚢 gestational sac；GS ヘルニア嚢 hernial sac ラトケ嚢 Rathke pouch 卵黄嚢 yolk sac 涙嚢 tear[lacrimal] sac / dacryocyst ☞嚢腫

のうえん 脳炎 encephalitis /ɪnsèfəláɪtɪs/ 亜急性硬化性全脳炎 subacute sclerosing panencephalitis；SSPE インフルエンザ脳炎 influenza encephalitis ウイルス性脳炎 viral encephalitis 単純ヘルペス脳炎 herpes simplex encephalitis；HSE 日本脳炎 Japanese encephalitis 辺縁系脳炎 limbic encephalitis 麻疹脳炎 measles encephalitis ▶脳炎ウイルス encephalitis virus

のうかしん 膿痂疹 impetigo ◀伝染性膿痂疹 contagious impetigo

のうかすいたい 脳下垂体 ☞下垂体

のうかん¹ 脳幹 brain stem, brainstem ◀聴性脳幹反応 auditory brain stem response；ABR 脳幹梗塞 brain stem infarction 脳幹死 brain stem death 脳幹出血 brain stem bleeding[hemorrhage] 脳幹損傷 brain stem injury 脳幹反射 brain stem reflex

のうかん² 納棺する place[put, lay] … in a coffin

のうきのうしょうがい 脳機能障害 brain dysfunction ◀高次脳機能障害 higher brain dysfunction 微細脳機能障害［損傷］minimal brain dysfunction[damage]；MBD

のうきょう 膿胸 thoracic empyema, pleural empyema, pyothorax ◀結核性膿胸 tuberculous empyema 陳旧性膿胸 old empyema 有瘻性膿胸 pyothorax[empyema] with fistula

のうきょけつ 脳虚血 brain ischemia, cerebral ischemia ◀一過性脳虚血発作 transient ischemic attack；TIA

のうげか 脳外科 ☞脳神経外科

のうけっかん 脳血管 cerebrovascular vessel, cerebral blood vessel ◀虚血性脳血管障害 ischemic cerebrovascular disorder ▶脳血管疾患 cerebrovascular disease；CVD 脳血管障害 cerebrovascular accident；CVA / cerebrovascular disorder 脳血管性認知症 cerebrovascular dementia 脳血管造影法 cerebral angiography；CAG

のうけっせん 脳血栓（症） cerebral thrombosis ☞血栓，脳卒中 ▶脳血栓塞栓症 cerebral thromboembolism

のうけつりゅう 脳血流 cerebral blood flow；CBF ▶脳血流シンチグラフィ cerebral perfusion[blood flow] scintigraphy

のうこうせっけっきゅう 濃厚赤血球 concentrated red （blood） cell；CRC, packed red blood cell

のうこうそく 脳梗塞 brain infarction,

cerebral infarction ☞脳卒中 ◆脳梗塞を起こす have a brain[cerebral] infarction / suffer a brain[cerebral] infarction ◀多発性脳梗塞 multiple cerebral infarction 陳旧性脳梗塞 old[previous] cerebral infarction 無症候性脳梗塞 asymptomatic cerebral infarction

のうざしょう 脳挫傷 brain contusion, cerebral contusion ◆階段から転落して脳挫傷を負う have[suffer] a brain contusion from falling down the stairs

のうし 脳死 brain death (形**brain-dead**), **cerebral death** ◆残念ですが，彼女は今脳死状態です I'm sorry, but she is now brain-dead. ◆もし彼女が脳死状態となってしまった場合，生命維持装置を外すことを希望なさいますか If she becomes brain-dead[In the event of brain death], do you want to have her life support removed [withdrawn]? ◆脳死を判定する determine and declare brain death ▶脳死患者 brain-dead patient 脳死臓器移植 organ transplant[transplantation] from a brain-dead donor[patient] 脳死判定(決定・確定)determination of brain death / (宣言・表明)declaration of brain death 脳死判定基準 brain death criteria / criteria for (the determination of) brain death

のうしつ 脳室 ventricle (形**ventricular**) ◀側脳室 lateral ventricle 第3〈4〉脳室 third〈fourth〉 ventricle ▶脳室開窓術 ventriculostomy 脳室拡大 ventricular enlargement 脳室穿刺 ventricular puncture 脳室ドレナージ ventricular drainage 脳室内出血 intraventricular bleeding[hemorrhage] 脳室腹腔シャント ventriculoperitoneal[VP] shunt

のうしゅ 嚢腫 cystoma ◀皮様嚢腫 dermoid cyst 卵巣嚢腫 ovarian cystoma

のうしゅく 濃縮 concentration (形**concentrated**) ▶濃縮乳 concentrated milk 濃縮尿 concentrated urine 濃縮物 concentrate

のうしゅじゅつ 脳手術 brain surgery [operation] ◀定位脳手術 stereotaxic [stereotactic] brain surgery

のうしゅちょう 脳腫脹 ☞脳浮腫

のうしゅっけつ 脳出血 brain hemorrhage, cerebral hemorrhage, bleeding in the brain ☞脳卒中 ◆脳出血を起こす have a brain[cerebral] hemorrhage / suffer a brain[cerebral] hemorrhage ◀高血圧性脳出血 hypertensive cerebral hemorrhage

のうしゅよう 脳腫瘍 brain tumor, cerebral tumor ◆脳腫瘍ができる have[develop] a brain tumor

のうじゅんかん 脳循環 brain circulation, cerebral circulation ▶脳循環障害 circulatory disturbance of the brain 脳循環代謝改善薬 cerebral circulation and metabolism improver 脳循環不全 cerebrovascular insufficiency

のうしょう 脳症 encephalopathy ◀ウェルニッケ脳症 Wernicke encephalopathy ウシ海綿状脳症 bovine spongiform encephalopathy；BSE / (狂牛病) mad cow disease 肝性脳症 hepatic encephalopathy 高血圧性脳症 hypertensive encephalopathy 高地脳症 high-altitude encephalopathy 進行性多巣性白質脳症 progressive multifocal leukoencephalopathy；PML 低酸素脳症 brain hypoxia 白質脳症 leukoencephalopathy ボクサー脳症 boxer's encephalopathy 無脳症 anencephaly

のうしんけい 脳神経 cranial nerve；CN ▶脳神経疾患 cranial nerve disease 脳神経損傷 cranial nerve injury ☞脳神経外科

のうしんけいげか 脳神経外科 neurosurgery (診療部門) **the department of neurosurgery, the neurosurgery department** ▶脳神経外科医 neurosurgeon / brain surgeon

のうしんとう 脳震盪 brain concussion ◆軽い脳震盪を起こす have[suffer] a mild brain concussion

のうせい 膿性(の) purulent, pus-like ▶膿性痰 purulent[pus-like] sputum 膿性分泌物 purulent[pus-like] discharge

のうせいまひ 脳性麻痺 cerebral palsy；CP

の

のうせきずいえき 脳脊髄液 cerebrospinal fluid；CSF ▶脳脊髄液圧 cerebrospinal fluid pressure 脳脊髄液検査 cerebrospinal fluid test 脳脊髄液漏 cerebrospinal fluid leakage

のうせきずいえん 脳脊髄炎 encephalomyelitis ◀急性散在性脳脊髄炎 acute disseminated encephalomyelitis；ADEM 脱髄性脳脊髄炎 demyelinating encephalomyelitis

のうせん 膿栓 pus plug

のうそう 脳槽 （くも膜下槽）subarachnoid cistern ▶脳槽造影法 cisternography 脳槽ドレナージ cisternal drainage

のうそくせん 脳塞栓（症） cerebral embolism, brain embolism, intracranial embolism ☞脳卒中 ◀心原性脳塞栓（症） cardiogenic cerebral[brain] embolism

のうそっちゅう 脳卒中 stroke, cerebral apoplexy, brain attack ◆脳卒中を起こしたことがありますか Have you ever had a stroke? ◆軽い脳卒中を起こす have a minor[mild] stroke／suffer a minor[mild] stroke ◆脳卒中の後遺症はありますか Do you have any lasting effects from the stroke? ◆この脳卒中で後遺症が出るかもしれません This stroke *may have aftereffects[may cause long-term damage]. ◀虚血性脳卒中 ischemic stroke 出血性脳卒中 hemorrhagic[bleeding] stroke

のうそんしょう 脳損傷 brain injury[damage] ◀外傷性脳損傷 traumatic brain injury；TBI 広汎性脳損傷 diffuse brain injury 微細脳損傷 minimal brain injury[damage] 無酸素性脳損傷 anoxic brain damage

のうたいしゃ 脳代謝 brain metabolism ▶脳代謝改善薬 brain metabolism enhancer／brain metabolic stimulant

のうていおんりょうほう 脳低温療法 brain hypothermia therapy

のうど 濃度 （液体の濃縮）concentration （効力）strength （密度）density （濃さ・粘り）consistency （水準・高さ）level ◆溶液を必要な濃度に薄める dilute the solution to the required concentration[strength] ◆濃度が高い〈低い〉be highly〈weakly〉concentrated／have a high〈low〉concentration ◀吸入酸素濃度 fractional concentration of inspiratory[inspired] oxygen；FiO₂ 血中アルコール濃度 blood-alcohol level[concentration] 血中濃度 blood level[concentration] 高〈低〉濃度 high〈low〉concentration 最小殺菌濃度 minimum bactericidal concentration；MBC 最小発育阻止濃度 minimum inhibitory concentration；MIC 酸素濃度 oxygen concentration ヘモグロビン濃度 hemoglobin concentration ☞薬物血中濃度

のうどう 能動（的な） active ▶能動運動 active movement 能動免疫 active immunity 能動輸送 active transport

のうどうみゃく 脳動脈 cerebral artery ◀後大脳動脈 posterior cerebral artery；PCA 前大脳動脈 anterior cerebral artery；ACA 中大脳動脈 middle cerebral artery；MCA ☞脳動脈瘤

のうどうみゃくりゅう 脳動脈瘤 cerebral aneurysm, brain aneurysm ▶未破裂脳動脈瘤 unruptured cerebral aneurysm ▶脳動脈瘤クリッピング cerebral aneurysm clipping 脳動脈瘤コイル塞栓術 endovascular coil embolization of a cerebral aneurysm 脳動脈瘤破裂 cerebral[brain] aneurysm rupture／rupture of a cerebral[brain] aneurysm

のうドック 脳ドック brain screening[checkup]

のうない 脳内（の） intracerebral ▶脳内血腫 brain[intracerebral] hematoma 脳内出血 intracerebral hemorrhage；ICH

のうナトリウムりにょうペプチド 脳ナトリウム利尿ペプチド brain natriuretic peptide；BNP

のうにょう 膿尿 pyuria

のうのうよう 脳膿瘍 brain abscess, cerebral abscess

のうは 脳波 brain wave, electroencephalogram；EEG ◆脳波を調べる check a *person's* brain waves ▶脳波計 electroencephalograph；EEG　脳波検査 electroencephalography；EEG / brain wave test　脳波パターン brain-wave pattern

のうふしゅ　脳浮腫　brain edema, cerebral edema　(脳腫脹)swelling of the brain, brain[cerebral] swelling　◆腫瘍の周りの脳浮腫によって麻痺が起きています The paralysis is due to swelling of the brain around the tumor.　◆脳浮腫を軽減させるためにステロイドを投与します I'm going to give you steroids to reduce *the swelling of the brain[the brain edema].

のうヘルニア　脳ヘルニア　brain herniation, cerebral herniation

のうほう¹　膿疱　pustule　(形pustular)，pus blister　◀掌蹠膿疱症 palmoplantar pustulosis　無菌性膿疱 sterile[aseptic] pustule　▶膿疱性乾癬 pustular psoriasis

のうほう²　囊胞　cyst　(形cystic)　◀肝囊胞 liver[hepatic] cyst　くも膜囊胞 arachnoid cyst　腎囊胞 kidney[renal] cyst　膵仮性囊胞 pancreatic pseudocyst　膵囊胞 pancreatic cyst　正中〈側〉頸囊胞 median 〈lateral〉cervical cyst　多囊胞腎 polycystic kidney disease；PKD[PCKD]　多囊胞(性)卵巣症候群 polycystic ovary syndrome；PCOS　多発性囊胞 multiple cysts　チョコレート囊胞 chocolate cyst　尿膜管囊胞 urachal cyst　ラトケ囊胞 Rathke cleft[pouch] cyst　卵巣囊胞 ovarian cyst　類皮囊胞 dermoid cyst　類表皮囊胞 epidermoid cyst　▶囊胞性線維症 cystic fibrosis

のうぼん　膿盆　kidney basin, emesis basin

のうやく　農薬　(殺虫剤)pesticide　(農芸用化学薬品)agricultural chemical　◀残留農薬 pesticide residue　▶農薬中毒 pesticide[agricultural chemical] poisoning

のうよう　膿瘍　abscess　◀肝膿瘍 liver[hepatic] abscess　歯槽膿瘍 alveolar abscess　腎周囲膿瘍 perirenal abscess　多房性膿瘍 multilocular abscess　脳膿瘍 brain abscess　肺膿瘍 lung[pulmonary] abscess　皮下膿瘍 subcutaneous abscess　腹腔内膿瘍 intraabdominal[intraperito-

neal] abscess　扁桃周囲膿瘍 peritonsillar abscess　▶膿瘍腔 abscess cavity　膿瘍切開 abscess incision　膿瘍排膿 abscess drainage / drainage of an abscess

のうりつ　能率(的な)　efficient　(名efficiency)　◆能率的な方法 an efficient way [method]　◆仕事の能率が以前より落ちたと思いますか Do you think you've become less efficient at work recently?

のうりゅう　脳瘤　encephalocele

のうりょく　能力　ability　(資質)faculty　(潜在的な能力)capacity　(実際的な能力)capability　(技能)skill, competence　(男性の性交能力)potency　◆体の動きをコントロールする能力を失う lose the ability to control *one's* body movements　◆毎日の仕事を行う能力を養う improve *a person's* ability to perform[carry out] daily tasks　◀運動能力 motor[athletic] ability　拡散能力 diffusion capacity　学習能力 learning ability　言語能力 language skills / linguistic competence /(言葉によるコミュニケーション能力)verbal communication skills　コミュニケーション能力 communication ability / communication skills / ability to communicate　作業能力 working[work] capacity[ability]　性的能力 sexual potency　責任能力 the ability to take responsibility for *one's* behavior [actions] /(刑事・民事上の責任能力)criminal responsibility　潜在能力 potential (capacity)　歩行能力 walking ability　予備能力 reserve capacity / functional reserve

ノーベルしょう　―賞　Nobel Prize　▶ノーベル医学生理学賞 Nobel Prize in Physiology or Medicine

ノーマライゼーション　normalization

のがす　逃す　miss　◆今治療しないと絶好の機会を逃すことになります If we don't treat it now, we'll miss[waste] an excellent opportunity.

ノカルジアしょう　―症　nocardiosis

のこり　残り　the rest, the remainder　(形remaining)

のこる　残る　stay, remain　(余っている)be

left

《居残る》 ◆しばらくここに残って下さい Please stay[remain] here for a while.

《残存する》 ◆使った後に残った点眼薬は捨てて下さい Please throw away the used container even if there is some eye drop solution remaining[left in it]. ◆薬はあと何日分残っていますか How many days' worth of medication *are left[do you have left]? ◆この切り傷は痕が残るかもしれません This cut may leave a scar. ◆尿意が残る感じがありますか Even after you've finished urinating, do you still feel that your bladder is not completely empty?

のせる　載せる　**put … on** ◆あごと額をこの台の上に載せて下さい Please put your chin and forehead on this support. ◆手を上げて頭の上に載せて下さい Please lift up your hands and put them on your head.

のぞく　除く

《取り除く》remove, get rid of （除外する）**rule out, exclude** ☞除外，除去 ◆障害物を除く remove[get rid of] an obstacle ◆他の原因を除く rule out[exclude] other causes

《…以外は》except (for) ◆木曜日と日曜日を除いていつでも院内にいます I'm in the hospital every day except Thursdays and Sundays. ◆コレステロールが高めであるのを除けば大丈夫です Except for a slightly high cholesterol level, you're (doing) fine.

のぞみ　望み　**hope** （実現の可能性が低い望み）**wish** ☞期待，希望 ◆(彼が)回復する望みはあります He has a good chance of recovering. / There is some hope of his recovery. ◆残念ですが，(彼女が)全快する望みはほとんどありません I'm afraid that there is little hope of her making a complete recovery. / I'm sorry, but it's unlikely that she'll recover completely. ◆どうぞ望みを捨てないで下さい Please don't give up hope. / You must keep your hope up. ◆申し訳ありませんが，お望み通りのことはできないのです We're sorry, but we can't give you what you want. ◆残念ですが，望み通りの効果は得られませんでした I'm sorry, but we were unable to get[achieve / obtain] the result we were hoping for.

のど　喉　**throat** /θróʊt/

《診察の基本表現》 ◆喉に何か問題がありますか Do you have any problems with your throat? ◆喉に不快感がありますか Do you have any discomfort in your throat? / Do you have an uncomfortable feeling in your throat?

《不快症状の表現》 ◆喉が痛みますか Do you have a sore throat? ◆つばを飲み込む時に喉が痛みますか Does your throat hurt when you swallow saliva? ◆喉が焼けるように痛む have a burning sensation in one's throat ◆何か物が喉につかえている〈引っかかっている〉感じがありますか Do you feel as if you've got something stuck〈caught〉in your throat? ◆喉に異物感がありますか Do you feel strange and uncomfortable in your throat? ◆食べ物がよく喉につかえますか Do you often choke on food? / Does food often get stuck in your throat? ◆鼻汁が喉に垂れますか Is the mucus from your nose draining into your throat? ◆喉が詰まる(何か物が引っかかっている)something gets stuck[caught] in the throat / (塊がある)have a lump in the throat ◆喉がかゆい have an itchy throat ◆喉がいがらっぽい the throat feels irritated / have an irritated throat ◆喉が渇く get[feel / become] thirsty

《処置の表現》 ◆喉にこのチューブを入れます I'm going to put[place / insert] this tube down your throat. ◆チューブが喉を通る時ごくんと飲むようにして下さい Please try to swallow the tube down in one gulp as it passes through your throat. ☞喉飴，喉ごし，喉仏

のどあめ　喉飴　**cough drop**[**sweet**]**, throat candy**

のどごし　喉ごし ◆喉ごしのよい食べ物 foods that go down smoothly / foods that can be swallowed easily

のどぼとけ 喉仏 Adam's apple

のばす 伸ばす・延ばす
《伸ばす》（縮んだものを伸ばす）stretch out （曲った物を真っすぐにする）straighten, make … straight （広げる・差し出す）extend （能力などを伸ばす）develop ◆足〈手〉を伸ばす stretch out one's legs〈hands / arms〉 ◆足を伸ばして下さい Please straighten [stretch out] your legs. ◆両腕を伸ばしたままにして下さい Please hold both your arms out straight. ◆背筋を伸ばす straighten one's back / make one's back straight ◆背筋を伸ばして座る〈立つ〉sit〈stand〉upright / sit〈stand〉up straight
《延期する》put off, postpone ☞延期 ◆経過によっては手術を延ばすこともあります Depending on how well you're doing, we may have to *put off[postpone] the surgery.

のびる 伸びる （縮んだものが伸びる）stretch （成長する）grow ◆膝の靱帯が伸びています You've stretched the ligaments in your knee. / The knee ligaments are stretched. ◆彼女は背が3 cm伸びています She has grown three centimeters.

のぼせ （顔面潮紅）hot flash, hot flush ◆のぼせることがありますか Do you ever have hot flashes?

のぼる 上る・登る go up, walk up, climb ◆階段〈坂〉を上る *go up[climb] stairs〈slopes〉

ノミ flea ◆ノミに刺される get[be] bitten by *a flea〈fleas〉 ◆ノミに刺された痕 a fleabite

のみあわせ 飲み合わせる take together ◆これらの薬の飲み合わせは大丈夫です〈よくありません〉These medications can〈cannot〉be taken together. ◆薬は飲み合わせによって相互作用のため副作用を起こすかもしれませんので，新しい薬を飲む前に必ずご相談下さい Certain medications, if taken together, may interact and cause harmful side effects, so be sure to check with me before taking a new medication.

のみぐすり 飲み薬 oral medication, internal medication ☞薬

のみこむ 飲み込む swallow ◆飲み込みにくいですか Do you have difficulty swallowing? ◆つばをゆっくり飲み込んで下さい Please swallow some saliva slowly. ◆つばをごくりと飲み込む swallow hard / swallow in one gulp ◆嚙まずに薬をそのまま飲み込む swallow the tablet whole without chewing ◆飲み込みにくいのは食べ物ですか，水分ですか Which do you have trouble swallowing, foods or liquids? ◆管が喉を通るとき，ごくんと飲み込むようにして下さい Please try to swallow the tube in one gulp as it passes down your throat.

のみほす 飲み干す drink up ◆ぐっと飲み干して下さい Drink it up quickly, please.

のみもの 飲み物 drink, beverage ◆何か冷たい飲み物をお持ちしましょうか Shall I bring you something cool[cold] to drink? ◆温かい飲み物 a warm[hot] drink ◆カフェインを含む飲み物 drinks containing caffeine / caffeinated drinks [beverages] ◆カフェイン抜きの飲み物 decaf / decaffeinated drinks[beverages] ◆カフェイン抜きのコーヒー decaf coffee

のむ 飲む
《水などを摂取する》drink （赤ん坊が乳を飲む）feed （乳を吸う）suck ◆水をお飲みになりますか Would you like to drink some water? ◆今は何も飲んではいけません You can't drink anything at the moment. ◆お子さんはミルクを普段どおり飲んでいますか Is your baby feeding as normal? ◆お子さんは母乳をうまく飲めないのですか Does your baby have difficulty sucking (milk)? ◆スープを飲む eat[have] soup /（直接カップから）drink soup
《酒を飲む》drink ◆お酒を飲みますか Do you drink (alcohol)? ◆ふだんはどんなお酒を飲みますか，ビール，ウイスキー，ワインですか What kind of alcohol do you usually drink, beer, whisky, or wine? ◆1週間にどのくらいお酒を飲みますか How much do you drink a week? ◆お酒の飲

み過ぎは体によくありません Too much drinking[Excessive drinking] is not good for your health. ◆お酒は適度に飲んで下さい Please drink alcohol in moderation.

《薬を服用する》take ☞薬 ◆今，何か薬を飲んでいますか Are you taking any medication at the moment? ◆熱を下げる薬を飲みましたか Did you take any drugs or medication to bring your fever down? ◆この薬は食後に飲んで下さい Please take this medication after meals. ◆この薬は起床後にコップ一杯の水で飲んで下さい Please take this medication with a full glass of water after waking up in the morning. ◆この薬は指示どおりに飲んで下さい Please take this medication exactly as directed[prescribed by your doctor]. ◆薬を飲み忘れる miss a dose of the medication

のり　糊　(接着剤)glue　(ペースト状の糊) paste ◀フィブリン糊 fibrin glue

のりおり　乗り降り　◆車の乗り降りはできますか Can you get in and out of cars?

のりもの　乗り物　vehicle　◆乗り物に酔う(車)get carsick[(飛行機)airsick／(船)seasick] ▶乗り物酔い motion[travel] sickness

のる　乗る・載る
《物の上に》stand on, get on　◆靴を脱いでこの体重計〈トレッドミル〉に乗って下さい Please take your shoes off and stand on this scale〈treadmill〉.
《乗り物に》get in, take, ride　◆車椅子に乗る get in a wheelchair. ◆車椅子に乗る手伝いをする help *a person* into a wheelchair.

ノルアドレナリン　noradrenaline

ノルウェー　Norway　(㊅Norwegian) ☞国籍 ▶ノルウェー人(の) Norwegian

のろい　slow　☞遅い，鈍い　◆彼の動作がのろくなったと感じますか Have you noticed that his movements have *become slower[slowed down]?

ノロウイルスかんせんしょう　―感染症
norovirus infection

ノンアルコール(の)　nonalcoholic, alco-

hol-free ▶ノンアルコール飲料 nonalcoholic drinks　ノンアルコールタイプ口内洗浄剤 alcohol-free (formula) mouthwash

ノンストレステスト　nonstress test；NST

ノンレムすいみん　―睡眠　nonrapid eye movement sleep, non-REM[NREM] sleep

は

は¹ 刃 (刀身)blade (刃先)edge ◆鋭利な刃で指を切る cut *one's* finger with a sharp blade

は² 波 wave

は³ 歯 tooth (複teeth 形dental 動歯が生える teethe /tíːð/)

《歯が抜ける・生える》 ◆歯が抜ける *one's* tooth falls[comes] out / (歯を失う)lose a tooth / (歯が抜けている)*one's* tooth is missing ◆前歯が1本抜けている one of the front teeth is missing / have a missing front tooth ◆歯が生える teethe / cut a tooth ◆赤ちゃんは歯が生え始めています Your baby is teething. / Your baby is cutting his〈her〉teeth. / Your baby's teeth are cutting in. ◆歯が生え変わる(乳歯が抜けて永久歯になる)the baby[milk] teeth fall out and the permanent teeth come in / (乳歯と永久歯が入れ替わる)the baby[milk] teeth are replaced by the permanent teeth ◆歯(乳歯)が生え揃う have a full set of baby teeth

《動作の表現》 ◆歯を磨く brush *one's* teeth ◆歯をどのくらいの頻度で磨きますか How often do you brush your teeth? ◆歯の正しい磨き方を学ぶ learn how to brush *one's* teeth properly[correctly] ◆歯にデンタルフロスを使う floss *one's* teeth / use dental floss ◆歯をほじる pick *one's* teeth ◆歯を食いしばる clench *one's* teeth

《診察の基本表現》 ◆歯の調子はどうですか How are your teeth? ◆歯に何か問題がありますか Do you have any problems with your teeth? ◆歯を診察しましょう I'm going to examine your teeth. ◆歯が痛みますか Do you have (a) toothache? / Do your teeth ache? ◆どの歯が痛むのですか Which tooth hurts[aches]? ◆冷たい物を飲むと歯がしみますか Do your teeth hurt[(刺すような痛みがあるか)Do you have

a stabbing pain in the teeth] when you drink something cold? ◆歯を磨く時歯茎から出血しますか Do your gums bleed when you brush your teeth? ◆最近, 歯の治療を受けましたか Have you recently had[received] any dental treatment?

《症状・異常の表現》 ◆歯がいい〈悪い〉have good〈bad / (虫歯)decayed〉teeth ◆歯の着色 staining of the teeth ◆歯が変色している *one's* tooth is[becomes] discolored / have a discolored tooth ◆歯にすき間がある have a gap between[in] the teeth / have gapped teeth ◆歯がぐらぐらする *one's* tooth is[feels] loose / have a loose tooth ◆歯が痛い have (a) toothache / *one's* tooth aches / have an aching tooth ◆歯がうずく have (a) throbbing toothache ◆歯がしみる(刺すような痛みがある)have a stabbing[sharp] pain in the teeth / (歯が過敏になっている)have sensitive teeth ◆奥歯が虫歯になっている *one's* back teeth are decayed / have decayed back teeth / have cavities in *one's* back teeth ◆歯の根の中の神経にまで炎症が及んでいる have an inflamed nerve root / have an inflammation that affects the nerve in the root of a tooth ◆歯の欠損 tooth defect ◆歯の損傷〈破折〉tooth injury〈fracture〉 ◆歯が欠けている *one's* tooth is broken / (歯の一部が欠けている)have a chipped[cracked] tooth / have a crack in *one's* tooth ◆…に歯をぶつける hit[bump] *one's* tooth against … ◆歯の詰め物〈クラウン〉がとれる a tooth filling〈crown〉*comes off[comes out] ◆魚の小骨が歯に挟まっています A small fish bone has got caught between your teeth.

《治療・処置の表現》 ◆歯を治療する treat a tooth ◆歯を削る drill a tooth ◆歯を抜く pull[extract] a tooth / (抜歯治療を受ける)have *one's* tooth pulled[taken] out ◆最近歯を抜きましたか Have you recently had any of your teeth pulled[taken] out? ◆歯を残す retain a tooth ◆歯に麻酔をかけます I'm going to numb (the area around) the tooth with (local) anesthesia. ◆歯の治療で麻酔をしたことがありますか Have you ever had anesthesia for a dental treatment? / Have you ever had dental anesthesia? ◆歯を矯正する straighten teeth ◆目的の位置まで歯を動かす move the teeth into the proper position ◆歯を修復する fix[repair] a tooth /（復元する）restore a tooth ◆歯に詰め物をする fill a tooth ◆歯にクラウンを被せる crown / cap / put a crown[cap] on a tooth ◆歯の詰め物（dental / tooth）filling ◆歯を漂白する bleach[whiten] *a person's* teeth ◆歯のプラークを除去する remove dental plaque

◀糸切り歯（犬歯）canine tooth /（尖頭歯）cuspid tooth　入れ歯（一揃いの）dentures /（1 本の）false[artificial] tooth　上の歯 upper tooth /（上の歯全体）the upper teeth　奥歯（臼歯）molar / back tooth　親知らずの歯（智歯）wisdom tooth　仮歯 temporary crown[dentures]　金歯 gold crown / gold-capped tooth　銀歯 silver crown / silver-capped tooth　差し歯 post crown　下の歯 lower tooth /（下の歯全体）the lower teeth　前歯 front tooth　虫歯（う歯）tooth decay / dental caries /（虫歯の穴）dental cavity　乱杭歯 irregular teeth / irregular set[alignment] of teeth /（1 本の）snaggletooth　☞歯医者, 歯型, 歯ぎしり, 歯茎, 歯並び, 歯ブラシ, 歯磨き

バー bar ◀移動用バー grab bar

ばあい 場合 （事例）case （時）time （状況）circumstances ★通例, 複数形で. ◆この薬はほとんどの場合によく効きます This medication works well in most cases. ◆場合によっては別の病室へ移らなければなりません Under[In] certain circumstances you may have to move to another room. ◆それは時と場合によります That depends. / It all depends. ◆予期しない副作用が見られる場合には連絡して下さい Please call[contact] us *in case[if]* you notice any unexpected side effects. ◆緊急の場合には in case of emergency

バーキットリンパしゅ ―腫 Burkitt lym-phoma

パーキンソン Parkinson （㊂parkinsonian）◀抗パーキンソン薬 antiparkinson (medication / drug / agent) ▶パーキンソン顔貌 parkinsonian facies　パーキンソン症候群 Parkinson[parkinsonian] syndrome / parkinsonism　パーキンソン振戦 parkinsonian tremor　パーキンソン病 Parkinson disease；PD　パーキンソン歩行 parkinsonian gait

はあく 把握する （つかむ）grasp （理解する）understand ◆状況を把握する grasp the situation ◆病状を把握する understand *the condition of[the situation with]* *one's* illness ▶把握反射 grasp[grasping] reflex

バージャーびょう ―病 Buerger disease （閉塞性血栓血管炎）thromboangiitis obliterans

パーセント percent,《英》per cent （割合）percentage ☞比率

パーソナリティ personality ☞人格 ◀妄想性パーソナリティ障害 paranoid personality disorder

ハート HAART （高活性抗レトロウイルス療法）highly active antiretroviral therapy

パート （勤務形態）part-time work[job] （人）part-time worker, part-timer （㊂part-time） ◆パートで働いていますか Do you work part-time? / Are you working part-time? / Are you a part-time worker[employee]?

パートナー partner ◆パートナーと暮らしていますか Do you live with a partner? ◆性行為のパートナー a sex partner ▶パートナードッグ（介助犬）service [assistance / partner] dog /（盲導犬）guide dog /（聴導犬）hearing dog (for deaf people)

はい1 肺 lung （㊂pulmonary /pʌ́lmənèri/㊂pneum(o)-/núːmoʊ/）★通例, pulmonary は医学用語として用いる. ◆肺の調子はどうですか How are your lungs? ◆肺に何か問題がありますか Do you have any problems with your lungs? ◆今までに肺の病気に罹ったことがありますか Have you ever had any lung disease(s) before? / (異常を指摘されたことがあるか)Have you ever been told that you have a problem with your lungs? ◆X線写真で右肺に影が認められます The X-ray shows a shadow on your right lung. ★on は「撮影された肺の上に」を表す. ◆CT で左の肺に空洞性病変がみられます The CT scan shows a hole-like[cavitary] lesion in your left lung. ★in は「肺の中に」を表す. ◆喫煙はあなたの肺に悪影響を及ぼします Smoking *is bad for[badly affects] your lungs. ◀石綿肺 asbestos lung / (pulmonary) asbestosis　加湿器肺 humidifier lung　塵肺 pneumoconiosis　蜂巣肺 honeycomb lung　無気肺 atelectasis ▶肺うっ血 pulmonary congestion　肺音 lung[respiratory] sounds ★通例, 複数形で.　肺拡散能 pulmonary diffusing[diffusion] capacity　肺ガス交換 pulmonary gas exchange　肺化膿症 pulmonary suppuration　肺虚脱 pulmonary collapse　肺血流シンチグラフィ pulmonary perfusion[blood flow] scintigraphy　肺サーファクタント pulmonary surfactant　肺挫傷 pulmonary contusion　肺出血 pulmonary hemorrhage　肺腫瘍 lung tumor　肺循環 pulmonary circulation　肺静脈 pulmonary vein　肺真菌症 pulmonary mycosis　肺性心 cor pulmonale　肺切除 pulmonary[lung] resection / (一側肺全切除)pneumonectomy　肺専門医 pulmonary (disease) specialist / pulmonologist / lung specialist　肺分画症 pulmonary sequestration　肺理学療法 lung [pulmonary] physiotherapy ☞肺アスペルギルス症, 肺アスペルギローマ, 肺アミロイドーシス, 肺移植, 肺炎, 肺活量, 肺がん, 肺気腫, 肺機能, 肺吸虫, 肺気量, 肺クリプトコッカス症, 肺結核, 肺血栓塞栓症, 肺高血圧, 肺梗塞, 肺サルコイドーシス, 肺疾患, 肺水腫, 肺生検, 肺線維症, 肺臓炎, 肺塞栓症, 肺損傷, 肺動静脈瘻, 肺動脈, 肺嚢胞, 肺膿瘍, 肺胞, 肺門, 肺野, 肺, 肺リンパ脈管筋腫症

はい²　胚　embryo /émbriòu/　☞胚移植, 胚細胞, 胚性幹細胞, 胚葉

ばい　倍　(2 倍) twice, double　(… 倍) times　☞2倍　◆3倍 three times

バイアス　bias　☞偏見

はいアスペルギルスしょう　肺アスペルギルス症　pulmonary aspergillosis　◀アレルギー性気管支肺アスペルギルス症 allergic bronchopulmonary aspergillosis；ABPA　侵襲性肺アスペルギルス症 invasive pulmonary aspergillosis；IPA　慢性進行性肺アスペルギルス症 chronic progressive pulmonary aspergillosis；CPPA

はいアスペルギローマ　肺アスペルギローマ　pulmonary aspergilloma

はいアミロイドーシス　肺アミロイドーシス　pulmonary amyloidosis

はいい　背位　☞仰向け, 背臥位

はいいしょく¹　肺移植 lung transplant [transplantation]　☞移植

はいいしょく²　胚移植 embryo transfer

はいいろ　灰色(の)　gray,《英》grey　(灰色がかった)grayish　(灰白色の)ashy　(濃い灰色の)dark gray　◆灰色の痰 gray phlegm

はいえき　排液　drainage（動drain）　◆管を胸腔に挿入し, 胸水を排液する insert a tube into the chest to drain (off) excess [the pleural] fluid　▶排液管 drainage tube　排液バッグ drainage bag

はいえん　肺炎　pneumonia /nu:móuniə/ ◆肺炎になる(肺炎に罹る)get[catch / contract] pneumonia / (肺炎を起こす)develop pneumonia　◆最近気管支炎や肺炎に罹りましたか Have you recently had[contracted] bronchitis or pneumonia?　◆インフルエンザが元で肺炎になっています The flu has developed into pneumonia. ◀異型肺炎 atypical pneumonia　院内肺炎 hospital-acquired[nosocomial] pneumonia　ウイルス性肺炎 viral pneumonia　過敏性肺(臓)炎 hypersensitivity pneumonitis　間質性肺炎 interstitial pneumonia　気管支肺炎 bronchial pneumonia / bronchopneumonia　器質化肺炎 organizing pneumonia　クラミジア肺炎 chlamydial pneumonia　好酸球性肺炎 eosinophilic pneumonia　誤嚥性肺炎 aspiration pneumonia　細菌性肺炎 bacterial pneumonia

市中肺炎 community-acquired pneumonia；CAP　術後肺炎 postoperative pneumonia　人工呼吸器関連肺炎 ventilator-associated pneumonia；VAP　胎便性肺炎 meconium pneumonia　ニューモシスチス肺炎 *Pneumocystic* pneumonia；PCP　ブドウ球菌肺炎 staphylococcal pneumonia　閉塞性肺炎 obstructive pneumonia　放射線肺(臓)炎 radiation pneumonia[pneumonitis]　マイコプラズマ肺炎 mycoplasma pneumonia　薬剤性肺(臓)炎 drug-induced pneumonitis　レジオネラ肺炎 *Legionella* pneumonia　連鎖球菌肺炎 streptococcal pneumonia
▶肺炎桿菌 *Klebsiella pneumoniae* ☞肺球菌

はいえんきゅうきん　肺炎球菌　pneumococcus（履pneumococci 履pneumococcal）(学名)*Streptococcus pneumoniae*
◀ペニシリン耐性肺炎球菌 penicillin-resistant *Streptococcus pneumoniae*；PRSP
▶肺炎球菌肺炎 pneumococcal pneumonia　肺炎球菌ワクチン pneumococcal conjugate vaccine；PCV

バイオテクノロジー　biotechnology, biotech

バイオリズム　biorhythm

はいかい　徘徊する　wander about, walk about　◀夜間徘徊 night[nighttime] wandering[walking]

はいがい　背臥位　supine position, face-up position　☞仰向け　◆背臥位になる lie on *one's* back

ばいかい　媒介する　(運ぶ)carry　(広げる)spread　(伝染・感染させる)transmit　(腰尾-borne)　◆この病気は蚊が媒介します This disease is carried[transmitted / spread] by mosquitoes.　◀蚊媒介疾患 mosquito-borne disease　昆虫媒介感染症 insect-borne infectious disease　食品媒介疾患 food-borne disease　ダニ媒介疾患 tick-borne disease　動物媒介疾患 animal-borne disease　▶媒介者 carrier　媒介動物 vector

はいかつりょう　肺活量　vital capacity；VC　◆肺活量を測定する measure *a per-*son's vital capacity　◀努力肺活量 forced vital capacity；FVC　予測肺活量 predicted vital capacity

はいがん　肺がん　lung cancer　◀III期の肺がん *third stage[stage three] lung cancer　◀小細胞肺癌 small cell lung cancer[carcinoma]；SCLC　非小細胞肺癌 non-small cell lung cancer[carcinoma]；NSCLC　▶肺がん検診 lung cancer screening / screening for lung cancer

はいきガス　排気ガス　exhaust（gas, fumes）★fumes は複数形で.　◀自動車排気ガス automobile[automotive] exhaust gas / auto exhaust[emissions]

はいきしゅ　肺気腫　pulmonary emphysema

はいきのう　肺機能　lung function, pulmonary function　◆肺機能に問題がある have problems with *one's* lung function　◆肺機能が低い have poor lung function / *one's* lung function is poor　◆術前に肺機能を検査しましょう Let's test[check] your lung function before the surgery. / Let's see[check] how well your lungs are working[functioning] before the surgery.　◆喫煙を続けると肺機能が徐々に低下します If you keep smoking, your lung function will gradually *get worse[decline].　◆禁煙することで肺機能の低下を遅らせることができます Stopping smoking can slow down the decline in your lung function.　◆肺機能を改善させる improve *one's* lung function　◀予測術後肺機能 predicted postoperative lung function
▶肺機能検査 lung[pulmonary / respiratory] function test / spirometric test

はいきぶつ　廃棄物　waste（material）
◆廃棄物を適正に処理する dispose of waste（materials）properly　◀医療廃棄物 biomedical[medical] waste；BMW　感染性廃棄物 infectious waste　産業廃棄物 industrial waste　放射性廃棄物 radioactive waste　未処理医療廃棄物 undisposed medical waste　有害廃棄物 hazardous waste　有毒廃棄物 toxic waste

はいきゅうちゅう　肺吸虫　lung fluke

◀ウェステルマン肺吸虫 *Paragonimus westermani* 宮崎肺吸虫 *Paragonimus miyazaki* ▶肺吸虫症 lung-fluke disease / paragonimiasis

はいきりょう　肺気量 lung volume[capacity] ◀全肺気量 total lung capacity；TLC ▶肺気量曲線 lung volume curve 肺気量分画 lung volume fraction / fraction of lung volume

はいきん　背筋 back muscle, dorsal muscle, muscle of the back ◆背筋を伸ばす straighten *one's* back（muscles） ◆背筋が弱ると姿勢が悪く不安定になります When the back muscles are weak, the posture becomes poor and unstable. ▶背筋力 back strength

はいぐうしゃ　配偶者 spouse /spáus/ （夫）*one's* husband （妻）*one's* wife ◆配偶者の有無（婚姻状況）marital status ◆配偶者はご存命ですか Is your husband ⟨wife⟩ alive and well? ◆配偶者が亡くなっている be widowed /（夫と死別した女性に対して）be a widow /（妻と死別した男性に対して）be a widower ◀非配偶者間人工授精 artificial insemination by donor；AID ▶配偶者間人工授精 artificial insemination by husband；AIH

はいくつ　背屈 dorsiflexion

はいクリプトコッカスしょう　肺クリプトコッカス症 pulmonary cryptococcosis

はいけい　背景 background ▶背景因子 background factor

はいけっかく　肺結核 pulmonary tuberculosis, tuberculosis of the lung ☞結核

はいけつしょう　敗血症 sepsis, septicemia（㊔septic, septicemic） ◆彼は敗血症を起こしかけています He is developing [getting] sepsis. ▶敗血症性ショック septic shock

はいけっせんそくせんしょう　肺血栓塞栓症 pulmonary thromboembolism；PTE

はいこうけつあつ　肺高血圧（症） pulmonary hypertension；PH ◀原発性肺高血圧症 primary pulmonary hypertension；PPH 肺動脈（性）肺高血圧症 pulmonary arterial hypertension；PAH

はいこうそく　肺梗塞 pulmonary infarction[infarct]

はいさいぼう　胚細胞 germ cell ▶胚細胞腫 germinoma 胚細胞腫瘍 germ cell tumor

はいサルコイドーシス　肺サルコイドーシス pulmonary sarcoidosis

はいしっかん　肺疾患 lung disease ◀間質性肺疾患 interstitial lung disease；ILD 拘束性肺疾患 restrictive lung disease びまん性肺疾患 diffuse lung disease 閉塞性肺疾患 obstructive lung disease 慢性閉塞性肺疾患 chronic obstructive pulmonary disease；COPD

はいしゃ　歯医者 （歯科医）dentist （歯科医院）the dentist, the dentist's, the dentist's office ◆歯医者に行く go to the dentist / see the dentist

はいしゅつ　排出 ☞排泄

はいじょ　排除する （取り除く）remove, get rid of （除外する）rule out, exclude ☞除外，除去，除く

はいしょうがい　肺傷害 ☞肺損傷

はいすいしゅ　肺水腫 pulmonary edema, lung edema ◆高地肺水腫 high-altitude pulmonary edema

はいせいかんさいぼう　胚性幹細胞 embryonic stem cell, ES cell

はいせいけん　肺生検 lung biopsy ☞生検 ◀開胸肺生検 open lung biopsy 経気管支肺生検 transbronchial lung biopsy；TBLB 経皮的肺生検 percutaneous lung biopsy

バイセクシャル bisexuality （両性愛者）bisexual

はいせつ　排泄 excretion, elimination （膿・分泌物）discharge （㊔excretory, eliminative ㊔excrete, eliminate, discharge 捨てる get rid（of）） ☞排尿，排便 ◆老廃物を体内から排泄する *get rid of[excrete] waste material from the body ◆排泄の介助をいたします Let me help you with using the toilet[（便器）bedpan]. ◆摂取量と排泄量を測る check[measure / monitor] *a person's* intake and output ◆術後2, 3日は床上排泄となります（便器や尿器を

使用する必要がある）You will need to use a bedpan or urinal for two or three days after the surgery. ◀尿排泄 urinary excretion 薬物排泄 drug excretion ▶排泄訓練(幼児の)toilet training /（排尿・排便障害の）bladder and bowel training 排泄行動 eliminative behavior 排泄習慣 bladder and bowel habits 排泄障害 elimination[excretory] disorder /（尿便失禁）bladder and bowel incontinence 排泄物 excreta / waste matter[material] excreted from the body ☞排泄管, 排泄性尿路造影

はいせつかん 排泄管 （excretory）duct

はいせつせいにょうろぞうえい 排泄性尿路造影 excretory urography

はいぜん 配膳 food delivery （service）, meal delivery （service）, serving trays of food ★通例，複数形で. ▶配膳室 hospital kitchen / food services room 配膳車 meal cart / meal[food] delivery cart

はいせんいしょう 肺線維症 pulmonary fibrosis, lung fibrosis ◀特発性肺線維症 idiopathic pulmonary fibrosis；IPF

はいぞうえん 肺臓炎 pneumonitis ◀過敏性肺臓炎 hypersensitivity pneumonitis ブレオマイシン肺臓炎 bleomycin pneumonitis 放射線肺臓炎 radiation pneumonitis

はいそく 背側（の）dorsal ☞背部

はいそくせんしょう 肺塞栓症 pulmonary embolism

はんそくまひ 半側麻痺 hemiplegia

はいそんしょう 肺損傷 lung injury ◀急性肺損傷 acute lung injury；ALI

バイタルサイン vital signs ★通例，複数形で. ◆バイタルサインを測りましょう I'm going to[Let me] take your vital signs. ◆バイタルサインは正常です Your vital signs are normal. ◆バイタルサインをみる take[check / monitor] *a person's* vital signs ◆バイタルサインを記録する record *a person's* vital signs

ばいち 培地 （culture）medium ◀寒天培地 agar medium

ばいてん 売店 （院内の）hospital shop, gift

shop ◆売店では洗面用具，パジャマなど様々な物を売っています They sell a variety of products including personal toiletries and pajamas at the hospital shop. ◆手術に必要な物を売店で買うことができます You can buy the things you need for your surgery at the hospital shop.

はいどうじょうみゃくろう 肺静脈瘻 pulmonary arteriovenous fistula （肺動静脈奇形）pulmonary arteriovenous malformation

はいどうみゃく 肺動脈 pulmonary artery ▶肺動脈圧 pulmonary arterial pressure 肺動脈カテーテル法 pulmonary artery catheterization 肺動脈狭窄 pulmonary artery stenosis 肺動脈血栓塞栓症 pulmonary artery thromboembolism 肺動脈楔入圧 pulmonary artery wedge pressure；PAWP 肺動脈性肺高血圧症 pulmonary arterial hypertension；PAH 肺動脈造影 pulmonary arteriography ☞肺動脈弁

はいどうみゃくべん 肺動脈弁 pulmonary valve ▶肺動脈弁狭窄症 pulmonary （valve）stenosis；PS 肺動脈弁膜症 pulmonary valve disease

ばいどく 梅毒 syphilis ▶梅毒血清反応 serologic test for syphilis；STS / serologic reaction for syphilis 梅毒トレポネーマ感作赤血球凝集試験 *Treponema pallidum* hemagglutination[TPHA] test

バイトブロック bite block

はいにょう 排尿 urination, micturition, voiding （🔊urinate, pass urine[water], void 🔊urinary）☞尿

《回数を尋ねる》 ◆1日に何回排尿しますか How many times a day do you urinate[pass urine]? ◆排尿回数はいつもより多いですか，少ないですか Do you have to urinate more frequently or less frequently than usual? ◆排尿のため夜中に起きますか Do you get up in the night to urinate[pass urine]? ◆夜中に何回排尿のために起きますか How many times a night do you get up to urinate?

《排尿の異常を尋ねる》 ◆排尿に問題があり

ますか Do you have any problems with urinating? /〔異常はあるか〕Have you noticed anything abnormal with your urination? ◆排尿時に痛みや不快感があります か Do you feel any pain or discomfort when you urinate[pass urine]? ◆排尿中に焼けるような感じがありますか Do you have any burning sensation *when you pass urine[during urination]? ◆排尿の最後に痛みがありますか Do you have (a) pain at the end of urination? ◆排尿が終わってから尿がポタポタ垂れますか Do you have any dribbling or leaking after you've finished urinating? ◆排尿が困難である have difficulty urinating ◆排尿の開始が難しい have difficulty starting to urinate ◆排尿を我慢するのが難しい have difficulty holding back urination ◆排尿をコントロールするのが難しい have difficulty *controlling *one's* bladder[with bladder control] ★bladder は膀胱.

◀平均排尿回数 average voiding rate ▶排尿回数 urinary frequency 排尿機能 bladder[urinary] function 排尿訓練〔幼児の〕toilet[potty] training /〔排尿障害の〕bladder training 排尿困難 urinary difficulty / difficulty (in) urinating /〔遷延性の〕urinary hesitancy 排尿時間 voiding time 排尿時灼熱感 urinary burning / burning[stinging] with urination 排尿失神 micturition syncope 排尿時膀胱尿道造影 voiding cystourethrography 排尿終末時〈初期〉痛 pain at the end〈beginning〉of urination / terminal〈initial〉micturition pain 排尿障害 urination disorder / urinary problem[disorder / disturbance] 排尿中断 interruption of *the urinary stream[micturition] 排尿痛 pain on urination / dysuria / painful urination

はいのう 排膿 drainage （略drain） ◆切開排膿 incision and drainage 膿瘍排膿 abscess drainage / drainage of an abscess ▶排膿管 drainage tube 排膿バッグ drainage bag

はいのうほう 肺嚢胞 pulmonary cyst
はいのうよう 肺膿瘍 lung[pulmonary]

abscess

はいはい 這い這いする crawl ☞這う
バイパス （側管）bypass （バイパス手術）
bypass surgery （略bypass） ◆移植片を使って心臓の詰まった血管のバイパス手術をする use grafts to bypass blocked blood vessels to the heart ▶冠動脈バイパス術 coronary artery bypass graft[grafting]; CABG ★CABG は cabbage /kǽbɪʤ/ と発音する. 静動脈バイパス venoarterial bypass

はいぶ 背部 back （略dorsal） ▶背部筋 back[dorsal] muscles / muscles of the back 背部痛 back pain / backache 背部損傷 back injury

パイプカット （精管切除）vasectomy
はいべん 排便 bowel movement /báʊəl -/; BM, defecation ☞便, 便通
《基本表現》 ◆排便する have a bowel movement / move[empty] the bowels / pass *a stool[stools] ◆排便を促す promote[stimulate] a bowel movement ◆排便を我慢する hold back *one's* bowel movements ◆排便のコントロールが難しい have difficulty *controlling *one's* bowels[with bowel control]
《排便習慣について尋ねる》 ◆1日に何回排便しますか How many times a day do you *move your bowels[empty your bowels / have a bowel movement]? ◆排便は規則正しいですか Are your bowel movements regular? / Do you have regular bowel movements?
《便通の異常について尋ねる》 ◆排便に問題がありますか Do you have any problems *moving your bowels[with your bowel movements]? /〔異常があるか〕Do you have any abnormal bowel movements? ◆排便が困難ですか Do you have difficulty *moving your bowels[passing stools]? ◆排便に変化がありましたか Have you noticed any changes in your bowel movements? ◆排便時に痛みや不快感がありますか Do you feel any pain or discomfort when you *have a bowel movement[empty your bowels]?

▶排便いきみ straining at stool / fecal straining　排便回数 stool[bowel movement] frequency　排便訓練(幼児の)toilet training /(排便障害の)bowel training　排便困難 difficulty moving *one's* bowels / defecation trouble　排便失神 defecation syncope　排便習慣 bowel habits　排便障害 defecation disorder　排便調節 bowel control　排便痛 pain on defecation / painful defecation　排便反射 defecation reflex

はいほう　肺胞　(pulmonary) alveoli (単 alveolus)　★通例，複数形で．(形alveolar)　◀気管支肺胞洗浄 bronchoalveolar lavage；BAL　びまん性肺胞傷害 diffuse alveolar damage；DAD　▶肺胞界面活性物質 alveolar surfactant　肺胞ガス交換 alveolar gas exchange　肺胞出血 alveolar hemorrhage　肺胞低換気症候群 alveolar hypoventilation syndrome　肺胞蛋白症 pulmonary alveolar proteinosis

ハイムリックしゅぎ　―手技　Heimlich maneuver

はいもん　肺門　pulmonary hilum, hilum of the lung (形hilar)　◀両側肺門リンパ節腫脹 bilateral hilar lymphadenopathy；BHL　▶肺門陰影 hilar shadow　肺門リンパ節 hilar lymph node

はいや　肺野　lung field[area]　▶肺野濃度 lung density

ばいやく　売薬　☞市販薬

はいよう¹　肺葉　pulmonary lobe, lung lobe, lobe of the lung　▶肺葉切除術(pulmonary) lobectomy

はいよう²　胚葉　germ layer　◀外胚葉 ectoderm　中胚葉 mesoderm　内胚葉 endoderm

はいよう³　廃用　disuse　▶廃用症候群 disuse syndrome　廃用性萎縮 disuse atrophy

ばいよう　培養　culture (形culture)　◀喀痰培養 sputum culture　血液培養 blood culture　細菌培養 bacterial culture　細胞培養 cell culture　組織培養 tissue culture　尿培養 urine culture　便培養 stool culture　▶培養検査 culture test[examination]

はいらん　排卵　ovulation (形ovulatory)　◆排卵は通常月経周期の 14 日目頃にあります Ovulation usually occurs around the fourteenth day of the menstrual cycle.　◆排卵を誘発する induce ovulation　▶排卵期 ovulation[ovulatory] phase　排卵期出血 ovulation bleeding　排卵周期 ovulation cycle　排卵障害 ovulation disorder　排卵誘発 ovulation induction　排卵誘発薬 ovulation-inducing medication[drug / agent]　排卵抑制 ovulation inhibition [suppression]

ハイリスク　high risk (形high-risk)　☞リスク　▶ハイリスク患者 high-risk patient　ハイリスク新生児 high-risk newborn　ハイリスク妊娠 high-risk pregnancy

はいりょ　配慮する　(注意を払う)pay attention to　(気をつける)take care of　(考慮する)be mindful of, be considerate to [toward(s), of] (形consideration)　◆患者さんの病状や好き嫌いに十分配慮した食事を提供いたします We serve meals, paying very close attention to each patient's condition and likes and dislikes.　◆あなたは栄養のバランスに配慮が必要です You need to be mindful of nutritional balance. / You need to take care *to eat[that you eat] a balanced diet.　◆テレビをご覧の際には同室の他の患者さんへの配慮をお願いします When you watch TV, please *show consideration for[be considerate of] the other patients in the room.　◆ご配慮いただきありがとうございます Thank you so much for your thoughtfulness [kind consideration].

はいリンパみゃっかんきんしゅしょう　肺リンパ脈管筋腫症　pulmonary lymphangioleiomyomatosis[LAM]

はいる　入る　《外から中に入る》come in[into], go in[into], enter, get in　★come in[into] は部屋にいる人の立場で表現する時に使う．　◆(部屋に入る時)中に入ってもよろしいですか May I come in?　◆キムさん，どうぞお入り下さい Mr Kim, please come (on) in.　◆手術

室に入る enter[go into] the operating room ◆右目に何かが入ったのですか Did you have something in your right eye? ◆傷口にごみが入る get some dust in *one's* wound

《含んでいる》（成分・栄養素を含む）**contain** （全体の一部として含む）**include** ◆食品にピーナツが入っているかどうか, 必ず原材料表示を確認して下さい Always check the list of ingredients to see if the food contains peanuts. ◆この軟膏には抗菌薬が入っています This ointment contains antibacterial agents. ◆この請求書には差額室料も入っています The special room charge is included in this bill.

《加わる》（加入する）**join** （参加する）**take part in, participate in** ◆糖尿病の患者会に入ることをお勧めします I recommend that you join[take part in] the diabetic patients' association. ◆国民健康保険に入っていますか Do you have National Health Insurance?

はいれつ 配列 **arrangement**

はう 這う **crawl** ◆お子さんは這いますか Is your baby crawling? ◆お子さんは這い始めましたか Has your baby started to crawl? ◆四つん這いする crawl (on *one's* hands and knees)

ハウスキーパー **housekeeper** （総称）**housekeeping staff**

ハウスダスト **house dust**

ハエ **fly**

はえかわる 生え変わる ◆多くの子どもは6歳頃から乳歯が抜けて永久歯に生え変わり始めます For most children, the baby teeth will start to fall out and the adult teeth will come in at around the age of six.

はえそろう 生え揃う ◆髪の毛が生え揃うには6か月から12か月かかるでしょう It will take six to twelve months for your hair to grow back completely. ◆お子さんは2歳までに歯が生え揃うでしょう By age two, your baby will have a full set of baby teeth. / By age two, all your baby's teeth will have come in.

はえる 生える **grow** ◆髪の毛は化学療法が終われば, たいてい生えてきます Hair usually grows back after chemotherapy. ◆舌に苔が生えている have a furred[coated] tongue / the tongue is[feels] furry ◆お子さんは歯が生え始めましたか Has your baby started teething[cutting his〈her〉teeth]?

はがす 剥がす （皮膚などをむく）**peel off** （引き裂く）**rip off, tear off** （取る）**take off, remove** ◆かさぶたを剥がしてはいけません Don't rip[peel] the scab off. ◆湿布を剥がす *take off[remove] the compress

はかせ 博士 ☞博士(はくし)

はがた 歯型・歯形 （歯科鋳型）**dental mold** （歯科印象）**dental impression**

はかばかしくない （速くない）**not ... quickly enough** （順調でない）**not ... well enough** （ほとんど改善していない）**show little improvement** ◆彼女の回復ははかばかしくありません She is not *getting better[recovering] quickly enough. / She is not doing well enough. / Her condition shows little improvement.

はかり 秤 **scale** ☞体重計

はかる 測る・計る・量る （大きさ・長さ・量などを）**measure** （重さを）**weigh** （体温・血圧などを）**take** （時間・速度を）**time** （数量・大きさなどを見積もる）**estimate** （調べる・検査する）**check, test** ☞測定 ◆身長と体重を計りましょう Let me measure your height and weight. / Let me weigh you and measure your height. ◆最近体重を計りましたか Have you weighed yourself recently? ◆熱〈血圧 / 脈〉を測りましょう Let me[I'm going to] take your temperature〈blood pressure / pulse〉. ◆腹囲を測りましょう Let me[I'm going to] measure *you around the waist[your waist / your abdominal circumference]. ◆毎日同じ条件で体重を測る measure *one's* weight under the same conditions every day ◆赤沈を測る check[test] *a person's* sedimentation rate

はがれる 剥がれる （取れる）**come off, fall off** （むける）**peel off** （薄片になって落ちる）**flake off** （☞flaky） （うろこ状になって落ちる）

scale off （ぼろぼろに崩れる）**crumble off**
◆表皮が剝がれやすい The outer skin is flaky. / The outer layer of the skin comes [peels] off easily. ◆この貼り薬は動いても剝がれません This medicated patch will not come off when you move. ◆治療しないと爪が剝がれ落ちるかもしれません If left untreated, the nail may become separated from the nail bed and eventually fall[crumble] off.

はきけ　吐き気　nausea /nɔ́ːziə/ （圏**nauseous**）☞**吐く** ◆吐き気がしますか Do you have any nausea? / Do you feel nauseous? / Do you feel like *vomiting [you're going to vomit]? ◆この薬を飲むと（副作用として）吐き気が起こることがあります This medication may *cause nausea [make you nauseous]（as a side effect）. ◆吐き気がひどい have[suffer] severe nausea ◆吐き気を和らげる薬を処方しましょう I'm going to prescribe a medication to relieve the nausea. ▶吐き気止め **anti-nausea medication[drug / agent]** / **anti-emetic** （medication / drug / agent）/ **antinauseant** （medication / drug / agent）

はぎしり　歯ぎしり　teeth grinding （睡眠時歯ぎしり）**sleep bruxism** （圏**grind** / **gráind / *one's* teeth**）◆眠っている時歯ぎしりすると言われたことがありますか Have you ever been told that you grind your teeth in your sleep?

パキスタン　Pakistan （圏**Pakistani** /pæ̀kɪstǽni/）☞**国籍** ▶パキスタン人（の） **Pakistani**

はく¹　吐く
《吐き出す》（嘔吐する）**vomit** /vámɪt/, **throw up, regurgitate** （咳とともに）**cough up** （唾とともに）**spit up** ◆食べた物を吐くことがありますか Do you ever vomit [throw up] after eating? ◆最近吐きましたか Have you vomited recently? ◆何回吐きましたか How many times[How often] did you vomit? ◆吐いた物は何でしたか What did you vomit? / What did the vomit look like? ◆どのくらいの量を吐きましたか How much did you vomit?

◆吐いた物の色は何色でしたか What color was the vomit? ◆多量に吐く vomit a large amount ◆無理に吐く induce vomiting ◆血を吐く（消化管から）vomit blood / （咳とともに）cough up blood / （唾とともに）spit up blood ◆血痰を吐く spit up bloody phlegm / （咳とともに）cough up bloody phlegm
《息を吐く》**breathe** /bríːð/ **out, exhale**
◆息を吸って，ゆっくり吐いて下さい Please breathe in, and then breathe out slowly. ◆息をゆっくり十分に吐いて下さい Please breathe out slowly and fully. / Please breathe out slowly, all the way.
◆鼻から吸ってゆっくり口から吐いて下さい Please inhale[breathe in] through the nose and exhale[breathe out] slowly through the mouth.

はく²　履く　put on （↔take off）（履いている）**wear** ◆ズボンを履いてもいいですか You can put your pants on now. ◆靴を履く put *one's* shoes on / put on *one's* shoes

はくい　白衣　white coat ▶白衣高血圧 white coat hypertension

ばくがとう　麦芽糖　malt sugar, maltose

はぐき　歯茎　gum, gingiva （圏**gingival**）☞**歯肉** ◆歯茎に何か問題がありますか Do you have any problems with your gums? ◆歯茎が痛みますか Do you have any pain in your gums? ◆歯を磨く時歯茎から血が出ますか Do your gums bleed when you brush your teeth? ◆歯茎が後退しています You have receding gums. / Your gums are receding. ◆歯茎が赤く腫れている *one's* gums are red and swollen / have swollen, red gums ◆歯茎から膿が出る have pus coming from the gums / the gums are oozing pus

はくし　博士　doctor, Doctor, Dr, Dr. （博士号）**PhD, Ph.D., doctorate** ★PhD は Doctor of Philosophy の略. ◆博士号をもつ医師 an MD, PhD / a medical doctor with a PhD degree ◀医学博士 PhD in medical sciences ▶博士課程 doctoral[PhD] program

はくしつ　白質　white matter（接頭leuk(o)-）◀大脳白質 cerebral white matter　▶白質ジストロフィー leukodystrophy　白質脳症 leukoencephalopathy

はくじょう　白杖　white cane, cane for the blind（周囲に視覚障害者であることを知らせるための）ID cane　☞杖

はくしょく　白色(の)　white　◆白色の分泌物(a) white discharge　◆乳白色の milky white / milky　◆灰白色の(白っぽい) whitish /（粘土色の）clay-colored /（薄い灰色の）light gray

はくせん　白癬　ringworm, tinea　◆足に白癬ができる have ringworm on *one's* leg　◀陰部白癬 ringworm of the groin / tinea cruris /（インフォーマルに）jock itch　爪白癬 ringworm of the nails / tinea unguium　足部白癬 athlete's foot / ringworm of the foot / tinea pedis　体部白癬 ringworm of the body / tinea corporis　頭部白癬 ringworm of the scalp[head] / tinea capitis

はくたい　白苔　fur, white coat　◀舌白苔 fur[white coat] on the tongue

はくだく　白濁　cloudiness（形cloudy）（角膜の）nebula（形nebulous）◆角膜の白濁 a corneal nebula / a faint cloudy spot on the cornea　◆尿の白濁 cloudy[nebulous] urine

はくちょうのくびへんけい　白鳥の首変形　swan-neck deformity

バクテリア　☞細菌

はくどう　拍動　pulsation（動pulsate, throb　形pulsating, throbbing）（鼓動）beat（動beat）◆心臓は元気に拍動しています The heart is beating strongly.　◆拍動性の頭痛 a pulsating[throbbing] headache　◆心尖拍動 apex beat　動脈拍動 arterial pulse

はくないしょう　白内障　cataract　◆白内障になる get[develop] cataracts　◆白内障は通常, 手術で治ります In most cases, cataracts can be cured by surgery.　◆白内障の手術をする(手術を受ける)have [undergo] cataract surgery /（手術を行う）perform cataract surgery　◀加齢白内障

age-related cataract /（老人性）senile cataract　ステロイド白内障 steroid cataract

はくはつ　白髪　white hair　（白髪混じり）gray hair

ばくはつ　爆発　explosion（動explode）◆怒りを爆発させる explode with anger / fly[burst] into a rage　▶爆発損傷 explosion injury　爆発的流行(感染症の広範囲にわたる発生)widespread outbreak

はくはん　白斑　white spot　（色素の欠如）leukoderma, vitiligo　（角膜の）leukoma, opaque white spot on the cornea　◀尋常性白斑 vitiligo vulgaris

はくはんしょう・はくばんしょう　白斑症・白板症　leukoplakia　◀外陰白斑症 vulvar leukoplakia　舌白板症 tongue[lingual] leukoplakia / smoker's tongue

はくひ　剥皮　peeling, decortication

はくひしょう　白皮症　albinism

はくへん　薄片・剥片　flake

はくもう　薄毛　thin hair

はくもうしょう　白毛症　poliosis

はくり　剥離　（分離）separation, detachment　（突然の剥離）abruption　（裂離）avulsion　（剝ぎ取り）stripping　（落屑）exfoliation　（擦過）abrasion　☞剥がれる　◀常位胎盤早期剥離 abruptio placentae　胎盤剥離 placental separation　網膜剥離 retinal detachment　▶剥離骨折 avulsion fracture

ばくりゅうしゅ　麦粒腫　sty /stáɪ/, stye, hordeolum　◆瞼に麦粒腫ができている have a sty on *one's* eyelid

ばくろ　曝露　exposure

はげ　禿げ　（禿げた箇所）bald patch　（丸く禿げた部分）bald spot　（禿げていること）baldness　（脱毛症）alopecia　☞脱毛, 禿げる　◆禿げがある have a bald patch[spot]

はげしい　激しい　（仕事・運動などがきつい）hard, strenuous　（痛みなどの症状が強い）severe, intense　（程度・勢いが強い）violent, extreme　（極度に激しい）excessive　◆今日は激しい運動を控えて下さい You shouldn't exercise hard today. / Please avoid hard[strenuous] exercise today.　◆激しい痛みがある have *(a) severe [(an) extreme] pain ◆激しい咳が出る have[get] *a violent[a severe / an intense] cough ◆(赤ん坊が)激しく泣く cry violently[excessively] ◆鼓動が激しい the heart pounds[throbs]

はげます 励ます （元気づける）cheer up （勇気づける）encourage

はげる¹ 剥げる ☞剥がれる

はげる² 禿げる （髪の毛が薄くなる）go[get, become] bald （毛を失う）lose *one's* hair （禿げた部分がある）have a bald patch [spot] ☞脱毛, 禿げ ◆若くして禿げる go bald prematurely

はけん 派遣（の） （臨時の）temporary （↔permanent) ◆派遣で働く work on a temporary basis ▶派遣社員 temporary office worker 派遣労働者 temporary worker[laborer]

はこう 跛行 limping, claudication ◀間欠性跛行 intermittent claudication

はこつさいぼう 破骨細胞 osteoclast

はこにわりょうほう 箱庭療法 sandplay therapy

はこぶ 運ぶ 《物・人を移動させる》（持って行く）carry （届ける・配達する）deliver （連れて来る）bring （連れて行く）take ☞搬送 ◆重い物を運ぶ carry heavy things ◆配膳車で食事を運ぶ deliver meals in[by] the meal delivery cart ◆彼女は当院に救急車で運ばれて来ました She was brought to this hospital by [in an] ambulance. / An ambulance brought her to this hospital. ◆患者は救急車で一番近い病院に運ばれました The patient was taken to the nearest hospital by[in an] ambulance. / An ambulance took the patient to the nearest hospital. 《状況が推移する》go ◆すべては順調に運んでいます Everything is going well[all right].

はさまる 挟まる （隙間に入って動かなくなる）get stuck ◆歯に魚の小骨が挟まったのですか Has a small fish bone gotten stuck between your teeth?

はさみ 鋏 scissors ★複数形で. ▶はさみ脚歩行 scissors gait はさみ姿勢 scis-

soring posture

パジェットびょう ―病 Paget disease ◀外陰パジェット病 Paget disease of the vulva 骨パジェット病 Paget disease of the bone 乳房外パジェット病 extra-mammary Paget disease 乳房パジェット病 mammary Paget disease

はしか 麻疹 ☞麻疹（ましん）

はじまる 始まる start （↔stop）, begin （↔end） （起こる）come on ◆診察は9時に始まります The examination will start [begin] at nine (o'clock). ◆その痛みはいつから始まりましたか When did the pain start[begin / come on]? ◆インフルエンザの流行がすでに始まっています Influenza[The flu] has already started[begun] to spread. / The influenza epidemic has already started[begun]. ◆陣痛が始まる go into labor

はじめ 初め beginning, start, onset （最初の first 元の original （最初に first, at first 元来は originally) ☞最初 ◆初めはうまくできなくても練習を続けていけば大丈夫です Even though you can't do well at the beginning[start], you'll improve by continuing this exercise. ◆初めのうちは少し痛みますが徐々に痛みはなくなるでしょう You may have (a) mild pain at first, but it will gradually go away. ◆陣痛の初めに at the onset of labor

はじめて 初めて（の） first （first) ☞最初 ◆この病院に来院したのは初めてですか Is this your first visit to this hospital? ◆このようなめまいを起こしたのは初めてですか Was this the first time for you to have this kind of dizziness? ◆初めて痛んだのはいつですか When did you first get this pain? / When did this pain first come on?

はじめまして 初めまして ◆(挨拶として) Nice to meet you. / Good to meet you. / Pleased to meet you.

はじめる 始める start （↔stop）, begin （↔end） （行動し始める）get started ◆化学療法は来週の月曜日から始めましょう Your chemotherapy[chemo] will start

next Monday. / We'll start giving you the chemotherapy[chemo] next Monday.
◆まず流動食から始めます You'll start off on a liquid diet. / We'll start you off on a liquid diet. ◆さあ，始めましょう Now, let's get started.

はしもとびょう 橋本病 Hashimoto disease, Hashimoto thyroiditis

パジャマ pajamas /pədʒá:məz/,《英》pyja-mas ★複数形で．1着のパジャマは a pair of pajamas という． ◆パジャマに着替えて下さい Please change into your pajamas. ◆授乳しやすいように前開きのパジャマを持ってきて下さい Please bring pajamas that button up at the front to make breastfeeding easier. ◆着替え用のパジャマを少なくとも1枚余分に持ってきて下さい Please bring at least one extra pair of pajamas to change into. ◆前開きのパジャマ button-front pajamas / pajamas that open at the front ◆パジャマの上着 a pajama top ◆パジャマのズボン paja-ma bottoms

はしゅ 播種 dissemination （🈩disseminated） ◀胸膜播種 pleural dissemina-tion 腹膜播種 peritoneal dissemina-tion ▶播種性血管内凝固 disseminated intravascular coagulation；DIC

ばしょ 場所 （所）place （正確な地点）spot, point （身体の一部）site, region （位置）location（🈩locate）（空間）space, room（🈩疑問文で where） ◆痛みはほかの場所に広がりますか Does the pain spread [move] *anywhere else[to another place]? ◆腫瘍の場所によっては胃を全摘しなくてはなりません Depending on the site[location] of the tumor, we might have to *remove the entire stomach[per-form a total gastrectomy]. ◆心電図室の場所は4階のエレベーターの反対側です The EKG Room is located on the fourth floor, across from the elevators. ◆ベッドの周りには所持品を全部置く場所がありません There isn't enough space around your bed to put all your belongings. ◆痛む場所はどこですか Where is the pain?

◆発疹が出た場所は体のどこですか Where on your body do you have the rash?

はしょうふう 破傷風 tetanus ◆破傷風に罹る get[contract] tetanus ◀ジフテリア・破傷風ワクチン diphtheria and teta-nus vaccine / DT vaccine ジフテリア・破傷風・百日咳混合ワクチン diphtheria, tetanus, and acellular pertussis vaccine / DTaP vaccine ▶破傷風菌 *Clostridium tetani* 破傷風抗毒素 tetanus antitoxin 破傷風トキソイド tetanus toxoid 破傷風ワクチン tetanus vaccine /（接種）tetanus vaccination

はしる 走る 《駆ける》run （急ぐ）rush ◆痛みが消えてからも当分は走ったり跳んだりは控えて下さい Please refrain from running or jumping for a while even after the pain has gone away.
《痛みなどを瞬間的に強く感じる》shoot ◆ビーンと走るような鋭い痛み a shooting pain

バス¹ （乗り物の）bus ◆バスで通勤する go to work by bus ◆バスに乗る get on the bus ◆バスを降りる get off the bus ▶バス停 bus stop

バス² （入浴の）bath ☞風呂 ▶バスタオル bath towel バスタブ bathtub バスルーム bathroom

はすい 破水 rupture of the membranes；ROM, breaking of the waters, amnior-rhexis ◆破水しましたか Have your waters broken? ◀人工破水 artificial rupture of the membranes 前期[早期]破水 premature rupture of the membranes；PROM

はずす 外す （取り外す）take off, remove （取り出す）take out ◆ID バンドは入院中外さないで下さい Please don't *take off [remove] your ID band during your stay in the hospital. ◆指輪を外す take off[re-move] *one's* ring ◆入れ歯を外す take out[remove] *one's* dentures ◆ギプスを外す take a cast off ◆人工呼吸器を外す remove[（コンセントを抜く）unplug /（電源を切る）disconnect] the ventilator / *remove the patient from[take the patient off] the ventilator

バスせんしょく　PAS 染色 PAS stain[staining]　（過ヨウ素酸シッフ染色）periodic acid-Schiff stain[staining]

バスト　（女性の胸回り）bust　▶バストパッド bust[breast] pad　☞バスト

バストバンド　（胸骨を支えるためのバンド）chest binder　（紐状の装着用バンド）chest strap　◆バストバンドをつける（装着する）put on a chest binder[strap]　（着用している）wear a chest binder[strap]

パスポート　passport

はずれる　外れる
《物が取れる》come off, come undone　◆このボタンがはずれそうです This button is *about to come off[coming loose].　◆この器具の取っ手ははずれやすいので丁寧に扱って下さい The handle of this instrument *comes off easily[easily comes undone], so please use it with care.
《脱臼する》dislocate, slip out of joint　◆肩の関節がはずれています You've dislocated your shoulder. / Your shoulder has slipped out of joint.

バセドウびょう　─病 Basedow disease, Graves disease

パソコン　personal computer；PC

バソプレシン　vasopressin；VP　（抗利尿ホルモン）antidiuretic hormone；ADH　▶バソプレシン受容体拮抗薬 vasopressin receptor antagonist

はだ　肌 skin　☞皮膚　◀乾燥肌 dry skin 鮫肌 rough skin /（魚鱗癬）ichthyosis 脂性肌 oily[greasy] skin 鳥肌 goose bumps[pimples] / gooseflesh / cutis anserina 敏感肌 sensitive[delicate] skin　▶肌荒れ（かさかさの乾燥した皮膚）rough dry skin /（ひび割れした皮膚）chapped skin　☞肌触り

パターン　pattern /pǽtən/　☞型　◆症状の出方に一定のパターンがありますか Do the symptoms *follow a set pattern[come on with a set pattern]?　◆睡眠のパターンに変化がありますか Have there been any changes in your sleeping patterns? /

Have your sleep patterns changed?　◀行動パターン behavior pattern　呼吸パターン breathing pattern　食行動パターン eating behavior pattern　睡眠パターン sleep pattern　▶パターン認識 pattern recognition

はだか　裸 nakedness （圏naked）　◆上半身裸になって，このガウンを着て下さい Please take off all your clothes from the waist up and put on this gown.　◆下半身裸になって，この検査着を履いて下さい Please take off all your clothes from the waist down and put on these exam shorts[pants].

はだぎ　肌着 ☞下着

はだし　裸足 bare feet　★複数形で．（圏barefoot）　◆裸足で歩く walk[go] barefoot / walk without (any) shoes (on)　◆裸足になって下さい（靴を脱いで）Please take your shoes off. / Please remove your shoes.

はたらき　働き　（仕事）work　（機能）function　（具体的な動き）action　（活動）activity　◆血液を送り出す心臓の働きが悪い The pumping function[action] of the heart is poor.　◆脳の働き brain activity[function]

はたらく　働く
《仕事をする》work, labor　★labor は肉体労働を表す．☞仕事　◆今働いていますか Are you currently working[employed]? / Are you working now? / Do you currently have a job?　◆週〈日〉に何時間働いていますか How many hours a week〈day〉 do you work?　◆最近働き過ぎですか Have you been working too hard[much] recently? / Have you been overworking yourself recently?　◆働き過ぎで病気になる get sick from overwork　◆工場で働く work in a factory　◆パートで働く work part-time / work on a part-time basis
《機能する》function, work　◆あなたの腎臓は正常に働いています Your kidneys are functioning normally.

はたんしゅっけつ　破綻出血 breakthrough bleeding

ハチ 蜂 （大型のスズメバチ）hornet （小型のスズメバチ）wasp （ミツバチ）bee ◆ミツバチに刺される get stung by a bee ◆スズメバチ刺傷によるアレルギー反応 allergic reactions *caused by[due to] hornet[wasp] stings ▶ハチ刺され（スズメバチ）hornet[wasp] sting / （ミツバチ）bee sting ハチ毒（スズメバチ）hornet[wasp] venom / （ミツバチ）bee venom ☞蜂蜜

はちがつ 8月 August; Aug. ☞1月

ばちじょう ばち状（の）clubbed ▶ばち爪 clubbed nail ばち指 clubbed finger[digit] / （親指の）clubbed thumb

はちぶんめ 八分目 ◆腹八分目にして下さい（適量に）You should *eat moderately[not eat too much].

はちみつ 蜂蜜 honey

はちょう 波長 wavelength

はついく 発育 （成長）growth （動grow）（発達）development （動develop 形developméntal）☞成長, 発達 ◆お子さんは順調に発育しています Your child is growing[developing] well. ◆発育が悪い（適切に育っていない）be not growing[developing] properly ◆発育が遅い〈早い〉grow[develop] slowly〈rapidly〉◆身体発育 physical development 胎児発育不全 fetal growth restriction ▶発育異常 growth abnormality 発育期 growth period[phase] / the period of growth 発育障害 growth disorder 発育状態 developmental condition 発育速度 growth rate 発育不全 underdevelopment / （低形成）hypoplasia / （無形成）aplasia 発育歴 developmental history

はつおん 発音する pronounce （図pronunciation）◆もっとゆっくり発音して下さい Please pronounce it more slowly. ◆お名前はどう発音するのですか How do you pronounce your name? ▶発音障害（構音障害）dyslalia

バッカルじょう ─錠 （口腔錠）buccal tablet

はっかん 発汗 sweating, perspiration ☞汗 ◆心因性発汗 mental sweating ▶発汗障害 sweating disorder

はつがん 発がん carcinogenesis （圏発がん性の carcinogenic, cancer-causing）◆発がん性のある化学物質 carcinogenic chemicals ▶発がん因子 carcinogenic[cancer-causing] factor 発がん物質 carcinogen / carcinogenic[cancer-causing] substance

ばっかん 抜管 extubation （↔intubation）◆気管から抜管する remove a tube from the windpipe

はっきり （明瞭に）clearly （相違が明らかに）distinctly （確かに）for sure, for certain, definitely ☞明らか, 明確, 明瞭 ◆私の声がはっきり聞こえますか Can you hear me clearly[distinctly]? ◆文字がはっきり見えますか, ぼやけていますか Can you see the letters clearly[distinctly], or do they look blurred? ◆この病気の原因ははっきりしていません The cause of this disease isn't clear. ◆はっきりとは言えませんが, 来週には退院できるでしょう I can't say *for sure[for certain], but you'll probably be able to leave the hospital next week. ◆お子さんはまだ意識がはっきりしませんか（意識が混濁しているか）Is your child still confused? ◆彼女は意識がはっきりしています She is fully conscious. ◆明日までにはっきりしたお返事をいただけますか Can I have a definite answer by tomorrow?

はっきんせいざい 白金製剤 platinum drug, platinum-based drug

パック pack ☞湿布 ◀温〈冷〉パック hot〈cold〉pack 氷パック ice pack

バックグランド background ☞背景

はっけっきゅう 白血球 white blood cell；WBC, leukocyte ◆白血球数が増加しています The number of white blood cells is increasing[rising]. ◆この治療で白血球数が減少します This treatment will cause *the number of white blood cells to go down[a decrease in the white blood cell count]. ◆白血球数を測定する measure the number of white blood cells / measure[check] *a person's* white blood cell counts ◀多核白血球 polymorphonuclear leukocyte　単核白血球 mononuclear leukocyte　ヒト白血球抗原 human leukocyte antigen；HLA　▶白血球減少（症）leukopenia / leukocytopenia　白血球除去赤血球 leukocyte-poor red cell；LPRC　白血球除去フィルター leukocyte depletion filter　白血球数 white blood cell count；WBC / leukocyte count　白血球増加（症）leukocytosis　白血球分画 differential leukocyte count

はっけつびょう　白血病　leukemia /luːkíːmiə/　◀急性骨髄性白血病 acute myeloid[myelogenous] leukemia；AML　急性リンパ性白血病 acute lymphocytic leukemia；ALL　成人Ｔ細胞白血病 adult T-cell leukemia；ATL　慢性骨髄性白血病 chronic myeloid[myelogenous] leukemia；CML　慢性リンパ性白血病 chronic lymphocytic leukemia；CLL

はっけん　発見する　（見つける）**find**（图finding）　（気づく・感知する）**detect**（图detection）　（新事実・未知の物を見出す）**discover**（图discovery）　◆がんを早期のうちに発見する find[detect] cancer in its early stages　◆首にしこりを発見する find a lump in[on] one's neck　◀医学上の発見 a medical discovery　◀偶発的発見 accidental[incidental] finding(s)　早期発見 early detection

はつげん　発現　（症状の）**manifestation**

はつご　発語　（話し言葉）**speech**　（発語・発声）**utterance**　◀不明瞭発語 slurred speech　▶発語失行 speech[verbal] apraxia　発語不能 aphasia

はっこう　発行する　（証明書などを）**issue**　◆すぐに診察券を発行しますので，ここでお待ち下さい We'll issue your hospital[patient] ID card right away, so please wait here.

はっさん　発散する　release, let off　◆ストレスを発散する release[let off]（one's）stress

ばっし¹　抜糸する　remove stitches, take out stitches（图removal of stitches, suture removal）　◆今日は抜糸しましょう I'm going to remove[take out] the[your]

stitches today.　◆抜糸してもらう have one's stitches out

ばっし²　抜歯　tooth extraction　☞歯

バッジ　badge　◆バッジを着けている wear a badge　◀時間外面会者バッジ after-hours visitor[visitors] badge　面会者バッジ visitor[visitors] badge

はっしょう　発症　（発病）**onset**（of a disease）　（病気の進展）**development**　（突発的発症）**outbreak**　（発疹の発症）**rash**　（勔始まる start　症状を現す develop）　勔起こる　◆頭痛はいつ発症しましたか When did the headache start?　◆この病気は感染してからすぐに発症します The symptoms of this disease develop immediately after infection.　◆急に発症する get[become] sick suddenly / fall[be taken] ill suddenly　◆めまいの突然の発症 sudden onset of dizziness　◆発疹の突発的な発症 a sudden rash / a rash outbreak

はっしん　発疹　☞発疹（ほっしん）

ばつずい　抜髄（法）　pulp extirpation, pulpectomy

はっせい¹　発生　《出来事が》**occurrence**（勔occur）　（感染症などの爆発的流行）**outbreak**（勔break out）　☞起こる　◆新型インフルエンザが発生するかもしれません A new strain of influenza [flu] might break out.　◆食中毒の発生 an outbreak of food poisoning　《生物の》**development**（勔develop　圀developméntal）　◀集団発生 mass outbreak[epidemic]　▶発生異常 developmental anomaly　発生遺伝学 developmental genetics　発生学 embryology　☞発生率

はっせい²　発声　（話す能力）**speech**（勔speak）　（声を出す能力）**voice**（圀vocal）　◆発声しにくいのは声帯にできたポリープのせいです It's a polyp on your vocal cords that's causing you to have difficulty speaking.　◀食道発声 esophageal speech　無喉頭発声 alaryngeal voice [speech]　☞発声障害

はっせいしょうがい　発声障害　voice disorder[disturbance], dysphonia　◀痙

攣性発声障害 spasmodic dysphonia；SD
心因性発声障害 psychogenic dysphonia

はっせいりつ　発生率　incidence（rate）
◆乳がんの発生率が高まっています The incidence of breast cancer *has risen[has become high]. ◆高い〈低い〉発生率 high〈low〉incidence

はったつ　発達　development（動develop 形developméntal）（成長）growth（動grow）　☞成長，発育 ◆お子さんは発達が少し遅れているようですが，心配はいりません Your child seems to be a little slow[behind] in his〈her〉development, but *there's no need to worry[you don't need to worry]. ◆順調に発達する develop *as expected[satisfactorily] ◆徐々に発達する develop gradually ◆発達が遅い develop slowly / be slow[behind] in *a person's* development ◆発達が遅れている have a developmental delay ◆子供の発達 child development ◆身体の発達 physical development ◆正常な発達 normal development ◆知能の発達 intellectual development ◀運動発達 motor development　言語発達 language[speech] development　精神発達 mental development　▶発達指数 developmental quotient；DQ　発達指標（目安）developmental milestone /（数標）developmental index　発達障害 developmental disorder　発達心理学 developmental psychology　発達性言語障害 developmental language disorder；DLD　発達段階[区分] the stage of development / developmental stage　発達年齢 developmental age　発達歴 developmental history

パッチ　patch　◀経皮（吸収）パッチ transdermal patch　▶パッチテスト patch test

はってん　発展　development（成長）growth（進行）progress　☞発達

パッド　pad　◀失禁用パッド（ベッド用の）incontinence（bed）pad / underpad　電極パッド electrode pad　バストパッド bust[breast] pad

バッド・キアリしょうこうぐん　―症候群 Budd-Chiari syndrome

はつねつ　発熱　fever /fíːvə/（動熱がある have a fever　体温が上がる develop a fever　熱っぽくなる become feverish）　☞熱
◆発熱のため今日は検査ができません You can't have the test today because *you have a fever[you're feverish]. ◆急に熱する develop a fever suddenly / develop a sudden fever

はつびょう　発病　☞発症

パップざい　―剤　☞湿布

パップ（スメア）テスト　Pap smear /-smíə/, Pap[Papanicolaou smear] test
◆前回のパップテストはいつ受けましたか When was your last Pap smear? ◆パップテストをしましょう Let's get[do] a Pap smear.

はつもうざい　発毛剤（育毛剤）hair-growing agent, hair restorer

ばていじん　馬蹄腎　horseshoe kidney

ハト　鳩　pigeon　▶鳩飼病 pigeon-breeder's lung　鳩胸 pigeon[chicken] chest / pigeon[chicken] breast / pectus carinatum

はな　鼻　nose（形nasal）（鼻孔）nostril
《日常動作の表現》◆鼻で息をする breathe through *one's* nose ◆鼻をかむ blow *one's* nose ◆鼻をすする sniffle ◆鼻を垂らす have a runny nose ◆鼻を拭く wipe *one's* nose ◆鼻をほじる pick *one's* nose
《診察の基本表現》◆鼻に何か問題がありますか Do you have any problems with your nose? ◆鼻を診察しましょう I'm going to examine your nose. ◆鼻で息を吸って下さい Please breathe in through your nose. ◆よく鼻が詰まりますか Do you often have a stuffy[congested] nose? / Does your nose often get stuffy[blocked]? ◆鼻の怪我をしたことがありますか Have you ever had any *nose injury[injury to your nose]?
《異常・症状の表現》◆鼻が詰まる have a blocked nose / *one's* nose is stuffed up ◆鼻がむずむずする（かゆい）have an itchy nose /（ちくちくする）*one's* nose tickles ◆鼻の異物 a foreign body in the nose / a

nasal foreign body　◆鼻の潰瘍 a nasal ulcer　◆鼻の腫瘍 a nasal tumor

☞鼻アレルギー，鼻風邪，鼻カニューラ，鼻くそ，鼻クリップ，鼻毛，鼻声，鼻汁，鼻血，鼻詰まり，鼻柱，鼻ポリープ，鼻指鼻試験

はなアレルギー　鼻アレルギー　nasal allergy

はなかぜ　鼻風邪　head cold

はなカニューラ　鼻カニューラ　nasal cannula

はながみ　鼻紙　☞ティッシュペーパー

はなくそ　鼻くそ　nasal mucus　◆鼻くそをほじる pick *one's* nose

はなクリップ　鼻クリップ　nose clip　◆鼻クリップを付ける put on[apply / attach] a nose clip / place a clip on the nose　◆鼻クリップを付けたままにしておく leave the nose clip attached

はなげ　鼻毛　nose hair, nasal hair, vibrissa　◆鼻毛を抜く pluck[pull out] *one's* nose hair

はなごえ　鼻声　nasal voice, twang　◆鼻声で話す speak with a twang / speak through *one's* nose

はなし　話　talk（圏talk）（話し合い）discussion（圏discuss）（会話）conversation（圏会話，話し合う）　◆彼はよくとりとめない話をしますか Does he often ramble in his talk?　◆まず少しお話をうかがいます I'd like to talk with you[We can talk] a little bit first.　◆ちょっとお話があるんですが May I talk to you for a moment?　◆治療計画についてお話をするのによい時だと思います I think this is a good time to talk about the treatment plan. / Now is the time to discuss the treatment plan.　◆彼女はよく昔の話をしますか Does she often talk about the old days?

はなしあいて　話し相手　someone to talk to[with]　◆話し相手になる keep *a person* company

はなしあう　話し合う　talk（about）, talk *things* over, discuss（相談する）consult（with）　☞議論　◆そのことは検査後に話し合いましょう Let's *talk about[discuss]

that after the test.　◆あなたの症状にどの治療法が適しているか話し合う必要があります We need to discuss which treatment options are suitable for your symptoms.　◆ご家族で話し合って下さい Please talk it over with your family.

はなじる　鼻汁　（鼻漏）nasal discharge, rhinorrhea　（粘液性の）nasal mucus　（鼻水）runny nose, watery nasal discharge　◆鼻汁が出ますか Do you have any discharge from the nose?　◆鼻汁がたくさん出ますか Do you have *a runny nose[a lot of discharge from your nose]? / Is your nose very runny?　◆鼻汁はどんな色ですか What color is the nasal discharge?　◆鼻汁は緑色ですか Is the discharge from your nose green?　◆鼻汁は喉のほうに垂れますか Does the nasal discharge drain into the throat?

鼻汁の性状

■色
●無色な colorless　●透明な clear　●白い white　●緑色の green　●緑色味を帯びた greenish　●黄色い yellow　●黄色味を帯びた yellowish

■性状
●水様性の watery　●薄くてさらさらした thin　●どろっとしてねばねばした thick and sticky　●膿のような pus-like　●血性の bloody　●血の付いた blood-stained　●かすかに血を帯びた blood-tinged

---

はなす¹　話す　（口をきく）speak　（話をする）talk　（告げる）tell　（相談する）consult　（話し合う）discuss　☞話，話し合う　《会話として話す・口をきく》　◆もう少し大きな声で話して下さい Could you speak a little louder?　◆もっとゆっくり話して下さい Could you speak more slowly. / Please speak more slowly.　◆うまく話せないのですか Do you have difficulty speaking[talking]?　◆話しかけても反応がないのですか Does she〈he〉not respond when you talk to her〈him〉?　◆お子さん

の話し方に感情的に反応しないようにして下さい Please try not to react emotionally to your child's way of talking.

《伝える・説明する》 ◆そのことについてもっと話してくれませんか Can you tell me more about that? ◆お話ししたいことがあるのですが I have something to *tell you [talk about with you]. / I'd like to have a word with you. ◆詳しいことは後でお話しします I'll tell you the details later on. / I'll explain in more detail later on. ◆率直に話す talk frankly[candidly] ◆簡潔に話す talk briefly

《話し合う・相談する》 ◆他に何かお話しすることがありますか Is there anything else you want to talk about? ◆悩み事があったらいつでも話して下さい Please feel free to tell me your troubles at any time. ◆担当の先生に話してみましたか Did you consult[talk to] your doctor? ◆今お話ししてもいいですか Is this a good time to talk?

《ある言語で会話する能力がある》 ◆日本語を話しますか Do you speak Japanese? ◆日本語を流暢に話す speak Japanese fluently / speak fluent Japanese

はなす² 離す （距離・間隔を空ける）keep ... away （別々に分ける）separate, keep ... apart ◆酸素濃縮器は火気から 2 m 離して置いて下さい Please keep the oxygen concentrator two meters away from heat and flame sources. ◆麻疹に罹っている子は他のきょうだい達から離して下さい A child with measles should be kept away from his〈her〉brothers and sisters.

はなす³ 放す let go (of), release ◆手を放して下さい Please let go (of it). / Please release your grip on it. ◆私の手を放さないで下さい Don't let go of my hand. ◆お子さんから目を放さないで下さい Please keep an eye on your child. ◆手が放せない be too busy / (予定などが詰まっている)be tied up

はなすじ 鼻筋 ☞鼻柱
はなたけ 鼻茸 ☞鼻ポリープ
はなぢ 鼻血 nosebleed, nasal bleeding, epistaxis ◆鼻血がよく出ますか Do you

often have nosebleeds? / Does your nose often bleed? ◆鼻血が出続けたことがありますか Have you ever had a series of nosebleeds? ◆鼻血を止める stop a nosebleed

はなづまり 鼻詰まり stuffy nose, blocked nose （鼻の充血）congested nose, nasal congestion （鼻閉）nasal obstruction[occlusion] ◆鼻詰まりを取る薬 a nasal decongestant

はなばしら 鼻柱 （眉間から鼻の先端までの部分）the bridge of the nose （左右の孔を分ける隔壁）the nasal septum, the septum of the nose

はなポリープ 鼻ポリープ nasal polyp ▶鼻ポリープ切除術 nasal polypectomy

はなみず 鼻水 ☞鼻汁(はなじる)
はなゆびはなしけん 鼻指鼻試験 nose-finger-nose test

はならび 歯並び set of teeth, row of teeth, teeth alignment[arrangement] ◆歯並びがいい(悪い) have even〈irregular / crooked〉teeth ◆歯並びを直す straighten *a person's* teeth / (患者が)have *one's* teeth straightened / (歯列矯正器をつける)put on (dental) braces / (歯列矯正器をつけている)wear (dental) braces

はなれる 離れる （去る）leave （別々になる）separate (from), be apart (from) （距離を空ける）stay clear (of), keep away (from) ☞離す ◆彼女は国を離れてから 7 年になります It's been seven years since she left her home country. ◆彼は家族と離れて東京で一人暮らしをしています He lives alone in Tokyo, away[apart] from his family. ◆AED のショックボタンを押す時は必ず患者から離れて下さい When you push the AED's shock button, make sure to *stay clear of[keep away from] the patient.

パニック panic （形panicky） ◆パニックに陥る get[go] into a panic / be thrown into a panic ◆パニック状態になる get panicky / be seized with panic ◆パニックになって泣きわめく scream and cry in panic ▶パニック症 panic disorder パ

ニック値 panic value　パニック反応 panic reaction　パニック発作 panic attack

ばにょうさん　馬尿酸　hippuric acid；HA

バニリルマンデルさん　―酸　vanillyl-mandelic acid；VMA

はねかえり　跳ね返り　rebound　▶跳ね返り現象 rebound phenomenon

ばねゆび　―指　trigger finger, snap finger, snapping finger　★親指ならば finger の代わりに thumb を用いる.

はは　母　mother, female parent（囲motherly, maternal）　◆未婚の母 *a single[an unmarried] mother　◆母方の祖母 one's grandmother on one's mother's side / one's maternal grandmother　◆母の愛情 motherly affection[love]

はば　幅　width（囲wide）　☞横　◆この酸素濃縮器は幅が 3 m です This oxygen concentrator is three meters wide[in width].　◆傷痕の幅はどのくらいですか How wide is the scar?　◆幅広い選択肢がある have a wide variety of options to choose from　◆腫瘍の幅は 1 cm です The tumor is one centimeter across.

ははおや　母親　☞母, 母親学級

ははおやがっきゅう　母親学級　class for expectant mothers　◆できれば母親学級に参加して下さい I recommend that if possible, you attend the classes for expectant mothers.

はばたきしんせん　羽ばたき振戦　flapping tremor

パパニコローせんしょく　―染色　Papanicolaou stain[staining], Pap stain[staining]

パピローマウイルス　papillomavirus　◀ヒトパピローマウイルス human papillomavirus；HPV

バビンスキーちょうこう　―徴候　Babinski sign

バビンスキーはんしゃ　―反射　Babinski reflex

はブラシ　歯ブラシ　toothbrush　◀電動歯ブラシ electric toothbrush

はみがき　歯磨き　tooth-brushing　◆食事の後は必ず歯磨きを行って下さい Make sure to brush your teeth after meals.　◆どのくらいの頻度で歯磨きやデンタルフロスをしますか How often do you brush and floss your teeth?　◀液体歯磨き mouthwash / dental rinse　練り歯磨き toothpaste　フッ化物配合歯磨き剤 fluoride dentifrice /（練り歯磨き）fluoride toothpaste /（洗口剤）fluoride mouthwash　▶歯磨き剤 dentifrice

ハム　HAM　（HTLV-1 関連脊髄症）HTLV-1 [human T-lymphotropic virus type 1] associated myelopathy

ハムストリングきん　―筋　hamstring muscles　★通例，複数形で.

はめる（身に着ける）put on　（身に着けている）wear　（ボタンを）button（up）　（はめ込む）put（in）, fit　◆指輪をはめる put on one's ring　◆シャツのボタンをはめる button（up）one's shirt / do up the buttons on one's shirt

はやあし　早足　fast walking, brisk walking　◆早足で歩く（早く歩く）walk fast[at a quick pace]

はやい¹　速い　（速度が）fast（↔slow）, rapid　（動きが）quick　◆脈が少し速いですね Your pulse is a little fast[rapid]. / You have a slightly fast[rapid] pulse.　◆緊張すると鼓動が速くなります When you're nervous, your heart beats rapidly[fast].　◆呼吸が速い *the breaths are[the breathing is] rapid[fast]　◆この病気は進行が速い This disease progresses[gets worse] quickly. / The progress of this disease is quick.

はやい²　早い　（時間的に早い）early　（回復などが早い）speedy　（時期的に早すぎる）premature, untimely（囲early, soon）　☞早く　◆退院するのはまだ早いでしょう It's too early for you to leave the hospital. /（まだ十分に回復していない）You haven't recovered enough to go home yet.　◆あきらめるのはまだ早いですよ It's too soon to give up.　◆射精が早い have premature ejaculation

はやおき　早起きする　get up early, rise early

はやく 早く **early** （近いうちに・まもなく）**soon** ☞早い ◆この薬は朝早く飲んで下さい Please take this medication early in the morning. ◆予定より早く赤ちゃんが産まれるかもしれません Your baby might *be born[come] earlier than expected. / You may have[deliver] your baby *earlier than expected[ahead of schedule]. ◆（手術後など）できるだけ早く起き上がって歩くようにして下さい Please try to get up and walk as soon as you can. ◆できるだけ早く治療を始めます We'll start the treatment *as soon as possible[as soon as we can]. ◆早く良くなりますように Get well soon. / I wish you a speedy recovery.

はやくち 早口 ◆早口で話す talk fast[rapidly] / speak fast[rapidly]

はやじに 早死に **early death, untimely death** ◆早死にする die young / die at an early age

はやね 早寝 ◆早寝する go to bed early

はやりめ はやり目 （流行性角結膜炎）**epidemic keratoconjunctivitis ; EKC**

はやる 流行る （一時的に流行っている）**go around** （急速に広まる）**spread quickly** （広がっている）**be widespread[prevalent]** ☞流行 ◆インフルエンザが流行っていますから、うつらないように気をつけて下さい There's flu going around, so please take care not to catch it. ◆この地域でノロウイルス感染症が流行っています A norovirus infection is going around in this area.

はら 腹 （胃・横隔膜から骨盤まで）**stomach** （腹部）**abdomen** ☞お腹, 腹部 ◆腹の具合が悪い have trouble[problems] with *one's* stomach / have stomach trouble / have an upset stomach ◀下腹 the lower abdomen わき腹 side of the abdomen / lateral region / flank

はらいもどす 払い戻す **refund, pay back** （償還する）**reimburse** （図**reimbursement**） ◆入院保証金は退院時に払い戻します The admission deposit will be refunded[We will refund the admission deposit] at the time of discharge from the hospital. ◆後から高額療養費の払い戻し（金）を受け

取ることができます High-cost medical-care expenses will be reimbursed later. / You'll be able to receive reimbursement for high-cost medical-care expenses later. ▶払い戻し金 refund / reimbursement

はらう 払う **pay** 《代価を渡す》支払う ◆カードで〈現金で〉払う pay *by credit card〈in cash〉 《意識を向ける》 ◆血圧にもっと注意を払って下さい Please pay more attention to your blood pressure.

はらおび 腹帯 ☞腹帯（ふくたい）

パラグアイ **Paraguay** （形**Paraguayan**） ☞国籍 ▶パラグアイ人（の） Paraguayan

パラコート **paraquat** ▶パラコート中毒 paraquat poisoning[intoxication]

パラシュートはんしゃ ─反射 **parachute reflex**

バラしん ─疹 **roseola** （特に小児の）roseola infantilis

パラチフス **paratyphoid fever**

パラノイア **paranoia** ☞妄想

はらばい 腹ばい ☞うつ伏せ

パラフィンほうまい ─包埋 **paraffin embedding**

はらまき 腹巻 ☞腹帯（ふくたい）

パラメディカル **paramedical**

パラメディック （救急救命士）**paramedic**

バランス **balance** （動**balance**） ☞均衡, 平衡 ◆バランスを保つのが難しいですか Do you find it difficult to *keep your balance[balance yourself]? ◆片足でバランスをとることができますか Can you balance yourself on one foot? ◆バランスを崩す lose *one's* balance ◆バランスのとれた食事 a well-balanced meal[diet] ◆栄養のバランスをとる eat a balanced diet / get a nutritional balance ◆左右のバランス the balance between left and right ◀座位バランス sitting balance ▶バランス感覚 sense of balance バランス訓練 balance training[exercise]

はり¹ 針 **needle** （ホチキスの）**staple** （縫合）**stitch** ◆針を刺す insert a needle ◆針を抜く take out a needle ◆傷口を5

針縫う put five stitches[staples] in the cut / sew up the cut with five stitches [staples] ◆針で刺すような痛み (a) stinging pain ◀注射針 injection[syringe] needle 毒針(昆虫などの) (poison) stinger ▶針穴瞳孔 pinhole[pinpoint] pupil 針刺し事故 needlestick accident 針生検(fine) needle biopsy

はり² 鍼 **acupuncture** ☞鍼灸(しんきゅう) ▶鍼師 acupuncturist / acupuncture practitioner 鍼治療 acupuncture therapy 鍼麻酔 acupuncture anesthesia

はり³ 張り ☞張る

バリアきのう ―機能 **barrier function**

バリアフリー(の) (段差などがない)**barrier-free** (障害者が利用しやすい)**accessible** (图accessibility) ◆バリアフリーの浴室 a barrier-free bathroom ◆家をバリアフリーに改装する remodel the house *to be barrier-free[for accessible living]

バリウム **barium** /bériəm/ (X線検査用のバリウム)**barium meal** (液)**barium liquid** (混合液)**barium mixture** ◆胃のX線検査でバリウムを飲む have[drink] a barium meal before a stomach X-ray ◆バリウムで便秘になることがあります Barium may cause constipation. ◆バリウムを体から出すため，水分を十分に摂って下さい Please drink lots of fluids to expel the barium from your body. ◀胃バリウム検査 barium meal (test) / (上部消化管検査) upper gastrointestinal[GI] series ▶バリウム造影剤 barium contrast medium バリウム注腸造影 barium enema；BE / contrast enema

はりぐすり 貼り薬 **patch** ☞湿布

はる¹ 張る (胃・腹が膨れる)**get[become] bloated, get[become] distended** (首・筋が硬くなる)**get[become] stiff** (腫れる)**get [become] swollen** ◆ガスでお腹が張っていますか Do you feel as if your abdomen is bloated[distended] with gas? / Does your abdomen feel bloated[distended] with gas? / (インフォーマルに)Do you feel gassy? ◆肩〈首〉が張る feel stiff in the shoulders〈neck〉/ have *stiff shoulders〈a

stiff neck〉 ◆乳房が乳で硬く張る the breasts become hard and swollen with milk

はる² 貼る (薬などを貼布する)**apply … to** (くっつける)**put[place] … on, attach … to** ◆冷湿布を肩に貼って下さい Please *apply a cold compress to[put a cold compress on] your shoulder. ◆胸に電極を貼ります I'm going to *attach electrodes to[put electrodes on] your chest. ◆バンドエイドを傷口に貼る put a Band-Aid on *one's wound

バルーン **balloon** ◆バルーン血管形成術とはバルーンカテーテルで狭くなった血管を拡げる治療法です Balloon angioplasty is a procedure in which a narrowed blood vessel is dilated[expanded] with a balloon catheter. ◀大動脈内バルーンパンピング intraaortic balloon pumping；IABP ▶バルーン拡張術 balloon dilatation バルーンカテーテル balloon catheter

バルサルバしけん ―試験 **Valsalva test**

バルサルバどう ―洞 **Valsalva sinus, sinus of Valsalva** ▶バルサルバ洞動脈瘤 aneurysm of the Valsalva sinus / Valsalva sinus aneurysm

バルサルバほう ―法 **Valsalva maneuver**

バルス **pulse** ☞脈 ▶パルス療法 pulse therapy ☞パルスオキシメータ

パルスオキシメータ **pulse oximeter** ◆このパルスオキシメータは血中の酸素レベルを測ります This pulse oximeter measures the level of oxygen in your blood.

バルトリンせん ―腺 **Bartholin gland**

パルボウイルス *Parvovirus* ◀ヒトパルボウイルス B19 感染症 human parvovirus B19 infection

はれ 腫れ **swelling, puffiness** ☞腫れぼったい, 腫れ物, 腫れる ◆体のどこかにしこりか腫れがありますか Do you have any lumps or swelling in any area of your body? ◆顔・手・足などの腫れは水分が体に溜まっている徴候かもしれません Puffiness of the face, hands, or legs may be a sign that your body is retaining too much fluid. ◆腫れはひどくなっています The swelling is getting worse. ◆腫れが引いてきています The swelling is *going down [decreasing / subsiding]. ◆腫れを取る relieve[get rid of / reduce] the swelling

バレーちょうこう ―**徴候** Barré sign

はれつ　破裂する　rupture, burst ☞破れる ◆血管が破裂しています The vessel has ruptured. ◆このくも膜下出血は脳動脈瘤の破裂によるものです This subarachnoid hemorrhage was caused by *an aneurysm in the brain that burst[a burst cerebral aneurysm]. ◆動脈瘤の破裂を予防する prevent an aneurysm from rupturing ◀再破裂 rerupture　子宮破裂 uterine rupture　食道静脈瘤破裂 rupture of the esophageal varices　大動脈瘤破裂 aortic aneurysm rupture　動脈瘤破裂 aneurysm rupture / rupture of an aneurysm　卵管破裂 tubal rupture

バレットかいよう ―**潰瘍** Barrett ulcer

バレットしょくどう ―**食道** Barrett esophagus

はれぼったい　腫れぼったい　swollen, puffy ☞腫れ ◆顔が腫れぼったく感じますか Does your face feel swollen at all? ◆目が腫れぼったい be puffy-eyed / have puffy eyes

はれもの　腫れ物 (腫れ上がった物) **swelling** (膿を持ったおでき) **boil** (しこり) **lump** ☞腫れ ◆首に腫れ物がある have a swelling[lump] on the neck ◆口の開いた腫れもの an open boil

はれる　腫れる　swell (up) (図**swelling**), **get**[**become**] **swollen** (大きくなる) **enlarge** ☞腫れ, 腫れぼったい, 腫れ物 ◆体のどこかが腫れていますか Have you noticed any swelling in any area of your body? ◆腫れた個所は痛みますか Are the swollen areas sore? ◆腫れてからどのくらい経ちますか How long have you had the swelling? ◆リンパ節が腫れています Your lymph nodes are swollen. ◆(注射の後などで)少し腫れるかもしれませんが, 心配ないでしょう You may have some slight swelling, but *it's nothing to

worry about[there's no need to worry]. ◆腫れたら冷やして下さい Please apply ice *if it becomes swollen[if it swells up]. ◆首〈わきの下〉が腫れている have a swelling *in one's neck〈under one's arms / in one's armpits〉 ◆爪の周囲の皮膚が腫れている The skin around the nails is swollen. ◆唇がひどく腫れる have severe swelling of the lips / have severely swollen lips

ハローベスト　halo vest (ハロー装具) **halo brace**

はん[1]　半　half ◆今 3 時半です It's three-thirty. / It's half past three (now). ◆彼は 3 歳半です He is three and a half (years old).

はん[2]　班 (チーム) **team** (グループ) **group** (特別な任務をもつ一団) **squad** ◆救護班 a rescue team[squad]

はん[3]　斑 (丸い点) **spot** (しみ状のもの) **blot** (小さい扁平な点・斑紋) **macula** ☞斑点 ◀カフェオレ斑 café-au-lait spot　死斑 livor mortis / postmortem lividity [staining]　皮下出血斑 petechiae　蒙古斑 mongolian spot　老人斑 age spot / senile lentigo / (肝斑) liver spot ☞黄斑, 紫斑, 斑状出血

ばん[1]　番
《順番》**turn** (順序) **order** ☞順番 ◆次はあなたの番です It's your turn next.
《番号》**number** ☞番号 ◆あなたの電話は何番ですか What's your telephone number? ◆グリーンさん, 2 番の部屋にお入り下さい Mrs Green, please enter room two.

ばん[2]　晩 (夕方から就寝まで) **evening** (夕方から明け方まで) **night** ◀今晩 this evening / tonight　昨晩 yesterday evening / last night　毎晩 every evening[night] / each evening[night]　明晩 tomorrow evening[night] ▶晩ご飯 evening meal / supper / dinner

パン　bread ◆ご希望があればパンをお出しします We can serve you bread, if you like. / You can have bread, if you prefer. ◆パンにしますか, ライスにしますか Which would you like, bread or rice?

はんい 範囲 (数量の幅)range (限界)limits ★通例，複数形で．(場所・部分)area (サイズ・規模)size (活動・理解力などの領域)scope (分野)field (期間)span (境界線)boundary ◆血圧は正常範囲内です Your blood pressure is within the normal range. ◆検査結果は正常範囲を超えています The test result is outside the normal range. ◆彼女のバイタルサインは正常範囲内です Her vital signs are within normal limits. ◆湿疹の範囲は広がっていますか Has the area of the rash *gotten larger[increased in size]? ◆関心の範囲 one's area of interest / the area of one's interest ◆調査の範囲 the scope of the investigation ◀活動範囲 scope[field] of activities 記憶範囲 memory span 許容範囲 permissible[acceptable / tolerance] limits

はんいんよう 半陰陽 genital ambiguity, hermaphroditism ◀仮性半陰陽 pseudohermaphroditism 真性半陰陽 true hermaphroditism

はんかいしんけい 反回神経 recurrent nerve ▶反回神経麻痺 recurrent nerve paralysis

はんかすいたいきのうていかしょう 汎下垂体機能低下症 panhypopituitarism；PHP

ハンガリー Hungary (囲Hungarian) ☞国籍 ▶ハンガリー人(の) Hungarian

はんきかん 半規管 semicircular canal [duct] (三半規管)three semicircular canals[ducts]

はんきゅう 半球 hemisphere /héməsfiə/ ◀小脳半球 cerebellar hemisphere 大脳半球 cerebral hemisphere 優位半球 dominant hemisphere

はんきょう 反響 (音の)echo (反応)response ▶反響動作 echopraxia

バンク bank ☞銀行

ばんぐみ 番組 program ◆お好きな番組は何ですか What's your favorite program? ◀スポーツ番組 sports program テレビ番組 TV[television] program ラジオ番組 radio program

バンクラデシュ Bangladesh (囲Bangladeshi) ☞国籍 ▶バングラデシュ人(の) Bangladeshi

はんけっきゅうげんしょう 汎血球減少 pancytopenia

はんげつばん 半月板 meniscus (圏menisci) ◀円板状半月板 discoid meniscus 外側〈内側〉半月板 lateral〈medial〉meniscus ▶半月板損傷 meniscus injury 半月板断裂 meniscus tear[rupture]

はんげんき 半減期 half-life ◆この薬の半減期はおよそ3時間です The half-life of this medication is about three hours. / This medication has a half-life of three hours. ◀長い〈短い〉半減期 a long〈short〉half-life

はんこう 反抗(的な) (造反的な)rebellious (挑戦的な)defiant (否定的な)negative ◆親に対して反抗的な態度をとる take a rebellious[defiant] attitude toward one's parent(s) ◆娘さんは今反抗期なのですね Your daughter is going through a rebellious stage[phase], isn't she?

ばんごう 番号 number ☞数字(囲み：数字の読み方) ◆診察券の番号を教えていただけますか Can you tell me your ID card number? ◆受付番号順に診察します Patients are seen in order of their check-in numbers. ◆番号をお呼びするまでここでお待ち下さい Please wait here until your number is called. ◆外線にかけるには0の番号を押して下さい Please dial 0[zero] for an outside line. ◀ID番号 ID[identification / identity] number 受付番号 check-in number 患者番号 patient number 緊急電話番号 emergency (phone) number 電話番号 telephone number 部屋番号 room number ▶番号札 number slip[ticket]

バンコーストしゅよう ―腫瘍 Pancoast tumor

バンコマイシン vancomycin ▶バンコマイシン耐性黄色ブドウ球菌 vancomycin-resistant *Staphylococcus aureus*；VRSA バンコマイシン耐性腸球菌 vancomycin-resistant *Enterococcus*；VRE

はんこん 瘢痕 scar（㊩scarred），cicatrix（㊩cicatricial）☞傷痕 ◆瘢痕のある皮膚 scarred skin ◆右足にケロイドの瘢痕がある have keloid scars on *one's* right leg ◆やけどの後の瘢痕 a burn scar / a scar from a burn ◀線状瘢痕 linear scar 肥厚性瘢痕 hypertrophic scar 瘢痕形成 cicatrization 瘢痕ケロイド scar[cicatricial] keloid 瘢痕拘縮 scar[cicatricial] contracture

はんこんすい 半昏睡 semicoma（㊩semicomatose, semiconscious）

はんざい¹ 半座位 semisitting position, Fowler position

はんざい² 犯罪 （法的な罪）crime（㊩criminal）（違反行為）offense （若者の非行）delinquency ☞罪 ◀青少年犯罪 juvenile crime[delinquency] / youth crime[delinquency] 性犯罪 sex crime[offense] ▶犯罪精神医学 criminal psychiatry

はんしゃ 反射 reflex ◆反射を調べましょう I'm going to check your reflexes. ◆膝を軽く叩いて反射を調べる check the reflexes by tapping *a person's* knee / check *a person's* *knee jerk[patellar reflexes] by tapping ◆反射神経がよい have good reflexes ◀アキレス腱反射 Achilles tendon reflex；ATR / ankle jerk [reflex] 咽頭反射 pharyngeal reflex 嚥下反射 swallowing reflex 咳嗽反射 cough reflex 下顎[咬筋]反射 jaw[mandibular / masseter] reflex / jaw jerk[reflex] 驚愕反射 startle reflex 血管迷走神経反射 vasovagal reflex 腱反射 tendon reflex 膝蓋腱反射 patellar tendon reflex；PTR / knee jerk[reflex] 条件反射 conditioned reflex；CR 上腕三頭筋反射 triceps (brachii) reflex / elbow jerk [reflex] 上腕二頭筋反射 biceps (brachii) reflex[jerk] 対光反射 light reflex 橈骨反射 radial reflex 脳幹反射 brain stem reflex 把握反射 grasp[grasping] reflex 排便反射 defecation reflex バビンスキー反射 Babinski reflex パラシュート反射 parachute reflex 病的反射 patho-

logic reflex 腹壁反射 abdominal wall reflex 閉口反射 jaw-closing reflex 防御反射 defense reflex モロー反射 Moro reflex 立毛筋反射 pilomotor reflex ▶反射異常 reflex disorder 反射運動 reflex movement 反射減弱 hyporeflexia 反射亢進 hyperreflexia

はんしゃかい 反社会的（な） antisocial ▶反社会的行為 antisocial behavior[act]

はんじょうしゅっけつ 斑状出血 （網膜の）blot bleeding[hemorrhage] （皮膚の）ecchymosis

ばんじょうむきはい 板状無気肺 discoid atelectasis, plate-like atelectasis

はんしょく 繁殖する multiply, grow ◆高温多湿の時は食物中の細菌が繁殖しやすくなります Bacteria in food multiply fast in hot and humid conditions.

はんしん 半身 （上下）half the body （左右）one side of the body ☞半側，片側（へんそく） ◆胸の診察をしますので上半身を脱いで下さい I'm going to[Let me] examine your chest. Please take off *your clothes from the waist up[your top things]. ◆下半身が麻痺している be paralyzed from the waist down ◆右半身が麻痺している be paralyzed on the right side of the body ◀下半身 the lower half[part] of the body / lower body 上半身 the upper half [part] of the body / upper body 左〈右〉半身 the left〈right〉side of the body ▶半身浴 half bath ☞半身不随

はんしんふずい 半身不随 partial paralysis, paralysis of one side of the body （半側麻痺）hemiplegia ◆右半身不随になっている be paralyzed on the right side of *one's* body

はんする 反する 《食い違う》（矛盾する）contradict, be inconsistent（with）（反対である）be contrary（to），be opposed（to） ◆その現象はこれまでの定説に反しています That phenomenon contradicts[is inconsistent with] the widely accepted theory. ◆私たちの予想に反して彼女は劇的に回復しました Contrary to our expectations, she made a dramatic recovery. 《規範などに合わない》（違反している）**be against** （規則・法律などを破る）**break, violate** ◆あなたの行為は病院の規則に反しています Your behavior is against the hospital （rules and） regulations. / With this behavior, you are breaking the hospital （rules and） regulations. ◆それは医の倫理に反しています It is medically unethical. / It is against[contrary to] medical ethics.

ばんせいいでん　伴性遺伝　**sex-linked inheritance** ◆この疾患は伴性遺伝です This disease is inherited through the sex chromosomes. ▶伴性遺伝病 sex-linked genetic disease

ハンセンびょう　―病　**Hansen disease, leprosy**

はんそう　搬送する　（連れて行く）**take** （連れて来る）**bring** （運ぶ）**carry** （輸送する）**transport** （図**transport, transportation**） （病院間を輸送する）**transfer** （図**transfer**） ◆彼女は救急車で病院の救急室に搬送されました She was taken[transported / transferred] by ambulance to the （hospital's） emergency room. / （運ばれて来た）She was brought to the （hospital's） emergency room by ambulance. ◆担架〈車椅子〉で患者を搬送する take[carry / transport] the patient *on a stretcher〈by wheelchair〉 ◀患者搬送 patient transport[transfer]　救急搬送 emergency transport[transfer]　母体搬送 maternal transport

ばんそうこう　絆創膏　（商標名）**Band-Aid**, 《英》**plaster, sticking plaster** （接着テープ）**adhesive tape** ◆切傷に絆創膏を貼る put *a Band-Aid[an adhesive tape] on the cut ◆この絆創膏を腕に貼りますから，2, 3分押さえていて下さい I'm going to put this Band-Aid on your arm, so could you hold it down for a few minutes?

はんそく　半側（の）　（片側の）**hemilateral** （一側性の）**unilateral** ☞半身, 片側（へんそく） ▶半側空間無視 hemispatial[unilateral spatial] neglect　半側麻痺 hemiplegia

はんたい¹　反対（の）　（反対側の）**opposite** （もう一方の）**other** （裏表が逆の）**reversed** ☞逆, 反論 ◆反対向きになって下さい Please turn over. / Please turn your body to the opposite side. ◆反対側の足を見せて下さい Let me look at the opposite leg. ◆反対側の視力を測りましょう Let me measure the vision[sight] in the other eye. ◆利き腕とは反対側に注射しましょう I'm going to[Let me] give you the injection in *the arm you don't write with [your nondominant arm]. ◆トイレは廊下の反対側にあります The restroom is *across from[opposite] the hallway. ▶反対咬合 reversed[opposite] occlusion

はんたい²　反対する　（不賛成である）**be opposed** （**to**） （図**opposition**）, **be against** （不服を唱える）**object** （**to**） （図**objection**） ◆彼女がその治療に反対する主な理由は費用です The main reason why she is opposed[Her main objection] to the treatment is *its cost[how much it costs]. ◆ご計画に反対したくはないのですが, 飛行機でのご旅行はもう少し待ったほうがよいでしょう I hate to object to your plan, but you should wait a while before traveling by plane. ◆喫煙には反対です I'm against smoking.

はんだん　判断する　（評価する）**judge** （図**judgment, judgement**） （決定する）**decide** （図**decision**） ◆適切な判断をくだす make an appropriate judgment ◆X線の結果から判断すると, 心配なことはありません Judging from the X-ray results, you have nothing to worry about. ◆あなたの判断にお任せします I'll leave it to you （to decide）. / I'll leave it to your judgment [decision]. ◆正しい判断をなさいましたね You made the right decision. ◆人を外見で判断する judge *a person* *by appearances[by his〈her〉 appearance]

はんちゅう　範疇　**category** /kǽtəgɔ̀:ri/ ◆非定型カルチノイドは悪性腫瘍の範疇に入ります Atypical carcinoid tumors are classified under the category of malignant tumors.

はんちょう 反跳 **rebound** ▶反跳圧痛 rebound tenderness　反跳現象 rebound phenomenon

はんちょうしつ 反張膝 **genu recurvatum, back-knee**

ハンチントンびょう ―病 **Huntington disease** （ハンチントン舞踏病）**Huntington chorea**

はんつき 半月 **half a month, a half month, two weeks** （🈟**semimonthly**）☞半年

はんてい 判定する （証明される）**prove** （判断する）**judge** ☞判断, 判明, 評価　◆インフルエンザ検査の結果は陽性の判定でした Your influenza test has proved positive.

ハンディキャップ **handicap**

パンデミック （世界的流行）**pandemic** ☞流行

はんてん¹ 斑点 （丸い点）**spot** （小さな点）**dot** （しみ・汚れ）**blemish** （小さなしみ状の点）**speck** （浮遊性の点）**floater** （小さい扁平な点・斑紋）**macula** ☞斑　◆痒みを伴う赤い斑点が背中にできる get[have] itchy red spots on *one's* back

はんてん² 反転 **inversion**

バンド **band** （腕輪）**bracelet** （バインダー）**binder** （ベルト）**strap, belt** （サポーター）**support** （固定具）**brace** ◆IDバンドを手首につける attach the ID[identification] band to *one's* wrist　◆胸郭バンドを着けている wear a chest strap[binder / band]　◆バンドで頭を締め付けられるような頭痛がある have a headache that feels like a tight band around the head　▶ゴムバンド rubber[elastic] band　ヘアバンド hairband　ヘルニアバンド hernia support [belt / brace]　リストバンド wristband

バンドエイド ☞絆創膏

はんとし 半年 **six months, half a year** （🈟**biannual, semiannual**）　◆半年以内にもう一度おいで下さい Please come and see me again within six months.　◆体調が完全に回復するにはおよそ半年かかるでしょう It'll take about half a year for you to recover completely.　◆患者会は半年ごと

に開かれます The patients' association is held *twice a year[every six months / biannually].

ハントしょうこうぐん ―症候群 ☞ラムゼイ・ハント症候群

ハンドル （取っ手・ドアノブ）**handle** （自転車・車椅子などの）**handlebars** ★複数形で。（自動車の）**steering wheel** ▶ハンドル外傷 （自転車などの）handlebar injury / （自動車の）steering wheel injury

はんのう 反応 （刺激・薬品などの作用で起こる現象）**reaction** （🈩**react** 🈟**reactive**） （現象に対する応答）**response** （🈩**respond**） （フィードバック）**feedback** ◆アレルギー反応を起こしたことがありますか Have you ever had an allergic reaction?　◆その薬に過敏に反応する *have a sensitivity[be sensitive] to the medication　◆反応を引き起こす trigger[bring on] a reaction　◆反応が遅い〈速い〉be slow〈quick〉to respond　◆瞳孔は開いていて光に反応しません The pupils are dilated and do not react[respond] to light.　◆大きな音に反応する respond to loud noises　◆肯定的な〈否定的な〉反応を与える give positive 〈negative〉feedback　◆連続した反応 a series of reactions　▶アレルギー反応 allergic reaction　炎症反応 inflammatory reaction　過剰反応 overreaction / overresponse　拒絶[拒否]反応 rejection （reaction）　心因反応 psychogenic reaction　潜血反応 occult blood reaction　遅延反応 delayed reaction[response]　ツベルクリン反応 tuberculin reaction　瞳孔反応 pupillary response[reaction]　防御反応 defense response[reaction]　有害反応 adverse reaction　陽性〈陰性 / 偽陰性 / 偽陽性〉反応 positive〈negative / false-negative / false-positive〉 reaction[response]　抑うつ反応 depressive reaction　連鎖反応 chain reaction　▶反応閾値 reaction threshold　反応時間 reaction[response] time　反応性うつ病 reactive depression 反応速度〈割合〉reaction rate / （スピード）reaction velocity　反応部位 reactive site

ばんのうやく 万能薬 **cure-all, panacea**

はんぱつ 汎発(性の) (全身性の)general-ized, universal (播種性の・散在性の)disse-minated (びまん性の)diffuse ▶汎発性[播種性]血管内凝固 disseminated intra-vascular coagulation ; DIC

ばんぱつ 晩発(性の) late, delayed ▶晩発性小脳皮質萎縮症 late cortical cer-ebellar atrophy ; LCCA 晩発性放射線障害 late[delayed] radiation injury

はんぷく 反復(性の) (何度も繰り返す)re-petitive (再発する)recurrent (時折起こる・間欠性の)episodic ◆反復性の痛み(a) recurrent pain ▶反復運動 repetitive movement 反復嘔吐 recurrent vomiting 反復刺激 repetitive stimulation 反復性緊張型頭痛 episodic tension-type head-ache 反復性群発頭痛 episodic cluster headache 反復性耳下腺炎 recurrent pa-rotitis 反復性疝痛 recurrent colic 反復性脱臼 recurrent dislocation 反復性腹痛 recurrent abdominal pain 反復流産 re-current abortion[miscarriage / preg-nancy loss]

はんふくがい 半腹臥位 semiprone (side) position

パンフレット (小冊子)brochure /broʊˈʃʊɚ/, pamphlet, booklet ★一般的には brochure を用いる。(1枚刷りのもの)leaflet ◆詳しくはこの糖尿病についてのパンフレットをお読み下さい For further information, please read this brochure on diabetes. ◆ご参考までに，これは食事療法についてのパンフレットです For your information [reference], here is a leaflet about diet therapy. ◆このパンフレットは無料です This brochure is free (of charge). ◆このパンフレットは入院準備について書いてあります This booklet[leaflet] gives details about how to prepare for your hospital stay.

はんぶん 半分 half (動半分に減らす halve) ◆薬の量を半分に減らす reduce the amount of the medication by half / halve the amount of the medication ◆錠剤を半分に割る cut[split / divide] the tablet in half ◆コップ半分の水で with half a cup of water

はんめい 判明する (明らかになる)be-come clear (結局…だとわかる)turn out, prove ◆検査結果から症状の原因が判明しました The cause of your symptom has become clear from the test results. ◆あなたの肺炎の原因となっている病原体はまだ判明していません The organism that's causing your pneumonia is still unclear. / We don't yet know what's causing your pneumonia. ◆血液検査の結果はまもなく判明します You'll get the results of the blood test soon. ◆ポリープは良性であることが判明しました The polyp proved [turned out] to be benign.

はんもう 半盲 hemianopsia, hemianopia (略half-blind, hemianopic) ◀同名半盲 homonymous hemianopia 両耳側半盲 bitemporal hemianopia 両鼻側半盲 bi-nasal hemianopia

はんりゅうどうしょく 半流動食 semili-quid diet ☞食事

はんろん 反論 (異議)objection (動ob-ject) (反駁)argument (動argue) ☞反対 ◆この記事に関しては，学会や専門医から反論が出ています The medical associ-ations and specialists (in the field) *argue against[object to] this article.

ひ¹ 比 ☞比較, 比率
ひ² 脾 spleen (㊅splenic) ☞脾臓 ◀副脾 accessory spleen
―ひ ―費 (出費・経費) expenses, costs (料金) fees, charges ★いずれも通例, 複数形で. ☞費用 ◀医療費 medical expenses[fees] 生活費 living expenses[costs] 入院費(料金) hospital expenses[fees / charges] / (請求書) hospital bill
ヒアルロンさん ―酸 hyaluronic acid
ビーアールエム BRM (生体応答修飾物質) biologic response modifier ▶BRM 療法 biologic response modifier therapy
ピーアイイーしょうこうぐん PIE 症候群 PIE syndrome (肺好酸球増多症候群) pulmonary infiltration with eosinophilia syndrome
ピーエイチ pH (水素イオン指数) potential [power] of hydrogen, hydrogen ion exponent
ピーエイチディー PhD, Ph.D. (博士) Doctor of Philosophy ☞博士(はくし)
ビーエスイー BSE (ウシ海綿状脳症) bovine spongiform encephalopathy (狂牛病) mad cow disease
ピーエスエイ PSA (前立腺特異抗原) prostate-specific antigen
ピーエスエス PSS (進行性全身性硬化症) progressive systemic sclerosis
ピーエスピーしけん PSP 試験 PSP test (フェノールスルホンフタレイン試験) phenolsulfonphthalein test
ビーエムアイ BMI (肥満度指数) body mass index ◆BMI は肥満度を測る指数で, 体重キログラムを身長メートルの二乗で割った数値です BMI is *a measure[an index] for estimating obesity, obtained by dividing weight in kilograms by height in meters squared. / BMI estimates obesity by dividing weight in kilograms by height in meters squared. ◆あなたの BMI は 32 で, これは肥満を示しています You have a BMI of thirty-two, which indicates obesity. / Your BMI of thirty-two indicates obesity. ◆18.5 未満の BMI は低体重とされます BMI of less than 18.5[eighteen point five] is considered underweight.
ビーがた B 型 (type) B (血液型) blood type B, type B blood, 《英》blood group B ☞血液型 ▶B 型インフルエンザ influenza (type) B B 型性格 type B personality ☞B 型肝炎
ビーがたかんえん B 型肝炎 hepatitis B, type B hepatitis ▶B 型肝炎ウイルス hepatitis B virus ; HBV B 型肝炎ワクチン hepatitis B vaccine
ピークフロー (ピーク呼気フロー) peak expiratory flow ; PEF ◆ピークフロー検査は肺からどのくらい速く空気が出せるかを測ります A peak flow test measures *how fast you can breathe air out of your lungs[(呼気の最大速度を) the maximum speed at which you can exhale air from your lungs]. ▶ピークフロー変動性 peak flow variability ピークフローメーター peak flow meter
ビーぐんれんさきゅうきん B 群連鎖球菌 group B streptococcus, group B strep ; GBS ▶B 群連鎖球菌感染症 group B strep[streptococcus] infection
ビーさいぼう B 細胞 B cell, B lymphocyte ▶B 細胞性悪性リンパ腫 B-cell malignant lymphoma
ピーシーアール PCR (ポリメラーゼ連鎖反応) polymerase chain reaction
ピーシーアイ PCI (経皮的冠動脈インターベンション) percutaneous coronary intervention
ビーシージー BCG (カルメット・ゲラン桿菌) bacille Calmette-Guérin ★一般的に英語圏では略語の BCG をあまり使わない. ◆BCG の予防接種を受ける have the tuberculosis vaccine / have a BCG shot [vaccine] / be vaccinated against tuberculosis ▶BCG 接種 BCG[antituberculosis] vaccination

ピーシーピーエス PCPS （経皮的心肺補助装置）percutaneous cardiopulmonary support

ピーティー PT （理学療法士）physical therapist, physiotherapist

ピーティーエスディー PTSD （心的外傷後ストレス障害）posttraumatic stress disorder

ピーティーシーアール PTCR （経皮経管的冠動脈再開通術）percutaneous transluminal coronary recanalization[revascularization]

ピーティーシーエイ PTCA （経皮経管的冠動脈形成術）percutaneous transluminal coronary angioplasty

ピーティーシーディー PTCD （経皮経肝胆道ドレナージ）percutaneous transhepatic cholangiodrainage

ピーティービーディー PTBD （経皮経肝胆汁ドレナージ）percutaneous transhepatic biliary drainage

ピービーエル PBL （問題解決型学習・問題基盤型学習）problem-based learning

ピープ PEEP （呼気終末陽圧）positive end-expiratory pressure

びいんとう 鼻咽頭 nose and throat, nasopharynx （形nasopharyngeal） ▶鼻咽頭エアウェイ nasopharyngeal airway 鼻咽頭炎 nasopharyngitis 鼻咽頭鏡 nasopharyngeal mirror

ひえいせい 非衛生(的な) （環境・設備の）unsanitary （清潔さ・疾病予防の）unhygienic （健康に悪い）unhealthy

ひえる 冷える get[become] cold （冷たく感じる）feel cold ◆手足がよく冷えますか Do your hands and feet often get cold? / Do you often have cold hands and feet?

ピエロ ☞クラウン

びえん 鼻炎 rhinitis /rɪnáɪtɪs/ ◀アレルギー性鼻炎 allergic rhinitis 季節性アレルギー性鼻炎 seasonal allergic rhinitis 急性〈慢性〉鼻炎 acute〈chronic〉rhinitis 通年性アレルギー性鼻炎 perennial allergic rhinitis 肥厚性鼻炎 hypertrophic rhinitis

びおん 鼻音 nasal sound, nasality ▶鼻

音症 rhinolalia / rhinophony

びおんとう 微温湯 lukewarm water, tepid water

びおんよく 微温浴 lukewarm bath, tepid bath

ひか 皮下(の) subcutaneous /sÀbkjuː-téimiəs/, hypodermic （直under the skin, below the skin） ▶皮下気腫 subcutaneous emphysema 皮下結節 subcutaneous nodule 皮下組織 subcutaneous tissue 皮下膿瘍 subcutaneous abscess ☞皮下脂肪, 皮下出血, 皮下注射

ひがい 被害 （損害）damage （損失・喪失）loss （損傷）injury ◆深刻な被害を及ぼす cause[do] serious damage ◆精神的な被害を受ける suffer psychological damage ◆騒音被害 noise damage ☞被害者, 被害妄想

ひがいきょうしきしんマッサージ 非開胸式心マッサージ closed-chest heart[cardiac] massage, external cardiac massage；ECM

ひがいしゃ 被害者 victim （動犠牲を強いるvictimize） ◆被害者意識を持つ feel victimized[(不等な扱いを受けたと感じる)unfairly treated] / have a feeling of *being victimized[being treated unfairly] ◀強姦被害者 rape victim セクシャルハラスメント被害者 victim of sexual harassment

ひがいほう 非開放(性の) closed ▶非開放性損傷 closed injury[wound]

ひがいもうそう 被害妄想 delusion of persecution, persecutory delusion

ひかえしつ 控室 waiting room ☞待合室

ひがえり 日帰り ◆この手術は日帰りでできます This surgery is a same-day procedure. / You can go home the day of this surgery. ▶日帰り手術(同日手術)day [same-day] surgery /(外来手術)outpatient[ambulatory] surgery 日帰り人間ドック one-day comprehensive physical [health] checkup

ひかえる 控える （量を減らす）cut down [back](on) （適度・適量にとどめる）be moderate （見合わせる・我慢する）refrain

(from) （避ける）avoid ☞差し控える，止める（やめる） ◆水分〈塩分〉を控えて下さい Please cut down on your water〈salt〉. / Be moderate in your water〈salt〉 intake.
◆飲酒は控えて下さい You should not drink alcohol. / Please refrain from drinking alcohol. ◆性行為は控えて下さい Please refrain from sexual activity. ◆激しい運動はしばらくの間控えて下さい Please avoid strenuous exercise for a while. / You shouldn't do any hard exercise for a while.

ひかぎゃく 非可逆（的な） irreversible

ひかく¹ 被殻 putamen （園putaminal）
▶被殻出血 putaminal bleeding[hemorrhage]

ひかく² 比較する compare ...（with, to）（図comparison 國比較的に comparatively 相対的に relatively） ◆この２つのＸ線写真を比較してみましょう Let's compare these two X-ray films. ◆前回の結果と比較して，今回はずっとよくなっています Compared with the last result, this one is much better. ◆この病気は比較的まれです This disease is comparatively rare.
◆このタイプの病気は進行速度が比較的遅い〈速い〉This type of disease develops at a relatively slow〈fast〉 speed. ◀無作為化比較試験 randomized controlled trial

ひかしぼう 皮下脂肪 subcutaneous fat ◆お腹に皮下脂肪がつく put on some *abdominal fat[fat around *one's* belly]
▶皮下脂肪型肥満 subcutaneous fat obesity

ひかしゅっけつ 皮下出血 bleeding under the skin (surface), subcutaneous bleeding[hemorrhage] （打撲による内出血斑）bruise /brúːz/ （園bruise） ☞痣，打ち身 ◆皮下出血を起こしやすいですか Do you bruise easily? / Do you bleed under the skin easily? / Do you tend to get blood spots under the skin? ◆（打撲などで）皮下出血を起こしている have a black-and-blue spot[mark] ▶皮下出血斑 petechiae

ひかちゅうしゃ 皮下注射 subcutaneous injection, hypodermic injection ☞注射
◆皮下注射をする give[administer] a subcutaneous[hypodermic] injection

ひかつどう 非活動（的な・性の） （不活発な）inactive （身体をあまり動かさない）physically inactive ◆非活動的なライフスタイル a physically inactive lifestyle / （座りがちな）a sedentary lifestyle

ひかねつけつえきせいざい 非加熱血液製剤 unheated blood product, non-heat-treated blood product

ひかり 光 （明かり）light （光線）ray （ぎらぎらした光）glare 園phot(o)- ☞明かり，光線 ◆光が見えますか Can you see a light? ◆目にペンライトの光を入れますが，真っ直ぐ前を見て下さい I'm going to shine this penlight into your eye(s), so please look straight ahead.
◆点滅する光を目で追いかけて下さい Please follow the flashing light with your eye. ◆光がまぶしい be sensitive to sunlight[light] / have problems with glare
◆光の周りに輪が見える see halos around lights ◆ちらちらする光 flickering lights ◆ぱっと走るような光 flashing lights ◆光の強度 light intensity ▶光アレルギー photoallergy 光アレルギー性接触皮膚炎 photoallergic contact dermatitis 光化学療法 photochemotherapy 光過敏症 photosensitive disorder 光過敏性てんかん photosensitive epilepsy；PSE 光凝固術 photocoagulation 光刺激 photic stimulation 光貼付試験 photopatch test

ひかんけつ 非観血（的な） （非侵襲的な）noninvasive ▶非観血的整復法 closed reduction 非観血的療法 noninvasive treatment

ひかんせん 非感染（性の） noninfectious （無菌性の）aseptic ▶非感染創 aseptic wound

ひかんてき 悲観的（な） pessimistic （↔optimistic） （消極的・否定的な）negative （↔positive） ◆病気のことを悲観的に考える be pessimistic about the disease / think pessimistically about the disease / have a pessimistic view of the disease

◆病気に対して悲観的な態度をとる have [take] a pessimistic[negative] attitude toward *one's* illness ◆悲観的な人生観 a pessimistic *view of[outlook on] life

ひきあげる 引き上げる **pull up** ☞捲る（まくる） ◆下着のシャツを引き上げる pull up *one's* undershirt

ひきうける 引き受ける （世話をする）**take care of** ◆あなたが診察中、お子さんのお世話を引き受けます I'm happy to take care of your child while the doctor sees [examines] you.

ひきおこしはんのう 引き起こし反応 traction response

ひきがね 引き金 **trigger** （動**trigger**） ◆喘息症状の引き金になったものがありますか Did anything trigger[(引き起こす] bring on] your asthma symptoms? / Was there any trigger for your asthma symptoms?

ひきこもり 引きこもり **shut-in** （社会からの隠遁）**recluse from society** （周囲との交流拒否）**social withdrawal** （解離）**dissociation** （外出拒否）**self-confinement at home, refusal to leave home**

ひきこもる 引きこもる （閉じこもる）**shut** *oneself* **up** （人目を避ける）**shut** *oneself* **off** （心を閉ざす）**withdraw** ◆何もしないで終日家に引きこもっている *shut oneself* up in *one's* home[stay at home] all day without doing anything ◆息子さんが引きこもるようになったきっかけは何ですか What made your son *withdraw into himself[withdraw from his family]?

ひきざん 引き算 **subtraction** ☞引く

ひきずる （物を引いて行く）**drag** （足を）**shuffle** （特に片足を）**limp** ◆足を引きずって歩く shuffle / drag *one's* foot ▶引きずり歩行 shuffling gait

ひきつぎ 引継ぎ **shift handover, patient handover** *between* **shifts[at shift change]** ◆勤務を交代する際に患者の引継ぎを行う share information about patients at shift change / transfer patient data between shifts ▶引継ぎ事項 matter to be handed over

ひきつぐ 引き継ぐ （責任を引き受ける）**take charge** （引き渡す）**hand over, hand on** ◆明日からは同僚の加藤医師が引き継ぎます From tomorrow, my colleague, Mr Kato, will take charge of your care. / From tomorrow, you'll be handed over to the care of my colleague, Dr Kato.

ひきつけ 痙攣、発作

ひきつづき 引き続き ◆引き続き原因究明に努めますので、もうしばらくお時間を下さい We're continuing to try to identify what's causing the problem, so please give me a little more time.

ひきつる 引きつる （激痛を伴って痙攣する）**get[have] a cramp, cramp** **(up)** （筋肉が短く繰り返しぴくぴくする）**have tics** **[spasms]** （急に突然ぴくっと収縮する）**twitch** （引っ張る）**pull** ◆筋肉が引きつったことがありますか Have you ever had any muscle cramps or twitching? ◆どの筋肉が引きつりますか Which muscle *cramps up[twitches]? ◆足の筋肉が引きつる get a cramp in (the muscles of) the leg / the leg muscles cramp up ◆無意識のうちに顔の筋肉がぴくぴく引きつる have involuntary *facial tics[spasms in the face] ◆まぶたが引きつる the eyelids twitch / have twitching (of the) eyelids ◆引きつるような感覚 a pulling sensation

ひきつれ 引きつれ ☞瘢痕

ひきぬく 引き抜く **pull out** ◆栄養管を引き抜く pull out the feeding tube

ひぎゃくたいじ 被虐待児 **battered child, abused child** ▶被虐待児症候群 battered child syndrome

ひきゅうしゅうせいほうごうし 非吸収性縫合糸 nonabsorbable suture

びきょう 鼻鏡 **nasal speculum** ▶鼻鏡検査 rhinoscopy

ひきょうどう 非共同(性の) **disconjugate, incomitant** ▶非共同眼球運動 disconjugate eye movement 非共同性斜視 incomitant strabismus

ひく 引く 《引っ張る》（上下・前後に引く）**pull** （軽く引き寄せる）**draw** ◆この取っ手を引くとキャ

ビネットが開きます Pull this knob and the cabinet will open. ◆あごを引く draw in *one's* chin ◆カーテンを引く draw [close] the curtain
《引き算する》**subtract** ◆100から7を引くといくつになりますか．If you subtract seven from one hundred, what do you get? / What's one hundred minus seven? ◆100から7を順番に引いて下さい Please count down from one hundred *by sevens [by subtracting seven each time].
《ペン・鉛筆などで描く》**draw** ◆線を引く draw a line
《症状が治まる》《鎮まる・軽減する》**go down, decrease, subside** 《よくなる》**get better** ◆腫れが引いてきています The swelling is *going down[decreasing / getting better]. ◆熱が引きました The fever has *gone down[subsided].
《風邪をひく》**catch, have** ◆風邪をひく catch[have] a cold

ひくい 低い 《数値が》**low** 《身長が》**short** 《音・声が》**low, low-pitched** ◆血圧が低い have low blood pressure / *one's* blood pressure is low ◆正常値〈平均〉より低い be lower than normal〈average〉 ◆カロリーの低い物を食べる eat low-calorie food ◆年齢の割に背が低い be short (in stature) for his〈her〉 age ◆低い音や声が聞き取りにくいですか Do you have difficulty hearing low[low-pitched] sounds and voices? ◆低い声で話す speak in a low voice ◆テレビの音を低くして下さい Please turn down the TV.

びくう 鼻腔 nasal cavity ◀後鼻腔 postnasal space ▶鼻腔栄養管 nasal feeding tube 鼻腔酸素カニューラ nasal oxygen cannula 鼻腔通気度検査 rhinometry 鼻腔内投与 intranasal administration ☞副鼻腔

ひげ 髭 《あご髭》**beard** 《口髭》**mustache,** 《英》**moustache** 《ほお髭》**whiskers** ★通例，複数形で．◆《顔の》ひげを剃る shave 《*one's*》face / have a shave ◆あごひげ《口ひげ》を剃る shave (off) *one's* beard 〈mustache〉 ◆ひげを剃りますから，動か

ないで下さい Please stay[be] still while I'm shaving your face. ◆ご自分でひげを剃りますか Will you shave yourself?
▶髭そり道具 shaving things[items] / (道具一式) shaving kit 髭そり用クリーム shaving cream[foam]

ひけいこうえいようほう 非経口栄養法 parenteral nutrition；PN

びけいせいじゅつ 鼻形成術 rhinoplasty 《インフォーマルに》**nose job**

ひけつ 秘訣 《秘密》**secret** 《鍵となるもの》**key** 《ヒント》**tip** ◆健康の秘訣は早寝早起きです The secret of good health is to go to bed early and to get up early in the morning.

ひけつえんしゃ 非血縁者(の) unrelated ▶非血縁者間骨髄移植 unrelated bone marrow transplant[transplantation]；UR-BMT 非血縁者間生体腎移植 unrelated living kidney transplant[transplantation]

ひけっかくせいこうさんきん 非結核性抗酸菌 nontuberculous mycobacterium；NTM ▶非結核性抗酸菌症 nontuberculous mycobacterial disease

ひケトン 非ケトン性(の) nonketotic

ひげんご 非言語(の) nonverbal ◆非言語メッセージを送る〈受け取る〉 send〈pick up / receive〉 nonverbal messages ◆非言語で意思の疎通を図る communicate nonverbally ◆非言語の合図を見逃す miss a nonverbal cue ▶非言語コミュニケーション nonverbal communication

ひけんしゃ 被験者 subject 《参加者》**participant**

ひこう¹ 肥厚 thickness, thickening 《形thickened》, **hypertrophy** 《形hypertrophic》 ◆肥厚した指〈足〉の爪 a thickened fingernail〈toenail〉 ◆胸膜肥厚 pleural thickening ▶肥厚性瘢痕 hypertrophic scar 肥厚性鼻炎 hypertrophic rhinitis 肥厚性幽門狭窄症 hypertrophic pyloric stenosis

ひこう² 非行 delinquency 《形delinquent》 ◆非行に走る子供たち children who turn to delinquency ◆非行の徴候を示す

show signs of delinquency ◀青少年非行 juvenile delinquency ▶非行少女〈少年〉female〈male〉juvenile delinquent

びこう 鼻孔 nostril ☞後鼻孔

びこうかい 鼻甲介 turbinate (bone), nasal concha

ひこうき 飛行機 airplane, plane ◆最近, 飛行機に乗りましたか Have you recently *flown in[traveled on] an airplane? ◆飛行機に酔う get airsick ▶飛行機酔い airsickness

ひこうしん 批糠疹 pityriasis ◀頭部批糠疹 pityriasis capitis /（ふけ）dandruff

びこきゅう 鼻呼吸 nasal breathing, nose breathing, breathing through *one's* nose

ピコグラム picogram ; pg

ひこつ 腓骨 fibula （⬚fibular, peroneal）, calf bone ▶腓骨骨折 fibular fracture / fracture of the fibula 腓骨神経麻痺 peroneal nerve paralysis

びこつ¹ 鼻骨 nasal bone ▶鼻骨骨折 nasal bone fracture / fracture of the nasal bone

びこつ² 尾骨 tailbone, coccyx （⬚coccygeal）, coccygeal bone ▶尾骨神経 coccygeal nerve 尾骨部 coccygeal region

ひざ 膝 knee /níː/ （⬚膝をつく kneel）（座った時の両太腿の部分）lap （膝蓋）patella, kneecap

《基本表現》 ◆膝を伸ばす extend[stretch out] *one's* knees ◆膝をすりむく scrape [graze / skin] *one's* knee ◆膝に負担をかける put stress on *one's* knees ◆膝をつく[ひざまずく]kneel (down) ◀転んで膝をつく fall onto *one's* knees ◆膝ががくんとする the knee buckles[gives way]

《診察の基本表現》 ◆膝に問題がありますか Do you have any *knee problems[problems with your knees]? ◆膝は痛みますか Do your knees[Does your knee] hurt? / Do you have any knee pain? / Do you have (any) pain in the knee(s)? ◆膝をつくのが難しいですか Do you have difficulty kneeling? ◆膝に水がたまっています Excess water[fluid] has *built up

[accumulated] in and around the knee (joints). ◆膝の水を抜くと一時的に楽になりますが, またたまるかもしれません We can drain[remove] the water[fluid] from the knee for quick relief, but it may build up again. ◆膝を曲げて, お腹の力を抜いて下さい Please bend your knees and relax your abdomen. ◆膝を軽く曲げて胸のほうにつけて下さい Please bend[flex] your knees slightly and bring them toward your chest. ◆膝を軽く叩いて反射を調べる check the reflexes by tapping *a person's* knee / check *a person's* *knee jerk[patellar reflex] by tapping

◀ジャンパー膝 jumper knee ▶膝当て knee pad /（サポーター）knee support 膝上切断 above-the-knee[AK] amputation 膝掛け lap blanket[throw] 膝関節 knee joint 膝義足 knee disarticulation prosthesis 膝下切断 below-the-knee[BK] amputation 膝装具 knee brace[orthosis] 膝立ち kneeling 膝副子 knee splint

ビザ visa ◆彼女のビザは切れています Her visa has expired. ◆ビザの有効期日が差し迫っているのですぐ更新して下さい Your visa is going to expire soon, so you should renew it *right away[as soon as possible]. ◆有効なビザ a valid visa

◀医療滞在ビザ visa for medical stay / medical stay visa 永住ビザ permanent-resident[residence] visa 学生ビザ student visa 観光ビザ tourist visa 再入国ビザ reentry visa 就労ビザ work[working] visa 短期滞在ビザ short-term (resident) visa 長期滞在ビザ long-term (resident) visa 入国ビザ entry visa

びさい 微細（な）（細かい・小さい）fine （最小の）minimal ◀微細運動 fine movement 微細運動技能 fine motor skill(s) 微細振戦 fine tremor 微細脳機能障害 minimal brain dysfunction；MBD 微細脳損傷 minimal brain damage[injury]

ひし 皮脂 sebum （⬚sebaceous） ▶皮脂欠乏 asteatosis 皮脂欠乏性湿疹 asteatotic eczema 皮脂腺 sebaceous gland(s)

ひじ　肘　elbow ◆肘を曲げる bend *one's* elbow(s) ◆肘を伸ばす straighten[stretch out] *one's* elbow(s) ◆肘の痛み (an) elbow pain /(a) pain in *one's* elbow ◀ゴルフ肘 golfer's elbow　テニス肘 tennis elbow　野球肘 baseball[(投手の) pitcher's] elbow ▶肘置き armrest　肘関節 elbow joint　肘関節脱臼 elbow dislocation　肘義手 elbow disarticulation prosthesis　肘杖 elbow crutch

ひしつ　皮質　cortex（臘cortical） ◀運動皮質 motor cortex　小脳皮質 cerebellar cortex　大脳皮質 cerebral cortex　副腎皮質 adrenal cortex ▶皮質運動〈感覚〉中枢 the cortical motor〈sensory〉center　皮質下出血 subcortical hemorrhage　皮質視床路 corticothalamic tract　皮質脊髄路 corticospinal tract

びじゃく　微弱(な)（弱い）**weak**（かすかな）**faint, feeble** ◆微弱な脈 a weak[faint / feeble] pulse ▶微弱陣痛 weak labor pains[contractions]

ひしゅ　脾腫　splenomegaly

ひじゅう　比重　specific gravity ◀高比重リポ蛋白 high-density lipoprotein；HDL / good cholesterol　低比重リポ蛋白 low-density lipoprotein；LDL / bad cholesterol　尿比重 urine specific gravity

びじゅう　☞鼻汁(はなじる)

びしゅっけつ　鼻出血　☞鼻血(はなぢ)

ひしょ　秘書　secretary ◀医療秘書 medical secretary

ひじょう[1]　非常　emergency ◆非常の際にはエレベーターではなく階段を使って下さい In case of (an) emergency, please use the stairs, not the elevators. ▶非常階段 emergency stairs / fire escape　非常口 emergency exit[door]　非常警報 emergency alert　非常ベル(火事の)fire alarm

ひじょう[2]　非常(に)　☞大変

びしょう　微小(な)　minimal（暖頭micr(o)-）◀微小癌 microcarcinoma　微小外科手技 microsurgery　微小血栓 microthrombus　微小循環 microcirculation　微小腺腫 microadenoma　微小変化型ネフローゼ症候群 minimal-change neph-

rotic syndrome；MCNS

びじょうかく　尾状核　caudate nucleus

ひじょうきん　非常勤(の)　part-time ☞パート ▶非常勤医 part-time doctor[physician] /(外部の病院からの)outside doctor[physician]

ひじょうみゃく　皮静脈　cutaneous vein, superficial vein

ひじょうひせいしゅよう　非上皮性腫瘍　nonepithelial tumor（間葉系腫瘍）**mesenchymal tumor**

ひしょくち　非触知(の)　nonpalpable, impalpable ▶非触知精巣 nonpalpable[impalpable] testis　非触知乳がん nonpalpable[impalpable] breast cancer

ひしん　皮疹　rash, exanthema（突発的に発生したもの）**eruption** ☞発疹(ほっしん) ◀麻疹様皮疹 measly rash

ひしんしゅう　非侵襲(的な)　noninvasive ▶非侵襲的陽圧換気 noninvasive positive pressure ventilation；NPPV

ヒスそく　―束　His bundle, bundle of His

ヒスタミン　histamine ◀抗ヒスタミン薬 histamine（receptor）antagonist / antihistamine

ヒスチジン　histidine ▶ヒスチジン血症 histidinemia

ヒステリー　hysteria（発作）**hysterics** ★複数形で.（臘hysterical, hysteric）◆ヒステリーを起こす get[become] hysterical / go into hysterics ◆ヒステリーを起こしている be in hysterics / be hysterical ◀転換ヒステリー conversion hysteria　不安ヒステリー anxiety hysteria ▶ヒステリー患者 hysteric　ヒステリー性格 hysterical personality　ヒステリー性失神 hysteric syncope　ヒステリー性失声症 hysteric aphonia　ヒステリー性難聴 hysterical hearing loss　ヒステリーてんかん hysteroepilepsy

ひステロイドけいこうえんしょうやく　非ステロイド系抗炎症薬　nonsteroidal antiinflammatory drugs；NSAIDs

ヒストプラズマしょう　―症　histoplasmosis

ヒスパニック　Hispanic（臘Hispanic）

びせい 鼻声 nasal voice, twang ☞鼻声
（はなごえ） ◀開鼻声 rhinolalia aperta 閉鼻声 rhinolalia clausa

びせいぶつ 微生物 microorganism, microbe（㊙microbial） ◀口腔微生物叢 oral microbial flora 病原微生物 pathogenic microorganism ▶微生物学 microbiology 微生物学者 microbiologist 微生物叢 flora

びせつ 鼻癤 nasal furuncle

びせんじょう 鼻洗浄 nasal douche[irrigation]

びぜんてい 鼻前庭 nasal vestibule

ひそ 砒素 arsenic ▶砒素中毒 arsenic poisoning

ひぞう 脾臓 spleen（㊙splenic） ▶脾臓梗塞 splenic infarction 脾（臓）損傷 splenic injury 脾（臓）摘出術 splenectomy

びぞう 微増 slight increase（㊙increase slightly）, small increase ◆血糖値が微増していますので，カロリーの摂りすぎに気をつけて下さい Your blood sugar level has slightly increased, so please watch your *caloric intake[calories].

びそく¹ 尾側（の） caudal（↔ rostral）

びそく² 鼻側（の） （両鼻側の）binasal

ひだ 襞 fold ◀（十二指腸の）縦ひだ longitudinal fold（of the duodenum）

ひたい 額 forehead, brow /bráu/ ◆あごと額を支持台につけて，光を見つめて下さい Please rest your chin and forehead on the support, and look at the light. ◆額を触りますがよろしいですか Is it all right[Do you mind] if I touch your forehead? ◆額に皺を寄せる knit[wrinkle] one's brow ◆額にかけて痛い It hurts across the forehead. ◆額に傷を負う（切り傷）have a cut[（打撲傷）bruise] on one's forehead ◆額の傷跡 a scar on the forehead

ひだい 肥大 （肥厚）hypertrophy（㊙hypertrophic） （腫大・拡大）enlargement（㊙enlarged） （㊙-megaly） ◆肥大した心臓 an enlarged heart ◆左心室が少し肥大しています Your left ventricle is slightly enlarged. ◀右室〈左室〉肥大 right〈left〉

ventricular hypertrophy 心肥大 cardiac hypertrophy / cardiomegaly 前立腺肥大 benign prostatic hyperplasia[hypertrophy]；BPH 扁桃肥大 tonsil hypertrophy / enlargement of the tonsils 末端肥大症 acromegaly ▶肥大型心筋症 hypertrophic cardiomyopathy；HCM 肥大心 hypertrophic heart 肥大扁桃 enlarged [swollen / hypertrophied] tonsil(s)

ひたいしょう 非対称 asymmetry（↔symmetry）（㊙asymmetric, asymmetrical）

ひだいしょう 非代償（の） decompensated, uncompensated ▶非代償性肝硬変 decompensated（liver）cirrhosis

ひたす 浸す （液体にどっぷりつける）soak （ちょっと浸す）dip （湿らす）moisten, wet ◆タオルをお湯〈氷水〉に浸して患部に当てるといいですよ You should soak the towel in warm〈iced〉water and apply it to the affected area.

ひだち 肥立ち （産後の）recovery after childbirth, convalescence after childbirth, postpartum recovery

ビタミン vitamin /váitəmin/ ◆ビタミンを摂る take vitamins ◆ビタミンや他のサプリメントを飲んでいますか Are you taking any vitamins or other supplements? ◆ワーファリン内服中は納豆，クランベリー，葉野菜などビタミンKを多く含む食品は摂らないで下さい While you are on warfarin, *please do not eat foods that contain large amounts of vitamin K [please avoid foods that are rich in vitamin K] such as natto, cranberries, or leafy, green vegetables. ◀活性型ビタミンD active vitamin D 脂溶性ビタミン fat-soluble vitamin 水溶性ビタミン water-soluble vitamin 総合ビタミン剤 multivitamin tablet[pill / supplement] 必須ビタミン essential vitamin ▶ビタミンA欠乏症 vitamin A deficiency ビタミンA過剰症 hypervitaminosis ビタミン強化食品 vitamin-enriched food ビタミンK依存性凝固因子 vitamin K-dependent coagulation[clotting] factor ビタミンK₂シロップ vitamin K₂ syrup ビタミン剤

vitamin tablet[pill]　ビタミンD依存性くる病 vitamin D-dependent rickets　ビタミンD欠乏性くる病 vitamin D-deficiency rickets　ビタミンD抵抗性くる病 vitamin D-resistant[-refractory] rickets　ビタミンB_6依存性痙攣 vitamin B_6-dependent seizure　ビタミンB_{12}欠乏性ニューロパチー neuropathy associated with vitamin B_{12} deficiency　ビタミン必要量 vitamin requirement　ビタミン補助食品 vitamin supplement

ひだり　左　the left (↔the right)　(関left 園 left)　◆左を見て下さい Please look to the left.　◆左上〈左下〉を見て下さい Please look at the upper〈lower〉 left-hand corner.　◆左の目を手で隠して下さい Please cover your left eye with your hand.　◆左を向いて下さい Please turn to *the left[your left].　◆左の腕に注射をする give the injection in the left arm　◆左手を使う use one's left hand　◆左半身が麻痺している the left side of the body is paralyzed / *be paralyzed[have paralysis] on the left side of one's body　◆左に曲がる turn left　☞左側, 左利き, 左向き

ひだりがわ　左側(に・の)　on one's[the] left side, in one's[the] left side　◆左側の痛み(a) pain on the left side　◆ナースステーションは左側です The nurses' station is on the left (side).

ひだりきき　左利き　be left-handed　◆右利きですか, 左利きですか Are you right-handed or left-handed?

ひだりむき　左向き(に)　on one's[the] left side　◆左向きに寝て下さい Please lie on your left side.　◆今度は左向きになって下さい(寝返りを打って) This time, please roll over onto your left side.

ひたん　悲嘆　grief　◆息子の死で悲嘆に暮れる be *grief-stricken[overcome with grief / crushed with grief] over the death of one's son

びちゅうかく　鼻中隔　nasal septum　(関 (nasal) septal)　▶鼻中隔矯正術 septoplasty　鼻中隔骨折 septal fracture　鼻中隔弯曲(症) (nasal) septal deviation

ひっかかる　(挟まる・からまる・くっつく) get[be] stuck, stick in, get[be] caught　◆何かが喉にひっかかった感じがする feel as if something is stuck[caught] in one's throat

ひっかく　引っ掻く　scratch　(かさぶた・吹き出物を引っ掻く) pick (at)　◆皮膚を引っ掻かないで下さい Please avoid scratching your skin.　◆かさぶたを引っ掻く pick at the scab　▶引っ掻き傷 scratch　引っ掻き痕 scratch mark

ひつぎ　柩　casket, coffin

ピックウィックしょうこうぐん　―症候群　pickwickian syndrome　(肥満低換気症候群) obesity hypoventilation syndrome

ピックびょう　―病　Pick disease

ひづけ　日付　date　(関日付を入れる date)　◆同意書に日付を入れるのを忘れないで下さい Please don't forget to date[put the date on] the consent form.

ひっこす　引っ越す　move (to, into)　◆引っ越しが原因でストレスを感じる feel stress due to moving　◆仙台に引っ越す move to Sendai　◆新しいアパートに引っ越す move to[into] a new apartment　▶引っ越しうつ病(house) moving blues / moving anxiety　引っ越し先(新住所) new address

ひっこめる　引っ込める　(息を吸い込んで) suck in (↔push out)　◆お腹を引っ込めて下さい Please suck in your stomach.

ひっす　必須(の)　(本質的になくてはならない) essential, indispensable　(絶対に必要な) imperative　☞必要, 不可欠　▶必須アミノ酸 essential amino acid　必須栄養素 essential nutrient　必須元素 essential element　必須脂肪酸 essential fatty acid　必須ビタミン essential vitamin

ひっぱる　引っ張る　(引く) pull　(無理やり引きずる) drag　(ぐいと引く) tug (on, at)　◆引っ張られるような感覚 a pulling[dragging] sensation　◆耳を引っ張る pull[tug] on[at] an ear

ひつよう　必要(がある)　(人が必要とする) need　(物・事が要求する) require　(関 necessary　不可欠な essential, indispensable)

◆水分を多く飲む必要があります You need to drink a lot of water. ◆今のあなたに必要なのは十分な休養です You need a good rest now. / What you need now is (to get) a good rest. ◆この薬は必要に応じて飲んで下さい Please take this medication *whenever you need it[as needed]. ◆尿検査が必要です You need to have a urine test. ◆手術を行うにはあなたの同意が必要です I need your consent to do this surgery. / Your consent is needed[necessary] for this surgery. ◆病気の回復にはもっと前向きになる必要があります For the sake for your recovery, you need to be more positive. /（前向きな態度が欠かせない）It's essential that you keep a positive attitude about your recovery. ◆すぐに手術をする必要はありません There's no need[hurry] to have surgery right away. ◆この入院説明書に必要な情報が載っています You'll find the necessary information in this admission brochure. ◆必要ならば，臨床心理士をご紹介いたします If (it's) necessary, we'll arrange for a clinical psychologist to come and see you. ▶必要条件 requirement / necessary condition ☞必要量

ひつようりょう　必要量　requirement, required quantity[amount], needs　★通例，複数形で．◆1日のビタミンCの必要量を満たす meet *one's* daily vitamin C requirements[needs] ▶1日必要量 daily requirement　栄養必要量 nutritional[dietary] requirement　ビタミン必要量 vitamin requirement

ひてい　否定する　（認めることを拒む）refuse（図refusal）（否認する）deny（図denial），say no（図negative）☞否認 ◆彼は若年性アルツハイマー病だという現実を否定しています He refuses to admit that he has early-onset Alzheimer disease. / He denies the reality of early-onset Alzheimer disease. ◆がんになったという事実を否定する deny the fact that *one* has cancer ◆物事を否定的に見る see things negatively ◆否定的な態度 a negative atti-

tude

ひていけい　非定型(の)　atypical ▶非定型[非結核性]抗酸菌 nontuberculous mycobacterium；NTM　非定型精神病 atypical psychosis　非定型肺炎 atypical pneumonia

びていこつ　尾骶骨　☞尾骨

ビデオないしきょう　─内視鏡　video endoscope

ビデオほじょかきょうくうきょうしゅじゅつ　─補助下胸腔鏡手術　video-assisted thoracic surgery；VATS

ひてきしゅつじゅつ　脾摘出術　splenectomy

ひてんけい　非典型(の)　not typical, atypical ◆あなたの症状は狭心症と考えるには非典型的です Your symptoms are not typical of angina.

ひでんりほうしゃせん　非電離放射線　nonionizing radiation ▶非電離放射線障害 nonionizing radiation injury[disorder]

ひどい　（病状が重い）severe, bad　（程度がひどい）terrible　（耐えがたい）unbearable　（苦しい・つらい）difficult, hard ◆ひどい痛みがある have (a) severe[terrible] pain / be in terrible[unbearable] pain ◆ひどく痛みますか Is the pain very bad? / Does it hurt a lot? ◆息切れは仰向けに寝るとひどくなりますか Do you find breathing more difficult when you're lying flat on your back? ◆咳がひどい have a bad cough ◆頭痛は徐々にひどくなっていますか Is your headache getting worse? ◆症状が前よりひどくなった時は連絡して下さい Please call us if your symptoms get worse.

ひといき　一息　《一呼吸》one breath ☞一気(いっき) ◆できるだけ勢いよく一息で吐いて下さい Please blow out as hard and fast as you can in one breath. 《少しの辛抱・努力》a little[bit of] patience, a little[bit of] effort ◆もう一息で検査はすべて終わります Just a little more patience and the test will be all over. 《一休み》a little rest, a break ◆この辺で一

ひとくい 非特異(の) nonspecific ▶非特異変化 nonspecific change 非特異免疫 nonspecific immunity 非特異療法 nonspecific therapy

ひとくち 一口 (一口の分量)mouthful (一飲み)gulp (一すすり)sip ◆一口ずつゆっくり食べて下さい Please eat slowly, one mouthful at a time. ◆薬を一口で飲む take the medication in one gulp ◆オレンジジュースを一口飲む take a sip [mouthful] of orange juice

ひどくもうそう 被毒妄想 poisoning delusion, delusion of poisoning

ヒトゲノム human genome

ひとごみ 人混み crowd ◆人混みを避ける avoid crowds ◆人混みを怖がる have a fear of crowds

ひとさしゆび 人差し指 first finger, index finger, forefinger ☞指

ひとしい 等しい (大きさ・数・量などが同じ)equal (まったく同じ)the same (そっくり)identical (圖ほぼ等しい about) ☞同じ, 同等 ◆あなたの卵巣腫瘍は鶏卵の大きさにほぼ等しいサイズです The tumor in your ovary is about the size of an egg. / The size of the tumor in your ovary is roughly that of an egg. ◆この2つの薬は成分が等しい These two medications are equal [the same] in terms of ingredients. / These two medications contain the same [identical] active ingredients.

ヒトじゅうもうせいゴナドトロピン 一絨毛性ゴナドトロピン human chorionic gonadotropin；hCG

ヒトせいちょうホルモン 一成長ホルモン human growth hormone；hGH

ヒトティーリンパきゅうこうせいウイルス１がた ―Tリンパ球向性ウイルス１型 human T-lymphotropic virus type 1；HTLV-1

ヒトはっけっきゅうこうげん 一白血球抗原 human leukocyte antigen；HLA

ヒトパピローマウイルス human papillomavirus；HPV ▶ヒトパピローマウイルスワクチン HPV vaccine

ヒトヘルペスウイルス human herpesvirus；HHV

ひとみ 瞳 (瞳孔)pupil ☞目

ひとみしり 人見知り stranger anxiety ◆お子さんは人見知りしますか Does your baby[child] have stranger anxiety? / Does your baby[child] cry when he〈she〉sees unfamiliar faces?

ヒトめんえきふぜんウイルス 一免疫不全ウイルス human immunodeficiency virus；HIV

ひとやすみ 一休み ☞一息(ひといき)

ひとり 一人・独り(で) alone, by *oneself*, on *one's* own ◆お一人でお住まいですか Do you live alone[by yourself]? / Are you living alone? ◆家に一人きりでいる時不安な気持ちにかられる feel anxious or nervous when *one* stays home alone ◆一人でできますか Can you manage[do it] *by yourself[on your own]? ◆一人で立つ〈歩く〉stand〈walk〉alone[without support / without help] ◆一人で服を着る dress *oneself* without support[help]

ひとりあそび 一人遊び・独り遊び ◆一人遊びをする play alone[by *oneself*]

ひとりあるき 一人歩き・独り歩き ◆一人歩きをする walk without support[help] / walk unaided

ひとりおやかてい 一人親家庭 single-parent family

ひとりぐらし 一人暮らし・独り暮らし single life ◆一人暮らしですか，それともご家族か友人とお住まいですか Do you live alone[by yourself], or with〈your〉family or friends?

ひとりごと 独り言 ◆独り言を言う talk to *oneself* / (ぶつぶつ言う)mutter to *oneself*

ひとりべや 一人部屋 private room, single room, room for one

ひない 皮内(の) intracutaneous (表皮の)intradermal ▶皮内検査 intracutaneous[intradermal] test 皮内出血 intradermal bruise 皮内注射 intracutaneous[intradermal] injection 皮内反応 intra-

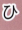

cutaneous reaction

ひなん 避難する （避難させる）evacuate （図evacuation） （避難する）escape ◆火災発生時に患者を避難させる evacuate patients in case of (a) fire ◆火災が発生しました．指示に従って避難して下さい A fire has broken out. Please evacuate the building as directed. ◀緊急避難所 (emergency) evacuation area ▶避難訓練（火災の）fire drill /（地震の）earthquake drill 避難命令 evacuation order

ビニールぶくろ 一袋 plastic bag

ひにょうき 泌尿器 urinary organs ★通例，複数形で．（図urologic） ▶泌尿器科（診療科）the department of urology / the urology department 泌尿器科医 urologist /（泌尿生殖器外科医）genitourinary surgeon 泌尿器科学 urology 泌尿器系 the urinary system 泌尿生殖器 the genitourinary[urogenital] organs

ひにん¹ 否認する deny （図denial） ☞否定 ◆自分の障害や病気を否認する deny one's problem or illness ◀病気否認 denial of illness

ひにん² 避妊 contraception （図contraceptive） （産児制限）birth control ◆避妊していますか Do you use[practice] birth control? /（経口避妊薬で）Are you *taking the pill[on the pill]? /（コンドームで）Do you use condoms for birth control? ◆どんな避妊具を使っていますか What kind of contraceptive device do you use? ◀緊急避妊ピル emergency contraceptive pills；ECP /（性交後ピル）morning-after pill 緊急避妊法 emergency contraception；EC 経口避妊薬 the pill ★通例，the をつけて．/ birth control pill / oral contraceptive；OC 子宮内避妊器具 intrauterine device；IUD / *birth control[contraceptive] ring ▶避妊具 contraceptive device 避妊用ゼリー contraceptive jelly 避妊用フィルム contraceptive film

びねつ 微熱 slight fever, mild fever, low-grade fever ☞熱 ◆微熱がある have a slight fever /（少し熱っぽい）be slightly feverish

ひねる 捻る twist （捻挫する）sprain ☞捻挫 ◆腰をひねる twist one's (lower) back / twist one's body at the waist ◆体をひねる twist one's body / twist around ◆首〈足首〉をひねる twist one's neck〈ankle〉

びねんまく 鼻粘膜 nasal mucosa ▶鼻粘膜誘発テスト nasal mucosa test

ひはいぐうしゃかんじんこうじゅせい 非配偶者間人工授精 artificial insemination by donor；AID

ひばく 被曝 exposure （動be exposed） ◆放射線の被曝を防ぐ shield … from exposure to radiation / prevent exposure to radiation ◆卵巣への被曝を防ぐためにお腹にこの鉛エプロンを載せます I'm going to [Let me] place this lead apron on your abdomen to *shield your ovaries from exposure to the radiation[prevent your ovaries from being exposed to the radiation]. ◀医療被曝 medical radiation exposure 体内被曝 internal exposure ▶被曝線量 exposure dose

ひばん 非番（の）off-duty ◆今日鈴木先生は非番です Dr Suzuki is off duty today. / Dr Suzuki has the day off today. ◆非番の医師 an off-duty doctor

ひび （小さな割れ目）small crack, narrow crack （図割れて亀裂がある cracked） （骨折などによる細いひび）hairline fracture （図fractured） ◆骨にひびが入っています There's a small[narrow] crack in the bone. / The bone is cracked. ☞ひび割れ

ひびく 響く （反響する）echo （振動する）vibrate ◆自分の声が響く感じがしますか Do you feel as if your voice is echoing [vibrating] in your ear(s) [head] when you speak?

ひびわれ ひび割れ crack （図亀裂がある cracked 荒れた chapped） ◆指にひび割れができる have cracked fingers ◆手がひび割れする one's hands get cracked [chapped] ◆ひび割れを起こした唇 chapped[cracked] lips

ひふ 皮膚 skin, cutis （図cutaneous 表皮の dermal） ☞肌

《基本表現》 ◆皮膚を掻く scratch the skin ◆皮膚をこする rub the skin
《診察の基本表現》 ◆皮膚に何か問題がありますか. 発疹, 変色, ひりひり感, かゆみ, 乾燥, 剥がれなどですか Do you have any problems with your skin? Any rash, discoloration, sore, itching, dryness, or flaking? ◆最近, 皮膚に何か変化がありましたか Have you noticed any changes in your skin? ◆(注射をする前に)アルコール綿で皮膚がかぶれたことがありますか Have you ever had a skin rash from using alcohol wipes before?
《症状の表現》 ◆皮膚が弱い have delicate [sensitive] skin ◆皮膚が荒れている(ざらざらした) have rough[(ひび割れた) chapped] skin / one's skin is[feels] rough [chapped] ◆皮膚がかゆい have itchy skin / one's skin *is itchy[itches] ◆皮膚に発疹が出る have a (skin) rash / one's skin breaks out in a rash ◆皮膚がみみず腫れを起こしている have welts on the skin ◆火傷で皮膚がむける the skin peels off as a result of burns ◆皮膚にあざがある have bruises[patches] on one's skin ◆皮膚に炎症を起こす irritate the skin / cause the skin to become irritated [inflamed] / cause skin irritation[inflammation] ◆皮膚が赤くすりむけて水膨れができている the skin is raw and blistered ◆黄疸で皮膚が黄色味を帯びる the skin becomes yellowish due to jaundice ◆皮膚の色 skin color ◆皮膚の変色 discoloration of the skin / skin color changes / changes in skin color ◆皮膚の黄染 yellowing of the skin / yellowish discoloration of the skin ◆皮膚のきめ[肌触り] skin texture ◆皮膚のしみ skin blemish / blemish on the skin

◀人工皮膚 artificial skin ▶皮膚科 the department of dermatology / the dermatology department　皮膚科医 dermatologist　皮膚潰瘍 skin ulcer　皮膚科学 dermatology　皮膚がん skin cancer　皮膚感覚 skin[cutaneous] sense[sensation] / (表在感覚) superficial sense[sensation]　皮膚カンジダ症 cutaneous candidiasis　皮膚緊満度 skin turgor　皮膚色素沈着 (skin) pigmentation　皮膚消毒 skin antisepsis[disinfection]　皮膚生検 skin biopsy　皮膚切開 skin incision　皮膚線条 stretch mark　皮膚掻痒症 cutaneous pruritus / skin itching　皮膚パッチテスト skin patch test　皮膚バンク skin bank　皮膚プリックテスト skin prick test　皮膚縫合 skin suture / skin suturing　☞皮膚移植, 皮膚炎, 皮膚筋炎, 皮膚疾患, 皮膚粘膜眼症候群, 皮(膚)弁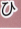

皮膚の色・性状

■ 皮膚の色
● 青い blue　● 青味がかった bluish　● 青銅色の bronze　● 青白い pale　● 青白さ(特に顔色の) pallor　● 赤い red　● 赤味がかった reddish　● 赤くなった reddened　● 赤紫の reddish purple　● 真っ赤な bright red　● 茶色の brown　● 薄い茶色の light brown　● 濃い茶色の dark brown　● 黄色の yellow　● 黄色味を帯びた yellowish　● 黄疸にかかったように黄色い jaundiced　● 灰色の gray　● 灰白色の ashen gray　● 濃い灰色の dark gray　● 灰色がかった grayish　● 黒い black　● 黒ずんだ darkened　● 変色した discolored

■ 皮膚の性状
● 健康的な皮膚 healthy[normal] skin　● 脂性の皮膚 oily[greasy] skin　● 萎縮した皮膚 atrophic skin　● 薄い皮膚 thin skin　● 肥厚した皮膚 thick[thickened] skin　● 炎症を起こしている皮膚 inflamed skin　● オレンジ皮様皮膚 orange peel skin　● かさぶただらけの皮膚 scabby skin　● 乾燥した皮膚 dry skin　● なめらかな皮膚 smooth skin　● ざらざらした皮膚 rough[scabrous / (さめ肌のような)dry and scaly] skin　● ひび割れた皮膚 cracked[chapped] skin　● じっとりとした皮膚 clammy skin　● しみだらけの皮膚 blotched skin　● 皺の寄った皮膚 wrinkled skin　● 損傷を起こした皮膚

broken skin ●たるんだ皮膚 slack[slackened] skin ●瘢痕のある皮膚 scarred skin ●ひりひりする皮膚（炎症を起こして）irritated skin ●敏感な皮膚 sensitive [delicate] skin ●吹き出物ができている皮膚 pimpled[pimply] skin ●まだら模様の皮膚 mottled skin ●やわらかい皮膚 soft skin ●硬くなった皮膚 hard[thick] skin

ひふいしょく 皮膚移植 skin graft[grafting] ◀全層皮膚移植 full-thickness skin graft[grafting]；FTSG 同種皮膚移植 allogenic skin graft[grafting] ▶皮膚移植片 skin graft

ビフィズスきん ―菌 Bifidobacterium bifidum

ひふえん 皮膚炎 dermatitis /də̀ːmətáɪtɪs/ ◀アトピー性皮膚炎 atopic dermatitis アレルギー性皮膚炎 allergic dermatitis おむつ皮膚炎 diaper dermatitis 海水浴皮膚炎 sea bather's dermatitis 化粧品皮膚炎 cosmetic dermatitis 脂漏性皮膚炎 seborrheic dermatitis 接触皮膚炎 contact dermatitis 日光皮膚炎 solar dermatitis / sun rash /（日焼け）sunburn 剝脱性皮膚炎 exfoliative dermatitis 放射線皮膚炎 radiation dermatitis / radiodermatitis

ピブカ PIVKA （ビタミンK欠乏時産生蛋白）protein induced by vitamin K absence

ひふきんえん 皮膚筋炎 dermatomyositis；DM

ひふくきん 腓腹筋 gastrocnemius (muscle), calf muscle, sural muscle

ひふくしんけい 腓腹神経 sural nerve

ひぶくれ 火脹れ burn blister

ひふしっかん 皮膚疾患 skin disease ◀湿疹性皮膚疾患 eczematous skin disease 水疱性皮膚疾患 bullous skin disease

ひふねんまくがんしょうこうぐん 皮膚粘膜眼症候群 mucocutaneous ocular syndrome （スティーブンス・ジョンソン症候群）Stevens-Johnson syndrome；SJS

ビブリオ Vibrio ▶腸炎ビブリオ Vibrio parahaemolyticus

ヒブワクチン Hib vaccine （インフルエンザ菌B型ワクチン）Haemophilus influenzae type B vaccine

ひぶんしょう 飛蚊症 floaters, muscae volitantes ★いずれも複数形で.

びふんむ 鼻噴霧 nasal nebulization ▶鼻噴霧器 nasal spray[nebulizer]

びへい 鼻閉 nasal obstruction[occlusion] （鼻詰まり）stuffy nose, blocked nose （うっ血した鼻）congested nose ☞鼻詰まり

ひべん 皮弁 skin flap, cutaneous flap ◀筋皮弁 myocutaneous[musculocutaneous] flap 筋膜皮弁 fasciocutaneous flap 大胸筋皮弁 pectoralis major myocutaneous[musculocutaneous] flap 有茎皮弁 pedicle flap 遊離皮弁 free flap

ひほうごうがたビリルビン 非抱合型ビリルビン unconjugated bilirubin

ヒポクラテス Hippocrates ▶ヒポクラテスの誓い the Hippocratic oath

ひほけんしゃ 被保険者 insured person

ひホジキンリンパしゅ 非ホジキンリンパ腫 non-Hodgkin lymphoma；NHL

ひまく 被膜 capsule（形capsular） （薄い膜）film

ひまつ 飛沫 （小さな水滴）droplet （水しぶき）spray ▶飛沫感染 droplet infection

ひまやくせいちんつうやく 非麻薬性鎮痛薬 nonnarcotic analgesic (medication, drug, agent)

ひまん 肥満 （病的な太りすぎ）obesity /oʊbíːsəti/（形obese）, corpulence （過体重）heavy weight（形overweight） （脂肪過多）excess[excessive] fat, adiposis ☞太る ◆甘いものを食べ過ぎると肥満になります You'll *put on weight[get obese] if you eat too many sweets. ◆肥満傾向である have a tendency to obesity ◀中心性肥満 central obesity 内臓脂肪型肥満 visceral fat obesity 皮下脂肪型肥満 subcutaneous fat obesity 病的肥満 morbid obesity ▶肥満児 overweight[obese] child 肥満度 degree of obesity 肥満度指数 body mass index；BMI / obesity index ☞肥満細胞

びまん びまん(性の) diffuse ▶びまん性甲状腺腫 diffuse goiter　びまん性軸索損傷 diffuse axonal injury ; DAI　びまん性肺疾患 diffuse lung disease　びまん性肺胞傷害 diffuse alveolar damage ; DAD　びまん性汎細気管支炎 diffuse panbronchiolitis ; DPB

ひまんさいぼう 肥満細胞 mast cell

ひみつ 秘密 secret （個人に関する秘密）privacy （機密保持）confidentiality （略con-fidential）◆秘密を守る keep a secret / protect *a person's* privacy ◆この場でのお話は秘密にいたします Everything we talk about here is confidential. ◆長寿の秘密 the secret of long life ▶秘密保持 protection of privacy / privacy protection

びもう 鼻毛 ☞鼻毛(はなげ)

ひやあせ 冷や汗 cold sweat ◆冷や汗が出る break out in a cold sweat / have [get] a cold sweat ◆冷や汗をかいている be in a cold sweat

ひゃくじゅうきゅうばん 119番 ◆119番で救急車を呼ぶ dial[call] one-one-nine for an ambulance

ひゃくとおばん 110番 ◆110番で警察を呼ぶ dial[call] one-one-zero for the police ★0はオーとも読む.

ひゃくにちぜき 百日咳 whooping cough /-kɔːf/, pertussis ◆百日咳に罹るcontract[catch / develop] whooping cough ◀ジフテリア・破傷風・百日咳混合ワクチン diphtheria, tetanus, and acellular pertussis vaccine / DTaP vaccine ▶百日咳菌 *Bordetella pertussis*　百日咳ワクチン pertussis[whooping cough] vaccine

ひゃくぶんりつ 百分率 percentage ☞比率

ひやけ 日焼け （ひりひり痛むほどの日焼け）sunburn （褐色の日焼け）suntan （動get sunburned[suntanned]）◆日焼けしないように日焼け止めクリームを塗る put on sunscreen[sunblock / sun cream] to prevent sunburn

ひやす 冷やす （適温に冷やす）cool （氷で冷やす）ice, apply ice （飲食物などを冷やす）chill ☞冷ます, 冷却 ◆腫れをとるために氷で冷やす apply ice to reduce the swelling / cool the swelling with ice to reduce it ◆熱い飲み物は冷やしてから飲んで下さい You should let hot liquids cool before drinking. ◆体を冷やす cool *one's* body ◆体を冷やさないようにして下さい (暖かくして) Please keep yourself warm. ◆オレンジジュースを冷蔵庫で冷やす chill the orange juice in the refrigerator ◆数分間やけどを流水で冷やす run cold water over the burn for several minutes ★run water は水を流す意. 　頭を冷やす calm [cool] down / (冷静さを保つ) keep *one's* cool

ひやとい 日雇い work for pay by the day, daily basis work ▶日雇い労働 day labor 日雇い労働者 day laborer

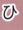

ヒューナーしけん ―試験 Huhner test （性交後試験）postcoital test ; PCT

ヒューヒューする whistle ◆呼吸をする時ヒューヒューする音を出す make a whistling sound when breathing

ひよう 費用 （料金・請求額）fees, charges （経費）expenses, costs ★いずれも通例, 複数形で. ☞ー費 ◆病院の費用は何で支払いますか How will you pay the hospital fees[charges]? ◀追加費用 additional expenses

ひょう¹ 表 （項目を順次並べた表）list （図表）chart （縦・横に配列した一覧表）table （予定表）schedule ◆これは妊娠中に飲んでもよい安全な薬の表です Here is a list of medications that are safe to take during pregnancy. ◀スケジュール表 schedule (chart / table)　料金表 price list / fee schedule / list of charges

ひょう² 票 （紙片）slip, sheet （用紙）form ◀受付票 outpatient check-in slip / numbered slip (given to patients in order of their arrival at the outpatient clinic)　質問票 questionnaire (sheet)　問診票 medical *history form[questionnaire / interview form]　予診票 preliminary medical history form　予約票 appointment slip

びよう 美容(の) （美顔用の）cosmetic

(美的な) aesthetic ▶美容矯正 cosmetic correction　美容外科 the department of cosmetic[aesthetic] surgery / the cosmetic[aesthetic] surgery department ☞美容整形

びょう　秒 second ◀1秒率 forced expiratory volume percentage in one[first] second / the ratio of forced expiratory volume in one[first] second to forced vital capacity；$FEV_{1.0}$ / FVC　1秒量 forced expiratory volume in one[first] second；$FEV_{1.0}$

ひょういもうそう　憑依妄想 possession delusion, delusion of possession

びょういん¹　病因　(病気の原因) cause of a disease　**(発症要因)** etiology of a disease　**(病原論・病因論)** pathogenesis ▶病因論 etiology

びょういん²　病院 hospital　**(診療所・医院)** clinic ☞巻末付録：病院関係者 ◆お子さんをすぐ病院に連れて来て下さい You must bring your child to (the) hospital at once. ★hospital は《米》では the を付けるが，《英》では付けないのが普通. ◆どこの病院でその手術を受けましたか Which hospital did you have the surgery at? ◆自宅近くの病院での治療を希望しますか Would you like to have the treatment at another hospital nearer your home? ◆250床の病院 a two-hundred-fifty-bed hospital
◀一般病院 general hospital　温泉病院 spa hospital　外来専門病院 day hospital　関連病院 affiliated hospital　救急病院 emergency hospital　教育病院 teaching hospital　公立病院 public[(地方自治体の)municipal / (地域の) community / (市立の) city] hospital　国立病院 national hospital　産科病院[産院] maternity hospital[clinic]　小児病院 children's hospital　精神科病院 psychiatric hospital　専門病院 special hospital　総合病院 general hospital　大学病院 university hospital　老人病院 geriatric hospital ▶病院関係者 hospital personnel[staff]　病院感染症 *hospital-acquired[nosocomial] infection　病院管理業務 hospital administration　病院規則 hospital rules[regulations]　病院食 hospital meals[food]　病院長 the director[president] of the hospital　病院ボランティア hospital volunteer

ひょうか　評価　(価値判断) evaluation (動evaluate)　**(査定)** assessment (動assess)　**(評点)** rating (動rate)　◆患者の全身状態を評価する evaluate[assess] the patient's general condition ◆痛みの数値評価尺度 *Numeric Rating Scale[NRS] for pain measurement ◀機能評価 functional assessment　行動評価 behavior assessment　再評価(検討し直し) reevaluation / (査定し直し) reassessment　心機能評価 evaluation[assessment] of heart[cardiac] function　体力評価 evaluation of physical fitness　疼痛評価 pain assessment　麻酔前評価 preanesthetic evaluation

びょうがテスト　描画テスト drawing test ◀時計描画テスト clock drawing test；CDT

びょうき¹　病気　(一般的に) illness, sickness　**(具体的な病名がつく病気)** disease
《基本表現》 ◆急性〈慢性〉の病気 *an acute〈a chronic〉disease ◆一般的な〈まれな〉病気 a common〈rare〉disease ◆悪性〈良性〉の病気 a malignant〈benign〉disease ◆重い〈軽い〉病気 a serious〈mild〉disease ◆長引く病気 a lingering[prolonged] illness ◆難治性の病気 an intractable disease ◆不治の病気 *a fatal[an incurable] disease ◆遺伝する病気 a hereditary[genetic] disease ◆先天的〈後天的〉な病気 *a congenital〈an acquired〉disease
《診察の基本表現》 ◆これまでに何か大きな病気に罹ったことがありますか Have you ever had any major illnesses? / Have you ever been seriously ill? ◆ご両親には何か病気がありますか Do your parents have any medical problems?
《患者の立場からの表現》 ◆病気になる get [become] sick[ill] / (病気を発症する) develop *a disease* / (病気を患う) have *an illness* ◆病気で苦しむ suffer from *a disease*

びょうき[1]

◆病気が重い〈軽い〉be seriously〈slightly〉sick ◆病気が良くなる〈悪くなる〉get better〈worse〉 ◆病気が回復する recover from *a disease* ◆病気を受容する〈否認する〉accept〈deny〉one's illness ◆病気と闘う fight against *a disease* / struggle[battle] with *a disease*

《医療者の立場からの表現》 ◆病気を発見する detect *a disease* ◆病気を治療する treat *a disease* ◆病気を治す cure *a disease* ◆病気を予防する prevent *a disease* ★イタリックの部分には具体的な病名を入れる.

▶病気休職 sick leave

びょうき[2] 病期 **stage** (病期分類)**staging** ◆あなたの肺がんの病期は1期です You have stage-one lung cancer. / Your lung cancer is at stage one.

びょうけつ 病欠 **sickness absence** (欠勤)**absence from work** *due to[because of] illness (欠席)**absence from school** *due to[because of] illness ◆病欠の連絡を入れる call in sick ◆病欠で休む take sick leave[days] ◆病欠の届けを出す submit a *sick note[doctor's note]

びょうげん 表現 **expression** (動**express**) (描写)**description** (動**describe**) ☞表す
◆これは日本語の慣用的な表現です This is a Japanese idiomatic expression. ◆曖昧な表現を避ける avoid using ambiguous expressions / avoid ambiguity of expression ◀感情表現 emotional expression

▶表現型 phenotype

びょうげん 病原 (病気の原因)**the cause** (of *a disease*) (病気の起源)**the origin** (of *a disease*) (病原論・病因論)**pathogenesis** (形**病原性の pathogenic**) ◀日和見病原体 opportunistic pathogen ▶病原性ウイルス pathogenic[disease-causing] virus 病原性細菌 pathogenic[disease-causing] bacteria 病原性大腸菌 pathogenic *Escherichia coli*[*E. coli*] 病原体 pathogen / disease-causing substance 病原体保有者 disease carrier 病原微生物 pathogenic microorganism

びょうざい 表在(性の) (表面的な)super-

ficial (浅い)**shallow** ☞表層 ▶表在感覚 superficial sense[sensation] 表在性潰瘍 superficial ulcer 表在性真菌症 superficial mycosis 表在痛 superficial pain

ひょうじ 表示する **indicate** (图**indication**) (感情などの表現)**express** (图**expression**) (計器の示す数値)**read** (图**reading**)
◆この薬は袋に表示してある通りに服用して下さい Please take this medication exactly as indicated on the package. ◆意思表示する express one's will ◆パルスオキシメータに表示される数値がいつもより低い時は早めに受診して下さい If the pulse oximeter indicates a lower than normal reading, come and see me earlier than usual. ◆受付番号がモニターに表示されましたら診察室にお入り下さい When your check-in number appears on the monitor, please come into the doctor's office.

びょうじ 病児 (乳幼児)**sick infant, ill infant** (小児)**sick child, ill child** (圈**children**) ▶病児保育 care for a sick infant[child]

びょうしき 病識 **awareness of** *one's* **disease[illness], insight into[about]** *one's* **disease[illness]** ◆彼には病識がない He has no awareness of his disease. / He is not aware that he is ill.

びょうしつ 病室 **hospital room, patient room** ◆あなたの病室は513号室です You'll be in room five hundred thirteen.
◆病室にご案内します I'll show you to your room. ◆貴重品は病室に置かないで下さい Please don't keep any valuables in your room. ◆病室が空いたらご連絡いたします We'll *get in touch with you[call you] when a bed becomes available.
◆内科病棟の病室に移る move[be transferred] to a room on the internal medicine ward ◆シャワートイレ付きの病室 a room with a shower and toilet ◆明るい病室 a bright[well-lit] room ◀隔離病室 isolation[quarantine] room 差額病室 special charge room / (一部のみ保険適用の部屋)room (that is) only partially covered by health insurance ▶病室着 hospital

gown

病室の種類

■一般病室 regular room
●個室 private room ●1人部屋 single [single-occupancy] room ●2人部屋 semiprivate[two-bed] room / room for two ●4人部屋 four-bed room / room for four ●大部屋 multiple-occupancy room / shared room / room shared by several patients

■特別室 special room /（高級な部屋）deluxe room

びょうじゃく 病弱（な） invalid （病気がちの）sickly （体が弱い）weak

ひょうじゅん 標準 （正常範囲）normal range （類normal） （一般的基準）standard （類standard） （平均）the average （類average） ◆あなたの赤ちゃんは体重が標準より少ない〈多い〉です Your baby's weight is below〈above〉the normal range for his 〈her〉age. ◆前立腺がんには標準的治療の選択肢がいくつかあります There are several standard treatment options for prostate cancer. ▶標準化 standardization 標準誤差 standard error ; SE 標準体重 standard (body) weight 標準的予防策 standard precautions 標準偏差 standard deviation ; SD

ひょうじょう 表情 （感情の表現）expression （顔つき）look ◆彼女は表情が乏しくなっています She *has little[doesn't have much] facial expression. / She doesn't show much expression on her face. ◆彼は顔の表情がなくなってこわばっています His face has become expressionless [blank] and fixed. ◆彼女は悲しそうな表情をしています She has[wears] a sad look [expression] on her face. / She looks sad. ◆表情を変える change one's expression ◆苦痛の表情を浮かべる one's face is in agony / one's agony shows on one's face ▶無表情 lack of facial expression / absence of expression on the face ▶表情減少 decreased expression

びょうしょう 病床 (hospital) bed / sickbed ☞ベッド ◆病床が200の病院 a two-hundred-bed hospital / a hospital with a capacity of two hundred beds ◀一般病床 general bed 療養病床 long-term care bed ▶病床監視装置 bedside monitor

びょうじょう 病状 （健康状態・容体）condition （一般的に人・物の状態）state (of a disease) （病気の進行）progress (of a disease) （特定の疾病の状態）pathologic condition ◆この病状では運動をしばらく控える必要があります With this condition, you shouldn't exercise for a while. ◆彼女の病状は安定しています Her condition is stable. / She is in stable condition. ◆彼の病状は好転しました His condition has improved. / He has taken a turn for the better. ◆残念ですが彼女の病状はかなり深刻です I'm afraid her condition is rather serious. ◆あなたはご自分の病状をどう理解していますか What do you understand [know] about your condition?

びようせいけい 美容整形（手術） cosmetic surgery, plastic and reconstructive surgery ◆顔の美容整形を行う perform [do] cosmetic *facial surgery[surgery on the face] ◆（患者が）鼻の美容整形手術を受ける have[undergo] cosmetic *nose surgery[surgery on the nose]

びょうぜんせいかく 病前性格 premorbid character

ひょうそ 瘭疽 whitlow, felon

ひょうそう 表層（の） superficial ☞表在 ▶表層性胃炎 superficial gastritis 表層火傷 superficial burn

びょうそう 病巣 lesion （病気の中心・発生箇所）focus （類focal） ☞病変 ◆コイン状の病巣 a coin lesion ◀初期病巣 primary[initial] lesion 転移性病巣 metastatic lesion ▶病巣感染 focal infection 病巣症状 focal symptom

びょうたい 病態 morbid condition, diseased condition ☞病状 ▶病態失認 anosognosia 病態生理学 pathophysiology / morbid physiology

ひょうてき　標的　target ▶標的細胞 target cell　標的臓器 target organ

びょうてき　病的(な) （病気による）**pathologic, pathological, diseased** （不健全な）**morbid** （異常な）**abnormal** （不健康な）**unhealthy** ▶病的骨折 pathologic fracture　病的状態 morbidity / diseased condition [state]　病的所見 pathologic findings　病的徴候 pathologic sign　病的肉芽 abnormal granulation　病的反射 pathologic reflex　病的肥満 morbid obesity

びょうとう　病棟 （入院患者用）**ward, floor** （まとまった部門として）**unit** ◆病棟をご案内しましょう I'll show you around the ward [floor].　▶隔離病棟 isolation[quarantine] unit[ward]　緩和ケア病棟 palliative care unit ; PCU　救急病棟 emergency unit[ward]　外科病棟 surgical ward[floor / unit]　産科病棟 maternity ward[floor / unit]　小児病棟 children's ward[floor / unit]　内科病棟 medical ward[floor / unit] / internal medicine ward[floor / unit]　閉鎖病棟 closed[(錠を下ろした)locked] ward[unit]　▶病棟管理 ward[floor / unit] supervision　病棟クラーク ward[floor / unit] clerk　病棟師長 ward[floor / unit] nursing supervisor　病棟助手 ward[floor / unit] assistant　病棟スタッフ ward[floor / unit] staff　病棟責任者 person in charge of the ward[floor / unit] / (取りまとめ役)unit coordinator

びょうにん　病人 （患者）**patient** （病気の人）**sick person, ill person** ▶病人役割行動 sick-role behavior　☞病人食

びょうにんしょく　病人食　diet[food] for sick people （患者用の）**diet[food] for patients** （調理法）**special recipe for sick people** ◆糖尿病患者用の病人食 a diet for patients with diabetes　◆化学療法を受けている患者の病人食 a special recipe for patients on chemotherapy

ひょうのう　氷嚢　ice pack, ice bag

ひょうのうしゅ　皮様嚢腫　dermoid cyst

ひょうはく　漂白する （脱色する）**bleach** （白くする）**whiten** ◆歯を漂白する bleach [whiten] *a person's* teeth　◀塩素漂白剤 chlorine bleach　▶漂白剤 bleach / bleaching agent

ひょうばん　評判 （世評）**reputation** （人気）**popularity** （囲**popular**）◆鈴木医師は腕がよいことで評判のよい先生です Dr Suzuki has a good reputation for being a skilled physician.　◆ご紹介する病院は質のよい医療を提供することで患者さんたちに評判がよいです The hospital I'm referring you to *is popular[has a good reputation]* among patients for its high quality services.

ひょうひ　表皮　epidermis （囲**epidermal, epidermic** 類表皮の **epidermoid**）**, the outer layer of the skin** ◆表皮が剝がれています The outer layer of the skin is coming [peeling] off. / (薄片状に剝がれている)The skin is flaky.　◀黒色表皮腫 acanthosis nigricans　類表皮嚢胞 epidermoid cyst　▶表皮内熱傷(表層火傷) superficial burn　表皮ブドウ球菌 *Staphylococcus epidermidis*　表皮母斑 epidermal nevus

びょうへん　病変　lesion ☞病巣　◀陥凹性病変 depressed lesion　境界病変 borderline lesion　局所性病変 local lesion　空洞性病変 cavitary lesion　前がん性病変 precancerous lesion　占拠性病変 space-occupying lesion ; SOL　飛び石状病変 skip lesion

ひょうほん　標本 （見本）**sample** （検体・試料）**specimen** ☞サンプル　◀無作為(抽出)標本 random sample　▶標本抽出 sampling

びょうめい　病名 ◆まだ病名は特定できません We can't identify the disease yet. / (診断できない)We can't diagnose the disease yet.　◆お父さんの死因となった病名を教えて下さい What was the name of the disease that caused your father's death?

ひょうめん　表面　surface （外側）**the outside** （囲表面的な・表在の **superficial** 外の・外部の **outside, external** 局部の **topical**）◆血は便の表面についていますか Is the blood on the surface of the stools?　◆皮膚の表面に触れる touch the surface of the skin　◆表面的な痛み *a superficial[an*

ひょうめん　　　　　　　　　　616　　　　　　　　　びょうれき

external] pain　▶表面麻酔 topical[surface] anesthesia

びょうり　病理　**pathology**　(形病理［学］の **pathologic, pathological**)　▶病理医 pathologist　病理解剖 autopsy　病理学 pathology　病理検査 pathologic examination　病理検査室 pathology lab[laboratory]　病理所見 pathologic findings　病理診断 pathologic diagnosis　病理組織学 pathologic histology　病理部 the department of pathology / the pathology department

びょうれき　病歴　**medical history**　(カルテ) **chart**　◀既往(病)歴 past medical history；PMH　現病歴 present (medical) history / history of (the) present illness；HPI / present illness；PI / history of (the) presenting complaint；HPC　▶病歴管理 medical record management　病歴聴取 (medical) history-taking

病歴聴取の基本表現

主訴を訊ねる

● どうなさいましたか How can I help you? / What can I do for you? / What's [What problems have] brought you along today?
● 呼吸〈お腹 / 耳〉に何か問題がありますか (Do you have) any problems with your breathing〈abdomen / ears〉?

症状について詳しく尋ねる

■症状の特徴
● どんなふうに痛みますか What does the pain feel like? / Can you describe the pain? / What kind of pain is it?
● 痛みはどのくらいひどいのですか How bad[severe] is it?
● 痛みは放散〈移動〉しますか Does it spread〈move〉*to other parts of the body [anywhere else]?
● 同じような痛みを経験したことがありますか Have you ever had this kind of pain before?

■発症時期・発症様式・経過

● いつ発症しましたか When did it start?
● 最初に気づいたのはいつですか When did you first notice it? / When did it first come on?
● どのくらい続いていますか How long have you had it? / How long has it been bothering you?
● どんな時に起こることが多いですか When does it usually come on?
● 夜〈朝〉の決まった時間帯ですか At a specific time *at night〈in the morning〉?
● 突然起こりますか，徐々にですか Does it come on suddenly or gradually?
● 毎回どのくらい続きますか How long does it last each time?
● 症状は一過性ですか，持続性ですか Does it come and go, or is it there all the time?
● どのくらいの頻度で起こりますか How often do you have it? / How often does it occur?
● 何回起こりましたか How many times have you had it?
● 軽快傾向ですか，悪化傾向ですか，変化なしですか Is it getting better, getting worse, or is there no change?

■誘発因子・増悪因子・緩和因子
● 何が原因で起こりますか〈起こりましたか〉What usually brings〈brought〉it on?
● 思い当たる誘因は何ですか What do you think is〈was〉causing it? / Can you think of anything that might be causing it?
● 症状を悪化させるものは何ですか What makes it worse? / Does anything make it worse?
● 症状を緩和させる〈消す〉ものは何ですか What makes it better〈go away〉? / Does anything make it better〈go away〉?

随伴症状・既往症・家族歴を尋ねる

● (頭痛の)ほかに気づいている徴候や症状がありますか Have you noticed anything else (with these headaches)?
● これまで罹った病気について教えて下さ

い Please tell me what other illnesses you've had.
●血縁のある方で糖尿病の人はいますか Does anyone in your immediate family have diabetes? / Do you know of any blood relative who has or had diabetes?

びよく 鼻翼(の) (nasal) alar (図the wing of the nose, ala of the nose, nosewing)
▶鼻翼呼吸 nasal alar breathing　鼻翼軟骨 alar cartilage

ひよりみ 日和見(の) opportunistic
▶日和見感染 opportunistic infection　日和見病原体 opportunistic pathogen

ひよわ ひ弱(な) ☞病弱

ひらく 開く
《開いた状態にする》open (図open) (血管・瞳孔などが) dilate (図dilated) ☞開ける
◆口を大きく開いて下さい Please open your mouth wide.　◆そのドアは開きません That door won't open.　◆心を開く open up to others / open one's mind (to others)　◆足を開いて立つ stand with one's legs apart　◆縫った傷口が開いた The stitches have come open[undone].
◆感染が落ち着くまで傷口は開いたままにしておきます I'm going to leave the wound open[傷口をふさがない] I won't close the wound] until the infection has *gone down[subsided].　◆子宮口が 5 cm 開いています Your cervix has dilated to five centimeters.
《開催する》hold　◆今度の土曜日に糖尿病患者のための勉強会を開きます We're holding[having] a study session for diabetic patients this coming Saturday.
《業務を開始する》open　◆会計窓口は 9 時に開きます The cashier window[counter] opens at nine in the morning.

ヒラメきん ─筋 soleus (muscle)

びらん 糜爛 erosion (図erosive) (潰瘍形成)ulceration ☞潰瘍, 爛れる　◆角膜びらん corneal erosion　口角びらん angular stomatitis　たこいぼびらん varioliform erosion　▶びらん性胃炎 erosive gastritis

ひりつ 比率 (割合)ratio, proportion

(率)rate　(百分率)percentage　◆入院患者に対する看護師の比率は 7:1 です The ratio of nurses to inpatients[The nurse-inpatient ratio] is one to seven.　◆この病気の発症の比率は人口 10 万人に対して約 20 人です The incidence rate of this disease is about twenty per one hundred thousand people.

ぴりぴり ◆ぴりぴりっとくる痛み(電撃性の) (an) electric shock-like pain ☞痛み

ひりひりする (体の一部・傷が痛む)smart (炎症を起こして痛む)feel[get, become] irritated (表面が焼けるように痛む)burn (チクチク・ぴりぴりする)tingle, sting ☞痛み
◆目がひりひりしますか Do your eyes smart[feel irritated]?　◆やけどがひりひりする The burn smarts[stings].　◆ひりひり感がありますか Do you have a burning [tingling] sensation?　◆体の片側にひりひりする痛みがある have (a) burning or tingling pain on one side of the body

びりょう 微量(の) very small amount [quantity] (of) (痕跡)trace (of) (接頭micro-)　◆微量の血液 a very small amount of blood / traces of blood　▶微量アルブミン尿 microalbuminuria　微量元素 trace element　微量元素欠乏症 trace element deficiency

ビリルビン bilirubin　◀間接型ビリルビン indirect bilirubin　高ビリルビン血症 hyperbilirubinemia　直接型ビリルビン direct bilirubin　▶ビリルビン尿 bilirubinuria

ピル (経口避妊薬)the pill　★通例, the を付けて. birth control pill　◆避妊用にピルを飲む take the pill to prevent pregnancy
◆ピルを飲んでいる be on the pill　◀低用量ピル low dose[dosage] pill

びるいかん 鼻涙管 nasolacrimal duct
▶鼻涙管閉塞 nasolacrimal duct obstruction

ヒルシュスプルングびょう ─病 Hirschsprung disease

ひるね 昼寝 nap (図nap)　◆ふだん昼寝をしますか Do you usually take a nap (during the day)? / Do you usually sleep during the day? ◆どのくらいの時間昼寝をしますか How long do you nap[take a nap] for? ◆15分程度の昼寝はリフレッシュに効果的です Taking fifteen minute or so naps is an effective way to *refresh yourself[make yourself feel refreshed].

ピルビンさん 　─酸　pyruvic acid

ひるま　昼間　daytime, day　◆昼間の耐えがたい眠気 excessive daytime sleepiness；EDS

ビルロートいせつじょじゅつ　─胃切除術　Billroth gastrectomy

ひれい　比例　proportion　(▶proportional)　◆あなたのコレステロール値は体重に比例して増加しています Your cholesterol levels are rising in proportion to your weight gain.　◆タバコの本数と肺気腫の重症度は必ずしも比例しません The severity of pulmonary emphysema is not necessarily proportional to the number of cigarettes smoked. /（対応しない）The number of cigarettes smoked does not necessarily correspond to the severity of pulmonary emphysema.

びれつ　鼻裂　cleft nose, nasal cleft

ひろい　広い　☞広範

ひろう　疲労　(倦怠感) tiredness (▶tire, tired)　(心身の激しい疲れ) fatigue /fətíːɡ/　(極度の疲労) exhaustion (▶exhausted /ɪɡzɔ́ːstɪd/)　☞疲れ, 疲れる　◆疲労していますか Are you tired[exhausted]?　◆疲労感がありますか Do you ever feel tired?　◆疲労しやすいですか Do you *get tired[tire] easily?　◆疲労がたまる fatigue builds up　◆疲労をとる *get over [recover from] one's tiredness[fatigue]　◆疲労感 sense of fatigue / feeling of being tired　◆精神的〈肉体的〉な疲労 mental〈physical〉 fatigue　◀易疲労性 easy fatigability　眼精疲労 asthenopia / eyestrain / eye fatigue　筋肉疲労 muscle fatigue　呼吸筋疲労 respiratory muscle fatigue　蓄積性疲労 accumulated fatigue　慢性疲労 chronic fatigue　慢性疲労症候群 chronic fatigue syndrome；CFS　▶疲労検査 fatigue test[survey]　疲労骨折 stress[fatigue] fracture

びろう　鼻漏　nasal discharge, rhinorrhea　☞鼻汁（はなじる）　◀後鼻漏 postnasal drip；PND

ひろがる　広がる・拡がる　(周囲に伸びる) spread　(放射状に広がる) radiate　(幅が拡がる) widen, broaden　(範囲・程度が拡張する) extend　☞広まる　◆痛みはほかの場所に拡がりますか Does the pain spread [move / travel] *anywhere else[to another place]?　◆乳がんはリンパ節に拡がっていました The breast cancer has *spread to[entered] the lymph nodes.

ひろげる　広げる・拡げる　(範囲・程度を拡張する) expand, extend, spread　(幅を) widen, broaden　(血管・瞳孔などを拡張する) dilate　◆消化管を拡げるために空気を入れる insert air to expand the GI tract　◆血管を拡げる dilate the blood vessels

ひろばきょうふ　広場恐怖(症)　agoraphobia；*fear of crowded or open spaces*

ひろまる　広まる　spread, go around　☞広がる　◆その病気はこの地域で急速に広まっています The disease has spread [gone around] quickly in this area.

ピロリきん　─菌　*Helicobacter pylori*　◆ピロリ菌による感染が消化性潰瘍の原因になることがあります *Helicobacter pylori* infection may cause peptic ulcers. / Peptic ulcers are sometimes caused by infection with *Helicobacter pylori*.

ピロリンさん　─酸　pyrophosphoric acid

ピン　pin　◆ピンでチクンと刺しますよ I'm going to prick you with a pin　◀ヘアピン hairpin / bobby pin

ビン　瓶　bottle　(口の広い瓶) jar　(容器) container　◀蓄尿瓶 urine storage container[bottle]　哺乳瓶 baby[feeding / nursing] bottle

びんかん　敏感（な）　sensitive, delicate　☞過敏　◆匂いに敏感になる become sensitive to smells　◀敏感肌 sensitive[delicate] skin

ピンク(の)　pink　(ピンクがかった) pinkish　◆ピンク色がかった痰 pinkish phlegm　▶ピンクリボン運動 Pink

ピンク（の）

Ribbon campaign

ひんけつ 貧血 anemia /əníːmiə/ （㊟anemic） ◆これまでに貧血になったことがありますか Have you ever had anemia? ◆少し貧血があります You're slightly anemic. / You have some slight anemia. ◆鉄分不足で貧血を起こす have anemia due to iron deficiency ◆貧血気味である feel anemic ▮悪性貧血 pernicious anemia 胃切除後貧血 postgastrectomy anemia 運動性貧血 exercise[exercise-induced] anemia 鎌状赤血球貧血 sickle cell anemia 巨赤芽球性貧血 megaloblastic anemia 再生不良性貧血 aplastic anemia 小球性低色素性貧血 microcytic hypochromic anemia 腎性貧血 renal anemia 正球性正色素性貧血 normocytic normochromic anemia 続発性貧血 secondary anemia 大球性正色素性貧血 macrocytic normochromic anemia 鉄欠乏性貧血 iron-deficiency anemia 妊娠性貧血 pregnancy anemia / anemia in pregnancy ファンコーニ貧血 Fanconi anemia 不応性貧血 refractory anemia；RA 溶血性貧血 hemolytic anemia 葉酸欠乏性貧血 folic acid deficiency anemia ▶貧血治療薬 antianemic （medication / drug / agent）

ひんこきゅう 頻呼吸 tachypnea

ひんし 瀕死（の） （死にかけている）dying （致死性の）fatal ◆彼女は依然として瀕死の状態です（危篤状態）She is still in （a） critical condition. ◆瀕死の患者 a dying patient ◆瀕死の重傷 a fatal injury

ひんしつ 品質 quality ▶品質管理 quality control；QC 品質保証 quality assurance；QA

ヒンズーきょう 一教 Hinduism ▶ヒンズー教徒 Hindu

ピンセット tweezers ★複数形で. 数える時には, 1本ならば a pair of tweezers, 2本ならば two pairs of tweezers という.

ひんたい 品胎 triplet ▶品胎児 triplets / （3人のうちの1人）triplet 品胎妊娠 triplet pregnancy

ひんど 頻度 frequency （㊟頻繁な frequent） ◆この異常は10万人に3人という頻度で起こります This abnormality occurs in three in[out of] one hundred thousand people. ◆どのくらいの頻度で痛みますか How often do you have the pain? / How often does the pain come on? ◆最も頻度の高い副作用 the most frequent side effect

---

頻度の表現

"How often …?"と尋ねて患者さんから返ってくる頻度の表現は様々あって, 人によりしばしば異なる. その中でもよく使われる一般的な表現のおおよその目安をあげると, 次のようになる.

always いつも ＞ usually たいてい ＞ （very） often しばしば ＞ frequently 頻繁に ＞ over and over 繰り返し ＞ sometimes 時々 ＞ seldom まれに

ピント ☞焦点

ひんにょう 頻尿 frequent urination[micturition], urinary frequency ☞尿

ひんぱく 頻拍 ☞頻脈 ◀回帰頻拍 reciprocating tachycardia 上室頻拍 supraventricular tachycardia；SVT 心室頻拍 ventricular tachycardia；VT 心房頻拍 atrial tachycardia；AT 発作性頻拍 paroxysmal tachycardia

ひんぱつ 頻発 ☞頻繁 ▶頻発月経 polymenorrhea

ひんぱん 頻繁（な） frequent （㊟often, frequently 何回も many times） ◆痙攣は頻繁に起こりますか Do you have the seizures often[frequently]? ◆頻繁に体位を変えて下さい Please try to change your position frequently. ◆同じことを頻繁に繰り返す repeat the same thing *over and over again[many times]

ひんみゃく 頻脈 frequent pulse, tachycardia （↔bradycardia） ☞頻拍 ◀洞頻脈 sinus tachycardia ▶頻脈性不整脈 tachyarrhythmia

ふ

ふ 負(の) （否定的・消極的な）negative
(↔positive) （マイナスの）minus (↔plus)
◆負の連鎖反応を起こす have[(引き起こす)
cause] a negative chain reaction ◆負の
制御 negative control ◆負の相関 a negative correlation ◆負の調節 negative
regulation ◆負のフィードバック negative feedback ◆負の要因 a minus[nega-
tive] factor

ファーストネーム first name, given
name ☞名前

ファイバースコープ fiberscope ◀胃
ファイバースコープ gastrofiberscope

ファイル file （動file）
《とじ込む》 ◆薬の副作用情報をファイルし
て保管する keep a file on information
about the side effects of a medication /
keep information about the side effects of
a medication on file ◆これまでの検査
データや医師からの説明文書をファイルし
ておく file past test result data and
physician's explanatory notes
《コンピュータ用語》 ◆ファイルを開く〈閉じ
る〉open〈close〉a file ◆ファイルを保存
する save a file ◆ファイルをダウンロード
〈アップロード〉する download〈upload〉a
file ◆ファイルを添付する attach a file
◀患者ファイル patient file 添付ファイル
attached file ▶ファイル名 file name

ファウラーたいい ―体位 Fowler position （半座位）semisitting position

ファクター factor ☞因子

ファックス fax （動fax） ◆申し訳ありませ
んが，検査結果のコピーをファックスでお送
りすることはできません I'm sorry, but we
can't *fax copies of test results[send you
copies of test results by fax].

ファブリびょう ―病 Fabry disease
（アルファガラクトシダーゼ欠損症）alpha-galac-
tosidase deficiency

ファローしちょうしょう ―四徴症 tet-
ralogy of Fallot；TF

ふあん 不安 （気がかり）concern （形con-
cerned） （心配）anxiety /æŋzáɪəti/ （形
anxious /æŋkʃəs/） （緊張・神経性の不安）
nervousness （形nervous） （落ち着かない気
分）uneasiness （形uneasy） （怖れ・恐怖）
fear ☞心配，悩み，悩む ◆何か不安なこ
とがありますか Are you concerned[anx-
ious] about anything? ◆手術を受けるこ
とに不安を感じますか Do you feel anxious
[nervous] about having the surgery? /
Are you afraid about (having) the surgery? ◆治療を続けることに経済的な不安
がありますか Is it financial concerns that
are making you wonder if you should
continue with the treatment? / Are you
unsure about continuing with the treatment because of financial concerns?
◆不安を感じるのはごく自然なことです It's
quite natural that you should feel uneasy
[anxious]. ◆漠然とした不安感をもつ
（はっきりした理由もなく）feel uneasy[anx-
ious / nervous] for no apparent reason /
（自分でも説明・理解できない）have inexpli-
cable anxiety ◆強い不安感にたびたび襲
われる have frequent attacks[bouts] of
intense anxiety / frequently suffer from
intense[strong] anxiety ◆不安を鎮める
calm[allay] *a person's* fear ◀抗不安薬
antianxiety medication[drug / agent] /
minor tranquilizer / anxiolytic 情動不安
restlessness 浮動性不安 free-floating
anxiety 予期不安 expectation anxiety
▶不安階層表 anxiety[fear] hierarchy
不安感 feeling(s) of anxiety[uneasiness]
不安管理トレーニング anxiety manage-
ment training 不安気分 anxious mood
不安発作 anxiety attack ☞不安症

ファンコーニしょうこうぐん ―症候群
Fanconi syndrome

ファンコーニひんけつ ―貧血 Fanconi
anemia

ふあんしょう 不安症 anxiety disorder
◀社交不安症[社交恐怖] social anxiety
disorder；SAD / social phobia 全般不安
症 generalized anxiety disorder；GAD

分離不安症 separation anxiety disorder

ふあんてい　不安定(な)　(容体などが一定でない)unstable, instable (図instability), labile (図lability)　(足元などがふらついた)unsteady (図unsteadiness), wobbly, shaky　(状況・事などが不確かな)unsteady, precarious, uncertain　(仕事・地位などが保証されない)insecure　(バランスが崩れた)unbalanced, imbalanced (図unbalance, imbalance)　◆血圧が不安定です Your blood pressure is unstable[not stable].　◆足元が不安定ですか Do you get[feel] unsteady[wobbly / shaky] on your feet? / Do your legs get wobbly?　◆精神的に不安定だ be emotionally unstable / be mentally unbalanced　◆不安定感がある(足元がふらつく感じ)have sensations of unsteadiness / (心理的に不安定な感じ・関節などがぐらぐらする感じ)have a sense of instability / (バランスがとれない感じ)have a sense of unbalance[imbalance]　◆収入が不安定である one's income is unsteady[precarious / uncertain] / have *an unsteady[a precarious] income　◀情動[情緒]不安定 emotional instability[lability]　▶不安定狭心症 unstable angina　不安定固視 unstable fixation　不安定歩行 unsteady gait

ぶい　部位　(部分・範囲)area, region　(体の部位・場所)site　(体の一部分)part　(位置)location　◆発疹がほかの部位に拡がっていますか Has the rash spread to other areas of your body?　◆手術の部位を剃る shave the surgical area　◆点滴部位が痛む the IV site hurts / the area where the IV was inserted hurts　◀キーゼルバッハ部位 Kiesselbach area　検査部位 the site[area] to be examined　骨折部位 fracture site / the site[location] of the fracture　手術部位 surgical site[area]　身体部位 part[region] of the body / body part[region]　注射部位 injection site[area]　反応部位 reactive site　付着部位 attachment site

ブイアールイー　VRE　(バンコマイシン耐性腸球菌)vancomycin-resistant enterococcus

フィート　foot (圏feet)；ft　☞巻末付録：単位の換算

フィードバック　feedback　◆フィードバックを与える give[provide] feedback　◆フィードバックを得る get[obtain] feedback　◀肯定的フィードバック positive feedback　否定的フィードバック negative feedback　▶フィードバック機構 feedback mechanism

ブイエスディ　VSD　(心室中隔欠損症)ventricular septal defect

フィットネスセンター　fitness (promotion) center

フィブリノゲン　fibrinogen

フィブリン　fibrin　▶フィブリン血栓 fibrin thrombus　フィブリン糊 fibrin glue

フィラデルフィアせんしょくたい　─染色体　Philadelphia chromosome：Ph

フィラリアしょう　─症　filariasis

フィリピン　the Philippines (圏Philippine)　☞国籍　▶フィリピン人 Filipino /fíləpíːnoʊ/　フィリピン人の Filipino / Philippine

フィルター　filter　◆エアコンのフィルターはこまめに掃除してください Please clean (any) air conditioner filters frequently.　◆下大静脈にフィルターを入れる implant[put / place] a filter into the inferior vena cava　◀下大静脈フィルター *inferior vena cava[IVC] filter　白血球除去フィルター leukocyte depletion filter

フィンランド　Finland (圏フィンランドの・フィンランド人の Finnish)　☞国籍　▶フィンランド人 Finn

ふうしん　風疹　(三日ばしか)rubella /ruːbélə/, German measles　☞予防接種　◀先天性風疹症候群 congenital rubella syndrome；CRS　麻疹・風疹混合ワクチン *measles and rubella[MR] vaccine　▶風疹ウイルス rubella virus　風疹抗体 rubella antibody　風疹ワクチン rubella vaccine

ブースター　(追加接種)booster (shot)　▶ブースター効果 booster effect

ふうどびょう　風土病　endemic disease

ふうにゅうたい　封入体　inclusion body

ふうふ　夫婦 husband and wife, married couple (既婚の married　婚姻の marital) ◆夫婦間の問題を解決する solve *one's* marital problems[difficulties] ▶夫婦カウンセリング marriage[marital] counseling　夫婦関係 marital relationship[relations]　夫婦間暴力 domestic violence /（夫による暴力）wife-beating ★インフォーマルな表現．夫婦げんか fight with *one's* husband〈wife〉/ marital quarrel　夫婦生活 married life /（特に性生活）sex life

プール　(swimming) pool ◆屋内温水プールで水中ウォークをする do water-walking[water-walk] in a heated indoor swimming pool ▶プール熱（プール性結膜炎）swimming pool conjunctivitis /（咽頭結膜熱）pharyngoconjunctival fever

フェイスマスク　face mask ☞マスク

フェイスリフト　facelift, face-lift

ふえいせい　不衛生（な） ☞非衛生

フェニルケトンにょうしょう　―尿症 phenylketonuria；PKU

フェノール　phenol (phenolic) ▶フェノール系消毒薬 phenolic disinfectant

フェノールスルホンフタレインしけん ―試験　phenolsulfonphthalein test, PSP test

フェリチン　ferritin

ふえる　増える　(重量が) gain (gain) (↔lose), put on　(数量が) increase (↔decrease), grow ☞増加，増殖，増やす，増す ◆最近，体重が増えましたか Have you gained[put on] weight recently? / Have you noticed any weight gain recently? ◆1週間で何kg増えましたか How many kilos have you gained[put on] in a week? ◆体重が増えすぎないように注意して下さい Please be careful not to *put on[gain] too much weight. / Please try to control your weight. ◆月経血量が増えた The menstrual flow has increased. ◆便〈尿〉の回数が増えた The bowel movements have〈Passing urine has〉become more frequent.

フェルティしょうこうぐん　―症候群

Felty syndrome

フェロモン　pheromone

ふおう　不応（性の）　refractory ▶不応期 refractory period　不応性貧血 refractory anemia；RA

フォークト・こやなぎ・はらだびょう　― 小柳・原田病　Vogt-Koyanagi-Harada disease, VKH disease

フォガーティカテーテル　Fogarty catheter

フォリイカテーテル　Foley catheter

フォルクマンこうしゅく　―拘縮　Volkmann contracture

フォローアップ　follow-up ◆フォローアップの受診 follow-up consultation ◆定期的なフォローアップ検査を3か月から6か月に1回受けて下さい Please take regular follow-up tests every three to six months.

フォン・ウィルブランドびょう　―病 von Willebrand disease；VWD

フォン・レックリングハウゼンびょう　― 病　von Recklinghausen disease

ふか　負荷　(圧迫) stress　(荷重) load　(義務・責任などの負担) burden ☞ストレス ◆体に軽い負荷をかける put some mild stress on *one's* body ◆怪我をした足に負荷をかけないよう注意して下さい Be careful not to put too much load on the injured leg. ◆運動負荷心電図をとりましょう We'd like you to do an exercise stress EKG. / We're going to take an exercise stress EKG. ▶圧負荷 pressure overload　右〈左〉心負荷 right〈left〉heart overload　後負荷 afterload　心身負荷 physical and mental burden　前負荷 preload　体重負荷運動 weight-bearing exercise　容量負荷 volume load ▶負荷量 loading dose ☞負荷試験，負荷心電図

ふかい[1]　深い　deep　(傷などが深刻な) serious　(熟睡の) sound ◆深い傷 a deep [serious] wound ◆潰瘍が深いと出血することがあります If an ulcer is deep, it can cause bleeding. ◆深い眠りに落ちる fall into a deep[sound] sleep ◆深い悲しみ (a) deep sorrow

ふかい²　**不快（な）**　（快適でない）**uncomfortable**　（嫌な）**unpleasant**　（すごく嫌なにおいの）**offensive**　（図苦痛 **discomfort**）
◆喉に痛みや不快な症状がありますか Do you have any pain or discomfort in your throat?　◆この処置は少し不快に感じるかもしれませんが，あっという間に終わります This treatment might be a bit uncomfortable, but it'll be over before you know it.
◆不快な経験をする have an unpleasant [uncomfortable] experience　◆不快なにおいがする have an unpleasant[offensive] smell / be bad-smelling　▶不快指数 discomfort index；DI /（温湿指数）temperature-humidity index；THI　☞不快感

ふかいかん　**不快感**　**discomfort, unpleasant feeling**　◆飲み込む時に喉に不快感がありますか Do you feel any discomfort in your throat when you swallow?　◆これまで胸に痛みや不快感がありましたか Have you ever had any pain or discomfort in your chest?　◀胸部不快感 chest discomfort　腹部不快感 abdominal discomfort

ふかぎゃく　**不可逆（性の・的な）**　**irreversible**　▶不可逆的損傷 irreversible damage[injury]　不可逆反応 irreversible reaction

ふかけつ　**不可欠（な）**　（本質的になくてはならない）**essential, indispensable**　（生命維持に不可欠な）**vital**　☞必須　◆適度な運動は健康に不可欠です Proper exercise is essential[indispensable] for good health.
◆ビタミンとミネラルは身体にとって不可欠な栄養素です Vitamins and minerals are essential[vital] nutrients for the body.

ふかこうりょく　**不可抗力（の）**　（避けられない）**unavoidable, inevitable**　（制御できない）**uncontrollable**　◆不可抗力の事故に遭う have an unavoidable accident

ふかさ　**深さ**　**depth**　◆昏睡の深さを測る measure the depth of coma

ふかし　**不可視（の）**　**invisible**　▶不可視光（線）invisible ray[light / radiation]

ふかしけん　**負荷試験**　（耐容試験）**tolerance test[testing]**　（ストレステスト）**stress test**　（荷重試験）**loading test**　◀運動負荷試験 exercise（tolerance）test[testing]　エルゴメーター負荷試験（bicycle）ergometer test / ergometry　荷重負荷運動 weight-bearing exercise　経口ブドウ糖負荷試験 oral glucose tolerance test；OGTT　トレッドミル負荷試験 treadmill test[testing]　ホルモン負荷試験 hormone stimulation test　水負荷試験 water loading test

ふかしんでんず　**負荷心電図**　**stress electrocardiogram[EKG], load electrocardiogram[EKG]**

ふかつ　**賦活（する）**　（活性化する）**activate**　（促進する）**stimulate**　☞活性化　◀免疫賦活薬 immunostimulant / immunostimulator　▶賦活剤 activator

ふかつか　**不活化（する）**　**inactivate**　（形不活化された **inactivated**）　◆アルコール消毒薬で多くの細菌は不活化されます Many bacteria can be inactivated by alcohol-based disinfectants.　▶不活化ワクチン inactivated[killed] vaccine

ふかづめ　**深爪**　◆深爪する cut a[one's] nail too short /（手指の）cut a[one's] fingernail *too short[（爪の下の組織まで）to the quick] /（足指の）cut a[one's] toenail *too short[to the quick]

ふかで　**深傷**　（ひどい傷）**severe wound**　（致命的な傷）**fatal wound**　◆深傷を負う be seriously wounded / suffer[have] a severe wound

ふかのう　**不可能（な）**　**impossible**　（非現実的な）**impractical**　◆アレルゲンを完全に避けるのはほとんど不可能です It's almost impossible to completely avoid allergens.　◆実行不可能なケアプラン an impractical care plan

ふかひ　**不可避（の）**　☞不可抗力

ふかんしょう　**不感症**　**frigidity**　（形frigid）　◀性的不感症 sexual frigidity

ふかんじょうさん　**不感蒸散**　**insensible perspiration**

ふかんぜん　**不完全（な）**　（不十分な）**incomplete**　（欠陥のある）**defective, imperfect**　（部分的な）**partial**　▶不完全右脚〈左脚〉ブロック incomplete right〈left〉bundle branch block；IRBBB〈ILBBB〉　不完全

寛解 incomplete remission　不完全骨折 incomplete fracture

ふきげん 不機嫌(な)　cross, grumpy　(気難しい)bad-tempered　◆今日彼女は寝不足で不機嫌です She's cross[grumpy / in a bad mood] today because she didn't get enough sleep.　◆息子さんは思い通りにならないと不機嫌になりますか Does your son get[become] bad-tempered when he doesn't have everything his own way?

ふきそく 不規則(な)　irregular　◆脈が不規則です Your pulse is irregular. / You have an irregular heartbeat. / Your heart skips beats.　◆不規則な生活をする live an irregular life / keep irregular hours　◆不規則な生活習慣を改める improve[fix] one's irregular daily routine

ふきでもの 吹き出物　☞痤瘡, にきび
ふきとる 拭き取る　wipe off[away]
ふきぬけこっせつ 吹抜け骨折　blow-out fracture

ぶきよう 不器用(な)　clumsy, awkward　◆手先が不器用だ be clumsy with one's hands　◆手先が不器用でよく物を落としますか Do you have clumsy hands and often drop things?　◆人付き合いが不器用ですか Do you feel[Are you] awkward with other people? / Do social situations make you feel awkward?

ふきんこう 不均衡　imbalance, disproportion, disequilibrium　(🄰unbalanced, imbalanced, disproportionate)　◆児頭骨盤不均衡 cephalopelvic disproportion; CPD　▶不均衡症候群 disequilibrium syndrome　不均衡発育 unbalanced growth

ふく¹ 服　clothes　★複数形で.　◆服を着る put one's clothes on / put on one's clothes / get dressed　◆服を着ている wear one's clothes　◆服を脱ぐ take one's clothes off / take off one's clothes / get undressed　◆服は上半身を脱いで下さい Please take[slip] your clothes off from the waist up. / Please take off your top things.　◆服を着ていいですよ You can get dressed now.　◆服を着たり脱いだりするのが難しい have difficulty getting dressed or undressed　◆ゆったりした服 loose-fitting[comfortable] clothes　◁妊婦服 maternity clothes[wear]　防護服 protective clothing　☞服装

ふく² 拭く　(拭きとる)wipe　(乾かす)dry　◆このタオルで顔を拭いて下さい Please wipe[dry] your face with this washcloth[towel].　◆(床上で)お体を拭きましょう I'm going to give you a bed bath.

フグ　fugu, puffer fish　▶フグ中毒 fugu poisoning　フグ毒 fugu toxin[poison]

ふくあつ 腹圧　abdominal (muscle) pressure　▶腹圧性尿失禁 stress (urinary) incontinence; SUI

ふくい 腹囲　abdominal circumference, waist circumference, waist size　◆腹囲を測りましょう Let me[I'm going to] measure *you around the waist[your abdominal circumference].　◆あなたの腹囲は 102 cm です You're one hundred (and) two centimeters around the waist. / Your abdominal circumference is one hundred (and) two centimeters.　▶腹囲測定 abdominal circumference measurement

ふくいんちょう 副院長　vice president

ふくがい 腹臥位　prone position, abdominal position, face-down position　☞うつ伏せ　◆腹臥位をとる lie prone / lie on one's front[stomach]

ふくがく 復学(する)　return to school, go back to school　◆復学をご希望されますか Would you like to return[go back] to school?　◆復学するには医師の許可が必要です You need your doctor's approval before you can return[go back] to school.

ふくくう 腹腔　abdominal cavity　(🄰腹部の abdominal　腹腔の celiac　腹膜の peritoneal)　◆脳室腹腔シャント ventriculo-peritoneal[VP] shunt　▶腹腔穿刺 abdominocentesis / abdominal paracentesis[puncture]　腹腔洗浄 peritoneal lavage / abdominal irrigation　腹腔動脈 celiac artery[arterial trunk]　腹腔内圧 intraabdominal pressure　腹腔内出血 intraabdominal hemorrhage　腹腔内注射

intraperitoneal injection　腹腔内膿瘍 intraabdominal[intraperitoneal] abscess　腹腔リンパ節 celiac lymph node　☞腹腔鏡

ふくくうきょう　腹腔鏡　laparoscope（腹腔鏡の laparoscopic）　▶腹腔鏡下手術 laparoscopic[keyhole] surgery　腹腔鏡下胆嚢摘出術 laparoscopic cholecystectomy；LAP-C　腹腔鏡検査 laparoscopy

ふくごう　複合（的な）　（複数の物が混合・結合した）combined　（異質な要素が組み合わさった）composite　（相互に関連する要素が集まった）complex　◀免疫複合体 immune complex；IC　▶複合移植 composite graft[grafting]　複合汚染 complex contamination / combined pollution　複合感覚 combined sensation　複合体 complex / composite　複合免疫不全症 combined immunodeficiency；CID

ふくこうがん　副睾丸　（精上体）epididymis　▶副睾丸炎 epididymitis

ふくこうかんしんけい　副交感神経　parasympathetic nerve　▶副交感神経作動[興奮]薬 parasympathomimetic (medication / drug / agent)　副交感神経遮断薬 parasympatholytic (medication / drug / agent) / parasympathetic blocking medication[drug / agent]

ふくこうじょうせん　副甲状腺　parathyroid gland　◀偽性副甲状腺機能低下症 pseudohypoparathyroidism　▶副甲状腺過形成 parathyroid hyperplasia　副甲状腺がん parathyroid cancer　副甲状腺機能検査 parathyroid gland function test　副甲状腺機能亢進症 hyperparathyroidism；HPT　副甲状腺機能低下症 hypoparathyroidism　副甲状腺腫 parathyroid adenoma　副甲状腺摘出術 parathyroidectomy　副甲状腺ホルモン parathyroid hormone；PTH　副甲状腺ホルモン関連蛋白質 parathyroid hormone-related protein；PTHrP

ふくざいじょうみゃく　伏在静脈　saphenous vein　▶伏在静脈移植片 saphenous vein graft；SVG

ふくざつ　複雑（な）　（繁雑に絡み合った）complicated　（相互に入り組んだ）complex　（2つ以上から成る）compound　（雑多な）mixed　◆職場の複雑な人間関係に悩んでいるのですか Do you have problems with complicated relationships at work?　◆両親に対して複雑な気持ちをもつ have mixed feelings[emotions] about *one's* parents　▶複雑骨折 compound fracture　複雑性尿路感染症 complicated urinary tract infection　複雑部分発作 complex partial seizure；CPS

ふくざつおん　副雑音　adventitious sound

ふくさよう　副作用　side effect　（有害反応）adverse effect[reaction], contrary effect　◆これまでに薬の副作用はありましたか Have you ever had[experienced] any side effects to medications?　◆この薬は肺に重篤な副作用を起こします This medication causes serious side effects in[to] the lungs.　◆この薬には軽い〈強い〉副作用があります This medication has some mild〈severe〉side effects.　◆この薬には副作用はほとんどありません This medication has very few side effects. / The side effects of this medication are quite rare.　◆この薬には胃の不調や便秘などの副作用があります The side effects of this medication include upset stomach and constipation. / This medication may cause side effects such as upset stomach and constipation.　◆副作用でご心配なことがあれば連絡して下さい Please call[contact] us if you're concerned about any side effects.　◆抗がん剤の副作用で脱毛する *have hair loss[lose *one's* hair] as a side effect of the anticancer medication　◆副作用は人によって異なります The side effects vary from person to person.　◆副作用は短期間続きますが, 治療が終われば徐々になくなるでしょう The side effects are short-term[temporary] and will gradually disappear[go away] once the treatment is over.　◆抗がん剤の副作用を最小限に抑える minimize the side effects of anticancer medication　◀医薬品副作用

ふくさよう adverse drug reaction；ADR　輸血副作用 blood transfusion side effects / side effects of blood transfusion　▶副作用情報 information about side effects / side effects information

ふくさんぶつ　副産物　byproduct, by-product　(派生物)outgrowth

ふくし¹　副子　splint（医splint）　◆怪我をした腕に副子を当てる splint the injured arm / apply a splint to the injured arm / place a splint on the injured arm　◀膝副子 knee splint

ふくし²　福祉　welfare（医補助的な assistive）　◆福祉関係の職業 a welfare-related profession / welfare work　◀医療福祉相談室 medical social work[services] office[unit]　介護福祉士 certified care worker　公共[社会]福祉 public[social] welfare　児童福祉 child welfare　社会福祉士 social worker；SW　精神保健福祉士 psychiatric social worker；PSW　老人福祉 welfare for the elderly / elderly welfare　▶福祉機器 assistive device[equipment]　福祉工学 assistive technology；AT　福祉サービス welfare service　福祉事務所(social) welfare office　福祉年金 welfare pension　福祉用具[用品] assistive technology products[goods]　☞福祉施設

ふくし³　複視　diplopia, double vision　◀単眼複視 monocular diplopia　両眼複視 binocular diplopia

ふくじ¹　副耳　accessory auricle, preauricular tag

ふくじ²　副次　☞二次

ふくしきこきゅう　腹式呼吸　abdominal breathing[respiration]　(横隔膜呼吸)diaphragmatic[diaphragm] breathing　☞呼吸(囲み：呼吸法)　◆腹式呼吸で深く呼吸をして下さい Breathe deeply using your diaphragm.　◆腹式呼吸の練習をする practice breathing deeply using the diaphragm

ふくししせつ　福祉施設　welfare facility　◀介護老人福祉施設 welfare facility for the elderly requiring long-term care　児

童福祉施設 child welfare facility

ふくしゃねつ　輻射熱　radiant heat

ふくしょう　復唱する　repeat　◆私の言葉を復唱して下さい Please repeat *after me[what I say].

ふくじん　副腎　adrenal gland, suprarenal gland　▶副腎過形成 adrenal hyperplasia　副腎偶発腫 adrenal incidentaloma　副腎クリーゼ adrenal crisis　副腎腫瘍 adrenal tumor　副腎静脈サンプリング adrenal venous sampling；AVS　副腎性器症候群 adrenogenital syndrome；AGS　副腎性女性化 adrenal feminism　副腎性男性化 adrenal virilism　副腎腺腫 adrenal adenoma　副腎摘出術 adrenalectomy　副腎白質ジストロフィー adrenoleukodystrophy；ALD　副腎不全 adrenal insufficiency　☞副腎髄質, 副腎皮質

ふくしんけい　副神経　accessory nerve, *cranial nerve[CN] XI

ふくじんずいしつ　副腎髄質　adrenal medulla　▶副腎髄質ホルモン adrenomedullary hormone

ふくじんひしつ　副腎皮質　adrenal cortex（医adrenocortical）　▶副腎皮質機能亢進症 adrenocortical hyperfunction　副腎皮質機能低下症 adrenocortical hypofunction / adrenocortical insufficiency　副腎皮質刺激ホルモン adrenocorticotropic hormone；ACTH / corticotropin　副腎皮質刺激ホルモン放出ホルモン corticotropin-releasing hormone；CRH　副腎皮質ホルモン adrenocortical[adrenal cortex] hormone；ACH / corticosteroid / corticoid

ふくすい　腹水　fluid in the abdominal cavity, ascites /əsáiti:z/, ascitic fluid　◆腹水がかなりたまっています There is an abnormal amount of fluid[water] in your abdomen. / A large amount of fluid[water] has *built up[accumulated] in your abdomen.　◆腹水を抜く drain the fluid from the abdominal cavity / drain the abdominal fluid　◀がん性腹水 cancerous ascites[ascitic fluid]　血性腹水 bloody[hemorrhagic] ascites　浸出性腹

水 exudative ascites　漏出性腹水 transudative ascites　▶腹水検査 ascites examination［analysis］

ふくすう　複数(の)　(2, 3の) a few　(5, 6の) several　(かなりの数の) a number of　◆複数の抗がん剤を組み合わせて治療します We're going to combine a few[two or more] chemotherapy drugs to treat your cancer.

ふくそう¹　服装　(衣服) clothes　(衣類) clothing　◆彼女は服装に無頓着です She's quite careless about her clothes. / She pays no attention at all to what she wears.　◆検査には動きやすい服装とウォーキングシューズでおいで下さい Please wear comfortable clothes and walking shoes for the test.

ふくそう²　輻輳　convergence　▶輻輳異常 convergence anomaly　輻輳（眼球）運動 convergence (eye) movement　輻輳眼振 convergence nystagmus

ふくぞう　複像　double image

ふくそく　腹側(の)　ventral (↔dorsal)

ふくたい　腹帯　abdominal belt[binder]　(包帯式の) abdominal bandage　(妊婦用の) maternity belt　◆腹帯を着ける put one's abdominal belt on / put on one's abdominal belt　◆腹帯を着けている wear an abdominal belt

ふくちょくきん　腹直筋　rectus abdominis (muscle)

ふくつう　腹痛　(胃・腹部の) stomachache　(腹部の) abdominal pain　☞痛み（囲み：痛みの表現）, お腹　◆腹痛がありますか Do you have any pain in your stomach or abdomen?　◆腹痛はどんな時に起こりますか When does the stomachache[abdominal pain] usually come on? / In what situations do you get the stomachache[abdominal pain]?　◆体位を変えると腹痛が治まりますか Does changing position help to relieve the stomachache? / Does the stomachache go away when you change position?　◆ひどい腹痛がある have a severe stomachache　◆腹痛を起こす get[develop] (a) stomachache　◀痙攣性腹痛 abdominal cramps　疝痛性腹痛 colicky abdominal pain　反復性腹痛 recurrent abdominal pain

ふくでんどうろ　副伝導路　accessory (conduction) pathway, bypass tract

ふくどく　服毒する　take poison　◆服毒自殺を図る try to *kill oneself [commit suicide] by taking poison　◆服毒死 death by[from] poisoning / poisoning death

ふくにゅう　副乳　accessory breast　▶副乳頭 accessory nipple

ふくはんのう　副反応　☞副作用

ふくひ　副脾　accessory spleen

ふくびくう　副鼻腔　(paranasal) sinus / sáinəs /　気圧性副鼻腔炎 barosinusitis　航空性副鼻腔炎 aerosinusitis　▶副鼻腔炎 sinusitis　副鼻腔気管支症候群 sinobronchial syndrome；SBS

ふくふ　覆布　drape

ふくぶ　腹部　abdomen /ǽbdəmən/, abdóminal region　☞お腹, 下腹部, 上腹部, 側腹部　◆腹部の超音波検査をしましょう I'm going to do an ultrasound of your abdomen.　◆腹部を触診する palpate the abdomen　▶腹部圧痛 abdominal tenderness　腹部硬直 abdominal rigidity　腹部腫瘤 abdominal tumor　腹部臓器 abdominal organ　腹部損傷 abdominal injury　腹部大動脈 abdominal aorta　腹部大動脈瘤 abdominal aortic aneurysm；AAA　腹部不快感 abdominal discomfort　腹部膨満 abdominal fullness[distension] / fullness in the abdomen

ふくへき　腹壁　abdominal wall　▶腹壁反射 abdominal wall reflex　腹壁ヘルニア abdominal[(腹側面の) ventral] hernia

ふくまく　腹膜　peritoneum (🔤peritoneal)　◀後腹膜腫瘍 retroperitoneal tumor　▶腹膜腔 peritoneal cavity　腹膜刺激徴候 peritoneal irritation sign / sign of peritoneal irritation　腹膜穿刺 peritoneal puncture[paracentesis]　腹膜中皮腫 peritoneal mesothelioma　腹膜播種 peritoneal dissemination　腹膜癒着 peritoneal adhesion　☞腹膜炎, 腹膜透析

ふくまくえん 腹膜炎　peritonitis /pèrə-tənáɪtɪs/　◀癌性腹膜炎 carcinomatous peritonitis　骨盤腹膜炎 pelvic peritonitis　穿孔性腹膜炎 perforative peritonitis　胆汁性腹膜炎 bile[biliary] peritonitis　糞便性腹膜炎 fecal peritonitis　癒着性腹膜炎 adhesive peritonitis

ふくまくとうせき 腹膜透析　peritoneal dialysis；PD　◀間欠的腹膜透析 intermittent peritoneal dialysis；IPD　自動腹膜透析 automated peritoneal dialysis；APD　連続携行式腹膜透析 continuous ambulatory peritoneal dialysis；CAPD

ふくむ 含む　《含有する》contain　《全体の一部として含む》include　◆カフェインを含む飲み物 caffeinated drinks[beverages] / drinks containing caffeine　◆発がん性物質を含む contain a cancer-causing substance　◆果物や野菜を多く含むバランスのとれた食事をして下さい Please eat a well-balanced diet that includes plenty of fruits and vegetables.　◆鉄分を多く含む食べ物を摂って下さい Please eat foods rich [high] in iron.　《口に入れておく》hold　◆この薬を飲みこむ前に口の中に 2, 3 分含んでいて下さい Please hold this medication in your mouth for a few minutes before swallowing it.

ふくめい 腹鳴　stomach rumbling, borborygmus

ふくやく 服薬　taking (a) medication [medicine]　☞薬, 服用　▶服薬指導 medication counseling[teaching]　服薬順守 medication[drug] compliance

ふくよう 服用する　take (a) medication [medicine]　☞薬, 服薬　◆今薬を服用していますか，または最近服用しましたか Are you taking or have you recently taken any drugs or medications?　◆この薬は指示どおりに服用して下さい Please take this medicine exactly as directed.　◆服用量（1 回の摂取量）a dose /（一定期間に摂取した積算量）a dosage　◆食前〈食後 / 食間〉服用（服薬指示）To be taken before〈after / be-tween〉meals　◀過剰服用 overdose / excessive intake　▶服用スケジュール dosing schedule

ふくらはぎ （腓腹筋）calf muscle, sural muscle, gastrocnemius muscle　◆ふくらはぎの痙攣 calf cramps

ふくらます 膨らます　（突き出す）push out　（頬・胸を息で膨らます）puff out, blow out　（ガスなどで膨張させる）inflate　◆お腹を膨らませて下さい Please *push out[inflate] your abdomen.　◆頬を膨らませて下さい Please *blow out[puff (out)] your cheeks.

ふくらむ 膨らむ　（腫れる）swell (out, up)　（顔などがむくむ）bloat　（拡張する）dilate　（範囲が広くなる）broaden

ふくれている 膨れている　（ガスなどで膨張した）be inflated　（腫れた）be swollen　（液体・ガスなどでむくんだ）be bloated　（拡張した）be dilated　（広くなった）be broadened

ふくろ 袋　bag　（小さな袋）pouch　（麻などの袋）sack　◆紙袋 a paper bag　◆ビニール袋 a plastic bag　◆入れ歯をはずしてこのビニール袋に入れて下さい Please remove your dentures and put them in this plastic bag.　◆採便袋 colostomy bag

ふくろみみ 袋耳　pocket ear

ふけ dandruff, scurf

ふけつ 不潔（な）　（汚い）dirty　（極端に汚い）filthy　（非衛生的な）unsanitary, insanitary　▶不潔恐怖症 mysophobia

ふけんこう 不健康（な）　（健康的でない）unhealthy　（体に悪い）unwholesome　☞不養生　◆不健康な生活を送る live an unhealthy life[lifestyle]　◆不健康な食品を控える *cut down[cut back] on unhealthy[unwholesome] food(s)

ふけんせい 不顕性（の）　（無症状の）silent, symptomless, asymptomatic, subclinical　（明白でない）inapparent　▶不顕性感染 silent[inapparent / asymptomatic / subclinical] infection　不顕性誤嚥 silent [asymptomatic / subclinical] aspiration

ふこう 不幸（な）　（恵まれない）unhappy　（運の悪い）unfortunate

ふさがる 塞がる　（詰まる）get[become]

ふさがる blocked[plugged, clogged]（up） （閉じる）close（up） （傷が治る）heal（up） ◆耳が塞がった感じがする feel as if the ears are blocked[plugged / clogged]（up） ◆傷は塞がった the wound has closed[healed]（up） ◆あいにく今週末は予定が塞がっています Unfortunately, my schedule is full this weekend.

ふさぎこむ 鬱ぎ込む become depressed

ふさぐ 塞ぐ （閉じる）close（up） （穴・管などを塞ぐ）fill, plug（up） （管などを遮る）obstruct, block ◆（縫合などにより）傷口を塞ぐ close（up）the cut[wound] ◆血栓が肺の血管を塞ぐ a blood clot obstructs[blocks] a vessel in the lung

ふし 父子 father and child ▶父子家庭 motherless family 父子関係 father-child relationship[relations]

ふじ 不治（の） （治療できない）incurable （致死性の）fatal

ぶじ 無事（に） （うまく）well （首尾よく）successfully （安全に）safely ◆彼女の手術は無事に終わりました Her surgery *went well[was successful].

ブジー bougie ◀尿道ブジー urethral bougie

ふしぎ 不思議（な） （奇妙な）strange （驚異の）wonderful, marvelous （興味深い）curious （説明できない）unaccountable

ふしぜん 不自然（な） unnatural （人為的な）artificial

ふしゅ 浮腫 （水腫）edema /ɪdíːmə/（🈩 edematous）（腫脹）（generalized） swelling ☞むくみ, むくむ ◀圧痕浮腫 pitting edema 黄斑浮腫 macular edema 血管（神経）性浮腫 angioedema / angioneurotic edema 喉頭浮腫 laryngeal edema 心原性浮腫 cardiac edema 腎性浮腫 renal edema 乳頭浮腫 optic disc edema / papilledema 脳浮腫 brain[cerebral] edema / cerebral swelling / swelling of the brain リンパ浮腫 lymphedema ▶浮腫性腫脹 edematous swelling

ふじゆう 不自由（な） （身体に障害がある）physically disabled[challenged] （麻痺した）paralyzed （機能が低下した）impaired ☞不便 ◆身体が不自由な人〈子供〉a person〈child〉with a physical disability[challenge] ◆彼は身体が不自由です He is physically disabled[challenged]. ◆歩行が不自由である have difficulty walking ◆半身麻痺で日常生活動作に不自由する have difficulty carrying out the activities of daily living due to paralysis on one side of the body ◆左足が不自由である（麻痺している）one's left leg is paralyzed ◆目〈耳〉の不自由な人 a blind〈deaf〉person / a visually〈hearing〉disabled[impaired] person ★blind や deaf には差別的なニュアンスはないが, the blind や the deaf は差別表現となる. ◆彼女は日本語が不自由です（上手に話せない）She can't speak Japanese properly[well]. /（自由に意思疎通できるほど上手でない）Her Japanese is not good enough to allow her to communicate freely.

ふじゅうぶん 不十分（な） （十分でない）not enough （量などが不足した）insufficient （本質的な物が不足した）deficient （不適切な）inadequate （不完全な）incomplete ☞不足 ◆不十分な説明 an inadequate explanation ◆不十分な情報 insufficient[inadequate] information

ふじゅん 不順 irregularity （🈩irregular） ◀月経不順 irregular periods[menstruation] / menstrual irregularity

ふじょ 扶助 （助け）assistance, help （主として公的な援助）aid ◀医療扶助 medical assistance

ふしょう 負傷 （事故による）injury （凶器などによる）wound ☞怪我

ふしょうかべん 不消化便 undigested food in stool

ふしょく 腐食 corrosion （🈩corrosive） ▶腐食作用 corrosive action 腐食性胃炎 corrosive gastritis 腐食性食道炎 corrosive esophagitis 腐食損傷 corrosive injury

ふしん¹ 不信 distrust （🈩distrustful） ◆スタッフに対して不信感を抱く be[feel] distrustful of the staff

ふしん² **不審** （疑問）doubt （形doubtful）
（悪い可能性への疑惑）suspicion （形suspicious） ◆この薬についてもしご不審な点がありましたら遠慮なくお尋ね下さい Feel free to ask me if *you have any doubts [you're suspicious] about this medication. ▶不審死 suspicious death / （原因不明の死）unexplained death

ふしん³ **不振**（な）poor, bad ◀学業不振 underachievement 学業不振児 underachiever 食欲不振 poor appetite / loss of appetite / anorexia

ふじん **婦人** woman ☞女性

ふじんか **婦人科** （婦人科学）gynecology /ɡàɪnɪkáləʤi/；GYN （形gynecologic, gynecological） （診療科）the department of gynecology, the gynecology department ☞産婦人科 ▶婦人科医 gynecologist 婦人科検診 gynecologic screening[checkup] 婦人科疾患 gynecologic[woman's] disease 婦人科診察［内診］gynecologic examination

ふずい¹ **不随** （麻痺）paralysis, palsy （形be[get, become] paralyzed） ☞麻痺 ◆右〈左〉半身不随である be paralyzed on the right〈left〉side ◆下半身不随になる become paralyzed from the waist down ◆首から下が不随である *be paralyzed [suffer paralysis] from the neck down ◀下半身不随 paralysis from the waist down / paraplegia 全身不随 full paralysis / paralysis of the whole body / （四肢麻痺）quadriplegia 半身不随（片麻痺）paralysis of *one side[half] of the body / hemiplegia

ふずい² **付随**（的な） （同時に起こる）accompanying （副次的に起こる）incidental （随伴する）concomitant ◆放射線治療に付随する問題点 problems accompanying [incidental to] radiation therapy

ふずいい **不随意**（の） involuntary ▶不随意運動 involuntary movement 不随意筋 involuntary muscle 不随意収縮 involuntary contraction

ふせい¹ **父性** paternity （形paternal）, fatherhood ▶父性愛 paternal[father's]

love 父性遺伝 paternal inheritance 父性行動 paternal behavior

ふせい² **不正**（な） （不適切な）improper （異常な）abnormal （典型と異なる）atypical （不規則な）irregular （機能不全に陥った）dysfunctional （悪い）bad （接頭mal-） ▶不正咬合 malocclusion / improper[abnormal] occlusion 不正性器出血 atypical[abnormal] genital bleeding 不正乱視 irregular astigmatism

ふせいみゃく **不整脈** arrhythmia, irregular pulse[heartbeat], unequal pulse [heartbeat] ◆不整脈がありますか Do you have an irregular pulse[heartbeat]? / Do you feel your heart beating irregularly? ◆不整脈はどのくらい続きますか How long does the irregular pulse last[go on for]? ◀抗不整脈薬 antiarrhythmic (medication / drug / agent) 徐脈性不整脈 bradyarrhythmia 心室性不整脈 ventricular arrhythmia；VA 心房性不整脈 atrial arrhythmia 洞不整脈 sinus arrhythmia 頻脈性不整脈 tachyarrhythmia

ふせぐ **防ぐ** （予防する）prevent （防御する）defend （保護する）protect ◆症状の悪化を防ぐ prevent *one's condition from getting worse ◆皮膚の乾燥を防ぐ prevent *the skin from drying[drying of the skin] ◆血栓を防ぐ薬 a medication to prevent *blood clot formation[blood clotting]

ふせっせい **不摂生** ☞不養生

ふせる **臥せる** be sick in bed

ふぜん **不全** （停止・障害）failure （不十分）insufficiency （機能障害）dysfunction, malfunction （遂行不能・機能不全）incompetence, incompetency （形incompetent 完全な状態でない incomplete, partial） ◀肝不全 liver[hepatic] failure[insufficiency] 冠不全 coronary failure[insufficiency] 呼吸不全 respiratory failure[insufficiency] 循環不全 circulatory failure 心不全 heart[cardiac] failure 腎不全 kidney[renal] failure 多臓器不全 multiple organ failure；MOF 洞不全症候群 sick sinus syndrome；SSS 脳循環不全 cerebrovascular insufficiency 発育不全 underdevelopment／(無形成)aplasia／(低形成)hypoplasia 副腎不全 adrenal insufficiency 勃起不全 erectile dysfunction；ED 免疫不全 immunodeficiency 免疫不全宿主 immunocompromised host 卵巣機能不全 ovarian insufficiency ▶不全強直 partial ankylosis 不全麻痺 paresis 不全流産 incomplete abortion

ふそく　不足　(欠乏)lack (圏lacking) (時間・人手などの不足)shortage (圏short) (必要な物の欠乏)deficiency (圏deficient) (接頭under-)　☞足りない　◆血液中に鉄分が不足すると鉄欠乏性貧血を起こします Lack of iron in the blood can lead to iron-deficiency anemia.　◆この症状は脳へ行く血流が不足して起こります This symptom occurs due to lack of blood flow to the brain.　◆あなたは栄養不足〈運動不足〉です You aren't getting[taking] enough nutrition〈exercise〉.　◆在宅で介護する人手が不足している suffer from a shortage of home[in-home] care workers　◀運動不足 lack of exercise　栄養不足 undernutrition／nutritional deficiency／hypoalimentation　活力不足 lack of energy[vitality]　酸素不足 oxygen deficiency／lack of oxygen (supply)／(低酸素症)hypoxia　授乳不足 underfeeding　睡眠不足 lack[shortage] of sleep　摂取不足 deficient intake　体力不足 lack of physical strength　注意不足 carelessness　鉄分不足 iron deficiency／lack of iron　ビタミン不足 vitamin deficiency／lack of vitamins

ふぞく　付属(の)　(提携している)affiliated (所属している)attached　◀大学付属病院 university[university-affiliated] hospital／hospital *affiliated with[attached to] the university

ふぞくき　(子宮)付属器　adnexa (uteri), appendages　◆通例，複数形で．　▶(子宮)付属器炎 adnexitis　付属器摘出術 adnexectomy

ブタ　豚　pig, swine　◆この食事には豚肉は含まれていません This meal does not contain pork.　◆豚肉を含まない食事 pork-free food[menu]　▶ブタインフルエンザ swine flu[influenza]

ふたい　不耐(性)　intolerance　◆果糖不耐症 fructose intolerance　牛乳不耐症 milk intolerance　乳糖不耐症 lactose intolerance

ふたえまぶた　二重瞼　double eyelid, eyelid with a fold　◆二重瞼の手術を行う perform[do] double eyelid surgery

ふたご　双子　twins (双子の1人)twin　☞双生児　◆双子の兄弟 twin brother(s)　◆双子の姉妹 twin sister(s)

ふたりべや　2人部屋　semiprivate room, two-bed room, room for two

ふたん　負担　(圧力)strain, stress (重荷)(extra) burden, load (作業量)workload (動支払う)pay　保険が補償の対象とする cover)　◆膝に負担をかける put[place] extra strain[stress] on the knees　◆腰に負担がかかっている be hard on *one's* back　◆心臓が肥大し負担がかかっている the heart is enlarged and overworked　◆この手術は体に負担が少ない This is a minimally invasive surgery.／This surgery causes less trauma to the body.　◆心臓の負担を減らす reduce the heart's workload　◆家事の負担を減らす *cut down on [reduce] *one's* housework　◆経済的な負担に耐える carry[bear] a financial burden　◆精神的な負担に苦しむ suffer (from) a psychological burden[load]　◆体に負担のかかるような活動をする do strenuous activities　◆医療費は全額が自己負担となります You'll have to pay all [one hundred percent] of your medical expenses[bills].／(健康保険の対象外)Your medical expenses are not covered by any health insurance.　◆医療費の3割が自己負担となります．残りの7割は保険が負担します You'll have to pay thirty percent of your medical expenses. The remaining seventy percent will be covered by insurance.　◆医療費の公費負担 public financial assistance for medical expenses　◀(患者)一部負担 partial copayment

患者負担金 medical expenses borne [paid] by the patient　自己負担 self[out-of-pocket] payment

ふだん　普段(の)　(いつもの)usual　(常態の)normal　(毎日の)everyday, daily　☞いつも, 通常, 普通　◆普段, 朝食に何を食べていますか What do you usually have[eat] for breakfast?　◆普段より尿の量は多いですか Are you urinating more than usual?　◆普段どおりの生活をしてもいいですよ You can *go about[carry on with] your normal daily activities.　◆手術後1か月もすれば普段の生活に戻れるでしょう You should be back to your normal life a month or so after the surgery.　◆普段の生活の中でできる運動をお勧めします I recommend (you try) an exercise you can do in your everyday[daily] life.

ふち　縁　(端)edge　(境界)border　(辺縁)margin　◆このほくろは縁が不規則になっています This mole has an irregular edge [border].　◆病変の縁 lesion borders / borders of the lesion

ふちゃく　付着する　attach　(図attachment)　(粘りつく)adhere (to)　(図adherent)　(くっつく)stick (to)　◆胎盤が子宮壁の下方に付着しています The placenta is attached to the lower part of the uterine wall.　◆血小板が血管の壁に付着すると血の塊ができます Blood clots are formed when platelets adhere[stick] to the wall of a blood vessel.　◆ガーゼに血液が付着しているので取り換えましょう There're some blood stains on the gauze, so I'm going to change it.　▶付着胎盤 adherent placenta　付着部位 attachment site

ふちゅうい　不注意(な)　careless　(図carelessness)　◆不注意による誤りを犯す make a careless mistake[error]　◆ごめんなさい. 電気を消し忘れたのは私の不注意でした I'm sorry, it was careless of me to forget to turn off the lights.

ふちょう　不調(な)　not well, unwell, ill　◆不調である(体調がすぐれない)do not feel well / feel unwell[ill] / be out of condition　◆体の不調を訴える complain that

one hasn't been feeling well / complain of feeling unwell[ill]　◆胃の不調 a stomach upset

ぶちょう　部長　(診療部の長)department head　(管理者)director　◆看護副部長 (the) vice director of nursing　看護部長 (the) director of nursing　外科部長(the) head of the surgery department　診療部長(the) medical director of physicians　薬剤部長(the) director of pharmacy

ふつう　普通(の)　(いつもの)usual　(常態の・正常な)normal　(ありふれた)common　(並みの・平均的な)fair, average　(通常の)regular　(特別ではない)ordinary　(一般の)general　☞いつも, 通常, 普段　◆普通, 吐き気は3日もすれば治ります The nausea will usually *clear up[go away] in a few days.　◆楽にして普通に呼吸して下さい Please relax and breathe normally[as you usually do].　◆月経の出血量は普通ですか Is your menstrual flow normal?　◆ご〈普通の風邪でご心配ありません It's just a common cold, nothing to worry about.　◆現在の気分はどうですか, よい, 普通, よくないですか How is your mood *at the moment[now], good, fair, or poor?　◆普通の状態に戻る *get back[return] to normal　◆普通以上〈以下〉である be above 〈below〉normal　◆普通食 regular[normal] diet / ordinary meal

フッかぶつ　フッ化物　fluoride　◆虫歯予防にフッ化物を歯に塗布する apply topical fluoride to the teeth to prevent tooth decay　▶フッ化物添加 fluoridation　フッ化物配合歯磨き剤 fluoride dentifrice / (練り歯磨き)fluoride toothpaste / (洗口剤)fluoride mouthwash

ふつかよい　二日酔い　hangover　◆二日酔いである be hangover / have a hangover　◆二日酔いをさます *get rid of[recover from] a hangover

ぶつかる
《衝突する》bump (into), hit　◆何かにぶつかりましたか Did you *bump into[hit] something?　◆自転車にぶつかったのですか Did you get hit by a bicycle?

《意見などが対立する》clash（over）, have a clash ◆治療方針に関して患者と家族の意見がぶつかっています The patient clashed with his〈her〉family members over which treatment plan he〈she〉should choose.

《かち合う》◆次の診察予定日が休日〈出張〉とぶつかっています The scheduled date for your next meeting with the doctor falls on a holiday〈day the doctor will be away on business〉.

ふっき　復帰する　go back（to）, get back（to）, return（to） ☞社会復帰 ◆仕事に復帰するおつもりですか Are you planning on *going back[returning] to work? / Do you intend to *go back[return] to work? ◆仕事に復帰するには担当医の許可が必要です You need your doctor's approval before you can return[go back] to work[your job]. ◆社会復帰する return to work〈after an illness〈injury〉〉/〈普通の生活に戻る〉return[get back] to normal life

ぶっきょう　仏教　Buddhism ▶仏教徒 Buddhist

ふっきん　腹筋　abdominal muscle ◆腹筋を鍛える strengthen *one's* abdominal muscles ◆腹筋運動をする do sit-ups

ぶつける　bump, hit ◆歯をぶつける bump *one's* teeth ◆車の天井に頭をぶつける hit[bump] *one's* head against[on] the car roof ◆転んで舗道に頭をぶつける fall and hit *one's* head on the pavement

ぶっしつ　物質 （一般的に）**substance** （素材）**material** （作用剤）**agent** ◆汚染物質 contaminant / pollutant / polluting substance　化学物質 chemical（substance / agent）危険物質 dangerous[hazardous] substance[material]　禁止物質 prohibited substance　抗酸化物質 antioxidant　阻害物質 inhibitor / inhibitory substance[agent]　大気汚染物質 air pollutant　発がん(性)物質 carcinogen / carcinogenic[cancer-causing] substance[agent]　放射性物質 radioactive substance[material]　有害物質 harmful substance[material]

有毒物質 toxic[poisonous] substance[material]

フッそ　フッ素　fluorine ☞フッ化物

ぶったいしつにん　物体失認　object agnosia

ぶつり　物理 （物理学）**physics** （形physical）◀生物物理学 biophysics ▶物理的アレルギー physical allergy　物理的環境 physical environment　物理的損傷 physical injury　物理療法[理学療法] physical therapy / physiotherapy；PT

ふていき　不定期(の)　irregular ☞不規則 ◆年に2, 3回不定期に会合をもちますので，ご参加ください Meetings are held irregularly, two or three times a year, so come and join them.

ふていしゅうそ　不定愁訴 （全身倦怠感）**general malaise[feeling of being unwell]** （原因が確認できない訴え）**unidentified complaint, complaint of unknown etiology[origin]** （非特異的な訴え）**nonspecific complaint** ▶不定愁訴症候群 unidentified clinical syndrome

ふてきおう　不適応　maladjustment ◀環境不適応 situational maladjustment　社会的不適応 social maladjustment

ふてきごう　不適合 （互換不能）**incompatibility** （形incompatible）（不一致）**incongruity** （形incongruent, incongruous）◀Rh型不適合 Rh incompatibility　ABO式血液型不適合 ABO incompatibility　血液型不適合 blood type incompatibility　血液型不適合妊娠 blood-type incompatible pregnancy / incompatibility of maternal and fetal blood types　血液型不適合輸血 incompatible blood transfusion ▶不適合義歯 incompatible dentures

ふてきせつ　不適切(な) （下手な・貧弱な）**poor** （目的にかなっていない）**inappropriate** （良くない）**not good** （的確でない）**not proper** ◆不適切な説明で申し訳ありません I apologize for my poor explanation. / I apologize for not explaining properly. ◆説明の中で不適切な表現があったことをお詫びいたします I apologize for having used an inappropriate expression in my explanation. ◆不適切な栄養摂取 poor nutrition

ふどう¹　**不同**　◆患者名は順不同です The names of the patients are in random order. ◆左右不同[非対照]の腕 asymmetrical arms　◆瞳孔不同 anisocoria ☞不同視

ふどう²　**不動(化)**　immobilization

ぶとう　**舞踏(様の)**　choreic　▶舞踏アテトーゼ運動 choreoathetoid movement / choreoathetosis　舞踏(様)運動 chorea / choreic[choreoid / choreiform] movement ☞舞踏病

ブドウきゅうきん　**―球菌**　staphylococcus　(㊋staphylococcal)　(学名)*Staphylococcus*　◀黄色ブドウ球菌 *Staphylococcus aureus*　表皮ブドウ球菌 *Staphylococcus epidermidis*　メチシリン感受性黄色ブドウ球菌 methicillin-susceptible *Staphylococcus aureus*；MSSA　メチシリン耐性黄色ブドウ球菌 methicillin-resistant *Staphylococcus aureus*；MRSA　▶ブドウ球菌エンテロトキシン staphylococcal enterotoxin；SE　ブドウ球菌感染症 staphylococcal infection / (口語的に) staph infection　ブドウ球菌食中毒 staphylococcal food poisoning　ブドウ球菌腸炎〈肺炎〉 staphylococcal enterocolitis〈pneumonia〉　ブドウ球菌皮膚剝脱症候群 staphylococcal scalded skin syndrome；SSSS

ふとうこう　**不登校**　school refusal, refusal to *go to[attend] school ☞登校拒否　◆お子さんが不登校になったきっかけは何かありましたか Was there any trigger that led to your child refusing to *go to [attend] school? / Did anything trigger your child's refusal to *go to[attend] school?　◆不登校の子供 a child who refuses to go to school

ふどうし　**不同視**　anisometropia　(㊋anisometropic)　▶不同視(性)弱視 anisometropic amblyopia

ぶどうしゅようけっかんしゅ　**―酒様血管腫**　port-wine stain[hemangioma]

ふどうせいふあん　**浮動性不安**　free-floating anxiety

ふどうせいめまい　**浮動性めまい**　(めまい感)dizziness　(頭部ふらふら感)lightheadedness ☞めまい

ふとうぞうし　**不等像視**　aniseikonia

ブドウとう　**―糖**　glucose　◀経口ブドウ糖負荷試験 oral glucose tolerance test；OGTT　▶ブドウ糖液 glucose solution　ブドウ糖錠剤 glucose tablet

ぶとうびょう　**舞踏病**　chorea　◀ハンチントン舞踏病 Huntington chorea　▶舞踏病様症候群 choreiform syndrome

ぶどうまく　**―膜**　uvea　▶ぶどう膜炎 uveitis

ふとうめい　**不透明(な)**　(液体・ガラスが透けて見えない)opaque　(↔transparent)　(不確かな)uncertain　◆胸部 X 線で左下肺に不透明な陰影がみられました Your chest X-ray shows an opaque shadow in the left lower lung.

ふともも　**太もも**　thigh /θάɪ/

ふとる　**太る**　gain weight　(↔lose weight), put on weight ☞肥満　◆太りすぎる get [become] overweight　◆太りすぎているbe overweight　◆今の体型はまだ太りすぎだと思いますか Do you still see[think of] yourself as overweight?

ふなよい　**船酔い**　seasickness　◆船酔いする get[become] seasick　◆船酔いしている be[feel] seasick

ぶなん　**無難(な)**　safer　◆飲酒は当分の間控えたほうが無難です It would be safer for you if you quit[stopped] drinking for the time being.

ふにん　**不妊**　infertility　(㊋infertile)　(絶対不妊)sterility　★sterile は機能的欠陥か断種を意味するきつい表現なので避けたい。◀男性不妊症 male infertility　卵管不妊 tubal infertility　▶不妊カップル infertile couple　不妊期間 infertile[infertility] period　不妊検査 infertility test　不妊[避妊]手術 sterilization　不妊相談 infertility consultation　不妊治療 infertility treatment

ふのう　**不能**　(機能不全)failure　(無能・無力)inability　(性的不能)impotence　(㊋元に戻せない)irreversible)　◆回復不能な脳損

傷 irreversible brain damage　◀嚥下不能 inability to swallow / aglutition　授乳不能(乳汁分泌不全) lactation failure / failure of lactation　性交不能 (sexual) impotence

ふはい　腐敗　putrefaction（囲putrefactive）, decay（囲decayed）　☞腐る　▶腐敗ガス putrefactive gas　腐敗菌 putrefactive bacteria　☞腐敗臭

ふはいしゅう　腐敗臭　putrid stench [smell]（囲foul-smelling）　◆腐敗臭のする便 foul-smelling stools

プバりょうほう　PUVA療法（ソラレン紫外線療法）psoralen–ultraviolet A therapy

ぶぶん　部分　part（囲partial）, portion （分割した部分）division, section　（位置・部位）site　（範囲）region　◆体の大部分 a large part[portion] of the body　◆肝臓を部分的に切除する remove part of the liver　◆肝臓の部分切除 partial *removal of the liver[hepatectomy]　◆一部分 a small part（of）　▶部分入れ歯 partial dentures　部分荷重 partial weight-bearing　部分かつら partial wig　部分寛解 partial remission　部分健忘 partial amnesia[memory loss] / (まだら健忘)lacunar amnesia　部分清拭 partial bed bath　部分切除 partial resection　部分前置胎盤 partial placenta previa　部分発作 partial seizure[epilepsy]

ふべん　不便　inconvenience（囲inconvenient）　◆通院が不便であれば，お近くの病院を紹介することもできます If our hospital is inconvenient for you, I can refer you to another hospital nearer your home.　◆何か不便なことがあれば，どうぞ遠慮なくおっしゃって下さい If you have [suffer] any inconvenience, don't hesitate to let us know.

ふぼ　父母　☞両親

ふほう　不法（な）　illegal, unlawful　▶不法移民 illegal immigrant　不法行為 illegal [unlawful] act　不法就労者 illegal[illegally employed] worker　不法滞在 illegal stay　不法滞在外国人 illegal foreign resident　不法入国者 illegal entrant

ふほうわ　不飽和（の）　unsaturated　◀一価不飽和脂肪酸 monounsaturated fatty acid　多価不飽和脂肪酸 polyunsaturated fatty acid；PUFA　▶不飽和脂肪酸 unsaturated fatty acid；UFA　不飽和鉄結合能 unsaturated iron-binding capacity；UIBC

ふまん　不満（苦情・訴え）complaint　（気に入らないこと）dissatisfaction（囲dissatisfied）, discontent　◆何か不満なことがあれば，どうぞ遠慮なくおっしゃって下さい If you are dissatisfied with any of our services[If you have any complaints about our services], please don't hesitate to let us know.　◆当病院のケアやサービスで何かご不満はございますか Do you have any complaints about the care or services provided at this hospital?　◀性的不満 sexual dissatisfaction　欲求不満 frustration

ふみなおりはんのう　踏み直り反応　placing reaction

ふみん　不眠　sleeplessness　（不眠症)insomnia　◆不眠はありますか Do you have any trouble sleeping? / Do you have any problem with insomnia[sleeplessness]? / Do you suffer from insomnia?　◆不眠はどのくらい続いているのですか How long have you been having trouble sleeping? / How long *have you had[have you been suffering from] insomnia?

ふめい　不明（の）（あきらかでない）unknown　（特定されない)undetermined　（説明のつかない)unexplained　◆原因不明の体重減少 unexplained weight loss　◆あなたの病気は原因不明です The cause of your illness is unknown[undetermined].　◆ご不明な点はスタッフにお尋ね下さい(質問や気掛かりなこと)Please ask the staff if you have any questions or concerns.　▶不明死 unexplained death / death of unknown cause(s)　不明熱 fever of unknown[undetermined] origin；FUO

ふめいりょう　不明瞭（な）（発音が）slurred, inarticulate　◆不明瞭に話す slur *one's* words　▶不明瞭言語 slurred

speech
ぶもん 部門 department, division, section ★後のものほど規模が小さくなる．(範疇)class, category (分野)field
ふやす 増やす (重量を)gain (↔lose), put on (数量を)increase (↔decrease) (倍増させる)double (増加させる)multiply (加える)add (to) ☞増える ◆体重を増やす gain[put on] weight ◆薬の量を増やす increase the medication dose ◆運動量を増やす increase the amount of exercise / get more exercise
ブユ black fly ▶ブユ刺症 allergic reaction(s) to black fly bites
ふゆう 浮遊する (浮く)float (揺れ動く)hover (医液体・気体の中に浮かんだ)suspended 空気・風で運ばれる airborne) ◀硝子体浮遊物 vitreous floater ▶浮遊感 floating[hovering] sensation / (頭部ふらふら感)lightheadedness 浮遊血栓 floating thrombus 浮遊歯 floating tooth 浮遊胆石 floating gallstone (懸濁)浮遊物質 suspended solid ; SS 浮遊粉塵 airborne [floating] dust
ふよう¹ 不用(の) (使用済みの)used (廃棄された)discarded ◆ご不用になった注射針は必ず当院にご持参下さい Please be sure to bring used needles to this hospital.
ふよう² 扶養する (支える)support (育てる)rear ◀児童扶養手当 child care benefit / child-rearing allowance ▶扶養家族 dependent 扶養手当 family allowance
ふようじょう 不養生 neglect of *one's* health ☞不健康 ◆これまでの不養生な生活を改めるには今が一番よい時です You have *neglected your health[been careless about your health], but now is the best time to change *your way of living [your lifestyle].
ふようせい 不溶性(の) insoluble

ブラ (pulmonary) bulla ▶感染性ブラ infectious bulla 気腫性ブラ emphysematous bulla
プラーク plaque ◆血管がプラークで詰まっています The blood vessels are blocked[clogged] by plaque. ◆プラークが歯にたまる Plaque collects[accumulates] on the teeth. ◆プラークを除去する remove[eliminate] plaque ◆プラークの増大 buildup of plaque ▶プラーク形成 plaque formation (歯の)プラークコントロール plaque control
プライバシー privacy ◆プライバシーには十分配慮いたします We'll respect and maintain your privacy. ◆プライバシーを守る protect *a person's* privacy ▶プライバシー保護 privacy protection
プライマリーケア primary care ▶プライマリーケア医 primary care physician
ブラインド blind, (window) shade ◆ブラインドを上げましょうか Shall I *pull up [open] the blinds? ◆ブラインドを下ろす draw[pull down / close] the blinds
ブラシ brush (医brush) ◆髪にブラシをかける brush *one's* hair ◀歯間ブラシ interdental brush 歯ブラシ toothbrush ヘアブラシ hairbrush ▶ブラシ細胞診 brush cytology
ブラジャー bra ◀授乳用ブラジャー nursing[breastfeeding] bra
ブラジル Brazil (医Brazilian) ☞国籍 ▶ブラジル人(の) Brazilian
プラス (数)plus (医plus) (↔minus) (有利な点)advantage (↔disadvantage) ◆個室には1日1万円プラス消費税の差額が必要です The charge for a private room will be an additional ten thousand yen a day, plus tax. ◆この手術のプラスとマイナス the advantages and disadvantages of this surgery
プラスチック plastic (医プラスチック製のplastic) ◆プラスチックの食器 plastic dishes[tableware] ▶プラスチック袋 plastic bag プラスチック包帯 plastic bandage
フラストレーション ☞欲求不満
プラスミノゲン plasminogen ◀組織プラスミノゲン活性化因子 tissue plasminogen activator ; tPA
プラスミン plasmin
プラセボ placebo /pləsíːboʊ/ ▶プラセボ効果 placebo effect プラセボ反応

placebo response

プラダー・ウィリーしょうこうぐん ―症候群 Prader-Willi syndrome；PWS

プラチナせいざい ―製剤 platinum drug, platinum-based drug

ふらつく feel unsteady ☞ふらふらする ◆じっと立っている時ふらつきますか Do you feel unsteady when you stand still? ◆まだ少し足元がふらつくので注意して下さい Be careful, because you'll still be a little unsteady on your feet.

ブラックアイ （眼瞼皮下出血）black eye （アライグマ眼）raccoon eye （パンダ眼）panda eye

ブラックアウト blackout ☞失神

フラッシュバック flashback ▶フラッシュバック現象 flashback phenomenon

ふらっとする （めまいがする）feel dizzy （頭がくらっとする）one's head swims （気を失いそうになる）feel faint ◆立ち上がる時ふらっとしますか Do you feel dizzy[faint] when you stand up?

ふらふらする （めまいがする）feel[get] dizzy （頭がくらくらする）feel[get] light-headed （気を失いそうになる）feel faint （足元が安定しない）feel[be] unsteady[shaky, wobbly] on one's feet, stagger （病気や疲労で力が入らない）feel[be] groggy ☞ふらつく ◆少しふらふらするかもしれません You may feel a little dizzy. ◆高熱で体が少しふらふらする feel[be] a little groggy because of a high fever

プラマーびょう ―病 Plummer disease

プラマー・ビンソンしょうこうぐん ―症候群 Plummer-Vinson syndrome；PVS

プラン plan ☞計画

フランス France （🈩フランスの・フランス人の French) ☞国籍 ▶フランス人(男性) Frenchman /（女性）Frenchwoman

ふり 不利（な）（不都合）disadvantage （不利な条件）handicap （🈩disadvantageous 状況などが望ましくない unfavorable) ☞不利益 ◆この治療で一番不利な点は入院が必要なことです The biggest disadvantage of this treatment is *that it requires hospitalization[the need for hospitaliza-

tion]. ◆不利な徴候 an unfavorable sign ◀社会的不利 social disadvantage [handicap]

フリードライヒうんどうしっちょうしょう ―運動失調症 Friedreich ataxia

フリーラジカル free radical

ふりえき 不利益 （不都合）disadvantage (🈩disadvantageous) ◆服薬を中断するとご自分が不利益を被ることになります It would be disadvantageous for you to *stop taking[discontinue] the medication.

プリオン prion ▶プリオン病 prion disease

ぶりかえす ぶり返す come back, return, relapse ☞再発 ◆痛みがぶり返してきましたか Is the pain beginning to *come back[return]?

フリクテン phlyctenula (🈩phlyctenular) ◀角膜フリクテン corneal phlyctenule ▶フリクテン角膜炎 phlyctenular keratitis　フリクテン結膜炎 phlyctenular conjunctivitis

プリズム prism

フリッカーけんさ ―検査 flicker test

フリッカーしやけい ―視野計 flicker perimeter

プリックテスト prick test

ブリッジ (dental) bridge (🈩bridge) ◆歯にブリッジをかける bridge a tooth / attach[place / fix] a bridge (between the teeth)

ふりょ 不慮（の）（偶然の）accidental （予期しない）unexpected ◆仕事中に不慮の事故で怪我を負う have an accidental injury at work ◆不慮の事態に備える prepare for an unexpected situation ◆不慮の死 an accidental death

ふりょう 不良（な）poor, bad （望ましくない）unfavorable (🈩頭mal-, under-, in-, un-) ◆治療成績が不良である have a poor treatment outcome ◀栄養不良 malnutrition / undernourishment　吸収不良症候群 malabsorption syndrome　血行不良 poor[bad] (blood) circulation　消化不良 indigestion / digestive disorder /

dyspepsia　予後不良 poor[unfavorable] prognosis　▶不良肢位 malposition　不良姿勢 malposture

プリン　purine　▶プリン体 purine body　プリン代謝 purine metabolism　プリン代謝拮抗物質 purine antagonist

ブリンクマンしすう　―指数 Brinkman index；BI

ふる　振る　（揺らす）shake　（手を振る）wave　◆ビンをよく振ってから使って下さい Please shake the bottle well before use.　◆お子さんはバイバイと手を振りますか Does your child wave bye-bye?

ふるえる　震える　shake（形shaky）（小刻みに震える）tremble, quiver　（寒さなどで身震いする）shiver　（がたがた震える・ぞくっとする）shudder　（筋肉などが無意識に震える）have a tremor　◆何もしていないのに手足が震えますか Do your hands and feet shake or tremble even though you're not doing anything?　◆寒気で震える shiver [shake] with (the) chills　◆声が震える speak in a trembling[quivering] voice　◆手が震える have shaky hands　◆手が震えるのは動作をしている時ですか，じっとしている時ですか Do you have *a tremor [shaking] while using your hands, or while your hands at rest?

フルオレセイン　fluorescein　▶フルオレセイン蛍光眼底血管造影 fluorescein fundus angiography / fundus fluorescence photography

ブルガダしょうこうぐん　―症候群 Brugada syndrome

ブルガリア　Bulgaria（形Bulgarian）☞国籍　▶ブルガリア人(の) Bulgarian

ふるきず　古傷　old wound　（傷跡）old scar

フルクトース　fructose

ふるさと　故郷　☞故郷(こきょう)

ブルセラしょう　―症 brucellosis

フルタイム　（仕事）full-time work[job]（働く人）full-time worker（形副full-time）☞常勤　◆フルタイムで働いていますか Do you work full-time? / Are you working full-time? / Are you a full-time worker

[employee]?

フルネーム　full name　☞名前(囲み：名前の確認と敬称)　◆フルネームをお聞かせ下さい Could you tell me your full name?　◆フルネームで署名して下さい Please sign your name in full. / Please sign your full name.

ブルンベルグちょうこう　―徴候 Blumberg sign　（反跳圧痛）rebound tenderness

フレイルチェスト　flail chest

プレコックスかん　―感 praecox feeling

プレッシャー　pressure　◆仕事でかなりのプレッシャーがかかっていますか Are you under a lot of pressure at work? / Is there a lot of pressure on you at work?　◆同僚から強いプレッシャーを受ける *be under [feel] intense pressure from *one's* fellow workers　◆精神的なプレッシャーを感じる feel emotional pressure / feel emotionally pressured　▶プレッシャーに弱い be vulnerable to pressure

ブレブ　（pulmonary）bleb　▶気腫性ブレブ emphysematous bleb

ふれる　触れる　touch　（曝される）be exposed (to)　☞触る(さわる)　◆点眼容器の先端が目に触れないようにして下さい Please be careful not to let the tip of the eyedropper touch your eyes.　◆化学物質に触れる be exposed to chemicals　◆日本文化に触れる come in contact with Japanese culture / be exposed to Japanese culture　◆動物と触れ合う interact with animals

フレンツェルめがね　―眼鏡 Frenzel glasses[goggles]　★複数形で.

ふろ　風呂　bath　☞入浴　◆24時間，シャワーやお風呂には入れません You won't be able to shower or *take a bath[bathe] for twenty-four hours.　◆お風呂に入ってもいいですよ You can have[take] a bath.　◆お風呂やシャワーはぬるま湯にして下さい Please take a bath or shower in lukewarm water.　▶風呂桶 (洗面器)washbasin / washbowl / (浴槽)bathtub　風呂場 bathroom

ブローカしすう　―指数 Broca index

ブローカしつご ―失語 Broca aphasia

ブローカちゅうすう ―中枢 Broca center （ブローカ野）Broca area （運動性言語中枢）motor speech center

プローブ probe ◆超音波のプローブを腔の中に入れる insert the ultrasound probe into the vagina ◀経腹壁走査プローブ transabdominal ultrasound probe

フローボリュームきょくせん ―曲線 flow-volume curve

プロカルシトニン procalcitonin

プログラム program （圏program） ◆今日からプログラムに基づいてリハビリを行っていきます From today, we're going to follow[begin] a program of rehabilitation exercises. ◀訓練プログラム training program 社会復帰プログラム return-to-work program リハビリテーションプログラム rehabilitation program

プロゲステロン progesterone

プロスタグランジン prostaglandin

プロステーシス prosthesis ◀陰茎プロステーシス penile prosthesis 乳房プロステーシス breast prosthesis / （インプラント）breast implant

ブロック block ◀脚ブロック bundle branch block 交感神経ブロック sympathetic nerve block 神経根ブロック nerve root block 神経ブロック nerve block 洞房ブロック sinoatrial[SA] block 二枝ブロック bifascicular block バイトブロック bite block 不全[不完全]ブロック incomplete[partial] block 房室ブロック atrioventricular[AV] block

フロッピーインファント floppy infant

プロテアーゼ （蛋白分解酵素）protease ▶プロテアーゼ阻害薬 protease inhibitor

プロテイン protein

プロテスタントきょうと ―教徒 Protestant

プロトコール protocol

プロドラッグ prodrug

プロトロンビン prothrombin ▶プロトロンビン時間 prothrombin time；PT

プロトンポンプそがいやく ―阻害薬 proton pump inhibitor；PPI

プロフィール profile /próufaɪl/ ◆患者のプロフィール a patient profile

プロラクチン prolactin；PRL ◀高プロラクチン血症 hyperprolactinemia 高プロラクチン血症性無月経 hyperprolactinemic amenorrhea ▶プロラクチン産生腺腫 prolactin-producing adenoma / prolactinoma

フロン chlorofluorocarbon；CFC ◀代替フロン alternative chlorofluorocarbon[CFC] ▶フロンガス CFC gas

ふわっとする ◆頭がふわっとする feel lightheaded

ふん 分 minute

ぶん 分
《分量》 ◆10日分の薬を処方しましょう I'm going to give you a prescription for ten days worth of medication.
《割り当て》 ◆これはあなたの分です This is yours. / This is for you.
《状態・様子》 ◆この分では血糖値は下がりません If you go on like this, your blood sugar level won't go down.

ぶんあつ 分圧 partial pressure ◀動脈血酸素分圧 partial pressure of oxygen in arterial blood；PaO₂ / arterial partial pressure of oxygen 動脈血炭酸ガス分圧 partial pressure of carbon dioxide in arterial blood；PaCO₂ / arterial partial pressure of carbon dioxide

ぶんいん 分院 branch hospital, the branch of a hospital

ぶんか¹ 分化 differentiation （↔undifferentiation 圏分化した differentiated） ◀細胞分化 cell differentiation 性分化 sex differentiation ▶分化細胞 differentiated cell 分化誘導因子 differentiation-inducing factor

ぶんか² 文化 culture （圏cultural） ◆日本で一番驚いた文化の違いは何でしたか What cultural differences have been most surprising for you in Japan? / What cultural differences have surprised you most in Japan? ◆異文化を学ぶ learn about a different[foreign] culture ◆異文化に接する come into contact with a different[foreign] culture ▶文化的特徴 cultural characteristic(s) 文化的背景 cultural background

ぶんかい 分解 （分離）separation（動separate）（解像度の分解能）resolution（動resolve）（物質・化合物の分解）degradation（動degrade）, breakdown（接尾-lysis）◀高分解能CT high-resolution CT[computed tomography]；HRCT 脂肪分解 lipolysis / breakdown of fats 蛋白分解 protein degradation / proteolysis / breakdown of protein 蛋白分解酵素 protease / proteolytic enzyme

ぶんかく 分画 （全体の一部分）fraction （隔離・分離）sequestration ◀血漿蛋白分画 plasma protein fraction；PPF 血漿分画製剤 plasma derivatives[products] 左室駆出分画 left ventricular ejection fraction；LVEF 肺気量分画 lung volume fraction / fraction of lung volume 肺分画症 pulmonary sequestration 白血球分画 differential leukocyte count

ぶんかつしょうしゃ 分割照射 fractionated irradiation

ぶんかつばらい 分割払い installment plan, partial payment plan ◆医療費を分割払いすることはできません You cannot pay your medical expenses by installments. ◆分割払いにする pay on the installment plan

ぶんき 分岐 （枝分かれ）branch（動branch）（特に2本に）fork（動fork）, bifurcation ◀気管分岐部 tracheal bifurcation

ぶんぎょう 分業 division of work （特に肉体労働の）division of labor ◀医薬分業 separation of physician and pharmacist functions / separation of the functions of the clinic and the pharmacy

ぶんきょく 分極 polarization ◀過分極 hyperpolarization 脱分極 depolarization

ふんごう 吻合 anastomosis（形anastomotic）◀端々吻合 end-to-end anastomosis ▶吻合器 (anastomosis) stapler 吻合部潰瘍 anastomotic ulcer

ふんこうかんせん 糞口感染 infection by the fecal-oral route, fecal-oral infection

ふんさいこっせつ 粉砕骨折 comminuted fracture

ぶんし¹ 分子 molecule（形molecular）◀低分子量 low molecular weight ▶分子生物学 molecular biology 分子標的薬 molecularly targeted drug 分子量 molecular weight；MW

ぶんし² 分枝(の) branched（☞分岐）▶分枝(鎖)アミノ酸 branched-chain amino acid；BCAA

ふんしゅつせいおうと 噴出性嘔吐 projectile vomiting

ぶんしょ 文書 （書面）writing （公的な書類）document, papers ★複数形で．（リーフレット）leaflet ☞書面 ◆この治療を行うにあたり，同意を文書でお出しいただくようお願いします You need to give your consent for[to] this treatment in writing. / We need your written informed consent before we can proceed with this treatment. ◆出生届の文書を出す report a child's birth in writing[written form] ◀(薬の)添付文書 (medication) information leaflet

ぶんしょうかんせいテスト 文章完成テスト sentence completion test；SCT

ふんじん 粉塵 dust ◆粉塵に曝される be exposed to dust ◀浮遊粉塵 floating [airborne] dust ▶粉塵吸入 dust inhalation 粉塵障害 dust hazard 粉塵マスク dust mask

ふんせき 糞石 stercolith, fecal stone, fecalith ◀虫垂糞石 stercolith of the appendix

ぶんせき 分析 analysis（動analyze）（定量分析）assay ◆血圧のデータを分析する analyze *a person's* blood pressure data ◀音声分析 phonetic analysis ゲノム分析 genome analysis 自己分析 self-analysis システム分析 systems analysis 自動分析 autoanalysis 精神分析 psychoanalysis 成分分析 constituent analysis 定性分析 qualitative analysis 定量分析 quantitative analysis 動脈血ガス分析

arterial blood gas analysis ▶分析装置 analyzer

ふんせんちゅうしょう 糞線虫症 strongyloidiasis

ふんそく 吻側(の) rostral (↔caudal)

ぶんたん 分担する （分け合う）share (図share) （分業する）divide work (図division of work) ◆家事を分担する share the housework chores ◆子育てを分担する divide childcare duties[responsibilities] / share the responsibility of taking care of the children

ふんにゅう 粉乳 powdered milk, dried milk ◀脱脂粉乳 dried skim milk 調整粉乳 formula (milk) / infant formula

ふんにょう 糞尿 feces and urine, urine and stool

ふんぬけいれん 憤怒痙攣 breath-holding spell[attack]

ぶんのう 分納 ☞分割払い

ぶんぴつ 分泌 （細胞・腺などからの分泌）secretion (図secrete, 図secretory) （排出）discharge /dísʃɑɚʤ/ (図dischárge) ◆ホルモンを分泌する secrete hormones ◆分泌を促進する increase[promote] secretion ◆分泌を抑制する suppress[inhibit] secretion ◀胃液分泌 stomach[gastric] secretion 膵液分泌 secretion of pancreatic juice 唾液分泌 salivary secretion / salivation 胆汁分泌 bile secretion 乳汁分泌 lactation / milk secretion 乳頭分泌 nipple discharge 粘液分泌 mucous secretion ホルモン分泌 hormone secretion ▶分泌液 secretion 分泌過多 hypersecretion 分泌型 IgA secretory IgA 分泌顆粒 secretory granule 分泌成分 secretory component ☞外分泌, 内分泌, 分泌物

ぶんぴつぶつ 分泌物 （排出物）discharge /dísʃɑɚʤ/ （細胞・腺などからの分泌液）secretion ◆乳首〈膣／傷口〉から分泌物が出ますか Do you have any discharge from your nipple(s)〈vagina／wound〉? / Have you noticed any nipple〈vaginal／wound〉discharge? ◆どんな分泌物ですか What does the discharge look like? ◆分泌物はどんな色ですか What color is the discharge? ◆分泌物はどんなにおいですか How does the discharge smell? ◆傷口からにおいのする分泌物が出る have a foul-smelling discharge from the wound ◀漿液性分泌物 serous discharge 膣分泌物 vaginal discharge 膿性分泌物 purulent[pus-like] discharge

---

分泌物の性状

■色
●透明な clear / transparent ●白い white ●乳汁のような milky ●乳白色の milky white ●黄色味を帯びた yellowish ●赤褐色の reddish brown ●赤い red ●緑色の green ●黄緑色の greenish yellow ●ピンクがかった pinkish

■性状
●さらさらした（水様性の）thin /（漿液性の）serous ●どろどろした thick ●ねばねばした sticky / viscous /（粘液性の）mucoid /（粘液膿性の）mucopurulent ●泡状の frothy / foamy ●膿のような pus-like / purulent ●チーズのようにどろどろの cheesy ●糊のような starchy ●血性の bloody

■臭い
●無臭の odorless ●悪臭の foul-smelling ●チーズのような cheesy ●酵母のような yeasty

---

ぶんぷ 分布 distribution ◀正規分布 normal distribution 線量分布 dose distribution ▶分布曲線 distribution curve

ふんべん 糞便 ☞便

ぶんべん 分娩 delivery, parturition （出産）childbirth, birth （陣痛）labor ☞お産, 出産, 陣痛 ◆分娩中〈後〉に何か問題がありましたか Did you have any problems during〈after〉your delivery? ◆分娩は正常でしたか Did you have a normal delivery? / Was your delivery normal? ◆無痛分娩を希望されますか Would you like to have a painless labor and delivery? ◆分娩を誘発する induce labor ◆分娩を促進する accelerate labor ◆分娩が始まる go into labor ◆分娩後に postpartum / after birth ◀鉗子分娩 forceps delivery　顔面位分娩 face presentation　吸引分娩 vacuum extraction delivery　筋腫分娩 myoma delivery　計画分娩 planned childbirth[delivery]　経腟分娩 vaginal delivery　稽留分娩 missed labor　骨盤位分娩 breech delivery[birth]　座位分娩 delivery in a sitting position / sitting position for[during] childbirth　自然分娩 natural childbirth[delivery]　自宅分娩 home childbirth[delivery]　正常分娩 normal childbirth[delivery] / eutocia　早期分娩 premature labor　多胎分娩 delivery of multiple fetuses / multiple births　墜落分娩 precipitate labor　無痛分娩 painless labor[delivery]　誘導分娩 induced labor[delivery]　▶分娩開始 labor onset　分娩監視装置 tocomonitor　分娩管理 management of labor and delivery　分娩後うつ病 postpartum depression　分娩骨折 birth fracture　分娩時〈分娩後〉出血 intrapartum〈postpartum〉bleeding[hemorrhage]　分娩持続時間 duration of labor　分娩室 delivery[birthing] room　分娩陣痛 labor pains　分娩遷延 prolonged labor　分娩[陣痛]促進薬 ecbolic〈medication / drug / agent〉　分娩胎位 labor presentation　分娩体位 posture in labor　分娩第一〈二／三／四〉期 first〈second / third / fourth〉stage of labor　分娩麻痺 obstetric[birth] palsy[paralysis]　分娩予定日 due date / expected date of delivery；EDD / expected date of confinement；EDC / probable date of confinement；PDC

ぶんぽう　分包する ◆粉薬は1回分ずつが分包されています The powder comes in single-dose packets[sachets]. ◆錠剤はすべて1回分ずつ分包したほうがよろしいですか Would you like to have all the pills in single-dose packets?

ふんまつ　粉末　powder ▶粉末薬 powdered medication[drug] / powder

ぶんまわしほこう　分回し歩行　circumduction gait

ふんむ　噴霧する　(液体を吹き付ける)**spray**（🈩spray）　(霧化させる)**nebulize**　◆息を吸うのに合わせて鼻腔内に薬を噴霧してください Spray the medicine into your nose as you breathe in. ◆人工唾液を処方しましょう。1日数回口内に噴霧することで口内を潤します I'll prescribe artificial saliva which can be sprayed into your mouth several times a day to keep it moist.　◀鼻噴霧 nasal spray　▶噴霧器 nebulizer　噴霧薬 aerosol　噴霧療法 nebulization / aerosol therapy

ふんもん　噴門　cardia（🈩cardiac, cardial）　▶噴門括約筋 cardiac sphincter /（胃食道括約筋）gastroesophageal sphincter /（下部食道括約筋）lower esophageal sphincter；LES　噴門形成術 cardioplasty / fundoplication　噴門弛緩症 chalasia

ぶんや　分野　(領域)**field**　(部門)**branch**　◀研究分野 field of study　専門分野 specialty / specialized field

ぶんよう　分葉　(脳・肺などの葉)**lobulation**（🈩lobular　分葉した lobulated）　(分節・区域)**segmentation**（🈩segmental　分葉した segmented）　▶分葉核球 segmented leukocyte　分葉構造 lobular pattern

ぶんり　分離　separation　(分裂)**split**　(物質などの)**isolation**　◆分離された細菌〈真菌〉の株 isolated bacterial〈fungal〉strain　◀脊椎分離症 spondylolysis　▶分離不安症 separation anxiety disorder

ふんりゅう　粉瘤　atheroma　★日本ではアテロームを粉瘤の意味で使用するが，欧米では一般に動脈硬化性粥腫を意味するので注意.

ぶんりょう　分量　(数量)**quantity**　(投与量)**dose, dosage**　★dose は1回の用量，dosage は一定期間にわたる用量.　☞量　◆薬の分量 the dose[dosage] of medication　◆降圧薬の分量を増やす〈減らす〉increase〈decrease〉the quantity of a[the] high blood pressure medication

ぶんるい　分類　classification（🈩classify）　(グループ分け)**grouping**（🈩group）　(型の区

分)**typing** ◆間質性肺疾患は，臨床病態からいくつかのカテゴリーに分類されています Interstitial lung diseases are classified into several categories according to their clinical manifestation. ◀国際疾病分類 International Classification of Diseases；ICD　重症度分類 classification of severity　組織型分類 histologic classification[typing]　病期分類 staging　▶分類学 taxonomy

ぶんれつ　分裂　(分割)**division**　(分離)**split**（略**split**）, **splitting** ◀核分裂 nuclear division / division of the nucleus /（細胞の）nuclear fission　減数分裂 meiosis　細胞分裂 cell division　体細胞分裂 somatic (cell) division　有糸分裂 mitosis　▶分裂爪 split nail

へ

ヘア hair （陰毛）pubic hair ☞髪，毛
▶ヘアクリーム hair cream　ヘアトニック hair tonic　ヘアバンド hairband　ヘアピン hairpin / bobby pin /〈英〉(hair) grip　ヘアブラシ hairbrush

ペアけっせい ―血清　paired serum

へいい 平易（な）（明白ではっきりした）plain （簡単な）simple （容易な）easy
◆平易な言葉で話す speak plainly[in plain language]　◆平易な言葉で説明する explain simply[in simple terms]　◆平易な英語 plain English

へいかつきん 平滑筋　smooth muscle
▶平滑筋細胞 smooth muscle cell　平滑筋腫 leiomyoma　平滑筋肉腫 leiomyosarcoma　★leio-は平滑を意味する．

へいきん 平均　average （㊫average　標準的・代表的な typical　数・量が平均の mean）◆平均して毎日どのくらいの量のお酒を飲みますか How much on average do you drink a day? / On average, how much do you drink a day?　◆睡眠時間は平均何時間ですか On average, how many hours of sleep do you get? / How many hours on average do you sleep?　◆初経年齢は平均して 12 歳です The average age for a girl to have her first period is twelve years. / The average age of the onset of menstruation is twelve years.
◆平均的な 1 日の食事内容を教えて下さい（典型的な）Please tell me what you eat on a typical day.　◆平均以上〈以下〉である be above〈below〉average　◆平均より高い〈低い〉be higher〈lower〉than average
▶平均血圧 average[mean] blood pressure　平均寿命 average life span　平均体重 average weight　平均値 the mean / mean value　平均排尿回数 average voiding rate　平均余命 average life expectancy / average expectation of life

へいけい 閉経　menopause （㊫meno-pausal）, the change of life　◆閉経していますか Have you already had[gone through] your menopause?　◆いつ閉経しましたか When did your periods stop? / When did you stop menstruating? / How old were you when you had your last period?　◆閉経の徴候 menopausal sign　◀早発閉経 premature menopause　▶閉経後骨粗鬆症 postmenopausal osteoporosis　閉経周辺期 perimenopause / perimenopausal period　閉経症候群 menopausal syndrome　閉経年齢 age of menopause

へいこう¹ 平衡　（安定・調和）balance （力などの釣り合い）equilibrium ☞均衡，バランス　◆心〈体〉の平衡を失う lose one's mental〈physical〉balance　◆心〈体〉の平衡を保つ keep[maintain] one's mental〈physical〉balance　◆平衡感覚の検査をしましょう Let's check your balance.　◆平衡感覚を失う lose one's sense of balance[equilibrium]　▶電解質平衡 electrolyte balance　▶平衡機能検査 *balance function[equilibrium] test　平衡障害 balance[equilibrium] disorder　平衡状態 equilibrium state / state of equilibrium

へいこう² 平行（な）　parallel （㊫parallel）◆床の白い線と平行にまっすぐ歩いて下さい Please walk straight, parallel to the white line on the floor.　▶平行線 parallel lines ☞平行棒

へいこう³ 並行（して）（一緒に・並んで）along with, in parallel with, side by side （同時に）at the same time, simultaneously　◆化学療法と並行して放射線治療を開始する予定です I'm planning radiation therapy *along with[in parallel with] chemotherapy. / I'm planning to start radiation therapy and chemotherapy *at the same time[simultaneously].

へいこうはんしゃ 閉口反射　jaw-closing reflex

へいこうぼう 平行棒　parallel bars ★複数形で．◆平行棒を使って訓練を始めましょう Let's start your training on the parallel bars.　◆平行棒の中に立って歩く

練習をする stand in the parallel bars and practice walking

べいこく　米国　America（圏American）（アメリカ合衆国）the United States of America, the United States ; the USA, the US　★ピリオドを付けて the U.S.A., the U.S. とも表記する．☞アメリカ

へいさ　閉鎖する　（閉じる）close（圏closure）（制限する）confine（圏confined）（遮断・閉めだす）occlude（圏occlusive）（口・穴をふさぐ）obturate　◆人工肛門は数か月後には閉鎖する予定です Your stoma should close (up)[We expect your stoma to close (up)] within a few months from now. ◆インフルエンザの流行で学級閉鎖になったのですか Is your class closed due to the flu outbreak?　◀学級〈学校〉閉鎖 class〈school〉closure　ストーマ閉鎖術 stoma closure　先天性胆道閉鎖症 congenital biliary atresia　僧帽弁閉鎖不全症 mitral (valve) insufficiency[incompetence]；MI　大動脈弁閉鎖不全症 aortic (valve) insufficiency[incompetence]；AI　瘻孔閉鎖 fistula closure / closure of a fistula　▶閉鎖空間 confined space　閉鎖[皮下]骨折 closed fracture　閉鎖式ドレナージ法 closed drainage system　閉鎖病棟 closed ward[unit] / locked ward[unit]

へいじつ　平日　weekday　◆院内のカフェテリアは平日午前 8 時 30 分から午後 6 時の営業となっております The cafeteria in the hospital is open (on) weekdays [Monday through Friday] from eight-thirty am to six pm.

へいじょう　平常(の)　（いつもの）usual（常態の）normal　◆普段　▶平常心(沈着さ) self-possession /（自制心）one's self-control, control of one's emotions

へいしょきょうふ　閉所恐怖(症)　claustrophobia　◆閉所恐怖症ですか Are you afraid[scared] of enclosed[confined] spaces?

へいせい　平静(な)　（落ち着いた）calm, composed（圏composure）（静かな）quiet　◆緊急事態に直面して平静でいる stay calm in the face of an emergency　◆心の平静さを保つ remain calm / keep[maintain] one's composure / keep one's cool　◆心の平静さを失う lose one's composure / lose one's presence of mind / lose one's cool　◆平静さを装う put on an appearance of composure　◆平静さを取り戻す regain[recover] one's composure

へいそく　閉塞する　（遮断する）block（圏blockage　圏blocked）（流れを遮る）obstruct（圏obstruction　圏obstructive, obstructed）（流路を塞ぐ）occlude（圏occlusive, occluded）（閉じる）close（圏closure　圏closed）　◆閉塞した血管を拡げる処置を行います I'm going to give you a treatment to dilate the blocked [obstructed / occluded] blood vessel.　◀冠動脈閉塞 coronary occlusion　気道閉塞 airway obstruction　耳管閉塞 tubal obstruction[occlusion]　胆道閉塞症 biliary obstruction　腸閉塞 ileus / intestinal [bowel] obstruction　鼻涙管閉塞 nasolacrimal duct obstruction　慢性閉塞性肺疾患 chronic obstructive pulmonary disease；COPD　▶閉塞隅角緑内障 angle-closure[closed-angle] glaucoma　閉塞性黄疸 obstructive jaundice　閉塞性換気障害 obstructive ventilator impairment　閉塞性血栓性血管炎 thromboangitis obliterans　閉塞性睡眠時無呼吸 obstructive sleep apnea；OSA　閉塞性動脈硬化症 arteriosclerosis obliterans；ASO　閉塞性肺炎 obstructive pneumonia　閉塞性肥大型心筋症 hypertrophic obstructive cardiomyopathy；HOCM

へいねつ　平熱　normal (body) temperature　◆平熱は何度ですか What's your normal body temperature?　◆平熱に戻っています Your temperature *is back [has returned] to normal.

へいはつ　併発する　（余病などで悪化させる）complicate（圏complications　★通例，複数形で）　◆痛風は高尿酸血症からよく併発する症状の 1 つです Gout is one of the common complications of hyperuricemia.　◆麻疹から脳炎を併発しています

The measles has developed into encephalitis. ◆余病を併発する develop complications ◆網膜症を併発した糖尿病 diabetes complicated by retinopathy

へいびせい　閉鼻声 rhinolalia clausa, nasal speech ☞鼻声(はなごえ)

へいよう　併用する (一緒に用いる)take[use] … together　(同時に用いる)take[use] … *at the same time[simultaneously]　(組み合わせて用いる)combine (図 combination) ◆この睡眠薬とアルコールを併用するのは危険です Taking this sleeping pill and alcohol together[at the same time] is dangerous. ◆他の薬を併用する際には必ず医師に確認して下さい When you take this together with other medications, be sure to check with your doctor. ◆2つの療法を併用する combine two treatments ◆併用禁忌の薬 contraindicated medications taken together[at the same time] ▶多剤併用化学療法 combination chemotherapy ▶併用効果 combined effect　併用療法 combination therapy[treatment] ∕ combined therapy[treatment]

ペイン　pain ☞痛み，疼痛 ▶ペインクリニック pain clinic　ペインコントロール pain control　ペインスケール pain (rating) scale

ペーシング　pacing ☞ペースメーカ ◀一時的〈恒久的〉ペーシング temporary〈permanent〉pacing　経皮的ペーシング transcutaneous pacing　心臓ペーシング (artificial) cardiac pacing ▶ペーシングカテーテル pacing catheter

ペース　pace ◆ご自分のペースで運動して下さい Please exercise at your own pace. ◆ペースを速める quicken[speed up ∕ increase] *one's* pace ◆ペースを遅くする slacken[slow down] *one's* pace ◆ゆっくりとしたペースで歩く walk at a slow pace ☞ペースメーカ

ペースメーカ　pacemaker ◆ペースメーカを装着している have a pacemaker implanted[put ∕ fitted ∕ installed ∕ inserted] in *one's* body ◆ペースメーカを埋め込む

implant[install] a pacemaker inside the body ◀一時的ペースメーカ temporary pacemaker　植込み型ペースメーカ implantable pacemaker　体外式ペースメーカ external pacemaker

ベータ　β, beta ◀A群β溶血性連鎖球菌 group A β-hemolytic *Streptococcus* ▶β カロテン β-carotene　β(受容体)刺激薬 β (-receptor) stimulant　β遮断薬 β-blocker　$β_2$ミクログロブリン $β_2$-microglobulin　βラクタマーゼ阻害薬 β-lactamase inhibitor　βラクタム系抗菌薬 β-lactam antibiotics

ベーチェットびょう　―病 Behçet disease ◀腸管ベーチェット病 intestinal Behçet disease

ペーハー　pH (水素イオン指数)potential of hydrogen, power of hydrogen, hydrogen ion exponent

ペーパータオル　paper towel ◆(超音波検査などで)このペーパータオルでゼリーを拭きとって下さい Please wipe the gel off with these paper towels.

へきうんどう　壁運動 wall motion ◆左室の壁運動異常 left ventricular asynergy ∕ asynergy of the left ventricle ◆梗塞部位の壁運動低下〈消失〉hypokinesis〈akinesis〉of the infarcted area ◀心臓壁運動 heart[cardiac] wall motion

へきざい　壁在(の) mural ▶壁在結節 mural nodule　壁在血栓 mural thrombus

へきそく　壁側(の) parietal ▶壁側胸膜 parietal pleura

へきちいりょう　僻地医療 medical care in remote[less populated] areas

ペグ　PEG (経皮内視鏡的胃瘻造設術)percutaneous endoscopic gastrostomy

ペグボード　peg board ◆このペグボードには穴が開いています．ペグを穴に入れる練習をしましょう Here's a peg board with several holes (in it). Let's practice inserting pegs into the holes.

へこみ　凹み dent, depression (乳房などのくぼみ)dimple ☞凹み(くぼみ) ◆むくんだ部位を指で押して離すと凹んだままですか When you press the swollen area with a finger and then remove it, does the dent [depression] remain for some time? ◆乳房の皮膚が凹んでいますか Does the skin on your breast appear dimpled? / Do you have a dimple in the skin of your breast? ◆乳首が凹んでいる(陥没している) have *an inverted[a turned-in / a retracted] nipple

ベジタリアン vegetarian ☞菜食主義者
▶ベジタリアン食 vegetarian food[meal]

ベスト best ◀最高，最善，最適 ◆ベストを尽くします I'll do the best I can. / I'll do all I can do. / I'll do my best. ◆ベストコンディションで手術に臨んで下さい I'd like you to be in *the best[top] condition for the surgery. ◆この治療法は今のところベストな選択肢です This treatment is the best option available.

ペスト plague ◀腺ペスト bubonic plague ▶ペスト菌 *Yersinia pestis*

へそ 臍 navel /néɪvl/, belly button, umbilicus (🔲umbilical) ◆お臍がじくじくしています The navel is wet and sticky. ◆臍の周り around *one's* navel ◀出臍 protruding navel ▶臍の緒 umbilical cord

べつ¹ 別(の) (もう１つの) another (他の) some other (異なる) different (余分の) extra ☞他 ◆別の病室に移っていただきます You'll be transferred to another room. ◆別の日にいらして下さい Please come and see me (on) another[some other] day. ◆そのことは別の機会に話しましょう Let's talk about it some other time. ◆別の治療法を試みます I'll try another[a different] treatment. ▶別料金 extra charge

べつ² 別(に)
《別々》《個別に》separately (離れて) apart ☞別居 ◆彼は親とは別に暮らしています He lives separately[apart] from his parents.
《特に》(in) particular, specifically ☞別条 ◆明日は別に予定はありません I have nothing (in) particular to do tomorrow. / I don't have anything particular[specific]

planned for tomorrow.

ベッカーがたきんジストロフィー 一型筋ジストロフィー Becker muscular dystrophy；BMD

ベッカーぼはん 一母斑 Becker nevus

べっきょ 別居する separate, get[become] separated (別居している)be separated (別々の家に住む) live apart[separately, in separate houses] ◆ご主人〈奥さん〉とは別居していますか Are you separated (from your husband〈wife〉)? / Do you live[Are you living] apart[separately] from your husband〈wife〉? ◆彼女は夫と別居してからうつになった She has become depressed since she separated from her husband. ▶別居結婚(単身赴任などの遠距離結婚)commuter marriage / (離婚前提の)legal separation

ペッサリー pessary

べつじょう 別条 ◆この症状は命に別条はありませんからご安心下さい This symptom is not life-threatening, so *don't worry[you don't need to worry].

ベッド bed ◆ベッドは電動式です Your bed is electronically operated. ◆ベッドの操作法をお教えします I'm going to show you how to operate your bed. ◆このボタンを押すとベッドを下げることができます You can lower your bed by pushing [pressing] this button. ◆ベッドの枕元を上げる raise the head of the bed ◆ベッドから降りないで下さい You must not get out of bed. ◆ベッドの上なら起き上がってもいいですよ You can sit up in bed. ◆トイレ以外はベッドで安静にしていて下さい Please stay in bed except for when you need to use the toilet. ◆ベッドから落ちる fall out of (the) bed ◆ベッドを整えましょう Let me make your bed. ◆現時点で空きベッドはありません We do not have any empty beds right now. / There are no beds available right now. ◀空きベッド vacant[unoccupied / empty] bed 介護ベッド nursing care bed 簡易ベッド(折り畳み式の)cot 差額ベッド(有料のベッド) extra-charge bed / pay bed / (特別室)

special（charge）room　新生児用ベッド（baby / hospital）bassinet　電動ベッド electric[electronically operated] bed　ベビーベッド（baby）crib[cot]　▶ベッドメイキング making the bed　ベッドランプ bedside lamp[light]　☞ベッドサイド, ベッド柵

ペット[1]　**pet**　◆ペットを飼っていますか Do you have any pets（at home）?　◆どんなペットを飼っていますか What kind of pets do you have?　◆ペットにアレルギーがありますか Are you allergic to pets?　▶ペット感染症 pet infection / infection caught from a pet

ペット[2]　**PET**　（陽電子断層撮影）**positron emission tomography**　◆PETはがんを検出する画像検査です A PET scan is an imaging test to detect cancer.　▶PETスキャン PET scan

ベッドサイド　**bedside**　◆ベッドサイドに座る sit at[by] the bedside　▶ベッドサイド教育 bedside teaching / teaching at the bedside　ベッドサイドテーブル bedside table　ベッドサイドマナー bedside manner

ベッドさく　─柵　**bed rail, bedside rail**　◆ベッド柵が上がっている時はご自分でベッドから降りないで，ナースコールボタンを押して下さい When the bedside rails are up, please do not get out of bed by yourself. Instead[In that case], please push[press] the nurse call button for help.　◆安全のためにベッドの柵を上げておきましょう For your safety, I'll put the bed rails up.　◆ベッドの柵を上げる〈下げる〉raise〈lower〉the bed rails

ペットボトル　**plastic bottle**

ヘッドホン　**headphones**　★複数形で.　◆このヘッドホンをつけて下さい Please put these headphones on.　◆ヘッドホンをつけて音楽を聴いて下さい Please wear headphones to listen to music. / Please listen to music with headphones on.

ヘッドレスト　**headrest**　◆このヘッドレストが頭を支えてくれます This headrest will support your head.

ベトナム　**Vietnam** /viètnɑ́:m/　（圏**Vietnamése**）　☞国籍　▶ベトナム人（の）Vietnamese

ペニシラミン　**penicillamine**　▶ペニシラミン腎症 penicillamine nephropathy

ペニシリン　**penicillin** /pènəsílin/　◆ペニシリンでアレルギー反応を起こしますか Are you allergic to penicillin? / Do you have a penicillin allergy?　▶ペニシリンショック penicillin shock　ペニシリン耐性肺炎球菌 penicillin-resistant *Streptococcus pneumoniae*；PRSP

ペニス　**penis** /pí:nɪs/　☞陰茎　◆ペニス，精巣，陰嚢に痛みがありますか Do you have any pain in your penis, testes, or scrotum?　◆ペニスがただれている have sores on *one's* penis　◆ペニスやその周りに痒いしこりがある have itchy lumps on and around *one's* penis　◆ペニスから透明な〈黄色い / 血性の〉分泌液が出る have a clear〈yellow / bloody〉discharge from *one's* penis

ヘノッホ・シェーンラインしはんびょう　─紫斑病　**Henoch-Schönlein purpura**；**HSP**

ヘバーデンけっせつ　─結節　**Heberden node**

ヘパリン　**heparin**　◆血液が固まらないようにヘパリンを投与します I'm going to put you on heparin, a medication that helps prevent blood clots.　◀低分子量ヘパリン low-molecular-weight heparin；LMWH　▶ヘパリン化 heparinization　ヘパリン加血 heparinized blood

ヘビ　蛇　**snake**　◆ヘビに咬まれる be bitten by a snake　◀毒ヘビ poisonous[venomous] snake　▶ヘビ咬傷 snake bite　ヘビ毒 snake venom

ベビー　**baby**　▶ベビーカー stroller / baby buggy /《英》pushchair　ベビーシッター babysitter　ベビーフード baby[infant] food　ベビーベッド（baby）crib[cot]

ヘビースモーカー　**heavy smoker**

ペプシノーゲン　**pepsinogen**

ペプシン　**pepsin**（圏**peptic**）　▶ペプシン活性 peptic[pepsin] activity　ペプシン消

化 peptic[pepsin] digestion
ペプチド peptide ◀心房性ナトリウム利尿ペプチド atrial natriuretic peptide; ANP　脳ナトリウム利尿ペプチド brain natriuretic peptide; BNP
ヘマトキシリン・エオジンせんしょく ―染色 hematoxylin-eosin stain[staining], HE stain[staining]
ヘマトクリット hematocrit; Hct
ヘモグロビン hemoglobin /híːməɡloʊbɪn/; Hb ◆ヘモグロビン値が正常より低い The hemoglobin level is below normal. ◆ヘモグロビン A1c 検査は血糖コントロールの重要な指標です The HbA1c test is an important marker of blood sugar control. ▶ヘモグロビン円柱 hemoglobin cast　ヘモグロビン濃度 hemoglobin concentration　☞ヘモグロビン尿
ヘモグロビンにょう ―尿 hemoglobinuria ◀発作性寒冷ヘモグロビン尿症 paroxysmal cold hemoglobinuria; PCH　発作性夜間ヘモグロビン尿症 paroxysmal nocturnal hemoglobinuria; PNH
ヘモクロマトーシス hemochromatosis
ヘモジデリン hemosiderin ▶ヘモジデリン沈着症 hemosiderosis
へや　部屋　room ◀相部屋になりますが，よろしいですか Is it all right with you *to share[if you share] a room with *another patient[other patients]?　相部屋 shared room　2 人部屋 semi private room / two-bed room / room for two　4 人部屋 four-bed room / room for four　大部屋 multiple occupancy room / shared room / room shared by several patients ▶部屋番号 room number
ペラグラ pellagra
へらす　減らす　reduce, decrease　(数値を) lower　(消費量を) cut down[back](on)　(体重などを) take off, lose　(苦痛・負担を) lighten ◆毎日のカロリー摂取量を減らす reduce[decrease] one's daily calorie intake ◆感染のリスクを減らす reduce [lower] the risk of infections ◆体重〈体脂肪〉を減らす lose[take off / reduce] one's weight〈body fat〉 ◆塩分を減らす cut down on salt ◆肉を減らす *eat less [cut down on] meat ◆タバコの本数を減らす smoke fewer cigarettes / cut down on smoking ◆アルコールの量を減らす drink less alcohol ◆経済的な負担を減らす lighten a person's financial burden [load]
ヘリウム helium
ヘリオトロープしん ―疹 heliotrope rash[eruption]
ヘリカルシーティ helical CT
ヘリコバクターピロリかんせんしょう ―感染症 *Helicobacter pylori* infection
ヘリコプター helicopter ◀ドクターヘリ air ambulance / *emergency medical service[EMS] helicopter / doctor helicopter
ベリリウム beryllium ▶ベリリウム中毒 beryllium poisoning

へる　減る　(徐々に減る) decrease　(体重が) lose　(量が) become less　(数が) become fewer ◆最近体重が減りましたか Have you recently lost weight? ◆体重はどのくらい減りましたか How much weight have you lost? ◆最近，月経の出血量が減っている The menstrual flow has decreased recently. ◆便の回数が減っている The bowel movements have become less frequent.
ベル　(call) bell　(警報器) alarm ◀非常ベル(火事の) fire alarm　ポケットベル pager / beeper　呼び出しベル call bell
ペルー Peru (㊅Peruvian)　☞国籍 ▶ペルー人(の) Peruvian
ペルオキシダーゼせんしょく ―染色 peroxidase stain[staining]
ベルギー Belgium (㊅Belgian)　☞国籍 ▶ベルギー人(の) Belgian
ベルげんしょう ―現象　Bell phenomenon
ヘルス health ◀メンタルヘルス mental health ▶ヘルスクラブ〈センター〉 health club〈center〉 ☞ヘルスケア
ヘルスケア health care, healthcare ▶ヘルスケアサービス health care services　ヘルスケアプラン health care plan　ヘルス

ヘルスケア　　　　650　　　　べん²

ケアワーカー health care worker

ヘルツ hertz；Hz

ベルト belt ◀拘束ベルト（腰の部分用）lap belt／（車椅子用）wheelchair belt　セーフティベルト safety belt

ヘルニア hernia /hˊɚːniə/（⊞**hernial** ヘルニアを起こした **herniated**）（ヘルニア形成）herniation ◆ヘルニアの手術を受ける have[undergo] surgery for a hernia ◆ヘルニアの手術を行う perform hernia（repair）surgery／perform surgery for repair of a hernia ◀陰嚢ヘルニア scrotal hernia　滑脱型（食道）裂孔ヘルニア sliding（esophageal）hiatal hernia　嵌頓ヘルニア incarcerated hernia　絞扼性ヘルニア strangulated hernia　臍ヘルニア umbilical hernia　鼠径ヘルニア inguinal hernia　大腿ヘルニア femoral hernia　椎間板ヘルニア slipped[herniated] disc／（intervertebral）disc hernia[herniation]　脳ヘルニア brain[cerebral] herniation　腹壁ヘルニア abdominal[（腹側面の）ventral] hernia ▶ヘルニア根治術 hernia repair（surgery）／hernioplasty　ヘルニア内容 hernia[hernial] contents　ヘルニア嚢 hernial sac　ヘルニアバンド hernia support[belt]

ヘルパー（ホームヘルパー）home care aide, home health aide,《英》home help ★英語の helper は手助けする人（助手・お手伝いさん）などを意味する.

ヘルパーティーさいぼう ―T 細胞 helper T cell

ヘルパンギーナ herpangina

ヘルペス herpes /hˊɚːpiːz/（⊞**herpétic**）◀陰部ヘルペス genital herpes　角膜ヘルペス corneal herpes　口唇ヘルペス cold sore／herpes labialis　帯状ヘルペス shingles／herpes zoster　単純ヘルペスウイルス herpes simplex virus；HSV／simplexvirus　単純ヘルペス脳炎 herpes encephalitis／herpes simplex encephalitis；HSE ▶ヘルペスウイルス herpesvirus[herpes virus]　ヘルペス後神経痛 postherpetic neuralgia；PHN　ヘルペス性口内炎 herpetic stomatitis

ベルまひ ―麻痺 Bell palsy（特発性顔面神経麻痺）idiopathic facial paralysis

ヘロイン heroin ☞麻薬 ▶ヘロイン依存 heroin dependence　ヘロイン嗜癖 heroin addiction　ヘロイン使用者 heroin user　ヘロイン常習者 heroin addict　ヘロイン中毒 heroin intoxication

ベロどくそ ―毒素 verotoxin, Vero toxin, Shigalike toxin

へん¹ 辺 part ☞辺り ◆胸のどの辺が痛みますか Where does your chest hurt?／Which part of your chest hurts?

へん² 片 piece（移植片）graft ◀植皮片 skin graft　翼状片 pterygium

へん³ 変（な）（不思議な・奇妙な）strange（普段と異なる）unusual（異様な）odd ◆喉に何かが詰まったような変な感覚を覚える have a strange sensation of something being stuck in the throat ◆変なにおい *odd smells[odors]

べん¹ 弁 valve（⊞**valvular**）（皮弁）flap ◆弁の欠陥 a valve defect ◆欠陥のある弁を修復する repair a defective valve ◆弁を生体弁に置き換える replace a valve with a tissue valve ◀回盲弁 ileocecal[Bauhin] valve　機械弁 mechanical（heart）valve　筋膜皮弁 fasciocutaneous flap　筋膜弁 fascial flap　三尖弁 tricuspid valve　静脈弁 venous valve　人工弁 artificial valve／valve prosthesis／（人工心臓弁）prosthetic heart[cardiac] valve　心臓弁 heart[cardiac] valve／valve of the heart　生体弁 tissue[biologic／bioprosthetic] valve　僧帽弁 mitral valve　大動脈弁 aortic valve　二尖弁 bicuspid valve　肺動脈弁 pulmonary valve ▶弁不全 valvular incompetence ☞弁狭窄, 弁形成術, 弁置換術, 弁閉鎖不全, 弁膜症

べん² 便 stool, feces（⊞**fecal**）★feces は患者との会話に用いないほうがよい.（便通）bowel movement /báʊəl-/；BM,《英》bowel motion 《排便の習慣・異常について尋ねる》 ◆いつもどのくらいの頻度で便をしますか How often do you move[empty] your bowels?／How often do you have a bowel movement? ◆今日，便が出ましたか Have you moved[emptied] your bowels today? / Have you had a bowel movement today? ◆最後に便が出たのはいつですか When did you last *have a bowel movement[empty your bowels]? ◆便をするのがつらいですか Do you have difficulty *moving your bowels[passing stools]? ◆便をする時痛みますか When you move your bowels, do you have any pain? ◆便を漏らすことがありますか Do you ever *leak stools accidentally[experience accidental stool leakage]?

《便の性状を尋ねる》 ◆便の形・色・量に変化がありましたか Have you noticed any changes in the shape, color, or amount of the stools? ◆どんな便ですか What do your stools look like? ◆便は硬めですか，軟らかめですか，それともゆるいですか Are the stools hard, soft, or loose? ◆便はどんな色をしていますか What color are your stools? / What's the color of your stools? ◆便の色は変わりましたか Has the color of your stools changed? ◆便に血や粘液が混じっていますか Is there any blood or mucus in your stools? ◆便のにおいはいつもと違いますか Do the stools have an unusual smell? ◆便をゆるくする loosen the bowels[stools] ◆血のついた便 blood-stained stools

《便検査の説明》 ◆便検査が必要です We need *a stool sample[a sample of your stools]. / We need to do[run] a stool test. ◆この容器に便を採って，次回持ってきて下さい Please put a stool sample in this container and bring it with you at your next visit.

◀血便 bloody stool 米のとぎ汁様便 rice-water stool[diarrhea] 脂肪便 fatty stool 宿便 stool[fecal] impaction 消化不良便 dyspeptic[undigested] stool 水様便 watery stool タール様便 tarry stool / melena 粘液便 mucous stool 粘血便 bloody mucous[mucoid] stool

▶便検査 stool test 便細菌叢 fecal flora ☞排便, 便意, 便器, 便座, 便失禁, 便潜血, 便通, 便培養, 便秘

便に関する表現

■色
●茶色 brown ●粘土色の clay-colored ●黄色がかった白の yellow-white ●白っぽい whitish / chalky ●白い white ●灰色の gray /《英》grey ●緑色がかった greenish ●赤みがかった reddish ●赤い red ●真っ赤な bright red ●黒っぽい dark ●黒い black ●炭のように黒い tarry black

■におい
●腐敗臭がする foul-smelling / offensive-smelling / bad-smelling ●酸っぱい臭いがする acidic / sour-smelling

■硬さ
●硬い hard / firm ●乾燥した dry ●半固体状の semisolid ●軟らかい soft ●ゆるい loose ●(粥のように)どろどろした mushy ●泥状の muddy ●下痢状の diarrheal ●液状の liquid ●水のような watery

■形状
●細い narrow ●鉛筆状の pencil-like ●リボン状の ribbon-like ●ウサギの糞のようなコロコロした rabbit-pellet-like ●固まっている (well-)formed ●かさが大きい bulky

へんい¹ 変異 （変動・変形）variation, variant (圏variant) （突然変異）mutation, mutant (圏mutant) ◀遺伝的変異 genetic variation 体細胞突然変異 somatic mutation 突然変異遺伝子 mutant gene ▶変異ウイルス mutant virus 変異型 variant

へんい² 偏位 （標準からの逸脱）deviation （位置が狂うこと）dislocation ◀眼球偏位 eye[ocular] deviation 水晶体偏位 lens dislocation ▶偏位角 angle of deviation

べんい 便意 defecation desire, urge to *have a bowel movement[defecate] ◆便意を催す have an urge to *empty one's bowels[have a bowel movement]

◆便をした後，まだ便意が残っていますか After you finish, do you still feel as if you need to move your bowels?

へんえん 辺縁(の) （末梢の）peripheral（図periphery） （端の）marginal（図margin） （辺縁系の）limbic（図limbus） ▶辺縁系脳炎 limbic encephalitis

へんか 変化する （完全に変わる）change（図change） （部分的に変わる）alter（図alteration） ☞変わる，変調，変動 ◆最近，血圧に変化がありましたか Has your blood pressure changed recently? / Has there been any change in your blood pressure recently? ◆最近，食習慣に変化がありましたか Have you noticed any change in your eating habits recently? ◆どんな変化ですか What kind of change is it? ◆体重の変化が激しいですか Does your weight fluctuate dramatically? ◆その症状は良くなっていますか，悪くなっていますか，それとも変化なしですか Is the symptom getting better, getting worse, or is there no change? ◆顔つきが変化する change in *one's* facial features ◀行動変化 behavior[behavioral] change 性格変化 personality change 体重変化 weight change ライフスタイルの変化 lifestyle change / change in lifestyle

へんかん 変換 （転換）conversion（図convert） （変化）change （図姿勢・体位の）positional, postural ◀体位変換 postural change 頭位変換性めまい positional[postural] vertigo ▶変換酵素 converting enzyme

べんき 便器 （差し込み式の）bedpan （椅子式の）(bedside) commode （トイレ内の）toilet (bowl) ◆便器をお使いになりますか(差し込み式の) Do you need to use the bedpan? ◆この椅子便器を使って下さい Please use this bedside commode. ◀ポータブル便器 portable toilet

べんきょうさく 弁狭窄 valvular stenosis ◀僧帽弁狭窄症 mitral (valve) stenosis；MS 大動脈弁狭窄症 aortic (valve) stenosis；AS

へんけい 変形 （歪み・奇形）deformity（図

deform） （彎曲）curvature（図curve） （形の変化）transformation（図transform） ◆指の変形にいつ気がつきましたか When did you notice that your fingers have *become deformed[changed shape]? ◀胸郭変形 thoracic deformity 手指変形 digital deformity スワンネック変形 swan-neck deformity 脊柱変形 spinal deformity[curvature] 足部変形 foot deformity 手の変形 hand deformity ボタン穴変形 buttonhole deformity ▶変形性関節症 osteoarthritis；OA / degenerative arthritis 変形性股関節症 hip osteoarthritis 変形性膝関節症 knee osteoarthritis

べんけいせいじゅつ 弁形成術 valve repair (surgery), valvuloplasty

へんけん 偏見 （先入観）prejudice （好みに基づく評価）bias ☞差別 ◆エイズ〈エイズ患者〉に対して偏見をもつ have a prejudice *about AIDS〈against people with AIDS〉 ◆ステロイドに対して偏見がある have a bias against steroids ◆性別に関する偏見 gender prejudice / prejudice based on gender ◆年齢への偏見 ageism / prejudice based on age ◀人種的偏見 racism / racial prejudice

へんこう 変更する （全面的に変える）change（図change） （部分的に変える）alter（図alteration） （一部修正する）modify（図modification） ☞変える，変わる ◆予約を変更したい場合には至急お知らせ下さい Let us know immediately if you'd like to change your appointment. ◆治療計画に変更はありません There's no change[alteration] in the treatment plan. ◆治療への反応を見ながら治療法を変更していきます We're going to modify the treatment plan based on your response to it. ◆手術の予定を今週の金曜日に変更します We'll reschedule the surgery for this Friday.

へんこうけんびきょうけんさ 偏光顕微鏡検査 polarization microscopy, polarized light microscopy

へんさ 偏差 deviation ◀標準偏差 standard deviation；SD ▶偏差値 deviation

べんざ 便座 toilet seat ◀温式便座 heated (warm) toilet seat 温水洗浄便座 toilet seat with warm-water bidet ★Washlet は和製英語(商標).

へんし 変死 (不自然な死)unnatural death, death from[by] unnatural causes (不審な死)suspicious death ◆変死体の身元確認をする identify the body of a person who died an unnatural death

へんじ 返事する answer (図answer), reply (to) (図reply) (応答する)respond (図response)
《呼びかけなどに応答する》◆名前を呼ばれたら返事をして下さい Please *answer me [respond] when I call your name./Please respond when your name is called. ◆来週までにお返事を下さい Please let me know your answer by next week. ◆よく考えてから返事して下さい I hope you'll think carefully before you reply.
《返信する》◆紹介していただいた先生宛に返事をお書きします I'll answer[reply to/send a reply to] your doctor's referral letter.

へんししょう 変視症 metamorphopsia
へんしつ 偏執(症) paranoia ☞妄想
べんしっきん 便失禁 fecal incontinence, bowel incontinence, loss of bowel control
べんしゅつ 娩出 expulsion (図expulsive) (分娩)delivery ◀胎盤娩出 placental delivery ▶娩出期 the expulsive stage[period] of labor 娩出力 expulsive force

べんじょ 便所 ☞トイレ
へんしょく¹ 変色 change in color, discoloration (図discolored) ◆皮膚と眼球結膜が黄色に変色している the skin and the whites of the eyes have become [turned] yellow / have (a) yellow discoloration of the skin and the whites of the eyes ◆皮膚の変色 discoloration of the skin / skin color changes / changes in skin color ◆変色した歯 discolored teeth

へんしょく² 偏食 unbalanced diet (好き嫌い)food likes and dislikes ★複数形で. ☞好き嫌い ◆偏食する have an unbalanced diet ◆偏食を直す *get over[overcome] one's food likes and dislikes/correct one's eating habits

へんしんもうそう 変身妄想 transformation delusion

ベンスジョーンズたんぱく ―蛋白 Bence Jones protein

へんずつう 片頭痛 migraine (headache) /máigrein-/ ◆片頭痛がする have [get] a migraine ◆片頭痛の前兆に気づく notice[recognize] the early (warning) signs of migraine ◆前兆を伴う〈伴わない〉片頭痛 migraine with〈without〉aura ▶片頭痛性格 migraine personality

へんせい¹ 変声 voice change, change of voice (思春期特有の声変わり)adolescent voice change, voice change in adolescence ▶変声期 the stage of adolescence[puberty] when the voice changes[breaks] 変声(期)障害 disturbance of adolescent voice change

へんせい² 変性 (障害を受けて細胞・組織が変化すること)degeneration (図degenerative) (蛋白・アルコールなどの性質が変化すること)denaturation (図denatured) ◀黄斑変性症 macular degeneration 脊髄小脳変性症 spinocerebellar degeneration; SCD 多系統変性症 multiple system degeneration 蛋白変性 protein denaturation 網膜色素変性症 retinitis pigmentosa; RP ▶変性関節疾患 degenerative joint disease; DJD

ベンゼン benzene ▶ベンゼン中毒 benzene poisoning

べんせんけつ 便潜血 fecal occult blood, occult blood in stools ▶便潜血検査 fecal occult blood test

へんそく 片側(性の) single-sided (一側性の)unilateral (図on one side 接頭hemi-) ☞半身, 半側 ◆痛みは片側性ですか Is the pain only on one side? ▶片側運動失調 hemiataxia 片側感覚消失 hemianesthesia 片側顔面攣縮 hemifacial spasm 片側失認 hemiagnosia 片側

身体失認 hemiasomatognosia 片側頭痛 hemicrania 片側性難聴 single-sided [unilateral] hearing loss 片側性副腎過形成 unilateral adrenal hyperplasia ☞片(側)麻痺

ベンゾジアゼピン benzodiazepine ▶ベンゾジアゼピン中毒 benzodiazepine poisoning[intoxication / overdose] ベンゾジアゼピン離脱症候群 benzodiazepine withdrawal syndrome

べんち 胼胝 callus

べんちかんじゅつ 弁置換術 valve replacement (surgery), implantation of a heart valve prosthesis

べんちゅう 鞭虫 whipworm ▶鞭虫症 trichuriasis

ベンチュリーマスク Venturi mask

へんちょう 変調 (変化) change (異常・常軌逸脱) aberration ☞変わる, 変化 ◆睡眠パターンの変調に気づく notice a change in one's sleeping patterns ◀記憶変調 memory change / change in memory 気分変調症 dysthymia / dysthymic disorder 精神変調 mental aberration

べんつう 便通 bowel movement / bávəl-/; BM ☞排便, 便 ◆便通に問題がありますか Do you have any problems with your bowel movements? ◆最近便通に変化がありましたか Have your bowel movements changed recently? ◆便通は規則的ですか Are your bowel movements regular? / Do you have regular bowel movements? ◆便通の回数はどのくらいですか How often do you have a bowel movement? / How often do you move [empty] your bowels? ◆便通は何日おきですか How many days apart do you have bowel movements? ◆手術後に便通がありましたか Have you moved your bowels since the surgery? ◆便通がない have no bowel movements ◆便通に異常がある have a problem with one's bowel movements ◆便通時に痛みがある have (a) pain when moving the bowels ◆便通時にいきむ strain when moving the bowels ◆便通を調節する control[regulate]

one's bowel movements ◆便通を促す promote a bowel movement

へんとう 扁桃(腺) tonsil (形tonsillar) ◆扁桃腺が腫れています You have swollen tonsils. / Your tonsils are swollen. ◆扁桃の手術を受ける have[undergo] tonsil surgery / (摘出術を受ける) have one's tonsils out ◀扁桃の手術を行う perform tonsil surgery / (摘出する) remove the patient's tonsils ◀口蓋扁桃 palatine[faucial] tonsil 耳管扁桃 tubal tonsil 舌扁桃 lingual tonsil 肥大扁桃 enlarged [swollen / hypertrophied] tonsil ▶扁桃陰窩 tonsillar crypt 扁桃周囲炎 peritonsillitis 扁桃周囲膿瘍 peritonsillar abscess 扁桃体 amygdaloid body 扁桃摘出術 tonsillectomy / tonsil removal surgery 扁桃肥大 tonsil hypertrophy / enlargement of a tonsil 扁桃誘発試験 tonsil provocation test ☞扁桃炎

へんどう 変動する (いろいろに変わる) vary (形variation) (大きく振れる) swing (形swing) (数値が上下する) fluctuate (形fluctuation) ☞変わる, 変化 ◆1日のうちで血圧が変動するのは珍しいことではありません It is not unusual for blood pressure to fluctuate[go up and down] during the day. ◆気分変動がある have mood swings ◆体重の変動が激しい one's weight fluctuates ◀日内変動(24時間変動) diurnal[daily] variation / (検査における精度) within-day[daily / intraday] precision / (病状の変動) daily[intraday] fluctuation 日差変動(検査における精度) between-day[day-to-day / interday] precision / (病状の変動) day-to-day[interday] fluctuation ピークフロー変動 peak flow variability

へんとうえん 扁桃炎 tonsillitis ◀咽頭扁桃炎 pharyngotonsillitis カタル性扁桃炎 catarrhal tonsillitis

べんなんかざい 便軟化剤 ☞緩下薬, 下剤

べんばいよう 便培養 stool culture

べんぴ 便秘 constipation (動get[become] constipated 便秘している be constipated) ◆便秘していますか Are you constipated? / Are you suffering from constipated? ◆便秘がちですか Do you tend to have[suffer from] constipation? / Do you often become constipated? ◆下痢と便秘を交互に繰り返しますか Do you have alternating diarrhea and constipation? / Do you have diarrhea alternating with constipation? ◆便秘しないように水分をたくさん摂って下さい Please drink plenty of fluids so as not to get constipated. ◆便秘を防ぐために繊維を多く含む食事をお勧めします I recommend *a diet rich in fiber[a high-fiber diet] to prevent constipation. ◆この薬を飲むと便秘になるかもしれません This medication may cause constipation. / This medication may make you constipated. ◆頑固な便秘 stubborn[obstinate] constipation ◁痙攣性便秘 spastic constipation 弛緩性便秘 atonic constipation 習慣性便秘 habitual constipation 閉塞性便秘 obstructive constipation ▶便秘薬［下剤］ laxative (medication / drug / agent)

へんぺい 扁平（な） flat ◆形が扁平である be flat (in shape) ▶扁平苔癬 lichen planus 扁平乳頭 flat nipple 扁平疣贅 flat wart / verruca plana ☞扁平上皮, 扁平足

べんへいさふぜん 弁閉鎖不全 valvular insufficiency[incompetence] ◁僧帽弁閉鎖不全症 mitral (valve) insufficiency [incompetence］；MI 大動脈弁閉鎖不全症 aortic (valve) insufficiency[incompetence］；AI

へんぺいじょうひ 扁平上皮 squamous epithelium ▶扁平上皮化生 squamous metaplasia 扁平上皮癌 squamous cell carcinoma 扁平上皮細胞 squamous cell

へんぺいそく 扁平足 flatfoot, flat foot (図flat-footed), fallen arch, pes planus ◆扁平足である have flatfeet / be flat-footed

べんべつ 弁別 （識別）discrimination ◁語音弁別検査 speech discrimination test

べんまくしょう 弁膜症 （心臓弁膜症） heart valve disease, valvular heart disease ◁三尖弁膜症 tricuspid valve disease 僧帽弁膜症 mitral valve disease 大動脈弁膜症 aortic valve disease 肺動脈弁膜症 pulmonary valve disease リウマチ性弁膜症 rheumatic valvular disease ▶弁膜症性心房細動 valvular atrial fibrillation

へんまひ 片麻痺 hemiplegia (図hemiplegic), paralysis of[on] one side of the body ◁顔面片麻痺 facial hemiplegia 痙性片麻痺 spastic hemiplegia 交差性片麻痺 crossed hemiplegia 交代性片麻痺 alternating hemiplegia ▶片麻痺歩行 hemiplegic gait

べんもう 鞭毛 flagella (図flagellum 図flagellar) ▶鞭毛運動 flagellar movement[beat]

ペンライト penlight ◆目にペンライトの光を当てる shine a penlight into *a person's eye(s)

べんり 便利（な） （都合が良い）convenient （役に立つ）useful, handy ◆寝巻は前開きのタイプが授乳に便利です Pajamas that open in the front are convenient (to wear) when nursing. ◆交通の便利が良い病院をご紹介しましょう Let me recommend a hospital that is convenient transportation-wise. ◆緊急用カードはお財布に入れておくと便利です You may find it useful[handy] to carry your medical alert card in your wallet.

ほ

ほいく 保育 day care, daycare ◀学童保育 after-school child care 集団保育 group day care[nursery] 乳児保育 infant care 病児保育 care for a sick infant [child] ▶保育器 incubator 保育士 child care worker / day care worker ☞保育園

ほいくえん 保育園・保育所 (child) day care (center), 〈英〉nursery (保育室) (child) day care room ◆子供を保育園に預ける put *one's* child in day care ◆保育園に通う go to day care ◆保育園に入っている be in day care ◀認可保育園 licensed day care center 無認可保育園 nonlicensed day care center

ほいん 母音 vowel

ほいんしゃ 保因者 carrier ☞キャリア ◆彼女は血友病の遺伝子の保因者です She carries a gene for hemophilia.

ほう 方 (方角) way, direction ☞方向 ◆こちらの方を見て下さい Please look [face] this way. ◆ドアの方を向いて下さい Please turn in the direction of the door.

ほういかいぼう 法医解剖 medicolegal autopsy

ほういがく 法医学 forensic medicine, legal medicine (医事法制の)medical jurisprudence

ぼういん 暴飲 overdrinking, excessive drinking, binge drinking ◆暴飲暴食する eat and drink excessively[too much] / overeat and overdrink / binge on food and drink

ぼうえい 防衛 defense (動defend) ☞防御, 防護 ◆免疫は有害物質に対する自然の防衛手段です The immune system is our body's natural defense against harmful substances. ◀過剰防衛 excessive self-defense 自己防衛 self-defense / self-protection / self-preservation 自己防衛本能 self-defense[self-protection]

instinct / instinct for self-defense[self-protection] ▶防衛機制 defense mechanism

ぼうえき 防疫 prevention of epidemics (伝染病対策)communicable diseases control

ぼうおん 防音 soundproofing, hearing protection ◆防音室で聴力検査をする perform a hearing test in a soundproof booth[room] ▶防音保護具 hearing protection device[equipment]

ぼうか 防火 fire prevention ▶防火装置 fire prevention equipment ▶防火訓練

ほうかい 崩壊 (関係などの断絶)breakdown (無秩序状態)chaos (体制などの破綻)collapse ◀学級崩壊 classroom chaos [collapse] 家庭崩壊 family breakdown 橋中心髄鞘崩壊症 central pontine myelinolysis；CPM ▶崩壊家族 broken family

ほうかくえん 胞隔炎 alveolitis

ぼうかくんれん 防火訓練 fire drill ◆防火訓練を行う conduct a fire drill

ほうかしきえん 蜂窩織炎 ☞蜂巣炎

ほうかつ 包括(的な) (広範囲にわたる)comprehensive (全てを含んだ)inclusive ▶包括医療 comprehensive medical care 包括支援センター comprehensive support center 包括払い(まとめ払い) bundled payment

ほうかはい 蜂窩肺 ☞蜂巣肺

ほうき 放棄 (世話を怠ること)neglect (遺棄)abandonment ◀育児放棄 child neglect

ぼうぎょ 防御 defense (保護)protection ☞防衛, 防護 ◀X線防御 X-ray protection 筋性防御 muscular defense ▶防御創 defense wound 防御反射 defense reflex 防御反応 defense reaction

ほうきょうじゅつ 豊胸術 breast implantation

ほうけい 包茎 phimosis /faimóusəs/ ◆男の赤ちゃんは亀頭の皮が剝けない包茎の状態が正常です Phimosis is normal in baby boys whose foreskin cannot be retracted over the tip of the penis. ◆包茎手術をしていますか Have you been circumcised? ◀仮性包茎 pseudophimosis 嵌頓包茎 paraphimosis / strangulation of the glans penis 真性包茎 true[genuine] phimosis ▶包茎手術 circumcision

ぼうけん　剖検　autopsy, postmortem examination ◆剖検所見 autopsy findings

ぼうご　防護　protection （圏protective） ☞防衛，防御 ◀放射線防護 radiation protection 放射線防護員 radiation protector ▶防護手袋 protective gloves 防護服 protective clothing 防護前掛け protective apron 防護マスク protective mask 防護眼鏡 protective glasses

ほうこう¹　方向
《方角》direction, way （位置）position ☞方 ◆進行方向を変える change *one's* direction ◆X線室はこちらの方向です（掲示）This way for the X-ray department. ◆（X線撮影などで）検査台がいろいろな方向に動きます The exam table will move you into different positions.
《方針》course, direction ☞方針 ◆今後は痛みを和らげる方向で進めていきます From now on, I'm going to shift the course of treatment to focus on relieving the pain. ◆がん治療の方向性はおっしゃる通りでよろしいと思います The directions you suggested for treating your cancer are all right with me.
◀垂直〈水平〉方向 vertical〈horizontal〉direction 縦方向 vertical[longitudinal] direction ▶方向感覚 sense of direction 方向見当識障害 directional disorientation 方向交代性〈方向固定性〉頭位眼振 direction-changing〈direction-fixed〉positional nystagmus

ほうこう²　芳香　aroma ▶芳香剤 air freshener / aromatic

ほうごう　縫合する （傷口などを縫い合わせる） sew （up）, stitch （up）, suture （修復する）repair （圏stitch, suture, repair 腰尾-rrhaphy） ◆この傷は縫合しなくてはなりません You'll need （to have） a few stitches in this wound. ◆傷口を5針縫合する *sew up[stitch up / suture / close] the cut[wound] with five stitches ◆会陰を縫合する place stitches in the perineum ◆胸骨を縫合する sew the breastbone together ◀アキレス腱縫合 Achilles tendon repair 血管縫合 angiorrhaphy 絹糸縫合 silk suture 腱縫合 tendon suture 靭帯縫合 syndesmorrhaphy 創縁縫合 wound suture 皮膚縫合 skin suture ▶縫合線離開 suture diastasis 縫合部 suture area[site] 縫合不全 suture[anastomotic] leakage 縫合用具 suture instrument ☞縫合糸，縫合針

ぼうこう¹　膀胱　（urinary） bladder （圏vesical 腰頭cyst(o)-, vesic(o)-） ◆これまで膀胱に何か問題がありましたか Have you ever had any problems with your bladder? ◆尿が出た後，膀胱はどんな感じですか，空になりますか，まだ残っている感じですか How does your bladder feel after you urinate? Does it feel empty or as if *it's still holding some urine[there's some urine still there]? ◆この管を膀胱に入れて尿を採ります Let me insert[put / place] this tube into your bladder and drain the urine. / I'm going to drain the urine from your bladder with this tube. ◆膀胱を空にする empty *one's* bladder ◀過活動膀胱 overactive bladder；OAB 痙性膀胱 spastic bladder 経尿道的膀胱腫瘍切除術 transurethral resection of a bladder tumor；TURBT 神経因性膀胱 neurogenic bladder 代用膀胱 substitute bladder 無緊張性膀胱 atonic bladder
▶膀胱括約筋 vesical sphincter 膀胱カテーテル bladder catheter 膀胱がん bladder cancer 膀胱感覚 bladder sensation 膀胱機能 bladder function 膀胱鏡検査 cystoscopy 膀胱訓練 bladder training 膀胱結石 bladder stone 膀胱砕石術 cystolithotripsy 膀胱刺激症状 bladder irritation[irritative] symptom 膀胱洗浄 bladder lavage[irrigation] 膀胱全摘除術 total cystectomy 膀胱造影法 cystography 膀胱直腸障害 bladder and rectal disturbance 膀胱内圧 intravesical pressure

膀胱内圧測定 cystometry　膀胱尿管逆流 vesicoureteral reflux；VUR　膀胱尿道鏡検査 cystourethroscopy　膀胱容量 bladder capacity　膀胱留置カテーテル indwelling bladder catheter　膀胱瘻造設術 cystostomy　☞膀胱炎

ぼうこう²　暴行　☞暴力　◆暴行手段に訴える use[resort to] violence　◀性的暴行 sexual violence[assault]

ぼうこうえん　膀胱炎　**cystitis** /sɪstáɪtɪs/, **bladder inflammation**

ほうごうがたビリルビン　抱合型ビリルビン **conjugated bilirubin**　▶非抱合型ビリルビン unconjugated bilirubin

ほうこうきん　縫工筋　**sartorius (muscle)**

ほうごうし　縫合糸　**surgical suture [stitch]**　▶吸収性〈非吸収性〉縫合糸 absorbable〈nonabsorbable〉suture

ほうごうしん　縫合針　**suture needle, surgical needle, sewing needle**

ほうこく　報告　**report**　（報告書）**(written) report**　☞レポート　◆事故について報告する give[make] a report on the accident　◆…の報告（書）を書く write a report on [about]...　◀インシデント報告 incident report　経過報告 progress report　検死報告 autopsy report　事故報告（医療事故の報告）accident[occurrence] report　疾病報告 disease report　症例報告 case report

ほうさん　放散する　**radiate**（図radiation）（広がる）**spread**　（移動する）**move**　◆痛みは体の他の部位に放散しますか Does the pain spread[move / radiate] to other parts of the body?　◆放散性の痛み a radiating pain

ほうし　胞子　**spore**　▶胞子嚢 sporangium / sporocyst

ほうし　帽子　**cap**　▶手術帽（子）surgical cap

ぼうしきゅうたいそうち　傍糸球体装置　**juxtaglomerular apparatus；JGA**

ぼうしつ　房室（の）　**atrioventricular**　▶房室回帰頻拍 atrioventricular[AV] reciprocating tachycardia；AVRT　房室解離 atrioventricular[AV] dissociation　房室接合部調律 atrioventricular[AV] junc-tional rhythm　房室接合部頻拍 atrioventricular[AV] junctional tachycardia　房室束 atrioventricular[AV] bundle　房室伝導 atrioventricular[AV] conduction　☞房室結節，房室ブロック

ぼうしつけっせつ　房室結節　**atrioventricular node, AV node**　▶房室結節リエントリー性頻拍 atrioventricular[AV] nodal reentrant tachycardia；AVNRT

ぼうしつブロック　房室ブロック　**atrioventricular block, AV block**　◀1度〈2度／3度〉房室ブロック first-degree〈second-degree / third-degree〉atrioventricular[AV] block　完全房室ブロック complete atrioventricular[AV] block

ほうしゃ　放射性（の）　（放射能のある）**radioactive**　▶放射性アレルゲン吸着試験 radioallergosorbent test；RAST　放射性廃棄物 radioactive waste　放射性物質 radioactive substance[material]　放射性免疫吸着試験 radioimmunosorbent test；RIST　放射性免疫測定法 radioimmunoassay；RIA　放射性ヨウ素 radioiodine / radioactive iodine　放射標識抗体 radiolabeled antibody　☞放射性同位元素，放射線，放射能

ほうしゃせいどういげんそ　放射性同位元素　**radioactive isotope, radioisotope；RI**　（放射性核種）**radionuclide；RN**　▶放射性同位元素治療 radioisotope[RI] therapy / radionuclide[RN] therapy

ほうしゃせん　放射線　**radiation**　（光線）**radioactive ray**　☞X線，レントゲン　◆がん組織に放射線を当てる *apply radiation to[irradiate] cancerous tissue　◆放射線を浴びる be exposed to radiation　◆正常細胞への放射線の被曝を防御する protect and shield normal tissues from exposure to radiation　◀介入的放射線医学 interventional radiology；IVR　診療放射線技師 medical radiation[radiologic] technologist；MRT　電離放射線 ionizing radiation　非電離放射線 nonionizing radiation　▶放射線医学 radiology　放射線科（診療科）the department of radiology / the radiology department　放射線科医

ほうしゃせん 659 **ほうたい**

radiologist　放射線感受性 radiation sensitivity / radiosensitivity　放射線検査 radiographic examination　放射線腫瘍医 radiation oncologist　放射線照射血液 irradiated blood　放射線照射効果 irradiation effect　放射線増感剤 radiosensitizer / radiosensitizing agent　放射線抵抗性 radioresistance　放射線被曝 radiation exposure　放射線滅菌法 radiation sterilization / radiosterilization　放射線量 radiation dose　☞放射線障害, 放射線診断, 放射線治療, 放射線防護

ほうしゃせんしょうがい　放射線障害 radiation injury[disorder, damage]　◀晩発性放射線障害 late[delayed] radiation injury　非電離放射線障害 nonionizing radiation disorder

> **放射線障害の表現**
> ●放射線潰瘍 radiation ulcer　●放射線口内炎 radiation stomatitis　●放射線宿酔 radiation sickness　●放射線食道炎 radiation esophagitis　●放射線腸炎 radiation enterocolitis　●放射線熱傷［火傷］radiation burn　●放射線肺臓炎 radiation pneumonitis　●放射線皮膚炎 radiodermatitis / radiation dermatitis

ほうしゃせんしんだん　放射線診断 radiodiagnosis　▶放射線診断医 diagnostic radiologist

ほうしゃせんちりょう　放射線治療 radiation therapy[treatment], radiotherapy　◀化学放射線治療 chemoradiotherapy / chemoradiation　定位放射線治療 stereotaxic[stereotactic] radiotherapy ; SRT

ほうしゃせんぼうご　放射線防護 radiation protection　▶放射線防護エプロン X-ray[radiation protection] apron / lead apron　放射線防護具 radiation protector

ほうしゃのう　放射能 radioactivity（形radioactive）　▶放射能汚染 radioactive contamination[pollution]

ほうしゅう　報酬 fee　◀診療報酬 medical fees / fees for medical services

ぼうしゅうざい　防臭剤　(脱臭剤)deodorant

ほうしゅく　縫縮 cerclage, circumferential suture　◀子宮頸管縫縮術 cervical cerclage / circumferential suture of the cervix

ほうしゅつ　放出する release（図release）　◆インスリンを放出する release insulin　▶放出因子 releasing factor　放出ホルモン releasing hormone

ぼうしゅようせいしょうこうぐん　傍腫瘍性症候群 paraneoplastic syndrome

ほうじょうきたい　胞状奇胎 hydatidiform mole, hydatid mole　◀全胞状奇胎 complete hydatidiform[hydatid] mole

ほうしょく　暴食 overeating, excessive eating, binge eating　☞暴飲

ほうしん¹　方針　(計画)plan　(方向)course　(方策)policy　◆治療方針を立てる map out a treatment plan / decide on the course of treatment　◆それが当病院の方針なので, 従っていただきたいのです That's the policy of this hospital, so I hope you'll follow[comply with] it.

ほうしん²　疱疹 herpes　☞ヘルペス

ほうしん　膨疹 wheal

ぼうしんけいせつ　傍神経節 paraganglion（図paraganglia）

ぼうじんマスク　防塵マスク dust mask

ぼうすい¹　房水 aqueous humor　▶房水循環 aqueous circulation　房水流 aqueous flow　房水流出 aqueous outflow

ぼうすい²　防水(の) waterproof（動防水加工する waterproof）　▶防水シート waterproof sheet　防水加工 waterproofing　防水剤 waterproofing agent

ぼうせいししょう　乏精子症 oligospermia, oligozoospermia

ほうせんきんるい　放線菌類 actinomycetes　★複数形で.　▶放線菌症 actinomycosis

ほうそうえん　蜂巣炎 cellulitis, phlegmon（形phlegmonous）　▶蜂巣炎性腸炎 phlegmonous enteritis

ほうそうはい　蜂巣肺 honeycomb lung

ほうたい　包帯 bandage（動bandage），dressing（動dress）　(吊り包帯)sling　◆足首に包帯を巻きましょう Let me bandage your ankle. / Let me wrap your ankle with a bandage. / Let me wrap a bandage around your ankle. ◆傷口に〈頭に〉包帯を巻く apply[put / place] a bandage *over the wound〈around *a person's head〉 ◆包帯を交換する change *a person's* bandage[dressing] /（新しいものに取り換える）replace the bandage with a new [fresh] bandage ◆包帯を濡らさないで下さい Please don't get the bandage wet. / Please keep the bandage dry. ◆包帯を取る remove[take off] the bandage ◆腕を包帯で吊る put *a person's* arm in a sling ◆包帯で腕を吊っている have *one's* arm in a sling / the arm is in a sling ◀圧迫包帯 pressure[compression] bandage 腕吊り包帯 arm sling　ガーゼ包帯 gauze bandage /（パッド）gauze pad /（巻包帯）gauze roll　ギプス包帯 plaster cast　サポート用[支持]包帯 support bandage　三角巾 triangular bandage　弾性[伸縮]包帯 elastic bandage　長下肢ギプス包帯 long leg cast；LLC　ネット包帯 net bandage　粘着包帯 adhesive bandage /（細長い絆創膏状のもの）adhesive strip /（接着テープ）adhesive tape　滅菌包帯 sterile[sterilized] bandage

ぼうだいどうみゃくリンパせつ　傍大動脈リンパ節　paraaortic lymph node

ぼうだいぶ　膨大部　ampulla ◀卵管膨大部 ampulla of the fallopian[uterine] tube

ほうち　放置する　（そのままにしておく）leave（alone）（見過ごす）neglect ◆車椅子をここに放置しないで下さい Please don't leave the wheelchair here. ◆事態をこのまま放置すると手遅れになります If you leave things as they are[If you don't do anything about the situation], it'll be too late. ◆子供を放置し虐待する親 parents who neglect and abuse their child〈children〉 ◀高齢者放置 elder neglect 小児放置 child neglect

ぼうちゅうざい　防虫剤　insect repellent, bug spray　（特に蛾の）moth repellent　（球状の）mothball ▶防虫剤中毒 *bug spray

[moth repellent] poisoning

ほうちゅうしょう　包虫症　hydatid disease　（エキノコックス症）echinococcosis

ぼうちょう　膨張　（腹部などの腫れ）distension（國distend）（ガスなどの膨らみ）inflation（國inflate）☞膨満 ◆腹部が膨張しています The abdomen is distended. ◀（肺の）過膨張 overinflation

ほうていでんせんびょう　法定伝染病　legally defined communicable disease

ぼうにょう　乏尿　（尿量減少）oliguria（國oliguric）（排尿緩慢）bradyuria ◀腎前性〈腎後性〉乏尿 prerenal〈postrenal〉oliguria ▶乏尿性急性腎不全 oliguric acute renal failure

ほうひ　包皮　the foreskin, prepuce（國preputial）　醖醤posth(o)- ◀亀頭包皮炎 balanoposthitis ▶包皮炎 posthitis 包皮垢 smegma preputii　包皮（環状）切除術 posthetomy / circumcision

ほうふ　豊富（な）　（豊かな）rich　（含有量の多い）high　（幅広い）extensive　（たくさんの）a great deal of, plenty of ◆食物繊維が豊富な野菜を食べるとよいでしょう You should eat vegetables rich[high] in dietary fiber. ◆星先生はこの手術に豊富な経験をお持ちです Dr Hoshi has extensive[a great deal of] experience with this surgery.

ぼうふ　防腐　antisepsis ◀死体防腐処置 embalming ▶防腐剤 antiseptic　防腐的処置 antiseptic treatment

ほうほう　方法　（やり方）way　（方式）method　（手順・手法）procedure ☞手段 ◆この病気の治療にはいくつか方法があります There are several *ways to treat [methods for treating] this disease. ◆どの治療方法を希望しますか Which treatment method do you prefer? ◆この方法でやってみて下さい Please try doing it (in) this way. ◆この方法がうまくいかない場合には別の方法をやりましょう If this procedure[method] doesn't work well, we'll try another. ◆私はこの方法が最善だと思います I think this is the best way. ◆問題解決のために様々な方法を試みる

try various ways to solve the problem ◆同じ方法で in the same way ◆違う方法で in a different way ◆効果的な方法 an effective way[method]

ほうまい 包埋 **embedding** ◀パラフィン包埋 paraffin embedding

ほうまつじょう 泡沫状(の) **foamy, frothy** ▶泡沫状痰 foamy[frothy] phlegm

ほうまん 膨満 (満杯)**fullness** (膨張)**bloating** (腫れ・腫大)**swelling** (腹部などの膨らみ)**distension** ◀胃膨満 gastric fullness 腹部膨満感 feeling of abdominal fullness[bloating / distension] / feeling of fullness[bloating] in the abdomen / sensation of abdominal distension

ほうもん 訪問する **visit** ◆退院後に訪問看護が必要ですか Do you need home visit nursing services after discharge from the hospital? ▶訪問[面会]カード visitor's pass 訪問介護 home-visit long-term care / visiting home care service 訪問看護 visiting nursing / home (health) nursing 訪問看護師 visiting nurse 訪問看護ステーション visiting nurses'[nurses] station (病児や障害児に対する)訪問教育 visiting teaching[teacher service] (for sick〈disabled〉children) 訪問クリニック home-based health care clinic 訪問指導 guidance by a visiting health worker 訪問診療 house call / home visit 訪問リハビリテーション home-visit rehabilitation / visiting rehabilitation

ほうりつ 法律 **law** (略legal) ◆法律を守る obey the law ◆法律を犯す break the law ◆法律に違反する be against the law ◆薬物の使用は法律で禁じられています(快楽用の麻薬)It's illegal[against the law] to use recreational drugs. / Recreational drug use is *prohibited by law [illegal].

ぼうりょく 暴力 **violence** (略violent) ◆暴力をふるう get[become] violent / use [commit] violence (against / toward) ◆身体・精神的な暴力を受ける suffer physical and psychological violence ◆子供に暴力をふるう use violence against children ◆暴力的になる turn violent ◀家庭内暴力 domestic violence；DV 校内暴力 school violence / (クラス内の) class violence / (大学内の) campus violence ▶暴力行為 violent behavior / (1回の行為) violent act, act of violence

ほうわ 飽和 **saturation** (略saturated) ◆血液中の酸素飽和度を測る measure the oxygen saturation of blood ◀動脈血酸素飽和度 arterial (blood) oxygen saturation；SaO_2

ほうわしぼうさん 飽和脂肪酸 **saturated fatty acid**；SFA

ほえき 補液 (脱水を改善させること)**rehydration** (水分を補うこと)**fluid replacement** ☞輸液 ◀経口補液剤 oral rehydration solution；ORS 経口補液療法 oral rehydration therapy；ORT 静注補液 intravenous fluid replacement

ほえる 吠える **bark** ◆犬が吠えるような咳 a barking cough

ほお 頬 **cheek** ◆頬がこけている have sunken cheeks / the cheeks are sunken ▶頬ひげ whiskers 頬骨 cheekbone

ボーエンびょう ―病 **Bowen disease**；BD (表皮内有棘細胞癌)**squamous cell carcinoma in situ**；SCC in situ

ポータブル **portable** ▶ポータブルテレビ portable television[TV] set ポータブルトイレ portable toilet / (室内便器) commode

ポートワインじょうけっかんしゅ ―状血管腫 **port-wine stain[hemangioma]**

ボーマンのう ―嚢 **Bowman capsule**

ホーム **home** ◀グループホーム group home 特別養護老人ホーム special nursing home for seniors[elderly people] 有料老人ホーム private residential home for seniors[elderly people] / (退職者の) (private) retirement home ▶ホームケア home care ホームタウン hometown ホームドクター family physician[doctor] ホームプログラム at-home program ホームヘルプサービス home care (and housekeeping) services ☞(ホーム)ヘルパー, ホームシック, ホームステイ

ホームシック(の) homesick ◆ホームシックになる get[become] homesick / (ホームシックにかかっている)be homesick

ホームステイ homestay ◆日本の家にホームステイしている stay with a Japanese family ◆ホームステイ先の家族と暮らしていますか Are you living with a homestay family?

ポーランド Poland (ポーランドの・ポーランド人の 圏Polish) ☞国籍

ポール・バンネルしけん —試験 Paul-Bunnell test

ポールマンぶんるい —分類 Borrmann classification

ほおん 保温する (温かく)keep … warm (熱く)keep … hot

ほか 他(の・に)
《別の・別に》 (その他の)other (もう1つの)another (異なる)different (圏else)
☞別 ◆他に何か症状がありますか Do you have any other symptoms? ◆他に何か気づいたことがありますか Have you noticed anything else? ◆(診察の最後に)他に何かおっしゃりたいことがありますか Is there anything else that you'd like to tell me? / (くだけた調子で)Anything else[And what else]? ◆質問はありますか Do you have any other questions? ◆その件については改めて他の日に話し合いましょう Let's talk about the matter *some other [another] day. ◆他に何か欲しいものがありますか Would you like[Do you want] anything else? / Is there anything else you'd like? ◆他の方法でやってみましょう Let's do it (in) another[a different] way
《…以外》except (for), but ◆ここには佐藤看護師の他に誰もいません There's no one here except[but] Nurse Sato. ◆血液検査は肝機能の他はすべて正常です Your blood test shows that everything except your liver function is normal.
《…に加えて》aside from, in addition to (同様に)as well as ◆彼女は英語の他にスペ

イン語も話します Aside from English, she also speaks Spanish. / She speaks Spanish as well as English. ◆薬による治療の他, 健康によい食事や規則的な運動をお勧めします In addition to taking the medication, I recommend you eat a healthy diet and get regular exercise.

ほかん¹ 補完(の) complementary ▶補完代替医療 complementary and alternative medicine；CAM

ほかん² 保管する keep ◆この薬は室温で〈冷蔵庫の中に〉保管して下さい Please keep this medication *at room temperature 〈in the refrigerator〉.

ほきゅう 補給する (手に入れる)get (供給する)supply (補う)supplement (圏supplement) ☞補う, 補充 ◆果物や野菜を食べて身体に必要なミネラルやビタミンを補給するとよいでしょう To get the minerals and vitamins your body needs, you should eat fruits and vegetables. ◆熱中症予防にはこまめに水分を補給して下さい Please drink plenty of water frequently [as often as possible] to prevent heatstroke. ◀栄養補給剤 dietary[nutritional] supplement 水分補給 hydration 鉄分補給剤 iron supplement

ほきょうしょくひん 補強食品 supplementary food, supplemental food

ほきんしゃ 保菌者 carrier ☞キャリア

ボクサーこっせつ —骨折 boxer's fracture

ボクサーのうしょう —脳症 boxer's encephalopathy

ぼくし 牧師 (病院付の)chaplain (プロテスタント教会の)pastor

ほぐす (軽くする)relieve (少なくする)lessen (緩める)loosen (up) (リラックスさせる)relax, ease (発散させる)release ◆肩の凝りをほぐす relieve[lessen] the stiffness in one's shoulders ◆こわばった筋肉をもみほぐす massage and loosen up one's stiff muscles ◆体をほぐす relax one's body / relieve the stiffness in one's body ◆緊張をほぐす release[relieve] one's (nervous) tension

ほくろ　黒子　mole ◆ほくろのサイズや色に変化がありましたか Have you noticed any changes in the size or color of the mole(s)? ◆首にほくろがある have a mole on *one's* neck ◆ほくろを取る remove a mole

ぼけ　呆け ☞認知症

ポケット　pocket ◆歯肉にポケットができている pockets have formed in *one's* gums ◀歯周ポケット periodontal pocket

ぼける¹ ☞ぼやける

ほけん¹　保険　insurance ☞健康保険
◆保険についてお伺いします I'd like to [Let me] ask you about your insurance. ◆日本の保険に入っていますか Do you have Japanese insurance? ◆保険に加入する join[enroll in] an insurance plan ◆当院では外国の保険は扱えませんので医療費全額を自費でお支払いいただきます I'm sorry, we can't accept foreign insurance at our hospital, so you'll have to pay all your medical expenses. ◆この薬には保険が使えません This medication is not covered by insurance. / Insurance does not cover the cost of this medication.
◀介護保険 long-term care insurance　健康保険 health insurance　公的保険 public health insurance　国民健康保険 National Health Insurance (system)　失業保険 unemployment insurance　社会保険 social insurance　傷害保険 accident insurance　生命保険 life insurance　任意保険 voluntary insurance　被保険者 insured person　民間医療保険 private medical insurance　旅行（傷害）保険 travel (accident) insurance　労働災害補償保険 workers' accident compensation insurance ▶保険給付 insurance benefits　保険〈保険外〉診療 health care services covered〈not covered〉by health insurance　保険保障範囲 insurance coverage　保険料 insurance premium ☞保険証

ほけん²　保健　health（公衆衛生）**public health** ◀介護老人保健施設 health care facility for the elderly requiring long-term care　精神保健 mental health　精神保健福祉士 psychiatric social worker；PSW　精神保健福祉センター mental health and welfare center　世界保健機関 the World Health Organization；WHO　地域保健 community health　老人保健 elderly health ▶保健衛生担当者 health officer　保健室 health office[center] /（学校の）school *health room[infirmary / sick room]　保健指導 health guidance ☞保健医療, 保健師, 保健所

ほけんいりょう　保健医療　health care ▶保健医療サービス health care service　保健医療施設 health care facility

ほけんし　保健師　public health nurse；PHN ◀学校保健師 school nurse　産業保健師 occupational health nurse；OHN

ほけんじょ　保健所　public health center ◆市町村の保健所で医療費の公費負担の申請をして下さい Please go to the local public health center and apply for public financial assistance for your medical expenses. ◆詳細については保健所に問い合わせて下さい Please check for details at the public health center. ◆結核の症例を保健所に届ける report a case of tuberculosis to the public health center

ほけんしょう　保険証　(health) insurance card, heath insurance certificate ◆保険証を持っていたら見せて下さい Do you have your insurance card with you? Please show it to me. ◆次回の来院の時には必ず保険証を持ってきて下さい Be sure to bring your insurance card next time you come. ◀国民健康保険証 National Health Insurance card

ほご　保護する　protect（图protection 图protective）（遮る）**shield**（图shield）☞守る ◆胃を保護する薬を処方する prescribe a medication to protect the stomach ◆太陽光線から皮膚を保護するために日焼け止めクリームを塗る wear (a) sunscreen[sunblock] to protect[shield] *one's* skin against the sun ◀過保護 overprotection　心筋保護 myocardial protection　プライバシー保護 protection

ほ

of privacy / privacy protection　母性保護 maternity protection[support]　▶保護眼帯 eye shield[patch]　保護具 protective device[equipment]　保護クリーム protective cream[(軟膏)ointment]　保護眼鏡 protective glasses　保護薬 protective agent ☞生活保護, 保護施設, 保護室, 保護者, 保護入院

ぼご **母語** **native language, mother tongue** ◆あなたの母語は何ですか What's your *native language[mother tongue]?

ほこう **歩行** **walking** (動walk) （足取り） **gait** ☞歩く ◆歩行に問題がありますか Do you have any difficulty walking? ◆歩行時に足の筋肉が痛みますか Do you get any leg (muscle) pain while walking? / Do your leg muscles ache when you walk?　◆歩行訓練が必要です You need to practice walking.　◆歩行訓練をしましょう Let's do walking exercise. / Let's start walking for exercise.　◆歩行には松葉杖が必要です You need crutches to help you walk.　◆歩行が不自由である have difficulty walking　◆歩行が遅い be slow in walking / *one's* walking is slow　◆歩行可能な患者 an ambulatory patient　◆荷重歩行 weight-bearing walking　つぎ足歩行 tandem gait[walking]　二点〈三点／四点〉歩行 two-point〈three-point / four-point〉 gait　松葉杖歩行 crutch gait[walking]　免荷歩行 non-weight-bearing walking　6分間歩行試験 six-minute walk test；6MWT　▶歩行介助 assistance with walking　歩行ギプス包帯 walking cast　歩行訓練 gait training[exercise] / walking exercise[practice]　歩行困難 difficulty (in) walking / walking difficulty　歩行障害 gait disturbance[abnormality]　歩行能力 walking ability　歩行補助具 walking aid / assistive[supportive] device for walking ☞歩行器

異常歩行 abnormal gait

●運動失調性歩行 ataxic gait　●外転歩行 abduction gait　●かかと歩行 heel gait　●加速歩行 festinating gait　●痙性歩行 spastic gait　●鶏歩 steppage[drop foot] gait　●小刻み歩行 short-stepped gait / brachybasia　●前傾歩行 frontal gait　●爪先歩行 tiptoe gait / walking on tiptoe　●動揺性歩行 waddling gait　●トレンデレンブルグ歩行 Trendelenburg gait　●パーキンソン歩行 parkinsonian gait　●はさみ脚歩行 scissor gait　●引きずり歩行 shuffling gait　●不安定歩行 unsteady gait　●分回し歩行 circumduction gait　●片麻痺歩行 hemiplegic gait　●歩行失行 gait apraxia　●麻痺性歩行 paralytic gait　●酩酊歩行 drunken gait　●よろめき歩行 staggering gait

ほこうき **歩行器** **walker** ◆歩行器か杖を使っていますか Do you use a walker or a cane?　◀椅子式歩行器 chair-type walker / wheeled walker with a seat

ほこうそ **補酵素** **coenzyme**

ぼこくご **母国語** ☞母語

ほごしせつ **保護施設** **public assistance institution**

ほごしつ **保護室** **seclusion room**

ほごしゃ **保護者** （後見人）**guardian** （親）**parent(s)** （乳幼児の世話人）**caregiver**

ほごにゅういん **保護入院** **hospitalization for** （medical） **care and protection**

ほこり **埃** **dust** ◆室内のほこりは時に喘息症状の誘因になります House dust can sometimes trigger asthma symptoms. ◆ほこりを吸い込まないようにマスクをして下さい Please wear a mask so as not to inhale[breathe in] dust.

ほじ **保持** （維持）**maintenance** （保護）**protection** （保存）**preservation** ☞保つ　◀開口保持器 mouth prop / bite block　カリウム保持性利尿薬 potassium-sparing diuretic　秘密保持 protection of privacy / privacy protection

ぼし[1] **母子** **mother and baby, mother and child** ☞母児 ◆母子ともにお元気です Both mother and baby are (doing) well.　◀周産期母子医療センター prenatal medical center　▶母子家庭 single mother family / fatherless family　母子関係 mother-child relationship[relations]　母子同室 rooming-in　母子保健センター mother and child health center　☞母子手帳

ぼし[2]　**母指・拇指**　（手の）thumb /θʌ́m/
▶母指圧痕像 thumbprinting　☞母指環

ぼし[3]　**母趾・拇趾**　（足の）big toe, hallux
◀外反母趾 hallux valgus　内反母趾 hallux varus

ぼじ　**母児**　☞母子　▶母児感染 fetomaternal infection　母児間輸血症候群 feto-maternal transfusion syndrome　母児血液型不適合妊娠 incompatibility of maternal and fetal blood types / maternal and fetal blood type incompatibility　母児免疫 maternal immunity / maternally acquired immunity

ほしい　**欲しい**　want　（丁寧に）would like　◆他に欲しいものがありますか Would you like[Do you want] anything else? / Is there anything else you'd like?　◆何かして欲しいことがありますか Is there anything you'd like me to do? / What would you like me to do?

ぼしきゅう　**母指球筋**　thenar eminence
▶母指球筋 thenar muscle

ホジキンリンパしゅ　—腫　Hodgkin lymphoma　◀非ホジキンリンパ腫 non-Hodgkin lymphoma；NHL

ほしつ　**保湿する**　（加湿する）humidify　（皮膚に潤いを与える）moisturize　◆皮膚が乾燥しすぎないように絶えず保湿して下さい You should always moisturize your skin to prevent it from drying out.　▶保湿器 humidifier　保湿機能 moisturizing function　保湿剤 moisturizer /（クリーム）moisturizing cream /（ローション）moisturizing lotion

ポジティブフィードバック　positive feedback

ぼしてちょう　**母子手帳**　mother and child health handbook, Boshi-techo
◆保健所で母子手帳を交付してもらって下さい Please get a Boshi-techo, a mother and child health handbook, at the health center.　◆母子手帳は妊娠の記録になりますので, 受診のたびに持ってきて下さい Please bring your Boshi-techo with you every time you come for your checkups because it will be used to record your pregnancy.

ポジトロンだんそうさつえい　—断層撮影　☞ペット

ほじゅう　**補充する**　（追加する）supplement　（图supplementation 图supplementary）, add（图addition 图additional）　（代用する）replace（图replacement）　☞補う, 補給　◆食事にビタミン剤を補充する supplement *one's* diet with vitamin pills　◆インスリンを補充する replace insulin　◀エストロゲン補充療法 estrogen replacement therapy；ERT　ステロイド補充療法 steroid replacement therapy　ホルモン補充療法 hormone replacement therapy；HRT　▶補充栄養 supplementary feeding　補充輸液療法 replacement fluid infusion therapy

ほじょ　**補助**　help　（脇役的な助け）assistance, assist（图assist 图assisted）　（公的な助け）aid　☞援助　◆歩行には松葉杖の補助を必要とする require the help[assistance] of crutches in order to walk　◀医療補助者 paramedic /（総称的に）the para-medical staff　栄養補助食品 dietary[nutritional] supplement　禁煙補助薬 anti-smoking[quit-smoking / stop-smoking] medication[drug / aid]　生殖補助医療 assisted reproductive technology；ART　ビデオ補助下胸腔鏡手術 video-assisted thoracic surgery；VATS　▶補助椅子（予備の椅子）spare chair /（調節付きの椅子）adjustable chair　補助化学療法 adjuvant chemotherapy　補助換気 assisted ventilation　補助人工心臓 ventricular assist system；VAS / ventricular assist device　☞補助具

ほしょう[1]　**保証**　guarantee（图guarantee）, assurance（图assure）　◆患者のプライバシーを守ることを保証する assure[guarantee] patient privacy　◀入院保証金 deposit upon admission　品質保証

ほしょう¹ quality assurance；QA ▶保証金deposit 保証書(written) guarantee ☞保証人

ほしょう² 保障 security ◀医療保障 medical security 社会保障給付 social security benefits

ほしょう³ 補償 compensation (動compensate) ◀障害補償給付 disability compensation benefits 傷病補償年金 injury and disease compensation pension 療養補償 medical compensation 労働災害補償保険 workers' accident compensation insurance

ほしょうにん 保証人 guarantor ◆入院にはどなたか保証人が必要です On admission to the hospital, you will need someone who can act as a guarantor for you. ◀連帯保証人 cosigner[co-signer] / joint guarantor

ほじょぐ 補助(装)具 assistive device, supportive device ◆歩く時杖などの補助具を使っていますか Are you using any assistive[supportive] devices such as a cane when you walk? ◀歩行補助具 walking aid / assistive[supportive] device for walking

ほじる pick ◆鼻をほじる pick *one's* nose

ほすい 補水 (水分供給) supply of water (脱水を改善させること) rehydration ☞補液

ほすうけい 歩数計 pedometer / pɪdάmətə/ ◆歩数計をつけて歩く walk with a pedometer

ホスゲン phosgene ▶ホスゲン中毒 phosgene poisoning

ポスト mailbox,《英》postbox

ホストファミリー host family

ホスピス hospice ◆ホスピスで最期を過ごす spend *one's* last days in a hospice ▶ホスピスケア hospice care

ホスファターゼ phosphatase ◀酸性ホスファターゼ acid phosphatase；ACP 前立腺酸性ホスファターゼ prostatic acid phosphatase；PAP

ほせい 補正する (訂正・修正する) correct (動corrected) (調整する) adjust (動adjusted) ▶補正カルシウム値 corrected

[adjusted] calcium level 補正値 corrected value

ぼせい 母性 maternity (形maternal) , motherhood ▶母性愛 maternal [mother's] love 母性遺伝 maternal inheritance 母性行動 maternal behavior 母性保護 maternity protection[support] 母性本能 maternal instinct

ほそい 細い 《径・幅が小さい》 (薄い・体が痩せた) thin (幅が狭い) narrow ◆細いカテーテルを血管内に挿入する insert a thin catheter into a vein ◆細くてリボン状の便 narrow, ribbon-like stool
《勢いがない・弱々しい》(量が少ない) small, light ◆彼女は食が細い She doesn't eat much. / She's a small[light] eater. ◆尿線が細くなっていますか Have you noticed any decrease in the size of your stream?

ほそく 補足する (もっと詳しく説明する) explain further (つけ加える) add (形additional) (補う) supplement (形supplementary) ◆今の説明に少し補足させて下さい Please let me *explain a little further about[add a little to] what I said just now. ▶補足説明 additional[supplementary] explanation

ほそめる 細める ◆物を見る時目を細める squint to see things

ほぞん 保存する (貯蔵する) store (图storage), keep (ファイルなどを取っておく) save (腐らないように保存する) preserve (图preservation, 形preserved) (保全・温存する) conserve (图conservation, 形conservative) ☞保管 ◆データを保存する save [store] data ◀精液保存 semen storage 凍結保存 cryopreservation ▶保存血液 stored[preserved / conserved] blood 保存食品 preserved food / (腐りにくい食品) nonperishable food 保存的治療 conservative treatment[therapy]

ほたい 補体 complement ▶補体価 complement activity[titer]

ぼたい 母体 mother's body (形maternal) ▶母体・胎児集中治療室 maternal-fetal intensive care unit；MFICU 母体

年齢 maternal age　母体搬送 maternal transport　母体保護法 Maternal Protection Law　母体免疫 maternal immunity

ボタン　button /bʌ́tn/　◆用事がある時はこのボタンを押して看護師を呼んで下さい Please push[press] this button to call the nurse when you need help.　◆パジャマのボタンをはずす〈かける〉undo〈do up〉the buttons on the pajamas　◀(緊急)呼び出しボタン(emergency) call button　▶ボタン穴変形 buttonhole deformity

ホチキス　stapler (動ホチキスで閉じる・留める staple)　(ホチキスの針)staple　◆傷口をホチキスで留めます I'm going to staple the cut[wound]. / I'm going to use a stapler to close the cut[wound].　◆ホチキスの針を取りましょう I'm going to remove[take out] the staples now.　◀医療用ホチキス medical stapler / (外科用の)surgical stapler

ほちょうき　補聴器　hearing aid　◆補聴器をつけていますか Do you wear a hearing aid?　◆補聴器を着ける〈外す〉*put on〈remove〉the hearing aid

ぼっき　勃起　(penile) erection (形erectile)　☞巻末付録：訊きにくい質問のコツ
◆勃起に問題がありますか Do you have any problems with erections? / Do you have any erection problems?　◆なかなか勃起しない have difficulty getting an erection　◆勃起が続かない have difficulty maintaining an erection during sexual activity　◆勃起が弱い have weak erections　◆勃起時に痛みがある have (a) pain during erection　▶勃起不全 erectile dysfunction；ED

ほっさ　発作　attack　(痙攣性の発作)seizure, spasm, convulsion　(周期的に起こる発作)paroxysm (形paroxysmal)　(再発性疾患の発作)episode　(ひとしきり続く発作)spell　◆心臓発作を起こしたことがありますか Have you ever had a heart attack?　◆めまいの発作をよく起こしますか Do you often have *dizzy spells[attacks of dizziness]?　◆発作が起こりそうな予兆がありますか Do you have any sign[warning]

that an attack is about to begin?　◆どのくらいの頻度で発作が起きますか How often do you have the attacks?　◆発作はどのくらい長く続きますか How long do the attacks last?　◆めまいは発作性ですか Does your dizziness come in attacks?
◆発作的な咳 a spasmodic cough　◆発作的に咳き込む have a coughing spell　◆軽い発作 a mild[minor] attack　◆重い発作 a severe[major / massive] attack　◆致命的な発作 a fatal attack　◀狭心症発作 anginal attack　痙攣発作 convulsive attack[seizure]　再発作(繰り返し起こる発作)recurrent attack / (第2の発作)second[another] attack　失神発作 fainting[syncopal] attack　心臓発作 heart attack / (心筋梗塞)myocardial infarction　喘息発作 asthma[asthmatic] attack　痛風発作 attack of gout / gouty attack　てんかん発作 epileptic seizure　パニック発作 panic attack　不安発作 anxiety attack　良性発作性頭位めまい症 benign paroxysmal positional vertigo；BPPV　▶発作後もうろう状態 postictal twilight state　発作性上室頻拍 paroxysmal supraventricular tachycardia；PSVT　発作性心房細動 paroxysmal atrial fibrillation；PAF　発作性心房頻拍 paroxysmal atrial tachycardia；PAT

ほっしん　発疹　(一般的に) rash, exanthema　(突発的に発生する)eruption　(斑点)spot　☞湿疹　◆体に発疹がありますか Do you have a rash anywhere? / Is there a rash anywhere on your body?　◆どんな発疹ですか What's the rash like? / What kind of rash is it?　◆皮膚に発疹が出る have a rash on one's skin / one's skin breaks out in a rash　◆かゆくて赤い発疹が出る have itchy, red spots　◆体中に発疹が出る have the rash all over one's body / one's body is covered in[with] *a rash[spots]　◆この軟膏を塗れば発疹が治まるでしょう This ointment will cure[clear up] your rash.　◆蕁麻疹(潰瘍)のような発疹 a hive-like〈ulcer-like〉rash　◀座瘡様発疹 acneiform[acnelike] eruption　水疱状発疹 blistery rash　突発性発

疹 roseola (infantilis) / exanthema subitum；ES 膿疱性発疹 pustular rash / rash composed of pus-filled lesions ▶発疹チフス(epidemic) typhus

ホッチキス ☞ホチキス

ホット **HOT** (在宅酸素療法)**home oxygen therapy**

ホットバイオプシー hot biopsy

ホットパック hot pack ☞温湿布，湿布

ボツリヌスきん ―菌 **botulinum** (学名) *Clostridium botulinum* ▶ボツリヌス毒素 botulinum toxin；BTX

ボディイメージ **body image** ◆娘さんは体重やボディイメージのことを気にしていますか Is your daughter concerned about her weight and body image?

ほてつ **補綴** **prosthesis** (形prosthetic) ◀歯科補綴学 prosthodontics / prosthetic dentistry ▶補綴物 prosthetic appliance

ほてり **火照り** **hot flush**[**flash**] ◆顔のほてりは更年期によく見られる症状です Facial flushing is a common symptom of menopause.

ほてる **火照る** **feel hot, have** (**hot**) **flushes**[**flashes**] ◆顔がほてって赤い have a flushed, red face / the face becomes flushed and red ◆顔がほてるような感じはありますか Does your face feel hot[flushed]?

ほどこす **施す** (与える)**give** (行う)**do** ◆救急処置を施す give emergency treatment ◆彼が救急車で病院に運ばれてきた時には手の施しようがありませんでした When the ambulance brought him to the hospital, *nothing could be done to save him[there was nothing we could do to save him].

ほにゅう **哺乳する** (乳を吸う)**suck** (乳を飲ませる)**nurse** (母乳を与える)**breastfeed** ◆授乳 ◆哺乳困難である(赤ちゃんが) have *difficulty (in) sucking[sucking difficulty] / (授乳するのが) have difficulty (with) nursing[breastfeeding] ▶哺乳力 baby's sucking power ☞哺乳瓶

ぼにゅう **母乳** **breast milk, mother's milk** ☞乳(ちち)，ミルク ◆母乳を与える

[飲ませる]breastfeed ◆お子さんを母乳で育てましたか Did you breastfeed your child? ◆母乳がよく出る have[produce] plenty of (breast) milk ◆母乳があまり出ない do not have[produce] enough (breast) milk / the breast milk supply is low ◆母乳を絞って貯める pump and store (breast) milk ◆母乳を絞り出す express (breast) milk ◆母乳指導を行う show *the mother* how to breastfeed the baby / give guidance on breastfeeding ◆母乳で育った子供 a breast-fed child ◀冷凍母乳 frozen breast milk ▶母乳栄養 breastfeeding (nutrition) 母乳搾乳器 breast pump 母乳性黄疸 breast milk jaundice

ほにゅうびん **哺乳瓶** **baby bottle, feeding bottle** ◆哺乳瓶を消毒する sterilize baby bottles ◆哺乳瓶で育てる bottle-feed *one's* baby

ほね **骨** **bone** ◆骨が完全につくには約3か月かかります It'll take about three months for the bone to heal completely. ◆骨がもろい The bones break easily. / The bones become brittle. ◆あごの骨がはずれる dislocate *one's* jaw / have a dislocated jaw ◆魚の骨が喉に引っかかる a fish bone gets stuck in *one's* throat ◆足の骨を折る break[fracture] *one's* leg / have a broken[fractured] leg ◆折れた骨を整復する set a broken[fractured] bone

ほはば **歩幅** **step** (**length**) (大股の1歩)**stride** ◆狭い歩幅で足を引きずって歩く walk with short and shuffling steps

ぼはん **母斑** **birthmark, nevus** (複nevi) ◀色素性母斑 pigmented nevus 獣皮様母斑 giant hairy nevus 青色母斑 blue nevus 表皮母斑 epidermal nevus ベッカー母斑 Becker nevus 疣贅状母斑 verrucous nevus ▶母斑細胞 nevus cell 母斑症 phacomatosis

ポビドンヨード povidone iodine

ほほ **頬** ☞ほお

ホメオスタシス homeostasis

ホモシスチンにょうしょう ―尿症 homocystinuria

ホモシステイン homocysteine

ホモセクシャル ☞同性愛

ぼやける (曇ってぼやける)get[become] cloudy (形・輪郭が不鮮明になる)get[become] blurred ◆物がぼやけて見える have cloudy[blurred] vision / the vision gets[becomes] cloudy[blurred] ◆ぼやけて見える箇所は視野のどの辺りですか Around where in your visual field do you have cloudy[blurred] vision? / What part of your visual field gets[becomes] cloudy[blurred]?

ほゆうしゃ 保有者 carrier ☞キャリア

ほよう 保養 (気晴らし)relaxation (休養) rest (病後の回復)recuperation, convalescence ▶保養地 health resort

ボランティア volunteer /vàləntíə/ (㊫voluntary /váləntèri/) ◆ボランティアが入院中のあなたを手助けいたします Volunteers are available to help you during your hospital stay. ◆ボランティアで働く work *on a voluntary basis[as a volunteer] ◆当院にはボランティアの通訳がおります A volunteer interpreter is available in this hospital. ◆ボランティアの仕事 volunteer work[activities] /《英》voluntary work ▶病院ボランティア hospital volunteer

ポリープ polyp /pálip/ (㊫polypous ポリープ状の polypoid) ◆喉にポリープが1つできていますが,悪性ではありません You have a polyp[A polyp has developed] in your throat, but it's not malignant. ◆このポリープは直径5 mm です This polyp is five millimeters across[in diameter]. / This polyp has a diameter of five millimeters. ◆約8 mm のポリープが2つあります You have two polyps, each about eight millimeters in size. ◆このポリープはキノコのような形をしています This polyp is shaped like a mushroom. / This polyp looks like a mushroom. ◆ポリープをとる remove[take out] the polyp(s) ◆レーズン大のポリープ a polyp the size of a raisin ◀悪性〈良

性〉ポリープ malignant〈benign〉polyp 胃ポリープ stomach[gastric] polyp 過形成性ポリープ hyperplastic polyp 化生性ポリープ metaplastic polyp 喉頭ポリープ laryngeal polyp 後鼻孔ポリープ choanal polyp 子宮頸管ポリープ uterine cervical polyp 声帯ポリープ vocal cord polyp 大腸ポリープ polyp of the large intestine /(結腸の)colonic polyp /(結腸直腸の)colorectal polyp 多発ポリープ multiple polyps 胆嚢ポリープ gallbladder polyp 直腸ポリープ rectal polyp / polyp of the rectum 鼻ポリープ nasal polyp 有茎性ポリープ pedunculated polyp ▶ポリープ様腫瘤 polypoid tumor ポリープ様声帯 polypoid vocal cord

ポリオ polio (急性灰白髄炎)acute poliomyelitis ◀経口ポリオウイルスワクチン oral poliovirus vaccine；OPV 不活化ポリオウイルスワクチン inactivated poliovirus vaccine；IPV ▶ポリオウイルス poliovirus

ポリグラフ polygraph

ホリスティックいりょう ―医療 holistic medical care

ポリソムノグラフィ polysomnography (終夜睡眠ポリソムノグラフィ)(overnight) polysomnography；PSG

ポリネシア Polynesia (㊫Polynesian) ▶ポリネシア人(の) Polynesian

ボリビア Bolivia (㊫Bolivian) ☞国籍 ▶ボリビア人(の) Bolivian

ポリペクトミー polypectomy ◀内視鏡的ポリペクトミー endoscopic polypectomy

ポリペプチド polypeptide ◀胃抑制ポリペプチド gastric inhibitory polypeptide；GIP

ポリポーシス polyposis ◀家族性大腸ポリポーシス familial polyposis coli；FPC / familial adenomatous polyposis；FAP

ポリメラーゼ polymerase ▶ポリメラーゼ連鎖反応 polymerase chain reaction；PCR

ボリューム volume /váljəm/ ◆ボリュームを上げる〈下げる〉turn up〈down〉the

volume / put the volume up〈down〉
◆ラジオのボリュームを下げていただけませ
んか Could you turn down the volume on
the radio? / Could you keep the radio
volume low?

ボルグスケール **Borg scale**

ホルターしんでんけい **―心電計** **Holter monitor** ◆患者に24時間ホルター心電計
を取り付ける attach a twenty-four-hour
Holter monitor to the patient / attach
[hook up] a Holter monitor to the patient
for twenty-four hours

ホルターしんでんず **―心電図** **Holter EKG[electrocardiogram]** ◆ホルター心
電図は24時間かけて心電図を記録する検
査です A Holter EKG is a test that records
your EKG for twenty-four hours. ◆ホル
ター心電図をとりましょう We're going to
do a Holter EKG. ◆これはホルター心電
図の日誌です．検査中の行動や症状を正確
に記録して下さい Here's a Holter monitor
diary form. Keep an accurate record of
your activities and symptoms during the
test.

ポルトガル **Portugal** (形Portuguese)
☞国籍 ▶ポルトガル人(の) Portuguese

ホルネルしょうこうぐん **―症候群**
Horner syndrome

ポルフィリンしょう **―症** **porphyria**
◀急性間欠性ポルフィリン症 acute intermittent porphyria；AIP

ホルマリン **formalin**

ホルムアルデヒド **formaldehyde**

ホルモン **hormone** (形hormonal) ◆ホル
モンを分泌する secrete hormones ◆更
年期になると女性ホルモンの生成が減少し
ます During menopause, the production
of female hormones decreases. ◀黄体形
成ホルモン luteinizing hormone；LH 黄
体形成ホルモン放出ホルモン luteinizing
hormone-releasing hormone；LH-RH /
(性腺刺激ホルモン放出ホルモン) gonadotropin-releasing hormone；GnRH 黄体ホ
ルモン luteal hormone 下垂体性性腺刺
激ホルモン pituitary gonadotropin 下垂
体前葉〈後葉〉ホルモン anterior〈posterior〉

pituitary hormone 環境ホルモン environmental hormone 甲状腺刺激ホルモ
ン thyroid-stimulating hormone；TSH
甲状腺刺激ホルモン放出ホルモン thyro-
tropin-releasing hormone；TRH 甲状腺
ホルモン thyroid hormone；TH 抗利尿
ホルモン antidiuretic hormone；ADH
子宮収縮ホルモン oxytocin；OXT 消化
管ホルモン gastrointestinal hormone 女
性ホルモン female (sex) hormone ステ
ロイドホルモン steroid hormone 性ステ
ロイドホルモン sex steroid hormone 性
腺刺激ホルモン gonadotropin；Gn 精巣
ホルモン testicular hormone 成長ホルモ
ン growth hormone；GH 成長ホルモン
放出因子[ホルモン] growth hormone-releasing factor；GRF / growth hormone-
releasing hormone；GH-RH 男性ホルモ
ン male (sex) hormone / androgen 蛋白
同化ホルモン protein anabolic hormone
副甲状腺ホルモン parathyroid hormone；
PTH 副腎皮質刺激ホルモン adrenocor-
ticotropic hormone；ACTH 副腎皮質ホ
ルモン adrenal cortex hormone；ACH
▶ホルモン産生腫瘍 hormone-producing
tumor ホルモン製剤 hormone preparation ホルモン負荷試験 hormone stimulation test ホルモン分泌 hormone secretion ホルモン補充療法 hormone re-
placement therapy；HRT ホルモン療法
hormone[hormonal] therapy

ホワイトニング (歯の)teeth whitening

ぼん **盆** **tray** (たらい状のもの)basin /
béisn/ ☞トレイ ◀嘔吐盆 emesis basin
膿盆 kidney[pus] basin

ほんいん **本院** (この病院)this hospital,
our hospital (分院と区別して)the main
hospital

ほんごく **本国** *one's* (own) country,
one's home country

ほんせきち **本籍地** permanent (residence) address ◆本籍地はどちらですか
What's your permanent (residence) address?

ほんだい **本題** the main topic[matter].
◆それでは今日の本題について話し合いま

しょう Now, let's talk about today's main topic[matter].

ほんたいせい 本態性(の) essential
▶本態性高血圧 essential hypertension 本態性振戦 essential tremor

ポンド pound；lb

ほんとうに 本当に ☞実に

ほんとうは 本当は ☞実は

ほんのう 本能 instinct (🈪instinctive)
◀自己防衛本能 self-defense[self-protection] instinct / instinct for self-defense[self-protection] 性本能 sexual instinct 母性本能 maternal instinct ▶本能行動 instinctive behavior

ほんばちょうりつ 奔馬調律 gallop rhythm

ポンプ pump ◀インスリンポンプ insulin pump 輸液ポンプ infusion pump

ボンベ cylinder ◀携帯用酸素ボンベ portable oxygen cylinder

ほんやく 翻訳 translate (🈪translation)
☞通訳 ◆英語に翻訳する translate into English ◆医療通訳が医師の言葉を英語に翻訳してくれます The medical interpreter will translate what the doctor says into English for you.

ま

マーカー marker ◀腫瘍マーカー tumor marker　前立腺がんマーカー prostate cancer marker

マーズ MERS （中東呼吸器症候群）Middle East respiratory syndrome

まいあさ 毎朝 every morning, each morning ☞毎回 ◆ふだん毎朝何時に目を覚ましますか What time do you usually wake up each morning?　◆毎朝起きたらすぐに体温を測って下さい Please take your temperature as soon as you get up every morning.

まいかい 毎回 （すべての回に）every time （各回に）each time　★「毎」を表す every と each は入れ替えて用いられることもあるが，every は「あらゆる・全ての」を意味し，each は「個別の・各々の」を意味する．◆運動する前には毎回ストレッチをして下さい Please stretch every time before exercising.　◆痛みは毎回どのくらい長く続きますか How long does the pain last each time?　◆錠剤は毎回 2 粒飲んで下さい Please take two tablets each time.

マイクログラム microgram；μg

マイクロサージェリー microsurgery

マイクロソーム microsome （㊤microsomal）◀甲状腺マイクロソーム抗体 thyroid microsomal antibody

マイクロは ―波 microwave ▶マイクロ波凝固療法 microwave coagulation therapy；MCT　マイクロ波手術 microwave surgery

マイコバクテリウム mycobacterium （㊤mycobacterial）（学名）*Mycobacterium* ▶マイコバクテリウムアビウムコンプレックス *Mycobacterium avium* complex；MAC　マイコバクテリウム感染症 mycobacterial infection

マイコプラズマ mycoplasma （学名）*Mycoplasma* ▶マイコプラズマ感染症 mycoplasma infection　マイコプラズマ抗体

mycoplasma antibody　マイコプラズマ肺炎 mycoplasma pneumonia

まいじかん 毎時間 every hour, each hour （㊤hourly）☞毎回

まいしゅう 毎週 every week, each week （㊤weekly）☞毎回 ◆毎週金曜日に every Friday　◆毎週 2 回 twice[two times] a week

まいしょく 毎食 every meal, each meal ☞毎回 ◆この薬を毎食後に服用して下さい Please take this medication after every[each] meal.

まいつき 毎月 every month, each month （㊤monthly）☞毎回 ◆毎月 1 回 once a month　◆毎月の診察 monthly consultation

まいとし 毎年 every year, each year （㊤annual, yearly）☞毎回 ◆毎年の健康診断を受ける have *an annual[a yearly] checkup　◆毎年 1 回 once a year / every year　◆毎年 2 回 twice[two times] a year

マイナートランキライザー minor tranquilizer

マイナス （数）minus （↔plus）（㊤minus）（不利な点）disadvantage （↔advantage）◆100 マイナス 7 はいくつですか What's one hundred minus seven?　◆気温がマイナス 20 度まで下がる the temperature falls[drops] to minus twenty degrees　◆この治療法のプラスマイナス the advantages and disadvantages of this treatment

まいにち 毎日 every day, each day （㊤everyday, daily）☞毎回 ◆毎日か 1 日おきに運動するとよいでしょう You should exercise every day or every other day.　◆毎日何時間眠りますか How many hours do you sleep each day?　◆毎日 3 回 three times a[every] day　◆毎日の生活 everyday[daily] life　◆毎日の運動 daily exercise

まいばん 毎晩 （夕方から就寝まで）every evening, each evening （夕方から夜明けまで）every night, each night （㊤nightly）☞毎回

まいふくし 埋伏歯 impacted tooth

▶埋伏智歯 impacted wisdom tooth

マイボームせん 一腺 meibomian gland

まいぼつじ 埋没耳 pocket ear

まいる 参る

《参じる》(相手の視点で)**come** (自分の視点で)**go** ☞来る ◆(ナースコールに応えて)すぐにまいります I'm coming right now. / I'll be right there. ◆また明日まいります I'll come to see you again tomorrow.

《弱る》 ◆精神的にまいっている be under a great deal of stress

マインドコントロール mind control

マウスケア mouth care, oral care

マウスピース mouthpiece ◆マウスピースを口にくわえて唇をしっかり閉じて下さい Please put the mouthpiece into your mouth and close your lips tightly around it. ◆口からマウスピースをはずす take the mouthpiece out (of the mouth)

まえ 前

《位置・場所が前》**front** ◆このガウンは前を開けて着て下さい Please put this gown on with the opening in the front. ◆首の前に小さなしこりがある have a small lump on the front of *one's* neck

《方向が前》**ahead, forward(s)** ◆真っ直ぐ前を見て下さい Please look straight ahead. ◆前を向いて立って下さい Please stand with your head facing forward. ◆腕を前に出す hold *one's* arm(s) out straight ahead ◆体を前に曲げる bend over / bend forward at the waist

《時間的に前》 《現在を基準として》**ago** (ある過去を基準として・漠然と)**before** (最後に)**last** ◆彼女は3か月前に日本に来ました She came to Japan three months ago. ★この場合は before を用いない. ◆お子さんは前より良くなっています Your child is getting better. / Your child is better than before. ◆彼は手術前すごく緊張していました He was very nervous before the surgery. ◆診察してから半年になります It's almost half a year since I saw you last. ◆痛みは前からあったのですか Have you had the pain for some time? ◆寝る前にたくさん水分をとる drink a lot of

water before going to bed ◆前よりよい〈悪い〉be better〈worse〉than before ◆前の院長 ex-president / former president ◆彼の前の妻 his ex-wife[former wife] ☞前開き, 前届み, 前掛け, 前歯, 前向き

まえあき 前開き ◆前開きのパジャマ pajamas that open in the front / button-front pajamas

まえかがみ 前届み (猫背)**stoop** (だるそうに肩を前に屈めること)**slouch** ◆前届みで歩く walk with a stoop

まえかけ 前掛け apron ◀防護前掛け protective apron

まえば 前歯 front tooth (圏teeth)

まえむき 前向き(な・に) (積極的な)**positive** (↔negative) ◆治療にもっと前向きになる必要があります You need to be more positive about the treatment. / It's essential that you take a positive approach toward[about] your treatment. ◆前向きに生きる live life positively / take a positive attitude toward life ◆前向きな態度でいる keep[maintain] a positive attitude (about / toward) ◆前向きに考える think positively

まかせる 任せる **leave … to** *a person* ◆そのことについての決定はあなたにお任せします I'd like to leave the decision to you. ◆その問題は担当看護師にお任せ下さい Please let your nurse take care of the problem.

まがる 曲がる

《進行方向を変える》**turn** ◆2つめの角を右に曲がって下さい Please turn right at the second corner. ◆超音波室は角を曲がったところにあります The ultrasound room is around the corner.

《上体を曲げた》**bent** (猫背になった)**stooped** (ねじれた・歪んだ)**crooked, twisted** ◆加齢で腰が曲がっている have a back that's bent[stooped] with age / *one's* back is bent[stooped] with age ◆曲がった鼻を直す fix a crooked[twisted] nose

マギルかんし 一鉗子 Magill forceps ★複数形で.

まく¹ 巻く （包むように巻きつける）**wrap （around）** （包帯でくくる）**bandage （up）** ◆腕にこの止血帯を巻きましょう Let me *wrap this tourniquet around[put this tourniquet on] your arm. ◆首にスカーフを巻く wrap a scarf around *one's* neck ◆捻挫した足首に包帯を巻く bandage a sprained ankle

まく² 膜(性の) **membranous** ▶膜性腎症 membranous nephropathy　膜性増殖性糸球体腎炎 membranoproliferative glomerulonephritis；MPGN

マグネシウム **magnesium** /mægníːziəm/ ▶低マグネシウム血症 hypomagnesemia　硫酸マグネシウム magnesium sulfate ▶マグネシウム欠乏症 magnesium deficiency　マグネシウム製剤 magnesium preparation

まくら 枕 **pillow** ◆枕をもう1つお持ちしましょうか Would you like another pillow? / Can I get you another pillow? ◆背に枕を当ててお座りになりますか Would you like to sit with your back propped up by pillows? ◆背中に枕を入れましょう Let me put a pillow behind your back. ◆枕に寄りかかって座る sit propped against pillows ◆右足の下に枕を入れる put a pillow under *one's* right leg ◆氷枕 ice pillow / ice pack [bag]　水枕 water pillow[cushion] ▶枕カバー pillowcase ☞枕元

まくらもと 枕元 **the head of the bed** （ベッドのそば）**bedside** ◆このボタンを押すとベッドの枕元が上がります If you push [press] this button, you can raise the head of the bed. ◆患者の枕元に座る sit at[by] the patient's bedside ◆枕元の明かり a bedside lamp[light]

まくる 捲る **roll up** ◆袖をまくって下さい Please roll up your sleeve(s). ◆ズボンをまくって膝を出す roll up the pant leg(s) and show *one's* knee(s)

マクログロブリンけつしょう ―血症 **macroglobulinemia**

マクロファージ **macrophage** ◀顆粒球 マクロファージコロニー刺激因子 granulo-

cyte macrophage colony-stimulating factor；GM-CSF　肺胞マクロファージ alveolar macrophage

まげる 曲げる **bend, flex** （傾ける）**tilt** （ねじる）**twist** ◆膝を曲げる bend[flex] *one's* knees ◆首を曲げる bend[twist] *one's* neck ◆体を前に曲げて下さい Please bend over[forward at the waist]. ◆体を左右に曲げて下さい Please bend[tilt] your body first to one side and then to the other (side). ◆体を後ろに曲げる bend backward

まさつ 摩擦する （こする）**rub** ☞擦れる ◆冷水摩擦をする rub the body with a cold, wet towel ☞摩擦音

まさつおん 摩擦音 **fricative, friction rub** [**sound**] ◀胸膜摩擦音 pleural friction rub

まじきり 間仕切り **partition**

まじる 混じる **mix** ◆便に血が混じっていますか Is there any blood in your stools? / Have you noticed any blood mixed in your stools? ◆尿に膿が混じりますか Is there any pus in your urine? / Have you noticed any pus in your urine? ◆痰に血液が混じっています Blood is mixed in with the phlegm. ◆血の混じった痰 blood-stained phlegm

ましん 麻疹 **measles** /míːzlz/, **rubeola** （圈麻疹様の）**measly** ★measles は通例，単数扱い．　予防接種 麻疹に罹る have [get / catch] (the) measles ▶麻疹ウイルス measles virus　麻疹脳炎 measles encephalitis　麻疹・風疹混合ワクチン measles and rubella vaccine / MR vaccine　麻疹様皮疹 measly rash　麻疹・流行性耳下腺炎・風疹ワクチン measles, mumps, and rubella vaccine / MMR vaccine　麻疹ワクチン measles vaccine

ます 増す （数・量が）**increase** /ɪnkríːs/ （圈 **íncrease**） （改善する）**improve** （圈 **impróvement**） （特に体重が）**gain** （圈 **gain**） ☞増える ◆息切れが増していますか Have you had increasing shortness of breath? ◆量が増す the volume increases / increase in volume ◆数が増す

the number increases / increase in number ◆食欲が増す *one's* appetite improves[increases] / have an increase [improvement] in appetite

マス **MAS** （胎便吸引症候群）meconium aspiration syndrome

まず ☞最初, 手始め

ますい 麻酔 anesthesia /ænəsθíːʒə/ （⚟ anésthetize ⚟anesthétic） ◆局所麻酔をする administer[give] local anesthesia / numb *the area* with local anesthesia ◆全身麻酔をする administer[give] general anesthesia ◆痛みがないように麻酔をします I'm going to *give you an anesthetic[put you under anesthesia] so there won't be any pain. ◆歯の周りに麻酔をします I'm going to anesthetize the area around the tooth. ◆麻酔についてご説明します Let me tell you about your anesthesia. / Let me go through your anesthesia with you. ◆手術は全身麻酔で行います We're going to perform the surgery under general anesthesia. ◆全身麻酔なので手術中は眠っていて痛みはありません You'll be having general anesthesia for this surgery, so it'll keep you asleep and pain-free throughout the surgery. ◆局所麻酔ですから手術中目が覚めているでしょう You'll have local anesthesia, so you'll be awake during the surgery. ◆2, 3時間で麻酔から覚めるでしょう You'll *wake up from[come out of] the anesthesia in a few hours. / The effects of the anesthesia will wear off in a few hours. ◆彼女はまだ麻酔がかかっています She's still under anesthesia. ◀ガス麻酔薬 gas anesthetic 吸入麻酔 inhalation anesthesia 局所麻酔 local anesthesia 局所麻酔薬 local anesthetic 硬膜外麻酔 epidural anesthesia サドルブロック麻酔 saddle block anesthesia 歯科麻酔 dental anesthesia 周囲浸潤麻酔 field block（anesthesia） 静脈麻酔 intravenous anesthesia 浸潤麻酔 infiltration anesthesia 脊髄くも膜下麻酔[脊椎麻酔] spinal anesthesia 全身麻酔 general anesthesia 伝達麻酔 conduction anesthesia 導入麻酔 induction of anesthesia 日帰り麻酔 outpatient[ambulatory] anesthesia 表面麻酔 topical[surface] anesthesia 冷凍麻酔 cryoanesthesia ▶麻酔（科）医 anesthesiologist 麻酔科 the department of anesthesiology / the anesthesiology department 麻酔回復室 postanesthesia care unit；PACU 麻酔学 anesthesiology 麻酔ガス anesthetic gas 麻酔合併症 complication(s) of anesthesia 麻酔器 anesthesia machine 麻酔記録 anesthesia chart[record] 麻酔前回診 preanesthesia round 麻酔前評価 preanesthesia evaluation 麻酔薬 anesthetic （medication / drug / agent）

まずい

《味が悪い》not good, bad ◆いつもの食事がまずいと感じますか Do you find that the foods you usually eat *don't taste good [taste bad]?

《不適切である》inadequate ◆私の説明がまずかったようです. 申し訳ありません It seems that my explanation was inadequate[（不明確な）unclear]. I'm sorry.

マスク mask ◆顔にこのマスクをかけます I'm going to slip[put] this mask over your face. ◆マスクをしている wear a mask ◆咳やインフルエンザの症状がある場合は, 必ずマスクを着用して下さい If you're coughing or have flu symptoms, be sure to wear a mask. ◀酸素マスク oxygen mask 鼻マスク nasal mask フェイスマスク face[facial] mask 粉塵マスク dust mask ベンチュリーマスク Venturi mask 防護マスク protective mask

マススクリーニング mass screening ◀新生児マススクリーニング検査 newborn mass screening

マスターベーション ☞自慰

マスト **MAST** （多抗原検索検査）multiple-antigen simultaneous test

マストさいぼう ―細胞 mast cell

まぜる 混ぜる mix （かき混ぜる）stir ◆この薬はジュースに混ぜて飲んでもいいですよ You can take this medication mixed with juice.

マゾヒズム masochism（圏masochistic）▶マゾヒスト masochist　マゾヒズム的性格 masochistic personality

また股　（両脚が分かれる部分）crotch　（鼠径，腿の付け根）groin　★crotch より上の部分を指す．◆股に痛みがある have (a) pain in the crotch (area) / *one's* crotch hurts　◆股がかゆい have (an) itching in *one's* crotch (area) / *one's* crotch itches　◆股擦れ a sore groin[crotch]

マダニ tick

マタニティ maternity　▶マタニティウェア maternity clothes[wear]　マタニティブルー maternity blues

まだら(の) mottled　（小さい空洞のような）lacunar　（圏斑点 spot　小さなしみ speckle）◆赤いまだら模様の発疹がある have a mottled red rash　▶まだら健忘 lacunar amnesia　まだら認知症 lacunar dementia

まちあいしつ　待合室 waiting room　（待合スペース）waiting area　（ロビー）lounge　◆順番が来たらお呼びしますので待合室でお待ち下さい We'll call your name when your turn comes. Till then, please wait [stay] in the waiting room.　◆手術の間ご家族は集中治療室の外にある待合室でお待ちいただきます During the surgery, family members will wait in the waiting area outside the intensive care unit.　◆ここはICU 患者様のご家族のための待合室です Please note this waiting area is for family members of ICU patients.　◀家族用待合室 the family waiting room[area]　救急外来待合室 the emergency (outpatient) waiting room[area]　小児科外来待合室 the pediatric outpatient waiting room　中待合室 inner waiting room；*waiting area just in front of the doctor's office*

まちいしゃ　町医者 general practitioner；GP

まちがい　間違い　（ミス）mistake　（誤り）error　☞誤り，間違う，ミス　◆不注意による間違いをする make a careless mistake　◆林先生が優秀な外科医であることは間違いありません There's no question that Dr

Hayashi is a good surgeon.　◆私の記憶に間違いがなければ，あなたのお母様も若い頃に乳がんに罹られたのですね If I remember correctly[right], your mother also had breast cancer when she was young.

まちがう　間違う　（ミスをする）make a mistake　（…を…と取り違える）mistake[take]… for …　（圏mistaken）　（誤った・不適当な）wrong　（圏by mistake, wrong）☞誤った，言い間違い，間違い，読み違える　◆ごめんなさい．間違えました I'm sorry, I made a mistake.　◆間違った診断をする wrongly [mistakenly] diagnose / make a wrong [mistaken] diagnosis　◆名前の綴りを間違える spell *a person's* name wrong　◆子供の病気を自分のせいだと自分を責めるのは間違っています It's *a mistake[wrong] to think that you're responsible for your child's illness.　◆このカプセルは吸入用ですので間違って飲んだりしないで下さい This capsule is (intended) for inhalation only. So don't take it by mouth by mistake.　◆来院する日時を間違えないように注意して下さい Please note[make a careful note of] the date and time of your next visit. / Please make sure not to mistake the date and time of your next visit.

まちじかん　待ち時間 wait(ing) time　（期間）wait(ing) period　◆今日の待ち時間はおよそ１時間になります The approximate[estimated] wait(ing) time today will be an hour.　◆待ち時間を短縮する minimize the wait(ing) time[period]　◆待ち時間は患者さんの病状で前後することがありますのでご了承下さい Please understand that wait(ing) times vary depending on the patient's medical condition.

まつ　待つ wait (for)　◆お呼びするまでここでしばらくお待ち下さい Please wait here for a while until your name is called.　◆順番をお待ち下さい Please wait your turn.　◆少々お待ち下さい Just a moment, please.　◆お待たせいたしました Thank you so much for waiting.　◆お

待たせしてすみません I'm sorry to have kept you waiting. / I'm sorry about the wait. ◆お電話をお待ちしております I'll be waiting for your call.

まっか **真っ赤(な)** bright red ◆便に真っ赤な血が付いている There is some bright red blood in the stools. / There are some bright red blood stains on the stools.

まっき **末期** final stage, last stage （不治の）terminal stage ☞終末期 ◆がんの末期である be in the final[terminal] stages of cancer ◀妊娠末期 the last days of pregnancy / the final[last] stage of pregnancy ▶末期医療 terminal[（緩和の）palliative /（ホスピスの）hospice]（medical）care 末期がん terminal[terminal-stage / end-stage] cancer 末期患者 patient with a terminal illness[disease] / terminal patient 末期症状 terminal symptom / symptoms of the final stages（of the disease）

マック MAC, *Mycobacterium avium* complex

マックバーニーてん **一点** McBurney point

まっくら **真っ暗(な)** pitch-dark ◆目の前が真っ暗になりましたか Did you black out? ★black out は一時的に気を失うこと.

まつげ **睫毛** eyelash ◀逆さまつげ ingrown eyelashes /（睫毛乱生）trichiasis

マッサージ massage （圏massage, give a massage）, rub （圏rub, give a rub） ◆マッサージをしましょう Let me give you a massage. ◆足をマッサージする rub *one's* leg(s) ◆背中のマッサージ a back massage[rub] ◀あんまマッサージ指圧師 massage and *finger pressure[shiatsu] practitioner /（男性の）masseur /（女性の）masseuse 心マッサージ heart[cardiac] massage フットマッサージ foot massage ▶マッサージ療法 massage therapy / massotherapy マッサージ療法士 massage therapist

まっさお **真っ青(な)** （顔色が）pale, white （色が）deep blue ◆顔が真っ青ですが，大丈夫ですか You look pale. Are you okay?

まっさかさま **真っ逆さま(に)** headfirst, headlong ◆真っ逆さまに木から落ちる fall headfirst[headlong] from a tree ◆プールに真っ逆さまに飛び込んで頭を打つ dive headfirst[headlong] into the pool and hit *one's* head

まっしょう **末梢(の)** peripheral ▶末梢血 peripheral blood 末梢血幹細胞移植 peripheral blood stem cell transplant[transplantation]；PBSCT 末梢循環障害 peripheral circulatory disturbance 末梢神経 peripheral nerve 末梢神経障害 peripheral neuropathy 末梢動脈疾患 peripheral arterial[artery] disease；PAD

まっすぐ **真っ直ぐ(に)** straight （圏straight 圏straighten） ◆真っ直ぐ前を見て下さい Please look straight ahead. ◆背筋を真っ直ぐにして座って〈立って〉下さい Please *sit up〈stand up〉straight. ◆背筋を真っ直ぐに伸ばす straighten *one's* back（up）/ make *one's* back straight ◆真っ直ぐに行く go straight ◆よろけて真っ直ぐ歩けない stagger and can't walk straight ◆真っ直ぐな姿勢 a straight posture

まっせつこつ **末節骨** distal phalanx ▶末節骨骨折 distal phalangeal fracture

まったく **全く** ☞全然

まったん **末端(の)** （遠位の）distal （接頭acr(o)-）▶末端肥大症（先端巨大症）acromegaly 末端部 distal part

まつばづえ **松葉杖** crutches ★複数形で. ☞杖 ◆松葉杖で歩く walk on crutches ◆松葉杖を使う use（a pair of）crutches ◆歩行には6週間松葉杖が必要です You will need to walk[be] on crutches for six weeks. ▶松葉杖歩行 crutch gait[walking]

―まで
《時間・期限》（までずっと）until, till （までには）by, by the time （…する前に）before （…へ・に）to ◆解熱するまで寝ていて下さい You should rest in bed until the fever goes away. ◆明日までにご連絡下さい Please *let me know[（電話で）give me a call and let me know] by tomorrow.

◆今週末まで金子先生は学会で出張しています Dr Kaneko will be away for[on] a conference until the end of this week. ◆夕食までには病室に戻ってきて下さい Please[I'd like you to] come back to your room *before dinner[by dinner time]. ◆午前中の受付時間は8時半から11時までです Our morning reception hours are from eight-thirty to eleven. 《範囲・限界》(up) to, as far as ◆手術室まで車椅子でお連れします I'll escort[take] you to the operating room in a wheelchair. ◆彼女は亡くなる直前まで意識がありました She was conscious up to the moment of (her) death. ◆できるところまで両腕をゆっくり伸ばして下さい Slowly extend your arms as far as *they'll go[you can]. ◆(作業後に)今日はここまでにしましょう That's all for today. / Let's call it a day.

まどぐち　窓口　window, counter　(受付) reception desk　◆会計窓口3番においで下さい Please come to (cashier) window number three. ◆窓口の事務員に訊いて下さい Please ask the clerk at the reception desk. ◆薬局の窓口 the pharmacy counter　◆検査室の窓口 the reception desk of an exam room　◀会計窓口 cashier window[counter]　時間外窓口 after-hours window[counter]　▶窓口係 clerk at the window[counter]

マナー　manner　◆マナーがいい have good manners / be well-mannered　◆マナーが悪い have bad[poor] manners / be bad-mannered

マニキュア　manicure　(⚫manicure)　(足の) pedicure　◆マニキュアをする manicure[(つやを出す) polish / do] one's nails　◆爪のマニキュアを落とす remove the nail polish　▶マニキュア液 nail polish /(英)nail varnish

まね　真似する　(同じようにする) do likewise　(模倣する) imitate　(まったく同じに真似る) copy　(例にならう) follow a person's example　◆私の口を見て真似して下さい Look at my mouth, and *copy the way I

move it[do likewise].

マネージャー　manager　◀ケアマネージャー care manager

マネジメント　management　☞管理

まばたき　瞬きする　blink　(意識的に瞬く) wink　◆少しの間、まばたきしないで下さい Please don't blink for just a second.

まひ　麻痺　paralysis /pəræləsɪs/　(⚫麻痺させる páralyze　⚫麻痺(性)の paralýtic), palsy /pɔ́:lzi/　(感覚の麻痺・しびれ) numbness /nʌ́mnəs/　(不全麻痺) paresis, partial paralysis　◆麻痺がありますか、もしくはありましたか Do you have or have you ever had any paralysis or numbness? ◆どこが麻痺していますか Where do you have the numbness[paralysis]? ◆意識を回復した後、体のどこかに麻痺の症状がありましたか Have you noticed any numbness[paralysis] in any part of your body since you regained consciousness? ◆突然顔や手足の片方に麻痺が起こる have sudden paralysis or numbness of the face, arm, or leg, on one side of the body　◆左半身が不完全に麻痺している be partially paralyzed on the left side of the body / have partial paralysis on one's left side　◆自動車事故で下半身が麻痺している be paralyzed from the waist down as a result of a car accident / the lower part of the body is paralyzed as a result of a car accident　◀運動麻痺 motor paralysis　感覚麻痺 sensory paralysis　完全麻痺 complete paralysis　顔面神経麻痺 facial (nerve) paralysis[palsy]　痙性麻痺 spastic paralysis　後(遺)麻痺 residual paralysis　四肢麻痺 quadriplegia　周期性四肢麻痺 periodic paralysis　小児麻痺 infantile paralysis[(急性灰白髄炎) poliomyelitis / polio]　進行性核上性麻痺 progressive supranuclear palsy；PSP　声帯麻痺 vocal cord paralysis　腸管麻痺 intestinal paresis　対麻痺 paraplegia　脳性麻痺 cerebral palsy；CP　不全麻痺 paresis / partial paralysis　片麻痺 hemiplegia　両麻痺 diplegia　▶麻痺症状 paralysis symptom　麻痺性イレウス paralytic ileus

麻痺性拘縮 paralytic contracture　麻痺性歩行 paralytic gait

まぶしい　眩しい　**glaring**（図**glare**）　◆明るい光がまぶしいですか Do you have any problems with glare? / Do bright lights bother your eyes?　◆日光〈光〉がまぶしい be sensitive *to the sun〈to light〉

まぶた　瞼　**eyelid**　図眼瞼　◆まぶたが腫れている have swollen eyelids / have puffy eyes　◆まぶたが痙攣する the eyelids spasm　◆まぶたがぴくぴく動く one's eyelids twitch / have a twitchy eye　◆まぶたが重くなる one's eyelids droop / have droopy[heavy] eyelids　◆上まぶたを裏返す turn[flip] a person's upper eyelid(s) inside out　◀上まぶた upper[top] eyelid　下まぶた lower[bottom] eyelid　一重〈二重〉まぶた single〈double〉 eyelids

マムシどく　―毒　**pit viper venom**

まめ　（水疱）**blister**　（たこ・胼胝）**callus**　（魚の目・鶏眼）**corn, clavus**　◆足にまめができる have[get] a blister on one's foot　◀血まめ blood blister

まもる　守る
《保護する・防ぐ》**protect**　（危険・危害などから守る）**shield**　☞保護　◆このカバーでX線からあなたの生殖器を守ります This cover will protect[shield] your reproductive organs from the X-rays.　◆患者を感染から守る protect the patient from infection
《従う》（指示などに従う）**follow**　（規則などを守る）**observe, abide by**　☞順守　◆担当医の注意事項を守って下さい Please follow your doctor's instructions.　◆病院の規則を守って下さい Please follow[observe / abide by] the hospital rules[regulations].
《ある状態を保つ》**keep**　◆秘密を守る keep one's word[promise]　◆あなたの個人情報については必ず秘密を守ります I'll keep your personal[private] information confidential[secure]. / All your personal[private] information will be (kept) completely confidential.　◆2, 3日安静を守って下さい Please *rest quietly[stay] in bed for a few days.

まやく　麻薬　（鎮痛・鎮静の）**narcotic**　（drug）　（違法薬物）（illegal）**drugs**　★通例, 複数形で.　（快楽を得るための薬物）**recreational drugs**　★通例, 複数形で.　◆麻薬を使う take[use] drugs　◆麻薬を常用している be on drugs　◆麻薬の常習癖がある have a drug habit / be a drug addict　◀合成麻薬 synthetic narcotic　非麻薬性鎮痛薬 nonnarcotic analgesic（medication / drug / agent）　▶麻薬常用[乱用] narcotic（drug）abuse　麻薬処方箋 narcotic prescription　麻薬性鎮痛薬 narcotic analgesic（medication / drug / agent）　麻薬中毒 narcotic（drug）addiction　麻薬中毒者（narcotic）drug addict　麻薬取締法 Narcotics Control Law

まゆ　眉　**eyebrow**　/áıbràʊ/　◆眉を上げて下さい Please raise your eyebrows.

まよなか　真夜中（に）　（漠然と深夜に）in the middle of the night　（午前0時ちょうどに）at midnight　◆真夜中に目が覚める wake up in the middle of the night

マラリア　**malaria**　◀熱帯熱マラリア falciparum malaria　▶マラリア原虫 malaria parasite

マリオットもうてん　―盲点　**Mariotte**（blind）**spot**

マリファナ　☞大麻

まるい　丸い　（円形の）**round, circular**　（球形の）**spherical**　◆丸い形をしている be round（in shape）　◆ここに15 mm大の丸い形をした異常陰影が見られます Here, you can see an abnormal shadow ; it's round and fifteen millimeters in size.

まるがお　丸顔　**round face**

マルク　（骨髄穿刺）**bone marrow puncture**　▶マルク針 bone marrow（aspiration / biopsy）needle

マルトース　（麦芽糖）**maltose, malt sugar**

マルトリンパしゅ　―腫　**MALT lymphoma**　（粘膜関連リンパ組織リンパ腫）**mucosa-associated lymphoid tissue lymphoma**

マルファンしょうこうぐん　―症候群　**Marfan syndrome**

まれ　稀（な）　（珍しい）**rare**（図**rarely**）　（通常と異なる）**unusual**　（普通ではない）**uncommon**　◆まれな病気 a rare disease　◆こ

の薬の副作用はかなりまれです The side effects of this medication are rather rare. ◆非常にまれですが，薬剤性肺炎などの合併症が生じることがあります Very rarely[In very rare cases], complications can occur, including drug-induced pneumonitis.

マレーシア Malaysia （形Malaysian）
☞国籍 ▶マレーシア人（の） Malaysian

マレットゆび ―指 （槌指） mallet finger （親指の） mallet thumb

マロリー・ワイスしょうこうぐん ―症候群 Mallory-Weiss syndrome

まわす 回す （向ける） turn （ひねる・向きを変える） twist （回転させる） rotate （ぐるぐる回す） circle ◆頭を右に回して下さい Please turn[twist] your head to the right. ◆首を回すと痛みますか When you turn[rotate] your neck around, does it hurt? ◆腕を前回し〈後ろ回し〉する circle one's arm *in front of〈behind〉 one's body / do forward〈backward〉 arm circles

まわり 周り・回り （周辺） circumference （圏around，《英》round） ☞周囲，周辺 ◆お腹周りを測りましょう Let me[I'm going to] measure *you around the waist[your waist circumference]. ◆目〈首〉の周りに発疹がある have a rash around the eyes〈neck〉 ◆首周りのサイズ one's collar size

まわりくどい 回りくどい roundabout ◆話し方がまわりくどい talk in a roundabout way

まわる 回る
《回転する》 turn （around，《英》round） （くるくる速く回る） spin （around，《英》round） （軸を中心に回る） rotate ◆目が回る feel[get] dizzy ◆部屋がぐるぐる回っているように感じますか Do you feel as if the room is spinning? ◆自分自身がぐるぐる回っているように感じますか Do you feel as if you're spinning around and around?
《回診する》 make (the) rounds (of) ◆もうすぐ医師が回ってきますのでベッドでお待ち下さい The doctors will be making (their) patient rounds soon, so please be waiting in bed. / The doctors will soon come in to see you, so please stay in your bed.

まんえん 蔓延する （広範囲に広まる） spread widely, go around （広まっている） be widespread （ある時期・地域に流行している） be prevalent （猛威を振るっている） be raging ☞流行る，流行 ◆インフルエンザが蔓延しています The flu epidemic *has spread widely[is widespread].

マンガン manganese ▶マンガン中毒 manganese poisoning

まんきさん 満期産 full-term birth ◆満期産でしたか Was the baby born at (full) term? ▶満期産児 full-term newborn / baby born at term

まんげつがんぼう 満月（様）顔貌 moon face （形moon-faced）

マンシェット cuff, manchette ◆血圧測定のために腕にこのマンシェットを巻きましょう Let me put this cuff on your arm to check your blood pressure.

まんしょう 満床 ◆あいにく当病院は満床です I'm afraid there are no beds available in this hospital. / Unfortunately, this hospital has no empty beds.

マンション （分譲マンション）condominium, condo （賃貸アパート）apartment （賃貸アパートの建物全体）apartment building [house] ☞アパート

まんせい 慢性（の） chronic （↔acute） （長期にわたる）long-term ◆慢性の咳 a chronic cough ◆慢性的な腰痛 (a) chronic low back pain ◆何か慢性的に不調な症状はありますか Do you have any chronic[long-term] health conditions? ◆慢性的な痛みが食欲不振や睡眠障害の原因でしょう Chronic pain may have caused your loss of appetite and sleep disturbances. ◆治療しないとこの症状は慢性化します If not treated, this symptom will become chronic. ▶慢性胃炎 chronic gastritis　慢性炎症 chronic inflammation　慢性肝炎 chronic hepatitis　慢性期 chronic stage[phase]　慢性硬膜下血腫 chronic subdural hematoma　慢性呼吸不

全 chronic respiratory failure　慢性腎臓病 chronic kidney disease；CKD　慢性心不全 chronic heart failure　慢性腎不全 chronic renal failure；CRF　慢性膵炎 chronic pancreatitis　慢性疼痛 chronic pain　慢性疲労症候群 chronic fatigue syndrome；CFS　慢性副鼻腔炎 chronic sinusitis　慢性閉塞性肺疾患 chronic obstructive pulmonary disease；COPD

まんぞく　満足　satisfaction（動満足させる satisfy　形満足した satisfied, happy　満足のいく satisfying　納得のいく satisfactory）　◆仕事に満足していますか Are you satisfied[happy] with your work?　◆私の説明でご満足いただけたでしょうか Has everything been explained[Have I explained everything] to your satisfaction?　◆満足のいく検査結果が得られました I'm glad to tell you that we could obtain satisfactory results.　◆満足した表情 a satisfied expression　◆食欲を満足させる satisfy *one's* appetite　◆食事にスパイスを使うことで満足感が得られると思います I hope you'll be able to satisfy your sense of taste by seasoning your food with spicy flavors.　◀患者満足度 patient satisfaction

まんなか　真ん中　（およその中心）the middle　（厳密に中心）the center　◆痛むのは真ん中ですか Is the pain in the middle?

まんぷく　満腹　full stomach　（飽満状態）satiety　◆満腹ですか Are you full?　◆いくら食べても満腹にならないのですか However much you eat, do you feel as if you're *never quite satisfied[still not full]?　▶満腹感 feeling of satiety / feeling full　満腹中枢 the satiety center

まんぽけい　万歩計　☞歩数計

マンモグラフィー　（乳房 X 線検査）mammography /mæmágrəfi/　（乳房 X 線写真）mámmogram　◆マンモグラフィーは X 線を使って乳房を調べる検査です A mammography is an X-ray examination of *a person's* breast.　◆以前マンモグラフィーを受けたことがありますか Have you ever had a mammogram?　◆マンモグラフィー

検査をしましょう I'm going to[Let me] perform[do] a mammography. / I think *you should have[we should do] a mammography.

み

み 身 body ◆身をかがめて下さい Please bend over[forward] at the waist. ◆身を起こす〈寝ている状態から〉rise from a lying position /〈ベッドから〉sit up in bed /〈座った状態から〉rise from a sitting position ☞身だしなみ，身につける，身の回り，身振り，身分，身元，身寄り

ミエリン myelin ▶ミエリン鞘 myelin sheath

みえる 見える
《見ることができる》〈見る〉**see** 《意識的に見る》**look at** （圏**visible**）☞見る ◆最近，物が見えにくいですか Do you have difficulty seeing things recently? ◆物がよく見えないのですか Do you have difficulty seeing things clearly? ◆遠くの物が見えにくいですか Do you have difficulty seeing things at a distance? ◆左目が見えない cannot see with *one's* left eye ◆物がぼやけて〈かすんで / 二重に / ゆがんで〉見えますか Is your vision cloudy〈blurred / double / distorted〉? / Do you have cloudy〈blurred / double / distorted〉 vision? ◆光が見えますか Do you see a light? ◆ぼんやり〈はっきり〉見える see dimly〈clearly〉 ◆X 線写真に異常な影が見えます An abnormal shadow *can be seen[is visible] on your X-ray film. ◆見える範囲の腫瘍をすべて摘除する remove all of the visible tumors
《…のように見える》**seem, look, appear** ◆このほくろは良性のように見えます This mole looks[appears / seems] benign. ◆傷は浅いように見えます The injury seems[appears] *rather slight[〈表面上の〉superficial]. / The injury doesn't seem to be deep.

ミエローマ myeloma
ミエログラフィ myelography
ミエロペルオキシダーゼ myeloperoxidase；MPO

ミオクローヌス myoclonus （圏**myoclonic**）◀動作時ミオクローヌス action myoclonus ▶ミオクローヌスてんかん myoclonus[myoclonic] epilepsy ミオクローヌス発作 myoclonic seizure

ミオグロビン myoglobin ▶ミオグロビン尿 myoglobinuria

みおとす 見落とす miss （見過ごす）**overlook** （圏**oversight**）◆見落としがないように再度チェックして下さい Please check again to make sure that you haven't missed[overlooked] anything. ◆うつ病の初期症状は見落としやすい It's easy to overlook[miss] the early signs of depression.

ミオパチー myopathy ◀眼筋ミオパチー ocular myopathy ステロイドミオパチー steroid myopathy 先天性ミオパチー congenital myopathy 代謝性ミオパチー metabolic myopathy 糖尿病性ミオパチー diabetic myopathy

みかく 味覚 sense of taste, taste sensation, gustatory sense, gustation ☞味 ◆味覚に変化が起きましたか Have you noticed any changes in your sense of taste? ◆味覚が鈍っていますか Has your sense of taste *gone dull[become dulled]? / Do the foods you eat tend to taste bland? ▶味覚異常 dysgeusia / impairment of the sense of taste 味覚検査 taste[gustation] test 味覚障害 taste disorder 味覚消失 gustatory anesthesia / loss of the sense of taste 味覚神経 taste nerve 味覚鈍磨 hypogeusia / decreased sensitivity to taste

みがく 磨く （ブラシをかける）**brush** （光沢を出す）**polish, shine** ◆歯を磨く brush *one's* teeth /〈英〉clean *one's* teeth ◆爪を磨く polish *one's* nails

みかくてい 未確定(の) （未解決の）**pending** （あいまいな）**indefinite** ◀診断未確定 not yet diagnosed

みかた 見方 ☞意見，見解，視点

みぎ 右 the right （↔the left）（圏**right** 圏**right**）☞右側，右利き，右向き ◆右を見て下さい Please look to your right. ◆右上

〈右下〉を見て下さい Please look at the upper〈lower〉right-hand corner. ◆右を向いて下さい Please turn to the right. ◆右の目を手で隠して下さい Please cover your right eye with your hand. ◆右の手を出して下さい Please hold out your right hand. ◆右の腕〈足〉を上げる raise *one's* right arm〈leg〉 ◆首を右に傾ける tilt *one's* head to the right ◆右を下にして寝る lie down on *one's* right side ◆右半身が麻痺している *be paralyzed[have paralysis] on the right side of *one's* body ◆右に曲がる turn right ◆右手にある be on[to] the right

みぎがわ 右側（に・の） on *one's*[the] right side, in *one's*[the] right side ◆右側が痛むのですか Is the pain on the right side? ◆右側のお腹が痛む have (a) right-side[sided] abdominal pain / have (an) abdominal pain in *one's* right side ◆原先生のオフィスは右側です Dr Hara's office is on the right side.

みぎきき 右利き be right-handed ◆右利きですか，左利きですか Are you right-handed or left-handed?

みぎむき 右向き（に） on *one's*[the] right side ◆右向きに寝て下さい Please lie on your right side. ◆（寝返りを打って）右向きになって下さい Please roll over onto your right side.

ミクロアルブミンにょう ―尿 microalbuminuria

ミクログロブリン microglobulin ◀β₂ミクログロブリン β_2-microglobulin

ミクロソーム ☞マイクロソーム

みけん 眉間 the space between the eyebrows, the middle of the forehead ◆眉間を軽く叩きますので，眼は開いたままにして下さい Please keep your eyes open while I tap on *the space between your eyebrows[the middle of your forehead]. ◆眉間に皺を寄せる knit *one's* brows

みこみ 見込み （希望）hope （可能性）chance, probability, possibility （実現の見込み）prospect ◆治る見込みがあります

You have a good chance of recovery. / There's a good hope of your recovery. ◆残念ですが，彼女が全快する見込みはあまりありません I'm afraid there's not much hope that she'll recover completely. / I'm afraid the prospect [chance / possibility] of her making a complete recovery is rather small. ◆回復の見込みは30％しかない have only a thirty percent chance of recovery

みこん 未婚（の） single, unmarried ◆未婚の母 a single mother / an unmarried mother ★single mother は離婚した子持ち女性も指す。 ▶未婚女性 single woman 未婚男性 bachelor

みさんぷ 未産婦 nullipara

みじかい 短い short（動shorten）, brief ◆短い期間 a short period ◆短い周期で on a short cycle ◆短い時間ならば痛みを我慢できそうですか Can you *put up with [stand] the pain if it's for a short (period of) time? ◆爪を短く切りすぎないようにして下さい Be careful not to cut your nails too short[（爪の下の組織まで）to the quick]. ◆気が短い be short[quick]-tempered / have a short[quick] temper

みじゅくじ 未熟児 premature baby[infant] ☞低出生体重児 ◆未熟児を産む give birth prematurely / give birth to a premature baby ▶未熟児網膜症 retinopathy of prematurity；ROP

みしょうか 未消化（の） undigested ◆未消化の食べ物を吐く vomit undigested food

みしょうにん 未承認（の） unapproved ▶未承認薬 unapproved medication [drug]

みしょち 未処置 ☞未治療

ミス mistake, error ★error のほうが格式ばった語。 ☞誤り，間違い ◆不注意なミスをする make a careless mistake ◆事務的なミス a clerical mistake[error] ◆人為的なミス (a) human error ◆最近，うっかりミスが多いですか Do you often make careless mistakes? ◆本当にすみません，私のミスでした I'm very sorry. It was my mistake. ◆今後はこのようなミスが起こらないように注意いたします From now on, I'll be more careful not to make the same mistake again. ◀医療ミス medical error / (医療過誤)medical malpractice

みず 水 water (🈨水のような watery) 〈お湯に対して〉cold water 〈水分・液体〉fluid, liquid ◇水分 ◆水を飲む drink water ◆水を飲み込む swallow water ◆肺に水がたまる water[fluid] *builds up[accumulates] in the lung ◆膝から水を抜く remove[drain] the water[fluid] from the knee(s) ◆水に溶ける物質 water-soluble substance ◆水のような鼻水 (a) watery nasal discharge ◆水のような便 watery stools ▶水制限 water restriction 水代謝 water metabolism 水中毒 water intoxication 水負荷試験 water loading test ☞水薬, 水枕

みすい 未遂(の) attempted ◆自殺未遂する attempt to kill *oneself* ◆未遂に終わった自殺(an) attempted suicide ◀自殺未遂 suicide attempt

みずいぼ 水いぼ (伝染性軟属腫)molluscum contagiosum；MC

みずぐすり 水薬 liquid medication ◆水薬を出す〈処方する〉give〈prescribe〉a liquid medication

みすごす 見過ごす ☞見落とす

みずぶくれ 水膨れ ☞水疱

みずぼうそう ☞水痘

みずまくら 水枕 water pillow[cushion]

みずむし 水虫 athlete's foot (足部白癬症)tinea pedis

みせいじゅく 未成熟(な) (未成熟の)immature (未発達の)undeveloped

みせいねんしゃ 未成年者 (法的に)minor (少年・少女)juvenile (🈨juvenile) ▶未成年者犯罪 juvenile crime

みせる¹ 見せる (提示する)show, let ... see ◆保険証を見せて下さい Please show me your insurance card. ◆お薬手帳を持っていたら見せて下さい Can I see[Let me see] your (personal) medication record if you have it with you?

みせる² 診せる (診察させる)let ... take [have] a look, let ... examine (受診する)see ◆すぐに眼科の専門医に診せたほうがいいでしょう You should see an ophthalmologist right away. ◆では, 背中を診せて下さい Well, let me take[have] a look at your back. / Well, let me examine your back.

みぞおち the pit of the stomach, epigastric fossa ◆みぞおちに痛みがある have (a) pain *in the pit of *one's* stomach[(胸骨の下に)just below the breastbone] ◆みぞおちの辺りがもたれる〈むかむかする〉have a sinking〈nauseous〉feeling in the pit of the stomach

みそっぱ 味噌っ歯 decayed milk teeth, decayed baby teeth

みだしなみ 身だしなみ (外見)(personal) appearance (自己管理)self-care (衣服などを整えること)(personal) grooming, grooming activity ◆彼女は身だしなみに無頓着です She takes no interest in *her appearance[(着るもの)what she wears]. / She doesn't care what she looks like. ◆身だしなみに気をつける *take care of [attend to] *one's* appearance ◆身だしなみに興味を失う lose interest in *one's* self-care[appearance]

みたす 満たす 《いっぱいにする》fill ◆ネブライザーのチャンバーにこの薬液を満たして下さい Please fill the nebulizer chamber with this (liquid) medication.
《満足させる》satisfy ◆空腹を満たす satisfy *one's* hunger
《条件に合う》meet ◆あなたの症状は関節リウマチの診断基準を満たしています Your symptoms meet the criteria for diagnosis of rheumatoid arthritis.

みたて 見立て diagnosis ☞診断

みだれる 乱れる (邪魔が入って乱れる)be disturbed (秩序なく混乱する)be in disorder (🈨不規則な irregular) ◆生活のリズムが乱れがちですか Do you have trouble keeping a daily routine? / Is the rhythm of your life often disturbed? ◆脈が乱れています Your pulse is irregular. / You have an irregular pulse.

みちりょう　未治療(の)　untreated　◆未治療の虫歯がある have untreated tooth decay

みっかばしか　三日ばしか　☞風疹

みつかる　見つかる　◆がんが早期のうちに見つかってよかったですね You are lucky that the cancer was found in its early stages.　◆退院後いいヘルパーさんが見つかるといいですね I hope you can find[get] a good home health aide after your discharge from the hospital.

みつご　三つ子　triplets　(3人のうちの1人)a triplet, one of the triplets

みつど　密度　density　◆高密度 high density　骨密度 bone mineral density；BMD　低密度 low density　▶密度計 densitometer　密度計測 densitometry

みつにゅうこくしゃ　密入国者　illegal entrant　(不法移民)illegal immigrant

ミツバチ　bee　☞蜂

みっぷうほうたいほう　密封包帯法　occlusive dressing technique

みてい　未定(の)　(日取りが決まっていない)not scheduled[fixed]　(未決定の)undecided　(不確定の)pending, uncertain　◆手術の日取りは未定です The date of the surgery hasn't been scheduled[fixed] yet.

みとおし　見通し　(展望)**outlook**　(見込み・将来性)**prospect**　◆今後の治療の見通しについて話し合いましょう Let's talk about the outlook for your treatment.　◆明るい見通し a bright prospect　◆暗い見通し a gloomy prospect

ミトコンドリア　mitochondria　(単mitochondrion)　(形mitochondrial)　▶ミトコンドリア脳筋症 mitochondrial encephalomyopathy

みとめる　認める
《受け入れる》**accept**　(過ちなどを)**admit**　◆彼はその状況を認めなかった He refused to accept the situation.　◆ミスを認めて謝る admit one's mistake and apologize
《許可する》**allow**　(正式に)**permit**　◆残念ですが，外泊は認められません I'm sorry, but you are not allowed to *go home for

the night[stay home overnight].
《認定する》**recognize**　(正式に)**approve**　◆この薬は喘息の標準的治療薬として認められています This medication is recognized[approved] as a standard treatment for asthma.
《所見を認識する》　◆検査の結果，異常は認められません The test results do not show *anything wrong with you[any abnormality].　◆インフルエンザの徴候が認められます There are signs of the flu. / Flu signs are present.

みどりいろ　緑色(の)　green　(緑色がかった)greenish　◆緑色の痰 green phlegm　◆緑色がかった便 greenish stools　◆黄緑色の分泌物 greenish yellow discharge

みとる　看取る　be at a person's deathbed　◆看護師の星と私がご主人の最期を看取りました Nurse Hoshi and I were at your husband's bedside when he died. / Nurse Hoshi and I cared for your husband on his deathbed.

ミドルネーム　middle name　☞名前

みなおす　見直す　(再考する)**reconsider, rethink**　(再検討する)**review**　◆生活習慣を見直して下さい Please reconsider[rethink] your daily habits or way of life.　◆治療計画を見直す review the treatment plan

みなみアフリカきょうわこく　南アフリカ共和国　South Africa　(形South African)　☞国籍　▶南アフリカ共和国人(の)South African

みなり　身なり　☞身だしなみ

みにつける　身につける
《習得する》**acquire**　(癖などをつける)**develop**　◆規則的な運動習慣を身につけて下さい You should get into the habit of doing regular exercise. / You should develop the habit of exercising regularly.　◆人工肛門の管理法を身につける acquire skills in caring for the stoma / learn how to care for one's stoma
《所持する》**carry**　◆発作が起きた時のために薬は常に身につけて下さい Please carry your medication with you at all times in

case of an attack.

《衣服などを着ける》**wear** ◆検査当日はゆったりした服を身につけておいで下さい Please wear loose-fitting clothes for the test. ◆身につけている装身具はすべて外して下さい Please remove[take off] all of your jewelry.

ミネソタためんじんかくもくろく —多面人格目録 **Minnesota Multiphasic Personality Inventory；MMPI**

ミネラル mineral ▶ミネラルウォーター mineral water　ミネラルコルチコイド mineralocorticoid

みのがす 見逃す miss ☞見落とす

みのまわり 身の回り ◆身の回りの品 *one's* belongings[things] ◆身の回りの世話をする look after *a person* / take care of *a person* ◆退院後身の回りの世話をしてくれる人はお近くにいますか Do you have someone nearby who can *look after you[take care of you] after your discharge from the hospital? ◆身の回りを整理する put *one's* affairs in order

みはる 見張る watch ◆誰かに常に見張られているような気がしますか Do you have the feeling of being constantly watched? / Do you feel as if you're being constantly watched?

みはれつどうみゃくりゅう 未破裂脳動脈瘤 unruptured cerebral aneurysm

みひらく 見開く 《眼を》**open** *one's* **eyes wide**

みぶり 身振り gesture（囮**gesture**）◆「さようなら」の身振りをする make a gesture of 'goodbye' / gesture[motion] 'goodbye' to *someone*

みぶん 身分 《身元》**identity** 《身分証明》**identification：ID**（囮**identify**）《公的な地位》**status** ☞身元 ◆身分を証明するものを見せて下さい（身分証）Please show me your ID. ◆身分を証明するものをお持ちですか Do you have any ID[identification] with you? / Are you carrying any (form of) ID[identification]? ▶身分証明 proof of identity　身分証明書 ID[identity / identification] card　身分証明書類

identity[identification] document / identity[identification] papers

みぶんか 未分化(の) undifferentiated（退形成性の）**anaplastic** ▶未分化癌 undifferentiated[anaplastic] carcinoma　未分化細胞 undifferentiated cell

みまい 見舞い visit ☞面会 ▶見舞い客 visitor

みまもる 見守る 《注意して見る》**keep** *one's* **eye** (**on**)**, watch** (**over**) 《様子を見る》**wait and see** ◆患者を見守る keep an eye on the patient ◆彼の病状を注意深く見守る keep a careful eye on his condition / watch his condition carefully ◆成り行きを見守る必要があります We'll have to wait and see how things turn out.

みまわる 見回る make[do, go on] *one's* **rounds** ◆平日は医師が毎朝見回ります The doctor makes her〈his〉rounds every weekday morning.

みみ 耳 ear 《聴力》**hearing**

《診察の基本表現》◆耳の具合はどうですか How are your ears? ◆耳に何か問題がありますか Do you have any problems with your ears? ◆お子さんがどちらかの耳を引っ張るのに気づきましたか Have you noticed your child tugging at one of his〈her〉ears? ◆お子さんは耳の感染症によくかかりますか Does your child often have ear infections? ◆耳を診察しましょう I'm going to examine your ears. ◆耳が炎症を起こしています The inside of the ear [The ear] is inflamed.

《聴こえ具合を尋ねる》◆耳の聞こえ方はどうですか How is your hearing? ◆最近，耳の聞こえ方に変化がありましたか。耳鳴りがしたり，音がこもって聞こえたりしますか Have you noticed any changes in your hearing? Any ringing or muffling in the ears? ◆耳はよく聞こえますか Do you hear well? / Is your hearing good? ◆両方の耳で同じように聞こえますか Do you hear the same in both ears? ◆耳が聞こえにくいのは高音のみ，低音のみ，それともあらゆる音ですか Do you have difficulty hearing high-pitched sounds only, low-pitched sounds only, or all sounds? ◆耳が遠くなりましたか Are you hard of hearing? ◆左耳がよく聞こえない can't hear well in *one's* left ear ◆耳がいい have good hearing / hear well / have good ears

《他の症状の表現》 ◆耳が痛い have *(an) earache[(a) pain in *one's* ear(s)] ◆耳の中から出血している be bleeding from the inside of the ear ◆耳が詰まった感じがする feel as if *one's* ears are blocked [plugged / clogged](up) ◆耳がかゆい *one's* ears are itchy / have itchy ears ◆耳に異物が入る get something in *one's* ear / get a foreign object stuck in the ear ◆耳に水が入る water enters the ear (canal) ◆耳に虫が入る an insect crawls [(飛び込む)flies] into the ear (canal) ◆耳に尖った物を入れる stick[insert] a sharp object in *one's* ear

◀折れ耳 folded ear /（たれ耳）lop ear 片耳 one ear / one of the ears カリフラワー耳 cauliflower ear ☞耳垢, 耳掻き, 耳障り, 耳栓, 耳たぶ, 耳だれ, 耳鳴り

みみあか 耳垢 **earwax, ear wax, cerumen** ☞耳垢(じこう) ◆外耳道は耳垢で詰まっています The ear canals are blocked with wax. ◆耳垢がたまる earwax builds up ◆耳垢を取る remove earwax / clean *one's* ears

みみかき 耳掻き **earpick** （綿棒）**cotton swab** ◆耳掻きをする clean *one's* ears ◆耳掻きはしばらくやめて下さい Please refrain from *using an earpick[cleaning your ears with a cotton swab] for a while.

みみざわり 耳障り（な）**unpleasant to the ear(s)** ◆耳障りな音（嫌な感じの）an unpleasant sound /（ギシギシときしむような）a grating sound /（ざわざわして癇に障る）a harsh sound

みみずばれ ─腫れ **welt**

みみせん 耳栓 **earplug, ear plug** ◆耳栓を着けている wear earplugs ◆耳栓をする *put in[insert] earplugs

みみそうじ 耳掃除 ☞耳掻き

みみたぶ 耳たぶ **earlobe**

みみだれ 耳だれ **ear discharge, otor-**

rhea ◆耳だれがありますか Do you have any discharge from your ear(s)?

みみなり 耳鳴り **ringing（sound）in the ears, tinnitus** ◆耳鳴りがしますか Do you have any ringing in the ear(s)? ◆耳鳴りが始まったのはいつですか When did the ringing[tinnitus] start? ◆耳鳴りが聞こえるのは片耳ですか, 両耳ですか, あるいは頭の中ですか Do you hear the ringing in one ear or both, or inside your head? ◆耳鳴りはどんな音ですか What does the ringing sound like? / What kind of ringing sound do you hear in your ear(s)? ◆耳鳴りはブーンブーンという音ですか Do you hear a buzzing sound[noise] in your ears? ◀高音性〈低音性〉耳鳴り high-pitched〈low-pitched〉tinnitus[ringing (in the ears)] 拍動性耳鳴り pulsatile tinnitus[ringing (in the ears)]

耳鳴りの音

耳鳴りの表現は文化によって, また人によって様々である. 英語圏では日本語に比べて擬音語で表現することが少ない. たとえ物理的には同じ音でも, 欧米人の耳は違う音として捉えて異なる表現を用いることがよくある. 以下, 代表的な耳鳴りの表現例を挙げる.

●一般的な耳鳴り音（鐘・呼び鈴などのような音）ringing（sound） ●カチカチ（時計のチクタク音）ticking（sound） ●カチッカチッ（クリック音）clicking（sound） ●キーキー（戸がきしむような音）creaking（sound） ●キーン / キキーッ（急ブレーキのような甲高い金属音）screeching（sound） ●ギシギシ（やすりでこすったようなきしみ音）grating（sound） ●ゴーゴー（滝の音・トンネルを通る時の轟音）roaring（sound） ●ザーザー（激しい流水音）rushing（sound） /（滝の音）waterfall（sound） ●チーチー（小鳥・虫が鳴く音）chirping（sound） ●ジージー（こおろぎが鳴くような音）cricket-like chirping [sound] ●シューシュー（蒸気の音・ヘビが出す音）hissing（sound） ●シュー / ヒュー（空気・水などが噴き出る音）whooshing（sound） ●チリンチリン / リンリン

（鈴などが出す音）tinkling (sound) ●ドクンドクン（拍動性の音）throbbing (sound) / pulsing[pulsating] (sound) ●パリパリ / バリバリ / カリカリ（煎餅を嚙み割るような音）crackling (sound) ●ヒューヒュー / ピーピー（口笛のような音）whistling (sound) ●ブーンブーン（ハエ・蜂の羽音）buzzing [humming] (sound)

みもと 身元 identity ☞身分 ◆身元を証明する prove *one's* identity ◆身元を保証してくれる人がいますか Do you have a guarantor? / Do you have someone who acts as a guarantor for you? ▶身元保証人（身元引受けの）guarantor / （人物証明の）reference / 《英》referee

みゃく 脈 pulse ◆脈を測りましょう Let me take[check] your pulse. ◆手首で脈をとる feel *a person's* pulse in[at] the wrist / feel *a person's* wrist pulse ◆脈は1分間に70です Your pulse is seventy a minute. / You gave a pulse of seventy beats a minute. ◆脈は60から70です Your pulse rate is between sixty and seventy. ◆脈が速くなりますか Do you feel your *heart beating fast[pulse quickens]? ◆脈が遅くなる the pulse slows down ◆脈が速い the pulse is fast[rapid / quick] ◆脈が遅い the pulse is slow ◆脈が弱い the pulse is weak [faint / feeble] ◆かすかに脈がある have a faint pulse / （脈が弱い）*one's* pulse is faint[weak / feeble] ◆脈は正常である the pulse is normal ◆脈はしっかりしている the pulse is steady ◆脈が規則的（不規則）である the pulse is regular〈irregular〉 ◆脈が途切れる the pulse becomes [is] intermittent / （跳ぶ）the heart skips beats ◀奇脈 paradoxical pulse　交互脈 alternating pulse　徐脈 infrequent pulse / bradycardia　速脈 quick[rapid] pulse　遅脈 slow pulse　二段脈 bigeminy / bigeminal pulse　頻脈 frequent pulse / tachycardia　不整脈 irregular [unequal] pulse / arrhythmia ▶脈圧 pulse pressure　脈なし病 pulseless dis-

ease / （大動脈炎症候群）aortitis syndrome ☞脈拍

みゃくかん 脈管 vessel （腟vascular） ◆腫瘍の脈管侵襲 tumor invasion into the vessels ▶脈管系 the vascular system

みゃくはく 脈拍 pulse ☞脈 ▶脈拍欠損 missing beat / pulse deficit　脈拍数 pulse rate

みゃくらくそう 脈絡叢 choroid plexus

みゃくらくまく 脈絡膜 choroid (membrane) ▶脈絡膜疾患 choroid disease

みやざきはいきゅうちゅう 宮崎肺吸虫 *Paragonimus miyazaki*

ミャンマー Myanmar （腟Burmese） ☞国籍 ▶ミャンマー人（の）Burmese

ミュンヒハウゼンしょうこうぐん ―症候群 Münchausen syndrome

みょうじ 名字 family name, surname （↔given name） （特に欧米人の姓）last name ☞名前

みより 身寄り relative

みらい 味蕾 taste bud, gustatory bud

ミリグラム milligram /mílɪɡræm/；mg ◆この薬の用量は0.5と0.25 mgの2種類あります This medication comes in 0.5- and 0.25-milligram tablets. / This medication comes in two strengths: 0.5 and 0.25 milligrams. ★point five and point two five または zero point five and zero point two five と読む.

ミリメートル millimeter /mílɪmìːtə/；mm ◆直径7 mmのポリープ a polyp of seven millimeters in diameter[size] ◆幅が5 mmです That's five millimeters across. ◀水銀柱ミリメートル millimeters of mercury；mmHg

ミリリットル milliliter /mílɪlìːtə/；ml, mL ◆お子さんは毎日ミルクを何ミリリットル飲みますか How many milliliters of milk [formula] does your baby take each day? ◆100 mLの水 one hundred milliliters of water

みる¹ 見る 《見る》 （目に入る）see （意識的に注意して見る）look (at), take a look (at) （テレビなどを）watch ☞見える ◆目を開けたまま

真っ直ぐ前を見て下さい Please keep your eyes open and look straight ahead. ◆近くの物を見る see[look at] things close at hand / see close[near] objects ◆遠くの物を見る see[look at] an object at a distance / see distant[faraway] objects ◆テレビをよく見ますか Do you often watch TV?
《観察する》see, observe ◆しばらく様子を見ましょう Let's wait for a while and see how things go[develop]. ◆私の見るところでは…In my opinion …
《世話をする》look（after）, take care（of）, care（for）◆入院中はどなたがお子さんの面倒を見ているのですか Who is looking after your child while you're in the hospital? ◆お勤めの間誰がお子さんの面倒を見ていますか Who *looks after[takes care of] your child while you're at work?

みる²　診る　(診察する)see, examine, look (at), take a look (at)　(診察してもらう) see　◆では背中を診ましょう Now, let me see[examine] your back.　◆しこりを見せて下さい Let me take a look at the lump. ◆かかりつけ医に診てもらいましたか Did you see your regular[family] doctor? ◆形成外科の専門医に診てもらって下さい Please see a plastic surgeon.　◆担当医がすぐに診ます Your doctor will *be with you[see you] shortly.

ミルク　milk　(粉ミルク) powdered milk, milk powder　(調整粉乳) formula（milk）(母乳) breast milk　(牛乳) cow's milk ☞乳(ちち), 乳(にゅう), 母乳　◆ミルクを飲む drink milk /（乳首から吸う）suck milk ◆ミルクを普通どおり飲みましたか Did he〈she〉have his〈her〉milk as normal? ◆ミルクの飲みは悪いですか(乳首からの吸いが弱い) Is his〈her〉sucking ability weak? / Is his〈her〉ability to suck milk weak? ◆ミルクを飲むのを嫌がりますか Does he〈she〉refuse to take milk?　◆ミルクで育てる(哺乳瓶で)bottlefeed a baby　◆ミルクで育った子供(哺乳瓶で)a bottlefed child
▶ミルクアルカリ症候群 milk-alkali syndrome　ミルクアレルギー milk allergy

みわける　見分ける　distinguish, differentiate　◆腫瘍が良性か悪性かを見分ける distinguish benign from malignant tumors / distinguish the difference between benign and malignant tumors ◆がんの種類を見分けるために腫瘍の生検をします I'm going to do a biopsy of the tumor to differentiate[determine] what type of cancer it is.
みんかん　民間(の)　private（↔public）(民間伝承の)folk　▶民間医療保険 private medical insurance　民間薬 folk remedy [medication]　民間療法 folk remedy
みんざい　眠剤　☞睡眠薬
みんせいいいん　民生委員　community welfare volunteer, district welfare volunteer, commissioned welfare volunteer

む

むいしき 無意識(の) (意識の無い)unconscious (不随意の)involuntary ◆無意識状態に陥る fall unconscious / fall into *an unconscious state[unconsciousness] ◆無意識の動作 involuntary movement ◆無意識に傷口を掻かないで下さい Be careful not to scratch (at) the wound unconsciously.

ムーンフェイス moon face

むえいとう 無影灯 shadowless lamp, operating light, surgical light

むえん 無塩(の) salt-free ☞減塩

むかい 向かい(に) (向こう側に)across from (横切って向こうに)across (反対側に)opposite ◆超音波検査室はレントゲン室の向かいです The ultrasound room is *across from[opposite] the X-ray room. ◆健診センターは通りを挟んで当病院の向かいにあります The health screening center is across the street from this hospital.

むがい 無害(の) (害を及ぼさない)harmless (良性の)innocent ◆金属の手術用クリップは身体に無害です Metal surgical clips are harmless to the body. ▶無害性(心)雑音 innocent murmur

むかえる 迎える
《連れて帰る》come and take ◆迎えに来てくれる人がいますか Is there someone who can come and take you home?
《過ごす》spend ◆自宅で〈ホスピスで〉最期を迎える spend *one's* last[final] days *at home〈in a hospice〉 ◆静かに死を迎える die peacefully / die a peaceful death / meet *one's* death calmly

むかし 昔 (過去)the past (昔の日々)the old days ☞過去 ◆昔のことを覚えている remember things that happened in the past ◆昔を思い出す remember[recall] the past ◆昔を懐かしむ miss the (good) old days / reminisce about the past[good old days]

むかつく
《吐き気がする》feel nauseous[sick, queasy] ◆胃がむかつく have an upset stomach / have a nauseous feeling in the stomach / feel sick (in *one's* stomach) / (吐きそうだ)feel *as if[like] *one* is going to throw up
《腹が立つ》get angry (いらいらする)get irritable ☞怒りっぽい, 怒る

むかりゅうきゅうしょう 無顆粒球症 agranulocytosis

むかんかく 無感覚(な) (しびれた)numb (鈍感な)insensible, insensitive ◆彼女は指先が無感覚になっています Her fingertips have become numb. ◆痛みに無感覚である be insensible to (the) pain

むかんけい 無関係(である) (関係ない)be not related (to) (妥当性がない)be irrelevant (to) (まったく関係がない)have nothing to do (with) ◆この症状は食事とは無関係です This symptom is not related to diet. ◆この病気は遺伝とは無関係です This disease has nothing to do with heredity.

むかんしょう 無汗症 anhidrosis

むかんじょう 無感情 ☞無関心, 無気力

むかんしん 無関心(な) (無頓着な)indifferent (to) (興味がない)uninterested (やる気のない)apathetic ☞無気力 ◆彼女は身だしなみに無関心です She is quite indifferent to[She takes no interest in] her appearance. ◆彼はこれまで楽しんでいたことに無関心になっています He has lost interest in the things he used to enjoy. ▶無関心状態 apathetic state

むガンマグロブリンけっしょう 無ガンマグロブリン血症 agammaglobulinemia

むき¹ 向き (位置)position (側面)side (方角)way, direction ☞体位(囲み：体位・動作の指示), 方向, 向く, 向ける ◆向きを変えて下さい Please turn around. ◆床ずれができないように体の向きを頻繁に変えて下さい Please change your position frequently to prevent bedsores. ◆体の向きを変えるのをお手伝いしましょう Let me help you *change your position[move onto your other side]. ◆右〈左〉向きに寝る lie on one's right〈left〉 side ◆横向きに眠る sleep on one's side ◆逆向き the opposite side[way / direction]

むき² 無機(の) inorganic (↔organic) ▶無機化合物 inorganic compound 無機水銀 inorganic mercury 無機物 inorganic matter[substance] 無機リン inorganic phosphorus 無機リン酸塩 inorganic phosphate

むきしつ 無機質 mineral ◀骨無機質 bone mineral

むきのうじん 無機能腎 nonfunctioning kidney

むきはい 無気肺 atelectasis （肺虚脱）collapsed lung, pulmonary[lung] collapse ◀板状無気肺 discoid[platelike] atelectasis 閉塞性無気肺 obstructive atelectasis

むきゅうかく 無嗅覚 anosmia

むきりょく 無気力 （無関心）apathy /ǽpəθi/ (形apathetic) （無感情）lack of feeling or emotion （無感動・嗜眠性）lethargy /léθədʒi/ (形lethárgic) （体力減退）loss of energy ☞無関心 ◆無気力な状態に陥る sink into apathy / lose all interest in anything ◆無気力な気分から抜け出す overcome one's apathy[apathetic mood] ◆疲れて無気力である be tired and lethargic / have no energy because of fatigue

むきん 無菌(の) sterile /stérəl/ (名sterility), germfree, aseptic ▶無菌室 clean[bioclean / germfree] room 無菌状態 sterility 無菌性髄膜炎 aseptic meningitis 無菌性膿疱 sterile[aseptic] pustule

むきんちょう 無緊張 atony /ǽtəni/ (形atónic) ▶無緊張性神経因性膀胱 atonic neurogenic bladder

むく 向く （体の向きを変える）turn （視線を向ける）look ☞体位(囲み：体位・動作の指示), 向き, 向ける ◆後ろを向いて下さい Please turn around. ◆こちらを向いて下さい(視線を)Please look this way. / (顔を)Please face this way. / (体を)Please turn over this way. ◆反対を向いて下さい Please turn over. ◆右〈左〉を向く turn to the right〈left〉 / look to one's right〈left〉 ◆上を向く look up[upward] ◆下を向く look down[downward] ◆正面を向く face forward / turn toward

むくみ 腫脹 (generalized) swelling (形swollen) (浮腫)edema /idíːmə/ ☞浮腫, むくむ ◆足にむくみが出たことはありますか Have you ever had any swelling in your legs[feet]? / Have your legs[feet] ever become swollen? ◆むくみが引く the swelling decreases[goes down] ◆むくみがひどくなる the swelling increases[gets worse] ◆足のむくみを診ましょう Let me[I'm going to] examine your legs for swelling. ◆足のむくみをとるには足を心臓より高く上げるとよいでしょう To reduce the leg swelling, you should raise your legs above the level of your heart.

むくむ 腫れる have swelling (形swollen) (顔などが)have bloating (形bloated) ☞浮腫, むくみ ◆足がむくんでいますか Are your legs swollen? / Do you have swollen legs? ◆体がどこかむくんでいますか Does any area of your body feel swollen? / Do you have any swelling[bloating] anywhere[in any part of your body]? ◆顔がむくんでいます Your face looks[is] swollen[bloated]. / You have a swollen[bloated] face. ◆むくんだ部位を押すと凹みはすぐに元に戻りますか, 凹んだままになっていますか After you press on the swollen area, does the dent[depression] spring back promptly or does it remain there?

むけいせい 無形成 aplasia
むけっかんや 無血管野 avascular area
むげっけい 無月経 amenorrhea, absence of menstruation ◀高プロラクチン血症性無月経 hyperprolactinemic amenorrhea 産褥無月経 puerperal amenorrhea 授乳性無月経 lactation amenorrhea ▶無月経乳汁漏出症候群 amenorrhea-galactorrhea syndrome

むける¹ 向ける （向きを変える）turn （意識などを集中させる）focus （注意・視線などを向ける）direct ☞体位(囲み：体位・動作の指示), 向き, 向く ◆両方の手のひらを上に向けて下さい Please turn both palms up. ◆こちらに顔を向けて下さい Please turn (your face) toward me. ◆体を逆方向に向ける turn one's body to the opposite side ◆ご自分の健康に注意を向ける必要があります You need to *focus your attention on[direct your attention to] your own health.

むける² 剥ける peel off （取れる）come off （薄片になって落ちる）flake off （うろこ状になって落ちる）scale off （ぼろぼろに崩れる）crumble off ☞剥がれる ◆彼の鼻の皮膚がむけています The skin on his nose is peeling. ◆火傷で皮膚がむける the skin peels off as a result of burns

むこう¹ 無効（な） no good （法的・正式な効力がない）invalid （効果のない）ineffective ◆このクレジットカードは無効です This credit card is invalid[not valid]. / （断られた）This credit card has been declined. ◆この薬は不整脈を抑えるのには無効でした This medication was ineffective[not effective] in suppressing the arrhythmia.

むこう² 向こう （向こう側）the other side （反対側）the opposite side ☞あちら, 向かい ◆トイレは廊下の向こう側にあります The restroom is on the other[opposite] side of the hallway.

むこうじょうちゅう 無鉤条虫 Taenia saginata, beef tapeworm

むこうずね 向こう脛 shin

むこうとうはっせい 無喉頭発声 alaryngeal voice[speech]

ムコールしょう ―症 mucormycosis

むこきゅう 無呼吸 apnea /ǽpniːə/, absence of breathing ◆睡眠中の無呼吸を指摘されたことがありますか Have you ever been told that you stop breathing while you sleep? ◆昼間の異常な眠気は睡眠中の無呼吸が原因である可能性があります Excessive daytime sleepiness may

be caused by absence of breathing during night-time sleep. ◀睡眠時無呼吸症候群 sleep apnea syndrome；SAS 中枢性睡眠時無呼吸 central sleep apnea；CSA 閉塞性睡眠時無呼吸 obstructive sleep apnea；OSA ▶無呼吸低呼吸指数 apnea-hypopnea index；AHI 無呼吸発作 apneic spell

ムコたとうしょう ―多糖症 mucopolysaccharidosis；MPS

むさくい 無作為（の） random （無作為化した）randomized ▶無作為化比較試験 randomized controlled trial；RCT 無作為化臨床試験 randomized clinical trial；RCT 無作為抽出 random sampling 無作為抽出標本 random sample 無作為割付 random allocation

むさんそ 無酸素（性の） （無酸素症による）anoxic （嫌気性の）anaerobic（↔aerobic） ▶無酸素（性）閾値 anaerobic threshold；AT 無酸素運動 anaerobic exercise / anaerobics 無酸素性脳障害 anoxic brain damage

むし¹ 虫 （昆虫）insect （小さな虫）bug （寄生虫など這う虫）worm ◆虫に刺される be bitten by *an insect[a bug] ▶虫アレルギー insect allergy / allergy to insects ☞虫下し, 虫刺され

むし² 無視する （注意を払わない）ignore, pay no attention (to) （気づかない）not take any notice (of) （軽視・放置する）neglect（図neglect） ◆担当医の忠告を無視する ignore[pay no attention to] one's doctor's advice ◆わずかに白血球が少なめですが, この程度は無視して大丈夫です Your white blood cells *are slightly low [have gone down slightly], but it's nothing you need to *worry about[take any notice of]. ◀半側空間無視 hemispatial[unilateral spatial] neglect

むし³ 霧視 blurred vision, blurry vision

むしくだし 虫下し （駆虫薬）antiparasitic (drug), anthelmintic

むしさされ 虫刺され insect bite[sting]

むしば 虫歯 tooth decay /díkéi/, dental caries （虫歯の穴）dental cavity ◆虫歯が

ありますか Do you have any *tooth decay [(dental) cavities]? ◆虫歯が痛む have (a) toothache caused by tooth decay ◆虫歯を治す repair tooth decay ◆虫歯に詰め物をする fill a cavity[decayed tooth] ◆規則的に歯を磨いて虫歯を防ぐ prevent tooth decay by brushing one's teeth regularly

むしぼう 無脂肪(の) **fat-free** ◆無脂肪の乳製品 fat-free dairy products

むしゅう 無臭(の) **odorless** ◆無臭の分泌物 odorless discharge

むじょうけん 無条件(に) (条件を付けずに)**unconditionally** (🔁**unconditional** 条件付けによるものでない **unconditioned**) (完全に)**completely** ◆ネット上の情報を無条件に信じるのは危険です It's dangerous to believe everything you read on the internet unconditionally. ◆そのご意見には無条件で賛成します I completely agree with that opinion. ▶無条件刺激 unconditioned stimulus 無条件反射 unconditioned reflex

むしょうこうせい 無症候性(の) (症状のない)**asymptomatic, symptomless, silent** (不顕性・潜在性の)**subclinical** ▶無症候性感染 silent[symptomless／asymptomatic／subclinical] infection 無症候性キャリア silent[asymptomatic／healthy] carrier 無症候性結石 silent[asymptomatic] stone 無症候性血尿 asymptomatic hematuria 無症候性心筋虚血 silent[asymptomatic／painless] myocardial ischemia 無症候性蛋白尿 asymptomatic proteinuria

むしょく 無色(の) **colorless**

むすう 無数(の) (多数の)**numerous** (数えきれない)**countless, innumerable** ◆彼の脳に無数の転移巣が見つかりました We've found numerous metastatic lesions in his brain.

むずかしい 難しい (困難な)**hard, difficult** (🔁**difficulty**) (深刻な)**serious** ◆立ち上がるのが難しい have difficulty standing up ◆彼が完治するのは難しいでしょう(可能性が低い)It is unlikely[(疑わしい)doubt-

ful] that he will recover completely.／It will be difficult for him to make a full recovery. ◆病状が以前より難しくなっています The symptom is more serious than before. ◆できることはすべてしましたが, 彼女はまだ非常に難しい状況にあります I did everything I could (do), but *she is still in (a) very serious condition[her condition is still very serious].

むずがゆい むず痒い feel itchy, itch ☞痒い, むずむず ◆足がむず痒い one's legs feel[are] itchy／one's legs itch

ムスカリン muscarine (🔁**muscarinic**) ▶ムスカリン受容体拮抗薬 muscarinic (receptor) antagonist ムスカリン様効果 muscarinic effect ムスカリン様作用 muscarinic action

むずかる (ぐずる)**fret** (ぐずっている)**be fretful**

むすこ 息子 son

むすぶ 結ぶ tie (縛る)**bind** ◆三角巾の両端を結ぶ tie the two ends of the triangular bandage together

むずむず(する) (かゆい)**feel itchy** (喉などがいがらっぽい)**tickle** (虫などが這っている感じがする)**have a crawling sensation** ◆夜に足がむずむずする感じがしますか Are you bothered by a crawling sensation in your legs at night? ◆鼻がむずむずする have an itchy nose／one's nose tickles ▶むずむず脚症候群 restless legs syndrome；RLS

むすめ 娘 daughter

ムスリム Muslim ☞イスラム教

むせい 夢精 wet dream (夜間遺精)**nocturnal emission**

むせいししょう 無精子症 azoospermia

むせきたんのうえん 無石胆嚢炎 acalculous cholecystitis

むせる choke (on, over) ◆食べ物や飲み物によくむせますか Do you often choke on your food or drink? ◆むせるような咳が出る have a choking cough

むだ 無駄(な) (意味がない)**meaningless** (役に立たない)**useless** ◆彼女に忠告しても無駄です It would be meaningless[useless] to give her any advice. / There's *no point[not much point] in giving her any advice.

むだん　無断(で)　(許可なしに)without permission　(通知なしに)without notice　◆病院を無断で外出する *go out of[leave] the hospital without permission[notice]　◆無断で仕事を休む be absent from work without notice　▶無断外泊 staying home overnight without (one's doctor's) permission

むちうち　鞭打ち　whiplash (injury)　▶鞭打ち損傷 whiplash injury

むちゃ　無茶(な)　(過度な)excessive　(理不尽な)unreasonable　▷無理　◆無茶な食事と飲酒 excessive[binge] eating and drinking　◆それは無茶な注文です That's an unreasonable request. / That's asking too much.　◆無茶な要求をする make unreasonable demands

むつう　無痛(の)　(痛みのない)painless　(無徴候の)silent, asymptomatic　(痛みが緩慢な)indolent　▶無痛性潰瘍 painless[silent / indolent] ulcer　無痛性甲状腺炎 painless[silent] thyroiditis　無痛性心筋虚血 painless[silent / asymptomatic] myocardial ischemia　無痛分娩 painless labor[delivery]

むどう　無動　akinesia (形akinetic)　▶無動発作 akinetic seizure　無動無言症 akinetic mutism

むとどけ　無届け(で)　☞無断

むなぐるしい　胸苦しい　feel tight[pressure] in one's chest　(息苦しい)be[feel, become, get] short of breath　◆胸苦しいのですか Does your chest feel tight? / Do you feel tight in your chest?　◆発作で胸苦しくなりましたか Did the attack make your chest feel tight? / Did you become short of breath because of the attack?

むなげ　胸毛　chest hair　◆手術前に胸毛を剃りましょう Let me shave your chest hair before the surgery.

むなしい　空しい・虚しい　(意味がない)meaningless　(空虚な)hollow, empty　(成果のない)fruitless　(役に立たない)useless

◆人生はむなしいと思いますか Do you feel as if life *is meaningless[has no meaning]? / Do you think that life is hollow [empty]?　◆むなしい努力をする make fruitless efforts / make efforts for nothing

むにょう　無尿　anuria, absence of urine production　◆いつから無尿の状態ですか Since when have you had no urine output?

むにんか　無認可(の)　(免許を受けていない)non-licensed　(法的に認可されていない)unauthorized　▶無認可保育園 non-licensed day care center

むね　胸　chest　(乳房)breast　(心臓)heart　☞胸部
《診察の基本表現》　◆胸が痛いのですか Do you have (any) *chest pain[pain in your chest]?　◆これまでに胸に痛みや不快感がありましたか Have you ever had (any) chest pain or discomfort?　◆階段を上がったり坂を上ったりする時胸が痛みますか Do you have chest pain when you *go up [climb up] stairs or slopes?　◆胸を出して下さい(上半身を脱ぐ)Please take off *your clothes from the waist up[your top things].　◆胸を拝見しましょう(乳房を)Let me examine your breasts.　◆胸の音を聴きましょう(肺音と心音を)I'm going to listen to your lungs and heart.　◆来週胸のX線写真を撮りましょう Let's take *a chest X-ray[an X-ray of your chest] next week.
《症状の表現》　◆胸が息苦しい be[feel] become / get] short of breath　◆胸が重苦しい(圧迫感)*feel pressure[(絞扼感)feel tight / (息が詰まるような感じ)have a stifling sensation] in one's chest　◆胸がつかえる(窒息しそうな感じがする)have a choking feeling　◆食べ物が胸につかえる(喉に)food gets stuck in the throat　◆胸がどきどきする one's heart beats fast[rapidly]　◆胸がむかむかする feel nauseous [queasy]　◆胸が焼ける get[have] heartburn
◀鳩胸 pigeon[chicken] breast　☞胸焼け

むねやけ　胸焼け　heartburn　◆胸焼け

ますか Do you have (any) heartburn? ◆胸焼けはどのくらい続いていますか How long have you had the heartburn? ◆胸焼けを鎮める relieve[alleviate] (one's) heartburn

むのうしょう 無脳症 anencephaly

むはいらん 無排卵 anovulation (形anovulatory) ▶無排卵性月経 anovulatory menstruation 無排卵性周期 anovulatory (menstrual) cycle

むひょうじょう 無表情(な) expressionless ◆彼は無表情な顔をしている He does not show any expression in his face. / He has *an expressionless face[(仮面のような顔)a masklike face / (ぼうっとした顔)a blank expression].

むぼうび 無防備(な) (保護されていない)unprotected (抵抗力がない)defenseless ◆無防備な性交の危険性 risks of unprotected sex

むゆうびょう 夢遊病 sleepwalking, somnambulism ▶夢遊病患者 sleepwalker

むゆけつしゅじゅつ 無輸血手術 surgery without blood transfusion

むよくせい 無抑制(の) uninhibited ▶無抑制性神経因性膀胱 uninhibited neurogenic bladder 無抑制尿失禁 uninhibited incontinence

むらがある (不安定な)unstable (まばらな)patchy ◆彼女は気分にむらがあります She is emotionally unstable. ◆むらのある脱毛 patchy hair loss

むらさき 紫(の) (赤みがかった)purple (青みがかった)bluish ◆唇と指の爪が紫色になる one's lips and fingernails turn[become] purple ◆皮膚に紫色のあざがある have purple bruises[patches] on one's skin

むり 無理
《無理だ》(不可能だ)impossible ◆その日に検査をするのは無理です It's impossible to do the test on that day. ◆赤ちゃんは小さすぎてその手術は無理です The baby is too small[young] to have the surgery.
《無理もない》(当然だ)natural ◆気が滅入

るのも無理はありません It's natural that you should feel depressed.
《無理をする》(やり過ぎる)overdo ◆疲れたら無理をしないで休息をとって下さい When you get tired, don't overdo yourself, but take some rest. ◆無理をしないように(頑張りすぎないように)Don't overdo things. / Don't push yourself too hard. / (働き過ぎないように)Don't work too hard. / (くだけた調子で「のんびりやろうよ」)Take it easy.
《無理やり…する》(強制する)force *a person* to do … ◆お子さんには無理やり食べさせないほうがいいですよ You shouldn't force your child to eat. ◆無理に吐く(誘発する)induce vomiting / make *oneself* vomit

むりょう 無料(の) free (of charge) ◆この小冊子は無料です．ご自由にお持ち下さい This brochure is free (of charge). Please feel free to take one. ◆院内の無料サービス free services in the hospital ▶無料胃がん検診 free stomach[gastric] cancer screening[checkup] 無料駐車区域 free parking area

むりょく 無力 (状況をどうすることもできないこと)helplessness (無能力)incompetence (無緊張・弛緩)atony 腰頭asthen(o)- ◀筋無力症 myasthenia 子宮頸管無力症 cervical incompetence 精子無力症 asthenozoospermia / asthenospermia ▶無力感 feeling of helplessness

ムンプス mumps /mʌ́mps/ ★mumpsは通例，単数扱い．(流行性耳下腺炎)epidemic parotitis ▶ムンプスウイルス mumps virus ムンプス精巣炎 mumps orchitis

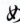

め 目・眼

《眼球・眼部》eye ◆黒目(虹彩)iris (and pupil) of the eye ◆目の異常 an eye problem[disorder / abnormality] ◆目の手術 eye surgery ◆目の奥に at the back of one's eye(s) / behind one's eye(s) ◆目の周りに around one's eyes

《診察の基本表現》 ◆目の調子はどうですか How are your eyes? ◆目に何か問題がありますか Do you have any problems with your eyes? ◆目が悪くなっていますか Is your eyesight failing? ◆目が疲れやすいのですか Do your eyes get tired easily? ◆右目がかすみますか Is the vision in your right eye blurred? / Do you have blurred [blurry] vision in your right eye? ◆目に怪我をしたことがありますか Have you ever had any *eye injuries[injuries to your eyes]? ◆目を診察しましょう I'm going to examine your eyes. ◆目を大きく開けて下さい Please open your eyes wide. ◆目を開けたまま真っ直ぐ前を見て下さい Please keep your eyes open and look straight ahead. ◆私の指〈点滅する光〉を目で追いかけて下さい Please follow *my finger〈the flashing light〉with your eyes. ◆目を閉じて下さい Please close your eyes. ◆両方の目を閉じて片足で立って下さい Please stand on one leg with your eyes closed. / Please close your eyes and stand on one leg. ◆目を固く閉じる close one's eyes tight(ly) ◆片目を閉じて見る look with one eye closed ◆目が炎症を起こしています Your eyes are inflamed. ◆右目が感染症にかかっているようです You seem to have an infection in the right eye. ◆目をこすらないで下さい Don't rub your eye(s). ◆長時間コンピュータ作業をするのは目によくありません It's not good for your eyes to stay on a computer very long. ◆コンピュータで目を酷使する strain[overtax / overwork] one's eyes using a computer ◆目を休ませる rest one's eyes / give one's eyes a rest

《視力・視野の異常》eyesight, vision ☞視野, 視力 ◆目がいい have good eyesight ◆目が悪い have poor[bad] eyesight ◆目が見えにくい have difficulty seeing (things) ◆目がぼやける have cloudy [blurred] vision / the vision becomes cloudy[blurred] ◆左の目が見えない be blind in the left eye ◆両方の目が見えない be totally blind ◆目が弱る the eyesight becomes weak ◆目が見えなくなる lose one's eyesight / go blind ◆暗い場所では目が見えない can't see in the dark ◆夜になると目が見えにくい have poor night vision ◆生まれつき目が見えない be born blind ◆目の不自由な人(盲目の)a blind person / (視力が低下している)a visually impaired[challenged] person

《その他の目の症状》 ◆目が赤い the eyes are red ◆目が充血している the eyes are bloodshot / (炎症を起こしている)the eyes are inflamed ◆目が痛む have (a) pain in the eye(s) / have (an) eye pain / the eyes hurt[ache] ◆目が乾く the eyes become[get] dry / (乾いている)the eyes are[feel] dry ◆目がゴロゴロする the eye feels gritty / have a gritty feeling in one's eye ◆目がしょぼしょぼする(目がかすむ)have bleary eyes / (まぶたが重く感じる)the eyelids feel heavy ◆目が疲れる the eyes get tired / (眼精疲労がある)have eye strain ◆目がまぶしい the eyes are dazzled by lights / (まぶしくなる)get dazzled by lights ◆目がかゆい the eyes are[feel] itchy ◆目がちくちくする the eyes sting[smart] ◆目がひりひりする the eyes become[are / feel] irritated ◆目にごみが入る get a speck of dust in one's eye / (ごみが入っている)have something in one's eye ◆疲れ目 tired eyes / (眼精疲労)eyestrain ◆涙目 watery [teary] eyes

《慣用表現》 ◆目が覚める(眠りから)wake up / (麻酔から)come out (of the anesthe-

sia）/（意識を取り戻す）recover consciousness ◆夜中に目が覚めますか Do you wake up *at night[during the night /（深夜に）in the middle of the night]? ◆目が回ったのですか Did you feel dizzy? ◆お子さんの病状から目を離さないようにします We're going to keep an eye on your child's condition. ◆腫瘍マーカーの値は目に見えてよくなっています Your tumor marker levels show marked improvement.
☞目医者, 目頭, 目薬, 目尻, 目つき, 目脂

―め ―目
《起点からの順番》◆妊娠は何週目ですか How many weeks pregnant are you? / How far along are you in your pregnancy? ◆左から2番目があなたの赤ちゃんです The second from the left is your baby.
《加減》◆塩分は控え目にして下さい Please cut down on your salt. / Please don't eat too much salt.

めいい 名医 excellent doctor[physician]
（熟練した・腕のいい）skilled doctor[physician]

めいかく 明確（な）（確かな）definite （明らかな）clear, clear-cut （明らかで正確な）clear and accurate （相違がはっきりした）distinct （具体的ではっきりした）specific
☞明らか, はっきり ◆これら2つの間には明確な因果関係があります There is a definite cause and effect relationship between these two. ◆あなたの既往歴について明確な情報が必要です We need to have clear and accurate information about your past medical history. ◆それらに明確な区別をつけることは難しい It is difficult to make a clear-cut distinction between them. ◆明確な指示を与える give specific instructions

めいさいしょ 明細書 itemized statement ◆明細書を発行する issue an itemized statement ◀診療報酬明細書 itemized medical bill / itemized billing statement of medical expenses /（健康保険金の請求書）*health insurance[medical billing]

claim 領収明細書 itemized receipt

めいしや 明視野 bright field

めいしゃ 目医者 ☞眼科

めいじる 命じる ☞指示

めいそう 瞑想 meditation（動meditate）

めいそうしんけい 迷走神経 vagus nerve（形vagal）▶迷走神経切離術 vagotomy 迷走神経痛 vagal neuralgia 迷走神経反射 vagal reflex 迷走神経麻痺 vagal paralysis

めいてい 酩酊する get[become] drunk（图drunkenness 图drunken）☞酔う ◆酩酊状態である be drunk / be in a drunken condition ★形容詞 drunken は名詞の前のみに用いる. ◆酩酊のあまり記憶を失う be so drunk as to lose *one's* memory ◀単純酩酊 ordinary drunkenness 病的酩酊 pathologic drunkenness ▶酩酊感 feeling of drunkenness 酩酊歩行 drunken gait

めいにゅうすい 迷入膵 aberrant pancreas

めいはく 明白（な）☞明確

めいふく 冥福 ◆お父様のご冥福をお祈りいたします I pray your father's soul may rest in peace.

めいめい 命名する name ◆赤ん坊をダニエルと命名する name the baby Daniel

めいりょう 明瞭（な）（明らかな）clear, plain （発音・言葉がわかりやすい）intelligible, articulate （相違がはっきりした）distinct ☞明らか, はっきり, 明確 ◆明瞭に話す speak clearly[intelligibly / articulately] ◆明瞭な英語で説明する explain in plain English ★plain English は「平易な英語」を意味する. ◀言語明瞭性 word intelligibility

めいる 滅入る ☞落ち込む

めいれい 命令 ☞指示

めいろ 迷路（内耳）labyrinth（形labyrinthine）◀骨迷路 bony labyrinth ▶迷路機能検査 labyrinthine function test 迷路障害 labyrinthine disturbance 迷路性眼振 labyrinthine nystagmus

めいわく 迷惑
《面倒・不便》（トラブル・面倒）trouble（動迷

惑をかける trouble) (不便) inconvenience (形 inconvenient) ◆ご迷惑をおかけして申し訳ありませんが隣の病室に移っていただけませんか I'm sorry to trouble you, but could you please move to the room next door? ◆もしご迷惑でなければ，予約日を月曜日から木曜日に変更していただけませんか If it isn't too much trouble[inconvenience], could you shift the date of your appointment from Monday to Thursday? ◆予約の時間が遅れご迷惑をおかけしたことをお詫びいたします We apologize for (the inconvenience caused by) the delay in your original appointment time.

《困らせること》 (気に障るもの) annoyance (動 annoy, bother) (迷惑な行為・人) nuisance ◆彼女の行為に同室の患者さんが迷惑しています Her behavior is annoying [bothering / a nuisance to] her roommates. / Her roommates are annoyed by her behavior. ◆院内での飲酒などの迷惑行為は一切ご遠慮願います Please absolutely refrain from (committing) nuisance behavior inside the hospital, such as consuming alcohol. ◆他の患者さんのご迷惑になりますのでテレビの音を小さくして下さい It's bothering the other patients, so could you please turn down the volume on your TV? / (掲示などで) In consideration of the other patients, please turn down the volume on your TV. ◆お見舞いの方は他の患者さんの迷惑にならないよう病棟ではお静かにお願いします We ask visitors to remain quiet on the wards to avoid disturbing the other patients.

メートル meter /míːtɚ/；m ◆休まずに何メートル歩けますか How many meters can you walk without taking a rest?

メープルシロップにょう ―尿 maple syrup urine ▶メープルシロップ尿症 maple syrup urine disease

メール (電子メール) email, e-mail, E-mail (動 email) ◆メールアドレスを教えて下さい What's your email address? / Please give[tell] me your email address. ◆詳細については後でメールします I'll email you (about) the details later. ◆お問い合わせはメールでお願いします．できるだけ早くお返事します Please email us (with) your inquiry, and we will get back to you as soon as possible. ◆彼にメッセージをメールで送る email the message to him / send the message to him by email ◆彼女からメールをもらう get[receive] an email from her

めがしら 目頭 the inner corner of the eye

めがね 眼鏡 glasses, eyeglasses, spectacles ★いずれも複数形で．数える時には a pair of glasses．◆ふだん眼鏡をかけていますか Do you usually wear glasses? ◆最近，眼鏡が合わなくなったと感じていますか Have you recently felt that your glasses aren't *working for[helping] you anymore? ◆眼鏡はいつ作りましたか When were your glasses made? ◆眼鏡を外して下さい Please *take off[remove] your glasses. ◆眼鏡をかけて下さい Please put on your glasses. ◆度の強い眼鏡をかける wear strong[high-strength / (レンズが厚い) thick] glasses ◆度の合った眼鏡を使う wear properly fitted glasses ◆眼鏡の度が合っていません The lenses are not the right strength for your eyes. ◆眼鏡を換える change (one's) glasses ◆眼鏡を処方する prescribe glasses ◆色付き眼鏡 colored[tinted] glasses ◀遠近両用眼鏡 (二重焦点眼鏡) bifocal glasses / (多焦点眼鏡) multifocal glasses 遠視用眼鏡 glasses for a farsighted person 矯正眼鏡 correcting glasses 近視用眼鏡 glasses for a nearsighted person 黒眼鏡 dark glasses 弱視用眼鏡 low-vision glasses 保護眼鏡 protective glasses 乱視用眼鏡 glasses for a person with astigmatism ▶眼鏡店 optician's

メキシコ Mexico (形 Mexican) ☞国籍 ▶メキシコ人 (の) Mexican

めぐすり 目薬 eye drops, eyedrops ★複数形で．(ローション) eye lotion (洗眼薬) eye wash, eyewash, collyrium ◆1日

2回両眼に目薬を1，2滴さして下さい Please apply[put] one or two eye drops to[into] both eyes twice a day. ◆目薬をさす時は目薬容器の先端が眼の表面に触れないようにして下さい Please try to avoid touching the surface of the eye(s) with the tip of the eyedropper.

めくる 捲る turn（over）（引っ繰り返す）flip ◆上まぶたをめくる turn[flip] *a person's* upper eyelid(s) inside out

メサコリンゆうはつしけん —誘発試験 methacholine challenge test

めざましどけい 目覚まし時計 alarm clock

めじり 目尻 the outer corner of the eye ◆目尻のしわ crow's feet

メス scalpel, surgical knife ◆患者の足にメスを入れる insert a scalpel into a patient's leg ◀電気メス electric[cautery] knife / electrotome レーザーメス laser knife[scalpel]

めずらしい 珍しい ☞稀

めせん 目線 ☞視線

メタノール methanol （メチルアルコール）methyl alcohol ▶メタノール中毒 methanol poisoning

メタボリックシンドローム metabolic syndrome

めだま 目玉 ☞眼球

メタンフェタミン methamphetamine ▶メタンフェタミン中毒 methamphetamine poisoning

メチシリン methicillin ▶メチシリン感受性黄色ブドウ球菌 methicillin-susceptible *Staphylococcus aureus*；MSSA メチシリン耐性黄色ブドウ球 methicillin-resistant *Staphylococcus aureus*；MRSA

めつき 目つき （顔つき）look （目の表情）expression in[of] the eyes

めっきん 滅菌 sterilization （動sterilize 形sterile 滅菌した sterilized）☞殺菌, 消毒 ◀ガス滅菌 gas sterilization 加熱滅菌 heat sterilization 乾熱滅菌 dry heat sterilization 高圧蒸気滅菌 high-pressure steam sterilization 蒸気滅菌器 steam sterilizer 超高温滅菌 ultrahigh

temperature sterilization 放射線滅菌 radiation sterilization ▶滅菌ガーゼ sterile gauze 滅菌ガウン sterile[sterilized] gown 滅菌器具 sterilizer 滅菌蒸留水 sterile distilled water 滅菌注射針 sterile[sterilized] needle 滅菌包帯 sterile[sterilized] bandage

メッセージ message ☞伝言 ◆鈴木先生に何かメッセージはありますか Do you have any message for Dr Suzuki? / May I take a message for Dr Suzuki?

メット MET （代謝当量）metabolic equivalent

めつれつしこう 滅裂思考 incoherent thinking[thought]

メニエールびょう —病 Ménière disease

めまい 眩暈 （めまい感）dizziness （形dizzy）,《英》giddiness（形giddy）★「めまい」は一般的によく使われるが医学的にはやや曖昧な言葉で，回転性のめまいから頭部ふらふら感までをいう。（回転性めまい）vertigo /vˈɜːtɪɡòʊ/ （頭部ふらふら感・浮遊感）lightheadedness ◆強いめまい severe dizziness ◆めまいがしますか Do you feel dizzy? ◆めまいの発作を起こしますか Do you have *dizzy spells[attacks of dizziness]? ◆これまでにめまいを起こしたことがありますか Have you ever had any dizziness[vertigo]? ◆めまいはどの位続きましたか How long did the dizziness[vertigo] last? ◆どんなめまいですか What is the dizziness like? ◆自分自身がぐるぐる回っているようなめまいですか Do you *feel as if[have the sensation that] you're turning or spinning around? / （メリーゴーランドに乗っているような）Does it feel as if you're on a merry-go-round? / （ボートに乗っているような）Does it feel as if you're on a boat? ◆周囲の部屋がぐるぐる回るようなめまいですか Do you feel as if the room is spinning around you? ◆急に立ち上がるとめまいがしますか Do you feel dizzy when you stand up quickly[suddenly]? ◆寝返りを打つとめまいがしますか Do you feel dizzy when you change your position in bed? ◆めまいは急な血圧低下によるものでしょう The dizziness is probably caused by a sudden drop in blood pressure. ◆思い当たる理由もないのにめまいが起きる become[get] dizzy for no apparent reason / suffer dizziness for no obvious reason ◆めまいを訴える complain of dizziness

◀回転性めまい rotary[rotatory] vertigo　高所めまい height vertigo　視性めまい visual[ocular] vertigo　耳性めまい aural[auditory] vertigo　心因性めまい psychogenic vertigo / dizziness of psychological origin　垂直めまい vertical vertigo　水平位めまい horizontal vertigo　前庭性めまい vestibular vertigo　浮動性めまい lightheadedness　良性発作性頭位めまい症 benign paroxysmal positional vertigo；BPPV　▶めまい外来 dizziness clinic　めまい感 dizzy feeling / feeling of dizziness

メモ memo　(短い記録) note　◆前もって質問をメモに書いておくとよいでしょう You'll find it helpful to write[jot] down your questions ahead of time.　◆ゆっくり話しますので，どうぞメモを取って下さい I'll try to speak slowly, so please go ahead and take notes of what I say.　▶メモ帳(はぎ取り式の) scratch[memo] pad / notepad　メモ用紙 scratch[memo] paper / notepaper

めもり 目盛り　(単位) unit　(測定器具などの) scale, graduation　(🔲目盛り付きの graduated)　◆3目盛り分の水薬を1日3回お子さんに飲ませて下さい Please give your child three units of this liquid medication, three times a day.　◆目盛り付きのスポイトで正確な量を測って下さい Please measure out the accurate[right] dose using the graduated syringe.

めやす 目安　(おおよその指針・基準) rough guide　(おおよその見積もり) rough estimate　(🔲about, around)　◆この表は1日に必要な摂取カロリーの目安を示しています This chart gives a rough guide[estimate] of (your) daily calorie needs.　◆1日の塩分摂取の目安 a rough estimate of daily salt

intake　◆入院期間の目安は2週間です You'll be staying in the hospital for about [roughly] two weeks.

めやに 目脂　eye discharge[mucus], discharge from the eyes　(かさぶた状の目やに) eye crust　◆目やにが出ますか Do you have any discharge from your eyes? ◆目やにがたまっている have excessive mucus in the eyes　◆朝起きると目やにがたまっている(目やにで目がくっついている) wake up with *one's* eyes glued together with crust

メラトニン melatonin

メラニン melanin　▶メラニン細胞 melanocyte　メラニン色素 melanin pigment

メラノーマ melanoma

メランコリー melancholia, melancholy

めん¹ 面

《物の表面》(表面) surface, face　(平面) plane　◆ざらざらした面 a rough surface　◆平らな面 *a flat[an even / a smooth] surface　◆でこぼこの多い面 *a bumpy[an uneven / a rough] surface

《状況などの側面》side, aspect　◆明るい面を見る look on the bright side　◆お金の面について話し合う talk about the financial aspect

◀横断面 transverse plane / cross section / transection　冠状面 coronal plane　矢状面 sagittal plane　心理面 psychological aspect　垂直面 vertical plane　水平面 horizontal plane　正中面 median plane　前頭面 frontal plane　内面 the inside / the interior / (内の表面) the inner surface

めん² 綿　cotton　(ウェットティッシュ) wipe　◀アルコール綿 alcohol wipe[(綿棒) swab]　消毒綿 antiseptic wipe[(綿棒) swab]　脱脂綿 absorbent cotton / (小さい球状の) cotton (wool) ball　▶綿製品 cotton goods[product(s)]　☞綿棒

めんえき 免疫　immunity　(🔲免疫をもった immune　免疫学的な immunologic, immunological)　◆多くの人は子供時代に罹った病気に免疫があります Many people are immune to childhood illnesses. / Many people have immunity against childhood illnesses. ◆ほとんどの人はそのウイルスに免疫を持っていないでしょう Few people will have immunity against the virus. ◆一般的に乳児は，生後 6 か月くらいまで母親からの免疫があるので病気にはほとんどかかりません Infants generally don't contract disease for about six months after birth due to immunity passed on from their mothers. ◆抗がん剤の投与で免疫力が低くなり，感染症に罹りやすくなります The anticancer drug will weaken your immune system and make you susceptible to infection. ◆このウイルスに感染すると生涯にわたる免疫がつきます Infection with this virus gives[confers] lifelong immunity. ◆はしかに免疫がある be immune to measles / have immunity against measles ◆その病気に免疫ができる become immune to the disease / develop immunity against the disease ◆免疫を高める boost[enhance / improve] immunity ◆免疫を下げる lower immunity ◆体の免疫システムを攻撃する attack the body's immune system ◆免疫システムが衰える the immune system declines[weakens] / have a weakened immune system ◀液性免疫 humoral immunity　獲得免疫 acquired immunity　蛍光免疫測定法 fluoroimmunoassay；FIA　酵素免疫測定法 enzyme immunoassay；EIA / enzyme-linked immunosorbent assay；ELISA　細胞性免疫 cellular immunity　自己免疫疾患 autoimmune disease　終生免疫 lifelong immunity　腫瘍免疫 tumor immunity　母児免疫 maternal immunity / maternally-acquired immunity　▶免疫異常 immunity disorder　免疫応答 immune response　免疫化学 immunochemistry　免疫学 immunology　免疫寛容 immunologic tolerance　免疫グロブリン immunoglobulin；Ig　免疫系 the immune system　免疫組織化学 immunohistochemistry　免疫調節薬 immunomodulator　免疫賦活薬 immunostimulant / immunostimulator　免疫複合体 immune complex；IC　免疫抑制薬 immunosup-

pressive drug；ISD / immunosuppressant　免疫療法 immunotherapy ☞免疫不全

めんえきふぜん　**免疫不全**　**immunodeficiency** ◀後天性免疫不全症候群 acquired immunodeficiency syndrome；AIDS　ヒト免疫不全ウイルス human immunodeficiency virus；HIV　▶免疫不全宿主 immunocompromised host

めんか　**免荷**　**non-weight-bearing**；**NWB** ▶免荷装具 non-weight-bearing orthosis　免荷歩行 non-weight-bearing walking

めんかい　**面会**　（見舞い・訪問）visit（動visit, see）（面接）interview ◆どなたにご面会ですか Who do you want to see[visit]? ◆キムさん，ご面会の方がいらっしゃっています Mr Kim, you have a visitor. / Mr Kim, there's someone who's come to see you. ◆すみませんが午前中は患者さんとの面会はできません I'm sorry, but visitors are not allowed in the morning. / I'm afraid patients won't be able to have visitors in the morning. ◆ご面会はご家族のみに限らせていただきます Visiting is restricted to family members only. / Visitors are restricted to family members only. ◆ご家族以外の方の面会は医師の許可がないとできません Visitors other than family members are not allowed without the doctor's permission. ◆集中治療室での面会は患者さん 1 人につき一度に 2 人までとなっております Each patient may have two visitors at one time in the ICU. / Two visitors per patient are allowed at one time in the ICU. ◆6 歳未満のお子さんの面会はご遠慮下さい Children under the age of six are not permitted to visit（patients）. ◆12 歳未満のお子さんの面会は大人が必ず付き添って下さい Children under the age of twelve must be accompanied by an adult when visiting. ◀時間外面会 after-hours visit ▶面会室 visitors room　面会ラウンジ visitors lounge ☞面会カード，面会時間，面会謝絶

めんかいカード　**面会(者)カード**　（面会許

可証) visitor pass, visitors pass （面会用バッジ) visitor badge, visitors badge ◆面会カードを総合案内で受け取って，お見舞いの前に病棟の看護師かスタッフにお出し下さい Please receive[pick up] a visitor pass at the General Information Desk and present it to a ward nurse or a member of staff before your visit.

めんかいじかん 面会時間 visiting hours ◆面会時間は，平日は午後3時から8時，日曜・祭日は午前10時から午後8時までです Visiting hours are from three pm to eight pm on weekdays and from ten am to eight pm on Sundays and holidays.

めんかいしゃぜつ 面会謝絶 ◆キムさんは面会謝絶です Mrs Kim is not allowed (to have) any visitors. ◆(張り紙) No visitors

めんきょ 免許 license （証明書）certificate ◀医師免許証 medical license / physician's license

めんせき 面積 （場所・地域の範囲）area （程度の範囲）extent （大きさ）size ◀体表面積 body surface area; BSA 熱傷面積 extent of the burn

めんせつ 面接 interview ☞面談

メンタル mental ▶メンタルテスト mental test メンタルヘルス mental health

めんだん 面談 （相談・協議）consultation （面接）interview （会合）meeting ◆次回の面談は，8月15日水曜日の午後3時からにしましょう Let's schedule *the next consultation[our next meeting] for Wednesday, August (the) fifteenth, at three in the afternoon. ▶面談室 consultation [interview / consulting] room

めんちょう 面疔 facial boil, furuncle

めんどう 面倒
《世話》care ◆家ではどなたがお父さんの面倒をみているのですか Who is *taking care of[looking after] your father at home? ◆面倒見のいい看護師 a caring nurse
《トラブル》trouble ◆面倒を起こす cause trouble ◆面倒なことになる get into trou-ble

めんぼう 綿棒 （cotton）swab, （商標名）Q-tip

めんぽう 面疱 comedo ☞にきび

モイスチャー moisture ▶モイスチャークリーム〈ローション〉moisturizing cream〈lotion〉/ moisture cream〈lotion〉/ moisturizer

もいちど もう一度 again ◆もう一度やってみて下さい Please try again. ◆もう一度言っていただけますか(I beg your) pardon? / Could you say that again?

もうがっこう 盲学校 school for the blind and visually impaired

もうけん 盲検法 blind test, masked test ◀二重盲検法 double-blind test

もうこう 毛孔 pore

もうこはん 蒙古斑 mongolian spot

もうこん 毛根 hair root

もうさいけっかん 毛細血管 (blood) capillary, capillary vessel ▶毛細血管拡張 telangiectasia 毛細血管拡張性運動失調 ataxia telangiectasia；AT

もうしおくり 申し送り ☞引継ぎ

もうしおくる 申し送る ☞引き継ぐ, 報告

もうしこむ 申し込む apply (for, to) (図)application (前もって通知する)notify ... in advance ◆介護保険は市の窓口で申し込んで下さい Please apply for long-term care insurance at the counter in the city office. ◆米飯ではなくパン食をご希望の場合，前日までに申し込んで下さい(24時間前までに)If you want to have bread instead of rice, please give us a day's notice. ◆入院の申し込みをする apply for admission to the hospital ◆申込用紙に記入する fill out[in] an application form ◀診察申込書(patient) consultation form 入院申込書 admission form / application form for admission

もうしつける 申し付ける ◆特別なご要望があればお申し付け下さい If you have any special requests[needs], please *let me know[tell me].

もうしゅうき 毛周期 hair cycle

もうじょうえい 網状影 reticular shadow

もうしわけ 申し訳(ない) (すまない)I'm〈We're〉sorry, excuse me〈us〉 ★excuseのほうが軽い謝り方. ☞謝る, すみません, 詫びる ◆大変申し訳ありません I'm very [awfully / terribly] sorry. ◆申し訳ありませんがご要望にはお応えできません I'm sorry, but we can't meet your request. ◆入院手続きが遅れており申し訳ありません Please excuse us for the delay in the admission procedures.

もうじん 盲人 blind person (視覚障害者) visually impaired[challenged] person ★the blind には差別的な響きがあるので blind people を用いるほうがよい.

もうせっけっきゅう 網赤血球 reticulocyte

もうそう 妄想 delusion (図delusional) (パラノイア)paranoia (図paranoid) ◀関係妄想 delusion of reference 誇大妄想 megalomania / delusion of grandeur 罪業妄想 delusion of guilt 嫉妬妄想 delusion of jealousy 心気妄想 hypochondriac delusion 注察妄想 delusion of observation 被害妄想 delusion of persecution / persecutory delusion 被毒妄想 delusion of poisoning 憑依妄想 delusion of possession 変身妄想 transformation delusion 物盗られ妄想 delusion of robbery 恋愛妄想 love delusion / erotomania ▶妄想型 paranoid type 妄想気分 delusional mood 妄想性障害 delusional disorder 妄想性パーソナリティ障害 paranoid personality disorder 妄想知覚 delusional perception 妄想着想 delusional intuition / sudden delusional idea 妄想反応 delusional reaction

もうちょう 盲腸 cecum ◀移動性盲腸 mobile cecum ▶盲腸炎 cecitis 盲腸切除術 cecectomy

もうてん 盲点 blind spot

もうどうけん 盲導犬 guide dog, (商標名) Seeing Eye dog

もうどく 猛毒(の) highly[deadly] poisonous, highly[deadly] toxic

もうのう 毛嚢 ☞毛包

もうはつ 毛髪 ☞髪, 毛

もうふ 毛布 **blanket** ◆もう一枚毛布をかけましょうか Would you like to have one more blanket? / Shall I put another blanket over you?

もうほう 毛包 **hair follicle** ▶毛包炎 folliculitis 毛包周囲炎 perifolliculitis

もうまく 網膜 **retina**（⌗**retinal**）◆光は水晶体を通して網膜に届きます Light passes through the lens to the retina. ▶網膜芽細胞腫 retinoblastoma 網膜色素変性症 retinitis pigmentosa；RP 網膜出血 retinal bleeding[hemorrhage] 網膜中心静脈〈動脈〉閉塞症 central retinal vein〈artery〉occlusion 網膜剝離 retinal detachment 網膜裂孔 retinal tear ☞網膜炎, 網膜症

もうまくえん 網膜炎 **retinitis** ◀サイトメガロウイルス網膜炎 cytomegalovirus retinitis

もうまくしょう 網膜症 **retinopathy** ◀糖尿病性網膜症 diabetic retinopathy 未熟児網膜症 retinopathy of prematurity；ROP

もうもく 盲目（の）**blind**（⌗**blindness**）☞盲人 ▶盲目的挿管 blind intubation

もうようたい 毛様体 **ciliary body** ◀虹彩毛様体炎 iridocyclitis

もうろう 朦朧 ◆意識がもうろうとしている（錯乱している）feel[be] confused /（意識が完全に戻っていない）be not fully conscious / be（only）half conscious /（見当識を失っている）be disoriented /（意識が混濁している）be delirious / be in a delirious state ◆今朝の記憶がもうろうとしている have only a dim[vague] memory of this morning ▶もうろう状態 twilight state / clouded[disordered] consciousness

もえつきしょうこうぐん 燃え尽き症候群 **burnout syndrome**

もぎかんじゃ 模擬患者 **simulated patient；SP**

もくてき 目的 （意図）**purpose** （具体的なねらい）**aim** （計画など達成可能な目標）**objective** （的を絞った目標）**target** ☞目標 ◆今日受診された目的は何ですか What's

brought you here today? ★purpose を用いて"What's the purpose of your visit today?"と訊くのは職務上の堅い表現になる. ◆この治療の主な目的は背中の痛みを和らげることです The main purpose[aim] of this treatment is to relieve your back pain. ◆日本に来られた目的は何ですか What's brought you to Japan? ★"What's the purpose of your visit to Japan?"はやや詰問調の響きがあるので避ける. むしろ「Did you come to Japan on business?（日本へは商用ですか）」「Have you come to Japan for sightseeing?（観光ですか）」などと具体的に訊いたほうがよい. ◆生きる目的がない have no purpose in life ◆社会復帰という目的を達成する achieve[meet / reach] the objective of *getting back to normal life[returning to work]

もくひょう 目標 （最終的な目標）**goal** （より具体的で達成可能な目標）**objective** （的を絞った目標）**target** ☞目的 ◆リハビリの短期的な目標と長期的な目標を設定しましょう Let's set short-term and long-term goals for your rehabilitation. ◆この治療はがん細胞を殺し腫瘍を小さくすることを主要な目標にしています The primary objective of this treatment is to kill（the）cancer cells and shrink（the）tumors. ◆目標を達成する achieve[reach] a goal ◀看護目標 nursing goal[objective] 最終目標 final[ultimate] goal 数値目標 numerical target 治療目標 therapeutic goal[objective] ▶目標設定 goal setting

もくようび 木曜日 **Thursday；Thurs.** ◆木曜日に on Thursday ◆木曜日ごとに on Thursdays

もし （もし…の場合には）**in case …, if …** ◆もし予期しない副作用が見られたら連絡して下さい Please call[contact] us *in case[if] you notice any unexpected side effects.

もたれる **sit heavy on** *one's* **stomach, feel heavy on** *one's* **stomach** ◆食べ物がもたれますか Does your food sit[feel] heavy on your stomach? /（消化不良がある）Do you have indigestion? ◆胃がもたれる感じがする have a heavy[sinking] feeling in the stomach ◆胃がもたれるような食事をする eat a heavy meal

もちあげる　持ち上げる　lift, raise ◆重い物を持ち上げる lift heavy things ◆頭を持ち上げる raise one's head ◆膝を伸ばしたまま足を持ち上げる lift one's leg(s) up, with the knee(s) straight

もちいる　用いる ☞使用，使う，利用

もちかえる　持ち帰る　take … home ◆このパンフレットを持ち帰ってじっくりご覧下さい Please take this brochure home and read it carefully.

もちこたえる　持ちこたえる　pull through ☞耐える ◆彼女は持ちこたえて回復すると思います I hope she'll pull through and recover.

もちだす　持ち出す
《持って外に出す》**take (out), carry (out)** ◆ロビーの新聞や雑誌の持ち出しはご遠慮下さい Please *do not take[refrain from taking] newspapers and magazines out of the lobby.
《話題に出す》**bring up** ◆この話を何度も持ち出して恐縮ですが，I hate to bring this up *again and again[repeatedly], but …

もちなおす　持ち直す　(回復する)**take a turn[change] for the better, improve** ☞回復 ◆彼の病状は持ち直して安定しています His condition has *taken a turn for the better[improved] and is stable.

もちもの　持ち物　one's things[belongings]　(私物)**personal belongings** ★いずれも複数形で. ◆持ち物にはすべて名前を付けて下さい Please put your name on all your belongings. / Please mark all of your things with your name. ◆持ち物をかごの中に入れる put one's things in the basket ◆入院中の持ち物は最小限にして下さい Please keep your personal belongings to a minimum during your hospital stay. ◆入院に必要な持ち物は入院案内のパンフレットを参考にして下さい Please read our admission brochure for information on what to bring to the hospital. ◆持ち物の管理はご自分の責任にてお願いします Belongings are kept (in the ward)

at your own risk.

もちろん　of course, sure, certainly　(ご遠慮なくどうぞ)**go ahead** ◆治療の選択肢はいくつかあります. もちろん手術はその1つです There are several treatment options. Of course surgery is one of them. ◆(許可を求められて)もちろんいいですよ Yes, of course. / Sure. / Certainly. / Go ahead.

もつ　持つ
《手で支えて持つ》**hold** ◆一人でコップを持てますか Can you hold the cup *by yourself[on your own]?
《持ってくる》**bring**　(持ち運ぶ)**carry** ☞持参 ◆飲んでいる薬をすべてお持ち下さい Please bring (with you) all the medications you are currently taking. ◆術後3か月から5か月の間は5 kg 以上の重いものを持たないで下さい For three to five months after the surgery, you shouldn't carry any heavy objects weighing over five kilos.
《所持する・所有する》**have** ◆健康保険証を持っていますか Do you have your health insurance card with you? ◆当院には医療通訳士の資格を持っているボランティアがいます We have licensed medical interpreters who work as volunteers.
《持ちこたえる》 ◆彼は春までもたないかもしれません He may not live[last] to the spring.

もっとも¹　(自然な)**natural**　(理にかなっている)**reasonable** ◆あなたが怒るのはもっともです It is only natural for you to get angry. ◆おっしゃることはもっともです What you say is quite reasonable. / What you say makes good sense.

もっとも²　最も　(最大の・に)**(the) most**　(最もよい・よく)**(the) best** ☞一番 ◆手洗いは菌の拡散を防ぐ最もよい方法です Washing your hands is the best way to prevent the spread of germs. ◆咳が最も多く出る時間帯はいつですか What time of day *do you cough most[is your cough worst]? ◆今最も恐れているのは敗血症です The condition I fear (the) most now is sepsis. ◆最も好きなスポーツは何ですか What sport do you like best? / What's your favorite sport?

もつれる （つまずく）trip（over *one's* feet）, stumble（over *one's* feet）（不明瞭に話す）have slurred speech［words］ ◆足がもつれて転ばないように気をつけて下さい Please be careful not to trip（over your feet）and fall. ◆彼は舌がもつれて明瞭に話せない He can't speak clearly because *he has slurred speech［his speech has become slurred］.

モデル model ◀動物モデル animal model

もどす 戻す
《元の状態にする》put … back, return ☞返す ◆車椅子は元の場所に戻して下さい Please put the wheelchair back where you found it. / Please return wheelchairs to their original location after usage.
◆話を首の腫れに戻しますが，初めて気づいたのはいつですか Let's return to talking about the swelling on your neck. When did you first notice it?
《嘔吐する》throw up, vomit, regurgitate ☞吐く

もとづく 基づく be based（on）◆エビデンスに基づく医療 evidence-based medicine；EBM ◆生命倫理に基づく医療 ethics-based medicine

もどる 戻る
《元の位置に戻る》come back, go back, return （戻っている）be back ☞帰る ◆検査が終わったらこちらに戻ってきて下さい Please come back here when the tests are finished. ◆すぐに〈1 時間で〉戻ってきます I'll be back soon〈within an hour〉.
◆自宅に戻る go home
《元の状態に復す》be［feel］back to, return （体力・意識などを取り戻す）regain, come to ◆平熱に戻りましたよ Your temperature *is back［has returned］to normal. ◆彼女は 1 時間もすれば意識が戻るでしょう She'll（start to）*regain consciousness［come to］in an hour or so. ◆2, 3 日したら元に戻れます You'll probably be［feel］

back to normal within a few days.

モニター （監視装置）monitor（動monitor）（監視）monitoring ◆監視 ◆彼女は昨夜脳卒中を起こし，状態を慎重にモニターしています She had a stroke last night, and we're monitoring her condition carefully［closely］. ◆彼の血圧を定期的にモニターする必要があります His blood pressure needs to be monitored regularly. ◆心電図モニターを装着する attach an EKG monitor to *a person's* body / put *a person* on an EKG monitor ◀観血的モニター invasive monitoring 血圧モニター blood pressure monitor 術中モニタリング intraoperative monitoring セルフモニタリング self-monitoring 胎児モニタリング fetal monitoring 薬物血中濃度モニタリング therapeutic drug monitoring；TDM ▶モニタリング装置 monitoring device / （設備）monitoring equipment / （機器）monitoring instrument

もの 物 things ★通例，複数形で. （何か）something, anything ★anything は疑問文・否定文で用いる. （物体）object ◆物を落とす drop things ◆物にぶつかる bump into things ◆近くの物が見えにくいですか Do you have difficulty seeing things close at hand? ◆物がぼやけて［かすんで］見えますか Do you have cloudy［blurred］vision? / Is your vision cloudy［blurred］? ◆物が二重に見えますか Are you seeing double? / Do you have double vision? ◆甘い〈辛い〉物はよく食べますか Do you often eat sweet〈hot〉things? ◆冷たい〈温かい〉物を飲む drink something cold〈hot〉 ◆物を噛む時痛みますか Does it hurt when you chew? ☞物覚え，物事，物忘れ

ものおぼえ 物覚え memory ☞記憶, 記憶力 ◆最近，彼は物覚えが悪くなりましたか Has he become forgetful recently? / Is his memory failing these days? ◆物覚えがいい have a good memory ◆物覚えが悪い have a poor［bad］memory

モノクローナルこうたい —抗体 monoclonal antibody

ものごと 物事 things ★複数形で. ◆物事をあるがままに受け止める take things as they are ◆物事を肯定的に見る see things from a positive *point of view [angle] ◆物事がうまくいかないのは自分のせいだと思いますか Do you blame yourself when things go wrong?

ものもらい (麦粒腫) sty, stye/stáɪ/, hordeolum ◆ものもらいがよくできますか Do you often have styes? ◆目にものもらいがある have a sty on *one's* eyelid

ものわすれ 物忘れ (忘れっぽさ) forgetfulness (動forget 形forgetful) (記憶喪失) memory loss ◆最近, 物忘れがありますか Have you been forgetting things recently? / Are you forgetful these days? ▶物忘れ外来 memory clinic

もむ 揉む (マッサージする) give a massage, massage (さする) give a rub, rub ◆肩を揉む give a shoulder massage / massage *a person's* shoulders ◆凝った筋肉を揉みほぐす massage and loosen up *a person's* stiff muscles

もも 腿 (大腿) thigh /θáɪ/ ◀内腿 inner thigh / the inside of the thigh

もやもやびょう もやもや病 moyamoya disease

もよおす 催す (衝動に駆られる) have an urge to (引き起こす) cause ◆突然尿意を催すことがありますか Do you have a sudden urge to urinate[go to the bathroom]? ◆眠気を催す become[feel] sleepy[drowsy] ◆この薬を飲むと吐き気を催すことがあります This medication may cause nausea. / This medication may make you nauseous[feel like vomiting]. ◆吐き気を催させるにおい a nauseating odor

もより 最寄り(の) the nearest ◆最寄りの保健所 the nearest health center

もらす 漏らす 《失禁する》 (しみ出す) leak (ぼたぼた落とす) dribble, drip (濡らす・お漏らしをする) wet ☞漏れる ◆尿を漏らすことがありますか Do you ever leak or dribble urine? ◆(子供に)お漏らししたの. 大丈夫だよ Did

you *have an accident[wet your pants]? Never mind! ★an accident は「パンツやシーツを汚す失敗」を意味する. ◆夜間に尿を漏らす wet the bed at night 《秘密などを外部に出す》 let out (身元・情報などを明らかにする) disclose ◆秘密を漏らす let out a secret ◆あなたの個人情報は誰にも漏らしません I won't disclose[tell] your personal information to anybody.

モラトリアム moratorium

モルヒネ morphine /mɔ́ːfiːn/ ▶モルヒネ依存 morphine dependence モルヒネ拮抗薬(オピオイド拮抗薬) opioid antagonist モルヒネ嗜癖 morphine addiction モルヒネ中毒 morphine poisoning[intoxication] モルヒネ中毒患者 morphine addict モルヒネ乱用 morphine abuse

もれる 漏れる (しみ出る) leak (図leak) (ポタポタ出る) dribble (特に気体・液体が漏れる) escape ☞漏らす ◆ガスが漏れているThere is a gas leak. / Gas is leaking. ◆抗がん剤が血管外に漏れると, 皮膚に強い傷害が生じることがあります Chemotherapy drugs may cause serious damage to the skin if the drip leaks outside the vein.

もろい (硬いものが砕けやすい) brittle (弱い) weak (壊れやすい) fragile ◆歳をとると骨がもろくなります The bones *break easily[become brittle] *with age[as we age]. ◆涙もろい feel tearful

モローはんしゃ ―反射 Moro reflex

モロッコ Morocco (形Moroccan) ☞国籍 ▶モロッコ人(の) Moroccan

モンゴル Mongolia (形Mongolian) ☞国籍 ▶モンゴル人(の) Mongolian

もんし 門歯 incursor, incisor tooth, incisive tooth (複teeth)

もんしん 問診 (medical) history-taking, interview, inquiry ◆問診票に記入して受付で登録して下さい Please fill out a health history questionnaire and register at our reception desk. ◆医師の診察前に, 看護師が問診させていただきます Before your doctor sees you, a nurse will *take your medical history[ask you questions regarding your medical history]. ▶問診票 medical history questionnaire[(interview) form]

もんだい **問題** (検討・解決を要する事柄) problem, matter (質問・疑問) question (面倒な事) trouble (困難) difficulty (不満・苦情) complaint ◆緊急の問題 an urgent problem ◆デリケートな問題 a delicate problem ◆胃に問題がありますか Do you have any problems with your stomach? ◆排尿に問題がありますか Do you have any problems[difficulty] urinating? ◆ご家族のどなたかに心臓に問題のある方がいますか Is there anybody in your family with heart trouble? ◆軽い貧血以外，特に大きな問題はありません Other than some mild anemia, I can't see anything seriously wrong. ◆この治療にはいくつか問題があります There are several difficulties with this treatment. ◆当病院のサービスで何か問題はありますか Do you have any complaints about this hospital's services? / Is there any problem with this hospital's services? ◆現在，その問題の解決に全力を注いでいるところです We are currently *focusing all our energy[concentrating] on solving the problem. ◆問題を抱える have a problem / have difficulties ◆問題を起こす cause trouble ◆問題に対処する deal [cope] with a problem ◆問題を解決する solve a problem / settle a matter ◆問題を処理する handle[deal with / manage] a problem ◆言葉に問題がある have language problems / have difficulty speaking ◆他の人とのコミュニケーションに問題がある have difficulty communicating with others ◀アルコール問題 alcohol problem 飲酒問題 drinking problem 家庭(内の)問題 domestic[family] problem 金銭問題 money problem / financial difficulties[problem / worries] 健康問題 health problem 社会問題 social problem 心理的問題 psychological problem 精神病的問題 psychiatric problem ▶問題患者 problem patient 問題行動 problem[abnormal] behavior 問題児 problem child 問題リスト problem list

もんみゃく **門脈** portal vein ▶門脈圧 portal vein pressure 門脈圧亢進症 portal hypertension 門脈循環 portal circulation 門脈造影 portography

モンローこう **―孔** Monro foramen, foramen of Monro (室間孔) interventricular foramen

やえば 八重歯 （重なった歯）double tooth （斜めに出た歯）oblique tooth
やがい 野外（の） outdoor, open-air（副 outdoors, out of doors） ☞屋外 ◆野外に出る際にはなるべく日光を避けるよう注意して下さい Whenever you go outdoors [out of doors], be careful to avoid exposure to the sun as much *as you can [as possible]. ▶野外活動 outdoor activities　野外スポーツ outdoor sports
やかん 夜間（に） （夜に）at night （夜のうちに） during the night, in the night（圏 nighttime, nocturnal） ☞夜中 ◆もし夜間に胸痛がひどくなるようでしたらすぐに救急外来に来て下さい If your chest pain gets worse *during the night[at night], come to the emergency room right away. ◆排尿するため夜間に何度も目を覚ますことがありますか Do you often wake up in the night to urinate? ◆夜間の勤務につく work the night shift / work on the night shift ▶夜間遺精 nocturnal emission /（夢精）wet dream　夜間介護 night[nighttime] care　夜間外来入口(hospital) night [nighttime] entrance /（救急の） emergency night[nighttime] entrance　夜間失禁 nocturnal incontinence　夜間せん妄 night[nocturnal] delirium　夜間当番医 night-duty doctor / doctor on night duty　夜間徘徊 night wandering[walking]　夜間頻尿 nocturia / nycturia
やきゅう 野球 baseball ▶野球肩 baseball shoulder　野球肘 baseball elbow /（ピッチャーの）pitcher's elbow
やきょう 夜驚（症） night terrors, sleep terrors ★通例, 複数形で.
やきん 夜勤 （交替制勤務）night shift （夜間当直）night duty （一般的に夜間の仕事）night work ◆週に何回夜勤がありますか How many times a week do you do night shifts? / How many night shifts per week do you work? ◆広田先生は今日夜勤です Dr Hirota is on night duty tonight. ◆夜勤で働く work (on) the night shift ◀準夜勤 evening shift ▶夜勤看護師 night-duty nurse / nurse on night duty
やく¹ 役 《務め》（仕事）job （役割）role, part ☞役割 ◆私の役はあなたに正確な情報を提供することです It is my job to provide you with accurate information. 《役立つ》（助けになる）help（圏help）, be helpful （有益である）be useful ◆この検査は腫瘍が悪性か否かを診断するのに役に立ちます This test is helpful[useful] in diagnosing whether the tumor is malignant or not. ◆何かお役に立てることがありますか Is there anything I can do for you? ◆お役に立てるならうれしく思います I'd be happy[glad] if I could help you. ◆お役に立てず申し訳ありませんでした I'm very sorry I wasn't able to help you.
やく² 約 （おおよそ）about, approximately （圏some） ◆頸椎捻挫は全治約1週間です The neck sprain will take about[approximately] a week to heal. / You'll recover from the neck sprain in a week or so. ◆当院のベッド数は約500床です There are some five hundred beds in this hospital.
やくえき 薬液 liquid medication
やくがい 薬害 drug-induced health damage[problem] ☞副作用
やくがく 薬学 pharmacy /fáə·məsi/ （薬理学）pharmacólogy
やくざい 薬剤 medication, drug, medicine ☞医薬品, 薬, 薬品, 薬物 ▶薬剤アレルギー drug allergy　薬剤感受性試験 drug susceptibility[sensitivity] test　薬剤性肝障害 drug-induced liver[hepatic] injury　薬剤耐性 drug resistance[tolerance]　薬剤耐性菌 drug-resistant bacterium　薬剤熱 drug fever　薬剤費 drug cost[price]　薬剤部 pharmaceutical department /（特に病院内の薬局・調剤室）dispensary　薬剤部長 (the) director of pharmacy ☞薬剤師

やくざいし 薬剤師 pharmacist
やくしょ 役所 (public) office ◀区役所 ward office 市役所(市の) city hall[office] / (地方自治体の)municipal office
やくしん 薬疹 drug eruption[rash] ◀固定薬疹 fixed drug eruption
やくそう 薬草 (medicinal) herb (圏herbal), drug plant ▶薬草治療薬 herbal medicine[medication / drug] 薬草療法 herbal medicine[remedy]
やくそく 約束
《取り決め》promise (圏promise, make a promise) ◆プライバシーを守ることをお約束します I promise to protect your privacy. ◆ベストを尽くすことを約束します I'll do my best, I promise. / I promise that I'll do my best. ◆禁煙すると約束してくれますか Will you promise to quit smoking? ◆約束を守る keep one's promise[word] ◆約束を破る break one's promise
《予約》appointment (面会などの約束)engagement ◆次の外来の約束は4週間後でいかがですか How about scheduling your next outpatient appointment for four weeks from today? ◆約束を取り消す cancel one's appointment[engagement]
やくだつ 役立つ ☞役
やくひん 薬品 medication, drug, medicine (化学薬品)chemicals ★通例, 複数形で. ☞医薬品, 薬, 薬剤, 薬物 ◀医薬品副作用 adverse drug reaction；ADR ▶薬品会社 drug[pharmaceutical] company
やくぶつ 薬物 (薬)medication, drug, medicine (薬効のある物質)medicinal substance (化学薬品)chemicals ★通例, 複数形で. (圏薬理的な pharmacologic, pharmacological 化学的な chemical) ☞医薬品, 薬, 麻薬, 薬剤, 薬品 ◆心筋梗塞の予防のために薬物治療を受けている be on medication to prevent against myocardial infarction / be taking medication for myocardial infarction prevention ◆(違法薬物の)薬物検査をする test a person for drugs / (血液〈尿〉で) test blood 〈urine〉 for the presence of illegal drugs ◆薬物を投与する give[administer] (a) medication ◀違法薬物 illegal drug[substance] 禁止薬物 prohibited[banned] drug[substance] 習慣性薬物 habit-forming drug[substance] / addictive drug[substance] ▶薬物依存 drug dependence[addiction] 薬物吸収 drug absorption 薬物相互作用 drug interaction 薬物代謝酵素 drug-metabolizing enzyme 薬物中毒(医薬品中毒)drug poisoning / poisoning by a drug / (麻薬などによる中毒) drug intoxication / (常用者) drug addict [abuser] 薬物動態 pharmacokinetics 薬物投与 medication / drug administration 薬物排泄 drug excretion 薬物有害反応 adverse drug reaction；ADR 薬物乱用 drug[substance] abuse 薬物療法 medication[drug] therapy / pharmacotherapy ☞薬物血中濃度

やくぶつけっちゅうのうど 薬物血中濃度 plasma drug level[concentration] ▶薬物血中濃度時間曲線下面積 the area under the plasma (drug) concentration-time curve；AUC 薬物血中濃度モニタリング therapeutic drug monitoring；TDM
やくめ 役目 role, part ☞役, 役割
やくよう 薬用(の) (薬剤添加の)medicated (薬効のある)medicinal ▶薬用化粧品 medicated cosmetics 薬用植物 medicinal plant[herb] 薬用石鹸 medicated [medicinal] soap
やくよく 薬浴 medicated bath
やくり 薬理(学) pharmacology (圏pharmacologic, pharmacological) ▶薬理遺伝学 pharmacogenetics 薬理学者 pharmacologist 薬理作用 pharmacologic[(薬効のある)medicinal] action
やくりょう 薬量 (1回の薬量)dose (一定期間にわたる薬量)dosage ☞薬, 用量
ヤグレーザー YAG laser, yttrium aluminum garnet laser
やくれき 薬歴 medication history
やくわり 役割 role, part ☞役 ◆規則正しい食生活は健康の維持に重要な役割を

果たします Eating *at regular times[regularly] plays an important role[part] in maintaining good health. ◀患者[病者]役割 sick role

やけど　火傷　（火・熱・薬品による火傷）**burn**　（熱湯・蒸気による火傷）**scald**　☞熱傷　◆やけどをしたのですか Did you *burn yourself[get burned]?　◆足に重度のやけどを負う have a severe[major / serious] burn on the leg.　◆顔と胸にⅢ度のやけどを負う have third-degree burns on the face and arm(s)　◆器具が熱くなっていますのでやけどに注意して下さい The instrument is hot, so be careful not to burn yourself.　◆軽度のやけど a mild[minor / light] burn　◆このやけどは軽いのでおそらく痕は残らないでしょう This is a light burn, so it probably won't leave a scar.　◆このやけどは皮膚の深いところまで及んでいます This burn extends deep into the skin.　◆手のやけどはひりひりしますか Does the burn on your hand smart?　◆やけどで皮膚がただれて痛む the skin becomes sore from the burn　◆やけどで皮膚が剥ける the skin peels as a result of the burn　◆やけどの水疱をつぶす break[pop] a burn blister　◆やけどの薬 a medication for burns /（軟膏）an ointment for burns / a burn ointment　◀低温やけど low-temperature burn

やける　焼ける　（やけどする・燃える）**burn, get burned**　（焼きつくような）**burning**）　（胸焼けする）**get[have] heartburn**　（日焼けする）**get sunburned**　（ほどよく日焼けする）**get (sun-)tanned**　◆排尿時に焼きつくような痛みがある have a burning pain when urinating　◆喉が焼けるように痛む have a burning sensation in *one's* throat　◆どんな食べ物で胸が焼けますか What foods give you heartburn?

やさい　野菜　vegetables　★通例，複数形で．◆毎日いろいろな種類の野菜を食べるとよいでしょう You should eat a variety of vegetables every day.　◆毎日1日につき5品目の野菜を食べて下さい You should eat five portions of vegetables a day.　◆繊維の多い野菜 high-fiber vegetables / vegetables high[rich] in fiber　◆裏ごしした野菜 strained vegetables　◀淡黄色野菜 light yellow vegetables　緑黄色野菜 dark-colored vegetables / dark green and [or] yellow vegetables

やさしい¹　優しい　（親切な・思いやりのある）**kind, good, nice**　（心が優しい）**kind-hearted**　（性格的に優しい）**good-natured**　（温厚な）**gentle**　（圖そっと **gently, softly** 暖昧…に配慮した **-friendly**）　◆患者に優しく接する be kind[good] to patients / care for patients kindly　◆彼女は優しい人です She is a nice person. / She is a kind-hearted[good-natured] person.　◆お子さんの背中を優しくさすって〈叩いて〉あげて下さい Please rub〈pat〉your child's back gently.　◆赤ちゃんに優しく話しかけてあげて下さい Please talk softly to your baby.　◆環境に優しい製品 eco-friendly products

やさしい²　易しい　（簡単な）**easy**（↔hard, difficult）（単純な）**simple**（↔complicated, difficult）（誰でもわかる平易な）**plain**　☞易い(やすい)　◆この機器は取り扱いがやさしいので心配いりません This device is easy to use[handle], so don't worry.　◆検査結果をやさしい言葉で説明する explain the test results in simple, plain words　◆できるだけやさしい英語で説明しますので，わからないところがあったら言って下さい I'll try to explain in plain English, so if there's anything you don't understand, let me know.

やしなう　養う　（扶養する）**support, provide for**　（育てる）**bring up, raise**　（能力をつける）**develop, build up**　◆彼は両親を入れて6人家族を養っています He is supporting[providing for] a family of six, including his parents.　◆大家族を養う have a large family to support[provide for]　◆体力を養う develop[build up] *one's* physical strength

―やすい　―易い　《楽・簡単》**be easy (to)**　☞易しい　◆この薬は飲み込みやすいです This medication

is easy to swallow.
《傾向》tend (to), be likely (to) （望ましくないことを起こす傾向）be prone (to) （影響・攻撃を受けやすい傾向）be susceptible[vulnerable] (to) （疾病素因）be predisposed (to, toward) ◆歳をとると夜トイレに起きやすくなります When people get older, they tend to get up more in the night to urinate. ◆一般に誤解されやすいのですが，この病気は移りません People are likely to misunderstand that, but this disease is not infectious[contagious]. ◆高齢の患者は特に副作用を起こしやすいのです Elderly patients are especially prone to side effects. ◆この薬は眠くなりやすいので服用後は車などを運転しないで下さい This medication can make you sleepy, so don't drive when taking it. ◆風邪を引きやすい be susceptible to colds / catch colds easily ◆感染症にかかりやすい be susceptible[vulnerable / predisposed] to infection

やすまる　休まる　（リラックスする）feel[be] relaxed （安心する）feel[be] at ease ◆あなたにとって心が休まるのはいつですか When do you feel relaxed?

やすみ　休み
《休暇》（休日）holiday （長期休暇）vacation （仕事からの休み）leave （勤務のない日）day off ☞休暇, 休日, 休む ◆いつも休みをどう過ごしていますか What do you usually do on holidays[your days off]? / How do you spend your days off? ◆このために仕事〈学校〉を何日休んでいますか How many days were you absent from work〈school〉 because of this? ◆今日星先生はお休みです Dr Hoshi *is off duty[is taking the day off] today.
《休息》rest （休憩）break ☞休養, 休む ◆1週間ほど休みをとったらいかがですか How about taking a good rest for a week? ◆疲れたでしょう。ひと休みしましょう You must be tired. Let's take a break[rest] now.

やすむ　休む
《休息する》rest, take a rest, have a rest （休憩する）take a break, have a break （リラックスする）relax ☞休養, 休まる, 休み ◆2, 3時間横になって休めば良くなるでしょう If you lie down and rest for a few hours, you'll feel better. ◆疲れたら無理をしないで2, 3日ゆっくり休んで下さい When you get[feel] tired, please don't overdo yourself, but take some good rest for *a couple of[a few] days. ◆ゆっくり休む take[have] a good rest / rest well ◆少し休む take a short break ◆食後はしばらくの間ゆっくり休んだほうがよいでしょう You should relax[take a good rest] for a while after eating a meal. ◆少なくとも週に2日はアルコールを飲まずに肝臓を休ませて下さい Please give your liver a rest[break] by having at least two alcohol-free days a week. ◆痛みは休むととれますか Does the pain disappear with rest? / Does rest relieve the pain?
《欠勤・欠席する》（日・期間を休む）take … off （休暇をとる）take leave （欠勤・欠席する）be absent (from), stay away (from) ☞休暇 ◆腰痛のため1日休む take a day off because of low back pain ◆仕事を少し休む take some time off work ◆病気休暇をとって仕事を休む take sick leave from work ◆学校を休む be absent from school / stay home from school ◆明日, 田中先生は休みます Dr Tanaka is off tomorrow. / Dr Tanaka will take tomorrow off.
《休業する》（閉める）close ◆土曜日の午後外来診療はお休みです The outpatient clinics[departments] are closed on Saturday afternoons.
《床に就く・眠る》go to bed, get into bed （休息する）have a rest （睡眠をとる）have a sleep ◆キングさん, お休みになる時間ですよ Mrs King, it's time for you to have a rest[sleep]. / （夜間に）Mrs King, it's time *for bed[to go to bed]. ◆いつも何時にお休みになりますか What time do you usually go to bed? ◆ぐっすりお休み下さい Have a good sleep. / Good night! / Sleep well! / （子供に「おやすみなさい」）Night-

やすむ　713　やめる¹

night. Sleep tight!　◆ゆうべはよくお休みになれましたか Did you sleep well (last night)? / Did you have a good night's sleep (last night)?

やすらか　安らか(な)　(穏やか・静かな) peaceful, quiet　(眠りなどが深い) sound　◆安らかに眠る sleep peacefully [soundly]　◆安らかな死を迎える die a peaceful[quiet] death / die peacefully

やすり　やすり file　爪やすり nail file

やせ　痩せ thinness　(ひどいやつれ) emaciation　(病気による衰弱) wasting　▶やせ願望 pursuit of thinness　やせ薬(体重減少を目的とした) weight-loss medication [drug] / diet pill

やせる　痩せる　(細くなる) get[become] thin　(体重を減らす) lose weight　(囲)細い thin　標準より体重が軽い underweight　ほっそりした slender, slim　◆1か月で5kg痩せる lose five kilos in a month　◆痩せ始めたのはいつ頃からですか About when did you start losing weight?　◆娘さんはかなり痩せていますが、ダイエットをしているのですか Your daughter seems to be rather thin[underweight]. Is she on a diet?　◆もっと痩せたいですか Do you want to be thinner?　◆痩せようとダイエットする go on a diet to lose[reduce one's] weight　◆痩せ過ぎる become too thin

やっか　薬価　medication fee, drug price, pharmaceutical price

やっきょく　薬局　pharmacy /fáː·məsi/, 《英》chemist, chemist's　(ドラッグストア) drugstore　(特に病院内の薬局・調剤室) dispensary　◆この処方箋を薬局の窓口にお出し下さい Please give this prescription in at the pharmacy counter.　◆この処方箋はどこの薬局でも調剤してもらえます You can have this prescription filled at any pharmacy.　◆処方箋を院外薬局へ持って行く take the prescription to an outside pharmacy　◀院外薬局 outside pharmacy　院内薬局 hospital pharmacy / dispensary　かかりつけ薬局 regular pharmacy

やっこう　薬効　(効きめ) medication effect　(意図した効能) medication efficacy

やとびょう　野兎病　tularemia, rabbit fever

やに　(タール) tar　(粘液) mucus　(分泌物) discharge　◆タバコのやに cigarette tar　◀目やに eye mucus[discharge] / (かさぶた状の目やに) eye crust

やにょう　夜尿(症)　bedwetting, nocturnal enuresis, nighttime enuresis　◆お子さんは夜尿がありますか Does your child wet the bed?

やぶる　破る　(規則などを破る) break, violate　(引き裂く) tear, rip　◆約束を破る break one's promise[word]　◆病院の規則を破る break[violate] the hospital rules

やぶれる　破れる　(破裂する) rupture, burst　(裂ける) tear, get torn　▶破裂　◆血管が破れて血が周辺の脳組織に流れ出ています The blood vessel has ruptured[burst] and the blood is spilling out into the surrounding brain tissue.　◆鼓膜が破れる one's eardrum ruptures / (破れている) have a ruptured eardrum

やまば　山場　(危機) critical moment [stage, period]　◆彼女の容体は今晩が山場です It will be a critical moment for her tonight. / She's going to be in the critical stage tonight.　◆山場を脱する come out of the critical stage / pass the immediate crisis.

やむ　病む　(病気になる) become[get] sick　(具合が悪い) be sick　(病気で苦しむ) suffer from　(心配する) worry (over, about)　☞病気　◆心臓を病んでいる have[suffer from] heart trouble　◆些細なことを気に病む worry over trifles

やめる¹　止める　(停止する) stop　(あきらめる) give up　(喫煙・習慣などをやめる) quit　(悪習などと手を切る) break　▶中止, 控える　◆副作用が出たら直ちに薬の使用をやめて連絡して下さい If you have any side effects, please stop the medication at once and contact[call] us.　◆今日はこのくらいでやめておきましょう Let's call it a day. / Let's stop here for the day.　◆タバ

コをやめる quit[give up] smoking ◆爪を嚙む癖をやめる break the habit of biting *one's* nails ◆間食をやめる stop eating between meals

やめる² 辞める quit, resign (from) （定年で退職する）retire ◆病気で学校を辞める quit school because of sickness ◆病気で仕事を辞める quit[resign from] *one's* job because of sickness

やもう 夜盲（症） night blindness （🈺 night-blind), nyctalopia

やりかた やり方 ☞方法

やりすぎ やり過ぎる overdo ◆ダイエットをやり過ぎですよ You're overdoing it a bit with your diet.

やる （する・行う）do, perform （試みる）try ◆できる限りのことはやりましたが彼女を助けることはできませんでした We did *everything we could[our best], but she couldn't be saved. ◆やればできますよ You can do it if you only try. ◆こんなふうにやってみて下さい Please do it like this. ◆もう一度やってみて下さい Please try again. ◆よくやりましたね．おめでとう！ You did it! Congratulations! / Congratulations! Well done!

やわらかい 軟らかい soft (↔hard) （柔軟な）flexible ◆便は硬めですか，軟らかめですか Are your stools rather hard or soft? ◆軟らかい食べ物 soft food

やわらぐ 和らぐ （治まる）ease, relieve ☞和らげる ◆この薬で痛みが和らぎましたか Has this medication eased[relieved] the pain? ◆2, 3日もすれば痛みが和らぐでしょう It'll be less painful in a couple of days. ◆このクリームで発疹のかゆみが和らぐでしょう This cream will relieve the itching from the rash.

やわらげる 和らげる （苦痛を徐々に軽くする）ease, relieve （痛みなどを少なくする）reduce, lessen （筋肉などをほぐす）relax ☞緩和，和らぐ ◆痛みを和らげる薬を出しましょう I'm going to give you something to ease[relieve] the pain. ◆肩の緊張を和らげる relax[relieve / ease / reduce] the tension in *one's* shoulders ◆筋肉の痛みやこわばりを和らげる reduce[relieve / ease] the pain and stiffness in *one's* muscles

ゆ

ゆ 湯
《温めた水》(熱い) hot water (温かい) warm water (生ぬるい) lukewarm[tepid] water (熱湯) boiling water ◆この薬はお湯で飲んで下さい Please take this medication with *warm water[a warm liquid]. 《風呂》bath ◆お湯加減はいかがですか How is the bath? / How's the temperature of the bath water? ◆熱すぎるお湯に入るのは体によくありません It's not good for you to take a bath that's too hot. ◆赤ちゃんをお湯に入れる give a baby a bath / bathe[give a bath to] a baby
◀足湯 footbath 産湯 baby's first bath 腰湯 hip bath / (座浴) sitz bath

ゆいごん 遺言 (遺言) will (臨終の言葉) *a person's* last[dying] words ★複数形で. ◆遺言を残す leave a will

ゆうい 有意(な) significant (図significance) ◆この研究結果は統計的に有意です This study result is statistically significant. ◆有意差 significant difference 有意水準 significance level / level of significance 有意性 significance

ゆういはんきゅう 優位半球 dominant hemisphere

ゆういん 誘因 cause (動cause) (引き金) trigger (動trigger) ☞原因 ◆めまいの誘因として思い当たることは何かありますか Can you think of anything that might be causing the dizziness? ◆この頭痛の誘因は何だと思いますか What do you think is causing this headache? ◆過度のストレスがあなたのうつ病の誘因となっているかもしれません Too much stress may be one of the causes of your depression. ◆ほこりが誘因で喘息の発作が起こることもあります Dust may trigger an asthma attack.

ユーイングにくしゅ ―肉腫 Ewing sarcoma

ゆううつ 憂鬱 depression (図気が滅入った depressed 気の滅入るような depressing) ☞鬱, 抑うつ ◆最近, 憂鬱な気分ですか Have you recently been[felt] depressed? ◆どんな時に一番憂鬱に感じますか In what situations[When] do you feel most depressed? ◆憂鬱な気分 a depressed mood ◆憂鬱な天気 depressing[(陰気な)gloomy] weather

ゆうえき 有益(な) (役に立つ) useful, beneficial (助けになる) helpful (役立つ情報を与える) informative ◆その方法はとても有益です That method is very useful. ◆腫瘍専門医は有益な助言を与えてくれるでしょう The tumor specialist will give you some useful[beneficial] advice. ◆訓練はあなたのリハビリにとって有益だったと思いますか Do you feel the training was helpful[useful] for your rehabilitation? ◆有益なウェブサイト an informative website

ゆうがい 有害(な) (害になる) harmful (良くない) bad (危険性のある) hazardous (都合の悪い・逆の) adverse ☞害 ◆喫煙の有害な影響 the harmful effects of smoking ◆有害な物に触れる be exposed to something harmful[hazardous] ◆過度の飲酒はあなたの病状に有害です Excessive drinking is *bad for[harmful to] your condition. ▶有害作用 adverse[harmful] effect 有害廃棄物 hazardous waste 有害反応 adverse reaction 有害物質 harmful substance[material] 有害薬物反応 adverse drug reaction ; ADR

ゆうがた 夕方 evening ◆夕方5時に at five in the evening ◆今日の夕方(に) this evening ◆明日の夕方(に) tomorrow evening

ゆうき¹ 勇気 courage (図courageous), bravery (図brave) ◆勇気ある決断をなさいましたね You made a courageous decision. / It was courageous of you to make that decision. ◆勇気を出して下さい Please be brave! / Please have courage.

ゆうき² 有機(の) organic (↔inorganic) ▶有機化合物 organic compound 有機水銀化合物 organic mercury compound 有機溶剤 organic solvent 有機リン化合物 organophosphorus compound 有機リン中毒 organophosphorus poisoning

ゆうぎ 遊戯 (遊び) play (娯楽) recreation (ゲーム) game ☞遊び ▶遊戯室 playroom / recreation room 遊戯療法 play therapy

ゆうきょくさいぼう 有棘細胞 prickle cell ▶有棘細胞癌 prickle cell carcinoma

ゆうけい 有茎 pedicle, peduncle (peduncular, pedunculated) ▶有茎移植 pedicle graft[grafting] 有茎性ポリープ pedunculated polyp 有茎皮弁 pedicle flap

ゆうこう 有効 (な)
《効果がある》effective (图effectiveness), good (活性の) active ☞効き目, 効く, 効果 ◆この薬は血圧を下げるのに有効です This medication *is effective[works well] for[in] lowering blood pressure. ◆この病気には有効な治療法がないのです There's no effective treatment for this disease. ◆この薬の有効性と安全性はすでに実証されています The effectiveness and safety of this medication have already been confirmed. ◆この薬の有効期限は 1 年です This medication is effective for one year.
《法的に効力がある》valid ◆処方箋の有効期間は発行した日を含め 4 日間です The prescription is valid for four days from and including the date of issue. ◆ビザの有効期限が迫っていますので, 早めに更新して下さい The expiration date on your visa is approaching[drawing near], so you should renew it *ahead of time[in advance]. ◆クレジットカードの有効期限が切れています Your credit card has already expired. ◆有効なビザ a valid visa
◀最少有効量 minimal effective dose ; MED ▶有効成分 active ingredient 有効量 effective dose ; ED

ゆうごう 融合 (固定) fusion (图fused) (同化・吸収) assimilation ☞癒合 ◀陰唇融合 labial fusion ▶融合腎 fused kidney

ゆうこうじょうちゅう 有鉤条虫 *Taenia solium*, pork tapeworm

ゆうさんそうんどう 有酸素運動 aerobic exercise, aerobics

ゆうしぶんれつ 有糸分裂 mitosis (图mitotic) ▶有糸分裂阻害剤 mitotic inhibitor 有糸分裂促進因子 mitogen

ゆうしょう 有償 ☞有料

ゆうしょく 夕食 dinner, supper, evening meal ☞食事 ◆夕食のお時間です It's time for your dinner. ◆夕食はいかがでしたか How did you enjoy your dinner? ◆夕食後 after dinner[supper]

ゆうじん 友人 friend ☞友達

ゆうずいしんけいせんい 有髄神経線維 myelinated[medullated] nerve fiber

ゆうせい 優性 (の) dominant (↔recessive) ◀常染色体優性遺伝 autosomal dominant inheritance ; AD ▶優性遺伝 dominant inheritance

ゆうぜい 疣贅 wart, verruca (图verrucous) ☞いぼ ◀陰部疣贅 genital[venereal] wart / (尖形コンジローマ) condyloma acuminatum ウイルス性疣贅 viral[virus] wart 脂漏性疣贅 seborrheic wart 足底疣贅 plantar wart 扁平疣贅 flat wart ▶疣贅状母斑 verrucous nevus

ゆうせいほごほう 優生保護法 (母体保護法) Maternal Protection Law

ゆうせん¹ 優先 priority /praɪɔ́ːrəti/, precedence ◆予約のある患者さんを優先的に診察しております During consultation hours, we give priority to those who have an appointment. / (予約なしの患者も受け付けているが) We welcome walk-in patients but give priority to those who have an appointment.

ゆうせん² 有線 (の) (インターネットに接続した) wired ▶有線 LAN wired LAN[local area network]

ゆうそう¹ 郵送する mail, send *in the mail[by mail] ◆診断書は郵送しますか, こちらに取りに来ますか Shall we mail the medical certificate to you, or will you come and pick it up at our office?

ゆうそう² 遊走 (の) (浮遊の) floating

ゆうそう² (移動性の)wandering, migratory (走化性の)chemotactic ▶遊走因子 chemotactic factor　遊走腎 floating[wandering] kidney　遊走精巣 migratory testis

ゆうつう　有痛(の)　painful (↔ painless) ▶有痛域 painful area　有痛性筋痙攣 painful muscle cramp[spasm]

ゆうどう　誘導する　(案内する)guide (連れて行く)take　(導く)lead (図誘導線 lead) (人工的に誘導する)induce (図induction induced) ◆火災など緊急事態発生の際には患者さんを安全な場所に誘導いたします In the event of a fire or other emergency, we'll guide[lead / take] patients to a safe area. ◆胸部誘導 chest lead　四肢誘導 limb lead　▶誘導体 derivative　誘導分娩 induced labor[delivery] / induction of labor[delivery]

ゆうどく　有毒(な)　poisonous, toxic ☞毒　◆有毒なガスを吸う inhale poisonous[toxic] gas　◆有毒化学物質 poisonous[toxic] chemicals　有毒ガス poison [toxic / poisonous] gas / (有毒煙) toxic smoke　有毒キノコ poisonous[toxic] mushroom　有毒昆虫 poisonous[toxic] insect　有毒植物 poisonous[toxic] plant　有毒廃棄物 toxic waste　有毒物質 toxic [poisonous] substance[material]

ゆうはつ　誘発する　(疾病・体の反応などを引き起こす)induce (図induction induced)　(刺激して反応などを引き起こす)provoke (図provocation, evocation 図provocative, evoked)　(原因となる)cause (引き金になる)trigger　◆排卵を人工的に誘発する artificially induce ovulation ◆ストレスがうつ状態を誘発することがあります Stress can induce[cause / trigger / lead to] depression. ◆眠気を誘発する薬 a medication to *induce sleep[make *a person sleepy*] ◆ストレスで誘発された頭痛 (a) stress-induced headache ◀運動誘発喘息 exercise-induced asthma；EIA　咳嗽誘発試験 cough provocation test　視覚誘発電位 visual evoked potential；VEP　陣痛誘発 induction of *labor contractions[(分娩)labor]　排卵誘発薬 ovulation-inducing drug[medication / agent]　扁桃誘発試験 tonsil provocation test　▶誘発因子(促進要因)precipitating factor /(反応などを引き起こす要因)provoking factor　誘発筋電図 evoked electromyogram　誘発試験 provocative[provocation] test　誘発点 trigger point

ゆうびょうりつ　有病率　prevalence

ユーブイ　UV　(紫外線)ultraviolet (ray) ◆UVカットのクリーム UV-blocking [sunblock] cream　▶UVケア UV (skin) protection

ゆうもん　幽門　pylorus (図pyloric) ◀肥厚性幽門狭窄症 hypertrophic pyloric stenosis　▶幽門狭窄症 pyloric stenosis / stricture of the pylorus　幽門形成術 pyloroplasty　幽門痙攣 pylorospasm　幽門腺 pyloric gland

ゆうよ　猶予　◆命にかかわるこの事態では一刻の猶予も許されません There's no time to lose in this life-threatening situation.

ゆうよう　有用(な)　☞役, 有益

ゆうり¹　有利(な)　(利点)advantage (図 advantageous)　(良い点)good point ◆この治療法の有利な点と不利な点をお話ししましょう Let me tell you the advantages and disadvantages of this treatment. ◆この手術の有利な点は術後に薬を飲み続ける必要のないことです The advantage[good point] of this surgery is that you don't have to continue taking medications after you've had it.

ゆうり²　遊離(性の)　free　▶遊離移植 *free graft[grafting]　遊離ガス像 free air [gas]　遊離サイロキシン *free thyroxine [fT₄]　遊離脂肪酸 free fatty acid　遊離トリヨードサイロニン *free triiodothyronine [fT₃]　遊離皮弁 free flap

ゆうりょう　有料　(代金の支払い)pay (図 pay 図有償の paid)　(料金)charge (図請求する charge)　◆インフルエンザ予防注射は有料です There is a charge[We charge] for flu shots. ◆通訳サービスは有料となっております Patients *must pay[are charged] for interpreting services. / We offer paid interpreting services. ▶有料

駐車場 pay parking lot　有料テレビ pay TV　有料ベッド pay bed　有料老人ホーム private residential home for seniors [elderly people] / (退職者の)(private) retirement home　有料ロッカー pay locker

ゆうろう 有瘻 fistula ☞瘻孔 ▶有瘻性膿胸 pyothorax[empyema] with fistula

ゆえき 輸液 infusion （点滴静注）intravenous drip, IV drip ◀経静脈高カロリー輸液 intravenous hyperalimentation；IVH /（完全静脈栄養）total parenteral nutrition；TPN　補充輸液療法 replacement fluid infusion therapy ▶輸液セット infusion set　輸液速度 infusion speed　輸液ポンプ infusion pump　輸液路確保 venous route establishment / establishment of a venous route

ゆかた 浴衣 yukata；*casual thin cotton kimono* ◆浴衣または前開きの寝間着をご用意ください Please have a yukata or button-front pajamas prepared[ready].

ゆがんだ 歪んだ （ねじれた）distorted （引きつった）contorted ◆物が歪んで見えますか Is your vision distorted? ◆痛みで顔が歪んでいます The face is contorted with pain.

ゆけつ 輸血 (blood) transfusion ◆輸血をしたことがありますか Have you ever had a blood transfusion? ◆輸血した後体調に変化がありましたか Did you have any problems after the blood transfusion? ◆手術中に輸血を行う場合があります There is some possibility you'll need a blood transfusion during the surgery. ◆宗教上の理由で輸血を拒否する refuse a blood transfusion for religious reasons ◀緊急輸血 emergency transfusion　血液型不適合輸血 incompatible blood transfusion　血小板輸血 platelet transfusion　自己血輸血 autotransfusion / autologous blood transfusion / transfusion of one's own blood　成分輸血 blood component transfusion　成分輸血製剤 blood component derivative　赤血球輸血 *red blood cell[erythrocyte] transfusion　全血輸血 whole blood transfusion　双胎間輸血症候群 twin-to-twin[twin-twin] transfusion syndrome；TTTS　胎児-母体間輸血症候群 fetomaternal transfusion syndrome　無輸血手術 surgery without blood transfusion ▶輸血感染症 transfusion[transfusion-transmitted] infection　輸血拒否 refusal of blood transfusion / refusal to receive a blood transfusion　輸血検査 blood transfusion test[testing]　輸血後肝炎 posttransfusion hepatitis　輸血事故 blood transfusion accident　輸血提供者 blood[transfusion] donor　輸血適応 indications for blood transfusion　輸血同意書 (informed) consent form for blood transfusion　輸血反応 blood transfusion reaction　輸血歴 (blood) transfusion history　輸血レシピエント［受血者］(blood) transfusion recipient

ゆごう 癒合 （固定）fusion (㌻fused)（同化・吸収）assimilation （粘着）adhesion ☞融合 ▶癒合歯 fused teeth　癒合椎 assimilation vertebra

ゆさぶられっこしょうこうぐん 揺さぶられっ子症候群 shaken baby syndrome；SBS

ゆさぶる 揺さぶる shake

ゆしせいなんこう 油脂性軟膏 grease, oleaginous ointment

ゆしゅつさいどうみゃく 輸出細動脈 efferent arteriole

ゆすぐ rinse ◆口をゆすぐ rinse out one's mouth

ゆせいかん 輸精管 ductus deferens, spermatic[deferent] duct ☞精管

ゆそう 輸送 transport, transportation （病院間の移動）transfer ☞搬送 ◀能動輸送 active transport

ユダヤじん ―人 Jewish person (㌻Jewish) ◆彼はユダヤ人です He's Jewish. ★Jew には差別的なニュアンスがあるので注意.

ゆたんぽ 湯たんぽ hot-water bottle[bag]

ゆちゃく 癒着 adhesion (㌻adhere (to) ㌻adhesive) ◆腹膜に癒着する adhere to the peritoneum ◆手術後，腹腔に癒着が

起こっています Adhesions have formed in the abdominal cavity after the surgery. ◀胸膜癒着術 pleurodesis 線維性癒着 fibrous adhesion 腸管癒着 intestinal adhesion 腹膜癒着 peritoneal adhesion ▶癒着性イレウス adhesive intestinal obstruction 癒着性炎症 adhesive inflammation 癒着性腹膜炎 adhesive peritonitis 癒着胎盤 adhesive placenta

ゆっくり 《急がないで》〈遅く〉**slowly**（↔fast）〈徐々に〉**gradually**（↔suddenly） ◆もう少しゆっくり話して下さい Please speak more slowly. / Could you speak a little more slowly? ◆痛みの起こり方はゆっくりですか Does the pain come on slowly[gradually]? ◆急がず，ゆっくりやって下さい There's no hurry. Take your time. ◆もっとゆっくりしたペースで at a slower pace 《くつろいで》 ◆今晩はゆっくりお休み下さい Please have a good night's rest tonight. ◆食事後ゆっくり休む take a good rest after (eating) a meal

ゆったり 〈ゆるい〉**loose** 〈快適な〉**comfortable** 〈リラックスした〉**relaxed** 〈広々とした〉**spacious** ◆この検査にはゆったりした服装でおいで下さい Please wear loose-fitting[comfortable] clothes for this test. ◆ゆったりした気分になる feel relaxed ◆ゆったりした病室 a spacious hospital room

ゆにゅう **輸入**(の) **afferent** 〈国外から持ち込まれた〉**imported** ▶輸入感染症 imported infectious disease 輸入脚症候群 afferent loop syndrome 輸入細動脈 afferent arteriole

ゆのみ **湯のみ** 〈一般的に〉**cup** 〈マグカップ〉**mug**

ゆび **指** 〈手の指〉**finger** 〈足の指〉**toe** /tóu/ 〈手の親指〉**thumb** /θʌ́m/ 〈足の親指〉**big[great] toe** 〈手・足の指〉**digit** (略**digital**) ◆どこが痛みますか．指で指して下さい Where is the pain? Please point to where it hurts (with one finger). ◆(イラストや文などを示しながら)お話しになりたいことを指で指して下さい Please point to what it is you want to say. ◆この器具に指を入れて下さい．血中の酸素量を測りましょう Please put your finger into this device. I'm going to[Let me] measure the amount of oxygen in your blood. ◆親指をしゃぶる suck *one's* thumb ◆右手の指の付け根の関節を痛める hurt the knuckles on *one's* right hand ◆手〈足〉の指の爪が彎曲している the fingernails〈toenails〉are curved ◆指の変形 digital deformity ◀薬指 ring[third] finger ★親指を入れず人差し指から数えて3番目の指になる．小指〈手の〉little finger /〈足の〉little toe 突き指 sprained finger〈〈親指〉thumb〉 槌指 mallet finger〈〈親指〉thumb〉 中指〈手の〉middle finger /〈足の〉middle toe ばち指 clubbed finger〈〈親指〉thumb〉 ばね指 trigger[snapping / snap] finger〈〈親指〉thumb〉 人指し指 index finger / forefinger ▶指切断 digital amputation /〈手の〉amputation of a finger〈〈親指〉thumb〉/〈足の〉amputation of a toe 指鼻試験 finger-to-nose test 指ブロック digital (nerve) block ☞指先，指しゃぶり，指輪

ゆびさき **指先** 〈手の〉**fingertip, the tip of a finger** 〈足の〉**the tip of a toe** 〈指先の腹〉**finger〈toe〉pad, the pad of a finger〈toe〉** ◆冷気に曝されると，白，青，そして赤くなるなど手や足の指先が変色することがありますか Have you noticed any color changes in the tips of your fingers or toes, for example, to white, blue, or red, in response to cold exposure? ◆手足の指先で感覚のおかしいところはありますか Do you have any abnormal or strange sensation in the tips of your fingers or toes?

ゆびしゃぶり **指しゃぶり** 〈親指の〉**thumb sucking** 〈手指の〉**finger sucking** ◆お子さんは今でも指しゃぶりをしますか(親指の) Does your child still suck his〈her〉thumb? ◆指しゃぶりの癖がある(親指の) have a thumb-sucking habit

ゆびわ **指輪** **ring** ◆指輪がきついですか Do your rings feel tight? ◆指輪をはずす take *one's* ring off / take off *one's* ring ◆指輪をはめる put *one's* ring on / put on

one's ring

ゆめ 夢 dream （悪夢）nightmare ◆夢を見る have a dream / dream ▶夢判断 dream interpretation

ゆるい 緩い （固まっていない）loose （動緩める loosen） （水のような）watery （軟らかい）soft (↔hard) ◆便がゆるい have loose [watery] stools

ゆるす 許す
《容認する》allow /əláu/ （許可する）permit ☞許可 ◆12歳未満のお子さんの面会は許されておりません Children under the age of twelve are not allowed[permitted] to visit patients.
《容赦する》forgive, pardon ◆私の不注意をお許し下さい Please forgive me for my carelessness.

ゆるめる 緩める （物理的に）loosen (↔tighten), relax （精神的に）relax, relieve ◆首や胸周りを締め付けている衣服をゆるめて下さい Please loosen any tight clothing around your neck and chest. ◆便をゆるめる薬 a medication to loosen the bowels ◆緊張した筋肉をゆるめる loosen[relax] *one's* tight muscles

よ

よい¹　良い
《好ましい》**good, fine**　《素晴らしい》**great, excellent**　《容易な》**easy**　☞いい, 良く
◆良いお知らせがあります I have some good news for you.　◆これまでの健康状態はどうでしたか. 良かったですか How has your health been up until now? Good?　◆よかった, LDL コレステロールが正常値以下まで下がりましたね Oh, good[great], your LDL cholesterol has dropped below normal.　◆それは良い考えですね That's a good[great] idea.　◆検査結果は良くないようです I'm afraid that the test results don't look good.　◆消化に良い食べ物 food that is easy to digest / easily digestible food
《忠告・助言》　◆正確な診断結果を出すために詳しく検査したほうがよさそうです To ensure an accurate diagnosis, I recommend that you *have a thorough examination[get yourself examined thoroughly].
《許可》　◆明日から歩いてもよいですよ You may walk starting tomorrow.

よい²　酔い
☞酔う　◀車酔い carsickness 乗り物酔い motion[travel] sickness 飛行機酔い airsickness 二日酔い hangover 船酔い seasickness　▶酔い止め antimotion-sickness medication[drug / tablet / pill]

よう¹　用
《すべきこと》**thing to do**　《仕事》**work, business**　◆何かご用ですか What can I do for you? / May[Can] I help you?　◆ほかにご用がありますか Is there anything else I can do for you?　◆ご用のある時には遠慮しないでコールボタンを押して呼んで下さい(援助が必要なら) If you need any help, don't hesitate to push[press] the call button and let us know.
◆用が済み次第そちらにうかがいます I'll be with you[I'll come and see you] as soon as I finish my work.

よう²　葉　**lobe**　◀右葉〈左葉〉 right〈left〉 lobe　上葉〈中葉 / 下葉〉 upper〈middle / lower〉 lobe　前頭葉〈後頭葉 / 側頭葉 / 頭頂葉〉 frontal〈occipital / temporal / parietal〉 lobe　分葉 lobulation / segmentation

よう³　癰　**carbuncle**

よう⁴　酔う　《酒に》**get[become] drunk**　《吐き気がする》**get[become] sick**　☞酩酊, 酔い　◆酔っ払うほど飲む drink enough to get drunk　◆酔っ払って意識を失う get drunk and pass out　◆悪酔いして気持ちが悪い(飲みすぎて) be[feel] sick from drinking (too much)　◆酔っ払い a drunk / a drunkard　◆バスに酔う get sick on buses
◆車〈飛行機 / 船 / 電車〉に酔う get carsick〈airsick / seasick / trainsick〉

ようあつかんき　陽圧換気　**positive pressure ventilation[respiration, breathing]**
◀間欠的陽圧換気 intermittent positive pressure ventilation；IPPV　呼気終末陽圧換気 positive end-expiratory pressure ventilation / PEEP ventilation　持続陽圧換気 continuous positive pressure ventilation；CPPV　非侵襲的陽圧換気 noninvasive positive pressure ventilation；NPPV

ようい¹　用意する　《準備する》**prepare (for), make preparations (for)**　《準備しておく》**get ready**　《手配する》**arrange (for), make arrangements (for)**　《提供する》**supply, provide**　☞準備, 手配　◆ご自分で食事の用意をしますか Do you cook for yourself? / Do you prepare meals (for) yourself?　◆用意はできましたか Are you ready?　◆キングさん, 夕食の用意ができました Mr King, dinner is ready.　◆診察券〈保険証〉をご用意下さい Please have your *hospital ID card〈insurance card〉 ready.　◆おむつはこちらで用意いたします We'll make arrangements for diapers[(成人用) incontinence underwear].　◆当院では検査着を用意しております Exam gowns will be supplied[provided] by the

hospital.

ようい² 容易(な) (楽な)easy (単純な)simple ☞簡単, 一易い ◆それは解決が容易な問題です It is *an easy[a simple] problem to solve. ◆彼女が事実を受け入れるのは容易ではないでしょう It won't be so easy for her to accept the fact.

よういく 養育する bring up, raise ☞育てる ▶養育費 cost of raising a child / child-care expenses

よういん 要因 factor (原因)cause ☞原因 ◆決定的な要因 a decisive factor ◆負の要因 a minus factor ◀外的要因 external factor / (外因子)extrinsic factor 気象要因 meteorological factor 体質要因 constitutional factor 内的要因 internal factor / (内因子)intrinsic factor

ようえき 溶液 solution

ようかい 溶解する (個体が液体の中で溶ける)dissolve (图dissolution) (個体が加熱で液化する)melt ☞溶かす, 溶ける ◀結石溶解療法 stone dissolution therapy 血栓溶解薬 thrombolytic (medication / drug / agent) 血栓溶解療法 thrombolytic therapy 線維素溶解 fibrinolysis 胆石溶解薬 gallstone-dissolving medication[drug / agent] 胆石溶解療法 gallstone dissolution therapy 粘液溶解薬 mucolytic (medication / drug / agent) ▶溶解度 solubility

ようかいご 要介護 (long-term) care needs, (long-term) care required [needed] ◆要介護度2の認定を受ける be certified as requiring care level two / be certified as a person with level-two care needs ▶要介護者(長期介護を必要とする人)person requiring long-term care / person with long-term care needs / (介護保険利用者)long-term care insurance recipient 要介護状態 condition requiring long-term care 要介護度 care (needs) level / the level of care needs 要介護度認定 certification of long-term care needs

ヨウかカリウム 一化カリウム potassium iodide

ようかくにん 要確認 (メモ書きなどで)

confirmation required[needed]

ようかんさつ 要観察 (メモ書きなどで)observation required[needed]

ようき 容器 container (点眼容器)eye-dropper ◆便を容器に入れる place[put] a stool sample in a container

ようきゅう 要求 (要望)request (強い要請)demand ☞要望 ◆彼女の要求に応じる meet[satisfy] her request[demand]

ようきん 腰筋 psoas (muscle) ◀小腰筋 psoas minor (muscle) 大腰筋 psoas major (muscle) 腸腰筋 iliopsoas (muscle)

ようぐ 用具 (機器)instrument, device (手仕事の道具)tool ☞器具, 道具

ようけつ 溶血 hemolysis (图hemolytic) ◀血管内溶血 intravascular hemolysis ▶溶血性黄疸 hemolytic jaundice 溶血性尿毒症症候群 hemolytic uremic syndrome；HUS 溶血性貧血 hemolytic anemia 溶血反応 hemolytic reaction ☞溶血性連鎖球菌

ようけつせいれんさきゅうきん 溶血性連鎖球菌 hemolytic streptococcus ▶溶血性連鎖球菌感染症 hemolytic streptococcal infection

ようけん 用件 ☞用

ようご¹ 用語 term (総称として)terminology (特定分野の語彙)vocabulary (言語)language (命名法)nomenclature ◆一般的な用語で病気を説明する(素人にも分かる言葉)explain the disease in layperson's terms ◀医学用語 medical term [terminology / language / vocabulary] 専門用語 technical term[word] / specialized vocabulary

ようご² 養護 (看病・看護)nursing (世話)care ◀特別養護老人ホーム special nursing home for seniors[elderly people] ▶養護学校[特別支援学校] special needs [education] school / school for children with special needs 養護教諭 school nurse 養護施設 (児童の)children's home / residential facility for children / (高齢者の)nursing home

ようこつ 溶骨(性の) osteolytic ▶溶骨

ようこつ

性病変 osteolytic lesion　溶骨性変化 osteolytic change

ようざい　溶剤　solvent

ようさん　葉酸　folic acid　▶葉酸欠乏 folic acid deficiency　葉酸欠乏性神経炎 folic acid deficiency neuropathy　葉酸欠乏性貧血 folic acid deficiency anemia　葉酸代謝拮抗薬 antifolate / folic acid antagonist

ようし[1]　用紙　(書式)form　(紙)paper　◆この用紙に記入して下さい Please fill out this form.　◀質問用紙 questionnaire　申込用紙 application form

ようし[2]　養子　adopted child　▶養子縁組 adoption　☞養子免疫

ようじ[1]　用事　☞用

ようじ[2]　幼児　(乳・幼児)infant　(よちよち歩きの子)toddler　(幼い子供)little child　(学齢前の子供)preschool child　☞ライフステージ　▶幼児期 infancy / early childhood / (学齢前)preschool period　幼児虐待 infant abuse　幼児語 baby talk / (小児語)child language

ようしえん　要支援　(long-term)support needs, (long-term) support required [needed]　▶要支援状態 condition requiring long-term[long-care] support　要支援度 support level / the level of support needs　要支援2 support (needs) level two

ようしき[1]　様式　(やり方)style　(型)pattern　◀生活様式 lifestyle / (暮らし方)way of living[life]

ようしき[2]　洋式(の)　Western-style　▶洋式トイレ Western-style toilet

ようしせんちりょう　陽子線治療　proton radiotherapy

ようしめんえき　養子免疫　adoptive immunity　▶養子免疫療法 adoptive immunotherapy

ようしゅ　用手(的な)　manual　☞徒手　▶用手人工呼吸法 manual artificial ventilation

ようじょう　養生する　☞休養

ようじょうにゅうとう　葉状乳頭　foliate papillae

ようしん　痒疹　prurigo　◀結節性痒疹 nodular prurigo

ようじん　用心する　☞注意

ようしんけい　腰神経　lumbar nerve　▶腰神経叢 lumbar plexus

ようじんけっせつ　謡人結節　singer's node[nodule]　(声帯結節)vocal (cord) nodule

ようす　様子　(容体)condition　(状況)situation　(徴候)sign　◆お子さんの様子を教えて下さい Can[Could] you tell me *how your child is[about your child's condition]?　◆出血している様子はありません There's no sign of bleeding.　◆しばらく様子を見ましょう Let's wait a while and see *how it goes[how things turn out / if anything develops / what happens].　◆彼女はすっかり落ち込んでいる様子です She looks[appears to be] very depressed.

ようすい　羊水　amniotic fluid　(口語)waters　▶羊水過少 oligohydramnios　羊水過多 polyhydramnios　羊水検査 amniotic fluid analysis　羊水混濁 meconium staining (of the amniotic fluid)　羊水穿刺 amniocentesis　羊水塞栓 amniotic (fluid) embolism

ようずい　腰髄　lumbar cord　▶腰髄症 lumbar myelopathy　腰髄損傷 lumbar cord injury

ようする　要する　(人が必要とする)need　(物・事が要求する)require　(時間がかかる)take　☞必要　◆十分な休息を要します You need a good rest.　◆この活動はかなりの体力を要します This activity requires [takes] a lot of energy.　◆この検査にはおよそ30分を要します This test will take about thirty minutes (to complete).

ようするに　要するに　(簡単に言うと)in short　(要約すると)to summarize, in summary　(肝心なことは)the point is …　◆要するに, 血圧のコントロールが必要です In short, you need to control your blood pressure.　◆要するに, あきらめずに続けることです The point is, you need to continue without giving it up.

ようせい¹ 陽性（の） positive（↔negative） ◆ツベルクリン検査の結果は陽性です You tested positive for tuberculin. / The result of your tuberculin test is positive. ◀偽陽性 false-positive 強陽性 strong[strongly] positive グラム陽性菌 gram-positive bacteria 弱陽性 weak[weakly] positive ▶陽性症状 positive symptom 陽性的中率 positive predictive value；PPV 陽性反応 positive reaction 陽性モデル positive model

ようせい² 要請する（頼む）request, ask （強く求める）demand（電話で呼ぶ）call ◆救急車を要請する request[call] an ambulance

ようせい³ 養成 ☞教育，訓練

ようせん 腰仙（の）lumbosacral ▶腰仙骨神経叢 lumbosacral plexus 腰仙髄損傷 lumbosacral spinal cord injury 腰仙部挫傷 lumbosacral strain

ようそ 要素（結果を生む要因）factor（成分・構成要素）component, element, constituent ☞要因，因子

ヨウそ 一素 iodine（㊙iodinated）☞ヨード ◀放射性ヨウ素 radioiodine / radioactive iodine ▶ヨウ素化合物 iodinated compound

ようだい 容体・容態 condition ◆現在のところ彼の容体は安定しています His condition is now stable. / He is now in (a) stable condition. ◆彼女の容体はかなり改善しています Her condition has improved a lot. / There has been some obvious improvement in her condition. ◆彼の容体は危機的状況を脱しました He's come out of the critical stage. / He's passed the immediate crisis. ◆彼女の容体が急変しました（急に悪化した）Her condition has taken a sudden turn for the worse. ◆彼の容体は思わしくありません（かなり深刻である）His condition is serious. / He is in (a) serious condition. / （不安定である）His condition is unstable.

ようちえん 幼稚園（5, 6歳児の）kindergarten（3, 4歳児の）nursery school ☞保育園

ようちゅうい 要注意 ◆血糖値は要注意です You should keep a check on your blood sugar. / Your blood sugar level requires *careful attention[（定期的な検査を要する）regular checkups]. ◆（掲示などで）要注意 Attention (Required)! / （重要なお知らせ）Important Notice

ようちりょう 要治療（メモ書きなどで）treatment required[needed], requiring treatment

ようつい 腰椎 lumbar vertebra, lumbar spine ▶腰椎骨折 lumbar fracture 腰椎症 lumbar spondylosis 腰椎穿刺 lumbar puncture 腰椎椎間板ヘルニア lumbar disc herniation 腰椎捻挫 lumbar sprain 腰椎麻酔 lumbar spinal anesthesia

ようつう 腰痛 lower[low] back pain；LBP, lumbago ◆慢性的な腰痛がある have chronic lower back pain ◆腰痛を楽にするストレッチ体操があります There are some stretching exercises you can do to relieve[ease] your lower back pain. ◆腰痛を悪化させるものは何ですか What makes the lower back pain worse? ▶腰痛体操 exercise for lower back pain

ようてん 陽転 positive conversion ◀ツベルクリン反応陽転 tuberculin conversion

ようでんし 陽電子 positron ▶陽電子断層撮影 positron emission tomography；PET

ようばい 溶媒 solvent

ようび 曜日 day (of the week) ◆今日は何曜日ですか What day (of the week) is it today? ◆月曜日に on Monday ◆月曜日ごとに on Mondays

ようひん 用品（必需品）supplies ★複数形で．（備品）equipment（品物・製品）item, goods ☞器具，道具 ◀看護用品 nursing supplies[equipment] 生理用品 sanitary goods[items]

ようふ 養父 foster father

ようぶ 腰部 lumbar region, lower back, low back ▶腰部交感神経節ブロック lumbar sympathetic nerve block 腰部硬膜外麻酔 lumbar epidural anesthesia 腰

ようぶ 部コルセット back[lumbar] brace[corset] 腰部脊柱管狭窄症 lumbar spinal canal stenosis 腰部脊椎症 lumbar spondylosis

ようふく 洋服 clothes ◆服 ◆（診察・検査が終わって）どうぞ洋服を着て下さい You can get dressed now.

ようぼ 養母 foster mother

ようほう 用法 （使い方）how to use （使用法・使用量）usage （使用の指示）directions for use ★direction は複数形で．（薬の投与）administration ◆薬

ようぼう¹ 容貌 （顔の特徴）facial features （表情）looks ★いずれも複数形で．（外見）appearance ◆容貌に変化がある have a change in one's facial features

ようぼう² 要望 （頼み）request （強い要請）demand （願い）wish ◆意向 ◆ご要望により明細書をお出しします Itemized statements are available on[upon] request. ◆申し訳ありませんが，ご要望にはお応えできません I'm sorry, but we can't meet[satisfy / comply with] your request [demand]. ◆食物アレルギーなど食事にご要望があればお知らせ下さい If you have any dietary requests[（必要性）needs] due to food allergies or other reasons, please let us know.

ようまく 羊膜 amnion, amniotic membrane, bag of waters

ようむいん 用務員 janitor

ようもうざい 養毛剤 （育毛剤）hair-growing agent, hair restorer

ようやく 要約 summary （動summarize） ☞要するに ◆要約しますと To summarize … / In summary … ◆看護要約 nursing summary 退院時要約 discharge summary

ようりょう¹ 用量 （1回の用量）dose （一定期間にわたる用量）dosage ☞薬 ◆処方された用量は必ず飲んで下さい Please be sure to take the prescribed dose. ◆この薬は飲み忘れても次の回の用量を2倍にしないで下さい Even if you miss one dose of this medication, please don't double the next dose. ◆低用量のアスピリン low-dose aspirin ◆1日用量 daily dose

▶用量反応関係 dose-response relationship

ようりょう² 容量 （容積）capacity （体積）volume ◀膀胱容量 bladder capacity ▶容量負荷 volume load

ようれんきん 溶連菌 ☞溶血性連鎖球菌

ヨーガ yoga ◆ヨーガをやる do[practice] yoga / do yoga exercises

ヨード iodine ☞ヨウ素 ◀低ヨード食 low-iodine diet 放射性ヨード療法 radio-iodine therapy[treatment] ▶ヨード液 iodine solution ヨード過敏症 iodine hypersensitivity ヨード剤 iodine preparation

よか 余暇 leisure (time), free time ◆いつも余暇をどう過ごしていますか How do you usually spend your leisure[free] time? / What do you usually do in your leisure[free] time? ▶余暇活動 leisure activities

ヨガ ☞ヨーガ

よき 予期する expect, anticipate （名expectation, anticipation） ☞予想，予測 ▶予期不安 expectation anxiety

よく¹ 良く ☞良い
《十分に》well （形good） （注意深く）carefully （完全には…でない）not quite ◆昨夜はよく眠れましたか Did you sleep well last night? ◆説明書をよく読んで下さい Please read the instructions carefully. ◆よく聞こえませんでした．もう一度おっしゃって下さい I didn't quite catch what you said. Could you say it again, please? 《しばしば》often, frequently ◆甘いものをよく食べますか Do you often eat sweets? 《よくぞ》 ◆よく頑張りましたね You did it! / You did well[great]! / Good for you! / （軽い口調で）Good job. 《良くなる・回復する》get well[better] （好転する）improve （前より気分がいい）feel better （症状などが消える）clear up ◆もうすぐ良くなりますよ You'll get better soon. / You'll soon be well again. ◆すぐに気分が良くなりますよ You'll feel better soon. ◆ごく普通の症状ですから2，3日も経てば良くなります It's quite a common

condition, so it should clear up in a few days or so. ◆彼女の容体は良くなっています She has improved[gotten better]. ◆脚の怪我はかなり良くなっています Your leg is healing well[nicely]. ◆傷口は良くなっています The wound has healed over. ◆早く良くなってね! Get well soon! ◆一刻も早く良くなることを願っています I hope you'll make a speedy recovery. ◆この薬は便通を良くしてくれます This medication helps[(促進する) promotes] bowel movements.

よく² 浴 bath ◀気泡浴 bubble bath 座浴 sitz bath　足浴 foot bath

よく³ 翌— next, following ◆翌週の金曜日には来られますか Can you come and see me next Friday? ◆翌朝 the next [following] morning

よくあつ 抑圧 repression, suppression

よくうつ 抑うつ depression（㊟depressive, depressed）☞鬱, 憂鬱 ▶抑うつ気分 depressed[depressive] mood　抑うつ状態 depressive state / state of depression　抑うつ反応 depressive reaction

よくしつ 浴室 bathroom ◆浴室は交代でお使いいただきます You can take turns using the bathroom.

よくじょう 翼状（の） winged, pterygoid ◀翼状針 winged needle　翼状突起 pterygoid process　翼状片 pterygium

よくせい 抑制する （作用・働きを抑止する） suppress, repress（㊟suppression, repression）（反応などを抑制・阻止する）inhibit（㊟inhibition）（拘束する）restrain（㊟restraint）（制御する）control（㊟control）（低下させる）depress（㊟depression）☞阻害 ◆がんの転移を抑制する suppress[inhibit] cancer metastasis ◆問題行動を抑制する control[restrain] problem behavior ◀血小板凝集抑制薬 antiplatelet aggregation　呼吸抑制 respiratory depression　骨髄抑制 myelosuppression　陣痛抑制 suppression of preterm labor　乳汁分泌抑制 lactation suppression　尿酸生成抑制薬 uric acid synthesis inhibitor　排卵抑制 ovulation inhibition[suppression]

免疫抑制薬 immunosuppressive（medication / drug / agent）/ immunosuppressant ▶抑制遺伝子 suppressor[repressor] gene　抑制因子 suppressor / repressor / inhibitor　抑制効果 inhibitory effect　抑制酵素 inhibitory enzyme　抑制試験 inhibition[suppression] test

よくそう 浴槽 bathtub

よくぼう 欲望 desire ☞欲求

よけつ 瘀血 ☞貯血

よこ 横
《傍ら・側》side ◆横向き ◆腕をこのように横に置いて下さい Please put your arms by your side, like this. ◆首をすばやく2, 3回横に振って下さい Please shake your head quickly from side to side two or three times. ◆首の横が痛む have (a) pain in the side of *one's* neck ◆右〈左〉横に on the right〈left〉side
《横になる》lie down ☞寝る ◆この検査台の上に横になって下さい Please lie down on this exam table. ◆横になると痛みがとれますか Does the pain go away when you lie down?
《横幅》（短いほうの幅）width（㊟wide）（長いほうの幅）length（㊟long）★英語では短いほうを横, 長いほうを縦とする. ◆ポリープのサイズは横2mm, 縦3mmです The (size of the) polyp is two millimeters wide[in width] and three millimeters long[in length].
《長軸に対して》（横断の）transverse（水平の）horizontal ▶横アーチ transverse arch　横軸 horizontal axis ☞横腹

よご 予後 prognosis（㊟prognostic） ◆この病気の予後は良好です This disease has a good prognosis. / The prognosis of this disease is good. ◆彼の予後は良くありません The likelihood of his recovering [His prognosis] is *not so good[rather bad / rather poor]. ▶予後因子 prognostic factor　予後不良 poor[unfavorable] prognosis　予後良好 favorable prognosis

よごす 汚す （一般的に）make … dirty （尿・便などで）soil （血液などのしみで）stain ☞汚れた ◆パジャマのズボンを汚す soil *one's* pajama bottoms

よこばら　横腹　(側腹部)the lateral abdominal region　(わき腹)side, flank

よこむき　横向き(に)　on[onto] *one's* side, sideways　☞横　◆横向きに寝て下さい Please lie on your side.　◆仰向けではなく，横向きに寝るとよいでしょう You should sleep on your side rather than on your back.　◆寝返りを打って横向きになる roll over onto *one's* side　◆横向きに立って下さい Please stand sideways.

よごれた　汚れた　(一般的に)dirty　(汗・尿・便などで汚れた)soiled　(しみが付いた)stained　☞汚い　◆汚れた洗濯物を洗う wash the dirty laundry　◆汚れたシーツを換える change soiled sheets

よしん　予診　(予備問診)preliminary (medical) history-taking　(予備的診察)preliminary examination　(予備的診断)preliminary diagnosis　▶予診票 preliminary medical history form

よせい　余生　the rest of *one's* life, *one's* remaining years　◆自国に戻って余生を送る return to *one's* country and *spend the rest of *one's* life[live out *one's* life] there

よそう　予想する　(期待する)expect　(図expectation)　(予測する)predict　(図prediction)　☞予測　◆予想外に(予想を上回って)above[beyond] *one's* expectations / (予想を下回って)below *one's* expectations　◆すべては予想通りに運びました Everything turned out as (we) expected.　◆予想以上に早く回復しています You're recovering quicker[more rapidly] than we expected.　◆予想に反して症状に顕著な改善が見られました Contrary to our expectations, there's been a marked improvement in the symptoms.　◆残念ですが，予想されたように悪性の腫瘍が見つかりました I'm sorry to have to tell you this, but we found a malignant tumor, as we had predicted.　◆予想しなかった妊娠 unexpected pregnancy

よそく　予測する　predict　(図prediction 図predictive, predicted)　foresee　☞予想　◆完治にどのくらいかかるか

を予測するのは難しいです It's difficult to predict how long it will take for you to make a complete recovery.　▶予測術後肺機能 predicted postoperative lung function　予測値 predictive value　予測肺活量 predicted vital capacity

よたよた　◆よたよた歩く(ふらふらと不安定に)walk unsteadily / stagger / (おぼつかない足取りで)walk with faltering steps

よだれ　涎　drool　(図drool), excessive salivation　(少量の)dribble　(図dribble)　◆口の片側からのよだれは顔面神経麻痺の徴候です Drooling on one side of the mouth is a sign of paralysis of the facial nerves.　▶よだれ掛け bib

よだん　予断　◆彼女の病状は深刻で予断を許しません Her condition is serious and there's no knowing *how things will develop[what will happen next].

よちょう　予兆　(前触れ)sign　(警告)warning　◆発作が起こりそうな予兆がある have a sign[warning] that an attack is about to begin

よちよち　◆よちよち歩く toddle　◆よちよち歩きの子供 a toddler　☞よたよた

よっきゅう　欲求　desire　◆欲求を満たす satisfy[fulfill] *one's* desire(s)　◆欲求を抑える control[suppress / stifle] *one's* desire(s)　◀性的欲求(欲望)sexual desire / (衝動)sexual impulse　☞欲求不満

よっきゅうふまん　欲求不満　frustration　(図frustrated)　◆欲求不満がたまる become[get] frustrated / (たまっている)be[feel] frustrated　◆欲求不満から暴飲暴食する eat and drink too much *out of[in] frustration

よっぱらう　酔っ払う　☞酔う

よつんばい　四つん這い　◆四つん這いで這う crawl *on *one's* hands and knees[on all fours] / (ずり這いする)creep　◆四つん這いになる get (down) *on *one's* hands and knees[on all fours]

よてい　予定　(スケジュール)schedule　(動schedule)　(計画)plan　(動plan)　(事前の手配)prearrangement　(動prearrange)　(予約・約束)appointment　(動appoint)　☞スケ

よてい | 728 | よびだし

ジュール

《予定表》 ◆経過観察のための検査と診察の来院予定をお渡しいたします I'm going to give you a schedule of follow-up visits for some tests and checkups. ◆予防接種の予定は市の広報をチェックして下さい Please check the vaccination schedule in [through] your local city bulletin.

《予定する》 ◆手術は冠動脈バイパス術を予定しています The surgery you're going to have is a coronary bypass. ◆手術日の予定を入れる schedule the date for *a person's* surgery ◆精密検査の予定を立てる schedule[set up a schedule for] a thorough examination ◆手術は火曜日の午前の予定です Your surgery is scheduled for Tuesday morning. ◆手術の予定を翌週に変更する reschedule the surgery for the next[following] week ◆予定の時間に必ず来て下さい Please be sure to come at the appointed time.

《予定がある・ない》 ◆あいにく明日は予定が入っています I'm sorry, but I've already made an appointment for tomorrow. ◆今週は予定が詰まっています I have a full [tight / busy] schedule (for) this week. / My schedule is full this week. ◆今週の土曜日は特に予定がありません I have nothing (particular) to do this Saturday. / I'm free this Saturday.

《予定通り》 ◆全ては予定通りに運びました Everything went as planned. ◆手術を予定通りに行う do[perform] *a person's* surgery on schedule ◆体重は予定通り減っていますか(期待通りに)Are you losing weight at the expected rate? ◆予定より早く〈遅く〉earlier〈later〉than expected / *ahead of〈behind〉schedule

▶予定手術 planned surgery 予定帳 appointment[schedule] book 予定表 schedule / (年間予定表)calendar ☞予定日

よていび 予定日 (出産期日)due date (妊娠満期日)term ◆予定日は3月10日です Your due date is March (the) tenth. ◆予定日はいつですか When is

your baby due? / When is your[your baby's] due date? ◆その男の子は予定日より3週間前の5月4日に生まれました The baby boy was born on May (the) fourth, three weeks ahead of *his due date [term]. ◀出産予定日 due date / (分娩予測日)expected[estimated] date of delivery;EDD / (出産予測日)expected date of confinement;EDC, probable date of confinement;PDC

よなか 夜中(に) (夜に)at night (夜間に)during the night, in the night (真夜中に)in the middle of the night ☞夜間 ◆排尿のため夜中に目が覚めますか Do you wake up during the night to urinate? ◆真夜中に目が覚める wake up in the middle of the night ◆夜中に何度もトイレに行く go to the bathroom several times during[in] the night

よなき 夜泣き nighttime crying ◆夜泣きしますか Does he〈she〉cry *at night[in the night]?

よにんべや 4人部屋 four-bed room, room for four

よび 予備(の) (品物がスペアの)spare (備蓄の)reserve (余分の)extra (下準備の)preliminary (テストケースとしての)pilot ◆予備の部品 spare parts ▶予備研究 preliminary study 予備診断 preliminary diagnosis 予備知識 preliminary knowledge 予備調査 pilot study[survey] 予備力 reserve capacity / functional reserve

よびかけ 呼びかけ ◆呼びかけに応えて目を開く open *one's* eyes in response to *a person's* voice

よびだし 呼び出し call ◆ベッドの枕元に呼び出しボタン,トイレには緊急の呼び出しボタンが付いています There's a call button at the head of the bed and an emergency call button inside the bathroom. ◆ご用の時は呼び出しボタンを押して下さい Please push[press] the call button when you need any help. ◆呼び出しベルを鳴らす ring the call bell ◆緊急呼び出し an emergency call[code]

よびょう　余病　☞合併症

よぶ　呼ぶ　**call**（呼んでくる・連れてくる）**get**　◆お呼びするまでここでお待ち下さい Please wait here until we call your name.　◆名前をお呼びしたら5番の部屋にお入り下さい When your name is called, please enter room five.　◆担当医を呼びましょう I'll call your doctor for you. / Let me get your doctor for you.　◆ご用がある時は遠慮せずにスタッフを呼んで下さい Please don't hesitate to call a staff member if you need any help.　◆（ナースコールに応えて）お呼びですか What can I do for you? / May I help you?　◆救急車を呼ぶ call an ambulance　◆ふだんお子さんをどう呼んでいますか（愛称を訊く）What name does your child go by?

よふかし　夜更かしする　**stay up late**（at night）, **sit up late**（at night）

よぼう　予防する　（防止する）**prevent**（図 **prevention** 図 **preventive, prophylactic**）（制御する）**control**（図 **control**）（保護する）**protect**（図 **protection**）　◆風邪を予防するために手洗いとうがいをして下さい Please wash your hands and gargle to prevent [protect against] colds.　◆感染の拡大を予防する prevent the spread of infection　◆動脈瘤の破裂を予防する prevent the aneurysm from rupturing　◀感染予防 prevention of infection / infection control　食中毒予防 prevention of food poisoning　床ずれ予防 bedsore prevention　▶予防医学 preventive medicine　予防照射 prophylactic irradiation　予防的治療 preventive treatment　☞予防策, 予防接種

よぼうさく　予防策　（防止策）**preventive measures**（用心のための対策）**precautionary measures, precautions**　★通例, 複数形で.　◆予防策を講じていますか Are you taking any preventive[precautionary] measures?　◆どんな予防策を講じていますか What precautions are you taking? / What preventive[precautionary] measures are you taking?　◀標準的予防策 standard precautions

よぼうせっしゅ　予防接種　（ワクチン接種）**vaccination**（圏 **vaccinate**）（ワクチン）**vaccine**（免疫をつけるための接種）**immunization, inoculation**（予防注射）（**preventive**）**shot**[**injection**,《英》**jab**]　☞ワクチン　◆これまでに何の予防接種を受けましたか What vaccinations[immunizations] have you had?　◆麻疹の予防接種を受けましたか Have you already been vaccinated for measles? / Have you already had *the measles vaccine[the vaccination for measles]?　◆4週間以内に何か他の予防接種を受けましたか Have you had any other vaccinations[immunizations] in the past four weeks?　◆予防接種を受けて具合が悪くなったことがありますか Have you ever had any problems with previous vaccines? / Have you ever felt sick after *being vaccinated[receiving a vaccination]?　◆赤ちゃんはポリオの予防接種が必要です Your baby needs to get[have] the polio vaccine. / Your baby needs to be vaccinated against polio.　◆次回の予防接種は4週間以上空けて受けて下さい You should wait at least four weeks before receiving the next vaccination.　◆今回のワクチンは不活化ワクチンなので, 次の予防接種まで1週間以上間隔を空けて下さい This vaccine is inactivated, so be sure to wait for at least one week before receiving another vaccination.　◆次回の予防接種は1年後です The next vaccination will be one year from now.　◆予防接種の情報は市の広報をチェックして下さい Please check[get / obtain] the information about vaccinations in[through] your local city bulletin.　◆今日はインフルエンザの予防接種をしましょう I'm going to *give you a flu shot[vaccinate you against the flu] today.　◆今日受けるインフルエンザ予防接種についての説明文を読んで理解しましたか Have you read and understood the vaccine information sheet about today's influenza vaccine?　◆あなたのかかりつけ医はインフルエンザ予防接種を受けてもよいと言いましたか Did your regular [family] doctor say you could get a flu shot? / Does your regular[family] doctor agree to your having the flu vaccination [shot]? ◆予防接種の効果や副反応を理解した上で，接種を希望しますか Now that you understand the benefits and side effects of the vaccine, do you still want to have the vaccination? ◆インフルエンザ予防接種の予診表 a flu vaccination questionnaire / a screening questionnaire for influenza vaccination ◀個別予防接種 individual vaccination　集団予防接種 mass vaccination[immunization]　初回予防接種 initial vaccination　追加予防接種 booster shot[injection] / booster[additional] vaccination　定期予防接種 routine vaccination[immunization]　任意予防接種 voluntary vaccination[immunization] ▶予防接種記録 vaccination record　予防接種証明書 certificate of vaccination　予防接種スケジュール vaccination[immunization] schedule

よぼうそち　予防措置 ☞予防策

よみかき　読み書き　reading and writing
　◆日本語の読み書きができますか Do you read and write Japanese? / Are you able to read and write in Japanese?

よみちがえる　読み違える （文字・内容を）**misread** （発音を）**mispronounce**

よむ　読む　read ◆サインする前にこの同意書をよく読んで下さい Please read this consent form carefully before signing it. ◆声に出して読む read aloud ◆声に出さずに読む read silently ◆お名前はどう読むのですか（どう発音するのか）How do you pronounce your name?

よめい　余命　life expectancy, expectation of life, *one's* **remaining days** ★複数形で．☞寿命 ◀平均余命 average life expectancy / average expectation of life

よやく¹　与薬　giving (a) medication ☞処方, 投薬, 投与 ▶与薬室 medication room

よやく²　予約 （診察・検査の）**appointment** （慟**make an appointment**） （部屋・座席の）**reservation** （慟**reserve**） ◆予約を受け付

ける accept an appointment ◆予約を確認する confirm an appointment ◆予約を守る keep an appointment ◆予約を変更する change[reschedule] an appointment ◆予約を延期する *put off[postpone] an appointment ◆予約を取り消す cancel an appointment ◆歯科医の予約がある have an appointment with a dentist / have a dentist's appointment ◆初診は予約した方のみになっております New patients are seen by appointment only. ◆予約した患者さんの診察が先になります Patients with appointments will be seen first. / The doctor will see patients with appointments first. ◆予約は必要ありません Appointments are not necessary. / No appointment is necessary. ◆予約のない患者さんも受け付けております We accept *patients without appointments[walk-in patients]. ◆再診の予約をする make a return appointment ◆受付で次回の予約をして下さい Please make an appointment for your next visit at the reception desk. / Please go to the reception desk to set up your next appointment. ◆次回の予約はいつがいいですか When is a good day for your next appointment? ◆予約のご希望日がありますか What days are good[best] for you [your appointment]? / Which day do you prefer? ◆外来の予約は来週の木曜日までいっぱいです I'm afraid there are no appointments available until next Thursday. ◆あなたの予約日は次の月曜日，5月 7 日です Your appointment is[You have an appointment] for next Monday, May (the) seventh. ◆検査当日は予約時間の 15 分前にご来院下さい Please come to the hospital fifteen minutes before your appointment on the day of the test. ◆予約の日に来られない場合はできるだけ早く電話して下さい If you cannot keep your appointment, please call us as soon as possible. ◆予約を取り消したり変更する場合には，少なくとも 24 時間前までに電話をして下さい Please call us at least twenty-four hours in advance to cancel or reschedule your appointment. ◀再診予約 follow-up[return] appointment 事前予約 advance appointment 電話予約 telephone appointment / appointment by phone ▶予約カード appointment card 予約時間 appointment time 予約制 appointment system 予約番号 appointment number 予約日 appointment date 予約票［券］appointment slip 予約表 appointment calendar

よりめ 寄り目 **crossed eyes** ☞斜視

よる 夜 （夜に）**at night** ☞夜間，夜中

よろける （転びそうになってつんのめる）**stumble** （よろよろ歩く）**stagger** （ふらついている・不安定になる）**be unsteady** (on *one's* feet) ◆よろけて転倒する stumble and fall ◆よろけて真っ直ぐ歩けない stagger and can't walk straight

よろこぶ 喜ぶ **be glad[happy]** (at, about, of) （大いに喜んで）**be delighted** (at, with) （快く…する）**be ready[willing]** (to …) ◆喜んで可能な限り何でもいたします I'm ready[willing] to do anything within my power for you. / I'll be glad[happy] to do anything within my power for you. ◆（頼み事をされて）喜んで With pleasure. / Certainly. / Sure.

よろしい 宜しい **all right, okay, OK** ◆よろしいですか(Is everything) all right? ◆それでよろしいですか Is that all right with you? ◆トレイを下げてもよろしいですか May I take your tray? ◆よろしかったらこの車椅子をお使い下さい You can use this wheelchair if you like[wish]. ◆よろしければドアを少し開けたままにしていただけませんか(嫌でなければ)If you don't mind, could you keep the door *slightly open[ajar]?

よろしく ◆どうぞよろしく Nice[Good / Pleased] to meet you. ★「お会いできてうれしい. よろしく」という意味がこめられている. / （改まって）How do you do? ◆斉藤先生によろしくお伝え下さい Please give my best regards to Dr Saito. ◆答えにくいこともお聞きするかと思いますが治療に必要なこ

となので，よろしくお願いします I know these questions may be difficult to answer, but I need to ask them to decide on your treatment plan. I hope you understand.

よろめき ☞よろける ▶よろめき歩行(ふらふら歩行)staggering gait / （ぐらついて倒れそうな歩行）toppling gait

よわい 弱い （機能などが劣った）**poor** （体力などがない）**weak** （かすかな）**faint, feeble** （傷つきやすい）**vulnerable** (to) ◆胃腸が弱い have (a) poor digestion / have a weak stomach ◆呼吸が弱い *the breaths are [the breathing is] weak ◆脈が弱い the pulse is weak[faint / feeble] ◆視力が弱い have poor eyesight[vision] / have weak eyes ◆プレッシャーに弱い be vulnerable to pressure

よわき 弱気(になる) （やる気をなくす）**lose heart** （悲観的になる）**be pessimistic** （落胆する）**be discouraged** ◆弱気にならないで下さい Please don't *lose heart[be pessimistic / be discouraged].

よわめる 弱める **weaken, lower** ◆感染症に対する抵抗力を弱める weaken[lower] the body's resistance to infectious diseases

よわる 弱る **become[get] weak** （弱っている）**be weak** ◆彼は足が弱っています His legs are weak. / He's weak in the legs. ◆彼女はベッドに起き上がることができないほど弱っています She is too weak to sit up in bed.

よんがた ４型・Ⅳ型 **type 4, type Ⅳ** ▶Ⅳ型アレルギー反応 type Ⅳ allergic reaction

よんき ４期 （第４の段階）**fourth stage, stage four** ☞期

よんきゃくづえ 四脚杖 **four-legged cane, quad cane, quad-point cane**

よんてんほこう 四点歩行 **four-point gait**

ら

らい 癩 Hansen disease, leprosy（⊞lep-rous）★一般的には Hansen disease が用いられる. ▶らい菌 *Mycobacterium leprae* らい結節 leproma

らいいん 来院する come to the hospital [clinic] ◆来院は今回が初めてですか Is this your first visit to this hospital[clinic]? ◆夜の 12 時以降は何も口にしないでご来院下さい Please come to the hospital without eating or drinking anything after midnight. ◆ご心配なことがあればいつでも来院して下さい Please come and see me whenever you have any concerns. ▶来院時死亡 dead on arrival；DOA 来院時心停止 cardiac arrest on arrival

らいげきし 雷撃死 death by lightning（strike）, lightning death

らいげきしょう 雷撃傷 lightning injury

らいげつ 来月 next month

らいしゅう 来週 next week ◆来週の月曜日 next Monday

ライしょうこうぐん ―症候群 Reye syndrome

ライス rice ☞ご飯

ライスりょうほう ―療法 RICE therapy ◆ライス療法はスポーツ外傷に対する応急処置のことです RICE therapy is an emergency treatment for sport[athletic] injuries. ◆ライス（療法）は, 受傷部位に対する安静, 冷却, 圧迫, 挙上の略語です RICE (therapy) *is the abbreviation for [stands for] rest, ice, compression, and elevation of the injured part of the body.

ライセンス license

ライソソーム lysosome

ライターしょうこうぐん ―症候群 Reiter syndrome

ライナック LINAC （直線加速器）linear accelerator

らいにち 来日する come to Japan （訪日する）visit Japan ◆来日したのはいつ〈何

年〉ですか When〈In what year〉did you come to Japan? ◆来日してからどのくらいになりますか How long have you been in Japan?

らいねん 来年 next year ◆来年の今ごろ〈来年 3 月に〉再受診して下さい Please come and see me again *about this time next year〈next March〉.

ライノウイルス rhinovirus （学名）*Rhinovirus*

らいびょう 癩病 ☞癩

ライフイベント life event

ライフサイクル life cycle

ライフスタイル lifestyle, way of life ◆ライフスタイルを変えることでこの病気のリスクを減らすことができます Lifestyle changes can lower the risk of this disease. ◆健康的なライフスタイル a healthy lifestyle ◆活動的なライフスタイル a physically active lifestyle ◆非活動的なライフスタイル（体を動かさない）a physically inactive lifestyle /（座りがちな）a sedentary lifestyle

ライフステージ stage of life, life stage

ライフステージ

人間の一生を区切る段階を表す呼び方は様々あって明確に決まっているとは言えない. その呼び方は, 用いる人・国・行政・関連機関によってそれぞれ異なる. 一般的な英語の呼称例を挙げるが, 日本語の呼称と必ずしも一致しないので注意する必要がある. （ ）内に目安となる年齢を示す.

- 新生児 neonate / newborn（birth to 28 days）
- 乳幼児 infant（1 month to 1 year）★よちよち歩きの toddler ということもある.
- よちよち歩きの小児 toddler（1〜3 years）
- 子供・小児 child（1〜12 years）
- 未就学児・学齢前の子供 preschooler（3〜6 years）
- 学齢児童・就学年齢の子供 child of school age（6〜18 years）
- ティーンエイジャー teenager（13〜19 years）
- 思春期・青年期の若者 adolescent（13〜

17 years)
- 妊娠・出産可能年齢の女性 childbearing age（15〜44 years）
- 前期成人 young adult（18〜24 years）
- 成人 adult（18 years〜）★adulthood を early adulthood（18〜44 years），middle adulthood（45〜64 years），late adulthood（65〜）とする分け方もある．
- 盛年・働き盛り the prime of life ★使い方は人によって異なる．
- 中年・中高年 middle age ★使い方は人によって異なる．
- 高齢者 elderly person／(一般に) older person[adult]★使い方は人によって異なる．
- 前期高齢者 (elderly) person aged 65 to 74 years
- 後期高齢者 (elderly) person aged 75 years and older

ライムびょう　―病　Lyme disease

ラウンジ　lounge　◀患者用ラウンジ patients lounge

ラオス　Laos（㈱Laotian）☞国籍　▶ラオス人(の) Laotian

ラおん　ラ音　rale(s)（副雑音）adventitious sounds（断続性の）**crackles ★複数形で使用されることが多い．◀湿性ラ音** moist rales[crackles]　**断続性ラ音** discontinuous sounds／crackles　**ベルクロラ音** Velcro rale(s)／(捻髪音) fine crackles　**連続性ラ音** continuous sounds

らがん　裸眼　the naked eye　◆左の視力は裸眼で 0.7 です（眼鏡をかけずに）The eyesight in your left eye is (zero) point seven without glasses.／You have 0.7 of naked vision in the left eye.　**◀裸眼視力** naked[(矯正なしの) uncorrected] vision[visual acuity]

らく　楽
《心身が安楽な》（快適な）**comfortable**（くつろいだ）**relaxed**　（気分が楽な）**easy**　（⑩安楽にする）**relax, ease, relieve）◆楽な姿**勢でお座り下さい Please sit in a comfortable[relaxed] position.　**◆どうぞ楽にして**下さい Please relax (your muscles).
◆楽にして動かないで下さい Please relax

and don't move.　**◆口で息をして楽にして**下さい Please breathe through your mouth and relax.　**◆そのことで気が楽に**なりましたか Did you feel a lot easier about it?　**◆無理をしすぎですよ．気持ち**を楽にしてはどうですか You're overdoing things. Take it easy.　**◆吐いた後は楽にな**りましたか（気分が良くなったか）Did you feel better after you vomited?　**◆痛みを楽に**する ease[relieve] one's pain　**◆痛みは体**位を変えると楽になりますか Does changing position(s) help ease[relieve] the pain?／Is the pain eased[relieved] by changing your (body) position?　**◆座っ**ていたほうが呼吸は楽ですか Do you find breathing easier when (you're) sitting?
《容易な》**easy**　（簡単な）**simple　◆まず楽に**達成できる目標を設定しましょう First, let's set a goal that you can easily achieve.
◆不安な気持ちを完全に取り除くのはそんなに楽なことではありません It isn't so easy to completely let go of worries and anxiety.

らくせつ　落屑　exfoliation, desquamation

らくたん　落胆する　☞失望

ラクツロース　lactulose

ラクトアルブミン　lactalbumin

ラクトース　lactose

ラクトフェリン　lactoferrin

ラクナこうそく　―梗塞　lacunar infarction

らくようげんしょう　落陽現象　setting sun phenomenon

らくらいし　落雷死　☞雷撃死

ラジウム　radium /réidiəm/　▶ラジウム療法 radium therapy

ラジオ　radio（set）◆ラジオを聴く listento the radio　**◆ラジオをつける〈切る〉turn**on〈off〉the radio　**◆ラジオの音量を下げ**る〈上げる〉turn down〈up〉the volume on the radio／put the radio on low〈high〉
▶ラジオ番組 radio program

ラジオアイソトープ　radioactive isotope, radioisotope；RI　（放射性核種）**radionuclide；RN　▶ラジオアイソトープ治療 ra**dioisotope[RI]　therapy／radionuclide

[RN] therapy

ラジオアレルゲンソルベントテスト （放射性アレルゲン吸着試験）radioallergosorbent test；RAST

ラジオイムノアッセイ （放射免疫測定法）radioimmunoassay；RIA

ラジオイムノソルベントテスト （放射性免疫吸着試験）radioimmunosorbent test；RIST

ラジオは ―波 radiofrequency wave, RF wave ▶ラジオ波焼灼療法 radiofrequency ablation；RFA

ラスト RAST ☞ラジオアレルゲンソルベントテスト

ラセーグちょうこう ―徴候 Lasègue sign

らせん 螺旋 helix （圏helical, spiral） ◀二重らせん double helix ▶らせん骨折 spiral fracture　らせんCT　helical CT [computed tomography]　らせん状視野 spiral (visual) field

ラダー ladder ▶がん性疼痛治療ラダー ladder for cancer pain relief

らっかさん 落下傘 parachute ▶落下傘反射 parachute reflex

らっかん 楽観（的な）optimistic (↔pessimistic)　（前向きな）positive (↔negative) ◆彼女の容体は楽観できません I'm afraid we can't be optimistic about her condition. / (まだ危機を脱していない) I'm afraid she is not yet out of danger.　◆病気のことを楽観的に考える be optimistic about *one's* illness / have an optimistic view of *one's* illness　◆将来に対して楽観的である be optimistic about *one's* future / have *an optimistic[a positive] attitude about *one's* future　◆楽観的な人生観 an optimistic view of life

ラッサねつ ―熱 Lassa fever

ラット rat

ラテックス latex /léiteks/　◆ラテックスゴムにアレルギーはありますか Are you allergic to latex rubber?　▶ラテックスアレルギー latex allergy　ラテックス過敏症 latex hypersensitivity　ラテックス凝集試験 latex agglutination test　ラテックス手袋

latex gloves　ラテックスフルーツ症候群 latex-fruit syndrome

ラトケのう ―嚢 Rathke pouch ▶ラトケ嚢腫瘍 Rathke pouch tumor　ラトケ嚢胞 Rathke cleft[pouch] cyst

ラベル label /léibəl/　◆ラベルを貼る put a label on / label　◆ラベルをはがす take a label off / remove a label

ラポール rapport /ræpɔ́ɚ/, bond of trust ◆患者とのラポールを築く have (a) good rapport with patients / establish[build / develop] (a) rapport with patients

ラマーズほう ―法 Lamaze method [technique]

ラムゼイ・ハントしょうこうぐん ―症候群 Ramsay Hunt syndrome；RHS

ラン LAN, local area network ▶無線〈有線〉LAN wireless〈wired〉LAN[local area network]

らんえんこう 卵円孔 oval foramen, foramen ovale

らんおう 卵黄 (egg) yolk ▶卵黄嚢 yolk sac　卵黄嚢腫瘍 yolk sac tumor

らんかん 卵管 fallopian[uterine] tube （圏tubal), salpinx （圏salpinges） ◀子宮卵管造影法 hysterosalpingography；HSG　配偶子卵管内移植 gamete intrafallopian transfer；GIFT ▶卵管炎 salpingitis　卵管鏡下卵管形成術 falloposcopic tuboplasty；FT　卵管峡部 isthmus of the fallopian tube / tubal isthmus　卵管結紮 tubal ligation　卵管采 fimbriae of the uterine[fallopian] tube / tubal fimbriae　卵管通過障害 fallopian tube obstruction [blockage / occlusion]　卵管通気法 tubal insufflation　卵管通水法 hydrotubation　卵管妊娠 tubal pregnancy　卵管破裂 tubal rupture　卵管不妊 tubal infertility　卵管膨大部 ampulla of the uterine[fallopian] tube

らんぐいば 乱杭歯 irregular[uneven, crooked] teeth, irregular set[alignment] of teeth　（1本の）snaggletooth

ランゲルハンスさいぼう ―細胞 Langerhans cell ▶ランゲルハンス細胞組織球症 Langerhans cell histiocytosis；LCH

ランゲルハンスとう ―島 islets of Langerhans ★複数形で.

らんさいぼう 卵細胞 egg cell ▶卵細胞質内精子注入法 intracytoplasmic sperm injection；ICSI

らんし¹ 卵子 egg, ovum（複ova）▶卵子銀行 egg bank 卵子提供 egg donation 卵子提供者 egg donor

らんし² 乱視 astigmatism /əstígmətìzm/（形astigmátic）, distorted vision ◆乱視がある have astigmatism / be astigmatic ◀不正乱視 irregular astigmatism ▶乱視表 astigmatism test chart[dial] 乱視用レンズ astigmatic lens

らんそう 卵巣 ovary（複ovarian）◆卵巣の手術をする operate on *a person's* ovary ◀多嚢胞卵巣症候群 polycystic ovary syndrome；PCOS ▶卵巣過剰刺激症候群 ovarian hyperstimulation syndrome；OHSS 卵巣がん ovarian cancer 卵巣奇形腫 ovarian teratoma 卵巣機能不全 ovarian insufficiency 卵巣茎捻転 ovarian torsion 卵巣周期 ovarian cycle 卵巣出血 ovarian bleeding[hemorrhage] 卵巣摘出術 ovariectomy / oophorectomy 卵巣嚢腫 ovarian cystoma 卵巣嚢胞 ovarian cyst 卵巣ホルモン ovarian hormone

らんそさいぼう 卵祖細胞 oogonium

ランチ lunch ☞昼食

ランドルトかん ―環 Landolt（broken）ring, Landolt C

ランバート・イートンしょうこうぐん ―症候群 Lambert-Eaton syndrome（ランバート・イートン筋無力症症候群）Lambert-Eaton myasthenic syndrome；LEMS

らんぱく 卵白 egg white ▶卵白アルブミン ovalbumin

ランプ lamp, light ◀紫外線ランプ ultraviolet lamp ベッドランプ bedside lamp[light]

ランブルべんもうちゅう ―鞭毛虫 *Giardia lamblia*[*intestinalis*] ▶ランブル鞭毛虫症 giardiasis

らんぽう 卵胞（ovarian）follicle（形follicular）▶卵胞期 follicular phase 卵胞刺激ホルモン follicle-stimulating hormone；FSH 卵胞ホルモン follicular hormone /（エストロゲン）estrogen

らんぼさいぼう 卵母細胞 oocyte, ovocyte

らんまく 卵膜 fetal membrane, extraembryonic membrane ▶卵膜剥離 stripping of the fetal membranes

らんよう 乱用・濫用（不適切な使用）improper use（使いすぎ）overuse（誤用）misuse（麻薬・アルコールなどの使用）abuse ◆睡眠薬の乱用 *improper use[misuse / overuse] of sleeping pills ◀コカイン乱用 cocaine abuse 麻薬乱用 narcotic（drug）abuse 薬物乱用 drug[substance] abuse

ら

り

リアルタイム real time ▶リアルタイム処理 real-time processing

リーシュマニアしょう ―症 leishmaniasis

リード・ステルンベルグさいぼう ―細胞 Reed-Sternberg cell

リウマチ rheumatism /rúːmətìzm/（㊟リウマチ性の rheumátic リウマチ様の rhéumatoid）☞関節リウマチ ◆リウマチを発症する develop rheumatism ◀悪性関節リウマチ malignant rheumatoid arthritis；MRA 回帰性リウマチ palindromic rheumatism；PR 関節リウマチ rheumatoid arthritis；RA 抗リウマチ薬 antirheumatic（medication / drug / agent）/（疾患修飾性抗リウマチ薬）disease-modifying antirheumatic drugs；DMARDs 若年性関節リウマチ juvenile rheumatoid arthritis；JRA ▶リウマチ因子 rheumatoid factor；RF リウマチ科 the department of rheumatology / the rheumatology department リウマチ学 rheumatology リウマチ患者 patient with rheumatism / rheumatic patient リウマチ結節 rheumatoid[rheumatic] nodule リウマチ性心疾患 rheumatic heart disease リウマチ性多発筋痛症 polymyalgia rheumatica；PMR リウマチ専門医 rheumatologist リウマチ熱 rheumatic fever

りえき 利益 good, benefit（㊟beneficial）◆激しい運動はあなたの利益にはなりません Strenuous exercise won't be of *much use[benefit] to you. ★be of use で役に立つを意味する. / Getting some strenuous exercise won't *do you any good[give you any benefit]. ☞利益相反

りえきそうはん 利益相反 conflict of interest

リエゾンせいしんいがく ―精神医学 liaison psychiatry

リエントリーひんぱく ―頻拍 reentrant

tachycardia, reentry tachycardia

りかい¹ 理解する understand ☞わかる ◆私の言うことが理解できますか Do you understand what I'm saying? ◆他人の言うことが理解できない have trouble understanding what other people say ◀相互理解 mutual understanding

りかい² 離開 diastasis ◀縫合線離開 suture diastasis

りがいかんけい 利害関係 ☞利益相反

りがくりょうほう 理学療法 physical therapy, physiotherapy；PT ▶理学療法士 *physical therapist[physiotherapist]；PT

りかん 罹患する contract（a disease）, catch（a disease）☞罹る ◀累積罹患率 cumulative incidence rate ▶罹患率 morbidity（rate）/（発症率）incidence（rate）

りきか 力価 titer

りきむ 力む strain（oneself）☞息む ◆便が固くて力まなければならないほどですか Do you have to strain to pass stools because they are very hard? ◆（検査などで）そんなに力まずに，力を抜いて下さい Don't strain yourself that much. *Relax your muscles[Let your body go limp].

リクライニング reclining ▶リクライニング椅子 reclining chair / recliner リクライニング車椅子 reclining wheelchair リクライニングシート reclining seat

リケッチア rickettsia（㊟rickettsial）（学名）Rickettsia ▶リケッチア感染症 rickettsial infection

リコペン lycopene

りこん 離婚 divorce（㊟divorce, get a divorce, get divorced）◆離婚していますか Are you divorced? ◆離婚してどのくらいになりますか How long have you been divorced〈from your husband〈wife〉〉?

リザーバーバッグ reservoir bag

りしょう 離床 ambulation ◀早期離床 early ambulation

りじんしょう 離人症 depersonalization

リスク risk ☞危険 ◆リスクを冒す run[take] a risk ◆リスクを避ける avoid

(running) a risk ◆リスクを減らす reduce a risk /〈最小限に抑える〉minimize a risk /〈下げる〉lower a risk ◆リスクを高める increase a risk ◆リスクは低い the risk is low[〈小さい〉slight] ◆リスクは高い the risk is high[〈大きい〉great] ◆リスクが上がる〈下がる〉the risk increases〈decreases〉 ◆肝臓がんを発症するリスク the risk[possibility] of developing liver cancer ◆肝臓がんのリスクファクター risk factors for liver cancer ◆この手術にはリスクが伴います There are risks involved in this surgery. ◆どんな手術にも多少のリスクが伴います Any surgery involves some risks. / There are some risks involved with any type of surgery. ◆この手技による死亡のリスクは 1% 以下です The risk of death for this procedure is less than one percent. ◆水痘にかかった人は帯状疱疹になるリスクがあります Anyone who has had chickenpox is at risk for shingles. ◆肺がんに罹るリスクは喫煙者で高くなります The risk of developing lung cancer is higher in people who smoke. / Smokers have a higher risk of developing lung cancer. ◆肥満は糖尿病のリスク要因の 1 つです Obesity is one of the risk factors for diabetes. ◀感染リスク risk of infection 喫煙リスク risk of[from] smoking ハイリスク患者 high-risk patient ハイリスク妊娠 high-risk pregnancy ▶リスクアセスメント risk assessment リスクファクター risk factor リスクマネジメント risk management

リステリアかんせんしょう ―感染症 listeria infection, listeriosis

リスト¹ list ◆リストにする list / make a list ◀メーリングリスト mailing list 問題リスト problem list

リスト² RIST ☞ラジオイムノソルベントテスト

リストカット wrist cutting ◆リストカットで自殺する *commit suicide[kill *oneself*] by cutting *one's* wrists

リストバンド wristband, (ID 情報が記載された)ID[identification, identity] bracelet ☞アイディーバンド ◆入院中はずっとリストバンドをはめていて下さい Please wear your wristband[ID bracelet] throughout your hospital stay.

リストラ restructuring ◆リストラされる(解雇される)*be fired[lose *one's* job] due to restructuring /〈一時的に解雇される〉be laid off ◆リストラされるのではないかとご心配ですか Are you concerned about *being fired[losing your job] because of restructuring?

リズム rhythm ◆生活のリズムが乱れていますか Has there been any disturbance in your daily rhythm? / Is your daily rhythm disturbed? ◀サーカディアンリズム circadian rhythm 心リズム cardiac rhythm バイオリズム biorhythm ▶リズム障害 dysrhythmia

りそう 理想(の) ideal ◆理想的には毎日 30 分散歩をするとよいでしょう Ideally you should *walk for thirty minutes[take a thirty-minute walk] every day. ◆理想的な体型 ideal (body) shape ◆理想体重 ideal (body) weight

リソソーム lysosome

りだつ 離脱 (薬物使用から身を引くこと) withdrawal (分離)detachment ◀アルコール離脱症候群 alcohol withdrawal syndrome コカイン離脱 cocaine withdrawal 大麻離脱 marijuana[cannabis] withdrawal ニコチン離脱症状 nicotine withdrawal symptoms ベンゾジアゼピン離脱症候群 benzodiazepine withdrawal syndrome

りだん 離断 disconnection ▶離断症候群 disconnection syndrome

りたんやく 利胆薬 cholagogue (胆汁分泌促進薬)choleretic (medication, drug, agent) (排胆薬)cholekinetic (medication, drug, agent)

リチウム lithium ▶リチウム腎毒性 lithium nephrotoxicity リチウム中毒 lithium poisoning

りつ 率 (割合・比率)rate, ratio (百分率)percentage, percent (発生率)incidence ◀1 秒率 the ratio of forced expiratory volume in one second to forced vital capacity；FEV$_1$／FVC　死亡率 death rate／mortality（rate）　体脂肪率 body fat percentage　発病率 incidence（rate）

りつい　立位　standing position　▶立位訓練 standing exercise／stand-up exercise　立位支持装具 standing brace

りっしょう　立証する　☞証明

りったい　立体（の）　（三次元の）three-dimensional　（暖調stere(o)-）▶立体感覚 stereognosis／stereognostic sense　立体視 stereopsis／stereoscopic vision　立体失認 astereognosis　立体内視鏡 stereoscopic［three-dimensional］endoscope

りつどう　律動（性の）　rhythmic, rhythmical　▶律動異常 dysrhythmia　律動性収縮 rhythmic contraction

リットル　liter／líːtə／；l, L　▶2 L の水 two liters of water

りつもうきん　立毛筋　arrector pili muscle, arrector muscle of hair　▶立毛筋反射 pilomotor reflex

りてん　利点　（良い点）good point　（有利な点）advantage　（↔disadvantage）☞有利

りとく　利得　gain, profit　◀疾病利得 gain from illness

リトマス　litmus　▶リトマス紙 litmus paper　リトマス試験 litmus test

リニアック　LINAC　（直線加速器）linear accelerator

リニメントざい　─剤　liniment

りにゅう　離乳　weaning　（暖調wean）, ablactation　◆いつ離乳を始めましたか When did you start weaning your baby off *breast milk［（調合乳）formula（milk）］? ◆お子さんは離乳が済んでいますか Has your baby already been weaned?　◆離乳すると徐々にお乳が出なくなります As you wean your baby off breast milk, your breasts will gradually stop producing milk.　▶離乳期 weaning period

りにゅうしょく　離乳食　weaning food, baby food　（固形食）solid food　◆離乳食を始める start a baby on solid food

りにょう　利尿　diuresis　（暖diuretic）◀強制利尿 forced diuresis　抗利尿ホルモン antidiuretic hormone；ADH　抗利尿ホルモン不適切分泌症候群 syndrome of inappropriate antidiuretic hormone secretion；SIADH　☞ナトリウム利尿ペプチド, 利尿薬

りにょうやく　利尿薬　diuretic（medication, drug, agent）◆これは利尿薬という, 尿の量を増加させる薬です This is a diuretic, a medication that helps to increase urination.　◀カリウム保持性利尿薬 potassium sparing diuretic　降圧利尿薬 antihypertensive diuretic（medication／drug／agent）

リネン　linen　（ベッドの）bed linen(s)　◆リネンを交換する change *a person's* bed linen　▶リネン室 linen room［closet］

リパーゼ　lipase

リハビリテーション　rehabilitation　（インフォーマルに）rehab／ríːhæb/　◆リハビリテーションのために作業療法を受ける必要があります You need to have some occupational therapy as part of your rehabilitation.　◆リハビリテーション計画を立てましょう Let's make［set up］your rehabilitation plan.　◆スコットさん, リハビリのお時間です Mrs Scott, it's time for your rehabilitation training.　◆一緒にリハビリテーションを頑張りましょう Let's work together on your rehabilitation.　◆これができれば, リハビリは卒業です Once you can do this, you'll be able to graduate from rehabilitation.　◆リハビリテーションを受ける receive rehabilitation　◆リハビリテーションに通う go for rehabilitation　◀外来リハビリテーション outpatient［ambulatory］rehabilitation　急性期リハビリテーション the acute phase［stage］of rehabilitation　呼吸リハビリテーション respiratory rehabilitation　在宅リハビリテーション home-based［in-home］rehabilitation／rehabilitation at home　社会リハビリテーション social rehabilitation　心臓リハビリテーション cardiac［heart］rehabilitation　ストーマリハビリテーション stoma［（人工肛門・人工膀胱）ostomy］rehabilitation　地域リハビリテー

ション community-based rehabilitation 認知リハビリテーション cognitive rehabilitation 訪問リハビリテーション home-visit rehabilitation / visiting rehabilitation ▶リハビリテーション医学 rehabilitation medicine リハビリテーション運動 rehabilitation exercise / exercise for rehabilitation リハビリテーション科 the department of rehabilitation / the rehabilitation department リハビリテーション看護 rehabilitation nursing リハビリテーション訓練 rehabilitation training リハビリテーション計画 rehabilitation plan / (プログラム) rehabilitation program リハビリテーション室 rehabilitation room リハビリテーションセンター rehabilitation center リハビリテーション専門医 rehabilitation physician / physiatrist / physician specializing in physical medicine and rehabilitation

リビドー libido

りびょう 罹病 ☞罹る, 罹患

リビングウィル living will （事前指示書） advance (health care) directive [decision] ◆リビングウィルをお持ちですか. もしあれば, そのコピーをご提出下さい Do you have a living will? If you do, please give us a copy of it.

リフト lift ◀車椅子用リフト wheelchair lift

リフレッシュ リフレッシュする refresh （形）リフレッシュした refreshed) ◆週末に自宅へ外泊してリフレッシュしましたか Are you (feeling) refreshed after staying home overnight on the weekend? / Was it refreshing to stay home overnight on the weekend? ◆シャーベットでリフレッシュしませんか How about a cup of sherbet as a refreshment?

リポイド lipoid ▶リポイドネフローゼ lipoid nephrosis

リボかくさん ―核酸 ribonucleic acid : RNA ◀デオキシリボ核酸 deoxyribonucleic acid : DNA

リポキシゲナーゼ lipoxygenase

リボソーム ribosome （形）ribosomal)

▶リボソーム RNA ribosomal RNA : rRNA

リポたとう ―多糖 lipopolysaccharide : LPS

リポたんぱく ―蛋白 lipoprotein : LP ◀高比重リポ蛋白 high-density lipoprotein / HDL / good cholesterol 中間型リポ蛋白 intermediate-density lipoprotein : IDL 超低比重リポ蛋白 very low-density lipoprotein : VLDL 低比重リポ蛋白 low-density lipoprotein : LDL / bad cholesterol

リボン ribbon ◆リボンをつけている wear a ribbon ◆髪にリボンをつける put a ribbon in *one's* hair ◆リボン状の便が出る pass ribbon-like stools

りゆう 理由 （訳）reason （原因）cause ◆受診の主な理由を話して下さい Please tell me the main reason you came to see me. ◆手術を拒否する理由は何ですか What's your reason for refusing the surgery? / What makes you refuse the surgery? ◆入院した理由は何でしたか Why were you admitted to the hospital? / What were you hospitalized for? ◆お母さんが亡くなられた理由をお聞かせ下さい What was the cause of your mother's death? / What did your mother die of? ◆生検でがんの可能性を排除できないという理由で手術が必要です You need to have surgery because we could not completely rule out the possibility of cancer from your biopsy. ◆健康上の理由でタバコをやめる quit smoking for health reasons ◆特に〈明らかな〉理由もなく憂鬱になる become [get] depressed for no particular 〈apparent〉 reason ◆個人的な理由で for personal reasons ◆家庭の理由で for family reasons ◆経済的理由で for financial [economic] reasons ◆特別な理由 a particular [special] reason ◆納得のいく理由 a convincing reason ◆法律上の理由 a legal reason ◆本当の理由 a real reason

りゅうがく 留学する （海外から日本に来る） come to Japan to study （外国へ行く）

study abroad, go abroad to study ◆なぜ留学先に日本を選んだのですか Why did you come to Japan to study? ▶外国人留学生 international[overseas / foreign] student　交換留学生 exchange student

りゅうかすいそ　硫化水素　hydrogen sulfide ▶硫化水素自殺 hydrogen sulfide suicide

りゅうかん　流感 ☞インフルエンザ

りゅうき　隆起　(突起物) **protuberance, prominence** ☞瘤 (こぶ), しこり, 腫瘤, 腫れ ◀オトガイ隆起 mental protuberance　喉頭隆起 laryngeal prominence /（一般的に）Adam's apple

りゅうこう　流行する　(一時的に流行る) **go around**　(ある地域・時期に広がっている) **be widespread[prevalent]**　(猛威を振るう) **rage**　(急速に広まる) **spread quickly** (☞ **epidemic**) ☞流行る ◆インフルエンザは関東で流行しています The flu is going around the Kanto district. / The flu is widespread[spreading quickly / raging] in the Kanto district. ◆すでにインフルエンザが大流行しています(流行の真っ盛りにある) The influenza epidemic is already in full swing. ◀爆発的流行 widespread outbreak　汎発性流行病 pandemic ▶流行性角結膜炎 epidemic keratoconjuctivitis；EKC　流行性耳下腺炎［ムンプス］mumps / epidemic parotitis

りゅうさん　硫酸　sulfuric acid ▶硫酸亜鉛 zinc sulfate　硫酸バリウム barium sulfate　硫酸マグネシウム magnesium sulfate

りゅうざん　流産　abortion　(一般的に) **miscarriage**　(死産) **stillbirth** ◆これまでに流産したことがありますか Have you ever had a miscarriage? ◆6週目で流産する have a miscarriage in *one's* sixth week ◀稽留流産 missed abortion　自然流産 spontaneous abortion　習慣流産 habitual abortion /（反復流産）recurrent abortion[pregnancy loss]　進行流産 inevitable abortion / abortion in progress　人工流産 induced[artificial] abortion　切迫流産 threatened[imminent] abortion

［miscarriage］不全流産 incomplete abortion

りゅうし　粒子　particle ◆吸入薬によって粒子径が異なるので, 別の吸入ステロイド薬を試してみましょう Let's try another inhaled corticosteroid because the particle size varies according to the different inhalant. ◀荷電粒子線治療 charged particle radiotherapy　重粒子線治療 heavy particle radiotherapy

りゅうしゅつ　流出　(液体・気体などの流出) **outflow**　(あふれ出すこと) **overflow**　(分泌物の排出) **discharge, drainage** ◀房水流出 aqueous (humor) outflow ▶流出口 outflow port　流出量 outflow

りゅうじょう　粒状(の)　(顆粒状の) **granular, granulated**　(小結節状の) **nodular** ▶粒状影 nodular shadow / granular shadow

りゅうち　留置する　(置く) **place** (in)　(差し込む) **insert, put** (in)　(埋める) **fill in, implant** (カテーテルを) **catheterize** (☞体内に留置の **indwelling**) ◆ステントを動脈に留置する place[put in] a stent in the artery ◆導尿のためカテーテルを膀胱に留置する place[put] a catheter in *a person's* bladder to drain the urine ◆カテーテルを通してコイルを動脈瘤に留置し, 破裂を予防します We're going to fill in the aneurysm with a coil to prevent it from rupturing；we'll insert the coil through a catheter. ◀ステント留置 stent placement / stenting　ドレーン留置 indwelling drainage　膀胱〈尿道〉留置カテーテル indwelling bladder〈urethral〉catheter ▶留置カテーテル indwelling catheter　留置スネア(取り外し可能な) detachable snare

りゅうちょう　流暢(に)　(よどみなく) **fluently** (☞ **fluent** ☞ **fluency**)　(容易に) **with ease** ◆彼女は日本語を流暢に話します She speaks Japanese fluently[with ease]. ◀言語流暢性 speech fluency /（単語の）word fluency

りゅうどうしょく　流動食　liquid diet ［food］ ◆流動食にする put *a person* on a liquid diet ◀半流動食 semiliquid diet

りゅうびじゅつ　隆鼻術　augmentation rhinoplasty

りゅうるい　流涙　lacrimation, increased tearing　◆いつ流涙が気になりましたか When did you first notice that your tears overflow onto your face? / (涙目になる) Since when did you notice that you have watery[teary] eyes?　▶流涙症 lacrimation / epiphora

りよう　利用する　use, make use (of), utilize　☞使用，使う　◆介護サービスを利用する use[make use of] a (long-term) care service　◆介護保険で患者が利用できるサービス services utilized by a patient under long-term care insurance　◆当院ではボランティアサービスが利用できます Volunteer services are available in this hospital.　☞利用者

りよう[1]　料　☞料金

りよう[2]　量　(統計・総量)amount　(薬量) dose, dosage　★dose は 1 回の用量，dosage は一定期間にわたり用いる量.　(分量・数量)quantity　(体積・容量)volume　(重量)weight　(月経などの流量)flow　(消費量)consumption　◆量が少ない be small in quantity　◆量が多い be large in quantity　◆少量の a little bit of / a small amount[quantity] of　◆大量の a lot of / a large amount[quantity] of / much / a great deal of / (薬量が)a large dose of / (喫煙量・飲酒量が)a heavy intake of / (過度の)excessive / (豊富な)abundant　◆出血の量が異常です The amount[volume] of bleeding is abnormal.　◆尿の量は毎回どのくらいですか How much urine do you pass each time? / How much do you urinate each time?　◆おりものの量が増えたのですか Have you noticed an increase in vaginal discharge? / Has the amount of your vaginal discharge increased?　◆薬の量を増やす increase the dose (of a medication)　◆砂糖の量を制限する limit the amount of sugar　◆タバコの量を減らす cut down[back] on smoking[the number of cigarettes smoked]　◆仕事の量を減らす cut back on *one's* work　◆薬の最

適な量 the optimal[optimum] dose of medication　◆多量の月経血 heavy menstrual bleeding[flow]　◆大量の輸血 massive blood transfusion　◀一日量 daily dosage　一回量 single dose　運動量 amount of exercise　酒量 alcohol consumption　尿量 urinary output[volume] / the volume of urine　必要量 requirement / required quantity[amount]

りょうあし　両足・両脚　(両下肢)both legs　(両方の足首から下の部分)both feet　☞足　◆仰向けに寝て両脚を伸ばして〈曲げて〉下さい Please lie on your back and *straight-en out both legs〈膝を曲げる〉bend your knees〉.　◆両足を揃えて〈開いて〉立って下さい Please stand with both feet together 〈apart〉.

りょういき　領域　(範囲)area, region　(分野)field　◆あなたの抱えている問題は私の専門外の領域ですので，専門医をご紹介しましょう Your problem is an area I don't know much about, so let me refer you to a specialist.　◀関心領域 area of interest　専門領域 specialty / specialized field　調節領域 control region

りょういく　療育　medical care and education　(for intellectually disabled children)　▶療育手帳 intellectual disability handbook

りょううで　両腕　both arms　◆軽く両腕を上げて下さい Please gently raise both your arms.　◆両腕をまっすぐ上に伸ばす stretch[extend] both arms straight upward

りょうかい　了解　(同意・承諾)consent　(承認・賛同)approval　(理解)understanding　(許可)permission　◆このことはあなたのご両親の了解をとらなければなりません We have to ask for your parents' consent [approval] on this matter.　◆了解しました All right. / OK. / I understand.

りょうかせい　両価性　ambivalence

りょうがわ　両側　both sides　☞両方　☞両側(りょうそく)　◆鼻血は両側から出ますか Are the nosebleeds from both sides? / Do you have the nosebleeds from

りょうがわ 742 **りょうほう**[1]

both sides? ◆首の両側にしこりがある have lumps on both sides of the neck

りょうがん 両眼 **both eyes**（⇒**binocular**）☞目, 両眼（りょうめ）▶両眼視野 binocular visual field 両眼視力 binocular vision[visual acuity] 両眼複視 binocular diplopia

りょうきん 料金（診療報酬など）**fee**（請求代金）**charge** ◀規定料金 standard[regulation] charge 差額料金（保険適応外）charge not covered by health insurance／（差額室料）special room charge 初診料（金）initial fee[charge] 処方箋料（金）prescription fee[charge] 診察料（金）doctor's[consultation] fee 調剤料金 dispensing fee 追加料金 additional charge[fee] 別料金 extra charge ▶料金表 fee schedule／list of charges／price list

りょうこう 良好（な）（よい）**good, fine**（満足のいく）**satisfactory**（期待できる）**favorable** ◆彼女の経過は良好です She's making good progress.／She's doing very well. ◆彼の術後経過は良好です His outcome after the surgery is good[satisfactory]. ◆すべて良好ですよ Everything is fine. ◆この病気の予後は一般的に良好ですのであまり心配なさらないように This disease generally has a favorable prognosis, so don't worry too much.

りょうしい 良肢位 functional position

りょうじそくはんもう 両耳側半盲 bitemporal hemianopsia[hemianopia]

りようしゃ 利用者（サービス使用者）**user**（福祉・心理などの相談者）**client**（受ող者）**recipient** ◀介護保険利用者 long-term care insurance recipient 車椅子利用者 wheelchair user 訪問介護サービス利用者 visiting home care service user

りょうしゅうしょ 領収書 receipt ◆これが領収書です Here's your receipt. ▶領収明細書 itemized receipt

りょうしん 両親 **one's parents**[father and mother] ◆ご両親はご健在ですか（存命か）Are your parents *still living[（健康か）in good health／（元気で生きているか）alive and well]? ◆ご両親はどのような原因で

亡くなられましたか What did your parents die of?

りょうしんがっきゅう 両親学級 parenting class, class for expectant[expecting] parents[mothers and fathers] ◆両親学級に参加する attend[take part in] parenting classes

りょうせい 良性（の）**benign**/bɪnáɪn/（↔malignant）◆良性腫瘍 benign tumor ◆良性ポリープと悪性ポリープの鑑別は困難です It's difficult to distinguish between benign polyps and malignant ones.

りょうせいほっさせいとういめまいしょう 良性発作性頭位めまい症 benign paroxysmal positional vertigo；BPPV

りょうそく 両側（の）（二重の）**double**（両方の）**bilateral** ☞両側（りょうがわ）▶両側性難聴 bilateral hearing loss 両側肺門リンパ節腫脹 bilateral hilar lymphadenopathy；BHL

りょうたん 両端 **two ends, both ends**（縁・へり）**(two) edges**（角）**(two) corners**（どちらの端も）**either end** ◆爪の両端を深く切りすぎないように気をつけて下さい Be careful not to cut the edges[corners] of the nails too deep. ◆トイレはこの廊下の両端にあります There are restrooms at either end of this hall. ◆包帯の両端を結ぶ tie *the two[both] ends of the bandage together

りょうて 両手 **both hands** ☞手 ◆両手をこのように動かして下さい Please move both your hands like this. ◆両手を頭上高く上げる raise both hands high above *one's head

りょうはし 両端 ☞両端（りょうたん）

りょうびそくはんもう 両鼻側半盲 binasal hemianopsia[hemianopia]

りょうほう[1] 両方 **both** ☞両側（りょうがわ）◆鼻血は両方，それとも片方の鼻から出ますか Does your nose bleed from both nostrils or from one? ◆両方の膝を立てて，お腹の力を抜いて下さい Please pull[bring] both your knees up, and relax your abdomen.

りょうほう² 療法 （長期間にわたる専門的治療）therapy （治療）treatment （一般的に流布している治療法）remedy ☞治療 ◆ホルモン療法を行う give[treat with] hormone therapy ◆エストロゲン補充療法を行っている be on estrogen replacement therapy ◆糖尿病患者の食事療法 diet therapy for patients with diabetes ◆化学療法の1クール a course of chemotherapy ◀維持療法 maintenance[support] therapy[treatment] インスリン療法 insulin therapy[treatment] 運動療法 exercise therapy 化学療法 chemotherapy 緩和的療法 palliative treatment[therapy] 外科療法 surgical treatment[therapy] 言語療法 speech therapy；ST 抗凝固療法 anticoagulant therapy 行動療法 behavior therapy 根治療法 radical[curative] therapy 作業療法 occupational therapy；OT 支持療法 supportive therapy 食事療法 diet[dietary] therapy 心理[精神]療法 psychotherapy 対症療法 symptomatic treatment[therapy] 放射線療法 radiation therapy / radiotherapy 民間療法 folk remedy 薬物療法 medication[drug] therapy / pharmacotherapy 理学療法 physical therapy[physiotherapy]；PT

りょうほうし 療法士 therapist ☞訓練士 ◀言語療法士[言語聴覚士] speech-language-hearing therapist；ST 作業療法士 occupational therapist；OT ストーマ療法士 enterostomal therapist；ET マッサージ療法士 massage therapist 理学療法士 physical therapist[physiotherapist]；PT

りょうまひ 両麻痺 diplegia ◆痙性両麻痺 spastic diplegia

りょうめ 両目 both eyes ☞目,両眼（りょうがん） ◆両方の目をぎゅっとつぶって下さい Please close both eyes tightly. ◆両目に黄斑変性がある have macular degeneration in both eyes

りょうよう 療養 （病気・怪我からの回復）recuperation （動recuperate），convalescence （形convalescent） （治療）medical treatment （医療・ケア）medical care ◆彼女はまだ療養中です She is still under medical treatment[care]. ◆療養できる施設を探す look for a facility where one can recuperate （from *one's* illness） ◀介護療養型施設 intermediate care facility / convalescent home 自宅療養 recuperation at home / home recuperation 長期療養 long-term medical care ◆療養給付 medical treatment benefits 療養病床 long-term care bed 療養補償 medical compensation ☞療養費

りょうようひ 療養費 medical （care） expenses ◆高額療養費 high-cost medical care benefits[expenses] 特定療養費 medical expenses for specified treatment and care 保険外併用療養費 authorized balance-billing of a patient for specific medical care not covered by a health insurance plan

りょくおうしょくやさい 緑黄色野菜 dark-colored vegetables, dark green and [or] yellow vegetables ★通例,複数形で. ◆健康のためには緑黄色野菜を毎日バランスよく食べて下さい To stay healthy, please eat a good balance of dark-colored vegetables every day.

りょくしょく 緑色（の） green （緑色を帯びた）greenish ▶緑色便 green[greenish] stool

りょくないしょう 緑内障 glaucoma ◆左目に緑内障がある have glaucoma in *one's* left eye ◀開放隅角緑内障 open-angle glaucoma ステロイド緑内障 steroid-induced glaucoma 正常眼圧緑内障 normal-tension glaucoma；NTG 続発緑内障 secondary glaucoma 閉塞隅角緑内障 closed-angle glaucoma

りょくのうきん 緑膿菌 pseudomonas （学名）*Pseudomonas aeruginosa* （俗称）blue pus bacillus ◀多剤耐性緑膿菌 multidrug-resistant *Pseudomonas aeruginosa*；MDRP ▶緑膿菌感染症 pseudomonas infection

りょけん 旅券 passport

りょこう 旅行 travel, trip （動travel, make

a trip) ◆海外旅行 overseas[foreign] travel / a trip abroad / an overseas trip ◆観光旅行 a sightseeing trip[tour] ◆最近, 日本国外へ旅行しましたか Have you recently traveled outside (of) Japan? ▶旅行者 traveler /（観光客など）tourist 旅行者下痢症 traveler's[travelers'] diarrhea 旅行（傷害）保険 travel（accident）insurance

リラックス ―する relax, become relaxed（圏relaxation）◆どうぞリラックスして下さい Please relax (your muscles). /（固くならないで）Please try not to tighten up. ◆リラックスできるようにお薬を差し上げましょう I'm going to give you a medication *to help you relax[that will make you feel relaxed]. ◆あなたはリラックスするために何をしますか What do you do to relax? ▶リラックス運動 relaxation exercise

りれきしょ 履歴書 curriculum vitae；CV, résumé /rézəmèɪ/

りろん 理論 theory（圏theoretical）▶理論値 theoretical value

リン phosphorus ◀高リン（酸）血症 hyperphosphatemia 低リン（酸）血症 hypophosphatemia 無機リン inorganic phosphorus 有機リン化合物 organophosphorus compound 有機リン中毒 organophosphorus poisoning

りんかく 輪郭 （外形）outline（圏outline）（特に体の外形）contour ◆治療のはっきりした輪郭を示す clearly outline the plan of treatment / give[show] a clear outline of the treatment ◆右目は物の輪郭がぼやけて見える have blurred vision in one's right eye ◆顔の輪郭 the contours of the face

りんきん 淋菌 gonococcus（圏gonococcal）（学名）Neisseria gonorrhoeae ◆淋菌感染症に罹る catch[contract] gonorrhea ▶淋菌感染症 gonococcal infection / gonorrhea 淋菌性膣炎 gonococcal vaginitis 淋菌性尿道炎 gonococcal urethritis；GU

リング ring ◀避妊リング（子宮内避妊器具）intrauterine device；IUD / birth control ring / contraceptive ring

りんげつ 臨月 the month of the baby's due date, the month the baby is due

りんごびょう ―病 （伝染性紅斑）erythema infectiosum, fifth disease

リンさん ―酸 phosphoric acid ☞リン ▶リン酸塩 phosphate

りんじ 臨時（の）（一時的な）temporary（パートの）part-time ◆これは臨時の処置です This treatment is only temporary. ▶臨時雇用者 part-time worker / part-timer / temporary worker 臨時措置 temporary measure(s)

リンししつ ―脂質 phospholipid

りんしたいけん 臨死体験 near-death experience；NDE

りんじゅう 臨終 （最期の瞬間）one's last moments ★複数形で. （死の床）one's deathbed （人生の終焉）end（of one's life）☞最期 ◆残念ですが, ご臨終です I'm sorry to say he〈she〉has passed away. ◆お母様のご臨終は安らかでした Your mother died[passed away] peacefully. / She died a peaceful[quiet] death. ◆彼女の臨終に立ち会う be with her *at her last moments[when she died] / be present at her deathbed ◆臨終が近い be nearing one's end[last moments]

りんしょう 臨床（の）clinical ▶臨床医 clinician 臨床医学 clinical medicine 臨床研究 clinical study[research] 臨床検討会 clinical conference 臨床工学 clinical engineering 臨床工学技士 clinical engineer；CE / medical engineer；ME 臨床実習 clinical training 臨床所見 clinical findings 臨床診断 clinical diagnosis 臨床心理学 clinical psychology 臨床心理士 clinical psychologist 臨床データ clinical data 臨床薬理学 clinical pharmacology ☞臨床検査, 臨床試験

りんじょう 輪状（の）（輪形の）annular, cricoid （円形の）circular ◀輪状暗点 annular[ring] scotoma 輪状軟骨 annular[cricoid] cartilage

りんしょうけんさ 臨床検査 clinical（laboratory）test, clinical（laboratory） testing ▶臨床検査技師 medical technologist；MT / clinical laboratory technician 臨床検査室(clinical) laboratory

りんしょうしけん 臨床試験 **clinical trial** [test] ◀無作為化臨床試験 randomized clinical trial；RCT

りんせつ[1] 鱗屑 **scale, squama**

りんせつ[2] 隣接(した) (建物が隣の)**next door** (隣り合った)**adjacent, adjoining** (近隣の)**neighboring** ◆当病院は隣接する健診センターと連携しています This hospital is affiliated with the health screening center next door.

リンパ lymph (㊗**lymphatic** リンパ球性の **lymphocytic** リンパ様の **lymphoid**) ◀急性リンパ性白血病 acute lymphocytic leukemia；ALL ヒトTリンパ球向性ウイルス1型 human T-lymphotropic virus type 1；HTLV-1 慢性リンパ性白血病 chronic lymphocytic leukemia；CLL ▶リンパ液 lymph リンパ行性転移 lymphogenous metastasis リンパ組織 lymphatic[lymphoid] tissue リンパ浮腫 lymphedema リンパ脈管筋腫症 lymphangioleiomyomatosis；LAM ☞リンパ管，リンパ球，リンパ腫，リンパ節

リンパかん ─管 **lymph vessel, lymphatic vessel** ◀癌性リンパ管症 carcinomatous lymphangitis ▶リンパ管侵襲 lymphatic permeation[invasion] リンパ管造影 lymphangiography

リンパきゅう ─球 **lymphocyte** (㊗**lymphocytic**) ◀異型リンパ球 atypical lymphocyte T〈B/NK〉リンパ球 T〈B/NK〉lymphocyte ▶リンパ球減少 lymphocytopenia / lymphopenia リンパ球刺激試験 lymphocyte stimulation test；LST / (リンパ球幼若化試験)lymphocyte transformation test；LTT リンパ球増多 lymphocytosis

リンパしゅ ─腫 **lymphoma** ◀悪性リンパ腫 malignant lymphoma エイズ関連リンパ腫 AIDS-related lymphoma T細胞リンパ腫 T-cell lymphoma B細胞リンパ腫 B-cell lymphoma 非ホジキンリンパ腫 non-Hodgkin lymphoma；NHL ホジ

キンリンパ腫 Hodgkin lymphoma MALT[粘膜関連リンパ組織]リンパ腫 MALT[mucosa-associated lymphoid tissue] lymphoma 濾胞性リンパ腫 follicular lymphoma

リンパせつ ─節 **lymph nodes** [glands] ★通例，複数形で. ◆首のリンパ節が腫れています The lymph nodes[glands] in your neck are swollen[(大きくなっている)enlarged]. / The lymph nodes[glands] in your neck have swollen up. ◆腫瘍はリンパ節に広がっています The tumor has spread[extended] to the lymph nodes. / The tumor has entered the lymph nodes. ◆リンパ節を摘出する remove[excise] lymph nodes ▶腋窩リンパ節 axillary lymph nodes 顎下リンパ節 submandibular lymph nodes 頸部リンパ節 cervical lymph nodes 鎖骨上窩リンパ節 supraclavicular lymph nodes 縦隔リンパ節 mediastinal lymph nodes センチネルリンパ節 sentinel lymph nodes 鼠径リンパ節 inguinal lymph nodes 肺門リンパ節 hilar lymph nodes 腹腔リンパ節 celiac lymph nodes 傍大動脈リンパ節 paraaortic lymph nodes ▶リンパ節炎 lymphadenitis リンパ節郭清術 lymphadenectomy / lymph node dissection リンパ節腫脹 lymph node enlargement[swelling] リンパ節生検 lymph node biopsy リンパ節転移 lymph node metastasis

りんびょう 淋病 ☞淋菌

りんり 倫理 **ethics** (㊗**ethical**) ◆患者の診療記録を世間に公開するのは医師の倫理に反します It is unethical for doctors[It violates medical ethics] to disclose patients' medical records to the public. ◆職業倫理にかなった行為 professional [ethical] conduct ◆生命倫理に基づく医療 ethics-based medicine ◀医療倫理 medical ethics 看護倫理 nursing ethics 職業倫理 professional ethics 生命倫理 bioethics ▶倫理委員会 ethics committee 倫理審査 ethics[ethical] review 倫理審査委員会 ethics[ethical] review board；ERB

る

るいえき　涙液　lacrimal fluid, tear fluid, tears　★通例，複数形で．　☞涙　▶人工涙液 artificial tears

るいかん　涙管　lacrimal duct, tear duct, tear canal　◀鼻涙管 nasolacrimal duct　▶涙管ブジー lacrimal bougie

るいかんがんしょう　類宦官症　eunuchoidism

るいじ　類似する　resemble（◫resemblance）, be similar（to）（◫similarity）　☞似る　◆摘出した脳腫瘍の組織像は肺がんの所見に類似しています The pathologic image of the resected brain tumor resembles that of lung cancer.　◆あなたの症状は甲状腺機能亢進症の徴候に類似しています Your symptoms are similar to the signs of hyperthyroidism.　▶類似化合物 analog / analogue　類似点 similarity / point of similarity[resemblance]

るいししつ　類脂質　☞リポイド

るいじょうひさいぼう　類上皮細胞　epithelioid cell

るいせき　累積（の）　cumulative　▶累積吸収線量 cumulative dose　累積効果 cumulative effect　累積死亡率 cumulative mortality[death] rate　累積生存率 cumulative survival rate　累積罹患率 cumulative incidence rate

るいせん　涙腺　lacrimal gland, tear gland

るいそう　るい痩　☞痩せ

るいてん　涙点　lacrimal point[opening, punctum]

るいのう　涙嚢　lacrimal sac, tear sac, dacryocyst　▶涙嚢炎 dacryocystitis

るいひのうしゅ　類皮嚢腫　dermoid cyst

るいひょうひのうしゅ　類表皮嚢腫　epidermoid cyst

ルーチン　routine /rùːtíːn/　▶ルーチン検査 routine test　ルーチン手技 routine technique

ループスじんえん　―腎炎　lupus nephritis

ループりにょうやく　―利尿薬　loop diuretic

ルーペ　loupe /lúːp/　(拡大鏡)magnifying glass

ルーマニア　Romania（㊟Romanian）　☞国籍　▶ルーマニア人（の）Romanian

ルーム　room　◀部屋　▶ルームチャージ (hospital) room charge　ルームメイト roommate

ルゴールえき　―液　Lugol solution

るすばんでんわ　留守番電話　answering machine　◆留守番電話にメッセージを残す leave a message on the answering machine

れ

れい¹ 礼 ☞感謝 ◆（感謝の言葉への返事）礼には及びません You're welcome. / Don't mention it. ◆ご協力をいただき厚く御礼申し上げます I really appreciate [Thank you very much for] your cooperation. ▶礼状 thank-you letter / letter of thanks

れい² 例 （代表例）example （個別の例）instance （図などによる例）illustration （事例）case （見本）sample ◆では例にならってご自分でやってみて下さい Now follow the example and try to do it yourself. ◆同様の例はよくあります There are a lot of similar cases. ◆例を挙げてみましょう Let me give you an example. ◆よくある例 a common example ◆典型的な例 a typical example[case] ◆過去の例からすると judging from previous instances[cases] ◆その一例としては To give an example, …

れいあんしつ 霊安室 （hospital）morgue,《英》(hospital) mortuary

れいがい 例外 exception （形exceptional） ◆これは例外的なケースです This is an exceptional[(普通でない) unusual] case. ◆今回だけは例外として外出を認めます We'll make an exception and give you permission to go out just this once. ◆申し訳ありませんが病院の規則に例外は認められません I'm sorry, but we cannot permit any exceptions to the hospital rules (and regulations).

れいかん 冷感 chills ★通例，複数形で. （冷感覚）cold sensation

れいきゃく 冷却 cooling （氷での冷却）icing ☞冷やす ◆身体冷却 body cooling ▶冷却効果 cooling effect 冷却水 cooling water 冷却装置 cooling apparatus / cooler

れいきゅうしゃ 霊柩車 hearse, funeral car[vehicle, coach]

れいしき 冷式（の） cold ▶冷式抗体 cold antibody 冷式自己免疫性溶血性貧血 cold autoimmune hemolytic anemia / cold AIHA

れいしっぷ 冷湿布 cold compress[pack, pad] ☞湿布 ◆冷湿布を首に貼る apply a cold compress to the neck / put a cold compress on the neck

れいすい 冷水 cold water ◆冷水摩擦をする rub *oneself* (down) with a cold wet towel

れいせい 冷静（な） calm, cool （図composure, cool） ◆冷静さを保つ stay [keep] calm[cool] / keep[maintain] *one's* composure[cool] ◆冷静さを失う lose *one's* composure[presence of mind] /（動揺する）be upset ◆冷静を装う put on an appearance of composure ◆冷静さを取り戻す regain[recover] *one's* *peace of mind[composure]

れいぞうこ 冷蔵庫 refrigerator （動冷蔵庫で冷やす refrigerate） ◆この薬は冷蔵庫の中で保管して下さい Please put[keep] this medication in the refrigerator.

れいとう 冷凍する freeze （形frozen） ☞凍結 ▶冷凍血液 frozen blood 冷凍食品 frozen food 冷凍母乳 frozen breast milk 冷凍麻酔 cryoanesthesia 冷凍焼け chilblains / perniosis

レイノー Raynaud ▶レイノー現象 Raynaud phenomenon レイノー病 Raynaud disease

れいはいどう 礼拝堂 chapel

れいパック 冷パック cold pack （氷の）ice pack ☞冷湿布

レイプ rape ◆レイプ被害者 a rape victim

れいぼう 冷房 air conditioning （エアコン）air conditioner ◆冷房システムは時にアレルギーや呼吸器疾患を引き起こすことがあります Air conditioning units sometimes cause allergies or respiratory diseases. ◆冷房を入れる〈切る〉turn [switch] the air conditioner on〈off〉 ◆冷房のきいた部屋 an air-conditioned room ▶冷房病 air-conditioner disease

レーザー laser /léɪzə/ ◆レーザーで顔のしみ[肝斑]を抜く remove liver spots from the face using laser treatment ◆網膜裂孔をレーザーで焼く treat retinal tears with laser therapy ◆レーザーポインターは目を傷めることがあります Laser pointers may sometimes cause eye injuries. ◀アルゴンレーザー argon laser 走査レーザー検眼鏡 scanning laser ophthalmoscope 炭酸ガスレーザー carbon dioxide laser ヤグレーザー *yttrium aluminum garnet [YAG] laser ▶レーザー眼障害 laser eye injury レーザー光凝固術 laser photocoagulation レーザー光線 laser beam[light] レーザー手術 laser surgery レーザー脱毛 laser hair removal レーザー治療 laser treatment[therapy] レーザーメス laser knife[scalpel]

レーシック LASIK（surgery） （レーザー角膜内切削形成術）laser-assisted in situ keratomileusis（surgery）

レーズン raisin ◆レーズンくらいの大きさのポリープ a polyp about the size of a raisin

れき ―歴 history （プロフィール）profile ◀家族歴 family history 既往歴 past（medical）history；PH 結婚歴 marital history 現病歴 present（medical）history／present illness；PI／history of the present illness；HPI／history of the presenting complaint；HPC 個人歴 patient profile 社会歴 social history 職業歴 occupational history 生活歴 life history 妊娠歴 obstetrical history 発育歴 developmental history 薬歴 medication history 輸血歴 history of blood transfusion

れきし 轢死 death due to being struck [hit] by a vehicle

れきねんれい 暦年齢 chronologic age, chronological age

レクリエーション recreation （形recreational） ▶レクリエーション療法 recreational therapy

レジオネラ legionella （学名）*Legionella* ▶レジオネラ感染症 legionella infec-

tion レジオネラ症 Legionnaires' disease／legionellosis レジオネラ肺炎 legionella pneumonia

レジデント resident ◀ジュニアレジデント junior resident シニアレジデント senior resident チーフレジデント chief resident

レシピエント recipient（↔donor） ◀輸血レシピエント（blood）transfusion recipient

レストレスレッグしょうこうぐん ―症候群 restless legs syndrome；RLS

レスパイトケア respite care

レズビアン lesbianism, female homosexuality （人）lesbian ☞同性愛

レスピレーター artificial respirator, mechanical respirator ☞人工呼吸器

レセプト ☞診療報酬明細書

レチノイド retinoid

レチノインさん ―酸 retinoic acid （ビタミンA酸）vitamin A acid

れっこう¹ 裂肛 anal fissure （出血性痔核）bleeding piles[hemorrhoids] ★複数形で．▶裂肛切除術 fissurectomy

れっこう² 裂孔 tear /téə/, hiatus /haɪéɪtəs/ （形hiatal） ◀滑脱型（食道）裂孔ヘルニア sliding（esophageal）hiatal hernia 網膜裂孔 retinal tear

れっしょう 裂傷 laceration, lacerated wound （裂け目）tear /téə/ （破裂）rupture ◆裂傷を負う have a laceration ◀会陰裂傷 perineal tear[laceration] 鼓膜裂傷 eardrum rupture 子宮頸管裂傷 cervical tear[laceration]

れっせい 劣性（の） recessive（↔dominant） ▶劣性遺伝 recessive inheritance 劣性遺伝子 recessive gene 劣性遺伝病 recessive hereditary disease 劣性形質 recessive trait[character]

れっとうかん 劣等感 inferiority complex（↔superiority complex）, sense of inferiority ◆自分の体形に対して劣等感を持つ have an inferiority complex about *one's* figure／feel inferior about *one's* figure

れっとうじょうちゅうしょう 裂頭条虫症 diphyllobothriasis

レットしょうこうぐん ―症候群 Rett

レットしょうこうぐん syndrome

レトロウイルス retrovirus （形retroviral）
▶レトロウイルス感染症 retrovirus[retroviral] infection

レニン renin ▶レニン-アンギオテンシン-アルドステロン系 the renin-angiotensin-aldosterone system

レノグラフィ renography

レビーしょうたい ―小体 Lewy body
▶レビー小体型認知症 Lewy body dementia / dementia with Lewy bodies；DLB

レビュー review ◀システムレビュー systems[systematic] review / review of systems；ROS ピアレビュー peer review

レプチン leptin

レプトスピラ *Leptospira* ▶レプトスピラ症 leptospirosis

レフレルしょうこうぐん ―症候群 Loeffler syndrome

レベル level ☞程度 ◆0 から 10 のスケールで，0 が痛みがなくて 10 が一番ひどい痛みとすれば，あなたの今の痛みのレベルは何ですか On a scale of zero to ten, with zero meaning no pain and ten being the worst pain, *how would you rate the pain [what's your pain level]? ◆低い〈高い〉ヘモグロビンのレベル a low〈high〉 hemoglobin level ◀意識レベル level of consciousness ストレスレベル stress level / level of stress 体力レベル energy level 聴力レベル hearing (threshold) level；HL 疼痛許容レベル pain tolerance level

レポート （報告書）report （論文）paper ☞報告 ◆レポートを書く write a report ◆レポートを提出する file[submit] a report ◆検査レポートのコピーを渡す *hand over[give] a copy of *a person's* examination report ◀インシデントレポート incident report オカレンスレポート occurrence report

レム REM （レム眼球運動）rapid eye movement ▶レム睡眠 REM sleep レム睡眠行動障害 REM sleep behavior disorder

れんあいもうそう 恋愛妄想 love delusion, delusion of love, erotomania

れんけい 連携 cooperation （組織の）affiliation （動affiliate） ◆当病院は隣接する画像センターと連携しています We work in close cooperation with the imaging center next door. / This hospital is affiliated with the imaging center next door.

れんごう 連合 （関連）association （形associated） （組み合わせ）combination ◀前頭連合野 frontal association area ▶連合運動 associated movement 連合反応 associated reaction

れんさ 連鎖 （相関関係）linkage （連続）chain ☞X 連鎖，連鎖球菌，連鎖反応

れんさきゅうきん 連鎖球菌 streptococcus, strep （形streptococcal） （学名） *Streptococcus* ◆連鎖球菌咽頭炎に罹る have (a) strep throat ◀A 群連鎖球菌 group A streptococcus；GAS B 群連鎖球菌 group B streptococcus；GBS 溶血性連鎖球菌 hemolytic streptococcus ▶連鎖球菌感染後糸球体腎炎 poststreptococcal glomerulonephritis 連鎖球菌感染症 streptococcal[strep] infection 連鎖球菌性肺炎 streptococcal pneumonia

れんさはんのう 連鎖反応 chain reaction ◆連鎖反応を示す show a chain reaction ◆負の連鎖反応を起こす cause a negative chain reaction ◆負の連鎖反応を断ち切る cut off a negative chain reaction

れんしゅう 練習する （実践する）practice （運動する）exercise （トレーニングする）train （名practice, exercise, training） ☞訓練 ◆腹式呼吸の練習をしましょう（横隔膜を使って深呼吸する）Let's practice deep breathing using the diaphragm. ◆手術前に深呼吸と咳の仕方を練習しておいて下さい Please do some deep breathing and coughing exercises before your surgery. ◆もう少し練習すれば歩けるようになります With a little more practice, you'll be able to walk.

れんしゅく 攣縮 （痙縮）spasm （形spasmodic, spastic） （収縮）contraction ◀冠動脈攣縮 coronary artery spasm 筋攣縮 muscle spasm 血管攣縮 vasospasm /

vascular spasm　血管攣縮性狭心症 vaso-spastic[coronary spastic] angina　線維束性攣縮 fasciculation　▶攣縮性斜頚 spasmodic torticollis

レンズ　lens（圏lenses）　◀凹レンズ con-cave lens　眼内レンズ intraocular lens；IOL　矯正レンズ corrective lens　コンタクトレンズ contact lens　ソフト（コンタクト）レンズ soft (contact) lens　透明レンズ clear lens　凸レンズ convex lens　二重焦点〈多焦点〉レンズ bifocal〈multifocal〉lens　ハード（コンタクト）レンズ hard (contact) lens　乱視用レンズ astigmatic lens

れんそう　連想する　（思い出させる）remind (of)　（関連づける）associate（圖associa-tion）　◆この絵を見て何を連想しますか What does this picture remind you of? / What comes to your mind when you see this picture?　◆自由連想法 free associa-tion　▶連想検査 association test

れんぞく　連続（して）　in a row　（切れ目なく続いて）consecutively, continuously（囫continue　圖continuity）　（順を追って続いて）successively　☞持続，続く　◆血糖値がここ 2 回の検査で連続して高い値を示しています Your blood sugar levels have gone up *in the last two consecutive tests.　◆5 日以上連続して熱が出たら，再び受診して下さい If you have the fever for more than five days in a row, please come and see me again.　◆1 週間以上連続して眠れなかったのですか Did the difficulty sleeping continue for more than a week?　◆抗菌薬を不必要に連続して服用するのはよくありません You shouldn't keep taking antibiotics continuously if you don't need them.　◆連続した（一連の）反応 a series of reactions　◆連続性を中断する break[interrupt] the continuity　▶連続[持続]携行式腹膜透析 continuous ambulatory peritoneal dialysis；CAPD　連続性雑音 continuous murmur　連続性ラ音 continuous (adventitious) sounds　連続装用コンタクトレンズ extended-wear contact lens

れんたいほしょうにん　連帯保証人　co-signer, co-signer, joint guarantor　☞保証人

レントゲン　roentgen　（X 線写真）X-ray, x-ray　☞X 線，放射線　◆念のため胸のレントゲンを撮りましょう Let me[I'm going to] take an X-ray of your chest just in case.　◆レントゲンを撮りますから放射線科へお連れします I'm going to take you to the radiology department for your X-ray.　◆これがあなたの胸のレントゲンです This is the X-ray of your chest.　◆レントゲン写真から判断すると，ご心配なことはありません Judging from the X-ray (films), you have nothing to worry about.　▶レントゲン技師 X-ray[radiologic] techni-cian / X-ray[radiologic] technologist　レントゲン検査 X-ray (examination)　レントゲン室 X-ray room

れんよう　連用　（切れ目なく連続して使用すること）continuous use　（いつまでも使用し続けること）prolonged use　◆この薬の連用は避けて下さい Please avoid taking this medication continuously. / Continuous use of this medication should be avoided.

れんらく　連絡する　（連絡を取る）contact, get in touch（with）　（電話をかける）call　◆2, 3 日中に症状が改善しない時は連絡して下さい Please call[contact] us if your symptoms do not improve within a few days.　◆副作用の疑いがある時には至急連絡して下さい Please contact[call] us im-mediately if you suspect any side ef-fects.　◆何かありましたらこちらからご連絡します We'll call[get in touch with] you if anything should happen.

れんらくさき　連絡先　（電話番号）contact number　（住所）contact address　◆ここに連絡先を記入して下さい（電話番号）Please write your contact number here.　◆緊急の連絡先は何番ですか What's your emergency contact number?　◆緊急連絡先はどなたですか Who should we con-tact in case of an emergency?　◀緊急連絡先（電話番号）emergency contact num-ber

ろ

ロイコトリエン leukotriene ▶ロイコトリエン受容体拮抗薬 leukotriene receptor antagonist；LTRA

ロイコプラキー leukoplakia ☞白斑症

ろう[1] 瘻 fistula ◀胃瘻造設術 gastrostomy 回腸瘻造設術 ileostomy 膵瘻 pancreatic fistula 腸瘻 intestinal fistula 動静脈瘻 arteriovenous fistula 尿管瘻 ureteral fistula 尿道瘻 urethral fistula 膀胱瘻造設術 cystostomy 有瘻性膿胸 pyothorax[empyema] with fistula ☞瘻孔

ろう[2] 聾(唖の) deaf ★deaf-mute には差別的なニュアンスがあるので，単に deaf を用いることが望ましい．▶ろう(あ)者 deaf (and speech-impaired) person ★総称としては deaf people と言う．☞聾学校，聾者

ろうか[1] 老化 (加齢)aging, senescence ☞加齢 ▶老化過程 aging process 老化現象 signs and symptoms of aging / condition caused by aging

ろうか[2] 廊下 hallway, hall, corridor ◆お手洗いは廊下の突き当たりにあります The restroom is at the end of the hallway.

ろうがっこう 聾学校 school for the deaf

ろうがん 老眼 (老視)presbyopia (老化による遠視)farsightedness due to aging ◆老眼ですね You've become farsighted due to old age. ▶老眼鏡(読書用の)reading glasses[spectacles] (for elderly people)

ろうご 老後 one's old age (余生)the rest of one's life (残りの歳月)one's remaining years ★複数形で.

ろうこう 瘻孔 fistula (瘻fistulous) ☞有瘻 ▶瘻孔性潰瘍 fistulous ulcer 瘻孔切開術 fistulotomy 瘻孔切除術 fistulectomy 瘻孔造影 fistulography 瘻孔閉鎖 fistula closure / closure of a fistula

ろうさ 労作 (努力・頑張り)effort (心身の酷使)exertion (瘻exertional) ▶労作性狭心症 effort[exertional] angina / angina of [on] effort 労作性胸痛 exertional chest pain / chest pain *on exertion[during exercise] 労作性呼吸困難 exertional dyspnea / dyspnea on exertion；DOE

ろうさい 労災 ☞労働災害

ろうし 老視 ☞老眼

ろうしゃ 聾者 person with a hearing impairment[disorder], deaf person, hard-of-hearing person ☞聾

ろうしゅつ 漏出 leak, leakage (濾出)transudation (瘻transudative) ☞漏れる ◀髄液漏出 cerebrospinal fluid leakage 胆汁漏出 biliary leak / bile leak[leakage] 蛋白漏出性胃腸症 protein-losing gastroenteropathy 乳汁漏出症 galactorrhea / lactorrhea ▶漏出液 transudate 漏出性胸水[腹水] transudative *pleural effusion ⟨ascites⟩

ろうじん 老人 elderly[older] person ⟨man, woman⟩, senior citizen (総称的に)elderly[older] people, senior citizens ★総称として the elderly も用いるが，この語は差別的に響くので，elderly[older] people や senior citizens を好む人が多い．また，日常会話では elderly より older がよく使われる．☞高齢者，ライフステージ，老年 ▶介護老人福祉施設 welfare facility for elderly people requiring long-term care 介護老人保健施設 health care facility for elderly people requiring long-term care ▶老人医療 medical care for elderly[older] people / medical elderly care 老人介護 elderly care / eldercare 老人虐待 elder abuse / abuse of older adults / (放置)elder neglect 老人差別 ageism / age discrimination 老人性難聴 age-related hearing loss 老人性白内障 senile cataract / (加齢白内障)age-related cataract 老人斑 age spots 老人病院 geriatric hospital 老人福祉 welfare for the elderly / elderly welfare 老人保健 health of the elderly / elderly health ☞老人ホーム

ろうじんホーム 老人ホーム (介護型の施設)nursing home[facility] (for seniors [elderly people]) (中程度のケア付き施設)

assisted living facility (for seniors[elderly people]) （自立型施設）retirement home, independent living facility (for seniors [elderly people]) ◀特別養護老人ホーム special nursing home for seniors[elderly people] 有料老人ホーム private residential home for seniors[elderly people] /（退職者の）(private) retirement home

ろうすい 老衰 senility ◆老衰で死ぬ die[pass away] of old age /（自然死する）die[pass away] of natural causes

ろうどう 労働 （一般的に）work （肉体労働）labor ☞作業, 仕事 ◀家事労働 housework / household work 重労働 hard labor 頭脳労働 brainwork / mental work 単純労働 unskilled labor 肉体労働 physical[manual] labor[work] ▶労働環境 work environment 労働基準監督署 Labor Standards Inspection Office 労働強度 work[labor] strength 労働時間 working hours[time] ☞労働災害, 労働者

ろうどうさいがい 労働災害 work-related accident[injury], workers' accident [injury], workplace accident[injury], occupational accident[injury], industrial accident[injury] ▶労働災害補償保険 workers' accident compensation insurance

ろうどうしゃ 労働者 （一般的に）worker （肉体労働者）laborer ◀外国人労働者 foreign worker[laborer]

ろうときょう 漏斗胸 funnel chest [breast], pectus excavatum

ろうねん 老年 old age （圏老衰の・老化している senile /síːnaɪl/）☞高齢者, ライフステージ, 老人 ▶老年医学 geriatrics / geriatric medicine 老年学 gerontology 老年看護 geriatric nursing 老年期 old age / senile period[stage] 老年期うつ病 senile depression / depression in elderly people 老年人口 elderly population 老年内科 the department of geriatrics / the geriatrics department 老年病専門医 geriatrician

ろうはいぶつ 老廃物 waste （matter, product）◆老廃物を体内から排出する

excrete waste matter from the body

ろうれい 老齢 old age ☞高齢者, 老人, 老年 ▶老齢年金 old-age pension

ろうろうかいご 老老介護 elder-to-elder home care, elderly care provided by an elderly family member

ローション lotion ◆このローションを患部に2, 3滴つけて下さい Please apply a few drops of this lotion to the affected area. ◀アイローション eye lotion スキンローション skin lotion 保湿ローション moisturizing lotion

ロールシャッハテスト Rorschach test

ロールプレイ role-playing （役割演技）role-play （圏role-play）▶ロールプレイング療法 role-playing therapy

ロールモデル role model

ローレルしすう 一指数 Röhrer index

ろか 濾過 filtration （圏filter）◀持続的血液濾過法 continuous hemofiltration；CHF 二重濾過血漿交換 double filtration plasmapheresis；DFPP ▶濾過圧 filtration pressure 濾過液 filtrate 濾過器 filter 濾過率 filtration fraction；FF

ろくおん 録音する record ◆会話を録音してもよろしいですか Would you mind if I record (ed) our conversation?

ろくがつ 6月 June；Jun. ☞1月

ろくなんこつ 肋軟骨 costal cartilage ▶肋軟骨炎 costochondritis

ログランクけんてい 一検定 log-rank test

ロシア Russia （圏Russian）☞国籍 ▶ロシア人 (の) Russian

ロジスティックかいきぶんせき 一回帰分析 logistic regression analysis

ろしゅつ 露出する expose （圏exposure）▶露出歯髄 exposed pulp 露出症 exhibitionism

ロスしゅじゅつ 一手術 Ross procedure [operation]

ロタウイルス rotavirus （圏rotaviral） （学名）*Rotavirus* ◆ロタウイルスに感染する get rotavirus ◆ロタウイルスに感染している be infected with rotavirus ◆彼の急性胃腸炎はロタウイルスによるものです His acute *stomach flu[gastroenteritis] is caused by rotavirus. / Rotavirus *is the cause of[has caused] his acute *stomach flu[gastroenteritis]. ▶ロタウイルス感染症 rotavirus[rotaviral] infection　ロタウイルス下痢症 rotavirus[rotaviral] diarrhea

ロッカー　locker　◆持ち物や貴重品は病室のロッカーに入れて下さい You can put your things and valuables in the locker in your room.　◀コインロッカー coin locker　有料ロッカー pay locker

ろっかん　肋間(の)　intercostal　▶肋間筋 intercostal muscle　肋間神経 intercostal nerve　肋間神経痛 intercostal neuralgia

ろっこつ　肋骨　(1本の)rib, costa (㊧costal)　(総称)the ribs, the costae　◆肋骨を折る break[fracture] *one's* rib(s)　◆肋骨を損傷する have a rib injury / injure[hurt] *one's* rib(s)　▶肋骨弓 costal margin[arch]　肋骨骨折 rib fracture

ろっぷんかんほこうしけん　6分間歩行試験　six-minute walk test；6MWT

ロビー　lobby　(休憩室)lounge　◆手術中は6階のロビーでお待ち下さい Please wait in the lobby on the sixth floor *during the surgery[while the surgery is going on].　◆ご面会はロビーでお願いします Visits should take place in the lobby. / (家族の面会は) Family members may visit in the lobby.

ろほう　濾胞　follicle (㊧follicular)　▶濾胞性結膜炎 follicular conjunctivitis　濾胞性扁桃炎 follicular tonsillitis　濾胞性リンパ腫 follicular lymphoma

ロボット　robot　◀介助ロボット care robot

ろれつ　◆彼はろれつが回らない(不明瞭に話す) His speech is slurred. / He slurs his words. / He can't speak clearly.

ろんぶん　論文　(研究論文)paper　(修士・博士などの学位論文)thesis　(特に博士論文)dissertation　(評論)essay　◆…に関する論文 a paper on[about] …

ロンベルグちょうこう　―徴候　Romberg

sign

ろんり　論理　logic (㊧logical)　◆論理的な結論を出す reach[draw] a logical conclusion / logically conclude

わ

わ　輪　環 (光の環) **halo** (円形) **circle** (丸状の輪) **ring** (ひも状の輪) **loop** ◆光の周りに輪が見えますか Do you see halos around lights?

ワーカホリック workaholic

わいしょう　矮小 (な) **small** (小型の) **dwarf, dwarfed, miniature** (顕頭極端に小さい **micro-**) ▶矮小陰茎 small penis / micropenis　矮小歯 dwarfed[dwarf] tooth　矮小腎 dwarf[miniature] kidney

わいせつ　猥褻 (な) (みだらな) **indecent** (卑猥な) **obscene** ▶わいせつ行為 indecent behavior[act]

ワイせんしょくたい　Y 染色体　Y chromosome

ワイヤー　wire ◆ワイヤーで胸骨をつなぎ合わせる *sew the breastbone back[hold the breastbone] together with wire ▶ワイヤーループ病変 wire-loop lesion

ワイルびょう　—病　Weil disease (レプトスピラ黄疸症) **leptospiral jaundice**

わかぎこっせつ　若木骨折　greenstick fracture

わかしらが　若白髪　prematurely gray hair, premature (hair) graying

わがまま　我儘 (な) (自分本位の) **selfish, self-centered** (甘やかされた) **spoiled**

わかもの　若者　young person (男性) **young man** (女性) **young woman** (総称的に) **young people, the youth** ☞ライフステージ

わかりにくい　分かりにくい　be hard to understand, be difficult to understand ◆わかりにくいことがあれば遠慮なく訊いて下さい If there's anything hard to understand[If there's anything you can't understand], please don't hesitate to ask me.

わかりやすい　分かりやすい　be easy to understand ◆この取扱い説明書はわかりやすい This instruction manual is *easy to

understand[user-friendly]. / This instruction manual is written in simple, plain words. ◆わかりやすい言葉で病気について説明する(一般人にわかる言葉で)explain the disease in layperson's terms / (患者・家族にわかるように)explain the disease so that patients and family members can understand easily

わかる　分かる (理解する) **understand** (知る) **know** (判明する) **prove to be, turn out to be**

《理解する》　◆すみませんが, 英語はわかりません I'm sorry, I don't understand English. ◆私の言うことがわかりますか Do you understand me[what I'm saying]? ◆あなたの言うことはわかりました I understand what you mean. / I understand what you want to say. ◆わからないことがあれば, どうぞ訊いて下さい If there is anything you don't understand, please ask us for help.

《判明する》　◆胸部 X 線上の陰影が良性か悪性かはまだわかっていません We don't yet know[It's not yet clear] whether the shadow on your chest X-ray is benign or malignant. ◆検査の結果は来週金曜日にわかります We'll know the test results next Friday. ◆その薬は効果がないことがわかりました That medication proved [turned out] to be ineffective.

《承知する》　◆わかりました(同意・理解を示して)I see. / I understand. ◆はい, わかりました(依頼などへの返事として)Yes, sure. / Yes, certainly.

わかれ　別れ　parting (別れの言葉) **goodbye** ☞別れる ◆別れを告げる say goodbye (to) ◆彼女に最期のお別れをするために会わせたい人がいますか Is there anyone you'd like to have with you to say final goodbyes to her? ◆(臨終の際に居合わせた家族に)お別れです It's time to say goodbye. / It's time for you to say your goodbyes.

わかれる¹　分かれる (分裂する) **divide** (**into**) (意見などが二分する) **split** (**into**) (分岐する) **branch** (**off**) ◆彼女の治療方針

に関して家族の意見が分かれています Her family members are divided over the treatment she should receive. / The opinions of her family members are divided [split] over what kind of treatment she should have.

わかれる² 別れる **part**（from）（別れを告げる）**say goodbye**（to）（離婚する）**get [be] divorced**（from），**divorce** *one's* husband〈wife〉 ☞別れ ◆明日ご帰国ですね。お別れするのが悲しいです You're returning to your country tomorrow, aren't you? I feel sad that I have to say goodbye to you. ◆彼女は3年前夫と別れました She got divorced from her husband three years ago. ◆現在，彼は妻と別れて暮らしている He and his wife are living apart at the moment. / He is living apart from his wife at the moment.

わき 腋 ☞腋の下

わきが 腋臭 （わきの下のにおい）**underarm odor, armpit odor** （体臭）**body odor** ◆わきがが強い have strong underarm odor ▶わきが症 axillary osmidrosis / hircismus わきが消臭剤 underarm deodorant

わきげ 腋毛 **underarm hair, the hair under** *one's* **arms** ◆腋毛を剃る shave under *one's* arms / shave *one's* armpits

わきのした 腋の下 **armpit, underarm, axilla**（略axillary）☞腋窩 ◆わきの下を触診します I'm going to feel[examine] your armpit(s). ◆わきの下が痛みますか Do you have any pain under your arm(s)? ◆わきの下にしこりがありますか Have you noticed any lump in your underarm area? ◆この体温計をピーッと鳴るまでわきの下にはさんで下さい Please keep this thermometer under your arm until it beeps.

わきばら 脇腹 （側腹部）**the lateral abdominal region** （横腹）**flank,** *one's* **side** ◆わき腹に痛みがある have (a) pain in *one's* side

ワクチン **vaccine** /vǽksíːn/（動vǽccinate 图vaccinátion）☞予防接種 ◆ポリオのワクチンを接種する vaccinate *a person* against polio ◆麻疹のワクチン接種(a) rubella vaccination ◆インフルエンザのワクチン接種 a flu shot ◀弱毒化ワクチン attenuated vaccine 生ワクチン live vaccine 不活化ワクチン inactivated[killed] vaccine

わけ 訳 ☞理由

わける 分ける （分類する）**classify** （分割する）**divide** （切り離す）**separate** /sépərèit/ （國部屋などが別の **separate** /sépərət/）★動詞と発音が異なることに注意. ◆がんの治療には，大きく分けて手術，放射線，化学療法があります Cancer treatment can be roughly classified into three types; surgery, radiation, and chemotherapy. ◆患者を3グループに分ける divide patients into three groups ◆感染症の患者の部屋を分ける put[place] patients with infectious diseases in separate rooms

ワゴン （配膳用などの）**wagon, cart**

わざと **on purpose, intentionally** ☞意図 ◆わざと答えを間違える give the wrong answer *on purpose[intentionally] ☞わざとらしい

わざとらしい （不自然な）**unnatural** （無理に作った）**forced** （気取った）**affected** ◆わざとらしい表情や振る舞いをしてしまうのは彼の病気のせいです It's his illness that's causing his unnatural[forced / affected] facial expression and gestures.

わざわざ ◆わざわざお越しいただいてありがとうございます Thank you for taking the trouble to come and see me.

わしで 鷲手 **claw hand, clawhand**

わしょく 和食 **Japanese dish[food]**

わずか （少しばかりの）**slight** （数の少ない）**a few** ◆その切り傷はわずかな傷痕を残すかもしれません The cut may leave a slight scar. ◆痛みはわずかにチクンとする程度です You'll just feel a slight prick[pricking pain]. ◆あとわずか数分の辛抱です Please *hold on[be patient] for just a few minutes more.

わずらう 患う ☞罹る

わすれる 忘れる **forget** ◆最近，彼女は忘れることがよくありますか Has she been forgetting things recently? ◆彼が忘れるのは最近の出来事ですか，それとも昔の出来事ですか Does he forget recent events or past events? ◆薬を飲み忘れないで下さい Please don't forget to take your medications. ◆忘れっぽい be forgetful

ワセリン petroleum jelly, (white) petrolatum （商標名）Vaseline

わたす 渡す （与える）**give** （手渡す）**hand** ◆署名した同意書は担当の医師あるいは看護師にお渡し下さい Please give [hand] the signed consent form to your doctor or nurse.

わびる 詫びる **apologize (for, to)** ☞謝る，すみません，申し訳 ◆病棟スタッフを代表してお詫びいたします Let me apologize to you on behalf of the ward staff. ◆お返事が遅れたことを心よりお詫びいたします I'm really sorry for not replying (to you) earlier. / （手紙の返事）I'm really sorry that I didn't write (to you) sooner.

わらい 笑い （笑い・笑い声）**laughter, laugh** （微笑）**smile** （含み笑い・くすくす笑い）**chuckle** （女の子などの甲高いくすくす笑い）**giggle** ☞笑う ◆笑いは百薬の長 Laughter is the best medicine. ◀強制[強迫]笑い forced[obsessive] laughing 作り笑い （無理に作った不自然な笑い）forced smile / （偽りの笑い）fake smile 独り笑い smiling [laughing / chuckling] to *oneself*

わらう 笑う （声を出して笑う）**laugh** （ほほ笑む・にこにこする）**smile** （くすくす笑う）**chuckle** （やや甲高い声でくすくす笑う）**giggle** ☞笑い ◆抑えきれずに笑う［笑い転げる］laugh uncontrollably ◆急に笑いだす（吹きだす）burst out laughing

わり 割 （百分率）**percent, percentage** ◆医療費を3割負担する pay thirty percent of *one's* medical expenses

わりあい 割合 **ratio, proportion** ☞比率

わりつけ 割付け ◀無作為割付 random allocation

わりに 割に （…にしては）**for** （…を考えると）**considering** ◆彼は年の割に背が高い

He is tall for his age. ◆彼女は年齢の割に状態がとてもよい She's in very good condition considering her age.

わる 割る 《壊す・砕く》**break** （縦に割る）**split** （分割する）**divide** ☞割れる ◆この錠剤は中央に小さな割れ目が入っていますので，半分に割って飲んで下さい This tablet has a little slit in the middle, so you can take it by breaking[splitting / dividing] it in half. 《薄める》（水を加える）**mix … with water** （希釈する）**dilute** ◆水薬を水で割る mix the liquid medication with water

わるい 悪い （よくない）**bad** （具合・状態が悪い）**ill, sick, wrong, poor** （弱い）**weak** （不都合な）**inconvenient** 《体調・状態がよくない》◆体調が悪い feel ill[bad] / be in poor[bad] condition ◆前より悪い get[feel] worse than before ◆健康状態が悪い be in poor[ill] health / be unhealthy ◆ご気分が悪かったらおっしゃって下さい Please let me know if you feel[get] sick. ◆どこかお悪いのですか What's the matter[problem]? / Can you tell me what the problem is? ◆胃の具合が悪いのですか Do you have any problems with your stomach? / Is there anything wrong with your stomach? ◆痛みは悪くなっていますか Is the pain getting worse? ◆（診察したところ）悪いところはありません I can't find anything wrong. / There doesn't seem to be anything wrong with you. ◆顔色が悪い look pale ◆血行が悪い have poor (blood) circulation 《能力などが劣る》◆目が悪い have poor[bad] eyesight ◆物覚えが悪い have a poor[bad] memory ◆ミルクの飲みは普通ですか，悪いですか Is his〈her〉ability to suck milk normal or weak? 《好ましくない》◆残念ですが，悪いお知らせです I'm afraid[I'm sorry,] I have some bad news for you. / I'm afraid the news isn't good. ◆治りがいまひとつ悪いようです You're recovering rather slowly. / Your recovery has been rather slow.

◆ご都合が悪いようでしたらおっしゃって下さい Please let me know if it's inconvenient for you. ◆機嫌が悪い be in a bad mood / be cross ◆ごめんなさい. 悪かったのは私のほうです I'm sorry, it was my fault. / I'm sorry, I was to blame (for it).

ワルダイエルいんとうりん ―咽頭輪
Waldeyer tonsillar ring

われめ **割れ目** （亀裂）crack （縦長で細い裂け目）split （細隙）slit （深い割れ目・裂溝）fissure （破れ目・裂孔）tear /téɚ/ （唇・口などの割れ目）cleft ☞割る

われる **割れる** （裂ける）split （折れる・壊れる）break ☞割る ◆頭が割れるように痛む have a splitting headache ◆爪が割れた The nails have become broken [split].

ワレンベルグしょうこうぐん ―症候群
Wallenberg syndrome （延髄外側症候群）lateral medullary syndrome

わんきょく **彎曲** （曲がった状態）clubbing, curvature （㊑clubbed, curved） （逸脱した状態）deviation （㊑deviated, deviant） ◆手の指〈足の指〉が彎曲している have clubbing of the fingers〈toes〉 ◆指の爪が彎曲している the fingernails are curved ◀鼻中隔彎曲症 nasal septal deviation / deviation of the nasal septum ▶彎曲足 clubfoot

わんしんけいそう **腕神経叢** brachial plexus ▶腕神経叢損傷 brachial plexus injury 腕神経叢麻痺 brachial plexus paralysis

わんとうどうみゃく **腕頭動脈** brachiocephalic artery[trunk]

わ

巻末付録①

悪い診断結果を伝える時

　悪い知らせは，プライバシーや患者の気持ちを十分に配慮して時と場を選んで慎重に伝える必要がある．外国人の患者は一人ひとり文化背景・個性・知識レベルが異なっているし，英語が母語であるとは限らない．できれば英語のわかる第三者（成人の家族，通訳，医療ソーシャルワーカーなど）に同席してもらうとよいだろう．言葉で伝えると同時に，患者とのアイコンタクトなど非言語的な情報の取得にも注意を払いたい．

❶ いきなり本題に入るのではなく，患者の気持ちや状態を確認する

　例えば，まず次のような言葉をかけ，患者の受け答えから，患者自身が持っている情報，置かれている精神状態，英語力や知識レベルなどを確かめる．

- こんにちは，医師の佐藤です．ホプキンズさんですね．　Hello, I'm Dr Sato. Are you Mr Hopkins?
- お待たせしました．　I'm sorry to have kept you waiting.
- 看護師の森が同席してよろしいでしょうか．　Is it all right if Nurse Mori sits with us?
- 今，ご気分はいかがですか．　How are you feeling now?
- 夜はよく眠れますか．　Can you sleep well at night?
- 食欲はどうですか．　How is your appetite?
- あなたの病状について（かかりつけ医の）林先生から何か聞いていますか．　What has Dr Hayashi (your regular doctor) told you about your condition?

❷ よくない知らせであるという前置きをして，悪い情報を伝える

図などを示しながら説明し，質問を受ける．

- 今日はこれまでの検査結果についてお話しさせていただきます．　Now, we're here to talk about what the test results showed.
- 実は，よくないお知らせがあります．　I'm afraid I have some bad news.
- 残念ですが，悪性リンパ腫です．　I'm sorry to have to tell you this, but you have malignant lymphoma.
- 残念ながら，がんが再発しています．　I'm sorry to have to tell you this, but the cancer has come back.

「残念ながら」という気持ちを示す表現としては，他に次のようなものがある．

- ・I'm sorry, but …
- ・I'm sorry to tell you that …
- ・I'm afraid that …
- ・Unfortunately, …　（遺憾なのですが）
- ・It's hard[difficult] for me to tell you this, but …　（申し上げにくいのですが）
- ・To be frank with you …　（率直に申し上げると）
- ・… as we expected　（予想されたように）

❸ 患者の気持ちに沿って共感を示す

　共感を示す表現には注意が必要である．例えば，"I know how you feel."（お気持ちはよくわかります）と言われると，「あなたに私の気持ちがわかるはずがない」と反発を抱く患者がいるかもしれない．

巻末付録

| ■お辛いでしょう． | This must be awful[terrible] for you. |
| ■さぞショックなことと思います． | I understand this must be a shock for you. |

❹ 今後の治療について話す

■セカンドオピニオンを受けたい場合は，遠慮なくおっしゃって下さい．	If you'd like to get a second opinion, please don't hesitate to let me know.
■この病気の治療としてはいくつか選択肢があります．例えば…．	There are several treatment options for this disease, such as …
■がんの専門医が後で詳しくご説明いたします．	We'll have a cancer specialist see you later and he'll〈she'll〉explain everything for you in detail.
■治療方針を決める前に慎重に考えましょう．	Let's think carefully before we decide on your treatment plan.
■長くかかるかもしれませんが，一緒に治療に取り組んでいきましょう．	This is going to be a long road, but I'd like you to know that we'll be working with you every step of the way.

❺ 延命治療について訊く

人工呼吸器の装着や胃瘻などについて，患者の意思を確認しておくとよい．

■もし不治あるいは末期の病状になった場合，延命治療を希望なさいますか．例えば…．	If you have an incurable and irreversible medical condition or if you have *a terminal [an end-stage] condition, would you like to have life support treatment, such as …?
■もし脳死状態になってしまった場合，生命維持装置を外すことを希望されますか．	If you become brain dead, would you like *to be taken off life support[to have life support removed]?
■リビングウィルや事前指示書をお持ちであれば，コピーをいただけますか．	If you have a living will or advance health care directive with you, could we have a copy of it?
■延命治療についてのご希望はいつでも撤回，変更ができます．	You can cancel or change your wish for life-support treatment at any time.
■苦痛を和らげる治療は最大限行うことをお約束いたします．	We promise that we'll try everything possible to relieve the pain and make you comfortable.

❻ 最後は，患者の立場になって話を締めくくる

■今後の生活で気がかりなことはありますか．	Do you have any concerns that this is going to affect your life?
■ここまでの話で何かご質問はありますか．	Do you have any questions for me〈about what I've told you〉?
■何かご質問があれば，担当医の関か私にご連絡下さい．	If you have any questions, please contact either Dr Seki (your doctor) or myself.
■ご質問を書きとめておくとよいかもしれません．	It may be helpful to write down any questions you have.
■来週の月曜日にお会いしましょう．	I'll see you next Monday.

参考 森島祐子，仁木久恵，Nancy Sharts-Hopko：『そのまま使える病院英語表現 5000』第 2 版．医学書院，2013.

巻末付録②

訊きにくい質問のコツ

患者がオープンに話すことをためらうような話題について質問する時には，プライバシーの確保や表現の選択に気を遣う必要がある．特に患者の性生活についての質問など，医師や看護師の中には苦手意識を持つ人が多い．

質問する必要があると判断した場合には，たとえ訊きにくいことでも，プロ意識を持って冷静に事実関係について尋ねる．その際，患者が不愉快な思いをしないよう配慮することが肝要である．患者が若者か，成人男性か，高齢者か，あるいは閉経前の女性なのかによっても質問の内容を変えなければならないだろう．大切なのは，個人的な価値観によって患者の性生活の内容に偏見を持たないということである．

❶ **いきなり本題に入るのではなく，まず質問が診察や治療に役立つ可能性について説明する．また，医療者側に守秘義務があることを伝える**

- これからあなたの性習慣についておうかがいします． / I'm going to ask about your sex life.
- 個人的な質問になるかと思いますが，診断や治療をする上で重要な質問なのです． / I know these questions are very personal, but they are important for diagnosis and treatment.
- 個人的な質問になるかと思いますが，この情報はあなたの治療に役立てるためのものです． / I know these questions are very personal, but this information will help me take better care of you.
- ここで話し合う内容は完全守秘扱いとさせていただきます． / Anything we discuss here will be completely confidential.

❷ **性生活について率直に尋ねる**

- 現在，性生活はありますか． / Are you currently sexually active?
- これまで性生活はありましたか． / Have you ever been sexually active?
- 性行為の相手は男性，女性，またはその両方ですか． / Are your partners men, women, or both?
- 先月〈この6か月間／一生を通じて〉，性行為の相手は何人いましたか． / How many partners have you had *in the past month〈in the past six months / in your life〉?
- 性交時に痛みがありますか． / Do you have any pain with intercourse?
- ご自分の性生活に満足していますか． / Are you satisfied with your sex life?
- 現在，性生活のことで何か問題がありますか． / Are you having any sexual difficulties at this time?
- 相手の方に何か問題がありますか． / Is your partner having any sexual difficulties?
- 直近に性行為をしたのはいつですか． / When was the last time you had intercourse?
- 避妊していますか． / Do you use contraception?
  - ――何を使っていますか． / What type do you use?
- 妊娠を考えていますか． / Are you trying to become pregnant?

★女性の患者には月経についての質問をする．「オルガズム」「自慰」「射精」「性交」「性行為」「性的」「性欲」「勃起」などの各見出し語も参照．

巻末付録

❸ 感染症について尋ねる

■ 性感染症の予防を講じていますか.

Do you take any precautions to avoid STDs [sexually transmitted diseases]?

——どんな予防法を講じていますか.

What precautions do you take?

■ これまでに性感染症にかかったことがありますか.

Have you ever had *an STD[a sexually transmitted disease]?

——それは何でしたか.

What was the problem?

■ HIV 感染の危険にさらされていますか, あるいはさらされたことがありますか(例えば輸血, HIV 感染者のパートナー, 注射針の共有など).

Do you have, or have you ever had, any risk factors for HIV (such as a blood transfusion, a partner with HIV infection, or sharing a needle)?

■ HIV 検査を受けたことがありますか.

Have you ever been tested for HIV?

——検査を希望しますか.

Would you like to be (tested for HIV)?

❹ 患者から質問を受ける

■ 性生活のことで何か気がかりなことがありますか.

Do you have any sexual concerns you'd like to discuss?

■ お訊きになりたいことがありますか.

Do you have any questions for me?

巻末付録③

単位の換算

　米国などでは，日本と異なる単位が広く使用されている．患者が体重，身長，体温を感覚的に捉えやすいように，換算式を知っておくと便利である．なお，1 以上の数字を発音する時は，kilograms, pounds, centimeters, inches, feet, degrees Celsius, degrees Fahrenheit のように単位は複数形となる．

❶ 重さ
■換算式　　◆1 キログラム[kg] ≒ 2.2 ポンド[lb]
　　　　　　◆1 ポンド[lb] ≒ 0.45 キログラム[kg]
　★概算　　50 kg≒110 lb / 60 kg≒132 lb / 70 kg≒154 lb / 80 kg≒176 lb

❷ 長さ
■換算式　　◆1 センチメートル[cm] ≒ 0.39 インチ[in]
　　　　　　◆1 インチ[in] ≒ 2.54 センチメートル[cm]
　　　　　　◆1 フィート[ft] = 12 インチ[in]
　★概 算　　150 cm≒59.1 in[4 ft　11 in] / 160 cm≒63.0 in[5 ft　3 in] / 170 cm≒66.9 in[5 ft　7 in] / 180 cm≒70.9 in[5 ft 11 in]

❸ 温度
■換算式　　◆華氏温度[°F] = (1.8×摂氏温度[°C])+ 32
　　　　　　◆摂氏温度[°C] = (華氏温度[°F]−32)×5/9
　★概算　　36 ℃≒96.8 °F / 37 ℃≒98.6 °F / 38 ℃≒100.4 °F / 39 ℃≒102.2°F / 40 ℃≒104 °F

巻末付録

巻末付録④

あいさつ

❶ 診察室で：初診のあいさつ

▶大人の患者に

医師や看護師は，相手の名前を確認すると同時に，自己紹介して患者に名前を知ってもらうことが大切である．それによって信頼関係が生まれる．できれば，立ち上がって迎え入れたり，握手するとよいだろう．

■こんにちは．私は医師の岸です．	Hello, I'm Dr Kishi.
■ナラヤンさんですね．	Are you Mr Narayan?
■ナラヤンさん，おはようございます．	Good morning, Mr Narayan.
■私は医師の岸です．	I'm Dr Kishi. / My name is Dr Kishi.
■看護師の山田です．	I'm Nurse Yamada. / My name is Ms〈Mr〉Yamada, your nurse〈for today〉.
■お待たせしました．	I'm sorry to have kept you waiting.
■お座りください．	Please *sit down[have a seat].
■どうなさいましたか．	How can I help you today? What can I do for you today?
■まずお話を聞かせて下さい．	First of all, tell me what's brought you here today.
■どなたの紹介ですか．	Who sent[referred] you here?
■紹介状をお持ちですか．	Do you have *a letter of referral[a referral letter]?

▶子供の患者に

■マイク君，こんにちは．医師の加藤です．★Hi のほうが親しみやすい言い方．	Hi[Hello], Mike. I'm Dr Kato.
■こんにちは，マイク君ですね．医師の加藤です．	Hi[Hello]. Are you Mike? I'm Dr Kato.
■まずお話をしましょう．	First of all, let's talk about what problems you've been having.

❷ 診察室で：再診のあいさつ

■ナラヤンさん，おはようございます．　Good morning, Mr Narayan.

★名前につける敬称：大人の患者の場合は，相手がファーストネームで呼んでほしいと言わない限り，Mr, Ms, Mrs, Miss, Dr（博士，医師）をつけて姓で話しかける．再診の時，ファーストネームで呼びかけたほうが親しみがわくと判断したときには，May I call you David?などと訊いてからにする．

■またお会いしてうれしく思います．　Nice to see you again.

★以前出会ったことのある人に再会した時には，meet ではなく see を用いる．

●今日，具合はいかがですか．　How are you today? / How do you feel today? / How are you feeling?

■前回の診察から具合はいかがですか．　How have you been since I last saw you?

■前回の治療〈薬〉は効果がありましたか．　Did the last treatment〈medication〉*work well for you[make you feel better]?

❸ 入院患者へのあいさつ

▶紹介のあいさつ

■ はじめまして，担当医の小田です．
Hello, I'm Dr Oda, your doctor.
Nice[Glad] to meet you.

> ★担当医は your doctor のみでよいが，attending doctor, doctor in charge ともいう．初対面の人には see ではなく，meet を用いる．

■ 私は…
I'm …
  1. 医師の荒川です.　　　　1. Dr Arakawa.
  2. 看護師の江口です.　　　2. Nurse Eguchi.
  3. 本日の担当看護師の小田です.　3. Ms〈Mr〉Oda, your nurse for today.

■ はじめまして，マケイさん.
Nice to meet you, Mrs McKay.

■ はじめまして，シムさん.
How do you do, Mrs Sim?

> ★How do you do? はフォーマルな表現.

■ こちらは…
This is …
  1. 同室の木村さんです.　　1. Mr Kimura, your roommate.
  2. 麻酔医の関先生です.　　2. Dr Seki, an anesthesiologist.

▶病室の往診時のあいさつ

■ キムさん，おはようございます.
Good morning, Ms Kim.

> ★Hello や Hi は朝，昼，夜にかかわらず一日中使える.

■ 調子はどうですか.
How are you doing?

■ 今日〈今朝〉ご気分はいかがですか.
How are you feeling today〈this morning〉?

■ ご気分は前よりよくなっていますか.
Are you feeling better?

■ ゆうべはよく眠れましたか.
Did you sleep well last night?

> ★欧米人のなかには How are you doing? と訊かれると，思わず Fine, thank you. や Pretty good, thanks. といった社交辞令的な返事をする人がいるので気をつける.

《子供の患者に》

■ スーザン，こんにちは.
Hello [Hi], Susan.

■ トム君，おはよう. さあ，起きて！
Good morning, Tom. Time to get up!
Rise and shine!

> ★ユーモラスな言い方.

▶退出時のあいさつ

■ もう行かなくてはなりません.
Well, I must be going now.

■ 失礼します. すぐに〈1時間以内に〉戻ってまいります.
Excuse me. I'll be back soon〈within one hour〉.

■ ジョーンズさん，さようなら.
Goodbye, Mr Jones.

■ ベイツさん，お休みなさい.
Good night, Mrs Bates.

■ それでは，またあとで.
(I'll) see you later.

■ 明日〈月曜日に〉またお会いします.
See you tomorrow〈on Monday〉.

■ お大事に.
Take care (of yourself).

《子供の患者に》

■ お休み.
Night-night.

■ ゆっくりお休み.
Sleep tight——hope the bedbugs don't bite!

> ★ユーモアを混じえて「床ジラミに噛まれないようにね」の意.

参考　森島祐子, 仁木久恵, Nancy Sharts-Hopko：『そのまま使える病院英語表現5000』第2版. 医学書院, 2013.

巻末付録⑤

電話応対の表現

❶ 電話をかける

■ もしもし，東京病院の看護師〈医師／受付係〉の佐藤ですが．
Hello, this is *Nurse Sato〈Dr Sato / Eriko Sato, the receptionist〉, (at) Tokyo Hospital.

★ Dr や Nurse などのタイトルがない時には，通例「姓」だけではなく，「ファーストネーム」も付けて言う．

■ グレイさんはいらっしゃいますか．
May I speak to Mr Gray, please?

■ グレイさんの奥様はいらっしゃいますか．
May I speak to *Mrs Gray[Mr Gray's wife], please?

▶ 相手が不在の場合

■ 電話があったことをお伝えいただけますか．
Could you tell him that I called?

■ 伝言をお願いできますか．
Could I leave a message for him?

■ 後でまたかけ直します．
I'll call 〈him〉 back later.

■ 折り返しお電話をいただけるようお伝え下さい．私の電話番号は03-3451…
Could you ask[tell] him to call me back?
My phone number is zero-three, three-four-five-one, …

★ 0 はアルファベットの O（オー）とも読む．

❷ 電話を受ける

■ おはようございます．東京病院の佐藤恵理子ですが，ご用件は何でしょうか．
Good morning, Tokyo Hospital. This is Eriko Sato. How can I *help you[be of assistance]?

■ こんにちは，北医師の診察室です．こちらは佐藤恵理子ですが，ご用件は何でしょうか．
Hello, Dr Kita's office. This is Eriko Sato speaking. How can I *help you[be of assistance]?

■ ご用件は予約のことですね．
I understand you're calling to make an appointment. Is that correct?

■ どちら様ですか．
Who's calling, please?
May I ask who's calling?

■ お名前をいただけますか．
Could I have your name, please?

■ お名前の綴りを教えて下さい．
How do you spell your name?
Could you please spell your name?

■ もう一度おっしゃって下さい．
I beg your pardon?
Could you say that again?

■ もう少しゆっくりお話しいただけますか．
Could you speak more slowly?

▶ 電話をつなぐ場合

■ 少々お待ち下さい．
Please hold for a moment.
Hold the line a moment, please.

- お待たせいたしました.

Thank you for holding.
Thank you for your patience.

- お電話を北先生〈内科病棟のナースステーション〉に回します.

Let me *put you through[transfer your call] *to Dr Kita〈to the nurses' station of the medical ward〉.

- もしもし, 医師の北ですが, どうされましたか.

Hello, this is Dr Kita. How can I help you?

▶ 呼び出した相手が不在の場合

- すみませんが, ただいま北先生はおりません.

I'm sorry. Dr Kita is not available right now.

- 北先生はオフィスにおりません.

Dr Kita is out of the office.

- 明日の午後2時過ぎにかけ直していただけませんか.

Could you call again tomorrow afternoon, after two?

- 看護師〈誰か他の者〉に変わりましょうか.

Would you like to speak to *a nurse 〈someone else〉?

- 折り返し電話をさせましょうか.

Shall I have him〈her〉 call you back?

- ご伝言はありますか.

Could [Can] I take a message?
Would you like to leave a message?

- 医師にご伝言を確かに申し伝えます.

I'll make sure that the doctor gets your message.

❸ 電話を切る

- ほかに何かありますか.

Is there anything else I can help you with?

- お電話ありがとうございました.

Thank you for calling[your call].

❹ その他の役に立つ表現

- 診察券の番号は何番ですか.

May I have your (hospital) ID card number, please?

- カルテを出しますので, ちょっとお待ちいただけますか.

Could you wait a moment while I pull up your medical chart?

巻末付録

巻末付録⑥

病院関係者

❶ 専門職
・医師 doctor / physician ☞専門医 ・内科医 internist / physician ・外科医 surgeon ・歯科医師 dentist ・口腔外科医 oral[dental] surgeon / maxillo-facial surgeon ・専門医 specialist ・一般医 generalist ・研修医 resident / house physician[doctor] ・担当医 doctor in charge / attending doctor[physician] ・看護師 nurse ・助産師 midwife ・保健師 public health nurse；PHN ・薬剤師 pharmacist ・社会福祉士 certified social worker；CSW ・医療ソーシャルワーカー medical social worker；MSW ・介護福祉士 certified care worker；CCW ・精神保健福祉士 psychiatric social worker；PSW ・臨床心理士 clinical psychologist ・栄養士 dietitian / nutrition-ist ・作業療法士 occupational therapist；OT ・理学療法士 physical thera-pist / physiotherapist；PT ・言語聴覚士[言語療法士]speech-language-hearing therapist；ST ・聴能訓練士 audiologist ・視能訓練士 orthoptist；ORT ・ストーマ療法士 enterostomal therapist；ET / stoma therapist ・義肢装具士 prosthetist and orthotist；PO ・診療放射線技師 medical radiation[radiologic] technologist[technician]；MRT ・臨床検査技師 clinical[med-ical] laboratory[lab] technician[technologist]；MLT ・聴覚検査技師 audiometrist ・検眼士 optometrist ・臨床工学技士 medical engineer；ME / clinical engineer；CE ・救急救命士 paramedic / emergency medical tech-nician；EMT ・歯科衛生士 dental hygienist ・歯科技工士 dental techni-cian

❷ サービス職
・看護助手 nursing assistant / nurse's aide ・介護員 hospital attendant /（男性の）orderly ・清掃員 the cleaning[housekeeping] staff / cleaner / clean-ing man〈woman〉 ・用務員 janitor / caretaker ・警備員 guard

❸ 事務職
・一般事務職員（general office）clerk ・受付事務職員 receptionist ・会計事務職員 cashier ・病棟事務職員 unit clerk

❹ 管理職
・院長 president / hospital administrator ・副院長 vice president ・診療部長 medical director for physicians ・医長（〜科の）the head of the … Depart-ment ・看護部長 director of nursing ・看護師長 nurse supervisor ・主任看護師 charge[head] nurse ・薬剤部長 director of pharmacy ・事務長 direc-tor of the administration department

❺ その他
・医学生 medical student ・看護学生 nursing student ・医療通訳 medical interpreter ・ボランティア volunteer ・牧師（病院付きの）(hospital) chaplain